Family Practice Guidelines

Second Edition

Jill C. Cash, MSN, APN, FNP-BC, is a Nurse Practitioner at Logan Primary Care in a rural health care setting in Southern Illinois. She is a Clinical Preceptor for Nurse Practitioner students in her practice for various Nurse Practitioner clinical programs.

Her previous experience includes High Risk Obstetrics as a Clinical Nurse Specialist in Maternal-Fetal Medicine at Vanderbilt University Medical Center. She has since then received her Family Nurse Practitioner Certification from the National Certification Corporation and has a special interest in Women's Health Care.

Ms. Cash is a member of the Illinois Society for Advanced Practice Nurses in Illinois; American Academy of Nurse Practitioners, American College of Nurse Practitioners; Association of Women's Health, Obstetrics, Neonatal Nursing; and Sigma Theta Tau International Honor Society of Nursing. She currently sits on the Board for Hospice for Southern Illinois, Board for The American Cancer Society, and the Board for Women for Health and Wellness in Southern Illinois.

She has authored several chapters in textbooks and is the co-author of *Family Practice Guidelines*.

Cheryl A. Glass, MSN, WHNP, RN-BC, is a Women's Health Nurse Practitioner who currently practices as a Clinical Research Specialist for KePRO in TennCare's Medical Solutions Unit in Nashville, Tennessee. She is also a Clinical Instructor at Vanderbilt University School of Nursing.

Previously, Ms. Glass has been a Clinical Trainer and Trainer Manager for Healthways. Her previous NP practice was as Clinical Research Coordinator on pharmaceutical clinical trials at Nashville Clinical Research. She also worked in a Collaborative Clinical OB Practice with the Director and Assistant Directors of Maternal-Fetal Medicine at Vanderbilt University Medical Center Department of Obstetrics-Gynecology.

The National Certification Corporation certifies Ms. Glass as a Women's Health Care NP. Cheryl is a member of the AANP, ACNP, and NPWH. She is the author of several book chapters and is co-author of *Family Practice Guidelines*. She has published five refereed journal articles. In 1999, Ms. Glass was named Nurse of the Year by the Tennessee chapter of the Association of Women's Health, Obstetric and Neonatal Nurses.

Family Practice Guidelines

Second Edition

Jill C. Cash, MSN, APN, FNP-BC

Cheryl A. Glass, MSN, WHNP, RN-BC

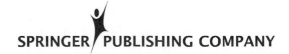

SPRINGER PUBLISHING COMPANY

Springer Publishing Company, LLC
11 West 42nd Street
New York, NY 10036
www.springerpub.com

Acquisitions Editor: Margaret Zuccarini
Production Editor: Gayle Lee
Cover Design: Steven Pisano
Project Manager: Laura Stewart
Composition: Apex CoVantage

ISBN: 978-0-8261-1812-7

E-book ISBN: 978-0-8261-1813-4

10 11 12 13 14/ 5 4 3 2 1

The author and the publisher of this Work have made every effort to use sources believed to be reliable to provide information that is accurate and compatible with the standards generally accepted at the time of publication. Because medical science is continually advancing, our knowledge base continues to expand. Therefore, as new information becomes available, changes in procedures become necessary. We recommend that the reader always consult current research and specific institutional policies before performing any clinical procedure. The author and publisher shall not be liable for any special, consequential, or exemplary damages resulting, in whole or in part, from the readers' use of, or reliance on, the information contained in this book. The publisher has no responsibility for the persistence or accuracy of URLs for external or third-party Internet Web sites referred to in this publication and does not guarantee that any content on such Web sites is, or will remain, accurate or appropriate.

Library of Congress Cataloging-in-Publication Data

Family practice guidelines / [edited by] Jill C. Cash, Cheryl A. Glass. — 2nd ed.
    p. ; cm.
  Includes bibliographical references and index.
  ISBN 978-0-8261-1812-7 (alk. paper) — ISBN 978-0-8261-1813-4 (e-book)
  1. Family nursing—Handbooks, manuals, etc. I. Cash, Jill C. II. Glass, Cheryl A. (Cheryl Anne)
[DNLM: 1. Family Practice—methods—Handbooks. 2. Primary Nursing Care—methods—Handbooks.
3. Diagnostic Techniques and Procedures—Handbooks. 4. Nurse Practitioners. 5. Physician Assistants. WY 49]
  RT120.F34F357 2011
  610.73—dc22   2010032172

Special discounts on bulk quantities of our books are available to corporations, professional associations, pharmaceutical companies, health care organizations, and other qualifying groups.

If you are interested in a custom book, including chapters from more than one of our titles, we can provide that service as well.

For details, please contact:
Special Sales Department, Springer Publishing Company, LLC
11 West 42nd Street, 15th Floor, New York, NY 10036-8002
Phone: 877-687-7476 or 212-431-4370; Fax: 212-941-7842
Email: sales@springerpub.com

Printed in the United States of America by Bang Printing.

To Rob,
my husband and life partner—
Thanks for your patience, understanding, and Dairy Queen trips late at night!
I will always love you.
—Jill

To my daughter and son, Kaitlin Cynthia and Carsen Ray—
You are my inspiration and joy. I love you!
—Mom

If one advances confidently in the direction of his dreams, and endeavors to live the life which he has imagined, he will meet with a success unexpected in common hours.

Henry David Thoreau

––––––––––––––––––

Ed,
I appreciate all of your patience and understanding while I took on this big endeavor.
I love you.
—Cheryl

Inspiration:
If you pursue what makes you happy, the rewards will be boundless.

Author unknown

Contents

SECTION II. PROCEDURES

SECTION III. PATIENT TEACHING GUIDES

Contributors

Julie Adkins, APN, FNP, BC
Certified Family Nurse Practitioner
UltiMed Plus
West Frankfort, Illinois

Rhonda Arthur, DNP, CNM, WHNP-BC, FNP-BC
Certified Nurse Midwife/Nurse Practitioner
Frontier School of Midwifery and Family Nursing
Hyden, Kentucky

Beverly R. Byram, MSN, FNP
Clinical Instructor
Vanderbilt University School of Nursing
Director, Ryan White Part D
Comprehensive Care Center
Nashville, Tennessee

Moya Cook, MSN, APN, FNP, BC
Certified Family Nurse Practitioner
Logan Primary Care
West Frankfort, Illinois

Debbie Croley, RN, MSN, GNP
Clinical Training Specialist
Healthways World Headquarters
Nashville, Tennessee

Lynn Followell, MS, APN-BC, CCRN
Certified Family Nurse Practitioner
Hospitalist
St. Mary's Good Samaritan Hospital
Mt. Vernon, Illinois

Elizabeth Parks, MS, PA-C
Family Practice Physician Assistant
Logan Primary Care
Herrin, Illinois

Christopher S. Shadowens, RN, PA-C
Family Practice Physician Assistant
Logan Primary Care
West Frankfort, Illinois

Kimberly D. Waltrip, APRN-BC
Clinical Instructor
Vanderbilt University School of Nursing
Nashville, Tennessee

Reviewers

Rhonda Arthur, DNP, CNM, WHNP-BC, FNP-BC
Certified Nurse Midwife/Nurse Practitioner
Frontier School of Midwifery and Family Nursing
Hyden, Kentucky

LeAnn Busby, RN, MSN, FNP
Nurse Practitioner
Nashville, Tennessee

Charlotte Covington, MSN, FNP-BC
Associate Professor at Vanderbilt School of Nursing
Nashville, Tennessee

Mary Jo Goolsby, EdD, MSN, NP-C, CAE, FAANP
Director of Research and Education
American Academy of Nurse Practitioners
Austin, Texas

Christopher S. Shadowens, RN, PA-C
Family Practice Physician Assistant
Logan Primary Care
West Frankfort, Illinois

Kimberly D. Waltrip, APRN-BC
Clinical Instructor
Vanderbilt University School of Nursing
Nashville, Tennessee

Preface

After working as an advance practice nurse at Vanderbilt University Medical Center, Jill Cash identified the need for an advanced practice nursing book that provided differential information for both symptoms and diseases. As novice nurse practitioners (although we had been nurses for years), we both identified the need for a quick reference that provided guidelines, procedures, and patient education. Assisted by many of our colleagues, *Family Practice Guidelines* was written and first published in 2000.

We have again asked our experienced physician assistant and nurse practitioner colleagues for assistance in revising this important resource suitable for advanced practice students, as well as novice and experienced health care providers. *Family Practice Guidelines, Second Edition* is this newly revised version. Throughout, information has been updated and is presented in a newly designed, user-friendly format that is more easily accessed using either the table of contents or the book index. Within the guidelines, more emphasis is placed on history taking, on the physical examination, and on key elements of the diagnosis. Web site links have been incorporated for use with PDAs. Highlighted page tips separate the book into different sections for easy identification. Updated dietary instructions are available in the Appendices, including a new addition—the Gluten-Free Diet—and are presented in handout format, making it easy for the patient to understand.

The book is organized into chapters using a body-systems format. The disorders included within each chapter are organized in alphabetical sequence for easy access. Running heads at the right top page make easier access possible. Disorders have been selected for inclusion based on those that are more commonly seen in the primary care setting.

NEW ORGANIZATION

The book is now organized into three major sections:

- Section I: "Guidelines" presents the 20 chapters containing the individual disorder guidelines.
- Section II: "Procedures" presents 18 procedures that commonly are conducted within the office or clinic setting.
- Section III: "Patient Teaching Guides" presents 138 Patient Teaching Guides that are now perforated for ease

of distributing to patients as a take-home teaching guide. For ease of reference, the Teaching Guides are organized by chapter content and can easily be associated with the disorder chapter by matching the Teaching Guide chapter number and title.

NEW TO THIS EDITION

One entirely new chapter has been added to present pain management guidelines for acute and chronic pain management and lower back pain management. Organization has been improved by clustering several guidelines into two new chapters to facilitate accessibility to important content. These two chapters include Chapter 6 "Nasal Guidelines" and Chapter 7 "Throat and Mouth Guidelines." Procedures include step-by-step descriptions and instructions for the novice practitioner.

NEW GUIDELINES

New guidelines have been added throughout, including:

- Chapter 4 "Eye Guidelines": Amblyopia and Blepharitis
- Chapter 10 "Gastrointestinal Guidelines": Celiac Disease, Elevated Liver Enzymes, Post-Bariatric Surgery Management, and Ulcerative Colitis
- Chapter 11 "Genitourinary Guidelines": Chronic Kidney Disease in Adults (CKD) and Interstitial Cystitis
- Chapter 13 "Gynecologic Guidelines": Bartholin Cyst or Abcess, Contraception, and Menopause
- Chapter 15 "Infectious Disease Guidelines": H1N1 Influenza A
- Chapter 16 "Systemic Disorders Guidelines": Vitamin D Deficiency
- Chapter 17 "Musculoskeletal Guidelines": Plantar Fasciitis
- Chapter 18 "Neurologic Guidelines": Migraine Headache and Multiple Sclerosis
- Chapter 19 "Endocrine Guidelines": Polycystic Ovarian Syndrome (PCOS)
- Chapter 20 "Psychiatric Guidelines": Attention Deficit Hyperactivity Disorder (ADHD), Violence Against Children, and Violence Against Older Adults.

NEW PROCEDURES

Three new procedures are included in Section II: Epley Procedure for Vertigo, the Clock-Draw Test, and Neurological Examination.

We believe that you will find that this thoroughly updated and easier-to-access second edition of *Family Practice Guidelines* will provide the quick-access reference that you have been searching for to use in your practice setting.

We appreciate your support of our first edition and know that you will value and utilize this new version of *Family Practice Guidelines*. You will no longer have to spend valuable office time searching for the information needed to provide quality patient care. It's included here, at your fingertips!

Jill C. Cash
Cheryl A. Glass

Acknowledgments

It has been a pleasure to work with the editorial staff and team at Springer Publishing Company.

To Margaret Zuccarini, Executive Acquisitions Editor: We are grateful to you for all of your talent and hard work on organizing the technical matters of this textbook. We greatly appreciate your patience through it all.

To Brian O'Connor: Thank you for your master skills at getting all of the initial paperwork done, calming us down, and reassuring us that all would work out in the end. Thanks for getting the files scanned and sent to us for revision in a timely manner.

To Elizabeth Stump, Assistant Editor: Thanks for coming to the rescue at the last minute for the incomplete files at the end!

To Laura Stewart, Project Manager, Apex Content Solutions, and Gayle Lee at Springer Publishing Company: Your expertise has been priceless. We really appreciate all of your assistance in the editorial process of our second edition.

Jill and Cheryl

Family Practice Guidelines

Second Edition

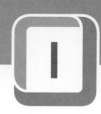

SECTION I

Guidelines

- Health Maintenance Guidelines *by Jill C. Cash and Elizabeth Parks*
- Pain Management Guidelines *by Moya Cook*
- Dermatology Guidelines *by Jill C. Cash*
- Eye Guidelines *by Jill C. Cash*
- Ear Guidelines *by Moya Cook*
- Nasal Guidelines *by Jill C. Cash*
- Throat and Mouth Guidelines *by Jill C. Cash*
- Respiratory Guidelines *by Cheryl A. Glass*
- Cardiovascular Guidelines *by Christopher S. Shadowens*
- Gastrointestinal Guidelines *by Cheryl A. Glass*
- Genitourinary Guidelines *by Cheryl A. Glass*
- Obstetrics Guidelines *by Jill C. Cash*
- Gynecologic Guidelines *by Rhonda Arthur*
- Sexually Transmitted Infections Guidelines *by Elizabeth Parks*
- Infectious Disease Guidelines *by Cheryl A. Glass*
- Systemic Disorders Guidelines *by Julie Adkins*
- Musculoskeletal Guidelines *by Julie Adkins*
- Neurological Guidelines *by Jill C. Cash*
- Endocrine Guidelines *by Lynn Followell*
- Psychiatric Guidelines *by Moya Cook, Jill C. Cash, and Cheryl A. Glass*

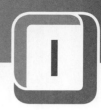
Health Maintenance Guidelines

Jill C. Cash and Elizabeth Parks

Health maintenance involves identifying individuals at risk for health problems and encouraging behaviors that reduce these risks. An important aspect of health maintenance is patient education, to include teaching individuals their risk factors for disease and also how to modify their behaviors to reduce their risks of comorbidities. This book contains Patient Teaching Guides that the practitioner may use for patient education; these forms are found in Section III "Patient Teaching Guides." They may be photocopied by the practitioner, filled in according to the patient's evaluation and needs, and given to the patient.

This chapter comprises tools that the practitioner can use in preventive health care assessment, which includes Web sites, screening guidelines, and suggestions for patient education and counseling.

PEDIATRIC WELL-CHILD EVALUATION

The Well-Child Care chart (Exhibit 1.1) is designed for use in newborns and young children up to the 5- to 6-year-old well-child exam. When complications arise, a detailed S.O.A.P. (Subjective, Objective, Assessment & Plan) note is required for documentation. The documentation should be kept in the front of the child's chart as an easy reference.

Growth charts for children are available in English and metric versions and multiple languages including English, Spanish, and French on the Centers for Disease Control and Prevention (CDC) Web site at http://www.cdc.gov/growthcharts/.

ANTICIPATORY GUIDANCE BY AGE

The anticipatory guidance tool (Exhibit 1.2) is provided as a quick reference for the practitioner from the child's initial visit at 1 month throughout his or her well-child visits until age 15. It is a list of topics that the practitioner should discuss with the caregiver. This information should be supplemented with booklets, teaching guides, and brochures for the caregiver.

NUTRITION

Proper nutrition is an essential part of maintaining health and preventing disease. Promote well-balanced diets for all patients with the emphasis of the prevention of obesity. Diet modification is an important part of disease or disorder management. Diet information is found in Appendix B "Diet Recommendations"; see also Tables 1.1, 1.2, 1.3, and 1.4 for more specific information.

The epidemic of obesity is the responsibility of all health care providers. Each office visit is an opportunity to evaluate the patient's weight, and discuss exercise. As the pain assessment becomes the "fifth vital sign" in the hospital setting, the body mass index becomes the "fifth vital sign" in the outpatient setting.

Teaching parents the correct serving sizes for children will help guide their children's eating habits for life. Dr. Debby Demory-Luce (2004) notes the rule of thumb for measuring portion sizes for fruits and vegetables is "one tablespoon per year of life" for children ages 1 to 6 years. Serving sizes for older children and adults are based on the food pyramids. Use the food pyramid to teach and reinforce proper nutrition. Some helpful Web sites about nutrition are:

A. The U.S. Department of Agriculture (USDA) food pyramid is located at http://www.mypyramid.gov/.
B. The U.S. Department of Agriculture (USDA) food pyramid for children is located at http://teamnutrition.usda.gov/kids-pyramid.html.
C. An interactive food pyramid is located at the Nutrition Exploration Web site at http://www.nutritionexplorations.org/kids/nutrition-pyramid.asp.
D. The Childhood Nutrition Web site is located at http://www.nourishinteractive.com/parents_area/healthy_family_nutrition_newsletter/portion_control_childhood_easy_weight_management_tips_reducing_kids_food_serving_sizes. This informative Web site gives helpful information such as:
   1. Serving sizes
   2. Parent tips tool
   3. Interactive nutrition tools
   4. A fun area for children with interactive nutrition games
   5. Healthy living tips ready for print

EXHIBIT 1.1 **Well-Child Care**

Name _____ DOB _____ Chart# _____

BIRTH HISTORY:

Mother's name _____ Age _____ G ____ P ____ Gestational age at delivery _____ weeks Birth weight _____ lbs _____ ounces

Apgar Scores: 5 minutes _____ 10 minutes _____

Delivery: Vaginal delivery or Cesarean _____ Pregnancy/Delivery complications: _____

	Initial visit	2 weeks	2 months	4 months	6 months	9 months	12 months	15 months	18 months	24 months	3 years	4 years	5 years
Date													
Height percentile													
Weight percentile													
Head circ. percentile													
Vital signs													
Labs													
Immunize													
Hepatitis B (Initial at birth)			#2		#3								
DTaP			#1	#2	#3			#4				#5	
IPV/OPV			#1	#2				#3				#4	
MMR							#1					#2	
Varicella							#1					#2	
Rotavirus			#1	#2	#3								
Hemophilus influenza B			#1	#2	#3		#4						
Pneumococcal													

	Initial visit	2 weeks	2 months	4 months	6 months	9 months	12 months	15 months	18 months	24 months	3 years	4 years	5 years
Influenza							#1			#2	#3	#4	#5
Hepatitis A							#1						
Feedings													
Denver Dev. Screen. Tool													
Physical exam date													
General appearance													
Skin													
Head/neck													
Eyes/ears													
Nose/throat													
Mouth/teeth													
Heart/lungs													
Abdomen													
Extremities													
Back													
Genitalia													
Neurologic													
Medication review													
Assessment plan													
Follow-up													

EXHIBIT 1.2 **Anticipatory Guidance**

INITIAL VISIT—2 WEEKS TO 1 MONTH

A. Safety

1. Infant should sleep on back or side
2. No toys, pillows in crib
3. Note sleeping patterns
4. Rear-facing car seat

B. Nutrition

1. Breast/bottle feeding
2. Feeding patterns
3. Advise caregiver not to prop bottle

C. Developmental

1. Handling fussy periods
2. Soothing techniques: music, reading

D. Medical Care

1. Use of thermometer
2. Fever
3. Vomiting
4. Diarrhea
5. Skin: Sun protection

E. Baby Care

1. Address questions and concerns from caregiver

F. Caregiver Concerns

1. Exhaustion
2. New role in family setting

G. Sibling Reaction

1. Anticipated jealousy and how to handle it

2 MONTHS

A. Safety

1. Review sleeping habits
2. Use rails on cribs
3. Do not leave child unattended on bed, changing table, and so on
4. Car seat safety

B. Nutrition

1. See Section III, Patient Teaching Guide for Chapter 1: Infant Nutrition

C. Parental Concerns

1. Childcare
2. Parents' time out

D. Immunizations

1. See CDC Recommended Immunization Schedule for Persons Aged 0 Through 6 Years—United States 2010 (Table 1.5)

4 MONTHS

A. Safety

1. Car seat safety
2. Choking, suffocation
3. Ways to assist in an emergency
4. Water safety: tubs, buckets, pools, and so on
5. Use of safety gates
6. Poison, poison control, use of ipecac
7. Covering electrical outlets

B. Nutrition

1. Begin solids (infant cereal)

C. Medical Care

1. Patterns of sleep
2. Digestive changes

4 MONTHS (continued)

D. Developmental

1. Putting hands together
2. Turning head
3. Squeal
4. Lift head up

E. Immunizations

1. See CDC Recommended Immunization Schedule for Persons Aged 0 Through 6 Years—United States 2010 (Table 1.5)
2. See CDC Catch-up Immunization Schedule for Persons Aged 4 Months Through 18 Years Who Start Late or Who Are More Than 1 Month Behind—United States 2010 (Table 1.6)

6 MONTHS

A. Safety

1. Review 4-month information
2. Current recommendations on use of walkers
3. Reinforce home safety
4. Security for chemicals, toxins, detergents
5. Use of cabinet and door locks, gates for stairs
6. High-chair safety
7. Car seat safety

B. Parental Concerns

1. Parents' time away
2. Childcare

C. Medical Care

1. Dental care
2. Footwear
3. Hematocrit

D. Developmental

1. No head lag
2. Turn to rattle noise
3. Reach toward object
4. Move toward toy

E. Immunizations

1. See CDC Recommended Immunization Schedule for Persons Aged 0 Through 6 Years—United States 2010 (Table 1.5)

9 MONTHS

A. Safety

1. Childproofing the home
2. Use of gates, locks, cabinet locks

B. Nutrition

1. See Section III, Patient Teaching Guide for Chapter 1: Childhood Nutrition
2. Foods and choking hazards
3. Easy snacks (Cheerios, crackers)

C. Developmental

1. Take two cubes
2. Verbal "mama"
3. Sit without support
4. Weight-bearing legs
5. Imitates sound
6. Setting limits with "no"

D. Medical Care

1. Elimination
2. Sleeping
3. Dental care

(continued)

EXHIBIT 1.2 **Anticipatory Guidance** *(continued)*

12 MONTHS

A. Safety

1. Accident prevention (poison control, windows, outlets, water)
2. Poison control

B. Nutrition

1. Introduction to cow's milk
2. Use of cup
3. Solid food intake

C. Developmental

1. Reading books
2. Playtime
3. Praising behavior
4. Stranger and separation anxiety
5. Encourage speech
6. Walking

15 MONTHS

A. Safety

1. Accident prevention review
2. Water safety
3. Choking hazards
4. Plastic bags
5. Electrical safety

B. Nutrition

1. Discuss feeding patterns and habits
2. Dental care and skin care

C. Developmental

1. Socialization skills
2. Speech
3. Bedtime routines
4. Reading
5. Music
6. Discipline

D. Immunizations

1. See CDC Recommended Immunization Schedule for Persons Aged 0 Through 6 Years—United States 2010 (Table 1.5)

18 MONTHS

A. Safety

1. Review 12 months

B. Developmental

1. Pretend play
2. Temper tantrums
3. Reinforce self-care
4. Self-comforting behavior
5. Peer interactions
6. Window safety

C. Immunizations

1. See CDC Recommended Immunization Schedule for Persons Aged 0 Through 6 Years—United States 2010 (Table 1.5)

24 MONTHS

A. Safety

1. Review 12 months
2. Crib to bed transition
3. Car seat and helmet safety
4. Water safety
5. Storage of hazardous household supplies

24 MONTHS *(continued)*

6. Poison control
7. Street safety
8. Playground (slides, swings, bikes, and so on)
9. Firearm safety
10. Climbing
11. Lighters and matches
12. Motorized toys

B. Nutrition

1. Fun foods to eat

C. Developmental

1. Peer interaction
2. Toileting habits
3. Common routines for eating
4. Bedtime
5. Story time
6. Praising good behavior

D. Medical Care

1. Dental care
2. Skin care
3. Hematocrit
4. Urinalyis
5. Lead screen
6. Elimination, stool, and voiding habits

3–4 YEARS

A. Safety

1. See topics at 24 months

B. Developmental

1. Pretend play
2. Fears
3. Fantasy
4. Sleeping habits (night terrors)
5. Setting realistic limits
6. Praising good behavior
7. Reading
8. Music
9. Childcare
10. Sibling relations

C. Medical

1. Dental
2. Vision
3. Hearing
4. Speech evaluation
5. Hemoglobin/hematocrit
6. TB skin test
7. Lead screen

5–6 YEARS

A. Safety

1. Review as discussed at previous visits
2. Safety with strangers

B. Developmental

1. School readiness
2. Sexual curiosities
3. Peer interactions
4. Good health habits (dental, diet, exercise, sleep)
5. Praise good behavior
6. Adult role models
7. Fears
8. Lying

(continued)

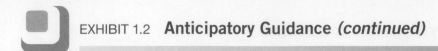

EXHIBIT 1.2 **Anticipatory Guidance** *(continued)*

5–6 YEARS *(continued)*

C. Medical

1. Dental
2. Vision
3. Hearing

D. Immunizations

1. See CDC Recommended Immunization Schedule for Persons Aged 0 Through 6 Years—United States 2010 (Table 1.5)

10 YEARS

A. Safety

1. Car and cycle safety
2. Pedestrian safety

B. Developmental

1. School adjustments
2. Social interactions
3. Communications skills
4. Health habits (same topics as ages 5–6)

C. Immunizations

1. See CDC Recommended Immunization Schedule for Persons Aged 7 Through 18 Years—United States 2010 (Table 1.7)

D. Medical

1. Hemoglobin, hematocrit, urinalysis
2. Vision
3. Hearing
4. Scoliosis
5. TB skin test

15 YEARS

A. Safety

1. Stranger awareness
2. Car and cycle safety

B. Developmental

1. Relationships with peers
2. Body image
3. Sexuality
4. Self-esteem
5. Peer pressure
6. Decision making
7. Role models
8. School adjustments
9. Extracurricular activities: sports, hobbies, exercise
10. Drug, alcohol, tobacco use
11. Suicide

C. Nutrition

1. Diet, healthy habits
2. See Section III, Patient Teaching Guide for Chapter 1: Adolescent Nutrition

D. Medical

1. CPR
2. Emergency numbers
3. Skin care
4. Vision
5. Hearing
6. Scoliosis
7. TB skin test
8. Hemoglobin, hematocrit

TABLE 1.1 Suggested Daily Food Guidelines for Toddlers

Food Items	Daily Amounts[a]	Comments/Rationale
Cooked eggs[b]	3–5 servings a week	Good source of protein; moderate use is recommended because of the high cholesterol content in egg yolks
Breads, grains, and cereals; whole-grain or enriched	4 or more servings (e.g., ½ slice of bread, ½ cup cereal, 2 crackers, ¼ cup noodles)	Provides thiamine, niacin, and, if enriched, riboflavin and iron Encourage the child to identify and enjoy a wide variety of foods
Fruit juices; canned fruit or small pieces of fruit	3 or 4 child-sized servings (e.g., ½ cup juice, ¼–½ cup fruit pieces)	Use those rich in vitamins A and C; also source of iron and calcium Self-feeding enhances the child's sense of independence
Vegetables	1 or 2 child-sized servings (e.g., ¼–⅓ cup)	Include at least 1 dark-green or yellow vegetable every other day for vitamin A
Meat, fish, chicken, casseroles, cottage cheese, peanut butter, dried peas, and beans	2 child-sized servings (e.g., 1 oz meat, 1 egg, ½ cup casserole, ¼ cup cottage cheese, 1–2 tbsp peanut butter)	Source of complete protein, iron, thiamine, riboflavin, niacin, and vitamin B_{12} Nuts and seeds should not be offered until after age 3 when the risk of choking is minimal
Milk, yogurt, cheese	4–6 child-sized servings (e.g., 4–6 oz milk, ½ cup yogurt, 1 oz cheese)	Cheese, cottage cheese, and yogurt are good calcium and riboflavin sources; also sources of calcium, phosphorus, complete protein, riboflavin, and niacin; also vitamin D if fortified milk is used
Fats and sweets	In moderation	May interfere with consumption of nutrient-rich foods; chocolate should be delayed until the child is 1 year old
Salt and other seasonings	In moderation	Children's taste buds are more sensitive than those of adults; salt is a learned taste, and high intakes are related to hypertension

[a]Amounts are daily totals and goals to be achieved gradually.
[b]New food item for the age group.

From *Broadribb's Introductory Pediatric Nursing*, by Markes, 1998. Philadelphia: Lippincott-Raven Publishers, p. 249.

TABLE 1.2 Foods to Meet the Nutritional Needs of the 6-Year-Old to 10-Year-Old

Food	Serving Size
Milk, vitamin D—fortified	2–3 cups
Eggs	3 or 4 per week
Meat, poultry, and fish	2–3 ounces (small serving)
Dried beans, peas, or peanut butter	2 servings each week If used as an alternative for meat, allow ½ cup cooked beans or peas or use 2 tbsp peanut butter for every 1 ounce of meat.
Potatoes, white or sweet (occasionally spaghetti, macaroni, rice, noodles)	1 small or ⅓ cup
Other cooked vegetables (green leafy or deep yellow)	3 or 4 servings per week ¼ cup is a serving size
Raw vegetables (salad greens, cabbage, celery, and carrots)	¼ cup
Vitamin C food (citrus fruit, tomato, and cantaloupe)	1 medium orange or equivalent
Other fruits	1 portion or more: 1 apple, 1 banana, 1 peach, 1 pear, ½ cup cooked fruit
Bread, enriched or whole-grain	3 slices
Cereal, enriched or whole-grain	½ cup
Additional foods	Butter or margarine, desserts, to satisfy energy needs

From *Broadribb's Introductory Pediatric Nursing,* by Markes, 1998. Philadelphia: Lippincott-Raven Publishers, p. 341.

TABLE 1.3 Suggested Number of Servings of Food Groups per Day

Food Group	Number of Servings per day
Milk/dairy	3 servings
Meat	2–3 servings
Fruits	3–4 servings
Vegetables	4–5 servings
Grains (breads and cereal)	9–11 servings

From *Serving sizes.* Childhood nutrition, n.d. Retrieved from http:www.nourishinteractive.com/parents_area/healthy_family_nutrition_newsletter/portion_control_childhood_easy_weight_management_tips_reducing_kids_food_serving_sizes

---

TABLE 1.4 Food Sources and Common Vitamins Missing From a Preteen or Adolescent Diet

Common Nutritional Vitamin Deficiencies	Food Sources for Vitamins
Vitamin A	Liver, whole milk, butter, cheese, yellow vegetables, green leafy vegetables, tomatoes, and yellow fruits
Vitamin D	Fortified milk, and fish liver oils
Vitamin B_6	Liver, kidney, chicken, fish, pork, eggs, whole-grain cereals, and legumes (beans)
Folic acid Vitamin B_9	Green leafy vegetables, liver, kidney, meats, fish, nuts, legumes, and whole grains (breads)
Calcium	Milk, hard cheese, yogurt, ice cream, small fish eaten with bones (e.g., sardines), dark-green vegetables, tofu, soybeans, and calcium-enriched orange juice
Iron	Lean meats, liver, legumes, dried fruits, green leafy vegetables, whole-grain and fortified cereals
Zinc	Oysters, herring, meat, liver, fish, milk, whole grains, nuts, legumes

From *Broadribb's Introductory Pediatric Nursing,* by Markes, 1998. Philadelphia: Lippincott-Raven Publishers, p. 395.

Height and weight are used to calculate body mass index (BMI). The mathematical calculation is BMI = kg/m^2; however, the Internet provides easy-to-use BMI calculators.

A. National Heart Lung and Blood Institute (NHLBI) includes a calculator in its Obesity Education Initiative: http://www.nhlbisupport.com/bmi/. This support site also includes patient information on risk assessment, weight control, and helpful recipes.

B. The Centers for Disease Control and Prevention (CDC) provides an online source for the calculation of BMI for children and teens: http://apps.nccd.cdc.gov/dnpabmi/Calculator.aspx.

The CDC's Web site also provides information on weight loss, physical activity, and parental tips.

Malnutrition and vitamin and mineral deficiency is commonly seen in the elderly population. Vitamins B$_6$, B$_{12}$, D, E, and folic acid and zinc, calcium, and iron are often deficient in the elderly diet, along with a protein and calorie deficiency. Using Zawenda's (1996) acronym WEIGHT LOSS can help you easily identify common causes of weight loss in the elderly.

WEIGHT LOSS

W: Wandering and not eating, due to forgetting to take time to eat

E: Emotional problems including depression

I: Impecuniosity (finances do not meet the needs to buy food and other things)

G: Gut problems

H: Hyperthyroidism or other endocrine abnormalities

T: Tremor or neurologic problems that make eating and holding utensils difficult

L: Low-salt, low-cholesterol diets avoided, often due to disliking the taste of recommended diets

O: Oral problems: edentulous, poor dental care, dentures not fitting, mouth disorders such as oral ulcers

S: Swallowing problems, difficulty swallowing or chewing food due to stroke or other impairment

S: Shopping or food preparation barriers, inability to purchase or prepare food and no resources for assistance

Identification of factor(s) contributing to an elderly patient's malnutrition assists you, the patient, and the patient's family in resolving them. Utilize your state's Area Agencies on Aging (AAA) for information on elder care resources in your area (Web sites not provided since they are state-specific).

EXERCISE

Physical exercise is a vital component of health maintenance. Exercise provides cardiovascular fitness and weight control, prevents osteoporosis through weight-bearing exercise, and decreases lipids. Exercise is important for flexibility, strength, and coordination. Exercise can also be used for both weight control and reduction. Approximately 3,500 calories must be burned to lose 1 pound of fat. So along with exercise, caloric intake must remain the same or decrease to result in weight loss.

Planning an Exercise Program

Exercise plans should be started after a health provider screens a patient, because heavy physical exertion may trigger an acute myocardial infarction. Factors most likely to influence risk are age, presence of heart disease, hypertension, and the intensity of the exercise planned. The medical history screening identifies individual and family history of problems, such as coronary heart disease, hypertension, and diabetes. Review health habits such as previous exercise or sedentary lifestyle, diet, and smoking.

Providers need to evaluate the patient using screening tests before prescribing an exercise program. Consider the patient's age and all comorbidities for additional tests.

A. Complete blood count

B. Blood glucose

C. Cholesterol screening

D. EKG (in patients older than 40 years)

E. Holter monitoring for arrhythmias

Persons with a heart murmur or other abnormal physical finding should defer exercise until the full nature of the disorder is evaluated. The best measure of an exercise work capacity is the determination of oxygen consumption at maximal activity, which is measured with a stress test. Hypertension, elevated resting blood pressures, and chronic obstructive lung disease are other factors that require attention prior to participation in exercise. Persons with hypertension should have a thorough evaluation, have antihypertensive agent(s) prescribed, and be monitored periodically during their prescribed graded exercise program.

Physical exercise is contraindicated in the presence of following conditions:

A. Congestive heart failure

B. Uncontrolled hypertension

C. Uncontrolled epilepsy

D. Uncontrolled diabetes

E. Atrioventricular (AV) heart block

F. Aneurysms

G. Ventricular instability

H. Aortic valve disease

Measurement of the heart rate during exercise is an easy and inexpensive method to evaluate cardiovascular fitness. Target heart rates vary by physical condition and a person's age. The following formula is used to evaluate target heart/aerobic activity level:

[220—(age of individual)] × 0.65 = Maximum heart rate range

Maximum heart rate × 0.65 = Minimum aerobic effect

Maximum heart rate × 0.85 = Maximum aerobic effect

Patient Education Before Exercise

All exercise program prescriptions should include frequency, duration, intensity, and when the exercise should be aborted. Persons should be educated on the signs and symptoms of heat exhaustion and should be advised when to seek first aid.

Exercise programs with aerobic activity at least three times a week on nonconsecutive days is the minimal amount of exercise individuals should set as a goal. The target heart rate should be sustained for 20 to 30 minutes for maximal cardiovascular effect.

Women engaged in regular physical exercise prior to pregnancy may safely continue exercise throughout pregnancy. The target heat rate for a pregnant woman during exercise should not exceed 140 beats per minute. Pregnancy activities should also be limited to low-impact aerobics and activities that do not require agility because a woman's center of balance changes throughout pregnancy, leaving the woman at risk for falling and injury.

Swimming is ideal for upper and lower body conditioning with low impact on joints. Swimming is not well suited for women at risk for osteoporosis, because it is not a weight-bearing exercise. Examples of weight-bearing exercise to help prevent osteoporosis include dancing, impact aerobics, and resistance training.

For exercise to benefit individuals, it must be continued lifelong. The health care provider should evaluate individual lifestyle and preferences in designing an exercise program. One exercise program can become boring over time and probably will not be continued. A variety of activities, class participation, and positive reinforcement help to keep physical activity fun as an integral part of a health maintenance program. See the Section III Patient Teaching Guide for this chapter, "Exercise."

Health care professionals who will be monitoring and prescribing exercise plans for large numbers of individuals are encouraged to seek special training and certification. The American College of Sports Medicine has a program that includes training for health care professionals.

OTHER PROVIDERS

It is the role of the primary care provider to ensure that the patient becomes a partner in preventive health measures to avoid disease comorbidities. The practitioner should refer the patient to see other health care providers to continue health maintenance.

A. Dental Care
1. Dental care should be routinely discussed.
2. Once teeth emerge, brushing should begin with a small soft brush.
3. In children, dental care should begin with soft, rubber brushes for gum care.
4. Encourage the child to brush teeth twice daily, to promote healthy habits.
5. Refer the patient to a dentist at 3 years, unless problems arise earlier.
6. Older child should be encouraged to use mouth guards with contact sports.
7. Encourage flossing when the child has the cognitive and developmental dexterity to use dental floss.
B. Vision Care
1. Begin initial vision screening for children at 3 years of age using the age-appropriate eye chart.
2. School screening should include a vision-screening component.
3. Refer patients to an optometrist for routine evaluation.

ADULT RISK ASSESSMENT FORM

The Adult Risk Assessment Form (Exhibit 1.3) should be used for all adult patients. It is used to evaluate a patient's risk for particular diseases. The practitioner should interview the patient, assessing for the risk factors listed on the Risk Assessment Form. The family history of first-degree relatives (parents, siblings, and children) should also be discussed, as many diseases are related to genetic factors. Keep a copy of the Risk Assessment Form in the front of the patient's chart, and update yearly or as needed. When complete, this tool can guide the practitioner in determining assessment needs of each patient.

ADULT PREVENTIVE HEALTH CARE

This flow sheet (Exhibit 1.4) helps the practitioner identify changes in the adult patient's risk factor status, make recommendations for health maintenance (e.g., immunizations, laboratory work, physical exams), and educate patients in prevention (Exhibit 1.5). Screening guidelines for each of these can be found in the associated chapters in this book, according to the national association recommendations (i.e., screening recommendations for mammograms were obtained from the American Cancer Society). The guide can be used as a quick reference for the practitioner to evaluate the patient's adherence to preventive measures. Keep a copy of this flow sheet and guide in the front of the patient's chart where they can be reviewed routinely and updated as necessary.

IMMUNIZATIONS

The Centers for Disease Control and Prevention (CDC) is the primary source for the current immunization schedules (see Tables 1.5–1.8). Consult its Web site for pocket-sized schedules, office printing and versions for Palm/Pocket–PCs handhelds. The download information for your iPhone, iTouch, Blackberry Storm, Palm Pre or PC, Palm OS, and Pocket PC is available on the CDC Web site at http://www.immunizationed.org/AnyPage.aspx?pgid=2.

IMMUNIZATIONS FOR TRAVEL

The Centers for Disease Control and Prevention (CDC) recommends certain vaccines to protect travelers from illnesses present in other parts of the world and to protect others upon your return to the United States. Vaccinations required are dependent on several factors:

A. Travel destination
B. Travel season
C. Age
D. Pregnancy or breastfeeding
E. Traveling with infants or children
F. Immunocompetent secondary to diabetes or HIV

EXHIBIT 1.3 **Adult Risk Assessment Form**

Name _____ DOB _____ Chart # _____

Allergies _____

Occupation _____

FAMILY HISTORY	
First-degree relatives with remarkable diseases (e.g., HTN, DM, CAD, Cancer & Thyroid)	
1.	6.
2.	7.
3.	8.
4.	9.
5.	10.

Assess the patient for the following risk factors:

A. Coronary Heart Disease
- ☐ High-fat/high-cholesterol diet
- ☐ Obese
- ☐ Elevated cholesterol level
- ☐ Stroke
- ☐ Hypertension
- ☐ Tobacco use

B. Lung Cancer
- ☐ High-fat/high-cholesterol diet
- ☐ Tobacco use

C. Cervical Cancer
- ☐ Early age of first intercourse
- ☐ Multiple sexual partners

D. Breast Cancer
- ☐ Nulliparous
- ☐ Primigravida after age 35
- ☐ High-fat diet

E. Colon Cancer
- ☐ History of polyps
- ☐ High-fat diet

F. Osteoporosis
- ☐ Less than 1 gram of calcium per day
- ☐ History of tobacco or alcohol use
- ☐ Sedentary lifestyle
- ☐ Thin, Caucasian
- ☐ Female gender

G. Glaucoma/Visual Impairment
- ☐ Family history of glaucoma
- ☐ Diabetes mellitus

H. Sexually Transmitted Infections/HIV
- ☐ Alcohol and drug use or abuse
- ☐ Multiple sexual partners
- ☐ Homosexual or bisexual partner
- ☐ History of intravenous drug use
- ☐ History of blood transfusion
- ☐ Exposed to or past history of STI

I. Substance Abuse
- ☐ Alcohol or drug use history
- ☐ Family history of substance abuse
- ☐ Stress or poor coping mechanisms
- ☐ Administer the **CAGE** Assessment:
  - ○ Do you feel you need to **C**ut down on drug/alcohol use?
  - ○ Are you **A**nnoyed by criticism?
  - ○ Do you feel **G**uilty about drinking (or drug use)?
  - ○ Do you ever have an **E**ye opener (morning drug or alcohol use to "get going")?

J. Accidents and Suicide
- ☐ Family history of suicide
- ☐ Alcohol or tobacco use
- ☐ History of depression
- ☐ High-stress or "hot-reactor" personality
- ☐ Male gender
- ☐ Alcohol use
- ☐ Previous suicide attempt
- ☐ Poor coping mechanisms or stress

K. Safety
- ☐ Does not use seat belt or car seat
- ☐ Drinks and drives
- ☐ Drives over the speed limit
- ☐ Does not wear safety helmet if driving motorcycle
- ☐ Inadequate number of smoke detectors or none in the home

EXHIBIT 1.4 **Adult Preventive Health Care Flow Sheet**

IMMUNIZATION SCHEDULE				
Immunization	**Date**	**Date**	**Date**	**Date**
Tetanus/diphtheria				
MMR				
TB (yearly)				
Hepatitis B				
Influenza (yearly)				
Pneumonococcal				
Other				
Other				

Assess patients for the following behaviors:

RISK ASSESSMENT				
Exam	**Date**	**Date**	**Date**	**Date**
Tobacco, amount				
Alcohol, amount				
Substance use				
Domestic violence				

Patients should be educated about any behavior modifications that can reduce their risk factors for health problems. The practitioner should note the date as well as the type of counseling given to a patient.

PATIENT EDUCATION				
Behavior Modification	**Date**	**Date**	**Date**	**Date**
Diet/exercise				
Tobacco/alcohol				
Injury prevention				
Skin protection				
Hormone replacement therapy				
Sexual practices				
Occupational hazards				
Self-exam: breast/ testicular				

EXHIBIT 1.5 **Adult Health Maintenance Guide**

Name _____ DOB _____ Chart # _____

Allergies _____ Occupation _____

The following tests should be performed according to the individual patient's risk factors, as part of preventive health care. The practitioner should fill in the date and result of each test and highlight any remarkable results.

Test	Date	Result	Date	Result	Date	Result	Date	Result
Height								
Weight								
BMI								
B/P								
Skin exam								
Oral cavity exam								
EKG								
TSH								
Lipid profile								
Urinalysis								
Rectal exam								
Hemoccult								
Colonoscopy								
PSA								
Testicular exam								
Pelvic exam/Pap smear								
Breast exam								
Mammogram								
STD/HIV								
Additionally, the practitioner should ensure that the patient receives other health care as needed. Assess patient's adherence to other preventive health care exams:								
Dental exam								
Vision/glaucoma exam								

TABLE 1.5 CDC Recommended Immunization Schedule for Persons Aged 0 Through 6 Years—United States 2010

Recommended Immunization Schedule for Persons Aged 0 Through 6 Years—United States • 2010
For those who fall behind or start late, see the catch-up schedule

Vaccine ▼ Age ▶	Birth	1 month	2 months	4 months	6 months	12 months	15 months	18 months	19–23 months	2–3 years	4–6 years
Hepatitis B[1]	HepB	HepB				HepB					
Rotavirus[2]			RV	RV	RV[2]						
Diphtheria, Tetanus, Pertussis[3]			DTaP	DTaP	DTaP	see footnote[3]	DTaP				DTaP
Haemophilus influenzae type b[4]			Hib	Hib	Hib[4]	Hib					
Pneumococcal[5]			PCV	PCV	PCV	PCV				PPSV	PPSV
Inactivated Poliovirus[6]			IPV	IPV	IPV	IPV					IPV
Influenza[7]					Influenza (Yearly)						
Measles, Mumps, Rubella[8]						MMR			see footnote[8]		MMR
Varicella[9]						Varicella			see footnote[9]		Varicella
Hepatitis A[10]						HepA (2 doses)				HepA Series	HepA Series
Meningococcal[11]										MCV	MCV

Range of recommended ages for all children except certain high-risk groups

Range of recommended ages for certain high-risk groups

This schedule includes recommendations in effect as of December 15, 2009. Any dose not administered at the recommended age should be administered at a subsequent visit, when indicated and feasible. The use of a combination vaccine generally is preferred over separate injections of its equivalent component vaccines. Considerations should include provider assessment, patient preference, and the potential for adverse events. Providers should consult the relevant Advisory.

1. Hepatitis B vaccine (HepB). (Minimum age: birth)

At birth:

• Administer monovalent HepB to all newborns before hospital discharge.

• If mother is hepatitis B surface antigen (HBsAg)-positive, administer HepB and 0.5 mL of hepatitis B immune globulin (HBIG) within 12 hours of birth.

• If mother's HBsAg status is unknown, administer HepB within 12 hours of birth. Determine mother's HBsAg status as soon as possible and, if HBsAg-positive, administer HBIG (no later than age 1 week).

After the birth dose:

• The HepB series should be completed with either monovalent HepB or a combination vaccine containing HepB. The second dose should be administered at age 1 or 2 months. Monovalent HepB vaccine should be used for doses administered before age 6 weeks. The final dose should be administered no earlier than age 24 weeks.

Committee on Immunization Practices statement for detailed recommendations: **http://www.cdc.gov/vaccines/pubs/acip-list.htm.** Clinically significant adverse events that follow vaccination should be reported to the Vaccine Adverse Event Reporting System (VAERS) at **http://www.vaers.hhs.gov** or by telephone, **800-822-7967.**

• Infants born to HBsAg-positive mothers should be tested for HBsAg and antibody to HBsAg 1 to 2 months after completion of at least 3 doses of the HepB series, at age 9 through 18 months (generally at the next well-child visit).

• Administration of 4 doses of HepB to infants is permissible when a combination vaccine containing HepB is administered after the birth dose. The fourth dose should be administered no earlier than age 24 weeks.

2. Rotavirus vaccine (RV). (Minimum age: 6 weeks)

• Administer the first dose at age 6 through 14 weeks (maximum age: 14 weeks 6 days). Vaccination should not be initiated for infants aged 15 weeks 0 days or older.

• The maximum age for the final dose in the series is 8 months 0 days.

• If Rotarix is administered at ages 2 and 4 months, a dose at 6 months is not indicated.

(continued)

TABLE 1.5 (continued)

3. **Diphtheria and tetanus toxoids and acellular pertussis vaccine (DTaP).** (Minimum age: 6 weeks)
   - The fourth dose may be administered as early as age 12 months, provided at least 6 months have elapsed since the third dose.
   - Administer the final dose in the series at age 4 through 6 years.

4. **Haemophilus influenzae type b conjugate vaccine (Hib).** (Minimum age: 6 weeks)
   - If PRP-OMP (PedvaxHIB or Comvax [HepB-Hib]) is administered at ages 2 and 4 months, a dose at age 6 months is not indicated.
   - TriHiBit (DTaP/Hib) and Hiberix (PRP-T) should not be used for doses at ages 2, 4, or 6 months for the primary series but can be used as the final dose in children aged 12 months through 4 years.

5. **Pneumococcal vaccine.** (Minimum age: 6 weeks for pneumococcal conjugate vaccine [PCV]; 2 years for pneumococcal polysaccharide vaccine [PPSV])
   - PCV is recommended for all healthy children aged younger than 5 years. Administer 1 dose of PCV to all healthy children aged 24 through 59 months who are not completely vaccinated for their age.
   - Administer PPSV 2 or more months after last dose of PCV to children aged 2 years or older with certain underlying medical conditions, including a cochlear implant. See MMWR 1997;46(No. RR-8).

6. **Inactivated poliovirus vaccine (IPV)** (Minimum age: 6 weeks)
   - The final dose in the series should be administered on or after the fourth birthday and at least 6 months following the previous dose.
   - If 4 doses are administered prior to age 4 years a fifth dose should be administered at age 4 through 6 years. See MMWR 2009;58(30);829-30.

7. **Influenza vaccine (seasonal).** (Minimum age: 6 months for trivalent inactivated influenza vaccine [TIV]; 2 years for live, attenuated influenza vaccine [LAIV])
   - Administer annually to children aged 6 months through 18 years.
   - For healthy children aged 2 through 6 years (i.e., those who do not have underlying medical conditions that predispose them to influenza complications), either LAIV or TIV may be used, except LAIV should not be given to children aged 2 through 4 years who have had wheezing in the past 12 months.

- Children receiving TIV should receive 0.25 mL if aged 6 through 35 months or 0.5 mL if aged 3 years or older.
- Administer 2 doses (separated by at least 4 weeks) to children aged younger than 9 years who are receiving influenza vaccine for the first time or who were vaccinated for the first time during the previous influenza season but only received 1 dose.
- For recommendations for use of influenza A (H1N1) 2009 monovalent vaccine see MMWR 2009;58(No. RR-10).

8. **Measles, mumps, and rubella vaccine (MMR).** (Minimum age: 12 months)
   - Administer the second dose routinely at age 4 through 6 years. However, the second dose may be administered before age 4, provided at least 28 days have elapsed since the first dose.

9. **Varicella vaccine.** (Minimum age: 12 months)
   - Administer the second dose routinely at age 4 through 6 years. However, the second dose may be administered before age 4, provided at least 3 months have elapsed since the first dose.
   - For children aged 12 months through 12 years the minimum interval between doses is 3 months. However, if the second dose was administered at least 28 days after the first dose, it can be accepted as valid.

10. **Hepatitis A vaccine (HepA).** (Minimum age: 12 months)
    - Administer to all children aged 1 year (i.e., aged 12 through 23 months). Administer 2 doses at least 6 months apart.
    - Children not fully vaccinated by age 2 years can be vaccinated at subsequent visits
    - HepA also is recommended for older children who live in areas where vaccination programs target older children, who are at increased risk for infection, or for whom immunity against hepatitis A is desired.

11. **Meningococcal vaccine.** (Minimum age: 2 years for meningococcal conjugate vaccine [MCV4] and for meningococcal polysaccharide vaccine [MPSV4])
    - Administer MCV4 to children aged 2 through 10 years with persistent complement component deficiency, anatomic or functional asplenia, and certain other conditions placing them at high risk.
    - Administer MCV4 to children previously vaccinated with MCV4 or MPSV4 after 3 years if first dose administered at age 2 through 6 years. See MMWR 2009;58:1042-3.

The Recommended Immunization Schedules for Persons Aged 0 through 18 Years are approved by the Advisory Committee on Immunization Practices (http://www.cdc.gov/vaccines/recs/acip), the American Academy of Pediatrics (http://www.aap.org), and the American Academy of Family Physicians (http://www.aafp.org). Department of Health and Human Services • Centers for Disease Control and Prevention

TABLE 1.6 CDC Catch-up Immunization Schedule for Persons Aged 4 Months Through 18 Years Who Start Late or Who Are More Than 1 Month Behind—United States 2010

Catch-up Immunization Schedule for Persons Aged 4 Months Through 18 Years Who Start Late or Who Are More Than 1 Month Behind—United States 2010

The table below provides catch-up schedules and minimum intervals between doses for children whose vaccinations have been delayed. A vaccine series does not need to be restarted, regardless of the time that has elapsed between doses. Use the section appropriate for the child's age.

PERSONS AGED 4 MONTHS THROUGH 6 YEARS

Vaccine	Minimum Age for Dose 1	Minimum Interval Between Doses			
		Dose 1 to Dose 2	Dose 2 to Dose 3	Dose 3 to Dose 4	Dose 4 to Dose 5
Hepatitis B[1]	Birth	4 weeks	8 weeks (and at least 16 weeks after first dose)		
Rotavirus[2]	6 wks	4 weeks	4 weeks[2]		
Diphtheria, Tetanus, Pertussis[3]	6 wks	4 weeks	4 weeks	6 months	6 months[3]
Haemophilus influenzae type b[4]	6 wks	4 weeks if first dose administered at younger than age 12 months **8 weeks (as final dose)** if first dose administered at age 12–14 months **No further doses needed** if first dose administered at age 15 months or older	4 weeks[4] if current age is younger than 12 months **8 weeks (as final dose)**[4] if current age is 12 months or older and first dose administered at younger than age 12 months and second dose administered at younger than 15 months **No further doses needed** if previous dose administered at age 15 months or older	8 weeks (as final dose) This dose only necessary for children aged 12 months through 59 months who received 3 doses before age 12 months	
Pneumococcal[5]	6 wks	4 weeks if first dose administered at younger than age 12 months **8 weeks (as final dose for healthy children)** if first dose administered at age 12 months or older or current age 24 through 59 months **No further doses needed** for healthy children if first dose administered at age 24 months or older	4 weeks if current age is younger than 12 months **8 weeks (as final dose for healthy children)** if current age is 12 months or older **No further doses needed** for healthy children if previous dose administered at age 24 months or older	8 weeks (as final dose) This dose only necessary for children aged 12 months through 59 months who received 3 doses before age 12 months or for high-risk children who received 3 doses at any age	
Inactivated Poliovirus[6]	6 wks	4 weeks	4 weeks	6 months	
Measles,Mumps, Rubella[7]	12 mos	4 weeks			
Varicella[8]	12 mos	3 months			
Hepatitis A[9]	12 mos	6 months			

(continued)

TABLE 1.6 *(continued)*

		PERSONS AGED 7 MONTHS THROUGH 18 YEARS		
Tetanus, Diphtheria/ Tetanus, Diphtheria, Pertussis[10]	7 yrs[10]	4 weeks	4 weeks if first dose administered at younger than age 12 months 6 months if first dose administered at 12 months or older	6 months if first dose administered at younger than age 12 months
Human Papillomavirus[11]	9 yrs	Routine dosing intervals are recommended[11]		
Hepatitis A[9]	12 mos	6 months		
Hepatitis B[1]	Birth	4 weeks	8 weeks (and at least 16 weeks after first dose)	
Inactivated Poliovirus[6]	6 wks	4 weeks	4 weeks	6 months
Measles, Mumps, Rubella[7]	12 mos	4 weeks		
Varicella[8]	12 mos	3 months if person is younger than age 13 years 4 weeks if person is aged 13 years or older		

1. **Hepatitis B vaccine (HepB).**
   • Administer the 3-dose series to those not previously vaccinated.
   • A 2-dose series (separated by at least 4 months) of adult formulation Recombivax HB is licensed for children aged 11 through 15 years.

2. **Rotavirus vaccine (RV).**
   • The maximum age for the first dose is 14 weeks 6 days. Vaccination should not be initiated for infants aged 15 weeks 0 days or older.
   • The maximum age for the final dose in the series is 8 months 0 days.
   • If Rotarix was administered for the first and second doses, a third dose is not indicated.

3. **Diphtheria and tetanus toxoids and acellular pertussis vaccine (DTaP).**
   • The fifth dose is not necessary if the fourth dose was administered at age 4 years or older.

4. **Haemophilus influenzae type b conjugate vaccine (Hib).**
   • Hib vaccine is not generally recommended for persons aged 5 years or older. No efficacy data are available on which to base a recommendation concerning use of Hib vaccine for older children and adults. However, studies suggest good immunogenicity in persons who have sickle cell disease, leukemia, or HIV infection, or who have had a splenectomy; administering 1 dose of Hib vaccine to these persons who have not previously received Hib vaccine is not contraindicated.
   • If the first 2 doses were PRP-OMP (PedvaxHIB or Comvax), and administered at age 11 months or younger, the third (and final) dose should be administered at age 12 through 15 months and at least 8 weeks after the second dose.
   • If the first dose was administered at age 7 through 11 months, administer the second dose at least 4 weeks later and a final dose at age 12 through 15 months.

5. **Pneumococcal vaccine.**
   • Administer 1 dose of pneumococcal conjugate vaccine (PCV) to all healthy children aged 24 through 59 months who have not received at least 1 dose of PCV on or after age 12 months.
   • For children aged 24 through 59 months with underlying medical conditions, administer 1 dose of PCV if 3 doses were received previously or administer 2 doses of PCV at least 8 weeks apart if fewer than 3 doses were received previously.
   • Administer pneumococcal polysaccharide vaccine (PPSV) to children aged 2 years or older with certain underlying medical conditions, including a cochlear implant, at least 8 weeks after the last dose of PCV. See MMWR 1997;46(No. RR-8).

6. **Inactivated poliovirus vaccine (IPV).**
   • The final dose in the series should be administered on or after the fourth birthday and at least 6 months following the previous dose.
   • A fourth dose is not necessary if the third dose was administered at age 4 years or older and at least 6 months following the previous dose.
   • In the first 6 months of life, minimum age and minimum intervals are only recommended if the person is at risk for imminent exposure to circulating poliovirus (i.e., travel to a polio-endemic region or during an outbreak).

7. **Measles, mumps, and rubella vaccine (MMR).**
   • Administer the second dose routinely at age 4 through 6 years. However, the second dose may be administered before age 4, provided at least 28 days have elapsed since the first dose.
   • If not previously vaccinated, administer 2 doses with at least 28 days between doses.

8. **Varicella vaccine.**
   - Administer the second dose routinely at age 4 through 6 years. However, the second dose may be administered before age 4, provided at least 3 months have elapsed since the first dose.
   - For persons aged 12 months through 12 years, the minimum interval between doses is 3 months. However, if the second dose was administered at least 28 days after the first dose, it can be accepted as valid.
   - For persons aged 13 years and older, the minimum interval between doses is 28 days.

9. **Hepatitis A vaccine (HepA).**
   - HepA is recommended for children aged older than 23 months who live in areas where vaccination programs target older children, who are at increased risk for infection, or for whom immunity against hepatitis A is desired.

10. **Tetanus and diphtheria toxoids vaccine (Td) and tetanus and diphtheria toxoids and acellular pertussis vaccine (Tdap).**
    - Doses of DTaP are counted as part of the Td/Tdap series
    - Tdap should be substituted for a single dose of Td in the catch-up series or as a booster for children aged 10 through 18 years; use Td for other doses.

11. **Human papillomavirus vaccine (HPV).**
    - Administer the series to females at age 13 through 18 years if not previously vaccinated.
    - Use recommended routine dosing intervals for series catch-up (i.e., the second and third doses should be administered at 1 to 2 and 6 months after the first dose). The minimum interval between the first and second doses is 4 weeks. The minimum interval between the second and third doses is 12 weeks, and the third dose should be administered at least 24 weeks after the first dose.

Information about reporting reactions after immunization is available online at **http://www.vaers.hhs.gov** or by telephone, **800-822-7967**. Suspected cases of vaccine-preventable diseases should be reported to the state or local health department. Additional information, including precautions and contraindications for immunization, is available from the National Center for Immunization and Respiratory Diseases at **http://www.cdc.gov/ vaccines** or telephone, **800-CDC-INFO** (800-232-4636).

Department of Health and Human Services • Centers for Disease Control and Prevention

TABLE 1.7   CDC Recommended Immunization Schedule for Persons Aged 7 Through 18 Years—United States 2010

Recommended Immunization Schedule for Persons Aged 7 Through 18 Years—United States • 2010
For those who fall behind or start late, see the schedule below and the catch-up schedule

Vaccine ▼ Age ▶	7–10 years	11–12 years	13–18 years
Tetanus, Diphtheria, Pertussis[1]		Tdap	Tdap
Human Papillomavirus[2]	see footnote 2	HPV (3 doses)	HPV series
Meningococcal[3]	MCV	MCV	MCV
Influenza[4]	Influenza (Yearly)		
Pneumococcal[5]	PPSV		
Hepatitis A[6]	HepA Series		
Hepatitis B[7]	Hep B Series		
Inactivated Poliovirus[8]	IPV Series		
Measles, Mumps, Rubella[9]	MMR Series		
Varicella[10]	Varicella Series		

Legend:
- Range of recommended ages for all children except certain high-risk groups
- Range of recommended ages for catch-up immunization
- Range of recommended ages for certain high-risk groups

This schedule includes recommendations in effect as of December 15, 2009. Any dose not administered at the recommended age should be administered at a subsequent visit, when indicated and feasible. The use of a combination vaccine generally is preferred over separate injections of its equivalent component vaccines. Considerations should include provider assessment, patient preference, and the potential for adverse events. Providers should consult the relevant Advisory Committee on Immunization Practices statement for detailed recommendations: **http://www.cdc.gov/vaccines/pubs/acip-list.htm.** Clinically significant adverse events that follow immunization should be reported to the Vaccine Adverse Event Reporting System (VAERS) at **http://www.vaers.hhs.gov** or by telephone, **800-822-7967.**

1. **Tetanus and diphtheria toxoids and acellular pertussis vaccine (Tdap).** (Minimum age: 10 years for Boostrix and 11 years for Adacel)
   - Administer at age 11 or 12 years for those who have completed the recommended childhood DTP/DTaP vaccination series and have not received a tetanus and diphtheria toxoid (Td) booster dose.
   - Persons aged 13 through 18 years who have not received Tdap should receive a dose.
   - A 5-year interval from the last Td dose is encouraged when Tdap is used as a booster dose; however, a shorter interval may be used if pertussis immunity is needed.

2. **Human papillomavirus vaccine (HPV).** (Minimum age: 9 years)
   - Two HPV vaccines are licensed: a quadrivalent vaccine (HPV4) for the prevention of cervical, vaginal and vulvar cancers (in females) and genital warts (in females and males), and a bivalent vaccine (HPV2) for the prevention of cervical cancers in females.
   - HPV vaccines are most effective for both males and females when given before exposure to HPV through sexual contact.
   - HPV4 or HPV2 is recommended for the prevention of cervical precancers and cancers in females.
   - HPV4 is recommended for the prevention of cervical, vaginal and vulvar precancers and cancers and genital warts in females.
   - Administer the first dose to females at age 11 or 12 years.
   - Administer the second dose 1 to 2 months after the first dose and the third dose 6 months after the first dose (at least 24 weeks after the first dose).
   - Administer the series to females at age 13 through 18 years if not previously vaccinated.
   - HPV4 may be administered in a 3-dose series to males aged 9 through 18 years to reduce their likelihood of acquiring genital warts.

3. **Meningococcal conjugate vaccine (MCV4).**
   - Administer at age 11 or 12 years, or at age 13 through 18 years if not previously vaccinated.
   - Administer to previously unvaccinated college freshmen living in a dormitory.
   - Administer MCV4 to children aged 2 through 10 years with persistent complement component deficiency, anatomic or functional asplenia, or certain other conditions placing them at high risk.

- Administer to children previously vaccinated with MCV4 or MPSV4 who remain at increased risk after 3 years (if first dose administered at age 2 through 6 years) or after 5 years (if first dose administered at age 7 years or older). Persons whose only risk factor is living in on-campus housing are not recommended to receive an additional dose. See *MMWR* 2009;58:1042–3.

4. **Influenza vaccine (seasonal).**
- Administer annually to children aged 6 months through 18 years.
- For healthy nonpregnant persons aged 7 through 18 years (i.e., those who do not have underlying medical conditions that predispose them to influenza complications), either LAIV or TIV may be used.
- Administer 2 doses (separated by at least 4 weeks) to children aged younger than 9 years who are receiving influenza vaccine for the first time or who were vaccinated for the first time during the previous influenza season but only received 1 dose.
- For recommendations for use of influenza A (H1N1) 2009 monovalent vaccine. See *MMWR* 2009;58:(No. RR-10).

5. **Pneumococcal polysaccharide vaccine (PPSV).**
- Administer to children with certain underlying medical conditions, including a cochlear implant. A single revaccination should be administered after 5 years to children with functional or anatomic asplenia or an immunocompromising condition. See *MMWR* 1997;46:(No. RR-8).

6. **Hepatitis A vaccine (HepA).**
- Administer 2 doses at least 6 months apart.

- HepA is recommended for children aged older than 23 months who live in areas where vaccination programs target older children, who are at increased risk for infection, or for whom immunity against hepatitis A is desired.

7. **Hepatitis B vaccine (HepB).**
- Administer the 3-dose series to those not previously vaccinated.
- A 2-dose series (separated by at least 4 months) of adult formulation Recombivax HB is licensed for children aged 11 through 15 years.

8. **Inactivated poliovirus vaccine (IPV).**
- The final dose in the series should be administered on or after the fourth birthday and at least 6 months following the previous dose.
- If both OPV and IPV were administered as part of a series, a total of 4 doses should be administered, regardless of the child's current age.

9. **Measles, mumps, and rubella vaccine (MMR).**
- If not previously vaccinated, administer 2 doses or the second dose for those who have received only 1 dose, with at least 28 days between doses.

10. **Varicella vaccine.**
- For persons aged 7 through 18 years without evidence of immunity (see *MMWR* 2007;56[No. RR-4]), administer 2 doses if not previously vaccinated or the second dose if only 1 dose has been administered.
- For persons aged 7 through 12 years, the minimum interval between doses is 3 months. However, if the second dose was administered at least 28 days after the first dose, it can be accepted as valid.
- For persons aged 13 years and older, the minimum interval between doses is 28 days.

The Recommended Immunization Schedules for Persons Aged 0 through 18 Years are approved by the Advisory Committee on Immunization Practices (**http://www.cdc.gov/vaccines/recs/acip**), the American Academy of Pediatrics (**http://www.aap.org**), and the American Academy of Family Physicians (**http://www.aafp.org**). Department of Health and Human Services • Centers for Disease Control and Prevention

TABLE 1.8 CDC Recommended Adult Immunization Schedule—United States 2010

Recommended Adult Immunization Schedule
UNITED STATES • 2010

Note: These recommendations must be read with the footnotes that follow containing number of doses, intervals between doses, and other important information.

Figure 1. Recommended adult immunization schedule, by vaccine and age group

VACCINE ▼ \ AGE GROUP ▶	19–26 years	27–49 years	50–59 years	60–64 years	≥65 years
Tetanus, diphtheria, pertussis (Td/Tdap)[1],*	Substitute 1-time dose of Tdap for Td booster; then boost with Td every 10 yrs				Td booster every 10 yrs
Human papillomavirus (HPV)[2],*	3 doses (females)				
Varicella[3],*	2 doses				
Zoster[4]				1 dose	1 dose
Measles, mumps, rubella (MMR)[5],*	1 or 2 doses			1 dose	
Influenza[6],*	1 dose annually				
Pneumococcal (polysaccharide)[7,8]	1 or 2 doses				1 dose
Hepatitis A[9],*	2 doses				
Hepatitis B[10],*	3 doses				
Meningococcal[11],*	1 or more doses				

Legend:

- ■ (light) For all persons in this category who meet the age requirements and who lack evidence of immunity (e.g., lack documentation of vaccination or have no evidence of prior infection)
- ■ (dark) Recommended if some other risk factor is present (e.g., on the basis of medical, occupational, lifestyle, or other indications)
- □ No recommendation

*Covered by the Vaccine Injury Compensation Program.

Report all clinically significant postvaccination reactions to the Vaccine Adverse Event Reporting System (VAERS). Reporting forms and instructions on filing a VAERS report are available at www.vaers.hhs.gov or by telephone, 800-822-7967.

Information on how to file a Vaccine Injury Compensation Program claim is available at www.hrsa.gov/vaccinecompensation or by telephone, 800-338-2382. To file a claim for vaccine injury, contact the U.S. Court of Federal Claims, 717 Madison Place, N.W., Washington, D.C. 20005; telephone, 202-357-6400.

Additional information about the vaccines in this schedule, extent of available data, and contraindications for vaccination is also available at www.cdc.gov/vaccines or from the CDC-INFO Contact Center at 800-CDC-INFO (800-232-4636) in English and Spanish, 24 hours a day, 7 days a week.

Use of trade names and commercial sources is for identification only and does not imply endorsement by the U.S. Department of Health and Human Services.

Figure 2. Vaccines that might be indicated for adults based on medical and other indications

VACCINE ▼ / INDICATION ▶	Pregnancy	Immuno-compromising conditions (excluding human immunodeficiency virus [HIV])[3–5,13]	HIV infection[3–5,12,13] CD4+ T lymphocyte count <200 cells/μL	HIV infection[3–5,12,13] CD4+ T lymphocyte count ≥200 cells/μL	Diabetes, heart disease, chronic lung disease, chronic alcoholism	Asplenia[12] (including elective splenectomy and persistent complement component deficiencies)	Chronic liver disease	Kidney failure, end-stage renal disease, receipt of hemodialysis	Health-care personnel
Tetanus, diphtheria, pertussis (Td/Tdap)[1,*]	Td	Substitute 1-time dose of Tdap for Td booster; then boost with Td every 10 yrs →							
Human papillomavirus (HPV)[2,*]	3 doses for females through age 26 yrs →								
Varicella[3,*]	Contraindicated	Contraindicated	Contraindicated	2 doses					
Zoster[4]	Contraindicated	Contraindicated	Contraindicated		1 dose				
Measles, mumps, rubella (MMR)[5,*]	Contraindicated	Contraindicated	Contraindicated	1 or 2 doses					
Influenza[6,*]	1 dose TIV annually								1 dose TIV or LAIV annually
Pneumococcal (polysaccharide)[7,8]		1 or 2 doses							
Hepatitis A[9]	2 doses								
Hepatitis B[10,*]	3 doses								
Meningococcal[11,*]	1 or more doses								

*Covered by the Vaccine Injury Compensation Program.

Legend:
- For all persons in this category who meet the age requirements and who lack evidence of immunity (e.g., lack documentation of vaccination or have no evidence of prior infection)
- Recommended if some other risk factor is present (e.g, on the basis of medical, occupational, lifestyle, or other indications)
- No recommendation

These schedules indicate the recommended age groups and medical indications for which administration of currently licensed vaccines is commonly indicated for adults ages 19 years and older, as of January 1, 2010. Licensed combination vaccines may be used whenever any components of the combination are indicated and when the vaccine's other components are not contraindicated. For detailed recommendations on all vaccines, including those used primarily for travelers or that are issued during the year, consult the manufacturers' package inserts and the complete statements from the Advisory Committee on Immunization Practices (www.cdc.gov/vaccines/pubs/acip-list.htm).

The recommendations in this schedule were approved by the Centers for Disease Control and Prevention's (CDC) Advisory Committee on Immunization Practices (ACIP), the American Academy of Family Physicians (AAFP), the American College of Obstetricians and Gynecologists (ACOG), and the American College of Physicians (ACP).

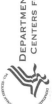

DEPARTMENT OF HEALTH AND HUMAN SERVICES
CENTERS FOR DISEASE CONTROL AND PREVENTION

(continued)

TABLE 1.8 (continued)

Footnotes

Recommended Adult Immunization Schedule—UNITED STATES • 2010

For complete statements by the Advisory Committee on Immunization Practices (ACIP), visit www.cdc.gov/vaccines/pubs/ACIP-list.htm.

1. **Tetanus, diphtheria, and acellular pertussis (Td/Tdap) vaccination**

Tdap should replace a single dose of Td for adults aged 19 through 64 years who have not received a dose of Tdap previously.

Adults with uncertain or incomplete history of primary vaccination series with tetanus and diphtheria toxoid-containing vaccines should begin or complete a primary vaccination series. A primary series for adults is 3 doses of tetanus and diphtheria toxoid-containing vaccines; administer the first 2 doses at least 4 weeks apart and the third dose 6–12 months after the second; Tdap can substitute for any one of the doses of Td in the 3-dose primary series. The booster dose of tetanus and diphtheria toxoid-containing vaccine should be administered to adults who have completed a primary series and if the last vaccination was received ≥10 years previously. Tdap or Td vaccine may be used, as indicated.

If a woman is pregnant and received the last Td vaccination ≥10 years previously, administer Tdap during the second or third trimester. If the woman received the last Td vaccination <10 years previously, administer Tdap during the immediate postpartum period. A dose of Tdap is recommended for postpartum women, close contacts of infants aged <12 months, and all health-care personnel with direct patient contact if they have not previously received Tdap. An interval as short as 2 years from the last Td is suggested; shorter intervals can be used. Td may be deferred during pregnancy and Tdap substituted in the immediate postpartum period, or Tdap can be administered instead of Td to a pregnant woman.

Consult the ACIP statement for recommendations for giving Td as prophylaxis in wound management.

2. **Human papillomavirus (HPV) vaccination**

HPV vaccination is recommended at age 11 or 12 years with catch-up vaccination at ages 13 through 26 years.

Ideally, vaccine should be administered before potential exposure to HPV through sexual activity; however, females who are sexually active should still be vaccinated consistent with age-based recommendations. Sexually active females who have not been infected with any of the four HPV vaccine types (types 6, 11, 16, 18 all of which HPV4 prevents) or any of the two HPV vaccine types (types 16 and 18 both of which HPV2 prevents) receive the full benefit of the vaccination. Vaccination is less beneficial for females who have already been infected with one or more of the HPV vaccine types. HPV4 or HPV2 can be administered to persons with a history of genital warts, abnormal Papanicolaou test, or positive HPV DNA test, because these conditions are not evidence of prior infection with all vaccine HPV types.

HPV4 may be administered to males aged 9 through 26 years to reduce their likelihood of acquiring genital warts. HPV4 would be most effective when administered before exposure to HPV through sexual contact.

A complete series for either HPV4 or HPV2 consists of 3 doses. The second dose should be administered 1–2 months after the first dose; the third dose should be administered 6 months after the first dose.

Although HPV vaccination is not specifically recommended for persons with the medical indications described in Figure 2, "Vaccines that might be indicated for adults based on medical and other indications," it may be administered to these persons because the HPV vaccine is not a live-virus vaccine. However, the immune response and vaccine efficacy might be less for persons with the medical indications described in Figure 2 than in persons who do not have the medical indications described or who are immunocompetent. Health-care personnel are not at increased risk because of occupational exposure, and should be vaccinated consistent with age-based recommendations.

3. **Varicella vaccination**

All adults without evidence of immunity to varicella should receive 2 doses of single-antigen varicella vaccine if not previously vaccinated or the second dose if they have received only 1 dose, unless they have a medical contraindication. Special consideration should be given to those who 1) have close contact with persons at high risk for severe disease (e.g., health-care personnel and family contacts of persons with immunocompromising conditions) or 2) are at high risk for exposure or transmission (e.g., teachers; child-care employees; residents and staff members of institutional settings, including correctional institutions; college students; military personnel; adolescents and adults living in households with children; nonpregnant women of childbearing age; and international travelers).

Evidence of immunity to varicella in adults includes any of the following: 1) documentation of 2 doses of varicella vaccine at least 4 weeks apart; 2) U.S.-born before 1980 (although for health-care personnel and pregnant women, birth before 1980 should not be considered evidence of immunity); 3) history of varicella based on diagnosis or verification of varicella by a health-care provider (for a patient reporting a history of or presenting with an atypical case, a mild case, or both, health-care providers should seek either an epidemiologic link with a typical varicella case or to a laboratory-confirmed case or evidence of laboratory confirmation, if it was performed at the time of acute disease); 4) history of herpes zoster based on diagnosis or verification of herpes zoster by a health-care provider; or 5) laboratory evidence of immunity or laboratory confirmation of disease.

Pregnant women should be assessed for evidence of varicella immunity. Women who do not have evidence of immunity should receive the first dose of varicella vaccine upon completion or termination of pregnancy and before discharge from the health-care facility. The second dose should be administered 4–8 weeks after the first dose.

4. Herpes zoster vaccination

A single dose of zoster vaccine is recommended for adults aged ≥60 years regardless of whether they report a prior episode of herpes zoster. Persons with chronic medical conditions may be vaccinated unless their condition constitutes a contraindication.

5. Measles, mumps, rubella (MMR) vaccination

Adults born before 1957 generally are considered immune to measles and mumps.

Measles component: Adults born during or after 1957 should receive 1 or more doses of MMR vaccine unless they have 1) a medical contraindication; 2) documentation of vaccination with 1 or more doses of MMR vaccine; 3) laboratory evidence of immunity; or 4) documentation of physician–diagnosed measles.

A second dose of MMR vaccine, administered 4 weeks after the first dose, is recommended for adults who 1) have been recently exposed to measles or are in an outbreak setting; 2) have been vaccinated previously with killed measles vaccine; 3) have been vaccinated with an unknown type of measles vaccine during 1963–1967; 4) are students in postsecondary educational institutions; 5) work in a health-care facility; or 6) plan to travel internationally.

Mumps component: Adults born during or after 1957 should receive 1 dose of MMR vaccine unless they have 1) a medical contraindication; 2) documentation of vaccination with 1 or more doses of MMR vaccine; 3) laboratory evidence of immunity; or 4) documentation of physician-diagnosed mumps.

A second dose of MMR vaccine, administered 4 weeks after the first dose, is recommended for adults who 1) live in a community experiencing a mumps outbreak and are in an affected age group; 2) are students in postsecondary educational institutions; 3) work in a health-care facility; or 4) plan to travel internationally.

Rubella component: 1 dose of MMR vaccine is recommended for women who do not have documentation of rubella vaccination, or who lack laboratory evidence of immunity. For women of childbearing age, regardless of birth year, rubella immunity should be determined and women should be counseled regarding congenital rubella syndrome. Women who do not have evidence of immunity should receive MMR vaccine upon completion or termination of pregnancy and before discharge from the health-care facility.

Health-care personnel born before 1957: For unvaccinated health-care personnel born before 1957 who lack laboratory evidence of measles, mumps, and/or rubella immunity or laboratory confirmation of disease, health-care facilities should consider vaccinating personnel with 2 doses of MMR vaccine at the appropriate interval (for measles and mumps) and 1 dose of MMR vaccine (for rubella), respectively.

During outbreaks, health-care facilities should recommend that unvaccinated health-care personnel born before 1957, who lack laboratory evidence of measles, mumps, and/or rubella immunity or laboratory confirmation of disease, receive 2 doses of MMR vaccine during an outbreak of measles or mumps, and 1 dose during an outbreak of rubella.

Complete information about evidence of immunity is available at www.cdc.gov/vaccines/recs/provisional/default.htm.

6. Seasonal Influenza vaccination

Vaccinate all persons aged ≥50 years and any younger persons who would like to decrease their risk of getting influenza. Vaccinate persons aged 19 through 49 years with any of the following indications.

Medical: Chronic disorders of the cardiovascular or pulmonary systems, including asthma; chronic metabolic diseases, including diabetes mellitus; renal or hepatic dysfunction, hemoglobinopathies, or immunocompromising conditions (including immunocompromising conditions caused by medications or HIV); cognitive, neurologic or neuromuscular disorders; and pregnancy during the influenza season. No data exist on the risk for severe or complicated influenza disease among persons with asplenia; however, influenza is a risk factor for secondary bacterial infections that can cause severe disease among persons with asplenia.

Occupational: All health-care personnel, including those employed by long-term care and assisted-living facilities, and caregivers of children aged <5 years.

Other: Residents of nursing homes and other long-term care and assisted-living facilities; persons likely to transmit influenza to persons at high risk (e.g., in-home household contacts and caregivers of children aged <5 years, persons aged ≥50 years, and persons of all ages with high-risk conditions).

Healthy, nonpregnant adults aged <50 years without high-risk medical conditions who are not contacts of severely immunocompromised persons in special-care units may receive either the intranasally administered live, attenuated influenza vaccine (FluMist) or inactivated vaccine. Other persons should receive the inactivated vaccine.

7. Pneumococcal polysaccharide (PPSV) vaccination

Vaccinate all persons aged ≥65 years with the following indications.

Medical: Chronic lung disease (including asthma); chronic cardiovascular diseases; diabetes mellitus; chronic liver diseases, cirrhosis; chronic alcoholism; functional or anatomic asplenia (e.g., sickle cell disease or splenectomy [if elective splenectomy is planned, vaccinate at least 2 weeks before surgery]); immunocompromising conditions including chronic renal failure or nephrotic syndrome; and cochlear implants and cerebrospinal fluid leaks. Vaccinate as close to HIV diagnosis as possible.

Other: Residents of nursing homes or long-term care facilities and persons who smoke cigarettes. Routine use of PPSV is not recommended for American Indians/Alaska Natives or persons aged <65 years unless they have underlying medical conditions that are PPSV indications. However, public health authorities may consider recommending PPSV for American Indians/Alaska Natives and persons aged 50 through 64 years who are living in areas where the risk for invasive pneumococcal disease is increased.

8. Revaccination with PPSV

One-time revaccination after 5 years is recommended for persons with chronic renal failure or nephrotic syndrome; functional or anatomic asplenia (e.g., sickle cell disease or splenectomy); and for persons with immunocompromising conditions. For persons aged ≥65 years, one-time revaccination is recommended if they were vaccinated ≥5 years previously and were younger than aged <65 years at the time of primary vaccination.

(continued)

TABLE 1.8 *(continued)*

9. Hepatitis A vaccination

Vaccinate persons with any of the following indications and any person seeking protection from hepatitis A virus (HAV) infection.

Behavioral: Men who have sex with men and persons who use injection drugs.

Occupational: Persons working with HAV-infected primates or with HAV in a research laboratory setting.

Medical: Persons with chronic liver disease and persons who receive clotting factor concentrates.

Other: Persons traveling to or working in countries that have high or intermediate endemicity of hepatitis A (a list of countries is available at wwww.cdc.gov/travel/contentdiseases.aspx).

Unvaccinated persons who anticipate close personal contact (e.g., household contact or regular babysitting) with an international adoptee from a country of high or intermediate endemicity during the first 60 days after arrival of the adoptee in the United States should consider vaccination. The first dose of the 2-dose hepatitis A vaccine series should be administered as soon as adoption is planned, ideally ≥2 weeks before the arrival of the adoptee.

Single-antigen vaccine formulations should be administered in a 2-dose schedule at either 0 and 6–12 months (Havrix), or 0 and 6–18 months (Vaqta). If the combined hepatitis A and hepatitis B vaccine (Twinrix) is used, administer 3 doses at 0, 1, and 6 months; alternatively, a 4-dose schedule, administered on days 0, 7, and 21–30 followed by a booster dose at month 12 may be used.

10. Hepatitis B vaccination

Vaccinate persons with any of the following indications and any person seeking protection from hepatitis B virus (HBV) infection.

Behavioral: Sexually active persons who are not in a long-term, mutually monogamous relationship (e.g., persons with more than one sex partner during the previous 6 months); persons seeking evaluation or treatment for a sexually transmitted disease (STD); current or recent injection-drug users; and men who have sex with men.

Occupational: Health-care personnel and public-safety workers who are exposed to blood or other potentially infectious body fluids.

Medical: Persons with end-stage renal disease, including patients receiving hemodialysis; persons with HIV infection; and persons with chronic liver disease.

Other: Household contacts and sex partners of persons with chronic HBV infection; clients and staff members of institutions for persons with developmental disabilities; and international travelers to countries with high or intermediate prevalence of chronic HBV infection (a list of countries is available at wwww.cdc.gov/travel/contentdiseases.aspx).

Hepatitis B vaccination is recommended for all adults in the following settings: STD treatment facilities; HIV testing and treatment facilities; facilities providing drug-abuse treatment and prevention services; health-care settings targeting services to injection-drug users or men who have sex with men; correctional facilities; end-stage renal disease programs and facilities for chronic hemodialysis patients; and institutions and nonresidential daycare facilities for persons with developmental disabilities.

Administer or complete a 3-dose series of HepB to those persons not previously vaccinated. The second dose should be administered 1 month after the first dose; the third dose should be administered at least 2 months after the second dose (and at least 4 months after the first dose). If the combined hepatitis A and hepatitis B vaccine (Twinrix) is used, administer 3 doses at 0, 1, and 6 months; alternatively, a 4-dose schedule, administered on days 0, 7, and 21–30 followed by a booster dose at month 12 may be used.

Adult patients receiving hemodialysis or with other immunocompromising conditions should receive 1 dose of 40 μg/mL (Recombivax HB) administered on a 3-dose schedule or 2 doses of 20 μg/mL (Engerix-B) administered simultaneously on a 4-dose schedule at 0, 1, 2 and 6 months.

11. Meningococcal vaccination

Meningococcal vaccine should be administered to persons with the following indications.

Medical: Adults with anatomic or functional asplenia, or persistent complement component deficiencies.

Other: First-year college students living in dormitories; microbiologists routinely exposed to isolates of Neisseria meningitidis; military recruits; and persons who travel to or live in countries in which meningococcal disease is hyperendemic or epidemic (e.g., the "meningitis belt" of sub-Saharan Africa during the dry season [December through June]), particularly if their contact with local populations will be prolonged. Vaccination is required by the government of Saudi Arabia for all travelers to Mecca during the annual Hajj.

Meningococcal conjugate vaccine (MCV4) is preferred for adults with any of the preceding indications who are aged ≤55 years; meningococcal polysaccharide vaccine (MPSV4) is preferred for adults aged ≥56 years. Revaccination with MCV4 after 5 years is recommended for adults previously vaccinated with MCV4 or MPSV4 who remain at increased risk for infection (e.g., adults with anatomic or functional asplenia). Persons whose only risk factor is living in on-campus housing are not recommended to receive an additional dose.

12. Selected conditions for which *Haemophilus influenzae* type b (Hib) vaccine may be used

Hib vaccine generally is not recommended for persons aged ≥5 years. No efficacy data are available on which to base a recommendation concerning use of Hib vaccine for older children and adults. However, studies suggest good immunogenicity in patients who have sickle cell disease, leukemia, or HIV infection or who have had a splenectomy. Administering 1 dose of Hib vaccine to these high-risk persons who have not previously received Hib vaccine is not contraindicated.

13. Immunocompromising conditions

Inactivated vaccines generally are acceptable (e.g., pneumococcal, meningococcal, influenza [inactivated influenza vaccine]) and live vaccines generally are avoided in persons with immune deficiencies or immunocompromising conditions. Information on specific conditions is available at www.cdc.gov/vaccines/pubs/acip-list.htm.

It is recommended that you contact the CDC prior to travel to get the latest update on recommended vaccinations. The CDC travel Web site is http://wwwnc.cdc.gov/travel/content/vaccinations.aspx.

REFERENCES

Centers for Disease Control and Prevention. (2010a). *CDC Catch-up Immunization Schedule for Persons Aged 4 Months Through 18 Years Who Start Late or Who Are More Than 1 Month Behind—United States 2010.* Retrieved March 13, 2010, from http://www.cdc.gov/vaccines/recs/schedules/downloads/child/2010/10_catchup-schedule-pr.pdf.

Centers for Disease Control and Prevention. (2010b). *CDC Recommended Adult Immunization Schedule—United States 2010.* Retrieved March 13, 2010, from http://www.cdc.gov/vaccines/recs/schedules/downloads/adult/2010/adult-schedule-bw.pdf.

Centers for Disease Control and Prevention. (2010c). *CDC Recommended Immunization Schedule for Persons Aged 0 Through 6 Years—United States 2010.* Retrieved March 13, 2010, from http://www.cdc.gov/vaccines/recs/schedules/downloads/child/2010/10_0-6yrs-schedule-pr.pdf.

Centers for Disease Control and Prevention. (2010d). *CDC Recommended Immunization Schedule for Persons Aged 7 Through 18 Years—United States 2010.* Retrieved March 13, 2010, from http://www.cdc.gov/vaccines/recs/schedules/downloads/child/2010/10_7-18yrs-schedule-pr.pdf.

Centers for Disease Control and Prevention. (2010e). *Vacations: What you need to know about vaccinations and travel: A checklist.* Retrieved March 13, 2010, from http://www.cdc.gov/travel/content/vaccinations.aspx.

Centers for Disease Control and Prevention. (n.d.). *BMI calculator for children and teens.* Retrieved March 13, 2010, from http://apps.nccd.cdc.gov/dnpabmi/Calculator.aspx.

Centers for Disease Control and Prevention. (n.d.). *Growth charts.* Retrieved March 13, 2010, from http://www.cdc.gov/growthcharts/.

Centers for Disease Control and Prevention. (n.d.). Immunization applications for PC/handhelds. Retrieved March 13, 2010, from http://www.immunizationed.org/AnyPage.aspx?pgid=2.

Childhood Nutrition. (n.d.). *Serving sizes.* Retrieved April 5, 2010, from http://www.nourishinteractive.com/parents_area/healthy_family_nutrition_newsletter/portion_control_childhood_easy_weight_management_tips_reducing_kids_food_serving_sizes.

Demory-Luce, D. (2004). *What's a child's portion for fruits and vegetables?* USDA/ARS Children's Nutrition Research Center at Baylor College of Medicine. Retrieved April 5, 2010, from http://www.bcm.edu/cnrc/consumer/archives/portionsizes.htm.

Mark, M. G. (1998). *Broadribb's Introductory Pediatric Nursing.* Philadelphia: Lippincott-Raven Publishers.

National Heart Lung and Blood Institute. (n.d.). *Obesity education initiative: BMI calculator.* Retrieved January 23, 2010 from http://www.nhlbisupport.com/bmi/.

Nutrition Exploration. (n.d.) *Interactive Pyramid.* Retrieved from http://www.nutritionexplorations.org/kids/nutrition-pyramid.asp.

U.S. Department of Agriculture. (n.d.) *Food pyramid.* Retrieved April 5, 2010. from http://www.mypyramid.gov/.

U.S. Department of Agriculture. (n.d.) *Food pyramid for children.* Retrieved April 5, 2010, from http://teamnutrition.usda.gov/kids-pyramid.html.

Zawenda, E. (1996). Malnutrition in the elderly. *Postgraduate Medicine, 100,* 208.

Pain Management Guidelines

Moya Cook

ACUTE PAIN

Definition

A. Acute pain is defined as pain that usually results from tissue injury; however, it may be experienced even with no identifiable cause. Acute pain usually resolves when the tissue injury heals. Most acute pain resolves in less than 6 weeks or less than 3 months.

Incidence

A. Acute pain is the most common reason for self-medication and presentation for treatment in the health care system. Acute pain is very individual and if not treated properly can have devastating physiological and psychological effects. Because pain is very subjective in nature, the patient care plan needs to be individualized to meet the patient's needs. Proper treatment of acute pain could prevent the development of some types of chronic pain syndromes.

Pathogenesis

A. Acute pain is usually the result of stimulation of the sympathetic nervous system.

Common Complaints

A. Pain at the specific site
B. Increased heart rate
C. Increased respiratory rate
D. Elevated blood pressure
E. Sweating
F. Nausea

Other Signs and Symptoms

A. Urinary retention
B. Dilated pupils
C. Pallor

Subjective Data

A. Elicit location of pain.
B. Note effects of pain on activity of daily living.
C. Note intensity of pain at rest and during activity.
D. List precipitating factors.
E. Identify alleviating factors.

F. Note the quality of pain.
G. Is there radiation of pain?
H. Rate pain on a pain scale (usually on the 1–10 scale with 1 being the least and 10 being the worst).

Adaptations need to be made to the assessment tool using the faces scale in children. Incapacitated or cognitively impaired patients may also need special consideration to evaluate their pain.

Physical Examination

A. Check temperature, pulse, respirations, and blood pressure.
B. Inspect
  1. Observe overall appearance.
  2. Note affect and ability to express self and pain.
  3. Note facial grimaces with movement.
  4. Note gait, stance, and movements.
  5. Inspect area at pain site.
C. Auscultate
  1. Auscultate heart and lungs.
  2. Auscultate neck and abdomen.
D. Palpate: Palpate affected area of pain.
E. Percuss
  1. Percuss chest.
  2. Percuss abdomen.
F. Musculoskeletal exam

When performing musculoskeletal exam, identify the location of pain, presence of trigger points, evidence of injury or trauma, edema, erythema, warmth, heat, lesions, petechiae, tenderness, decreased range of motion, pain with movement, crepitus, laxity of ligaments or cords, spasms, or guarding.

  1. Perform complete musculoskeletal exam, concentrating on area of pain.
  2. Assess deep tendon reflexes (DTRs).
G. Neurologic exam
  1. Perform complete neurologic exam.
  2. Identify change in sensory function, skin tenderness, weakness, muscle atrophy, and/or loss of deep tendon reflexes.

Diagnostic Tests

A. **No diagnostic testing is required unless clearly indicated to rule out organic cause of pain.** If organic disease is suspected diagnostic testing may include:
   1. CT imaging
   2. MRI
   3. Blood chemistries
   4. Radiographic X-ray
   5. Lumbar puncture
   6. Ultrasound
   7. EKG/echocardiogram

Differential Diagnosis

The differential diagnoses depend on the location of the acute pain.

A. Head
   1. Migraine
   2. Cluster headache/migraine headache
   3. Temporal arteritis
   4. Intracranial bleeding or stroke
   5. Sinusitis
   6. Dental abscess
B. Neck
   1. Meningitis
   2. Muscle strain/sprain
   3. Whiplash injury
   4. Thyroiditis
C. Chest
   1. Pulmonary emboli
   2. Myocardial infarction
   3. Pneumonia
   4. Costocondritis
   5. Angina
   6. GERD/esophagitis
D. Abdomen
   1. Peritonitis
   2. Appendicitis
   3. Ectopic pregnancy/uterine pregnancy
   4. Endometriosis
   5. PID
   6. Peptic ulcer
   7. Cholelithiasis
   8. Colitis/diverticulitis
   9. Constipation
   10. Gastroenteritis
   11. Irritable bowel syndrome
   12. UTI, kidney stone, pyelonephritis
   13. Prostatitis
E. Musculoskeletal
   1. Muscle sprain/strain/tear
   2. Skeletal fracture
   3. Viral infection
   4. Gout
   5. Vitamin D deficiency

Plan

Acute pain is a symptom, not a diagnosis. Try to identify the cause or source of the acute pain depending on the location. If the pain is organic in nature make the appropriate referral. The overall goal is to treat the acute pain appropriately.

A. **Visceral pain:** treatment of choice is corticosteroids, intraspinal local anesthetic, NSAIDS, and opioids.
B. **Somatic pain:** acetaminophen, cold packs, corticosteroids, localized anesthetics, NSAIDS, opioids, and tactile stimulation.
C. **Neuropathic pain:** tricyclic antidepressants, using Amitriptyline as the first-line treatment for neuropathic pain. Anticonvulsants like carbamazepine (Tegretol), phenytoin (Dilantin), and valproic acid (Depakene) can be useful in treating neuropathic pain. Other treatments include local anesthetics, tramadol (Ultram), and glucocorticoids.

Follow-up

A. Once organic cause of pain has been ruled out, initial follow-up is 48–72 hours after onset.
B. Ensure the patient has access to care on a regular schedule.

Consultation/Referral

If the acute pain is organic, make the appropriate referral to a specialist.

CHRONIC PAIN

Definition

A. Chronic pain is a nociceptive sensation that persists for months or even years beyond the usual healing time and is out of proportion with the pathologic stressors causing it.

Incidence

Pain syndromes are commonly seen in clinical practice and are the third most widespread health problem in the United States. Chronic pain costs the American people about $65 billion a year in health care expenses, disability costs, and lost productivity. Chronic pain patients have a better than 50% chance of becoming addicted to drugs. As the U.S. population continues to age and the average life expectancy is increasing, the primary care provider will be providing care for more chronic diseases and handling more chronic pain patients.

A. Women are affected more than men by 2:1.
B. Onset is usually in the fourth, fifth, or sixth decades and is often associated with marked functional disability.

Pathogenesis

A. Pain and nociception are not synonymous. Nociception is explained neurologically as a sensory process. Pain is a perceptual process that is influenced by the patient's affective and cognitive functions.

Predisposing Factors

A. Age 30–50 years
B. Female gender
C. History of having seen many physicians
D. Frequent use of several nonspecific medications
E. Depression
F. Personality, including moods, fears, expectations, coping efforts, and resources

Common Complaints

A. Specific to site of pain
B. Emotional distress related to fear, maladaptive or inadequate support systems, and other coping resources

C. Treatment-induced complications
D. Overuse of drugs
E. Inability to work
F. Financial complications
G. Disruption of usual activities
H. Sleep disturbances
I. Pain becomes primary life focus

Other Signs and Symptoms

A. Pain lasts longer than 6 months.
B. There may be anger and loss of faith or trust in the health care system. This type of patient frequently takes too many medications, stays in bed a great deal, has seen many physicians, has lost skills, and experiences little joy in either work or play.

Subjective Data

A. Elicit a clear description of the onset, location, quality, intensity, and time course of pain and any factors that aggravate or relieve it.
B. Determine the extent to which the patient is suffering, disabled, and unable to enjoy usual activity.
C. Assess whether the patient's behavior seems appropriate to the disease or injury, or if there is evidence of symptom amplification for any psychological or social reasons. **The intensity of the chronic pain is often out of proportion to the pathologic state causing it.**
D. Obtain a complete review of systems including nausea, numbness, weakness, insomnia, loss of appetite, dysphoria, or malaise.
E. Obtain a complete family and social history.
F. Obtain the patient's medical history relevant to the pain including diagnosis, testing, treatments, and outcomes.
G. Assess the patient's understanding of the pain and what can be done to relieve it.

Physical Examination

A. Check temperature, pulse, respirations, and blood pressure.
B. Inspect
   1. Observe overall appearance.
   2. Note affect and ability to express self and pain.
   3. Note facial grimaces with movement.
   4. Note gait, stance, and movements.
   5. Inspect area at pain site.
C. Auscultate
   1. Auscultate heart and lungs.
   2. Auscultate neck and abdomen.
D. Palpate: Palpate affected area of pain.
E. Percuss
   1. Percuss chest.
   2. Percuss abdomen.
F. Musculoskeletal exam

When performing musculoskeletal exam, identify the location of pain, presence of trigger points, evidence of injury or trauma, edema, erythema, warmth, heat, lesions, petechiae, tenderness, decreased range of motion, pain with movement, crepitus, laxity of ligaments or cords, spasms, or guarding.

   1. Perform a complete musculoskeletal exam, concentrating on the area of pain.

G. Neurologic exam
   1. Perform complete neurologic exam.
   2. Note the patient's affect and mood. Administer a depression test.
   3. Identify change in sensory function, skin tenderness, weakness, muscle atrophy, and/or loss of deep tendon reflexes.

Diagnostic Tests

A. **None is required unless clearly indicated to rule out organic cause of pain.**
   1. Remember that pain previously diagnosed as chronic pain syndrome can be organic and vice versa. Organic causes must always be evaluated and excluded.
B. Consider using depression tool such as the Beck Depression Inventory. This tool can be administered at a subsequent appointment to follow the patient's symptoms.

Differential Diagnosis

A. Pain disorder
B. Pain related to a disease with no cure
C. Somatization disorder
D. Conversion disorder
E. Hypochondriasis
F. Depression
G. Chemical dependency
H. Fibromyalgia

Plan

A. General interventions
   1. Treatment is multidimensional and should not be focused on pharmacological treatment alone.
   2. Offer hope and potential for improvement of pain control and improvement of function but *not* cure.
   3. The pain is real to the patient, and acceptance of the problem must occur before a mutually agreed on treatment plan can be initiated.
   4. Depression is a common emotional disturbance in chronic pain patients and is treatable. Screening with the Beck Depression Inventory or other screening tool is suggested.
   5. Identify specific and realistic goals for therapy such as a good night's sleep, being able to go shopping, or being able to return to work.
   6. Carefully assess the level of pain using available tools such as a daily pain diary or other pain assessment scales.
   7. Avoid pain reinforcement such as sympathy and attention to pain. Provide positive response to productive activities. Improving activity tolerance assists in desensitizing the patient to pain.
   8. Shift the focus from the pain to accomplishing daily assigned self-help tasks. The accomplishment of these tasks functions as positive reinforcement.
   9. Consider alternative approaches to pain control such as the following:
      a. Cognitive behavioral training such as problem solving, guided imagery, hypnosis, controlled breathing exercises, attention diversion, meditation, yoga exercises, and progressive muscle relaxation (PMR) to help relax major muscle groups.

b. Occupational therapy.
c. Vocational therapy.
d. Physical therapy such as noninvasive techniques, transcutaneous electrical nerve stimulation (TENS), hot or cold therapy, hydrotherapy, traction, massage, bracing, exercise.
e. Myofascial release treatments.
f. Individual and family therapy or counseling.
g. Anesthetic or neurosurgical procedures.
h. Acupuncture and music therapy have also been shown to improve quality of life in patients with chronic pain.
B. Patient teaching: See the Section III Patient Teaching Guide for this chapter, "Chronic Pain."
C. Pharmaceutical therapy
1. Monitoring patients receiving narcotic treatment with random urine comprehensive drug screens can assist the practitioner with narcotic abuse and proper use of narcotic medication. If narcotic addiction is present, pursue detoxification as soon as possible.
2. NSAIDs provide relief and reduce local tissue irritation.
3. All therapies need a 2- to 3-week trial to adequately evaluate therapy.
4. Tricyclic antidepressants are extremely useful in the management of chronic pain. Patients who are not depressed obtain excellent pain relief with tricyclic antidepressants such as Amitriptyline and doxepin.
5. Anticonvulsants are useful in controlling some neuropathic pain: carbamazepine (Tegretol), phenytoin (Dilantin), and valproic acid (Depakene). **Patients need to be monitored monthly for hepatic dysfunction and hematopoietic suppression.**
6. Phenothiazines in conjunction with tricyclics have been used in the treatment of chronic pain. These drugs are not considered a primary therapy and are often associated with unacceptable side effects.
7. Benzodiazepines and barbiturates are not useful in the treatment of chronic pain.
8. Diphenhydramine HCl (Benadryl) or hydroxyzine HCl (Atarax) is an appropriate choice for patients requiring mild sedation.
9. Severe anxiety should be treated with antidepressants.
10. Opiates are generally not used in the treatment of benign chronic pain.
11. New research has identified that some hormone replacements may assist in the treatment of chronic pain. Treatment with hormones would require laboratory testing and/or a referral to an endocrinologist.

Follow-up

A. See patients every 4–6 weeks for evaluation.
B. Ensure the patient has access to care on a regular schedule.
C. These brief visits should be regular so that care is not perceived to be dependent on escalation of symptoms.

Consultation/Referral

A. Consider patient referral to a pain clinic if pain control is not adequate.

B. Consult with a physician if referral is needed for psychological counseling or pain clinic assessment, or if substance abuse is suspected.

⬛ LOWER BACK PAIN

Definition

Painful conditions of the lower back may be categorized as follows:

A. Potentially serious disorders: acute fractures, tumor, progressive neurologic deficit, nerve root compression, and cauda equine syndrome
B. Degenerative disorders: aging or repetitive use, degenerative disease, and osteoarthritis
C. Nonspecific disorders: benign and self-limiting with unclear etiology

Incidence

A. Lower back pain is commonly seen in patients from ages 20–40.
B. Approximately 70%–80% of people experience back pain at one point in their lifetime.

Pathogenesis

A. Pain arises from fracture, tumor, nerve root compression, degenerative disk, osteoarthritis, and strain of the ligaments and musculature of the lumbosacral area.

Predisposing Factors

A. Trauma causing ligament tearing; stretching of vertebra, muscles, tendons, ligaments, or fascia
B. Repetitive mechanical stress
C. Tumor
D. Exaggerated lumbar lordosis
E. Abnormal, forward-tipped pelvis
F. Uneven leg length
G. Chronic poor posture due to inadequate conditioning of muscle strength and flexibility, improper lifting techniques causing excessive strain, poor body mechanics
H. Inadequate rest
I. Emotional depression

Common Complaints

A. Pain in the lower back area may range from discomfort to severe back pain, with or without radiation.

Other Signs and Symptoms

A. Ambulating with a limp
B. Limited range of motion
C. Posture normal to guarded

Subjective Data

A. Ask the patient to discuss the origin of pain. How has the pain progressed or changed since the initial injury?
B. Ask the patient to point to an area where pain is felt.
C. Have the patient describe the pain. Is it radiating, with sharp, shooting pain down to the lower leg and feet?
D. Ask: What makes the pain worse or better? Have the patient list current medications or therapies used for pain, noting results of treatment.

E. Investigate occurrence of systemic symptoms such as fever and weight loss.

F. Explore patient's past medical history. Note previous trauma or overuse, TB, arthritis, cancer, and osteoporosis.

G. Inquire about symptoms such as dysuria, bowel or bladder incontinence, muscle weakness, paresthesia, and loss of sensation.

H. Ask the patient about precipitating factors such as athletics, heavy lifting, driving, yard work, occupation, sleep habits, or systemic disease.

I. Use a pain scale to describe the worst pain and the best pain levels.

Physical Examination

A. Check temperature, pulse, blood pressure, and respirations.

B. Inspect
   1. Observe general appearance; note discomfort and grimacing on movement and/or examination.
   2. Distraction may distinguish pain behavior from actual pathology.
   3. Note evidence of trauma with bruises, cuts, and fractures.
   4. Note posture and gait.

C. Palpate
   1. Palpate spine and paravertebral structures, noting point tenderness and muscle spasm. Palpation elicits paravertebral tenderness and generalized tenderness over lower back to upper buttocks.
   2. Examine abdomen for masses.
   3. Extremities: Palpate peripheral pulses.

D. Perform neurologic examination
   1. Identify sensation and pain distribution.
   2. Determine motor strength and evaluate whether muscle strength is symmetrical: upper extremity resistance is equal bilaterally.
   3. Test deep tendon reflexes and dorsiflexion of big toe.

E. Check sensation of perineum to rule out cauda equina syndrome.

F. Perform tractions tests: straight leg raises, crossed leg raise, Yeoman Guying, Patrick's test. Musculoskeletal findings include the following:
   1. Straight leg raising and dorsiflexion of foot on affected side may reduce lower back discomfort.
   2. Elevate each leg passively with flexion at hip and extension of knee. Positive straight leg raise is radicular pain when leg is raised 30°–60°.
   3. Crossed leg raises: test is positive when pain occurs in leg not being raised.
   4. Yeoman Guying: unilateral hyperextension in prone position identifies lumbosacral mechanical disorder.
   5. Patrick's test: place heel on opposite knee and apply lateral force; check for hip or sacroiliac disease.
   6. Range of motion: increased pain with extension often indicates osteoarthritis. Increased pain with flexion often indicates strain or injured disk.

G. Pelvic exam: Consider pelvic and rectal exam, if indicated. If the patient has fallen on the coccyx, a rectal exam is needed to check for stability.

Diagnostic Tests

A. CBC, erythrocyte sedimentation rate, serum calcium, alkaline phosphatase, urinalysis, and serum immuno-electrophoresis when inflammatory, neoplastic, diffuse bone disease, or renal disease is suspected.

B. Radiography of spine.

C. Consider the following tests:
   1. MRI to rule out disk disease and tumors.
   2. Bone scan to rule out cancer.

Differential Diagnoses

A. Back pain secondary to musculoskeletal pain
B. Herniated intervertebral disease
C. Sciatica
D. Fracture
E. Tumor
F. Abdominal aneurysm
G. Pyelonephritis
H. Metabolic bone disease
I. Gynecologic disease
J. Peripheral neuropathy
K. Depression
L. Prostatitis
M. Spinal stenosis
N. Osteoarthritis
O. Osteoporosis

Plan

A. General interventions
   1. The patient should continue physical activity. Tell him or her to let pain be his or her guide.
   2. For acute muscle strain, have the patient apply local cold packs 20–30 min several times a day for the first 24 hours. Thereafter, hot packs may be used.
   3. Chronic or recurrent pain may be treated with either ice or heat applications, whichever gives relief.

B. Patient teaching
   1. Give accurate information on the prognosis for quick recovery such as continuing light physical activity, doing back-strengthening exercises, and avoiding overuse of medications.
   2. Improvement occurs in most cases in a few weeks, although mild symptoms may persist.
   3. Provide handouts on back exercises; see the Section III Patient Teaching Guide for this chapter, "Back Stretches."
   4. After intense pain abates, the patient may perform low-back exercises for range of motion and strengthening, and isometric tightening exercises of abdominal and gluteal muscles.
   5. Teach patient knee-chest exercises. Have him or her place his or her back against the wall and contract abdominal and gluteal muscles 5–10 repetitions 4–6 times per day.
   6. Encourage the patient to walk daily.
   7. Teach him or her relaxation techniques.
   8. Encourage the patient to modify work hours and job tasks.
   9. Refer the patient for therapeutic massage or physical therapy as needed.

10. Obesity is often related to decreased exercise and poor physical fitness with reduced trunk muscle strength and endurance. Obese patients may experience back pain with normal activity.

C. Pharmaceutical therapy
1. Analgesics: acetaminophen 350–650 mg every 4–6 hours. Maximum dose is 4,000 mg a day. Inquire of any other current medications and/or OTC preparations containing acetaminophen.
2. NSAIDs: unless contraindicated due to GI symptoms or cardiovascular disease.
    a. Aspirin: 325–650 mg every 4–6 hours.
    b. Ibuprofen: 200–800 mg every 6–8 hours. Maximum dose is 3.2 g a day under the care of the provider, otherwise 1.2 g a day.
    c. Naproxen: 500 mg initially, followed by 250 mg every 6–8 hours.
    d. Piroxicam (Feldane): 20 mg every day.
    e. Meloxicam (Mobic): 7.5–15 mg daily.
    f. Celebrex: 100–200 mg twice a day.
    g. Nabumetone (Relafen): 500 mg twice a day (maximum dose of 2,000 mg per day).
3. Muscle relaxants
    a. Cyclobenzaprine HCl (Flexeril): 10 mg three times daily.
    b. Carisoprodol (Soma): 350 mg four times daily.
    c. Methocarbamol (Robaxin): 1.5 g every day initially, then 750–1,000 mg every day.
    d. Orphenadrine citrate (Norflex): 100 mg twice a day.
    e. Metaxalosne (Skelaxin): 800 mg 3–4 times a day.

Follow-up

A. If pain is severe or unimproved, follow-up in 24 hours.
B. If pain is moderate, reevaluate patient in 7–10 days.
C. See patient in 4–6 weeks to reevaluate condition and behavioral changes.
D. Recurrences are not uncommon but do not indicate a chronic or worsening case.

Consultation/Referral

A. Consult with a physician when considering red-flag diagnoses such as cauda equina syndrome, herniated disk, widespread neurologic involvement, carcinoma, or significant trauma.
B. Referral to a physician is needed for patients who note significant morning stiffness with a gradual onset prior to age 40, with continuing spinal movements in all directions, and involving some peripheral joints, iritis, skin rashes indicating inflammatory disorders such as ankylosing spondylitis, and related disorders.

Individual Considerations

A. Pregnancy: Pregnancy is often associated with low back discomfort. This is due to the redistribution of body weight. As weight increases in the abdominal area with the growing fetus, patients tend to compensate by changing posture and tilting the spine back.
B. Adults: For patients older than age 50 presenting with no prior history of backache, consider differential diagnosis of neoplasm. The most common metastasis seen is secondary to the primary site of breast or prostate, or to multiple myeloma. Pain most prominent in a recumbent position rarely radiates into the buttock or leg.

REFERENCES

Costead, L., & Banasik, J. (2005). *Pathophysiology* (3rd ed.). St. Louis: Elsevier Saunders.

Dunphy, L., Brown, J., Porter, B., & Thomas, D. (2007). *Primary care: The art and science of advanced practice nursing* (2nd ed.). Philadelphia: F. A. Davis Company.

Institute for Clinical Systems Improvement. (2008). *Health care guidelines: Assessment and management of acute pain* (6th ed.). Retrieved March 20, 2010, from http://www.icsi.org/pain_acute/pain__acute__assessment_and_management_of__3.html.

Institute for Change Systems Improvement. (2008, November). *Health care guidelines: Low back pain/adult.* Retrieved March 20, 2010, from www.icsi.org/guidelines.

Michigan Quality Improvement Consortium. (n.d.). *Management of acute low back pain.* Retrieved March 22, 2010, from www.guidelines.gov.

National Guideline Clearinghouse. (2007). *Assessment and management of pain.* Retrieved March 20, 2010, from www.guidelines.gov.

National Guideline Clearinghouse. (2008). *Management of acute low back pain.* Retrieved March 20, 2010, from www.guidelines.gov.

National Guideline Clearinghouse. (2009). *Managing chronic non-terminal pain including prescribing controlled substances.* Retrieved March 20, 2010, from www.guidelines.gov.

Spearling, N., March, L., Bellamy, N., Bodguk, N., & Brooks, P. (2005). Management of acute musculoskeletal pain. *APLR Journal of Rheumatology, 8.* Retrieved March 20, 2010, from EbscoHost Database.

Tennant, F. (2010). Hormone replacements and treatments in chronic pain. *Practical Pain Management, 10*(1): 36–40.

Dermatology Guidelines

Jill C. Cash

ACNE ROSACEA

Definition
A. A multifactorial vascular skin disorder, acne rosacea is characterized by chronic inflammatory processes in which flushing and dilation of the blood vessels occur on the face. It is manifested in four stages of pathologic events.

Incidence
A. Acne rosacea affects approximately 13 million people in the United States.

Pathogenesis
A. Rosacea is a functional vascular anomaly with a tendency toward recurrent dilation and flushing of the face. This results in inflammatory mediator release, extravasation of inflammatory cells, and the formation of inflammatory papules and pustules.

Predisposing Factors
A. Tendency to flush frequently
B. Exposure to heat, cold, or sunlight
C. Consumption of hot or spicy foods and alcoholic beverages
D. Some topical medications, astringents, or toners

Common Complaints
A. **Papules, pustules, and nodules. Hallmarks for diagnosis are the small papules and papulopustules. Many presenting erythematous papules have a tiny pustule at the crest. No comedones present.**
B. Periodic reddening or flushing of face.
C. Increase in skin temperature of face.
D. Face flushing in response to heat stimuli (hot liquids) in mouth.

Other Signs and Symptoms
A. Periorbital erythema
B. Telangiectasia, paranasally and on cheeks
C. Rhinophyma
D. Plethoroconjunctivitis with erythematous eyelid margins
E. Conjunctivitis: diffuse hypereremic type or nodular

F. Keratitis: lower portion of cornea, associated with pain, photophobia, and foreign body sensation

Subjective Data
A. Ask the patient to describe the location and the onset. Was the onset sudden or gradual? How have the symptoms continued to develop?
B. Assess if the skin is itchy or painful.
C. Assess for any associated discharge (blood or pus).
D. Complete a drug history. Has the patient recently taken any antibiotics or other medications?
E. Determine whether the patient has used any topical medications, astringents, toners, or new skin-care products.
F. Rule out any possible exposure to industrial or domestic toxins, insect bites, and possible contact with venereal disease or HIV.
G. Ask the patient about close contact with others with skin disorders.
H. Identify whether exposure to heat, cold, or sunlight provokes the symptoms.
I. Ask whether eating or drinking hot or spicy foods or consumption of alcoholic beverages provokes the symptoms.

Physical Examination
A. Check temperature, pulse, respirations, and blood pressure.
B. Inspect
   1. Inspect skin, focusing on face and scalp.
   2. Inspect nose and paranasal structures.
   3. Inspect eyes, eyelids, conjunctiva, and cornea. **An ocular manifestation, rosacea keratitis, may cause corneal ulcers to develop.**

Diagnostic Tests
A. None.
B. Consider skin biopsy to rule out sarcoidosis, if suspected.

Differential Diagnoses
A. Acne rosacea
B. Acne vulgaris

C. Steroid-induced acne
D. Perioral dermatitis
E. Seborrheic dermatitis
F. Lupus erythematosus
G. Cutaneous sarcoidosis

Plan

A. General interventions: Identify any causative or provocative factors: heat, cold, hot or spicy foods, alcoholic beverages, sunlight.
B. Patient teaching: See the Section III Patient Teaching Guide for this chapter, "Acne Rosacea."
C. Pharmaceutical therapy.
   1. Drug of choice: tetracycline 500–1,000 mg twice to four times daily for 2–4 weeks.
   2. Others: erythromycin 500 mg twice daily until clear, minocycline (Minocin), 50–200 mg daily divided into 2 doses, doxycycline (Vibramycin) 100 mg daily, ampicillin, and metronidazole (Flagyl, Protostat). Start at higher dose and taper to maintenance dose.
      a. Topical antibiotics. Apply topical metrogel twice daily after cleansing skin.
      b. Do no use topical steroids. Topical steroids may worsen irritation.
      c. Other topical antibiotics: Clindamycin (Cleocin T), erythromycin twice daily.
   3. Refractory cases may respond to isotretinoin (Accutane).

Follow-up

A. Follow-up in 2 weeks to evaluate therapy.
B. See patients every 2–4 weeks for evaluation until maintenance is reached.
C. Relapses are common following discontinuance of antibiotics; repeat treatment.

Consultation/Referral

A. Consult or refer the patient to a dermatologist if there is no improvement, or if the patient is unable to reach maintenance.
B. Provide an immediate referral to an ophthalmologist for treatment and follow-up if the eye is involved.

Individual Considerations

A. Adults: Tinted sulfacetamide (Sulfacet-R) lotion may be used by fair-skinned patients to cover erythema.

ACNE VULGARIS

Definition

A. Acne vulgaris is a disorder of the sebaceous glands and hair follicles of the skin that are most numerous on the face, back, and chest. The sebaceous glands become inflamed and form papules, pustules, cysts, open or closed comedones, and/or nodules on an erythemic base. In severe cases, scarring can result.

Incidence

A. Nearly 80%–90% of all adults experience acne during their lifetime. Acne vulgaris, commonly seen in adolescence, may even extend into the third or fourth decade of life.

Pathogenesis

A. Sebum is overproduced and collects in the sebaceous gland. Sebum, keratinized cells, and hair collect in the follicle. With *Propionibacterium acnes* present, the duct becomes clogged, and lesions (noninflammatory and/or inflammatory) evolve.

Predisposing Factors

A. Age (adolescence)
B. External irritants to skin (makeup, oils, equipment contact on skin)
C. Hormones (oral contraceptives with high progestin content)
D. Medications (lithium, halides, hydantoin derivatives, rifampin)
E. Hot, humid weather

Common Complaints

A. Outbreak of pimples on face, chest, shoulders, and back that do not resolve with over-the-counter (OTC) treatment.
B. Acne rosacea: telangiectasia, flushing, and rhinophyma present.

Other Signs and Symptoms

A. Mild: comedones open (blackhead) and closed (whitehead)
B. Moderate: comedones with papules and pustules
C. Severe: nodules, cysts, and scars

Subjective Data

A. Elicit the age of onset of outbreak, duration, and course of symptoms.
B. Determine what makes the lesions worse or better.
C. Ask whether there are certain times of the month or year when lesions are better or worse.
D. Identify the patient's current method of cleanser or moisturizer treatment.
E. Ask if the patient has ever been treated by a provider for this problem. If so, determine the treatment and results of the treatment.
F. Assess whether other family members have this same problem.
G. Ask the patient for a description of the patient's environment and occupation.
H. Explore with the patient any current stress factors in his or her life.

Physical Examination

A. Check temperature, blood pressure, and pulse.
B. Inspect
   1. Observe skin for location and severity of lesions.
   2. Rate severity of lesions as mild, moderate, or severe.
      a. Mild: Few papules/pustules, no nodules
      b. Moderate: Several papules/pustules, rare nodules
      c. Severe: Many papules/pustules with many nodules
   3. Take a picture of areas of affected skin for chart and document date. Use this for future appointments as a reference to compare results for follow-up visits.

Diagnostic Tests

A. No tests are generally required.
B. Culture lesions to rule out gram-negative folliculitis with patients on antibiotics.
C. Consider hormone testing if other primary causes of acne considered (FSH, LH, testosterone levels).

Differential Diagnoses

A. Acne vulgaris
B. Acne rosacea
C. Steroid rosacea
D. Folliculitis
E. Perioral acne
F. Drug-induced acne

Plan

A. General interventions
   1. Document location and severity of lesions. Assess quality of improvement at each office visit.
   2. The primary goal of treatment is prevention of scarring. Good control of lesions during puberty and early adulthood is required for best results. Anticipate ups and downs during the normal course and treatment.
B. Patient teaching
   1. See the Section III Patient Teaching Guide for this chapter: "Acne Vulgaris."
   2. Instruct the patient on proper cleansing routine. The patient should wash affected areas with mild soap (Purpose, Cetaphil) twice a day and apply medications as directed.
   3. Warn the patient that washing face more than two to three times a day can increase oil production and cause drying.
   4. Discuss current stressors in the patient's life and discuss treatment options.
   5. Recommend exercise routine 3–5 days a week.
   6. Recommend oil-free sunscreens. UV light is beneficial; however, there is a need to use with caution when retinoids and tetracycline have been prescribed.
C. Pharmaceutical therapy: **It may take up to 1–3 months before results are visible when using these medications.**
   1. Mild: treatment of choice is topical. Use one of the following:
      a. Benzoyl peroxide, 2.5%, 5%, 10%, begin with 2.5% at bedtime. May graduate to 5% or 10% twice daily, if needed, as tolerated.
      b. T-Stat, apply to dried areas twice daily. Avoid eyes, nose, and mouth creases.
      c. Topical Tretinoin 0.1% (Retin-A Micro), use at bedtime. Apply 20–30 min after washing skin.
         i. With Retin-A use, the patient may see a flare of rapid turnover of keratin plugs.
         ii. Instruct the patient to avoid abrasive soaps.
         iii. Warn the patient regarding photosensitivity.
      d. Desquam E, use at bedtime. Wash face with soap, then apply Desquam E.
   2. Moderate: Use one of the above topical medications in addition to one of the following oral medications:

a. Tetracycline 500 mg twice daily for 3–6 weeks, for adolescents older than 14 years. As condition improves, begin tapering medication to 250 mg twice daily for 6 weeks, then to daily or to every other day.
   i. Instruct the patient to take tetracycline on an empty stomach and to avoid dairy products, antacids, and iron.
   ii. Warn the patient about photosensitivity. This medication may be used as a maintenance dose at 250 mg daily or every other day for those patients who break out after discontinuing antibiotic therapy. No drug resistance is seen with tetracycline.
b. Erythromycin 250 mg four times per day after meals or topical erythromycin 2%, solution or gel, twice daily or clindamycin (Cleocin T), solution, pads, or gel, twice daily. Erythromycin resistance has been seen.
c. Minocycline 100 mg twice daily. When this is effective, taper to 50 mg twice daily.
   i. Have the patient drink plenty of fluids.
   ii. CNS side effects (headaches) have been seen.
d. Bactrim single strength twice daily, if the above regimens do not work well. Bactrim works well if others fail because it is effective for gram-negative folliculitis.
e. Oral contraceptives with higher doses of estrogen have also been effective for girls.
   3. Severe: Medications as prescribed per dermatologist.

Follow-up

See patients every 6–8 weeks for evaluation:

A. Mild: adjust dose depending on local irritation.
B. Moderate (oral and topical medications)
   1. Adjust dose according to irritation.
   2. Taper oral antibiotics with discretion and/or continue topical medications.
   3. Oral antibiotics may be tapered and discontinued when inflammatory lesions have resolved.

Consultation/Referral

A. Consult with a physician if treatment is unsuccessful after 10–12 weeks of therapy or if acne is severe.
B. The patient may need dermatology consultation.

Individual Considerations

A. Pregnancy
   1. Acne may flare up or improve during pregnancy.
   2. Medications preferred during pregnancy are topical agents.
   3. **Teratogens include tretinoin, tetracycline, and minocycline.**
      a. **When using teratogenic medications, contraception must be practiced to avoid pregnancy to prevent severe fetal malformations.**
      b. **Begin contraception 1 month prior to starting the medication and 1 month after finishing the medication.**

BENIGN SKIN LESIONS

Definition
A benign skin lesion is a cutaneous growth with no harmful effects to the body. Benign lesions must be distinguished from the following:

A. Basal cell carcinoma: nodular tumor with pearly surface, telangiectasia on surface, and depressed center or rolled edge.
B. Squamous cell carcinoma: irregular papule, with scaly, friable, bleeding surface.
C. Malignant melanoma: asymmetric papule, with irregular border, of two or more colors, and greater than 6 mm in diameter.

Incidence
A. Benign lesions are common to all races, and they are seen primarily in the adult and elderly populations.

Pathogenesis
A. The course varies, depending on the specific type of lesion.

Predisposing Factors
A. Sun exposure in the adult and elderly populations
B. Dermatosis papulosa nigra: common in African Americans and Asians

Common Complaints
A. New lesion of the skin.

Other Signs and Symptoms
A. Seborrheic keratosis: waxy papule with a stuck-on appearance is seen in adults on sun-exposed areas; they appear symmetric, 0.2–3.0 cm in size, with a well-demarcated border and of a variety of colors (tan, black, brown).
B. Dermatosis papulosa nigra: hyperpigmented mole located on face or neck; a pedunculated papule that is symmetric, 1–3 mm in diameter.
C. Cherry angioma: vascular papule, red to purple, located on trunk in adults; begins in early adulthood; 1- to 3-mm diameter papules that do not blanch.
D. Solar lentigines (liver spots): tan maculae on sun-exposed areas in elders, especially on face and hands; border is irregular, and the size varies.
E. Senile sebaceous hyperplasia: enlarged sebaceous glands that appear as yellow papules on sun-exposed areas, especially on face in elders; papules have central umbilication, and their size varies.
F. Keratoacanthoma: sun-exposed area lesion, smooth, skin-colored or reddish appearance dome-shaped papule at first, then may turn and grows to 1–2 cm in a few weeks, with crusted interior.

Subjective Data
A. Identify when the patient first discovered the lesion.
B. Determine whether the lesion has changed in size, shape, or color.
C. Ask if the patient has discovered more lesions.
D. Elicit information regarding a family history of skin lesions or cancer.

Physical Examination
A. Temperature
B. Inspect
 1. Observe skin; note all lesions and evaluate each for asymmetry, border, color, diameter, evolving changes, and/or elevation change.
 2. Note the patient's skin type.

Diagnostic Tests
A. Benign lesions do not require any tests.
B. If unsure regarding possible malignancy, a biopsy is recommended.

Differential Diagnoses
A. Benign skin lesion:
 1. Seborrheic keratosis
 2. Dermatosis papulosa nigra
 3. Cherry angioma
 4. Solar lentigines
 5. Senile sebaceous hyperplasia
 6. Keratoacanthoma

Plan
A. General interventions
 1. Reassure the patient that lesions are benign. No treatment is required unless the patient chooses to have the lesion removed for cosmetic purposes.
 2. Lesions may be removed using cryotherapy if they are bothersome for the patient.
B. Patient teaching: See the Section III Patient Teaching Guide for this chapter, "Skin Care Assessment."
C. Pharmaceutical therapy:
 1. Topical 5-fluorouracil, 5% imiquimod cream (Aldara) or topical diclofenac gel may be used for benign lesions.

Follow-up
A. Routine skin exams should be performed yearly.

Consultation/Referral
A. Immediately refer patient to a dermatologist if malignancy is suspected or confirmed by biopsy.

Individual Considerations
A. Adults: Skin lesions begin to appear in early adulthood. Encourage patients to monitor lesions over time.
B. Geriatrics: Benign lesions are commonly seen in the elderly population.

ANIMAL BITES, MAMMALIAN

Definition
A. Bites of any mammalian animal to the human can be potentially dangerous. Human bites are included.

Incidence
A. Account for 1–3.5 million ER visits each year.
B. About 80%–90% of bites are dog bites.
C. About 6% of bites are cat bites.
D. From 1%–15% are human bites.
E. Children and the elderly are especially prone.

Pathogenesis
A. Mechanical trauma and break to skin and/or underlying structures.
B. Infection from transmission of bacteria
1. *Pasteurella multocida* is primarily associated with cat bites, but may also be associated with dog bites.
2. *Staphylococcus aureus,* Staphylococcus epidermis, and Enterobacter species can be transmitted with dog and cat bites.
3. *Streptobacillus moniliformis* can be transmitted with rat and mice bites.
4. *Streptococcus, Staphylococcus,* and Eikenella can be transmitted with human bites.
5. Human bites can transmit diseases: actinomycosis, syphilis, tuberculosis, hepatitis B, and potentially HIV.
C. Rabies, an acute viral infection, may be transmitted by means of infected saliva or by an infected animal licking mucosa of an open wound. It is rarely contracted by means of airborne transmission, but this has been reported to occur in bat-infested caves.

Predisposing Factors
A. Children and the elderly
B. Entering an animal's territorial space and/or surprising an animal

Common Complaints
A. Bitten
B. Pain
C. Redness
D. Swelling

Subjective Data
A. Ask: What person or type of animal bit the patient?
B. Ask: Was this a provoked or unprovoked attack?
C. Did the patient identify and contact the owner of the animal?
D. Ask: What was the behavior of the animal: unusual, strange, or ill-appearing?
E. Ask: How much time has elapsed from being bitten to seeking treatment?
F. Has the patient started any self-treatment?
G. What is the patient's tetanus immunization status?
H. Review for any prior rabies immunizations.
I. Does the patient know if the animal was a domestic animal? Is the animal's vaccination status known?
J. If the bite is of human origin, determine if it is a closed-fist injury or plain bite.

Physical Examination
See Table 3.1.

Diagnostic Tests
Refer to Table 3.1.

Differential Diagnoses
A. Animal bite: dog, cat, human, and so forth.
1. Cat bites more frequently become infected.
2. Bites on the hand have the highest infection rates. Bites on the face have the lowest infection rates.
B. Cellulitis and abscesses.
C. High-risk potential for rabies from the following:
1. Skunks, foxes, raccoons, and bats are primary carriers.

TABLE 3.1 Bites

Animal	Signs and Symptoms	Physical Exam—Check temperature for all animal bites	Diagnostic Tests
Dog	Crush injury, lacerations and abrasions.	Inspect site, underlying structures, and distal neurovascular, motor, and sensory function. Palpate area. If wound is over 24 hr old check any signs of cellulitis, lymphangitis.	If infected: culture for anaerobes and aerobes.
Cat	Puncture wounds, may be deep.	Determine depth and extent of wound. Check for foreign bodies. If wound is over 24 hr old check any signs of cellulitis, lymphangitis.	If sepsis suspected: test blood, abscess, pus, and tissue for aerobes and anaerobes.
Rat and squirrel	Laceration, abrasions. More superficial in nature.	Check for signs of infection, if wound is over 24 hr old. Check any signs of cellulitis, lymphangitis.	
Human	Crush injury, laceration. Wound of hand (closed-fist wound).	Check for signs of infection, if wound is over 24 hr old. Check any signs of cellulitis, lymphangitis. Also, examine for fractures, air in the joint, subchondral bone defects, osteomyelitis. Examine for full range of interphalangeal and metacarpophalangeal joints.	As above. Also, take X-ray film of structures underlying bite.

2. Rabbits, squirrels, chipmunks, rats, and mice are seldom infective for rabies.
3. Properly vaccinated animals seldom are infective.

Plan

A. General interventions
1. Control bleeding.
2. Wound care:
   a. Immediately wash wound copiously with soap and water.
   b. Irrigate wound with saline, benzalkonium chloride (Zephiran), or 1% povidoneiodine (if the patient is not allergic to iodine).
   c. May use water pik.
   d. Use 150–1,000 mL of solution.
   e. Direct stream on entire wound surface.
   f. Scrub entire surrounding area.
   g. Debride all wounds.
   h. Trim any jagged edges to prevent cosmetic and/or functional complications.
   i. Cover with dry dressing.
3. Do not suture wounds with high risk for infection:
   a. Hand bites, closed-fist injuries.
   b. Bites older than 6–12 hours.
   c. Deep or puncture wounds.
   d. Bites with extensive injury of surface or underlying structures.
4. Rabies control measures:
   a. Consult with the local health department regarding risk of rabies in the area.
   b. The domestic animal should be identified, caught, and confined for 10 days of observation. If the animal develops any signs of rabies, it should be destroyed and its brain tissue analyzed. No treatment is necessary if results are negative.
   c. The wild animal should be caught and destroyed for brain tissue analysis. No treatment is necessary if results are negative.
   d. If the bat or wild carnivore cannot be found, rabies prophylaxis is instituted.
B. Patient teaching: Instruct the patient how to keep site free from infection.
C. Pharmaceutical therapy
1. Antibiotic prophylaxis is controversial, but it is generally recommended for wounds involving subcutaneous tissues and deeper structures.
   a. Prescribe amoxicillin, clavulanate acid (Augmentin) 500–875 mg every 12 hours; for children, prescribe 25–45 mg/kg/dose in two divided doses for 3–7 days. Available as 200 mg/5 mL and 400 mg/5 mL liquid.
   b. Alternatively, prescribe erythromycin (E-Mycin) 250 mg four times daily for 3–7 days; for children, prescribe erythromycin (Eryped) 30–50 mg/kg/day in four divided doses for 3–7 days.
2. Tetanus prophylaxis
3. Rabies prophylaxis
   a. Active immunization: human diploid cell vaccine (HDCV), 1 mL, is given intramuscularly on first day of treatment, and repeat doses are administered on days 3, 7, 14, and 28.
   b. Passive immunization: rabies immunoglobulin (RIG) (human) should be used simultaneously with first dose of HDCV; recommended dose of RIG is 20 IU/kg. Approximately one-half of RIG is infiltrated into wound, and the remainder is given intramuscularly.

Follow-up

A. Evaluate wound and change dressing in 24–48 hours.
B. Reevaluate as indicated. If the patient is on immunoprophylaxis and has no signs of infection, see in 1 week.
C. Instruct the patient to return immediately for any signs of infection.

Consultation/Referral

A. Refer all patients with bites of ears, face, genitalia, hands, and feet.
B. Consult with a doctor if suspicion of rabies is involved.
C. Contact the local health department.
D. Wounds involving tendon, joint, or bone require hospitalization and surgical consultation.

Individual Considerations

A. Pregnancy: Use appropriate antibiotic management.

INSECT BITES AND STINGS

Definition

A. Bites and/or stings on the skin come from commonly encountered insects: bees, hornets, wasps, mosquitoes, chiggers, ticks, fleas, and fire ants.

Incidence

A. Bites are seen in all age groups, more commonly in summer months.

Pathogenesis

A. Some bites elicit local tissue inflammation and destruction due to proteins and enzymes in the poison or venom of the insect.
B. IgE-mediated allergic reactions (immediate or delayed) may occur.
C. Serum-sickness reaction may appear 10–14 days after a sting with venom. Toxic reactions can also occur from multiple stings yielding large inoculation of poison or venom.
D. With tick bites, exposure to the Rocky Mountain Spotted Fever, Lyme disease, Ehrlichiosis, and Babesiosis disease may occur.

Predisposing Factors

A. Exposure to areas of heavy insect infestations
B. Warm weather months
C. Outdoor exposure with barefoot, bright clothes
D. Use of perfumes and/or colognes
E. Previous sensitization

Common Complaints

A. Local reaction: pain, swelling, and redness at site after insect bite

B. Toxic reaction: local reaction plus headache, vertigo, gastrointestinal symptoms (nausea, vomiting, diarrhea), syncope, convulsions, and/or fever

Subjective Data

A. Did patient see what bit or stung him or her?
B. If the patient felt the bite or sting, was he or she bitten or stung once or multiple times?
C. How long ago did it occur?
D. Where was the patient when the injury occurred (environment)?
E. Has the patient ever been bitten or stung before? If so, did he or she have any reaction then? If so, what was the treatment?

Physical Examination

A. Check temperature, pulse, respirations, and blood pressure. Observe overall respiratory status.
B. Inspect
   1. Inspect site of injury for local reaction; note erythema, rash, or edema.
   2. Perform ears, nose, and throat exam.
C. Auscultate: Assess heart and lungs.
D. Palpate
   1. Palpate injured site.
   2. Assess nodes for lymphadenopathy.
   3. Perform abdominal exam, if appropriate.

Diagnostic Tests

A. None is required.
B. Consider taking skin scrapings to evaluate under microscope.
C. Consider culture if infection is suspected.

Differential Diagnoses

A. Insect bite
   1. Bees, hornets, wasps: Local pain, redness, pruritus, and swelling occur at site. Red papules and wheals appear, enlarge, and then subside within hours. Delayed hypersensitivity occurs within 7 days with enlarged, local reaction with fever, malaise, headache, arthralgias, and lymphadenopathy. Toxicity can occur. Anaphylaxis may be seen with generalized warmth and urticaria, erythema, angioedema, intestinal cramping, bronchospasm, laryngospasm, shock, and collapse.
   2. Ticks: Local redness, swelling, itching; enlarged area of redness and swelling may occur.
   3. Mosquitoes and chiggers: Local redness, swelling, and itching occur. Delayed reaction can include edema and burning sensation.
   4. Fleas: Local redness, swelling, and itching occur. Usually papules noted in a zigzag pattern, especially on legs and waist. Note hemorrhagic puncta surrounded by erythematous and urticarial patches.
   5. Body lice: Small noninflammatory red spots, intensely pruritic, are found on waist, shoulders, axilla, and neck. Note linear scratch marks. Note secondary infection.
   6. Scabies: Pruritus is the dominant symptom. Note inflammation and burrows in skin with papules and vesicles, especially in the webs of the hands and feet.
   7. Fire ants: Papules appear and turn to pustules within 6–24 hours after bite. Watch for localized necrosis with scarring. Urticaria and angioedema can occur.
B. Allergic reaction.

Plan

A. General interventions. **Anaphylaxis: Activate EMS immediately.**
   1. With all bites and stings, treat anaphylaxis first.
   2. Local reactions: Treat with analgesic of choice. Apply ice packs to site for approximately 10 min. Elevate affected extremities.
   3. Delayed reactions: Administer antihistamines as needed. Consider corticosteroid use.
   4. Routine wound care: Cleanse wound. Remove stinger. If it's a painful sting, apply a cotton ball soaked in meat tenderizer or sodium bicarbonate paste.
   5. Debride as necessary.
   6. For imbedded insects, apply petroleum jelly, nail polish, or alcohol over site for 30 min and wait for insect or tick to withdraw.
   7. Hospitalize the patient for severe reactions.
B. See the Section III Patient Teaching Guide for this chapter, "Insect Bites and Stings."
C. Pharmaceutical therapy
   1. Antihistamines
      a. Children
         i. Two years old: 2–6 years: diphenhydramine 6.25 mg every 4–6 hours
         ii. Older child: 6–12 years: diphenhydramine 12.5–25 mg every 4–6 hours
      b. Adult: diphenhydramine (Benadryl) 50 mg every 6 hours as needed
   2. Mild anaphylaxis
      a. Epinephrine 1:1,000 (aqueous) administered subcutaneously. Usual dose is as follows:
         i. Children: 0.01 mg/kg, may repeat in 4 hours if needed
         ii. Adults: 0.3 mg IM , may repeat if needed
   3. Oral antihistamines for next 24 hours. (Atarax)
      a. Children: Hydroxyzine hydrochloride (Atarax) 2–4 mg/kg/day divided into three doses
      b. Adults: Hydroxyzine hydrochloride (Atarax) 10–25 mg four times daily
   4. Severe anaphylaxis
      a. Epinephrine 1:1,000 (aqueous), given subcutaneously (see Mild anaphylaxis, above)
      b. Oxygen 2–4 L as needed
      c. Albuterol (Ventolin) 5 mg/mL per dose by nebulizer
         i. Children: 0.1–0.15 mg/kg in 2 mL of saline
         ii. Adults: 2.5 mg (0.5 mL of 0.5% solution) in 2 mL saline
   5. Self-treatment for anaphylaxis (emergency treatment kits)
      a. Ana-Kit contains a preloaded syringe.
      b. Epipen and Epipen Junior Auto-Injectors are spring-loaded automatic injectors. Children: 0.01 mg/kg intramuscularly in thigh. Adults: 0.3 mg intramuscularly in thigh.

Follow-up

A. Follow-up in 2 weeks to evaluate effectiveness of treatment. If symptoms worsen prior to this, reevaluation is needed.

Referral/Consultation

A. Consult with physician when anaphylaxis occurs.

Individual Considerations

A. Pediatrics: Children are at a higher risk than adults for complications of a reaction.
B. Geriatrics: Elderly adults are at high risk for complications of reactions.

CANDIDIASIS

Definition

A. A fungal infection of the mucous membranes and/or skin, candidiasis is caused by the *Candida albicans* fungus.

Incidence

A. It occurs frequently in women, children, and the elderly population.

Pathogenesis

A. An overgrowth of *Candida albicans* occurs when mucous membranes and/or skin are exposed to moisture, warmth, and an alteration in the membrane barrier.

Predisposing Factors

A. Immunosuppression
B. Use of antibiotics
C. Hyperglycemia
D. Chronic use of steroid
E. Frequent douching by women
F. Adults who wear dentures

Common Complaints

A. Oral: persistent white patch on the tongue or roof of mouth may be slightly reddened with or without crevices on the tongue.
B. Vaginal: thick, white, "cottage-cheese-like" vaginal discharge with or without vaginal itching
C. Genital: bright, red rash with well-demarcated lesions advancing to pustules or erosions in genital or diaper area
D. Males: erythemic rash that may advance to erosions seen on male genitalia. Scrotum may be involved.

Subjective Data

A. Question the patient about onset, duration, and location of lesions.
B. Determine whether the patient has a history of previous infections.
C. Inquire into medical history and current medications.
D. Rule out the presence of any other current medical conditions.

Physical Examination

A. Check temperature, pulse, respirations, and blood pressure.
B. Inspect.

1. Assess skin and mucous membranes for discharge and lesions.
2. Observe location and severity of lesions.

C. Palpate: palpate lymph nodes in neck and groin.

Diagnostic Tests

A. Vaginal and genital infections need to be evaluated for STDs, especially if the patient is sexually active with multiple partners.
B. Specimens to consider include wet prep/Potassium Hydroxide 10% solution (KOH), gonorrhea/chlamydia.

Differential Diagnoses

A. Oral Candidiasis
   1. Leukoplakia
   2. Stomatitis
   3. Formula (for newborns)
B. Diaper area
   1. Candidiasis
   2. Contact dermatitis
   3. Bacterial infection
C. Genital area
   1. Candidiasis
   2. Bacterial infection
   3. Bacterial vaginosis
   4. Chlamydia
   5. Gonorrhea
   6. Trichomoniasis

Plan

A. Patient teaching
   1. Use your medication on your skin to help with symptoms.
   2. Do not scratch. Keep fingernails short.
B. Pharmaceutical therapy: Choose *one* of the following pharmaceutical therapies:
   1. Oral
      a. Nystatin (Mycostatin) oral suspension 100,000 U/mL, 2 ml for infants, 4–6 ml for older children and adults, four times daily for 7–10 days.
      b. Gentian violet aqueous solution, 1% for infants, 2% for adults, 1–2 times per day.
      c. Lotrimin buccal troches, five times per day for 2 weeks, only for adults.
   2. Diaper
      a. Nystatin cream, 3–4 times per day for 7–10 days.
      b. Mycolog II, apply sparingly to skin twice daily until resolved.
   3. Vaginal
      a. Clotrimazole 1% cream, 5 g intravaginally for 7–14 days.
      b. Miconazole 2% cream, 5 g intravaginally for 7 days (OTC).
      c. Terconzaole 0.8% cream, 5 g intravaginally for 3 days.
      d. Terconazole 80 mg vaginal suppository, at bedtime for 3 days.
      e. Fluconazole (Diflucan) 150 mg, oral tablet one time.
      f. Other preparations available in stronger or weaker doses.

Follow-up
A. None indicated unless not resolved or complications arise.

Consultation/Referral
A. Consult a physician if not resolved within 2 weeks.

Individual Considerations
A. Pregnancy
1. Most effective medications for pregnant women are clotrimazole, miconazole, and terconazole.
2. Recommend a full 7-day course of treatment during pregnancy.
B. Adults
1. Consider immunosuppression in all adults with oral candidiasis (HIV, diabetes, chemotherapy, leukemia).
2. Adults with oral lesions need to be assessed for leukoplakia, especially if the patient has a history of smoking or using chewing tobacco.

CONTACT DERMATITIS

Definition
A. Contact dermatitis is a cutaneous response to direct exposure of the skin to irritants (irritant contact dermatitis) or allergens (allergic contact dermatitis).
1. Irritant contact dermatitis is a nonimmunologic response of the epidermis.
2. Allergic contact dermatitis is an immunologic response after one or more exposures to a particular agent.

Incidence
A. Occurs in all ages. People who work with chemicals daily and wash their hands numerous times a day have a higher incidence of irritant dermatitis. Irritant contact dermatitis is seen in the elderly due to dry skin.

Pathogenesis
A. Irritant contact dermatitis is caused by an alteration of the outer layer of the dermis due to exposure to chemicals; lotions; cold, dry air; soaps; detergents; or organic solvents.
B. Allergic contact dermatitis is caused by an alteration in the epidermis when, after exposure to an allergen, the immune system responds by producing inflammation of the cutaneous tissue. Common allergens include poison ivy, poison oak, sumac, nickel jewelry, hair dye, rubber and leather chemicals (latex gloves), cleaning supplies, harsh soaps, detergents, and topical medicines.

Predisposing Factors
A. Occupation (hairdresser, nurse, housecleaner, and so forth)
B. Jewelry
C. Activities in yard or woods

Common Complaints
A. Irritation of the skin, ranging from redness to pruritic inflammation, with possible progression of blisters.

1. Poison oak, ivy, and sumac induce classic presentation: lesions (vesicles) and papules on an erythemic base presenting in a linear fashion with sharp margins.
2. Diffuse pattern with erythema may be seen when oleoresin is contacted from pets or smoke from burning fire.
B. Exposure to some type of irritant known to the patient. Round or annular lesions may have an internal cause such as a drug reaction.

Other Signs and Symptoms
A. Chronic
1. Erythema with thickening.
2. Scaling.
3. Fissures.
4. Inflammation. With chronic dermatitis, lichenification may occur with scales and fissures.
B. Diaper dermatitis: prominent red, shiny rash on buttocks and genitalia.
C. Candidiasis diaper rash.
1. Bright red rash with satellite lesions at margins.
2. Inflammation and excoriations present.
3. Creases may be involved.

Subjective Data
A. Ask the patient when irritation began and how it has progressed.
B. Elicit history of exposure to allergens.
C. Question the patient regarding activity and skin contact with irritants prior to outbreak (cleaning agents, walking in woods, hobbies, change in soap/laundry detergent, shaving cream, lotions, and so forth).
D. List occupation and family history of allergens.
E. Review medication list including prescription, over-the-counter, and herbal to evaluate an interaction.
F. List medications used to relieve symptoms and results.

Physical Examination
A. Temperature
B. Inspect
1. Inspect skin, noting types of lesions and location of lesions. **Note the pattern of inflammation. The shape of irritation may mimic the shape of the irritant, such as the skin under a ring or watch, for example.**
2. Determine progression of lesions.
3. Differentiate between primary and secondary lesions.

Diagnostic Tests
A. Consider none if source is known.
B. Wet mount (KOH, saline) to rule out fungal infection if candidiasis is suspected.
C. Culture pustules.
D. Patch test to rule out allergic contact dermatitis.

Differential Diagnoses
A. Irritant contact dermatitis
B. Allergic contact dermatitis
C. Diaper dermatitis
D. Candidiasis

E. Tinea
F. Drug reactions
G. Pityriasis rosea
H. Scabies

Plan

A. General interventions
1. Irritant contact dermatitis: removal of irritating agent.
a. Topical soaks with saline or Burow's solution (1:40 dilution) for weeping areas.
b. Lukewarm baths (not hot), oatmeal (Aveeno) baths, as needed.
c. For dry erythematous skin, Eucerin or Aquaphor ointments to rehydrate skin.
d. Remind the patient to avoid scratching skin and to keep nails short.
e. Suggest use of mild soaps and cleansers.
2. Allergic contact dermatitis:
a. Instruct the patient to avoid contact with agent.
b. Have the patient wash with cool water immediately after exposure.
c. Lukewarm baths with oatmeal (Aveeno) 3–4 times per day.
d. Tell the patient to apply calamine lotion after baths.
3. Diaper dermatitis:
a. Instruct parent to change the patient's diaper frequently, cleaning with water only, and allow skin to air dry 15–30 min four times a day. Tell parent not to use lotions or powders, but to apply zinc oxide (Desitin ointment or powder, or Happy Hiney) with each diaper change.
b. If candidiasis diaper rash presents, for treatment refer to the "Candidiasis" section in this chapter.
B. Patient teaching: See the Section III Patient Teaching Guide for this chapter, "Dermatitis."
C. Pharmaceutical therapy
1. Irritant contact dermatitis: hydrocortisone 2.5% ointment 3–4 times per day for 2 weeks.
2. Allergic contact dermatitis
a. Hydrocortisone 2.5% ointment 3–4 times per day for 1–2 weeks after blistering stage.
b. High-potent steroids: fluocinonide 0.05%) (Lidex) ointment 3–4 times per day. Not to be used on face or skin folds.
c. Hydroxyzine 25–50 mg four times daily, diphenhydramine HCl (Benadryl) 25–50 mg four times daily. For children, 0.5 mg/kg/dose three times daily as needed.
d. If rash is severe (face, eyes, genitalia, mucous membranes), consider prednisone 60–80 mg/day to start, and taper over 10–14 days.
e. Triamcinolone acetonide (Kenalog) 40–60 mg by IM injection.
3. Secondary infections: erythromycin 250 mg four times daily or amoxicillin, clavulanate acid (Augmentin) 875 mg twice daily for 10 days.
4. Candidiasis
a. Miconazole nitrate 2% cream, miconazole powder, or nystatin cream.
b. Clotrimazole (Lotrimin) or ketoconazole (Nizoral) cream 3–4 times per day for 10 days.
c. If inflammation is present along with yeast, use Mycolog II.
d. If secondary bacterial infection is present, use mupirocin (Bactroban) ointment three times daily for 7–10 days.

Follow-up

A. None required if case is mild.
B. See patient again in 2–3 days for severe cases, or phone to assess progress.

Consultation/Referral

A. Consult with a physician when steroid treatment is necessary or if worsening symptoms develop despite adequate therapy.

Individual Considerations

A. Pregnancy: If medications are necessary during pregnancy, consider gestational age of fetus and category of medication.
B. Pediatrics: For infants and children, consider hydroxyzine (Atarax) 0.5 mg/kg/dose three times daily as needed for severe pruritus.
C. Elderly: Patients may only exhibit scaling as the prominent irritation rather than erythema and inflammation. Topical medications (neomycin, vitamin E, lanolin) and acrylate adhesives are common causes of contact dermatitis.

⬛ ECZEMA OR ATOPIC DERMATITIS

Definition

A. This pattern of skin inflammation has clinical features of erythema, itching, scaling, lichenification, papules, and vesicles in various combinations. Currently, the term *eczema* is used interchangeably with *dermatitis*. Most common variants are atopic dermatitis and atopic eczema. Classification is by cause, either endogenous or exogenous.

Incidence

A. Overall prevalence of all forms of eczema is about 18:1000 in the United States.
B. With atopic dermatitis, 60% of those affected become afflicted between infancy and 12 years of age. It is more common in boys.

Pathogenesis

A. Eczema is characterized by a lymphohistiocytic infiltration around the upper dermal vessels. Seen is epidermal spongiosis or intercellular epidermal edema and inflammation.

Predisposing Factors

A. Family history of atopic triad: dermatitis, asthma, and allergic rhinitis
B. Exposure to allergen
1. Common foods: cow's milk, nuts, wheat, soy, and fish
2. Common environmental allergens: dust, mold, cat dander, and low humidity
C. Exposure to topical medications, most commonly neomycin, lanolin, and topical anesthetics like benzocaine

Common Complaints

Skin changes:

A. Itching, impossible to relieve
B. Dryness
C. Discoloration, lichenification, and scaling
D. Thickening
E. Associated bleeding and oozing skin

Other Signs and Symptoms

A. Primary lesions, papules, and pustules that may lead to excoriation.
B. Lesions commonly seen on trunk, face, and antecubital and popliteal fossae of children. Adults will have lesions on face, trunk, neck, and genital area.
C. Other common features include infraorbital fold (Dennie sign), increased palmar creases, facial erythema, and scaling.

Subjective Data

A. Determine whether the onset was sudden or gradual.
B. Ask the patient if the skin is itchy or painful.
C. Assess if there is any associated discharge (blood or pus).
D. Ask if the patient has recently taken any antibiotics, other oral drugs, or topical medications.
E. Ask the patient about use of soaps, creams, or lotions.
F. Assess for any preceding systemic symptoms (fever, sore throat, anorexia, vaginal discharge).
G. Ask the patient about recent travel abroad.
H. Rule out insect bites.
I. Rule out any possible exposure to industrial or domestic toxins.
J. Elicit what precipitates itching.

Physical Examination

A. Temperature
B. Inspect
   1. Inspect skin for lesions.
   2. Recognize bacteria-infected eczema; *Staphylococcus aureus* is the most common pathogen. It appears with acute weeping dermatitis; crusted, and small, superficial pustules.

Diagnostic Tests

A. Culture skin lesions to determine viral, bacterial, or fungal etiology.
B. Blood work: Serum IgE is elevated with atopic dermatitis.

Differential Diagnoses

A. Atopic dermatitis, acute or chronic
B. Contact dermatitis, acute or chronic
C. Seborrheic dermatitis
D. Ichthyosis vulgaris
E. Infections
F. Neoplastic disease
G. Immunologic and metabolic disorders

Plan

A. General interventions
   1. Frequently treat the dry skin with emollients (Aquaphor, Eucerin).
   2. Pat, don't rub skin.
   3. Children: only bathe every 2–3 nights. Avoid excessive use of soap and water when bathing.
   4. Avoid wool products and lanolin preparations.
   5. Keep fingernails cut short to prevent scratching/scarring skin.
   6. May need to treat secondary bacterial infections as appropriate.
   7. Eliminate trigger foods one at a time for 1 month at a time to see improvement. Begin with eliminating cow's milk products. Consider soy-based foods instead.
   8. Allergy testing may be considered if symptoms continue.
   9. Ointments are usually recommended over creams for moisturizing.
B. Patient teaching: See the Section III Patient Teaching Guide for this chapter, "Eczema."
C. Pharmaceutical therapy
   1. Atopic: acute, adult
      a. Wet dressings with Burow's solution changed every 2–3 hours.
      b. Potent topical corticosteroid: betamethasone valerate 0.1% 2–3 times daily.
      c. Antihistamine of choice: Cetirizine HCl (Zyrtec) or diphenhydramine HCl (Benadryl).
      d. Severe cases: Oral steroid: prednisone 1 mg/kg (40–60 mg/day) tapered over 2–3 weeks.
   2. Atopic: acute, infants and children
      a. Hydrocortisone: infants and children: 2.5% ointment twice daily; 1% on face and intertriginous areas.
      b. Adolescents: triamcinolone acetonide 0.1% (Aristocort) ointment, apply thinly twice daily for 2–3weeks. **Precautions should be given regarding possibility of hypopigmentation of skin even with short-term use of steroids on skin.**
      c. Antihistamines for itching
         i. Infants and children: may use hydroxyzine (Atarax) 0.5 mg/kg/dose three times daily as needed or diphenhydramine HCl (Benadryl). For those 2–6 years: 6.25 mg every 4–6 hours. For those 6–12 years: 12.5–25 mg every 4–6 hours.
         ii. Adolescents: may use hydroxyzine 25–50 mg/dose every 4–6 hours or diphenhydramine HCl (Benadryl).
         iii. Atopic: chronic, adult: short course of potent topical corticosteroid (betamethasone dipropionate (Diprolene) or clobetasol propionate (temovate) twice daily for 7 days.
   3. Antibacterial treatments for secondary bacterial infections: *Staphylococcus aureus*
      a. Augmentin 875 mg by mouth twice a day for 10–14 days.
      b. Keflex 500 mg by mouth four times a day for 10–14 days.
      c. Erythromycin 500 mg by mouth four times a day for 10–14 days *or*
      d. Dicloxacillin 250 mg every 6 hours for 10 days.

Follow-up

A. See patient in office in 1–2 weeks, and then every month until condition is stabilized.
B. Monitor the patient for superimposed staphylococcal infection; may use oral erythromycin or dicloxacillin.
C. Patient may be seen every 3–6 months thereafter for patient education updates.

Consultation/Referral

A. Eczema herpeticum (herpes simplex type 1) may progress rapidly. Refer the patient to a dermatologist.
B. Refer the patient to a dermatologist if skin eruptions are severe or fail to respond to conservative treatment.

Individual Considerations

A. Pregnancy: Avoid oral steroids.
B. Children: Teach patients to apply emollients when they have an itch rather than scratching. The goal is to control the rash and symptoms.
C. Young adults and elderly: Nummular eczema is commonly seen, characterized by coin-shaped vesicles and papules seen on extremities and/or trunk.

ERYTHEMA MULTIFORME

Definition

A. This dermal and epidermal inflammatory process is characterized by symmetric eruption of erythematous, iris-shaped papules ("target" lesions), and vesicobullous lesions.

Incidence

A. Erythema multiforme accounts for up to 1% of dermatology outpatient visits.
B. Children under 3 years and adults older than age 50 are rarely affected.
C. It may occur in seasonal epidemics.
D. Approximately 90% of cases of erythema multiforme minor follow a recent outbreak of HSV-1.

Pathogenesis

A. The disorder is thought to be an immunologic reaction in the skin, possibly triggered by circulating immune complexes.

Predisposing Factors

A. Infections: recurrent herpes simplex virus (HSV), mycoplasmal infections, and adenoviral infections
B. Drugs: sulfonamides, phenytoin, barbiturates, phenylbutazone, penicillin
C. Idiopathic: greater than 50%; consider occult malignancy

Common Complaints

A. Rash with intense pruritus
B. Nonspecific upper respiratory infection (URI) followed by rash

Other Signs and Symptoms

A. Primary: maculas, papules, plaques
B. Secondary: erythema, dull red targetlike lesions blanch to pressure; distribution is symmetric, primarily on flexor surfaces. **Classic target lesions develop abruptly and symmetrically and are heaviest peripherally; they often involve palms and soles.**
C. Swelling of hands and feet
D. Painful oral lesions
E. Photoeruption pattern
F. Constitutional symptoms are frequently weakness and malaise

Subjective Data

A. Ask if the patient has ever been diagnosed with erythema multiforme.
B. Determine whether the onset of symptoms was sudden or gradual.
C. Assess for any associated discharge (blood or pus).
D. Identify the location of the symptoms.
E. Complete a drug history. Has the patient recently taken any antibiotics or other drugs? Question the patient regarding use of any topical medications.
F. Determine presence of any preceding systemic symptoms (fever, sore throat, anorexia, vaginal discharge).
G. Rule out any possible exposure to industrial or domestic toxins.
H. Question the patient concerning any possible contact with venereal disease.
I. Ask the patient about any close physical contact with others with skin disorders.
J. Elicit information concerning any possible exposure to HIV.
K. Rule out sources of chronic infection, neoplasia, or connective tissue disease.

Physical Examination

A. Check temperature, pulse, respirations, and blood pressure.
B. Inspect
   1. Inspect skin for lesions.
   2. Inspect mouth and mucous membranes for lesions.
C. Palpate: Palpate abdomen for masses and tenderness.
D. Auscultate: Auscultate heart, lungs, and abdomen.
E. Neurologic exam.

Diagnostic Tests

A. Punch biopsy of skin
B. CBC
C. Urinalysis

Differential Diagnoses

A. Erythema multiforme
   1. Erythema multiforme minor: pruritus, swelling of hands and feet, painful oral lesions.
   2. Erythema multiforme major: fever, arthralgias, myalgias, cough, oral erosions with severe pain.
B. Urticaria.
C. Viral exanthems.
D. **Stevens-Johnson syndrome (SJS): Stevens-Johnson syndrome (SJS) is a severe systemic reaction with fever, malaise, cough, sore throat, chest pain, vomiting, diarrhea, myalgia, arthralgia, and severe skin manifestations with painful bullous lesions on mucous membranes.**
E. Pemphigus vulgaris.
F. Bullous pemphigoid.

G. Other bullous diseases.

H. Staphylococcal scalded skin syndrome (SSSS).

Plan

A. General interventions
1. Identify and treat precipitating causes or triggers.
2. Burow's solution may be used for mild cases as needed.
3. Oral lesions may be treated with saline solution, warm salt water, and/or Mary's mouth wash (Benadryl, lidocaine, and Kaopectate).
4. Remove any suspected drugs.
5. Provide adequate pain relief if skin or oral lesions are painful. Lesions remain fixed at least 7 days.
6. Maintain nutrition and fluid replacement for this hypercatabolic state.
7. Consider chronic viral suppression therapy for recurrent herpes simplex viral infections.

B. Patient teaching: See the Section III Patient Teaching Guide for this chapter, "Erythema Multiforme."

C. Pharmaceutical therapy
1. Potent topical corticosteriods: betamethasone dipropionate 0.05% or clobetasol propionate 0.05% twice daily for up to 2 weeks. Avoid use on face and groin.
2. Open lesions should be treated like open burn wounds. Stop offending medications that may cause blistering of wounds and treat with steroids.
3. Systemic corticosteroids: Prednisone 50–80 mg daily in divided doses, quickly tapered.

Follow-up

A. See the patient in office in 1–2 days to evaluate initial treatment.

Consultation/Referral

A. If patient has recurrent or chronic infection, refer him or her to a physician.

B. Immediate consultation and/or hospital admission is critical if Stevens-Johnson syndrome is suspected.

Individual Considerations

A. Pediatrics: Systemic corticosteroids may increase risk of infection and prolong healing. Use low- to mid-potency topical corticosteroids.

FOLLICULITIS

Definition

A. Folliculitis is a bacterial infection of the hair follicle.

Incidence

A. A very common disorder, folliculitis occurs in all ages and is seen more frequently in males.

Pathogenesis

A. Bacterial organisms (most common *Staphylococcus aureus*) invade the follicle wall and cause an infectious process.

Predisposing Factors

A. Break in the skin tissue

B. Use of razors on skin

C. Poor hygiene

D. Diabetes

Common Complaints

A. Outbreak of pustules on the face, scalp, or extremities that do not resolve despite proper hygiene and care.

Other Signs and Symptoms

A. Tenderness and itching at site

B. Furuncle (abscess): a deep pustule, tender, firm or fluctuant, found in groin, axilla, waistline, buttocks

C. Carbuncle: a group of follicles coalescing into one larger, painful, infected area; may see fever and chills

D. Excoriated folliculitis: chronic thickened, excoriated papules or nodules

Subjective Data

A. Elicit the initial outbreak of lesions and onset and progression of lesions.

B. Identify what makes the lesions better or worse.

C. Ask the patient what medications, soaps, or lotions he has used on the lesions.

D. Complete a medical history. Ask if the patient has had an outbreak similar to this before.

E. Describe systemic symptoms if they have occurred (fever, chills, and so forth).

F. Does the patient have a beard, shave his face, or use a razor frequently?

G. Is there a recent history of use of a hot tub? (Commonly seen 1–4 days after use of hot tub, whirlpool or swimming pool use).

H. Does the patient wear tight pants/jeans or use oils that clog pores in the groin area?

I. Is the patient currently being treated with antibioitics for acne? (may see flare of gram-negative folliculitis with chronic use of antibioitics).

Physical Examination

A. Check temperature, pulse, respirations, and blood pressure.

B. Inspect: Assess skin for lesions and describe.

C. Palpate: Palpate lesions and associated lymph nodes.

Diagnostic Tests

A. Culture and sensitivity to verify appropriate antibiotic coverage

B. Gram stain

C. KOH/wet prep

D. Culture hair if fungi suspected (tinea of scalp)

Differential Diagnoses

A. Folliculitis

B. Acne vulgaris

C. Ingrown hair follicle

D. Keratosis pilaris

E. Contact dermatitis

Plan

A. General interventions: Warm moist compresses to site for comfort.

B. Patient teaching

1. See the Section III Patient Teaching Guide for this chapter, "Folliculitis."
2. If razors are used on the area, have the patient use clean sharp razors, throw old razors away, and not share razors. Avoid use of irritating creams or lotions on affected area.
3. Encourage proper hygiene, frequent washing of hands and skin with antibacterial soap.
4. Warm compresses 3–4 times a day encouraged at site for 15–20 min.
5. Bleach bath (1/2–1 cup of bleach to 20 L water) reduces spread of staph infection.

C. Pharmaceutical therapy
1. Mild cases: mupirocin (Bactroban) ointment to affected area three times daily until resolved.
2. *Staphylococcus aureus*
   a. Dicloxacillin (Dynapen) 250 mg by mouth four times daily for 10–14 days.
   b. Erythromycin 250 mg by mouth four times daily for 10–14 days.
   c. Cephalexin (Keflex) 500 mg by mouth twice daily for 10–14 days.
3. *Pseudomonas aeruginosa*
   a. Ciprofloxacin (Cipro) 500 mg by mouth twice daily for 10 days.
   b. Ofloxacin 400 mg by mouth twice daily for 10 days.
4. Antistaphylococcal antibiotics
   a. Cephalexin 250–500 mg four times a day (children 25–50 mg/kg/d bid)
   b. Clindamycin 150–300 mg four times a day (children 8–16 mg/kg/day in 3–4 doses/day)
   c. Dicloxacillin 125–500 mg four times a day (children 12.5 mg/kg/day four times a day)
   d. Erythromycin 250–500 mg four times a day (children 30–50 mg/kg/day four times a day)
5. Bacteria caused by organisms other than Staphylococcus may be treated for an extended period of time, 4–8 weeks. These areas may include axilla, chest, back, beard, and groin.
6. Severe cases may be treated with oral antibiotics with topical permethrin every 12 hours every other night for a 6-week period or itraconzaole 400 mg daily, isotretinoin 0.5 mg/kg/day for up to 4–5 months with UVB light therapy. Consider dermatology referral for severe cases.

Follow-up
A. If not resolved in 2 weeks, further evaluation is needed.
B. Severe cases, in which carbuncles are not improved with treatment of antibioitic therapy, may warrant incision and drainage.
C. Continue to follow every 2 weeks until resolved.
D. Test for diabetes mellitus if severe cases.

Consultation/Referral
A. Refer the patient to a physician for testing for immunodeficiency if severe cases occur or if resistance is seen.
B. Dermatology referral.

HAND-FOOT-AND-MOUTH SYNDROME

Definition
A. This is a viral infection caused by coxsackievirus Al6, with vesicular lesions present on the hands, feet, and oral mucosa.

Incidence
A. Hand-foot-and mouth syndrome is most commonly seen in preschool children.

Pathogenesis
A. Enteroviruses invade the intestinal tract of humans and are spread to others by fecal-oral and/or oral-oral (respiratory) routes. The incubation period is approximately 4–6 days.

Predisposing Factors
A. Childhood
B. Confined households or day-care centers, camps
C. Seasonal: summer and fall most common

Common Complaints
A. Generalized rash, with lesions on the tongue, gums, and roof of the mouth
B. Lesions (vesicles) also present on the hand, feet, and buttocks

Other Signs and Symptoms
A. Fever
B. Sore throat
C. **Some enteroviruses have been associated with severe consequences such as meningitis, encephalitis, and others. The family should monitor symptoms carefully.**

Subjective Data
A. Question the patient regarding onset, duration, and progression of symptoms and lesions.
B. Determine whether any family member or other contact person had similar symptoms.
C. Identify areas where the child comes in contact with numerous children (child care facility, nurseries at church, school, and so forth).
D. If not noted in presenting symptoms, ask the patient regarding upper respiratory symptoms (sore throat, fever, headache, runny nose, cough, and so forth).

Physical Examination
A. Check temperature, pulse, respirations, and blood pressure.
B. Inspect: Inspect skin, ears, nose, and oral cavity for lesions.
C. Palpate
   1. Palpate abdomen and lymph nodes in neck.
   2. Assess for meningism.
D. Auscultate: Auscultate lungs and heart.

Diagnostic Tests
A. Usually none; consider cultures of oral lesions if secondary bacterial infection is suspected.

Differential Diagnoses
A. Hand-foot-and-mouth syndrome
B. Pharyngitis

C. Pneumonia
D. Meningitis
E. Meningococcemia: exanthem, petechial rash

Plan

A. General interventions: Supportive treatment. Warm saline gargles, acetaminophen (Tylenol) as needed for discomfort, and increased fluids. Popsicles are useful to soothe oral lesions, especially for small children.
B. Patient teaching: Reinforce good oral and body hygiene. The virus may be harbored in the gastrointestinal tract for long periods of time.
C. Pharmaceutical therapy
  1. None is recommended.
  2. Acetaminophen (Tylenol) as needed for fever and malaise.

Follow-up

A. None recommended unless symptoms worsen or do not resolve in 7–10 days.

Consultation/Referral

A. Refer to physician for any symptoms related to meningitis or encephalitis.

Individual Considerations

A. Pediatrics: Seen primarily in the pediatric population.

HERPES SIMPLEX VIRUS TYPE 1

Definition

Herpes simplex type 1 (HSV-1) viral infection of the cutaneous tissue manifests itself by vesicular lesions on the mucous membranes and skin. Herpes simplex virus type 1 is most often associated with oral lesions (mouth, lips), and herpes simplex virus type 2 is associated with genital lesions. The virus appears in three stages:

A. Primary
B. Latency
C. Recurrent infections

Incidence

A. HSV-1 is seen in patients of all ages and in equal numbers of males and females.
B. The infection rate is estimated to be 30,000:100,000–70,000:100,000.

Pathogenesis

A. Viral infection can be transmitted from a vesicular lesion or fluid (saliva) containing the virus to the skin or mucosa of another person by direct contact, with an incubation period of 2–14 days. Trigeminal ganglia are the host of the oral virus. The virus can be reactivated, whereupon it travels along the affected nerve route and produces recurrent lesions. Common sites of infection are the lips, face, buccal mucosa, and throat.

Predisposing Factors

A. Immunocompromised patients
B. Prior HSV infections
C. Exposure to virus

Common Complaints

A. Painful lips, gums, and oral mucosa

Other Signs and Symptoms

A. Primary lesion: fever, blisters on lips, malaise, and tender gums
B. Recurrent episodes: fever blisters with prodrome of itching, burning, tingling sensation at site before vesicles appear

Subjective Data

A. Ask questions regarding location, onset, and duration of lesions.
B. Elicit description of prodromal symptoms.
C. Ask the patient if systemic symptoms occur with vesicular outbreak.
D. Determine when the initial outbreak of lesions occurred (commonly seen in childhood).
E. Inquire whether the patient has been exposed to anyone with similar lesions.
F. If the lesion(s) is recurrent, ask the patient if stress, skin trauma, or sun exposure stimulates outbreak of fever blisters.

Physical Examination

A. Check temperature, pulse, respirations, and blood pressure.
B. Inspect: Inspect skin, note location, appearance, and stage of vesicles.
C. Palpate: Palpate lymph nodes for lymphadenopathy.

Diagnostic Tests

A. Viral cultures

Differential Diagnoses

A. Herpes simplex virus 1.
B. Impetigo (Impetigo appears as amber-colored vesicular lesions with crusting).
C. Stomatitis (Stomatitis appears as erythemic or erosion lesions in the mouth and lips).
D. Herpes zoster (Herpes zoster causes vesicles that run along a single dermatome).
E. Stevens-Johnson syndrome.
F. Herpangina: Vesicles can be noted on the soft palate, tonsillary area, and uvula area, usually caused by the coxsackievirus.

Plan

A. General interventions:
  1. Comfort measures. Ice may be used to reduce swelling as needed.
  2. Blistex may be applied as needed and lip ointment with SPF 30 or greater when exposed to sunlight.
B. Patient teaching
  1. **Educate the patient regarding the disease process of HSV-1.**
  2. Instruct patient to wash hands frequently.
  3. Suggest proper care of lips to prevent drying and to reduce pain.
  4. Educate regarding transmission of virus to others.
  5. Teach patient to expect recurrences at variable times.

C. Pharmaceutical therapy: **Precautions should be used when administering medication to patients who are immunocompromised and who have a history of renal insufficiency.**
1. Lidocaine 2% as needed for comfort.
2. Diphenhydramine (Benadryl) elixir may be used to rinse mouth as needed.
3. Acetaminophen (Tylenol) as needed for pain.
4. Campho-Phenique application as needed.
5. Initial episode: acyclovir 200 mg by mouth five times per day for 7–10 days or until resolved.
6. Recurrent episodes: Begin one of the following when prodrome begins or within 2 days of onset of lesions to get maximum effect.
   a. Acyclovir 200 mg by mouth five times per day for 5 days.
   b. Acyclovir 800 mg by mouth twice daily for 5 days.
7. Other alternatives antivirals: dosage depends on renal function
   a. Famciclovir (Famvir)
   b. Valacyclovir (Valtrex)
8. Suppressive therapy
   a. Acyclovir 200 mg by mouth 2–5 times per day for 1 year.
   b. Acyclovir 400 mg by mouth twice daily for 1 year.

Follow-up
A. None needed if resolved without complications.

Consultation/Referral
A. Refer the patient to a physician if treatment is unsuccessful or further complications arise.

Individual Considerations
A. Pediatrics: Initial outbreak commonly occurs in childhood.

HERPES ZOSTER, OR SHINGLES

Definition
A. Herpes zoster is a viral infection manifested by painful, vesicular lesions on the skin, limited to one side of the body, following one body dermatone.

Incidence
A. Infection may occur at any age; however, it is more common in older adults and the elderly. It occurs in 10%–20% of the U.S. population.

Pathogenesis
A. After the primary episode of chickenpox (varicella-zoster), the virus remains dormant in the body. Herpes zoster occurs when the varicella virus has been stimulated and reactivated in the dorsal root ganglia, producing the clinical manifestations of herpes zoster as discussed below. Duration of infection usually lasts 14–21 days, but may be longer in elderly or debilitated patients.

Predisposing Factors
A. Adulthood
B. Immunocompromised patients
C. Spinal cord trauma or injury

Common Complaints
A. Prodrome: itching, burning, tingling, or painful sensation at lesion sites
B. Active: malaise, fever, headache, pruritic rash on the skin

Other Signs and Symptoms
A. Lesions: clusters of vesicles on an erythemic base that burst and produce crusted lesions; commonly seen on the chest and back area. Distribution of lesions typically appears along a single dermatome.
B. Motor weakness (may be seen in approximately 5% of patients)

Subjective Data
A. Determine onset, location, and progression of rash.
B. Ask the patient about prodromal symptoms: burning, itching, tingling, or painful sensation at site prior to lesions breaking out.
C. Evaluate patient status regarding immunosuppressive agents, diseases, and so forth.

Physical Examination
A. Check temperature, pulse, respirations, and blood pressure.
B. Inspect
   1. Observe skin for lesions, noting characteristics and distribution.
   2. Inspect ears, nose, and throat.
C. Auscultate: Auscultate heart and lungs.

Diagnostic Tests
A. Usually none.
B. Culture vesicular lesions.
C. Consider Tzanck smear.
D. Young patients with herpes zoster: Consider and test for HIV.

Differential Diagnoses
A. Herpes zoster
B. Varicella
C. Poison ivy
D. Herpes simplex virus
E. Contact dermatitis
F. Coxsackievirus
G. Postherpetic neuralgia

Plan
A. General interventions: Comfort measures. Instruct the patient to apply wet dressings (Burow's solution) on site for 30–60 min at least four times a day. Calamine lotions may be used as needed; oatmeal (Aveeno) bath for comfort; acetaminophen (Tylenol) as needed for malaise, temperature, and comfort.
B. Patient teaching
   1. See the Section III Patient Teaching Guide for this chapter, "Herpes Zoster (Shingles)."
   2. Tell the patient the rash usually lasts approximately 2–3 weeks.
   3. Instruct the patient to monitor himself or herself for postherpetic neuralgia.

4. Instruct the patient to call if symptoms worsen or do not improve, or if lesions become infected.
5. Emphasize to the patient that the virus is easily transmitted to vulnerable persons.

C. Pharmaceutical therapy
1. Antiviral medications should be initiated within 24–48 hours after outbreak.
   a. Acyclovir (Zovirax) 800 mg every 4 hours while awake for 7–10 days.
   b. Famciclovir (Famvir) 500–750 mg by mouth three times daily for 7 days.
   c. Valacyclovir (Valtrex) 1,000 mg by mouth three times daily for 7 days.
2. Acetaminophen (Tylenol) or ibuprofen as needed for pain or discomfort.
3. Narcotics may be used for severe pain as needed.
4. Postherpetic neuralgia.
   a. Poster-herpetic neuralgia may be treated with narcotics.
   b. Long-term medications may be needed for control of pain.
      i. Gabapentin 100–600 mg three times daily.
      ii. Amitriptyline 25 mg every bedtime or other low-dose tricyclic antidepressants.
5. If secondary infection occurs of the skin, apply silver sulfadiazine (Silvadene) topically to site until resolved.
6. Use of steroids is controversial. Corticosteroids may be used with caution. May increase risk of dissemination.

Follow-up

A. As needed for complications.
B. Monitor the patient for complications: postherpetic neuralgia, Guillain-Barré syndrome, motor weakness, secondary infection, meningoencephalitis, ophthalmic and facial palsy, corneal ulceration, and so forth.

Consultation/Referral

A. Consult with physician if secondary infection occurs or if secondary complications arise.

Individual Considerations

A. Pregnancy: Acyclovir is in category C drug classification. The safety and efficacy of the use of the antiviral medications during pregnancy needs to be considered.
B. Pediatrics: Shingles is rarely seen in children.
C. Elderly
1. Postherpetic neuralgia occurs in approximately 15% of patients. It is commonly seen in the elderly patient.
2. Viral infection is seen in older adults.
3. The virus is contagious for those who have not had the chickenpox.

IMPETIGO

Definition

A. Impetigo is a bacterial infection of the skin most commonly caused by *Staphylococcus aureus* or *Streptococcus pyogenes,* or both.

Incidence

A. It occurs equally in males and females and is most commonly seen in children, especially children from 2–6 years of age.

Pathogenesis

A. An alteration in the skin integrity allows bacterial invasion into the epidermis, causing an infection. Small, moist vesicles ranging from red macules to honey-colored crusts or erosions occur singly or grouped together. Most common organisms are *Staphylococcus aureus* and group A β-hemolytic streptococci.

Predisposing Factors

A. Poor hygiene
B. Warm climates
C. Break in the skin

Common Complaints

A. Tender sores around the mouth and nose area in which the lesions continue to spread and worsen, despite over-the-counter medication treatment.

Subjective Data

A. Elicit onset, progression, duration, and location of lesions.
B. Ask the patient whether he or she has had contact with any other child or person with similar lesions.
C. Assess whether the patient exhibits any other symptoms, especially systemic symptoms (fever, malaise, and so forth).
D. Elicit what treatment has been tried, if any.

Physical Examination

A. Check temperature, pulse, respirations, and blood pressure.
B. Inspect
1. Examine skin, noting types of lesions and skin involvement.
2. Examine ears, nose, mouth, and throat.
C. Auscultate: Auscultate lungs and heart.

Diagnostic Tests

A. None required
B. May perform culture if recurrent or resistant to treatment

Differential Diagnoses

A. Impetigo
B. Varicella
C. Folliculitis
D. Erysipelas
E. Herpes simplex
F. Second-degree burns
G. Pharyngitis or tonsillitis: throat erythema, with tonsillary hypertrophy and exudate present; lymph nodes: adenopathy of anterior cervical chain
H. Ecthyma: severe case of impetigo with lymphadenitis

Plan

A. General interventions
1. Crusted lesions may be removed with thorough, gentle washing three to four times daily.

2. Impetigo must be adequately treated and resolved to prevent postinfection complications such as the following: post-streptococcal acute glomerulonephritis, cellulitis, ecthyma, and bacteremia.
B. Patient teaching: Encourage good hand washing and hygiene to reduce spreading infection.
C. Pharmaceutical therapy
  1. If few lesions noted without involvement of face or cellulitis: mupirocin (Bactroban) ointment to site four times daily for 10 days.
  2. Systemic antibiotics
     a. Children: dicloxacillin 12.5–25 g/kg/day four times daily for 10 days.
     b. Adults: dicloxacillin 125–250 mg four times daily for 10 days.
     c. Children: erythromycin 30–60 mg/kg/day four times daily for 10 days.
     d. Adults: erythromycin 250 mg by mouth four times daily for 10 days.
  3. Other effective antibiotics include cephalexin, cefaclor, cephradine, cefadroxil, and amoxicillin.

Follow-up
A. Schedule appointment in 10–14 days to determine resolution of infection.

Consultation/Referral
A. Consult a physician if complications arise or if resolution is not complete with antibiotic therapy.

LICE (PEDICULOSIS)

Definition
Pediculosis (lice) is an infestation of the louse on human beings in one of three areas:

A. Head (pediculosis capitis)
B. Pubic area (*Phthirus pubis*)
C. Body (pediculosis corporis)

Incidence
A. Pediculosis capitis is most common in children. It is estimated that head lice infestations occur in the school systems anywhere from 10%–40% of the time.
B. They are more commonly found in girls than boys.
C. *Phthirus pubis* infestation is more common in adults.
D. Lice affect all demographics: social, racial, and economic groups.

Pathogenesis
A. Head and body lice are transmitted by direct contact from person to person, that is, through sharing hats, combs, brushes, and so forth. The parasite hatches from an egg, or nit. Once hatched, the lice live on humans by sucking blood through the skin. The average adult louse lives 9–10 days. The nits appear as small white eggs on the hair shaft. Nits are very difficult to remove and survive up to 3 weeks after removal from the host. Body lice lay nits in the seams of clothing.
B. Pubic lice are found at the base of the hair shaft, where they lay nits. Pubic lice are transmitted through sexual contact.

Predisposing Factors
A. Head and body lice: exposure to crowded public areas, such as schools; inability to clean and launder clothing, bed linens, and so forth
B. Pubic lice: sexual contact with infected people
C. Poor hygiene

Common Complaints
A. Head lice: severe itching and scratching of the head, neck area, and commonly behind the ears
B. Body lice: severe itching on the body, which may lead to secondary infections of the skin
C. Pubic lice: severe itching of genital area

Other Signs and Symptoms
A. Excoriated skin from intense scratching.
B. Visible lice or nits in hair, body, or clothing.
C. Papules with an erythemic base may develop on the genital area, axilla, chest, beard, or eyelashes.
D. *Phthirus pubis* or nits or lice are found on eyelashes of children.

Subjective Data
A. Inquire as to exposure to anyone known to have lice.
B. Identify whether the patient attends a crowded environment such as school, day care, and so forth.
C. Ask if lice and nits have been seen by the patient or guardian.
D. Determine onset, duration, and course of symptoms. Ask: When were lice or nits first discovered?
E. Assess whether the patient has been symptomatic (itching, scratching).
F. Inquire about social habits of cleaning, laundry, and so forth.

Physical Examination
A. Temperature to rule any secondary infection.
B. Inspect
  1. Inspect hair, body, pubic area, and clothing seams for nits or lice.
  2. Note excoriation of skin.
  3. Examine eyelashes of children.
  4. Examine skin for secondary bacterial infection.

Diagnostic Tests
A. None
B. Culture excoriated area if secondary bacterial infection suspected

Differential Diagnoses
A. Lice
B. Scabies

Plan
A. General interventions
  1. Treat immediately with appropriate pediculicides (see pharmaceutical therapy).
  2. After treatment, it is imperative to remove each nit and louse; use fine-tooth comb for nit removal.
  3. Evaluate entire family for lice.
  4. Treat secondary bacterial infection as needed.

B. Patient teaching
1. See the Section III Patient Teaching Guide for this chapter, "Lice (Pediculosis)."
2. Specific instructions need to be given to clients on how to get rid of lice and nits.
3. Reinforce good hygiene; teach children not to share combs, brushes, hats, and hair accessories.
C. Pharmaceutical therapy
1. Pediculosis capitis: lindane (Kwell), synergized pyrethrins (Rid) (0.3%).
2. Permethrin (Nix) treatment; see directions on bottle.
3. Apply, repeat in 24 hours, then again in 1 week.
4. Pediculosis corporis: Apply lindane (Kwell) to skin and allowed to remain on skin for several hours. Irritation to the scalp or skin may be caused from overuse of the pediculicide treatments.
5. *Phthirus pubis:* lindane (Kwell) or per-methrin (Nix), apply to pubic area as directed.
6. **Lindane (Kwell) toxicity may occur from ingestion or overuse and is exhibited by headaches, dizziness, and convulsions.**
7. Eyelash manifestation: after removing nits, apply petroleum jelly to lashes three to four times a day for 8–10 days. **Eyelashes should never be treated with pediculicides.**

Follow-up
A. None recommended.
B. Some schools and institutions require follow-up to evaluate whether infestation is resolved before admitting the child back into the classroom.

Consultation/Referral
A. If lice are a repeated problem, contact social services or the health department to have a visiting nurse or aide visit the home to evaluate home conditions and to teach the family how to prevent infestations.

Individual Considerations
A. Pregnancy: Lindane (Kwell) is contraindicated during pregnancy.
B. Pediatrics
1. Head lice commonly seen in school-aged children.
2. Lindane (Kwell) should not be used in infants.

LICHEN PLANUS

Definition
A. Lichen planus is a relatively common acute or chronic inflammatory dermatosis. It affects skin and mucous membranes with characteristic flat-topped, shiny, violaceous (purplish color) pruritic papules with lacy lines on the skin, and milky-white papules in the mouth.

Incidence
A. Lichen planus accounts for 0.1%–1.2% of office visits to dermatologists.
B. It exhibits no racial preference.

Pathogenesis
A. Etiology is unknown, although it is possibly a cell-mediated immune response. Most cases remit within 7 years. Lesions may heal with significant postinflammatory hyperpigmentation.

Predisposing Factors
A. Severe emotional stress.
B. Drugs may induce lichenoid plaques.

Common Complaints
A. Rash with or without pruritus
B. Primary lesions: small, flat-topped papules that are polygonal, lightly scaly, and violaceous
C. Secondary lesions: erythema, scales, and erosions

Other Signs and Symptoms
A. Distribution: volar aspect of wrists, ankles, mouth, genitalia, and lumbar region
B. Wickham's striae (white, lacelike pattern on surface)
C. Scalp: atrophic skin with alopecia
D. Nails: destructions of nail fold and bed, especially in large toe
E. Men: lesions of glans penis
F. Women: erosive lesions of labia and vulva

Subjective Data
A. Determine whether the onset was sudden or gradual.
B. Ask the patient to describe if the skin is itchy or painful.
C. Assess lesions for any associated discharge (blood or pus).
D. Identify the location(s) of the problem.
E. Complete a drug history. Ask the patient if he or she has recently taken any antibiotics or other drugs. Ask if he or she has used any topical medications, lotions, or other creams.
F. Determine the presence of any preceding systemic symptoms (fever, sore throat, anorexia, or vaginal discharge).
G. Rule out insect bites.
H. Identify any possible exposure to industrial toxins, domestic toxins, or color-film-developing chemicals.
I. Ask if the patient has had any possible sexual contacts with HIV or sexually transmitted infections (STIs).
J. Ask if the patient has had close physical contact with others with skin disorders.

Physical Examination
A. Check temperature, pulse, respirations, and blood pressure.
B. Inspect
1. Inspect skin and note lesion distribution.
2. Inspect mucous membranes: buccal mucosa, tongue, and lips.
3. Examine hair and nails.
4. Observe genitalia.

Diagnostic Tests
A. A drop of mineral oil accentuates papule.
B. If necessary to confirm diagnosis, deep shave or punch biopsy of developed lesions.
C. HIV or STI testing if indicated.

Differential Diagnoses
A. Lichen planus
B. Lichenoid drug eruptions
C. Leukoplakia
D. Chronic graft-versus-host disease
E. Candidiasis (thrush)
F. Lupus erythematosus
G. Contact dermatitis
H. Bite trauma
I. Secondary syphilis

Plan
A. General interventions: Discontinue any suspected drug agent.
B. Patient teaching: See the Section III Patient Teaching Guide for this chapter, "Lichen Planus."
   1. Instruct patients that the disease may be chronic; most cases resolve spontaneously.
   2. Encourage the patient to avoid severe emotional stress.
   3. Encourage the patient to avoid scratching and prevent secondary infection.
   4. Reassure the patient that lichen planus is not contagious.
C. Pharmaceutical therapy
   1. Oral antihistamines: hydroxyzine hydrochloride 10–50 mg four times daily as needed for pruritus, or Cetirizine HCl (Zyrtec) 10 mg daily.
   2. Medium- to high-potency topical corticosteroids
      a. Mouth lesions: fluocinonide 0.05%, ointment or gel, two or three times daily.
      b. Body lesions: betamethasone dipropionate (Diprolene) 0.05%, Triamcinolone (Kenolog) or other class 1 cream or ointment, two times daily. **Caution patients about steroid atrophy.**
      c. Genital lesions: desonide cream 0.05% twice daily initially, although higher-potency creams may be necessary. Topical corticosteroids should be used on genitalia in short bursts only.
      d. Hypertrophic lesions: intralesional injections, such as injecting triamcinolone 5–10 mg/mL, 0.5–1 mL per 2-cm lesion, are helpful for pruritus relief. Use cautiously in dark-skinned patients because of risk of hypopigmentation.
   3. Oral prednisone is rarely used, but if necessary use with a short course only and taper.

Follow-up
A. See the patient in 1 week for evaluation of treatment.

Consultation/Referral
A. Refer the patient to a dermatologist if there is no response to initial treatment.

Individual Considerations
A. Pregnancy: Use caution with medications prescribed.
B. Pediatrics: For severe itching, consider oral antihistamine.

PITYRIASIS ROSEA

Definition
A. Pityriasis rosea is an acute, self-limiting, benign skin eruption characterized by a preceding "herald patch" that is followed by widespread papulosquamous lesions.

Incidence
A. Pityriasis rosea is relatively common, with more than 75% of cases in individuals from 10–35 years of age.
B. Slightly higher incidence in women than men.
C. Incidence is higher during the spring and autumn.

Pathogenesis
A. Disease is idiopathic; some evidence exists to support viral origin or autoimmune disorder.

Predisposing Factors
A. Recent acute infection.

Common Complaints
A. Rash: Salmon, pink, or tawny-colored lesions generally concentrated in lower abdominal area, but may develop on arms, legs, and rarely on the face.
B. Mild pruritus.

Other Signs and Symptoms
A. Earliest lesions may be papular, but may progress to 1- to 2-cm oval plaques.
B. Long axes of oval lesions run parallel to each other, hence the term "Christmas tree distribution."
C. Preceding herald patch (2–10 cm with central clearing) closely resembles ringworm; usually abruptly appears a few days to several weeks prior to the generalized eruptive phase.

Subjective Data
A. Elicit information about occurrence of initial, single, 2- to 10-cm round-to-oval lesion.
B. Question the patient as to known contacts with similar symptoms. Small epidemics have been identified in fraternity houses and military bases.

Physical Examination
A. Temperature to rule out any infection
B. Inspect
   1. Examine all body surfaces with patient unclothed.
   2. Look for characteristic lesions and distribution.
   3. Check the mucous surfaces, palms, and soles, which are usually spared by pityriasis rosea.

Diagnostic Tests
A. Generally none required; however, KOH wet preparation may be useful to distinguish herald patch from tinea corporis.
B. Serology to rule out syphilis, if applicable.
C. If unable to identify herald patch, a serologic test for syphilis should be ordered because syphilis may be clinically indistinguishable from pityriasis rosea.
D. White blood count normal; no specific lab markers for pityriasis rosea.

Differential Diagnoses

A. Pityriasis rosea
B. Nummular eczema
C. Tinea corporis
D. Tinea versicolor
E. Viral exanthems
F. Drug eruptions
  1. Captopril
  2. Bismuth
  3. Barbiturates
  4. Clonidine
  5. Metronidazole
G. Secondary syphilis
H. Lichen planus

Plan

A. General interventions
  1. Direct sunlight to point of minimal erythema hastens disappearance of lesions and decreases itching. Ultraviolet B (UVB) light in five consecutive daily exposures can decrease pruritus and shorten rash, particularly if administered within the first week of eruption.
  2. Not proven to be contagious and relatively harmless, so isolation is not required.
B. Patient teaching
  1. See the Section III Patient Teaching Guide for this chapter, "Pityriasis Rosea."
  2. Advise patients disease is self-limiting and clears spontaneously in 1–3 months.
C. Pharmaceutical therapy
  1. Generally none is required, but for itching the following recommendations exist: group V topical steroids and oral antihistamines as per usual dosing.
  2. Prednisone 20 mg twice daily for 1–2 weeks in rare cases of intense itching.

Follow-up

A. None is required unless secondary infection (impetigo) develops. Disease may recur in approximately 2% of patients.

Consultation/Referral

A. Consult or refer the patient to a physician when disease persists beyond 3 months.

Individual Considerations

A. Pregnancy: Disease has not been shown to affect fetus.
B. Pediatrics: Rash more frequently affects face and distal extremities. Impetigo may result from scratching or poor hygiene.
C. Geriatrics: Disease rarely seen in geriatric patients. Strongly consider other differential diagnoses, particularly drug reactions.

PRECANCEROUS OR CANCEROUS SKIN LESIONS

Definition

A. Potentially malignant or malignant cutaneous cells form precancerous or cancerous skin lesions, respectively.

Incidence

A. There are approximately 700,000 new cases of basal cell and squamous cell carcinomas reported each year. Approximately 32,000 of these cases per year are found to be malignant melanoma.
  1. Squamous cell carcinoma accounts for 20% of all skin cancers, and it occurs mostly in the middle-aged and elderly populations.
  2. Basal cell carcinoma is the most common form of skin cancer, with approximately 400,000 new cases per year in the United States. It is often seen in the sixth or seventh decade of life.
  3. Malignant melanoma accounts for less than 5% of all skin cancers and is responsible for more than 60% of deaths due to skin cancer. Melanoma is frequently seen in younger people, with the median age being in the low 40s.

Pathogenesis

A. Squamous cell carcinoma (SCC): Abnormal cells of the epidermis penetrate the basement membrane of the epidermis and move into the dermis, producing squamous cell carcinoma. This often begins as actinic keratosis that undergoes malignant change.
B. Basal cell carcinoma (BCC): Abnormal cells of the basal layer of the epidermis expand. The surrounding stroma support the basal cell growth. Ultraviolet rays (sunlight) are the major contributor to BCC. BCC is a slow-growing tumor that rarely metastasizes.
C. Malignant melanoma: Abnormal cells proliferate from the melanocyte system. Initially, the cells grow superficially and laterally into the epidermis and papillary dermis. After time, the cells begin growing up into the reticular dermis and subcutaneous fat. Malignant tumors occur due to the inability of the damaged cells to protect themselves from the long-term exposure of the ultraviolet rays.

Predisposing Factors

A. Advanced age (older than age 50).
B. Median age of 40 years for malignant melanoma.
C. Exposure to ultraviolet light (sun exposure).
D. Fair complexion.
E. Smokers (damaged lips).
F. Skin damaged by burns and/or chronic inflammation.
G. History of blistering sunburns before 18 years of age increases risk.

Common Complaints

A. New lesions found on the skin
B. Ulcer that does not heal

Other Signs and Symptoms

A. Squamous cell carcinoma: skin lesions seen in sun-exposed areas or skin damaged by burns or chronic inflammation; lower lip lesions common; firm, irregular papules with scaly, bleeding, friable surface like sandpaper; grows rapidly
B. Basal cell carcinoma: tumor seen on face and neck; nodules greater than 1 cm that appear shiny, pearly color with telangiectasia; center caves in

C. Malignant melanoma: asymmetrical tumor of skin with irregular border, variation in color, greater than 6 mm in diameter; can metastasize to any organ

D. Bowen's disease (squamous cell carcinoma in situ): chronic, nonhealing erythemic patch with sharp, irregular borders; occurs on skin and/or the mucocutaneous tissue; resembles eczema but does not respond to steroids

Subjective Data

A. Have the patient identify when lesion was first noted.

B. Ask the patient to describe any changes in size, color, or shape of the lesion.

C. Determine whether the patient has noted any new lesions.

D. Ascertain any family history of malignant melanoma.

E. Determine the patient's history of skin exposure to the sun or any other ultraviolet rays.

F. Ask the patient about smoking history. If the patient smokes, ask how many packs per day.

Physical Examination

A. Temperature

B. Inspect
  1. Examine skin for lesions.
  2. Note surface, size, shape, border, color, and diameter of lesion.
  3. Examine scalp and ears for lesions.

Diagnostic Tests

A. Biopsy suspicious lesions.

Differential Diagnoses

A. Squamous cell carcinoma

B. Basal cell carcinoma

C. Malignant melanoma

D. Actinic keratosis

E. Solar lentigo

F. Seborrheic keratosis

G. Common nevus

H. Leukoplakia

Plan

A. General interventions
  1. Monitor progress of lesions detected.
  2. Biopsy any suspicious lesions.

B. Patient teaching
  1. See the Section III Patient Teaching Guide for this chapter, "Skin Care Assessment."
  2. Educate patients regarding importance of early identification of lesions and monthly assessment of skin.

C. Pharmaceutical therapy: None indicated.

Follow-up

A. If diagnosis made, follow with examination every month for 3 months, twice a year for 5 years, then yearly.

Consultation/Referral

A. Refer all patients to the dermatologist if skin cancer is suspected.

Individual Considerations

A. Pediatrics: Teach parents to use SPF 30 or greater on pediatric patients exposed to the sun.

B. Geriatrics: The elderly are at high risk for skin lesions. Monitor them closely.

PSORIASIS

Definition

A. A common benign, chronic, inflammatory skin disorder, psoriasis is characterized by whitish scaly patches commonly seen on the scalp, knees, and elbows.

Incidence

A. Disease occurs in 1%–3% of the world population.

B. Psoriasis affects 2–8 million people in the United States.

C. It occurs at any age.
  1. Peaks of onset seen in adolescence
  2. Young adult (16–22 years old)
  3. Adult (57–60 years old)

Pathogenesis

A. Etiology is unknown; this is a multifactorial disease with a definite genetic component. Hyperproliferation of the epidermis and inflammation of the epidermis and dermis are seen, with epidermal transit time rapidly increased (six- to ninefold). A T-lymphocyte-mediated dermal immune response may be due to microbial antigen or autoimmune process.

Predisposing Factors

A. Family history

B. Drugs that exacerbate condition
  1. Lithium
  2. β-blockers
  3. Nonsteroidal anti-inflammatory drugs (NSAIDS)
  4. Antimalarials
  5. Sudden withdrawal of systemic or potent topical corticosteriods

C. Stress (common triggering factor)

D. Local trauma or irritation

E. Recent streptococcal infection

F. Alcohol use

G. Tobacco use

H. HIV association; suspected if onset is abrupt

Common Complaints

A. Dry scaly rash

Other Signs and Symptoms

A. Pruritic and/or painful lesions.

B. Silvery scales on discrete erythematous plaques
  1. Onset commonly occurs as a guttate form with small, scattered, teardrop-shaped papules and plaques after a streptococcal infection in a child or young adult.
  2. Larger, chronic plaques occur later in life.

C. Lesions are commonly seen on scalp, elbows, knees, but may involve any area of the body.

D. Glossitis or geographic tongue: small pits or yellow-brown spots (oil spots).

E. Positive Auspitz Sign: punctate bleeding points with removal of scale.
F. Onycholysis.
G. Stippled nails and pitting; approximately 50% of patients have nail involvement.
H. Periarticular swelling of small joints of fingers and toes. **Joint pain and involvement signals psoriatic arthritis.**
I. Pustular variant with predominant involvement of hands and/or feet including nails.

Subjective Data

A. Question the patient regarding any predisposing factors listed above to identify risk factors.
B. Ask the patient if there have been changes in the course of symptoms.
C. Ascertain whether the symptoms worsen in winter and clear in summer.
D. Determine site of lesion and whether the onset is sudden or painful.
E. Ask the patient to describe the skin: is it itchy or painful?
F. Assess lesions for any associated discharge (blood or pus).
G. Ask if the patient is using any new soaps, creams, or lotions.
H. Rule out any exposure to industrial or domestic toxins.
I. Ask the patient about any possible contact with venereal disease (STDs).
J. Review whether there was close physical contact with others with skin disorders.
K. Elicit information regarding any preceding systemic symptoms (fever, sore throat, and anorexia).

Physical Examination

A. Check temperature, pulse, respirations, and blood pressure.
B. Inspect
   1. Inspect skin; note type of lesion and distribution. Assess oral mucosa, nails, and nail beds.
   2. Assess joints.
C. Palpate: Palpate joints for tenderness.

Diagnostic Tests

A. None is indicated unless HIV infection is suspected, in which case run HIV test.
B. If joint inflammation is present, consider rheumatoid factor, erythrocyte sedimentation rate (ESR), and uric acid.
C. If there is a history of streptococcal infection, order antistreptolysin O titer (ASOT).

Differential Diagnoses

A. Psoriasis
B. Scalp: seborrheic dermatitis
C. Body folds: candidiasis
D. Trunk: pityriasis rosea, tinea corporis
E. Hand dermatitis
F. Squamous cell carcinoma
G. Cutaneous lupus erythematosus

Plan

A. General interventions
   1. This is a chronic disorder that requires long-term treatment, a high degree of patient involvement, and therapy that is simple and inexpensive.
   2. Aim of treatment is control, not cure.
   3. Exposure to sunlight may be beneficial. However, a small percentage of patients worsen with exposure to sunlight.
   4. Sequence of agents for involvement of less than 20% body surface is as follows:
      a. Emollients (Eucerin cream or Aquaphor cream).
      b. Keratolytic agents (Salicylic acid gel or ointment).
      c. Topical corticosteroids: use lowest potency to control disease.
      d. Calcipotriene ointment: vitamin D analogue (calcipotriene ointment 0.005%).
      e. Anthralin: use as short-contact therapy 1%–3%.
      f. Coal tar (Estar, PsoriGel): use in conjunction with topical steroids or anthralin. May apply at bedtime or in the morning for 15 min and then shower off.
      g. Medicated shampoos: useful for scalp psoriasis, in conjunction with topical steroids and other treatments.
B. Patient teaching
   1. See the Section III Patient Teaching Guide for this chapter, "Psoriasis."
   2. Help the patient understand the chronic nature of this disease characterized by flares and remission. Teach stress monitoring and control. Assist with coping techniques.
   3. A trial of a gluten-free diet may be tried to help symptoms. See Appendix B: "Gluten-Free Special Diet."
C. Pharmaceutical therapy: If disease is not controlled with first agent, then an alternative agent may be tried.
   1. Mild-to-moderate disease: topical steroids as first-line therapy.
   2. Emollients to start treatment (e.g., Eucerin Plus lotion or cream, Lubriderm Moisture Plus, Moisturel).
   3. Scalp: use coal tar shampoo (Zetar, T/Gel, Pentrax) in place of regular shampoo two times per week.
      a. Apply lather to scalp, allow to soak for 5 minutes, and then rinse.
      b. If scale is very thick, use P and S Liquid (OTC). Massage in at night and wash out in morning.
   4. For additional treatment as needed, apply triamcinolone acetonide 0.1% (Kenalog 0.1%) lotion or equivalent to scaly, stubborn areas once or twice daily until controlled. **Avoid face.**
   5. Dovonex scalp solution: apply on dry scalp as directed.
   6. Face and skin folds: hydrocortisone cream 1%, apply sparingly up to 4 weeks, preferably no more than 2 weeks. If lesions are unresponsive, consider increasing to 2.5% and taper quickly with improvement.

7. Body, arms, and legs: use triamcinolone acetonide 0.025% (Aristocort A) cream twice daily up to 2 weeks. **Avoid normal skin.**
8. For thick plaques, try Keralyt gel (6% salicylic acid), then corticosteroids.
9. Coal tar (Estar gel) once or twice daily in combination with corticosteroids.
10. Anthralin (Dritho-Creme) is beneficial as alternate to steroid lotion for scalp psoriasis. **Avoid sunlight.**
11. Vitamin D_3 analogue: (Calcipotro), twice daily up to 8 weeks, is comparable to midpotency corticosteroids. **Avoid face and skin folds.**

Follow-up
A. See patients in 2–3 weeks to evaluate treatment.
B. Follow-up in 2 months to monitor side effects.
C. Follow-up must be individualized for each patient.

Consultation/Referral
A. Medical management: for involvement greater than 20% of body, refer the patient to a dermatologist for the following:
  1. Light therapy with ultraviolet A or B. UVB light therapy is often used in conjunction with keratolytic agents.
  2. Synthetic retinoids: etretinate or acitretin.
  3. Low-dose cyclosporine or Azulfidine.
B. Refer patients with extensive disease, psoriatic arthritis, or inflammatory disease to a physician or dermatologist.
C. Cases of generalized pustular psoriosis of exfoliative erythroderma should be referred immediately to a dermatologist.
D. All systemic therapies should be given under supervision of a dermatologist.

SCABIES

Definition
A. Scabies is a contagious skin infestation by the mite *Sarcoptes scabei.*

Incidence
A. Scabies occurs mainly in individuals in close contact with many other individuals, such as school children or nursing home residents. It is rare among African Americans.

Pathogenesis
A. Scabies is transmitted through close contact with an individual who is infested with the mite *Sarcoptes scabiei.* Transmission may occur through sexual contact or contact with mite-infested clothing or sheets. The fertilized female mite burrows into the stratum corneum of a host and deposits eggs and fecal pellets. Larvae hatch, mature, and repeat the cycle.
B. A hypersensitivity reaction is responsible for the intense pruritus.

Predisposing Factors
A. Close contact with large numbers of individuals
B. Institutionalization
C. Poverty
D. Sexual promiscuity

Common Complaints
A. Intense itching, worse at night
B. Skin excoriation
C. Generalized pruritus
D. Rash

Other Signs and Symptoms
A. Mites burrow in finger webs, at wrists, in the sides of hands and feet, axilla buttocks, and in penis and scrotum in males.
B. Discrete vesicles and papules, distributed in linear fashion.
C. Erythema.
D. Secondary infections due to scratching or infection (pustules and pinpoint erosions).
E. Nodules in covered areas (buttocks, groin, scrotum, penis, and axilla), which may have slightly eroded surfaces that persist for months after mites have been eradicated.
F. Diffuse eruption that spares face.

Subjective Data
A. Elicit information regarding housing conditions, close contact or sexual contact with potentially infected individuals.
B. Question the patient regarding onset, duration, and location of itching.

Physical Examination
A. Temperature
B. Inspect
  1. Examine all body surfaces with patient unclothed.
  2. Use a magnifying lens to identify characteristic burrows in finger webs, wrists, and penis.
  3. Inspect adult pubic area for lesions.

Diagnostic Tests
A. Three findings are diagnostic of scabies:
  1. Microscopic identification of *S. scabei* mites
  2. Eggs
  3. Fecal pellets (scybala)
B. Burrow identification: Ink the suspected area with a blue or black felt-tipped pen, then wipe with an alcohol swab. The burrow absorbs the ink, while the surface ink is wiped clean.
C. A tiny black dot may be seen at the end of a burrow, which represents the mite, ova, or feces, and can be transferred by means of a 25-gauge hypodermic needle to immersion oil on a slide for microscopic identification.
D. Place a drop of mineral oil on a suspected lesion, scrape lesion with a #15 blade, and transfer the shaved material to a microscope slide for direct examination of the mite under low power.

Differential Diagnoses
A. Scabies
B. Atopic dermatitis
C. Insect bites

D. Pityriasis rosea

E. Eczema

F. Seborrheic dermatitis

G. Syphilis

H. Pediculosis

I. Allergic or irritant contact dermatitis

Plan

A. General interventions
1. Implement comfort measures to reduce pruritus.
2. Treat secondary infection(s) with antibiotics.
3. Household members should be treated simultaneously as a prophylactic measure and to reduce the chance of reinfection.
4. The patient should be advised that pruritus may continue for up to a week even with a successful treatment due to local irritation.

B. Patient teaching: See Section the III Patient Teaching Guide for this chapter, "Scabies."

C. Pharmaceutical therapy
1. First line of therapy, due to its low toxicity, is 5% permethrin (Elimite cream) applied to all body areas from neck down and washed off in 8–14 hours. One application is highly effective, but some dermatologists recommend retreatment in 1 week.
2. Alternative therapy is lindane (Kwell) cream, applied to all skin surfaces from the neck down and washed off in 8–12 hours. Some dermatologists retreat in 7 days.
3. A single oral dose of the anthelmintic agent ivermectin (200 µg/kg) has been shown to be effective and to rapidly control pruritus in healthy patients and HIV patients.
4. Diphenhydramine (Benadryl) 25–50 mg may be given by mouth every 4–6 hours if indicated for pruritus. Other nonsedating antihistamines may be used. Toxicity is usually a result of patient overtreatment (failure to follow prescribed regimen). Advise the patient of this danger.

Follow-up

A. Follow-up in 2 weeks to assess treatment response.

Consultation/Referral

A. Consult or refer the patient to the physician if, at 2-week follow-up, pharmaceutical therapy has been ineffective.

Individual Considerations

A. Pregnancy
1. Permethrin is preferred over lindane in pregnant and/or lactating women due to decreased toxicity.
2. Patient should be warned of its potential to cause neurotoxicity and convulsions with overuse (more than two treatments).

B. Pediatrics
1. Infants and toddlers often have more widespread involvement that can include the face and scalp.
2. Vesicular lesions on palms and soles are more commonly seen.
3. Drug of choice is permethrin 5% cream, apply over the head, neck, and body, avoiding the eyes. The cream should be removed by bathing in 8–14 hours.

4. Lindane should not be used in infants and toddlers.
5. Infants and children with underlying cutaneous disease, malnutrition, prematurity, or a history of seizure disorders should be treated with special caution due to their increased risk of toxicity.

C. Partners: All intimate contacts within the last month and close household and family members should be treated.

D. Geriatrics
1. The elderly tend to have more severe pruritus despite fewer lesions.
2. They are at risk for extensive infections due to an age-related decline in immunity.
3. The excoriations may become severe and may be complicated by cellulitis.

⬚ SEBORRHEIC DERMATITIS

Definition

A. A common chronic, erythematous, scaling dermatosis, seborrheic dermatitis occurs in areas of the most active sebaceous glands, such as face and scalp, body folds, and presternal region.

Incidence

A. Seborrheic dermatitis is very common.

B. Incidence is higher in HIV-infected individuals.

Pathogenesis

A. Etiology is unknown. There is a possibility that it is hormonally dependent, has a fungal (*Pityrosporum ovale* or *Candida albicans*) component, is neurogenic, or may reflect a nutritional deficiency.

B. Currently it is identified as an inflammatory disorder that most probably results from a dysfunction of sebaceous glands.

Predisposing Factors

A. Possible link between infantile and adult forms

B. Possible familial trend

C. High association with HIV-infected individuals

Common Complaints

A. Infants: "cradle cap"

B. Adults: "dandruff," dry flaky scalp

C. Rash with "sticky flakes"

Often no presenting complaints are found on a routine physical exam.

Other Signs and Symptoms

A. Variable pruritus, often increased with perspiration and winter

B. Oily, flaking skin around ears, nose, eyebrows, and eyelids

C. Red, cracking skin in body folds; axilla; groin; or anogenital, submammary, or umbilical areas

D. Primary lesions: plaques

E. Secondary lesions: erythema, scales, fissures, exudate, and symmetric eyelid involvement

F. Distribution pattern in infants: scalp and diaper area

G. Distribution area in adults: scalp, eyebrows, paranasal area, nasolabial fold, external auditory canal, chest, and groin

H. Secondary impetigo in children

Subjective Data

A. Identify location, onset, and progression of symptoms.
B. Ask the patient to describe symptoms. Ask if the skin is itchy or painful.
C. Assess lesions for any associated discharge (blood or pus).
D. Elicit information regarding use of topical medications, soaps, creams, or lotions.
E. Determine whether there were any preceding systemic symptoms (fever, sore throat, anorexia, or vaginal discharge).
F. Rule out any possible exposure to industrial or domestic toxins.
G. Ask the patient to identify what improves or worsens this condition.

Physical Examination

A. Check temperature, pulse, respirations, and blood pressure.
B. Inspect
  1. Inspect skin; note areas of lesions and distribution.
  2. Assess eyes for blepharitis.
  3. Inspect ears and nose.
C. Palpate: Palpate skin, noting texture and moisture.

Diagnostic Tests

A. None required.
B. Consider possible skin biopsy to rule out other conditions.

Differential Diagnoses

A. Seborrheic dermatitis
B. Atopic dermatitis
C. Candidiasis
D. Dermatophytosis
E. Histiocytosis X
F. Psoriasis vulgaris
G. Rosacea
H. Systemic lupus erythematosus
I. Tinea capitis
J. Tinea versicolor
K. Vitamin deficiency
L. HIV disease

Plan

A. General interventions
  1. Shampooing is the foundation of treatment.
    a. Infants: Rub petroleum jelly into scalp to soften crusts 20–30 min before shampooing.
    b. Shampoo daily with baby shampoo using a soft brush.
    c. Toddlers or adolescents: Shampoo every other day with antiseborrheic shampoo (Selsun Blue, Exsel, or Nizoral).
  2. If skin does not clear after 1–2 weeks of treatment, it is appropriate to use ketoconazole 2% cream.
  3. Seborrheic blepharitis
    a. Hot compresses plus gentle debridement with cotton-tipped applicator and baby shampoo twice a day.
    b. For secondary bacterial infection, sulfacetamide sodium 10% (ophthalmic Sodium Sulamyd).

4. Continue treatment for several days after lesions disappear.
B. Patient teaching: See the Section III Patient Teaching Guide for this chapter, "Seborrheic Dermatitis."
C. Pharmaceutical therapy
  1. Most shampoos should be used two times per week. Those with coal tar can be used three times per week.
  2. Medicated shampoos
    a. Coal tar (Denorex, T/Gel, Pentrax, Tegrin) shampoo, apply as directed.
    b. Salicylic acid (Ionil Plus, P and S) shampoo, apply as directed.
    c. Selenium sulfide (Exsel, Selsun Blue) shampoo used daily.
    d. Ketoconazole 2% (Nizoral) cream, apply to affected area twice daily for 4–6 weeks.
    e. Combination shampoos: coal tar and salicylic acid (T/Sal); salicylic acid and sulfur (Sebulex). These shampoos may be used one to two times a week, alternating with other shampoos during the week. Always apply corticosteroids as thin layer only; avoid eyes.
  3. Topical corticosteroid lotions or solutions: use in combination with medicated shampoo if 2–3 weeks of treatment with shampoo alone fails.
  4. Adults: Scalp
    a. Start with medium potency, for example, betamethasone valerate 0.1% lotion 20–60 mL twice daily.
    b. If treatment is not effective in 2 weeks, increase potency, for example, fluocinonide 0.05% solution 20 or 60 mL twice daily, or fluocinolone acetonide 0.01% oil 120 mL nightly with shower cap.
    c. As dermatitis is controlled, decrease to mild potency, for example, hydrocortisone 1%–2.5% lotion 60 or 20 mL once or twice daily.
  5. Adults: Face or groin
    a. Low-potency agents, for example, hydrocortisone 1% cream or desonide 0.05% cream once or twice daily.
    b. Consider lotion for eyebrows for easier application.
  6. Recalcitrant disease
    a. Add ketoconazole 2% cream (15, 30, or 60 g) every day.
    b. Sulfacetamide sodium 10%, with sulfur 5%, lotion 25 g once or twice daily.
  7. New therapy: topical τ-linoleic acid (Borage) oil.

Follow-up

A. Tell the patient to call the office in 5–6 days to report progress.
B. Have the patient return to the office if no improvement is seen.

Consultation/Referral

A. Refer the patient to a dermatologist if the condition does not clear in 10–14 days.

Individual Considerations

A. Pregnancy: Ketoconazole is not recommended.
B. Pediatrics
   1. Avoid using tar preparations on infants.
   2. Use baby shampoo only.
   3. If lesions are inflammatory, use topical steroids no stronger than hydrocortisone 0.5%–1.0% twice daily.
   4. Betamethasone valerate (Valisone) lotion may be used daily for scalp only if other treatments fail.
   5. Be aware of potential for emotional distress in adolescents.
   6. Treat with antiseborrheic shampoo every other day for adolescents.

⬡ TINEA CORPORIS (RINGWORM)

Definition

A. Tinea corporis (ringworm) is a fungal infection of the skin tissue (keratin) commonly seen on the face, trunk, and extremities.

Incidence

A. Ringworm is a fairly common fungal infection seen in adults and children.

Pathogenesis

A. The causative fungal species varies, depending on the location of the infection. Three common organisms include *Epidermophyton*, *Microsporum*, and *Trichophyton*.
B. The infection can be obtained from other people, animals (puppies, kittens), and the soil.

Predisposing Factors

A. Exposure to person or facilities (e.g., locker rooms) infected with the fungus
B. Poor nutrition
C. Poor health
D. Poor hygiene
E. Warm climates
F. Immunosuppression

Common Complaints

A. Scaly, itchy patch of skin, often circular in shape

Other Signs and Symptoms

A. Tinea capitis: erythema, scaling of scalp, with hair loss at site asymptomatic
B. Tinea corporis: circular, erythematous, well-demarcated lesion on the skin with hypopigmentation in center of lesion; usually pruritic
C. Tinea cruris: well-demarcated scaling lesions on groin (not scrotum) or thigh; usually pruritic
D. Tinea pedis: scaly, erythemic vesicles on feet, between toes, and in arch, with extreme pruritus
E. Tinea unguium (onychomycosis): thickening and yellowing of toenail or fingernail, often with other fungal infection or alone

Subjective Data

A. Ask the patient onset, duration, and progression of patch or rash on skin.
B. Assess the patient for other areas of skin involvement.
C. Ask if the lesion is pruritic.
D. Inquire as to the patient's exposure to anyone with similar symptoms.
E. Determine whether the patient has a history of similar lesions.
F. Query the patient regarding predisposing factors.
G. Review with the patient what remedies were used and with what results.

Physical Examination

A. Temperature
B. Inspect
   1. Examine all areas of skin.
   2. Note type of lesions present.

Diagnostic Tests

A. Obtain scrapings of the border of the lesion for evaluation
   1. KOH
   2. Wet prep
   3. Fungal cultures

Differential Diagnoses

A. Tinea corporis
B. Dermatitis
C. Alopecia areata
D. Psoriasis
E. Contact dermatitis
F. Atopic eczema

Plan

A. General interventions
   1. Identify type of lesion.
   2. Identify other infected family members or sexual partners for treatment.
B. Patient teaching
   1. See the Section III Patient Teaching Guide for this chapter, "Ringworm."
   2. Reinforce medication regimen for 4- to 8-week period for resolution.
C. Pharmaceutical therapy
   1. Tinea capitis
      a. Adults: griseofulvin 500 mg by mouth per day for 4–8 weeks.
      b. Children: griseofulvin 10–20 mg/kg/day for 4–8 weeks. **Griseofulvin is best absorbed with high-fat foods.**
      c. Ketoconazole (Nizoral) may also be used.
   2. Tinea corporis, pedis, and cruris: use wet dressings with Burow's solution along with one of the following:
      a. Clotrimazole 1% (Lotrimin) cream, or econazole nitrate 1% cream, twice daily for 14–28 days.
      b. Terbinafine 1% cream (Lamisil), topical, apply once or twice daily for 1–4 weeks. Not recommended for children.
   3. Onychomycosis: Successful treatment is difficult.
      a. Itraconazole (Sporanox) 100 mg, two tablets by mouth twice daily for 7 days. Repeat in one month, then repeat again in one more month.

Monitor liver function tests (LFTs) at 6 weeks after starting medication.

  b. Terbinafine 1% cream (Lamisil)
    i. Fingernail: 250 mg once daily for 6 weeks.
    ii. Toenail: 250 mg daily for 12 weeks.

Follow-up

A. A 2- to 4-week follow-up is recommended to evaluate progress.
B. Monitor LFT at 6 weeks and if Itraconazole (Sporanox) is continued longer.

Consultation/Referral

A. Consult a physician if the infection has not improved.

Individual Considerations

A. Pregnancy: Oral antifungal medications are not recommended during pregnancy.
B. Pediatrics
  1. Tinea capitis is common in children 2–10 years old. When hair has been lost, regrowth takes time.
  2. Tinea pedis is common in adolescents.
  3. Tinea unguium is common in adolescents, but rare in children.
C. Adults
  1. Tinea capitis is rare in adults.
  2. Tinea cruris is more common in obese males, but rare in females.
  3. Tinea pedis is common in adults.
  4. Tinea unguium is seen in adults.

TINEA VERSICOLOR

Definition

A. Tinea versicolor is a fungal infection of the skin, which may be chronic in nature. It is most commonly seen on the upper trunk; however, it may spread to extremities.

Incidence

A. Tinea versicolor is seen most frequently in adolescents and young adults.

Pathogenesis

A. This is a fungal infection of the skin caused by an overgrowth of *Pityrosporum orbiculare,* part of the normal skin flora.
B. Discoloration of the skin is seen, forming round or oval maculae, which may become confluent.
C. Maculae range from 1 cm to very large, greater than 30 cm.

Predisposing Factors

A. Immunosuppressive therapy
B. Pregnancy
C. Warm temperatures
D. Corticosteroid therapy

Common Complaints

A. Scaly rash on the upper trunk with occasional mild itching

Other Signs and Symptoms

A. Annular maculae with mild scaling
B. Asymptomatic or pruritic
C. Pink, white, or brown color rash

Subjective Data

A. Ascertain when and where the rash began.
B. Have the patient describe how the rash has changed.
C. Assess the patient for any associated symptoms with the rash, such as itching, burning, and so forth.
D. Identify what products the patient has used on the skin to treat rash and with what results.
E. Elicit information regarding a history of similar rashes.
F. Query the patient regarding current medications.
G. Review any medical history for comorbid conditions.

Physical Examination

A. Temperature
B. Inspect
  1. Inspect skin and note type of lesion.
  2. Examine other areas of skin for similar lesions.

Diagnostic Tests

A. Wet prep/KOH.
B. Wood's lamp: Wood's light is useful in examining skin to determine extent of infection. Inspection of fine scales with Wood's lamp reveals scales with a pale yellow-green fluorescence that contains the fungus.
C. Culture lesion: When obtaining sample scraping, obtain sample from edge of lesion for best sample of hyphae. (Hyphae and spores have a "spaghetti and meatball" appearance.)

Differential Diagnoses

A. Tinea versicolor
B. Tinea corporis
C. Pityriasis alba
D. Pityriasis rosea: herald patch is clue to diagnosis
E. Seborrheic dermatitis
F. Vitiligo

Plan

A. General interventions: Apply medication as directed.
B. Patient teaching
  1. See the Section III Patient Teaching Guide for this chapter, "Tinea Versicolor."
  2. Because causative species is a normal inhabitant of skin flora, recurrence is possible.
  3. Skin pigmentation returns after infection is cleared up. This may take several months to resolve.
C. Pharmaceutical therapy
  1. Selenium sulfide 2.5% (Selsun Blue).
    a. Apply to skin at bedtime one time. Shower off in the morning.
    b. Apply Selsun Blue to skin lesions, wait 30 min, then shower off for 12 days.
    c. Treatment may need to be used monthly until desired results are obtained. **Encourage use of Selsun Blue on entire body surface except for face and head.**

2. Other medications used
   a. Clotrimazole 1% cream twice daily for 4 weeks.
   b. Ketoconazole (Nizoral) cream daily for 14 days.
   c. Ketoconazole (Nizoral) 200 mg by mouth once daily for 3 days, for adults only. **When using ketoconazole (Nizoral) as treatment, caution the patient regarding liver damage with toxicity.**

Follow-up
A. None required if resolution occurs.
B. Monitor LFTs every 6 weeks if on Ketoconazole.

Consultation/Referral
A. Consult with a physician if current treatment is unsuccessful.

Individual Considerations
A. Pediatrics: Commonly seen in adolescents.
B. Adults: Commonly seen in young adults.

WARTS

Definition
A. A wart is an elevation of the epidermal layer of the skin (skin tumor). Warts are caused by the Papillomavirus.

Incidence
A. Warts occur in people of all ages, more commonly in children and early adulthood.
B. By adulthood, 90% of all people have positive antibodies to the virus.
C. Warts are seen more frequently in females than males.

Pathogenesis
A. A circumscribed mass develops on the skin that is limited to the epidermal layer. The virus, papillomavirus, is located within the nucleus of the cell.
B. The virus may be transmitted by touch and is commonly seen on the hands and feet.
C. Most warts resolve without treatment within 12–24 months.

Predisposing Factors
A. Skin trauma
B. Immunosuppression
C. Exposure to public showers, pools, locker rooms, and so forth

Common Complaints
A. Bump on the skin or specific area of the body (hands, feet, arms, and legs)
B. Usually painless unless present on the bottom of the foot

Other Signs and Symptoms
A. Common wart (verruca vulgaris): flesh-colored, irregular lesion with rough surface; black dots in center of lesion occasionally seen, which is thrombosed capillaries; can occur on any body part
B. Filiform wart (verruca filiformis): thin, threadlike, projected papule on face, lips, nose, or eyelids

C. Flat wart (verruca plana): flat-topped, flesh-colored papule, 1–3 mm in diameter, with smooth surface; seen in clusters or in a line, on face and extremities
D. Plantar wart (verruca plantaris): firm papula, 2–3 cm in diameter, indented into skin with verrucous surface; painful with ambulation, when placed on ball or heel of foot
E. Venereal warts: see STDs in Chapter 14

Subjective Data
A. Determine onset, location, and duration of tumor.
B. Elicit information regarding a history of previous warts.
C. Identify with the patient what treatment has been used in the past and what the results were. Question the patient regarding length of time OTC medications were used, and how aggressive he or she was with the treatment.

Physical Examination
A. Temperature
B. Inspect
   1. Assess skin for lesions, noting location, appearance, size, and surface texture of tumor.
   2. Examine the entire body for other lesions.

Diagnostic Tests
A. None indicated.

Differential Diagnoses
A. Wart
   1. Verruca vulgaris.
   2. Filiform wart.
   3. Verruca plana.
   4. Verruca plantaris.
B. Seborrheic keratosis.
C. Callus.
D. Molluscum contagiosum: flesh-colored group of firm papules found on the face, trunk, and/or extremities. A white core may be expressed from lesion. Lesion may be successfully removed by curettage or cryotherapy.

Plan
A. General interventions
   1. Identify type of wart.
   2. Conservative treatment is recommended for children.
B. Patient teaching: See the Section III Patient Teaching Guide for this chapter, "Warts."
C. Pharmaceutical therapy
   1. Common wart: after soaking and filing wart with a nail file, apply one of these:
      a. Salicylic acid 17% (Compound W) gel twice daily for up to 12 weeks, if needed. Keep site covered with adhesive.
      b. Duct tape is very effective.
      c. Cryotherapy with liquid nitrogen to site. Repeat every 3–4 weeks until resolved. Apply adhesive tape over site and keep covered.
   2. Flat wart or filiform wart
      a. Retinoic acid, apply to site twice daily for 4–6 weeks.

    b. Aldara (imiquimod) 5% cream may be applied by the patient at home. Although labeled use is for genital warts, the patient may consider off-label use at bedtime and wash off after 6–8 hours every other day until resolved.

  3. Plantar wart: salicylic acid 40% (Mediplast), apply over wart. Remove in 24–48 hours, and remove dead skin with stone or by scraping. Repeat every 24–48 hours until wart is removed. May take up to 6–8 weeks.

Follow-up
A. Follow the patient every 4–6 weeks until resolved.

Consultation/Referral
A. If diagnosis is unclear, refer the patient to a dermatologist for surgical excision and biopsy.

Individual Considerations
A. Pediatrics: Warts are commonly seen in young school-aged children.

WOUNDS

Definition
A. Wounds are breaks in the external surface of the body.

Pathogenesis
A. Wounds can be caused by any one of innumerable objects that breach the skin. Lacerations and abrasions typically heal by a three-stage process of clotting, inflammation, and skin cell proliferation. The most common pathogens of wound infections are *Staphylococcus aureus* and β-hemolytic streptococcus.

Predisposing Factors
A. Exposure to accidental or intentional injury
B. Accident prevention failure
C. High-risk behaviors
D. Conditions that predispose to poor wound healing
  1. Diabetes
  2. Corticosteroid therapy
  3. Immunodeficiency
  4. Advanced age
  5. Undernourishment

Common Complaints
A. Bleeding
B. Pain
C. "Cut" in the skin integrity

Other Signs and Symptoms
A. Signs and symptoms of infection: Deep wounds and dirty wounds have increased risk for infection.
B. Soft tissue damage: Wounds with tissue necrosis have increased risk for infection.

Subjective Data
A. Elicit the patient's description of how the wound occurred, including where and when the injury was sustained.
B. Ascertain how much time elapsed until treatment. If 6 hours have elapsed, bacterial multiplication is likely.
C. Ask if the patient is currently immunized for tetanus.
D. Complete a drug history; include any allergies to medications, anesthetics, or dressings.
E. Ask if the patient is taking any medications, especially steroids or anticoagulants.
F. Assess iodine and sulfa drug allergies before starting treatment.
G. Review with the patient whether there is anything significant in the past medical history that may interfere with the healing process (e.g., immunodeficiency).

Physical Examination
A. Check temperature, pulse, respirations, and blood pressure.
B. Inspect
  1. Inspect wound.
  2. Measure wound for size and depth. Wounds with untidy edges may heal more slowly and with disfigurement.
  3. Assess underlying bony structures.
  4. Inspect for foreign objects.
C. Palpate
  1. Palpate extremities for neurovascular function and sensation.
  2. Palpate tissue distal to wound.
  3. Palpate lymph nodes surrounding injured area.
D. Neurologic exam: Assess motor function distal to wound.

Diagnostic Tests
A. Culture wound site if it appears infected.
B. Take X-ray films for deep or crushing wounds.

Differential Diagnoses
A. Wound, minor
B. Nonaccidental self-inflicted injury
C. Self-inflicted injury
D. Domestic violence

Plan
A. General interventions
  1. Wounds that require open-wound management
    a. Abrasions and superficial lacerations
    b. Wounds with great amount of tissue damage
    c. Wounds more than 6 hours old
    d. Contaminated wounds
    e. Large area of superficial skin denudation
    f. Puncture wounds
  2. For wounds that do not require sutures:
    a. Cleanse wound well with warm water and soap; remove all dirt and foreign bodies.
    b. Forceful irrigation may be needed; use fine-pore sponge (Optipore) with a surfactant, such as poloxamer 188 (Skin Clens). If wound edges easily approximate, apply steri-strips.
    c. Dry, sterile dressings (Telfa, Duoderm, or Opsite) may be used.
  3. If inflammation is present, soak and wash for 15–20 min 3–4 times per day. Cover with clean, dry dressing. **Do not use steri-strips.**

4. For wounds that require sutures:
    a. Clean with warm water and soap. Irrigate with sterile saline solution.
    b. Anesthetize with 1%–2% lidocaine (Xylocaine). Do not use solution with epinephrine at fingertips, nose, or ears. Probe wound for any remaining foreign bodies. Approximate wound edges.
    c. Suture with technique appropriate to site:
        i. Skin sutures: nonabsorbable material (e.g., nylon, Prolene, silk).
        ii. Subcutaneous and mucosal sutures: absorbable material (e.g., Dexon, Vicryl, or plain or chromic gut).
        iii. Extremities: 4–0 nylon.
        iv. Soles of feet: 2–0 nylon.
    d. Cover with clean, dry dressing; change after first 24 hours.
    e. Suture removal is based on location:
        i. Head and trunk: 5–7 days.
        ii. Extremities: 7–10 days.
        iii. Soles and palms: 7–10 days.
    f. Tetanus prophylaxis (see Chapter 1).
B. Patient teaching: See the Section III Patient Teaching Guide for this chapter, "Wounds."
C. Pharmaceutical therapy
    1. Control pain with acetaminophen (Tylenol) or ibuprofen, as needed.
    2. Topical antibiotic ointments: Polysporin, bacitracin, and mupirocin.
    3. Oral antibiotics for prophylaxis
        a. Amoxicillin, clavulanate acid (Augmentin)
            i. Adolescents: 250–500 mg twice daily.
            ii. Children: 25–45 mg/kg/day twice daily for 7–10 days. Available as 200 mg/5 mL or 400 mg/5 mL liquid.
        b. With penicillin allergy, use erythromycin.
            i. Adolescents: (E-Mycin) 250 mg four times daily for 7–10 days.
            ii. Children: (Eryped) 30–60 mg/kg/day four times daily for 7–10 days. Available as 200 mg/5 mL or 400 mg/5 mL liquid.
    4. Other alternatives: cephalexin (Keflex), cefadroxil (Duricef), ciprofloxacin.
    5. Tetanus toxoid 0.5 mL by IM injecton in deltoid, if no booster has been administered in the last 5 years.

Follow-up
A. Have the patient return for evaluation and dressing change in 24–48 hours.

Consultation/Referral
Refer the patient to a physician for wounds of the type listed here.
A. Facial wounds
B. Subcutaneous tissue penetration
C. Functional disturbance of tendons, ligaments, vessels, or nerves
D. Grossly contaminated wounds
E. Wounds requiring hospitalization or aggressive antimicrobial therapy for evidence of pyogenic abscess, cellulitis, and ascending lymphangitis
F. Wounds diagnosed with Methicillin Resistant Staphylococcus Aureus (MRSA) should be treated with the following oral antibioitics: Trimethoprim Sulfamethoxazole (Bactrim), Minocycline or Doxycycline, Clindamycin, Rifampin (should be used in combination with one of the previous antibiotics) and Linezolid. Antibiotics not recommended due to high resistance include: beta lactams, fluoroquinolones, Dicloxacillin and Cephalexin. Treating the nares with Bactroban ointment twice a day and having the patient use hibiclens soap for showering will help to prevent recurrent infections. For severe cases of infection, the patient requires hospitalization for aggressive antibiotic treatment.

XEROSIS (WINTER ITCH)

Definition
A. Xerosis, often called "winter itch," is dry skin.

Incidence
A. Xerosis occurs in 48%–98% of patients with atopic dermatitis.
B. It occurs more frequently in elderly patients.

Pathogenesis
A. Dry skin may fissure, appear shiny and cracked, and leave subsequent inflammatory changes.

Predisposing Factors
A. Frequent bathing with hot water and harsh soaps
B. Cold air
C. Low humidity
D. Central heating or cooling
E. Alcohol use
F. Poor nutrition
G. Cholesterol-lowering drugs
H. Systemic disease manifested by thyroid, renal, or hepatic disease; anemia; diabetes; or malignancy

Common Complaints
A. Dry, rough skin, especially on legs.

Other Signs and Symptoms
A. Pruritic, scaling skin, particularly on legs, with cracks and/or fissures.
B. Pruritus may be associated with a systematic disorder. **Itching of scabies is particularly intense at night.**
C. Plaques 2–5 cm in diameter.
D. Erythema.
E. Wheal-and-flare response typical of urticaria.

Subjective Data
A. Obtain the patient's description of the onset of symptoms and whether it was sudden or gradual.
B. Ask the patient to identify any discomfort. Ask if the skin is itchy or painful.
C. Assess lesions for any associated discharge (blood or pus).
D. Determine whether the patient has recently ingested any new medicines (antibiotics, cholesterol-lowering medications, or other drugs), alcohol, or new foods.
E. Ask the patient about use of any topical medications.
F. Identify any preceding systemic symptoms (fever, sore throat, anorexia, or vaginal discharge).

G. Ask the patient about bathing in hot water.
H. Review the patient's full medication history for comorbid conditions.

Physical Examination

A. Check temperature, pulse, respirations, and blood pressure.
B. Inspect: Inspect skin for lesions, noting texture of skin.
C. Palpate
   1. Palpate abdomen for masses and hepatosplenomegaly.
   2. Palpate lymph nodes.

Diagnostic Tests

A. There are no diagnostic tests for Xerosis.

Differential Diagnoses

A. Xerosis
B. Scabies
C. Atopic dermatitis

Plan

A. General interventions
   1. Hydration and lubrication of skin.
   2. Assess for and treat secondary infection.
B. Patient teaching
   1. See the Section III Patient Teaching Guide for this chapter, "Xerosis (Winter Itch)."
   2. Avoid alkaline soaps: use Dove, Basis, or soap substitute, such as Cetaphil or Aquanil.
C. Pharmaceutical therapy
   1. Apply emollient cream or lotion (Sarna, Lac-Hydrin, or Eucerin).
   2. Use OTC skin lubricants (petroleum jelly, mineral oil, or cold cream).
   3. Topical corticosteroid
      a. Triamcinolone 0.025% 2–4 times daily or 0.1% 2–3 times daily, apply sparingly.
      b. Hydrocortisone 1% or 2.5% 2–4 times daily, apply thin film.
   4. Systemic antihistamine to control pruritus, such as diphenhydramine (Benadryl) 25–50 mg every 4–6 hours as needed.

Follow-up

A. Follow-up as indicated until resolved.

Consultation/Referral

A. Consult or refer the patient to a dermatologist if no improvement is seen.

Individual Considerations

A. Pediatrics: Avoid corticosteroid preparation, or use low-potency corticosteroid only.
B. Geriatrics: Monitor the patient for possible skin breakdown and/or ulceration.

REFERENCES

Beacham, M. D., & Bruce, E. (1993). Common dermatoses in the elderly. *American Family Physician, 47,* 1445–1450.

Belkengren, R., & Sapala, S. (1995). Pediatric management problems. *Pediatric Nursing, 21,* 164–165.

Dambro, M. R. (1995). *Griffith's five minute clinical consult* (pp. 564–565). Baltimore: Williams & Wilkins.

Dambro, M. R. (1997). *Griffith's five minute clinical consult.* Baltimore: Williams & Wilkins.

Drago, F., Parodi, A., & Rebora, A. (1995). Persistent erythema multiforme: Report of two new cases and review of literature. *Journal of the American Academy of Dermatology, 33,* 366–369.

Edmunds, M. W., & Mayhew, M. S. (1996). *Procedures for primary care practitioners* (pp. 71–73). St. Louis: Mosby.

Farber, E. M. (1995). Therapeutic perspectives in psoriasis. *International Journal of Dermatology, 34,* 456–460.

Fihn, S. D., & McGee, S. R. (1982). *Outpatient medicine* (pp. 89–90, 93–94). Philadelphia: W. B. Saunders.

Fitzpatrick, T. T., Johnson, R. A., Polano, M. K., Suurmend, D., & Wolff, K. (1992). *Color atlas and synopsis of clinical dermatology common and serious diseases* (2nd ed., pp. 10–12, 40–51, 54–55, 242–245, 474–477). New York: McGraw-Hill.

Fleischer, Jr., A. B. (1993). Pruritus in the elderly: Management by senior dermatologists. *Journal of the American Academy of Dermatology, 28,* 603–609.

Gaunder, B. (1986). Insect bites and stings: Managing allergic reactions. *Nurse Practitioner, 11,* 16–28.

Goldstein, B. C., & Goldstein, A. D. (1997). *Practical dermatology* (2nd ed., pp. 84–86, 174–175, 178–183, 183–186, 503). St. Louis: Mosby Year-Book.

Griffith, H. W. (1995). *Instructions for patients* (5th ed.). Philadelphia: W. B. Saunders.

Habif, T. P. (1990). *Clinical dermatology.* St. Louis: Mosby.

Halevy, S., & Shai, A. (1993). Lichenoid drug eruptions. *Journal of the American Academy of Dermatology, 29,* 249–255.

Hansen, R. C. (1996). Scabies: Tips for diagnosing and cautions about treatment. *Modern Medicine, 64,* 27.

Hazin, R., Abuzetun, J., & Khatri, K. (2009). Derm diagnoses you can't afford to miss. *The Journal of Family Practice, 58,* 298–306.

Hoole, A. J., Pichard, Jr., C. G., Quimette, R. M., Lohr, J. A., & Greenberg, R. A. (1995). *Patient care guidelines for nurse practitioners* (4th ed., pp. 59–60, 87–88). Philadelphia: J. B. Lippincott.

Janniger, C. K., & Schwartz, R. A. (1995). Seborrheic dermatitis. *American Family Physician, 52,* l49–155, 159–160.

Jerrard, D. A. (1996). ED management of insect stings. *American Journal of Emergency Medicine, 14,* 429–433.

Lebwohl, M., Abel, E., Zanolli, M., Koo, J., & Drake, L. (1995). Topical therapy for psoriasis. *International Journal of Dermatology, 34,* 613–684.

Perkins, P. (1996). The management of eczema in adults. *Nursing Standard, 10,* 49–53.

Phillips, T. J. (1996). Current treatment options in psoriasis. *Hospital Practice, 30,* 155–157, 161–164, 166.

Reisman, R. E. (1994). Insect stings. *New England Journal of Medicine, 331,* 523–527.

Sams, Jr., W. M., & Lynch, P. J. (1996). *Principles and practice of dermatology* (2nd ed., pp. 341–359, 404–405, 441–445, 810–812, 881–882). London: Churchill Livingstone.

Scheinfield, N. (2009). Two generalized red rashes. *The Clinical Advisor, 12,* 75–76, 79–80.

Scheinfield, N. (2010). Skin disorders in older adults. *Consultant, 50,* 60–66.

Singleton, J. K. (1997). Pediatric dermatoses: Three common skin disruptions in infancy. *Nurse Practitioner, 22,* 32–33, 37, 43–44.

Thiboutot, D. M. (1994). Acne rosacea. *American Family Physician, 50,* 1691–1697, 1701–1702.

Tintinalli, J. E., Ruiz, E., & Krome, R. L. (1996). *Emergency medicine: A comprehensive study guide* (pp. 319–321). New York: McGraw-Hill.

Venables, J. (1995). The management and treatment of eczema. *Nursing Standard, 9,* 25–28.

Weston, W. L. (1996, February). What is erythema multiforme? *Pediatric Annals, 25*(2), 106–109.

Wilkin, J. K. (1994, March). Rosacea: Pathophysiology and treatment. *Archives of Dermatology, 130*(3), 359–362.

Zajac, M.H.S., & Jacobson, A. (2009). Impetigo: Taking on a common skin infection. *The Clinical Advisor, 12,* 30–34.

Zuber, T. J. (1997, February 15). Rosacea: Beyond first blush. *Hospital Practice (Office Edition), 32*(2), 188–189.

Zug, K. A., & McKay, M. (1996). Eczematous dermatitis: A practical review. *American Family Physician, 54*(4), 1243–1250, 1253–1254.

CHAPTER 4

Eye Guidelines

Jill C. Cash

AMBLYOPIA

Definition
A. Amblyopia is a decrease in the visual acuity of one eye. It is commonly seen in young children and cannot be corrected by either glasses or contact lenses.

Incidence
A. Amblyopia is most commonly diagnosed in children and occurs in approximately 2.5% of the population.

Pathogenesis
Amblyopia has numerous causes, including:

A. Congenital defect.
B. Develops from a corneal scar or cataract.
C. Occurs from an uncorrected high refractive error, which causes visual blurring.
D. Develops when each eye has a different refractive error that leads to blurred vision.
E. Strabismic amblyopia may also occur due to the loss of vision in the eye that turns inward or outward.

Predisposing Factors
A. One parent with amblyopia

Common Complaints
A. Decreased vision—complains of sitting close to the TV, sitting in the front row of a classroom, or having trouble in sports seeing the ball, and so on.
B. Vision that does not correct with either glasses or contact lenses
C. Wandering eye and frequent eye squinting

Other Signs and Symptoms
A. Rubbing the eye frequently
B. Tired eyes

Subjective Data
A. Elicit onset of visual changes, noting course of symptoms and severity.
B. Assess for pain or any new injury or trauma to the eye.
C. Inquire regarding new events or changes in health history, including contact lenses, glasses, illnesses, and cataracts.
D. Review patient and family history of amblyopia.

Physical Examination
A. Inspect eyes.
   1. Note extraocular movements of eyes.
   2. Examine sclera, pupil, iris, and fundus.
   3. Examine eyes for red reflex.
B. Assess vision based on age, using Snellen chart for children older than 3 years.
C. Visual fields may be assessed with a parent holding the child in lap.

Diagnostic Tests
A. None

Differential Diagnoses
A. Amblyopia
B. Organic brain lesion

Plan
A. All children need to have a visual exam prior to starting school.
B. Recommend exam by ophthalmologist for children with strabismus and for those with a family history of amblyopia.
C. Measures for refractive correction or patching of the stronger eye are usually performed to encourage the weak eye to develop.
D. Without treatment, the weaker eye will not correct itself.
E. Surgery may be required for abnormal positioning of the eye.

Follow-up
A. Follow-up with an ophthalmologist.

Consultation/Referral
A. Refer the patient to an ophthalmologist for evaluation and treatment.

Individual Considerations
A. None

BLEPHARITIS

Definition
A. Blepharitis is dryness and flaking of the eyelashes, resulting from an inflammatory response of the eyelid.

Incidence
A. The exact incidence is not known, however, blepharitis is commonly seen.

Pathogenesis
A. Seborrheic: excessive shedding of skin cells and blockage of glands occur.
B. *Staphylococcus:* most common bacteria found, responsible for bacterial infection of lid margin.
C. Commonly seen with inadequate flow of oil and mucous into the tear duct.

Predisposing Factors
A. Diabetes
B. Candida
C. Seborrheic dermatitis
D. Acne rosacea

Common Complaints
A. Burning and itching
B. Lacrimal tearing
C. Photophobia
D. Recurrent eye infections, styes or chalazions
E. Dry, flaky secretions on lid margins and eyelashes

Other Signs and Symptoms
A. Seborrheic blepharitis: lid margin swelling and erythema, flaking, nasolabial erythema, and scaling
B. *Staphylococcus aureus* blepharitis: erythema/edema, scaling, burning, tearing, itching, and recurrent stye or chalazia
C. May have dandruff of scalp and eyebrows

Subjective Data
A. Elicit onset and duration of signs and symptoms.
B. Note sensations of itching, burning, or pain in the eye.
C. Ask: What makes signs and symptoms worse? What makes signs and symptoms better?
D. Any change in soaps, creams, lotions, or shampoos?
E. Has the patient had similar signs and symptoms in the past?
F. Note any visual change or pain since the last eye exam.
G. Note contributing factors involved, if present.

Physical Examination
A. Inspection
    1. Inspect eyes, noting extraocular movements of eyes.
    2. Examine sclera, pupil, iris, and fundus.
    3. Examine eyes for red reflex.
    4. Note erythema or edema on lid margin; note dryness, scaling, and flakes.
    5. Assess vision based on age, using Snellen chart for children older than 3 years.
    6. Visual fields may be assessed with a parent holding the child in lap.

Diagnostic Tests
A. None

Differential Diagnoses
A. Blepharitis
    1. *Staphylococcus aureus*
    2. Seborrheic
B. Conjunctivitis
C. Squamous cell carcinoma
D. Stye
E. Upper respiratory infection
F. Sinusitis

Plan
A. Wash eye with antibacterial soap and water. May use gentle baby shampoo.
B. Apply warm compresses to eye for comfort daily for approximately 10–20 min.
C. Apply bacitracin or erythromycin ophthalmic ointment to margin of eye at bedtime, taking care not to contaminate the medication bottle.
D. Stop use of contacts until eye is healed.
E. Refer all patients with recurrent blepharitis for evaluation with an eye specialist.
F. Oral antibiotics: Tetracycline 250 mg by mouth, four times a day for 4 weeks. Alternative: Doxycycline 100 mg by mouth, twice a day, or oxacillin 250 mg four times a day.
G. May consider long-term treatment with Doxycycline if infections reoccur.

Follow-up
A. Recommend follow-up with primary provider in 1–2 weeks.
B. Encourage good hygiene for prevention of recurrent episodes.

Individual Considerations
A. Pediatrics: Tetracycline is not recommended for children younger than 8 years.

CATARACTS

Definition
A. A cataract, opacity of the crystalline lens of the eye, causes progressive, painless loss of vision (functional impairment). Pre-senile and senile cataract formation is painless and progresses throughout months and years. Cataracts are frequently associated with intraocular inflammation and glaucoma.

Incidence
A. Cataracts are the most common cause of blindness in the world.
B. Ninety-five percent of people older than age 60 have cataracts without visual disturbance.
C. Fifty percent of people older than age 75 have significant visual loss due to cataracts.

Pathogenesis
A. Age-related changes of the lens of the eye result from protein accumulation, which produces a fibrous thickened lens that obscures vision.

Predisposing Factors
A. Age
B. Trauma
C. Medications (e.g., topical or systemic steroids, major tranquilizers, or some diuretics)
D. Medical diseases (e.g., diabetes mellitus, Wilson's disease, hypoparathyroidism, glaucoma, congenital rubella syndrome, chronic anteri, or uveitis)
E. Chronic exposure to ultraviolet B light
F. Down syndrome
G. Low antioxidant vitamin use
H. Alcohol use

Common Complaints
A. Decreased vision
B. Blurred or foggy vision, "ghost" images
C. Inability to drive at night

Other Signs and Symptoms
A. Initial visual event can be a shift toward nearsightedness.
B. Visual impairment can be more marked at distances, with abnormal visual acuity exams.
C. Severe difficulty with glare.
D. Altered color perception.
E. Frequent falls or injuries.

Subjective Data
A. Review the onset, course, and duration of visual changes, including altered day or night vision and nearsighted versus farsighted vision.
B. Assess whether involvement is in one or both eyes.
C. Determine what improves vision—use of glasses or use of extra light.
D. Review the patient's medical history and current medications.
E. Review the patient's history for traumatic injury.
F. Discuss the patient's occupation and leisure activities to determine exposure to ultraviolet rays.

Physical Examination
A. Inspect
  1. Conduct a funduscopic examination.
    a. Check red reflex and opacity.
      i. A bright red reflex is seen in the normal eye.
      ii. Cataract formation is seen by the disruption of the red reflex.
      iii. Lens opacities appear as dark areas against the background of the red-orange reflex.
    b. Examine color of opacity. For brunescent cataracts, the nucleus acquires a yellow-brown coloration and becomes progressively more opaque.
    c. Check retinal abnormalities, hemorrhage, scarring, and drusen.

Diagnostic Tests
A. Check visual acuity.
B. Check peripheral vision.
C. Perform slit-lamp exam to determine the exact location and type of cataract.

Differential Diagnoses
A. Cataracts
B. Glaucoma
C. Age-related macular degeneration (macular degeneration causes vision loss that is symptomatically similar to cataracts)
D. Diabetic retinopathy
E. Temporal arteritis

Plan
A. General interventions
  1. Monitor the patient for increased interference of visual impairment on his or her lifestyle.
  2. Cataracts do not need to be removed unless there is impairment of normal, everyday activities.
  3. Surgery is the definitive treatment; however, modification of glasses may improve vision adequately to defer surgery. Contact lenses are optically superior to glasses.
B. Patient teaching
  1. Prevention is important. Teach the patient to use protective eyewear to prevent trauma.
  2. Use sunglasses to prevent the penetration of ultraviolet B rays.
  3. Wear a hat with a visor.

Follow-up
A. Surgical removal is indicated if the visual disturbance is interfering with the patient's life, such as causing falls or prohibiting reading.

Consultation/Referral
A. Refer patient for ophthalmologic consultation.
B. Patients should be followed by an ophthalmologist to monitor the cataract for increased size and progressive visual impairment.
C. Contact social worker or community resources as needed.

CHALAZION

Definition
A. Chalazion is a chronic lipogranulomatous inflammation of a meibomian gland located in the eyelid margin. Inflammation occurs from occlusion of the ducts.

Incidence
A. The incidence is unknown.

Pathogenesis
A. Meibomian glands secrete the oil layer of the tear film that covers the eye. When the glands become blocked, the oil or lipid extrudes into the surrounding tissue causing the formation of a nodule.

Predisposing Factors
A. Chalazion may occur as a secondary infection of the surrounding tissues.

Common Complaints
A. Swelling, nontender palpable nodule, usually pea-size, inside lid margin or eye
B. Discomfort or irritation due to swelling

Other Signs and Symptoms
A. Tearing.
B. Feeling of a foreign body in the eye.
C. If infection is present, the entire lid becomes painfully swollen.

Subjective Data

A. Review onset of symptoms, their course and duration, and any concurrent visual disturbance.
B. Question the patient regarding possible foreign body or trauma to the eye.
C. Elicit the quality of pain or tenderness of the eyelid.
D. Review past eye problems and the treatment received.

Physical Examination

A. Temperature
B. Inspect
   1. Inspect the eye, sclera, and conjunctiva for a foreign body.
   2. Check for red- or gray-colored subconjunctival mass.
C. Palpate
   1. Palpate eyelid for masses and tenderness.
   2. Check for preauricular adenopathy. Usually a hard, nontender nodule is found on the middle portion of the tarsus, away from the lid border; it may develop on the lid margin if the opening of the duct is involved. Some chalazia continue to increase in size and can cause astigmatism by putting pressure on the eye globe.
   3. Chalazia may become acutely tender; however, note the difference between the chalazia and the stye, which is found on the lid margin.

Diagnostic Tests

A. Check visual acuity.

Differential Diagnoses

A. Chalazion
B. Chronic dacryocystitis
C. Hordeolum
D. Blepharitis
E. Xanthelasma

Plan

A. General interventions
   1. Small chalazia do not usually require treatment.
   2. Warm, moist compresses may be applied for 15 min four times a day.
B. Patient teaching: Instruct patient regarding compresses and hand washing.
C. Pharmaceutical therapy
   1. Sulfacetamide sodium (Sulamyd) ophthalmic ointment 10%, four times daily, for 7 days for bacterial infection.
   2. Tobradex Opthalmic drops: 1–2 drops every 2 hours for first 24–48 hours then every 4–6 hours. Reduce dose as condition improves. Treat for 5–7 days as needed. Not recommended in children younger than 2 years.
   3. Intrachalazion corticosteroid injection by an ophthalmologist.

Follow-up

A. For large infected chalazia, evaluate the patient every 2–4 weeks.

Consultation/Referral

A. If the chalazion does not resolve spontaneously, incision and curettage by an ophthalmologist may be necessary.

CONJUNCTIVITIS

Definition

A. Conjunctivitis is inflammation of the conjunctiva.

Incidence

A. Viral conjunctivitis is the most common type; conjunctivitis occurs in 1%–12% of newborns.

Pathogenesis

Primarily three types of conjunctivitis are seen:

A. Bacterial (*Haemophilus influenzae, Streptococcus pneumoniae, Staphylococcus aureus, Neisseria gonorrhoeae,* and *Chlamydia*)
B. Viral (adenovirus, coxsackievirus, and ECHO viruses)
C. Allergic (seasonal pollens or allergic exposure)

Predisposing Factors

A. Contact to conjunctivitis
B. Exposure to sexually transmitted infection (STI)
C. Other atopic conditions (allergies)

Common Complaints

A. Red eyes
B. Eye drainage
C. Itching (with allergic conjunctivitis)

Other Signs and Symptoms

A. Bacterial
   1. Fast onset, 12–24 hours of copious purulent or mucopurulent discharge
   2. Burning, stinging, or gritty sensation in eyes
   3. Crusted eyelids upon awakening, with swelling of eyelid
   4. Usually starts out unilaterally; may progress to bacterial infection
   5. Bacterial conjunctivitis may present as beefy red conjunctiva
B. Viral
   1. Symptoms may begin in one eye and progress to both eyes
   2. Tearing of eyes
   3. Sensation of foreign body
   4. Systemic symptoms of upper respiratory infection (runny nose, sore throat, sneezing, fever)
   5. Preauricular or submandibular lymphadenopathy
   6. Photophobia, impaired vision
   7. Primary herpetic infection: vesicular skin lesion, corneal epithelial defect in form of dendrite, uveitis
C. Allergic
   1. Itchy, watery eyes, bilateral
   2. Seasonal symptoms
   3. Edema of eyelids without visual change
   4. With allergic conjunctivitis hyperemia of eyes is always bilateral, and giant papillae on tarsa may be seen
   5. May also see eczema, uriticaria, and asthma flare

Subjective Data

A. Elicit onset, duration, and course of symptoms.
B. Question patient regarding presence of discharge upon awakening.

C. Elicit changes in vision since symptoms began.

D. Determine whether there has been any injury or trauma to the eye.

E. Assess whether these symptoms have appeared before.

F. Rule out exposure to anyone with conjunctivitis.

G. Ask patient about any new events, such as use of contact lenses or change in contact lenses or solutions.

H. Review patient and family history of allergies.

Physical Examination

A. Check temperature, pulse, respirations, and blood pressure.

B. Inspect
1. Observe eyes for color and foreign objects. Perform complete eye exam.
2. Note lid edema.
3. Assess pupillary reflexes.
4. Examine skin.
5. Inspect ears, nose, and throat.

C. Auscultate
1. Auscultate heart and lungs.

D. Palpate
1. Palpate preauricular lymph nodes and anterior and posterior cervical chain lymph nodes.

Diagnostic Tests

A. Gram's stain testing for discharge/exudate extracted from eyes if gonococcal infection is suspected and/or all neonates.

B. Culture for chlamydia, if suspected.

C. Perform fluorescein stain of eye if foreign body suspected or corneal abrasion/ulceration suspected.

D. Test visual acuity with Snellen chart. Assess peripheral vision and extraocular movements (EOMs).

Differential Diagnoses

A. Conjunctivitis

B. Corneal abrasion

C. Blepharitis

D. Drug-related conjunctivitis

E. Herpetic keratoconjunctivitis

F. Iritis

G. Gonococcal or chlamydial conjunctivitis

Plan

A. General interventions
1. Patient education: See Section III Patient Teaching Guide for this chapter, "How to Administer Eye Medications."
   a. Cool compresses to affected eye should be performed several times a day.
   b. Clean eyes with warm moist cloth from inner to outer canthus to prevent spreading infection.
   c. Encourage good hand washing with antibacterial soap.
   d. Instruct on the proper method on instilling medication into eye. Give patient teaching guide on "How to Administer Eye Medications."
   e. Instruct the female patient to discard all eye makeup, including mascara, eyeliner, and eye shadow, worn at the time of the infection.
2. Bacterial conjunctivitis is contagious until 24 hours after beginning medication.

3. Viral conjunctivitis is contagious for 48–72 hours, but it may last up to 2 weeks.

B. Pharmaceutical therapy
1. Bacterial
   a. Drug of choice is erythromycin (Ilotycin) ophthalmic ointment 0.5% in each eye four times daily for 7 days.
   b. Trimethoprim/polymixin B sulfate (Polytrim) ophthalmic ointment in each eye four times daily for 7 days.
   c. Sulfacetamide sodium (Sulamyd) or garamycin (Gentamicin) ophthalmic solution: 2 drops in each eye every 4 hours while awake for 7 days.
   d. If using aminoglycoside or neomycin ointments or drops, use caution and monitor closely for reactive keratogonjunctivitis.
2. Viral
   a. Antiviral medications
      i. Trifluridine 1% drops: 1 drop every 2 hours while awake; no more than 9 drops per day. May then go to 1 drop every 4 hours for 7 days. Not recommended for children younger than 6 years.
      ii. Oral antiviral medications (trifluridine, valacyclovir) may be used for herpes simplex keratitis. Herpes zoster ophthalmicus is often treated with acyclovir, famciclovir, or valacyclovir and lessens symptoms if started within 72 hours of onset of symptoms.
3. Allergic
   a. Topical antihistimines/mast cell stabilizer.
      i. Azelastine HCl (Optivar): Not recommended for those younger than 3 years. For those older than 3 years, 1 drop to the affected eye twice a day.
      ii. Olopatadine HCl (Pataday) 0.2%: Not recommended for those younger than 3 years. For those older than 3 years, 1 drop to the affected eye daily.
      iii. Olopatadine HCl (Patanol) 0.1%: Not recommended for those younger than 3 years. For those older than 3 years, 1 drop twice a day to the affected eye.
   b. Mast cell stabilizer.
      i. Cromolyn sodium (Crolom) ophthalmic solution for children older than 4 years, 1–2 drops 4–6 times daily.
   c. Topical NSAID.
      i. Ketorolac tromethamine (Acular) 0.5%: Not for use in children younger than 3 years: 1 drop four times a day. This is used for severe symptoms of atopic keratoconjuncitivits.
   d. Artificial tears 4–5 times daily.
   e. Oral antihistimines may be used in severe cases. (Loratadine or diphenhydramine HCl.)
4. Concurrent conjunctivitis and otitis media should be treated with a systemic antibiotic; no topical eye antibiotic is needed.

Follow-up

A. If resolution occurs within 5–7 days after proper treatment, follow-up is not needed.

B. If patient continues to have symptoms or if different symptoms appear, then follow-up with the primary provider is recommended.

Consultation/Referral
A. Consult or refer patient to physician if patient is not responding to treatment.
B. Refer if patient is suspected of having periorbital cellulitis.

Individual Considerations
A. Pediatrics: In neonates, consider gonococcal and chlamydial conjunctivitis.
B. Partners: Check partners for gonorrhea and chlamydia when adolescent or adult presents with gonococcal or chlamydial conjunctivitis.

CORNEAL ABRASION

Definition
A. A corneal abrasion is the loss of epithelial tissue, either superficial or deep, from trauma to the eye.

Incidence
A. In the United States, approximately 2.4 million eye injuries occur annually.
B. Corneal abrasions account for approximately 10% of new admissions to eye emergency units.

Pathogenesis
A. Trauma occurs to the epithelial tissue of the cornea.

Predisposing Factors
A. Trauma to the eye caused by a human fingernail, tree branches, wood particles, children's toys, and sports injuries
B. A history of surgical trauma, causing globe weakening

Common Complaints
A. Sudden onset of eye pain
B. Foreign-body sensation in the eye
C. Watery eye
D. Mild photophobia

Other Signs and Symptoms
A. Change in vision
B. Redness, swelling, inability to open the eye

Subjective Data
A. Elicit onset, duration, and course of symptoms; note any past history of similar symptoms.
B. Question the patient regarding visual changes (blurred, double, or lost vision, or loss of a portion of the visual field).
C. Question the patient regarding the mechanism of injury and how much time has elapsed since the injury (minutes, hours, or days). Ask: What is his or her occupation, and what sports are involved? Were goggles being worn and are they routinely worn during the sport or activity?
D. Review the patient's history of exposure to herpetic outbreaks.
E. Determine the degree of pain, if any, headache, photophobia, redness, itching, or tearing.

F. Ascertain whether the patient wears contact lenses or glasses and for what length of time.
G. Ask if the patient has tried any treatments before presentation to the office. If so, what?
H. Rule out the presence of any other infections, such as sinus infection. **Conjunctival discharge signifies an infectious etiology.**

Physical Examination
A. Check vital signs: temperature, pulse, and blood pressure.
B. Inspect
  1. Observe *both* eyes.
  2. Test visual acuity and pupil reactivity and symmetry.
  3. Observe cornea surface with direct illumination, noting shadow on surface of iris.
  4. Evert eyelids for cornea inspection.
  5. Inspect for foreign body and remove if indicated.
  6. Fluorescein stain as indicated.
C. Funduscopic exam.

Diagnostic Tests
A. Perform fluorescein stain test: **An epithelial defect that stains with fluorescein is the hallmark symptom.**

Differential Diagnoses
A. Corneal abrasion.
B. Corneal foreign body.
C. Acute angle glaucoma.
D. Herpetic infection (HSV): HSV is associated with decreased corneal sensation.
E. Recurrent corneal ulceration.
F. Ulcerative keratitis.
G. Corneal erosion.

Plan
A. General interventions
  1. Superficial corneal abrasions do not need patching.
  2. For deeper abrasions, apply a patch that prevents lid motion for 24–48 hours.
  3. Pressure patch is no longer recommended.
B. Patient teaching
  1. Discuss the use of protective eyewear and prevention of future ocular trauma for the patient with a history of use of power tools or hammering.
  2. See the Section III Patient Teaching Guide for this chapter, "How to Administer Eye Medications."
  3. Advise that the patient should not use/wear contact lenses until the eye is completely healed.
C. Pharmaceutical therapy
  1. Antibiotic drops or ointment. **Never instill antibiotic ointment if there is a possibility of a perforation. Patch the eye and refer the patient to a physician or ophthalmologist.**
    a. Adults and children: sulfacetamide sodium ophthalmic solution 10% (Sulamyd), 1–2 drops instilled into the lower conjunctival sac every 2–3 hours during the day; may instill every 6 hours during the night.
    b. Sulfacetamide's sodium (Sulamyd) ophthalmic solution, or ointment interacts with gentamicin. Avoid using them together.

  c. PABA derivatives decrease sulfacetamide's action. Wait 1/2–1 hour before instilling sulfacetamide.

  d. Sulfacetamide precipitates when used with silver preparations. Avoid using them together.

2. Adults and children: polymyxin B sulfate (Polytrim) 10,000 μ, bacitracin zinc 500 μ/g ophthalmic ointment (Polysporin), a small ribbon of ointment applied into the conjunctival sac one or more times daily or as needed.

3. Adults and children: erythromycin ophthalmic ointment 0.5% (Ilotycin), 1-cm ribbon of ointment applied into the conjunctival sac up to 6 times daily, depending on the severity of infection.

4. Bacitracin 500 μ/g ointment, 1/2-inch ribbon twice a day to four times a day for 7 days.

5. Erythromycin 0.5% ointment, 1/2-inch ribbon twice a day to four times a day for 7 days.

6. Analgesics: Topical analgecis should be used sparingly. Diclofenac (Boltaren) 0.1% solution to eye four times a day as needed, or Ketorolac (Acular) 0.5 solution in eye four times a day as needed.

7. Avoid use of home prescriptions that will interfere with the healing process.

Follow-up

A. Reevaluate the patient within 24–48 hours. Cornea usually heals within 24–48 hours.

B. Ophthalmic ointment or drops should be continued for 4 days after re-epithelialization occurs to help in the healing process.

C. If the patient is still symptomatic in 48 hours, consider referral to an ophthalmologist.

Consultation/Referral

Immediate referral to an ophthalmologist is required for large or central lesions or deep or penetrating wounds.

Individual Considerations

A. Pregnancy: Retinal detachment should be considered as a source of eye pain and visual loss, especially in a woman with severe pregnancy-induced hypertension.

B. Pediatrics: Encourage protective eyewear for sports including hockey, soccer, baseball, and basketball.

DACRYOCYSTITIS

Definition

A. Infection or inflammation of the lacrimal sac, or dacryocystitis, can be acute or chronic.

B. Dacryocystitis is usually secondary to obstruction.

Incidence

A. The incidence is unknown.

Pathogenesis

A. Bacterial infection of the lacrimal sac usually is caused by *Staphylococcus* or *Streptococcus*.

Predisposing Factors

A. Nasal trauma

B. Deviated septum

C. Nasal polyps

D. Congenital dacryostenosis

E. Inferior turbinates

Common Complaints

A. Pain in the eye

B. Redness

C. Swelling

D. Fever

E. Tearing

Other Signs and Symptoms

A. Purulent exudate may be expressed from the lacrimal duct.

Subjective Data

A. Elicit the onset, course, and duration of symptoms. Are symptoms bilateral or unilateral?

B. Review the patient's activity when the symptoms began, to determine if etiology is chemical, traumatic, or infectious.

C. Review other presenting symptoms such as fever and discharge.

D. Review the patient's history for previous episodes. Note treatments used in past.

E. Review history for a recent herpetic infection or fever blister.

F. Review ophthalmologic history.

G. Review medications.

Physical Examination

A. Check temperature, pulse, and blood pressure.

B. Inspect

 1. Assess both eyes.

 2. Check peripheral fields of vision, and sclera.

 3. Evaluate conjunctiva for distribution of redness, ciliary flush, and foreign bodies.

 4. Inspect lid margins: Evaluate for crusting, ulceration, and masses.

C. Palpate: Palpate lacrimal duct. Discharge can be expressed from the tear duct with the application of pressure. See Figure 4.1.

Diagnostic Tests

A. Check visual acuity.

B. Culture discharge for *Neisseria* if suspected.

Differential Diagnoses

A. Dacryocystitis

B. Chalazion

C. Blepharitis

D. Xanthoma

E. Bacterial conjunctivitis

F. Hordeolum

G. Foreign body

Plan

A. General interventions

 1. Warm, moist compresses at least four times per day.

 2. Instruct female patients to discard old makeup including mascara, eyeliner, and eye shadow used prior to infection.

B. Patient teaching: Application of compresses, hand washing, and proper cleaning. See the Section III Patient Teaching Guide for this chapter, "How to Administer Eye Medications."

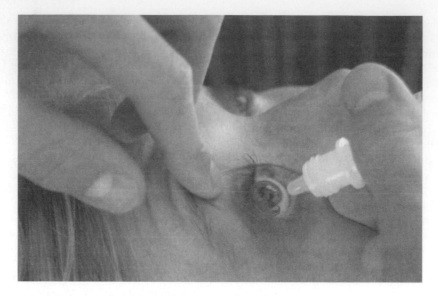

Figure 4.1 How to instill eye drops into the eye.

C. Pharmaceutical therapy
  1. Dicloxacillin 250 mg by mouth four times daily for 7 days
  2. Erythromycin 250 mg by mouth four times daily for 7 days

Follow-up
A. Follow-up in 2 weeks if symptoms are not resolved.

Consultation/Referral
A. Refer the patient to an ophthalmologist for irrigation and probing if needed.
B. Lab studies are generally performed by an ophthalmologist.

DRY EYES

Definition
A. Insufficient lubrication of the eye, or dry eyes, is due to a deficiency of any one of the major components of the tear film.
B. Defects in tear production are uncommon, but may occur in conjunction with systemic disease. Presence of systemic disease should be evaluated.

Incidence
A. Increased incidence of dry eyes in the elderly is due to decreased rate of lacrimal gland secretions.

Pathogenesis
A. Decreased production of one or more components of the tear film results in dry eyes. The tear film comprises three layers:
  1. An outermost lipid layer, excreted by the lid meibomian glands
  2. A middle aqueous layer, secreted by the main and accessory lacrimal glands
  3. An innermost mucinous layer, secreted by conjunctival goblet cells
B. A defect in production of the aqueous phase by lacrimal glands causes dry eyes or keratoconjunctivitis sicca. The condition most often occurs as a physiologic consequence of aging, and it is commonly exacerbated by dry environmental factors. It may also develop in patients with connective tissue disease.
C. In Sjögren's syndrome, the lacrimal glands become involved in immune-mediated inflammation.
D. Mucin production may decline in the setting of vitamin A deficiency.
E. Loss of goblet cells can occur secondary to chemical burns.

Predisposing Factors
A. History of severe conjunctivitis
B. Eyelid defects such as fifth or seventh cranial nerve palsy, incomplete blinking, exophthalmos, and lid movement hindered by scar formation
C. Drug-induced conditions including use of anticholinergic agents
  1. Phenothiazine
  2. Tricyclic antidepressants
  3. Antihistamines
  4. Diuretics
  5. Isotretinoin (Accutane)
D. Systemic disease such as rheumatoid disease, Sjögren's syndrome, and neurologic disease
E. Environmental factors such as heat (wood, coal, gas), air conditioners, winter air, and tobacco smoke
F. Use of contacts
G. Increasing age
H. Lipid abnormalities

Common Complaints

A. Ocular fatigue
B. Foreign-body sensation in the eye
C. Itching burning, irritation, or dryness sensation in the eye

Other Signs and Symptoms

A. Photophobia.
B. Cloudy, blurred vision.
C. Rainbow of color around lights. Acute angle-closure glaucoma can present with a red, painful eye; cloudy, blurred vision and a rainbow of color around lights; dilatation of the pupil; nausea and vomiting.
D. Bell's palsy, signs of stroke, or other conditions that affect the blinking mechanism.

Subjective Data

A. Elicit onset, duration, and frequency of symptoms.
B. Note factors that worsen or alleviate symptoms.
C. Note medical history for systemic conditions and strokes.
D. List current medications, noting anticholinergic drugs and isotretinoin (Accutane) use.
E. Note whether the patient wears contact lenses or glasses, and ask for what length of time.
F. Review occupational and home exposure to irritants and allergens.
G. Assess whether the patient produces tears. Note eye drainage amount, color, and frequency.
H. Review history of any previous ocular disease, surgeries, and so forth.

Physical Examination

A. Check temperature, pulse, respirations, and blood pressure.
B. Inspect
  1. Observe and evaluate *both* eyes.
  2. Conduct a detailed eye exam: check the eye, lid, and conjunctiva for masses and redness.
  3. Check pupil reactivity and corneal clarity. The corneal reflex should be checked if there is concern about a neuroparalytic keratitis or facial nerve palsy.
  4. Complete a funduscopic exam. Check for completeness of lid closure as well as position of eyelashes.
  5. Examine mouth for dryness.
  6. Inspect skin for butterfly rash.
C. Palpate
  1. Palpate lacrimal ducts for drainage.
  2. Invert upper lid and check for foreign body or chalazion.
  3. Check sinuses for tenderness.
  4. Palpate thyroid.
  5. Palpate joints for warmth and redness or inflammation.

Diagnostic Tests

A. Perform Schirmer's test. Use Whatman no. 41 filter paper, 5 mm by 35 mm. A folded end of filter paper is hooked over the lower lid nasally, and the patient is instructed to keep his or her eyes lightly closed during the test. Wetting is measured after 5 min, less than 5 mm is usually abnormal.

Differential Diagnoses

A. Dry eyes.
B. Stevens-Johnson syndrome.
C. Sjögren's syndrome: Chronic dry mouth, dry eyes, and arthritis triad suggest Sjögren's syndrome. Facial telangiectasias, parotid enlargement, Raynaud's phenomenon, and dental caries are associated features. Patients complain first of burning and a sandy, gritty, foreign-body sensation, particularly later in the day.
D. Systemic lupus erythematosus.
E. Scleroderma.
F. Ocular pterygium.
G. Superficial pemphigoid.
H. Vitamin A deficiency.

Plan

A. General interventions
  1. If no ocular disease is present, reduce environmental dryness by use of a room humidifier for a 2-week trial.
  2. Apply artificial tear substitutes and nonprescription drops.
  3. Consider stopping medications being used that may be contributing to the source of dry eye symptoms.
  4. Caution should be used when using OTC allergy medications, if allergy is a contributing cause. Topical antihistimines may exacerbate the condition over time.
B. Patient teaching: See the Section III Patient Teaching Guide, "How to Administer Eye Medications."
C. Pharmaceutical therapy
  1. Topical artificial tears 1 or 2 drops four times daily; preferably one without preservatives (i.e., Theratears, Dry eye therapy, Tears Naturale).
  2. Drops may be instilled as often as desired.

Follow-up

A. Reevaluate the patient in 2 weeks.

Consultation/Referral

A. Refer the patient to an ophthalmologist if symptoms are unrelieved at the 2-week follow-up.
B. Make an immediate referral for red eye, visual disturbance, or eye pain.

Individual Considerations

Geriatrics:

A. The rate of lacrimal gland secretions diminishes with aging; therefore, the elderly are at an increased risk for developing dry eye.
B. Ace-inhibitors may reduce the risk of dry eye syndrome in some patients. Consider treatment with ace-inhibitors for hypertension as appropriate in clients.

EYE PAIN

Definition

A. Sensation of pain may affect the eyelid, conjunctiva, or cornea.

Incidence

A. Unknown. Pain in the eye is most often produced by conditions that do not threaten vision.

Pathogenesis

A. The external ocular surfaces and the uveal tract are richly innervated with pain receptors. As a result, lesions or disease processes affecting these surfaces can be acutely painful.

B. Pathology confined to the vitreous, retina, or optic nerve is rarely a source of pain.

Predisposing Factors

A. Eyelids: inflammation such as hordeolum (stye), trichiasis (in-turned lash), and tarsal foreign bodies.

B. Conjunctiva: viral and bacterial conjunctivitis or allergic conjunctivitis; toxic, chemical, and mechanical injuries.

C. Cornea: keratitis (inflammation of the cornea) accompanying trauma, infection, exposure, vascular disease, or decreased lacrimation; microbial keratitis from contact use. If blood vessels invade the normally avascular corneal stroma, vision may become cloudy. Severe pain is a prominent symptom; movement of the lid typically exacerbates symptoms.

Common Complaints

A. Eye pain (sharp, dull, deep): The quality of the pain needs to be considered. Deep pain is suggestive of an intraocular problem. Inflammation and rapidly expanding mass lesions may cause deep pain. Displacement of the globe and diplopia may ensue.

B. Eye movement may cause sharp pain due to meningeal inflammation (the extraocular rectusmuscles insert along the dura of the nerve sheath at the orbital apex). Most cases are idiopathic, but 10%–15% are associated with multiple sclerosis.

Other Signs and Symptoms

These symptoms may be unilateral or bilateral.

A. Eyelids
1. Tenderness
2. Sensation of foreign body
3. Redness
4. Edema
B. Conjunctiva
1. Mild burning
2. Sensation of foreign body
3. Itching (allergic)
C. Cornea
1. Burning.
2. Foreign-body sensation.
3. Considerable discomfort.
4. Reflex photophobic tearing.
5. Blinking exacerbates pain.
6. Pain relieved with pressure holding the lid shut. With a foreign body or a corneal lesion, pain is exacerbated by lid movement and relieved by cessation of lid motion.
D. Sclera: redness
E. Uveal tract (uveitis or iritis)
1. Dull, deep-seated ache and photophobia.

2. Profound ocular and orbital pain radiating to the frontal and temporal regions accompanying sudden elevation of pressure (acute angle-closure glaucoma).
3. Vagal stimulation with high pressure may result in nausea and vomiting.
4. Usual history of mild intermittent episodes of blurred vision preceding onset of throbbing pain, nausea, vomiting, and decreased visual acuity.
5. Halos around light.
F. Orbit
1. Deep pain with inflammation and rapidly expanding mass lesions
2. Eye movement causing sharp pain due to meningeal inflammation
G. Sinusitis: secondary orbital inflammation and tenderness on extremes of eye movement

Subjective Data

A. Review the onset, duration, and course of symptoms. Inquire regarding the quality of pain.
B. Review any predisposing factors such as trauma or a foreign object. Ask: Was the onset sudden or gradual?
C. Note reported changes in visual acuity or color vision.
D. Note aggravating or alleviating factors.
E. Determine whether the eye pain is bilateral or unilateral.
F. Review history for herpes, infections, and toxic or chemical irritants.
G. Review history for glaucoma and previous eye surgeries or treatments.
H. Assess the patient for any other symptoms such as migraine headache, sinusitis, or tooth abscess.
I. Inquire whether the patient has lost a large amount of sleep.
J. Inquire whether he or she has been exposed to a large amount of UV light or sunlight (vacation, tanning beds).
K. Review history for any other medical problems such as lupus, sarcoidosis, or inflammatory bowel disease.

Physical Examination

A. Inspect
1. Evaluate *both* eyes.
2. Test visual acuity and color vision.
3. Observe for extraocular movements.
4. Check the eye, lid, and conjunctiva for masses and redness.
5. Check pupil reactivity and corneal clarity.
6. Conduct a funduscopic exam for disc abnormalities.
7. Perform ear, nose, and throat exam.
B. Palpate
1. Palpate lacrimal ducts for drainage.
2. Palpate sinus for tenderness.
3. Invert upper lid and check for foreign body or chalazion.

Diagnostic Tests

A. Fluorescein stain
B. Measurement of intraocular pressure

Differential Diagnoses

A. Eye pain.
B. Hordeolum.

C. Chalazion.

D. Acute dacryocystitis.

E. Irritant exposure.

F. Conjunctival infection.

G. Corneal abrasion.

H. Foreign body.

I. Ulcers.

J. Ingrown lashes.

K. Contact lens abuse.

L. Scleritis.

M. Acute angle-closure glaucoma. With acute angle-closure glaucoma, fixed, midposition pupil, redness, and a hazy cornea may be present.

N. Uveitis.

O. Referred pain from extraocular sources such as sinusitis, tooth abscess, tension headache, temporal arteritis, and prodrome of herpes zoster.

Plan

A. General interventions
 1. The initial task is to be sure that there is no threat to vision.
 2. Treatment modality depends on the underlying cause of eye pain.

B. Patient teaching: See the Section III Patient Teaching Guide for this chapter, "How to Administer Eye Medications."

C. Pharmaceutical therapy: Medication depends on the underlying cause.

Follow-up

A. Follow-up depends on the underlying cause.

Consultation/Referral

A. Any change in visual acuity or color vision requires an urgent ophthalmologic consultation.

EXCESSIVE TEARS

Definition

A. Excessive tears disorder is an overproduction of tears. Complaints vary from watery eyes to overflowing tears that run down the cheeks, a condition known as epiphora.

Incidence

A. The incidence is unknown.

Pathogenesis

A. The most common cause is reflex overproduction of tears (as occurs in the elderly) due to a deficiency of the tear film.

B. Lacrimal pump failure and obstruction of the nasolacrimal outflow system are other causes of excessive tears.

C. Canalicular infections may be caused by *Actinomyces israelii* (Streptothrix) and *Candida*.

Predisposing Factors

A. Blepharitis (inflammation of the eyelid)

B. Allergic conjunctivitis (infectious or foreign body)

C. Exposure to cold, air conditioning, or dry environment

D. Lid problems: impaired pumping action of the lid motion due to seventh nerve palsy or conditions that stiffen the lids such as scars or scleroderma

E. Lid laxity from aging or ectropion (sagging of the lower lid)

F. Sinusitis

G. Atopy

H. Age: increased incidence in the elderly due to an over-production of tears by the lacrimal gland

I. Congenital obstruction

Common Complaints

A. Watery eyes or tears running down cheeks are common complaints.

Other Signs and Symptoms

A. Unilateral tearing: obstructive etiology

B. Bilateral tearing: environmental irritants

Subjective Data

A. Inquire about onset, course, and duration of symptoms. Note frequency of excessive tearing.

B. Ascertain whether this a new symptom or whether the patient has a past history of similar complaints. Ask: How was it treated, and what was the response to treatment(s)?

C. Determine severity. Do the tears run down the cheek?

D. Ascertain whether tearing is unilateral or bilateral.

E. Review common environmental predisposing factors.

F. Question the patient regarding vision changes.

G. Review medical history.

H. Review recent history for sinus infections or drainage, facial fractures, and surgery.

Physical Examination

A. Inspect
 1. Evaluate *both* eyes.
 2. Observe the lid structure and motion.
 3. Conduct a dermal exam to rule out butterfly rash.

B. Palpate
 1. Apply gentle pressure over the lacrimal sac to check drainage.
 2. Invert upper lid to check for foreign body.
 3. Palpate face for sinus tenderness.

Diagnostic Tests

A. Culture any drainage expressed from the lacrimal sacs.

Differential Diagnoses

A. Excessive tears.

B. Dendritic ulcer: Early symptoms are tears running down cheeks associated with a foreign-body sensation.

C. Congenital glaucoma.

D. Dacryocystitis (purulent discharge).

E. Reflex tearing caused by dry eyes.

F. Blepharitis.

Plan

A. General interventions
 1. Eliminate identifiable irritants.
 2. Treatment is mainly aimed at the underlying condition (i.e., ocular infection).

3. Dacryocystitis is treated with hot compresses at least four times a day and systemic antibiotics.
B. Patient teaching: Instruct the patient on the application of compresses.
C. Pharmaceutical therapy
1. None is required for diagnosis of excessive tears without infections pathology.
2. Dacryocystitis
a. Erythromycin 250 mg four times daily for 7 days.
b. Dicloxacillin 250 mg four times daily for 7 days.

Follow-up
A. See patient in 48–72 hours to evaluate symptoms, especially if antibiotic therapy was needed.

Consultation/Referral
A. Patients unresponsive to treatment should be promptly referred to an ophthalmologist.
B. Consider referral for lid malposition or nasolacrimal duct obstructions.

Individual Considerations
A. Pediatrics: Nasolacrimal duct obstruction. Approximately 6% of newborns are diagnosed with a congenital obstruction within the first weeks of life. With moist heat and massage, many resolve spontaneously

GLAUCOMA, ACUTE ANGLE-CLOSURE

Definition
A. This ocular emergency is caused by elevations in intraocular pressure that damage the optic nerve leading to loss of peripheral fields of vision, and it can lead to loss of central vision and result in blindness.

Incidence
A. Acute angle-closure glaucoma is the second leading cause of blindness in the United States. Approximately 5%–15% of the patient population develops glaucoma.

Pathogenesis
A. The essential pathophysiologic feature of glaucoma is an intraocular pressure that is too high for the optic nerve. Increased intraocular pressure increases vascular resistance, causing decreased vascular perfusion of the optic nerve and ischemia. Light dilates the pupil, causing the iris to relax and bow forward. As the iris bows forward, it comes into contact with the trabecular mesh-work and occludes the outflow of aqueous humor, resulting in increased intraocular pressure.

Predisposing Factors
A. Narrow anterior ocular chamber
B. Prolonged periods of darkness
C. Drugs that dilate the pupils (i.e., anticholinergics)
D. Advancing age
E. African American heritage
F. Family history
G. Trauma
H. Neoplasm
I. Corticosteroid therapy
J. Neovascularization

Common Complaints
A. Ocular pain
B. Blurred vision, decreased visual acuity, "cloudiness" of vision
C. "Halos" around lights at night
D. Neurologic complaints (headache, nausea, or vomiting)

Other Signs and Symptoms
A. Red eye with ciliary flush.
B. "Silent blinder" causes extensive damage before the patient is aware of visual field loss.
C. Dilated pupil.
D. Hard orbital globe.
E. No pupillary response to light.
F. Increase intraocular pressure (normal intraocular pressure is 10–20 mmHg).

Subjective Data
A. Review the onset, course, and duration of symptoms; note visual changes in one or both eyes.
B. Review medical history and medications.
C. Review family history of glaucoma.
D. Determine whether there has been any difficulty with peripheral vision, any headache photophobia, or any visual blurring.
E. In children, ask about rubbing of eyes, refusal to open eyes, and tearing.
F. Rule out presence of any chemical, trauma, or foreign bodies in the eye.
G. Review any recent history of herpes outbreak.
H. Ask the patient whether this has ever occurred before, and if so, how it was treated.

Physical Examination
A. Blood pressure
B. Inspect
1. Examine both eyes.
2. Rule out foreign body.
3. Inspect for redness, inflammation, and discharge.
4. Check pupillary response to light.
5. Redness noted around iris, dilated pupil, and cornea appears cloudy.
C. Palpate: Palpate the globe of the eye.
D. Funduscopic exam: This may reveal notching of the cup and a difference in cup-to-disc ratio between the two eyes.

Diagnostic Tests
A. Check visual acuity and peripheral fields of vision.
B. Measure intraocular pressure with a tonometer.

Differential Diagnoses
A. Acute angle-closure glaucoma
B. Acute iritis
C. Acute bacterial conjunctivitis
D. Iridocyclitis
E. Corneal injury
F. Foreign body
G. Herpetic keratitis

Plan
A. General interventions

1. Severe attacks can cause blindness in 2–3 days. **Seek medical attention immediately to prevent permanent vision loss.**
2. Frequency of attacks is unpredictable.
B. See the Section III Patient Teaching Guide for this chapter, "How to Administer Eye Medications."
C. Pharmaceutical therapy: **Must be instituted by an ophthalmologist.**
   1. Acetazolamide (Diamox) 250 mg orally
   2. Pilocarpine (Pilocar) 4% every 15 min during acute attack
D. Surgical intervention
   1. Surgery is indicated if intraocular pressure is not maintained within normal limits with medications or if there is progressive visual field loss with optic nerve damage.
   2. Surgical treatment of choice is peripheral iridectomy—excision of a small portion of the iris whereby the aqueous humor can bypass the pupil.

Follow-up
A. Annual eye exams by an ophthalmologist are necessary to monitor intraocular pressure and treatment efficacy.

Consultation/Referral
A. All patients should be referred to an ophthalmologist *immediately* for measurement of intraocular pressure, acute management, and possible surgical intervention (laser peripheral iridectomy).

Individual Considerations
A. Pediatrics: Infants with tearing, rubbing of eyes, and refusal to open eyes should be referred to a pediatric ophthalmologist for immediate care.
B. Adults
   1. Women normally have slightly higher intraocular pressures than men.
   2. Asians may have higher intraocular pressures than African Americans and Caucasians.
   3. Individuals older than age 40 should have their intraocular pressure measured periodically. Every 3–5 years is sufficient after a stable baseline is established for the patient.
C. Geriatrics: Incidence increases with age, usually in those older than age 60.

HORDEOLUM (STYE)

Definition
A. Hordeolum is an infection of the glands of the eyelids (follicle of an eyelash or the associated gland of Zeis [sebaceous] or Moll's gland [apocrine sweat gland]), usually caused by *Staphylococcus aureus.*
B. If swelling is under conjunctival side of eyelid, it is an internal hordeolum.
C. If swelling is under the skin of the eyelid, it is an external hordeolum.

Incidence
A. The incidence is unknown; it is more common in children and adolescents than adults.

Pathogenesis
A. Acute bacterial infection of the meibomian gland (internal hordeolum) or of the eyelash follicle (external hordeolum) is usually caused by *Staphylococcus aureus.*

Predisposing Factors
A. Age: More common in the pediatric populaiton.

Common Complaints
A. Eye tenderness
B. Sudden onset of a purulent discharge

Other Signs and Symptoms
A. Redness and swelling of the eye.

Subjective Data
A. Review the onset, course, and duration of symptoms.
B. Determine whether there is any visual disturbance.
C. Note whether this is the first occurrence. If not, ask how it was treated before.
D. Evaluate how much pain or discomfort the patient is experiencing.
E. Review the patient's history for chemical, foreign body, and/or trauma etiology.
F. Review the patient's medical history and medications.

Physical Examination
A. Inspect
   1. Examine both eyes; note redness, site of swelling, and amount and color of discharge.
   2. Evert the lid and check for pointing.
   3. Assess sclera and conjunctivae for abnormalities.
   4. Inspect ears, nose, and throat.
B. Palpate
   1. Palpate eye for hardness and expression of discharge.
   2. Evaluate for preauricular adenopathy.

Diagnostic Tests
A. Test visual acuity.
B. Discharge can be cultured, but usually treated presumptively.

Differential Diagnoses
A. Hordeolum.
B. Chalazion: The main differential diagnosis is chalazia, which point on the conjunctival side of the eyelid and do not usually affect the margin of the eyelid.
C. Blepharitis.
D. Xanthoma.
E. Bacterial conjunctivitis.
F. Foreign body.

Plan
A. General interventions: Contain the infecting pathogen. Crops occur when the infectious agent spreads from one hair follicle to another.
B. Patient teaching
   1. See Section III Patient Teaching Guide for this chapter, "How to Administer Eye Medications."
   2. Reinforce good hand washing.
   3. Patients should discard all eye makeup including mascara, eyeliner, and eye shadow.

C. Pharmaceutical therapy
1. Sulfacetamide sodium (Sulamyd) ophthalmic ointment 10%, 0.5–1.0 cm placed in the conjunctival sac four times daily for 7 days.
2. Sulfacetamide sodium (Sulamyd) 10% opthalmic drops, 2 drops instilled every 3–4 hours for 7 days.
3. Polymyxin B sulfate and bacitracin zinc (Polysporin) ophthalmic ointment, 0.5–1.0 cm placed in the conjunctival sac four times daily for 7 days.
4. If crops of styes occur, some clinicians recommend a course of tetracycline to stop recurrences (consult with a physician).

Follow-up

A. Have patient telephone or visit the office in 48 hours to check response.
B. If crops occur, diabetes mellitus must be excluded. Perform blood glucose evaluation.

Consultation/Referral

A. Hordeolum may produce a diffuse superficial lid infection known as "preseptal cellulitis" that requires referral to an ophthalmologist.
B. If hordeolum does not respond to topical antimicrobial treatment, refer the patient to an ophthalmologist.

Individual Considerations

A. None

STRABISMUS

Definition

Strabismus is an eye disorder in which the optic axes cannot be directed toward the same object due to a deficit in muscular coordination. It can be nonparalytic or paralytic.

A. *Esotropia* is a nonparalytic strabismus in which the eyes cross inward.
B. *Exotropia* is a nonparalytic strabismus in which the eyes drift outward. Exotropia may be intermittent or constant.
C. Pseudostrabismus gives a false appearance of deviation in the visual axes.

Incidence

A. Strabismus occurs in approximately 3% of the population.
B. Esotropia (nonparalytic strabismus) is the most common ocular misalignment representing more than half of all ocular deviations in the pediatric population. Accommodative esotropia occurs between 6 months and 7 years with an average age of 2.5 years, and it may be intermittent or constant.
C. Intermittent exotropia is the most common type of exotropic strabismus and is characterized by an outward drift of one eye, most often occurring when a child is fixating at distance.

Pathogenesis

A. *Paralytic strabismus* is related to paralysis or paresis of a specific extraocular muscle. *Nonparalytic strabismus* is related to a congenital imbalance of normal eye muscle tone causing focusing difficulties, unilateral refractive error, nonfusion, or anatomical difference in the eyes.

Predisposing Factors

A. Familial tendencies
B. Congenital defects

Common Complaints

A. Crossing of the eyes
B. Turning in of the eyes
C. Photophobia
D. Diplopia

Other Signs and Symptoms

A. The patient's head or chin tilts, or the patient closes one eye, to focus on objects.

Subjective Data

A. Describe the onset, duration, and progression of symptoms.
B. Review any history of eye problems. Ask: How were they corrected?
C. Determine whether the patient, if a child, has reached the age-appropriate milestones in development.
D. Does the patient make faces or move his or her head to see better (tilting the head or chin to improve acuity or to correct diplopia)?
E. Rule out any eye damage, surgery, and so forth.

Physical Examination

A. Inspect: Observe alignment of lids, sclera, conjunctiva, and cornea.
B. Check pupillary response to light, size, shape, and equality.
C. Check the red reflex.

Diagnostic Tests

A. Test visual acuity.
B. Perform the cover-uncover test: In this test, the "lazy eye" drifts out of position and snaps back quickly when uncovered.
C. Corneal light reflex (Hirschberg's) test: Perform the Hirschberg's test for symmetry of the pupillary light reflexes to help detect strabismus. Normally, the light reflexes are in the same position on each pupil, but not with strabismus (positive Hirschberg's test).
D. Test extraocular movements (EOMs): If a nerve supplying an extraocular muscle has been interrupted or the muscle itself has become weakened, the eye fails to move in the direction of the damaged muscle. If the right sixth nerve is damaged, the right eye does not move temporally. This is paralytic strabismus.

Differential Diagnoses

A. Strabismus
B. Pseudostrabismus
C. Ocular trauma
D. Congenital defect

Plan

A. General interventions
1. When poor fixation is present, patch the stronger, dominant eye to promote vision and muscle strengthening in the weaker eye.
B. Patient teaching: Reinforce the need to consistently wear an eye patch, especially with children.
C. Pharmaceutical therapy: None.

Follow-up
A. Monitor progress with eye patch.
B. Surgical intervention depends on the degree of deviation.

Consultation/Referral
A. Additional testing should be done by an ophthalmologist.
B. Pseudostrabismus (a false appearance of strabismus when visual axes are really in alignment) is one of the most common reasons a pediatric ophthalmologist is asked to evaluate an infant.

Individual Considerations: Pediatrics
A. Use the tumbling or illiterate E to test children; for preschoolers, use the Allen picture cards.
B. In very young children, test visual acuity by the assessment of developmental milestones: looking at mother's face, responsive smile, reaching for objects. By 3–5 years of age, most children can cooperate for performance of accurate visual acuity screening tests.
C. The eyes of the newborn are *rarely aligned* during the first few weeks of life. By the age of 3 months, normal oculomotor behavior is usually established, and an experienced examiner may be able to document the existence of abnormal alignment by that time.

SUBCONJUNCTIVAL HEMORRHAGE

Definition
A. Subconjunctival hemorrhage presents as blood patches in the bulbar conjunctiva.

Incidence
A. Frequently seen in newborns, subconjunctival hemorrhage may also be seen in adults after forceful exertion (coughing, sneezing, childbirth, strenuous lifting).

Pathogenesis
A. This disorder is believed to be secondary to increased intrathoracic pressure that may occur during labor and delivery or with physical exertion.

Predisposing Factors
A. Local trauma
B. Systemic hypertension
C. Acute conjunctivitis
D. Vaginal delivery
E. Severe coughing
F. Severe vomiting

Common Complaints
A. Red-eyed appearance without pain.

Other Signs and Symptoms
A. Bright red blood in plane between the conjunctiva and sclera
B. Usually unilateral
C. Normal vision

Subjective Data
A. Identify onset and duration of symptoms.
B. Elicit information about trauma to the eye; is it due to severe coughing or vomiting?
C. Identify history of conjunctivitis or hypertension.

Physical Examination
A. Check temperature, pulse, respirations, and blood pressure (rule out hypertension).
B. Inspect
   1. Observe eyes.
   2. Inspect ears, nose, and mouth.
   3. Inspect skin for bruises or other trauma.
   4. Assess for signs of trauma or abuse. **Blood in the anterior chamber (hyphema) can result from injury or abuse.**
C. Other physical examination components dependent on etiology.

Diagnostic Tests
A. Perform visual screening.
B. Test extraocular movement (EOMs) and peripheral vision.

Differential Diagnoses
A. Subconjunctival hemorrhage
B. Systemic hypertension
C. Blood dyscrasia
D. Trauma to eye
E. Conjunctivitis
F. Hyphema
G. Abuse

Plan
A. General interventions: Reassure the patient. The hemorrhage is not damaging to the eye or vision, and the blood reabsorbs on its own over several weeks.
B. Teach safety to prevent trauma to the eye.
C. Pharmaceutical therapy: None.

Follow-up
A. If subconjunctival hemorrhage recurs, evaluate the patient further for systemic hypertension or blood dyscrasia.

Consultation/Referral
A. Consult or refer the patient to a physician if hyphema is noted, if glaucoma is suspected, or if the patient has additional eye injuries.

Individual Considerations
A. Pediatrics: Common in newborns after vaginal delivery.
B. Adults: Always measure blood pressure to rule out systemic hypertension.
C. Geriatrics
   1. Always measure blood pressure to rule out systemic hypertension.
   2. Consider evaluation for blood dyscrasia.
   3. Check clotting times if patient is taking warfarin (Coumadin).

UVEITIS

Definition
A. Uveitis, also known as iritis, is inflammation of the uveal tract (iris, ciliary body, and choroid) and is usually accompanied by a dull ache and photophobia due to the irritative spasm of the pupillary sphincter.

Incidence

A. The true incidence is unknown. Approximately 15% of patients with sarcoidosis present with uveitis.

Pathogenesis

A. The cause is unknown. Underlying causes include infections, viruses, and arthritis.

Predisposing Factors

A. Collagen disorders
B. Autoimmune disorders
C. Ankylosing spondylitis
D. Sarcoidosis
E. Juvenile rheumatoid arthritis
F. Lupus
G. Reiter's syndrome
H. Behcet's syndrome
I. Syphilis
J. Tuberculosis
K. AIDS
L. Crohn's disease

Common Complaints

A. Eye pain: painless to deep-seated ache
B. Photophobia
C. Blurred vision with decreased visual acuity
D. Black spots

Other Signs and Symptoms

A. Unilateral or bilateral symptoms
　1. Unilateral: the pupil is smaller than that of the other eye because of spasm.
B. Ciliary flush
C. Pupillary contraction
D. Nausea and vomiting with vagal stimulation
E. Halos around lights
F. Hypopyon (pus in anterior chamber)
G. Limbal flush with small pupil

Subjective Data

A. Elicit the onset, course, duration, and frequency of symptoms. Are symptoms bilateral or unilateral?
B. Identify the possible causal activity or agent (chemical, traumatic, or infectious etiologies).
C. Review the patient's history of previous uveitis and other ophthalmologic disorders.
D. Review any associated fever, rash, weight loss, joint pain, back pain, oral ulcers, or genital ulcers.
E. Review full medical history for comorbid conditions.

Physical Examination

A. Check temperature, pulse, respirations, and blood pressure.
B. Inspect
　1. Assess both eyes for visual acuity and peripheral fields of vision.
　2. Check sclera and conjunctiva.
C. Other physical components to be completed related to comorbid conditons.

Diagnostic Tests

A. Slit-lamp test: Slit-lamp examination reveals cells in the anterior chamber and "flare," representing increased aqueous humor protein. Inflammatory cells, called "keratici precipitates," can collect in clusters on the posterior cornea.
B. Flashlight examination: Flashlight examination shows a slightly cloudy anterior chamber in the uveitic eye.

Differential Diagnoses

A. Uveitis: Uveitis is usually idiopathic, but it may be associated with many systemic and ocular diseases.
B. Acute angle-closure glaucoma.
C. Retinal detachment.
D. Central retinal artery occlusion.
E. Endophthalmitis.

Plan

A. General interventions: Treat underlying cause as indicated.
B. **Provide immediate referral to an ophthalmologist due to possible complications of cataracts and blindness.**
C. Patient teaching: Inform the patient that recurrent attacks are common and also require immediate attention.
D. Pharmaceutical therapy:
　1. **Medications given per ophthalmologist.**
　2. Uveitis and colitis often flare simultaneously; oral steroids are effective for both.

Follow-up

A. The patient with uveitis needs a follow-up with an ophthalmologist; recurrent attacks are common.

Consultation/Referral

A. The patient should be referred *immediately* to an ophthalmologist for evaluation and intervention.

Individual Considerations

A. None

⬛ RESOURCES

American Academy of Ophthalmology
415-561-8500

American Council of the Blind
1155 15th Street NW, Suite 1155
Washington, DC
800-424-8666; 202-467-5081
3 PM to 5:30 PM (eastern standard time), Monday through Friday
e-mail: ncrabb@access.digex.net

American Foundation of the Blind
212-502-7600

American Printing House for the Blind
1839 Frankfort Avenue
PO Box 6085
Louisville, KY 40206-6085
800-223-1839; 502-895-2405

AT&T National Special Needs Center
2001 Route 46, 3rd Floor Parsippany, NJ 07054
800-872-3883; 800-833-3232 TDD 8:30 AM to 6:30 PM (eastern standard time), Monday through Friday

Books on Tape
PO Box 7900
Newport Beach, CA 92658-7900
800-626-3333

Glaucoma Research Foundation
415-986-3162

Guide Dog Foundation for the Blind
371 E Jerico Turnpike
Smithtown, NY 11787
800-548-4337
9 AM to 5 PM (eastern standard time), Monday through Friday
e-mail: guidedog@guidedog.org

National Service for the Blind and Physically Handicapped
National Library of Congress
1291 Taylor Street NW
Washington, DC 20542
800-424-8567; 202-794-8650
8 AM to 4:30 PM (eastern standard time), Monday through Friday
e-mail: nls@loc.gov

National Society to Prevent Blindness
National Center for Sight

500 E Remington Road, Suite 200
Schamberg, IL 60173
800-221-3004
8 AM to 5 PM (central daylight time), Monday through Friday
e-mail: 7477.100@Compuserve.com
Vision Foundation
617-926-4232

REFERENCES

Behrman, R., & Kliegman, R. (1994). *Nelson essentials of pediatrics.* Philadelphia: W. B. Saunders.

Behrman, R., & Vaughan, V. (1996). *Nelson textbook of pediatrics.* Philadelphia: W. B. Saunders.

Duguid, G. (1997). Red eye: Avoid the pitfalls. *The Practitioner, 241,* 188–195.

Fukuyama, J., Hayasaka, S., Yamada, K., & Setogawa, T. (1990). Causes of subconjunctival hemorrhage. *Ophthalmologica, 200,* 63–67.

Jackson, W. B. (1993). Differentiating conjunctivitis of diverse origins. *Survey of Ophthalmology, 38,* 91–104.

King, R. (1993). Common ocular signs and symptoms in childhood. *Pediatric Clinics of North America, 40,* 753–766.

Rucker, L. (Ed.). (1997). *Essentials of adult ambulatory care.* Baltimore: Williams & Wilkins.

Ruppert, S. (1996). Differential diagnosis of pediatric conjunctivitis. *Nurse Practitioner, 21,* 12–26.

Ear Guidelines

Moya Cook

⬛ ACUTE OTITIS MEDIA

Definition
A. Acute otitis media is inflammation of the middle ear associated with a collection of fluid inside the middle ear.

Incidence
A. Acute otitis media may occur at any age. It is most commonly seen in children.
B. Over two-thirds of children have had at least one episode of otitis media by 3 years of age.
C. One-third of children have had three or more episodes by 3 years of age.
D. One-third of all pediatric visits are for otitis media.

Pathogenesis
A. Obstruction of the eustachian tube can lead to a middle ear effusion. Contamination of this middle ear fluid often results from a backup of nasopharyngeal secretions. The most common bacterial pathogens are *Streptococcus pneumoniae, Haemophilus influenzae,* and *Moraxella catarrbalis.*

Predisposing Factors
A. Age less than 12 months
B. Recurrent otitis media (three or more episodes in the last 6 months)
C. Previous episode of otitis media within the last month
D. Medical condition that predisposes to otitis media (i.e., Down's syndrome, AIDS, cystic fibrosis, cleft palate, and craniofacial abnormalities)
E. Native American heritage
F. Smoking in the household
G. Day-care attendance
H. Bottle propping
I. Family history of allergies

Common Complaints
A. Ear pain
B. Pulling ears
C. Fever may or may not be present

Other Signs and Symptoms
A. Sleeplessness within past 48 hours
B. Decreased appetite
C. Increased fussiness
D. Acute hearing loss
E. Upper respiratory infection symptoms
F. Mastoiditis presenting with a swollen and red mastoid
G. Perforated tympanic membrane (sudden pain followed by drainage)
H. Cholesteatoma (saclike structure in the middle ear accompanied by white, shiny, greasy debris)

Subjective Data
A. Elicit onset and duration of symptoms.
B. Inquire whether the patient recently had (or has concurrently) a URI.
C. Determine whether the patient has any change in hearing.
D. Assess the patient for any drainage from the ear(s).
E. Question the patient or his or her caregiver regarding risk factors.
F. Identify the patient's history of otitis media.

Physical Examination
A. Check temperature, pulse, respirations, and blood pressure.
B. Inspect
   1. Observe ears for red or opaque membrane.
   2. Observe ears for decreased or absent tympanic membrane mobility.
   3. Inspect nose, mouth, and throat.
C. Auscultate: Auscultate heart and lungs.

Diagnostic Tests
A. Tympanogram shows flat or type B curve.
B. Hearing test should be done in patients with persistent otitis media (greater or equal to 3 months duration).
C. Consider CBC if the patient appears toxic with a high fever.

Differential Diagnoses
A. Acute otitis media
B. Otitis media with effusion

C. Red tympanic membrane secondary to crying (differentiated from acute otitis media by mobility with pneumatic otoscopy)

D. URI

E. Mastoiditis

F. Foreign body in the ear

G. Otitis externa

Plan

A. General intervention: Pain relief with acetaminophen.

B. Patient teaching: See the Section III Patient Teaching Guide for this chapter, "Child With Acute Otitis Media."

C. Pharmaceutical therapy
   1. Drug of choice: amoxicillin 40–50 mg/kg/day divided into three daily doses for 10 days.
   2. Trimethoprim with sulfamethoxazole 8 mg/kg/day of trimethoprim (40 mg/kg/day of sulfamethoxazole) divided into two daily doses for 10 days.
   3. Erythromycin with sulfisoxazole 40 mg/kg/day of erythromycin (150 mg/kg/day of sulfisoxazole) (Pediazole) divided into four daily doses for 10 days. **Do not use in children under 2 months of age.**
   4. If the patient is asymptomatic and acute otitis media is found on exam, consider observation without antibiotics (follow-up in 48 hours).
   5. Other antibiotics (if first-line antibiotic fails): amoxicillin and clavulanate acid (Augmentin), cefixime (Suprax), azithromycin (Zithromax), and cefprozil (Cefzil).
   6. For persistent otitis media (3 months or longer), consider using an antibiotic for 21 days. **Residual otitis media may need treatment with additional amoxicillin or β-lactamase-resistant antibiotic.**

Follow-up

A. Check the patient in 2–4 weeks or if fever and complaints persist for more than 48 hours after antibiotic is begun.

Consultation/Referral

A. Consult or refer the patient to a physician if he or she is less than 6 weeks of age, appears septic, or has mastoiditis.

B. A patient with persistent otitis media with a hearing loss of 20 dB or more should be referred to an otolaryngologist.

Individual Considerations

A. Pregnancy: Do not use sulfa medications (sulfonamides) in pregnant clients at gestation.

B. Pediatrics
   1. Children 6 weeks old or younger: Consider a blood culture and lumbar puncture if septicemia is suspected. The patient may need IV antibiotics depending on culture results. Do not use sulfa medications (sulfonamides) in children less than 2 months old.
   2. In older children, consider decongestants for nasal congestion. Antihistamines are not recommended.

C. Geriatrics: Elderly patients may present with otitis media with effusion secondary to blocked eustachian tube and URI.

⬛ CERUMEN IMPACTION

Definition

A. Cerumen impaction, or earwax buildup, can cause conductive hearing loss or discomfort.

Incidence

A. Cerumen impaction occurs in patients of all ages. It is commonly seen in the elderly. The incidence in nursing home patients is 40%.

Pathogenesis

A. Wax builds up in the external canal. With age, the normal self-cleaning mechanisms of the ear fail. Cilia, which have become stiff, cannot remove cerumen and dirt from the ear canal. The pushing of cotton swabs, paper clips, bobby pins, and so forth into the ear canal may also impact cerumen.

Predisposing Factors

A. Aging (decreased function of ear cilia)

B. Use of hearing aids

C. Use of cotton swabs to clean ear canals

Common Complaints

A. Dryness and itching of ear canal

B. Dizziness

C. Ear pain

D. Hearing loss

Subjective Data

A. Elicit onset and duration of symptoms.

B. Elicit history of cerumen impaction.

C. Question the patient regarding the method of cleaning ears.

Physical Examination

A. Check temperature, pulse, respirations, and blood pressure.

B. Inspect
   1. Observe ears for thick, light to dark brown wax occluding the auditory canal.
   2. Observe tympanic membrane if possible. Perforated tympanic membrane is associated with otitis media.
   3. Inspect nose and throat.

C. Auscultation: Auscultate heart and lungs.

Diagnostic Tests

A. Conductive hearing loss of 35–40 dB.

B. Rinne tuning fork test reveals bone conduction greater than air conduction in affected ear (abnormal).

Differential Diagnoses

A. Cerumen impaction.

B. Foreign body in the ear canal.

C. Otitis externa: White, mucuslike ear discharge is associated with otitis externa.

Plan

A. General interventions
   1. Remove impaction by means of lavage or curettage.
   2. Document the patient's hearing before and after removal of cerumen.

B. Patient teaching
  1. See the Section III Patient Teaching Guide for this chapter, "Cerumen Impaction."
  2. Instruct the patient not to clean ears with cotton swabs, bobby pins, and so forth.
C. Pharmaceutical therapy
  1. Drug of choice: Debrox, mineral oil, or olive oil 2–3 drops in the ear every day for 1 week to loosen the cerumen before lavage or curettage. **Do not use Debrox if perforation of tympanic membrane is suspected.**
  2. For prevention, have the patient use the above softeners for 2–3 days. Then have him or her use one capful of hydrogen peroxide in the ear twice daily, allow it to bubble for 5–10 min, then turn head to allow it to run out.

Follow-up
A. No follow-up is needed unless indicated. Recurrence is common.

Consultation/Referral
A. Consult or refer the patient to a physician when cerumen cannot be cleared.

Individual Considerations
A. Geriatrics: Cerumen impaction is very common in the elderly due to atrophic cilia and dry epithelium in the ear canal.

HEARING LOSS

Definition
Impaired hearing (complete or partial hearing loss) results from interference with the conduction of sound, its conversion to electrical impulses, or its transmission through the nervous system. There are three types of hearing loss:

A. Conductive hearing loss
B. Sensorineural hearing loss
C. Combined conductive and sensorineural loss

Incidence
A. Hearing loss is present in 10%–15% of patients; approximately 30 million Americans have some degree of hearing impairment.

Pathogenesis
A. *Conductive hearing loss* presents with a diminution of volume, particularly low tones and vowels. It may be caused by one of the following:
  1. Otosclerosis disorder of the architecture of the bony labyrinth fixes the footplate of the stapes in the oval window.
  2. Exostoses are bony excrescences of the external auditory canal.
  3. Glomus tumors are benign, highly vascular tumors derived from normally occurring glomera of the middle ear and jugular bulb.
B. *Sensorineural hearing loss* characteristically produces impairment of the high-tone perception. Affected patients can hear people speaking, but they have difficulty deciphering words because discrimination is poor. It may be caused by one of the following:
  1. Presbycusis is hearing loss associated with aging and is the most common cause of diminished hearing in the elderly; onset is bilateral, symmetric, and gradual.
  2. Noise-induced hearing loss is due to chronic exposure to sound levels in excess of 85–90 dB.
  3. Drug-induced hearing loss can be caused by aminoglycoside antibiotics, furosemide, ethacrynic acid, quinidine, and aspirin.
  4. Meniere's disease produces a fluctuating, unilateral, low-frequency impairment usually associated with tinnitus, a sensation of fullness in the ear, and intermittent episodes of vertigo.
  5. Acoustic neuroma is a benign tumor of the eighth cranial nerve (rare).
  6. Sensorineural hearing loss is generally bilateral and symmetric, and it may be genetically determined.
  7. Sudden deafness can derive from head trauma, skull fracture, meningitis, otitis media, scarlet fever, mumps, congenital syphilis, multiple sclerosis, and perilymph leaks or fistulas.

Predisposing Factors
A. Acoustic or physical trauma
B. Ototoxic medications (such as gentamicin and aspirin)
C. Changes in barometric pressures
D. Recent URI
E. Pregnancy
F. Otosclerosis
G. Nasopharyngeal cancer
H. Serous otitis media
I. Cerumen impaction
J. Foreign body in the ear

Common Complaints
A. Partial hearing loss
B. Total hearing loss
C. Difficulty understanding the television, phone conversations, and people talking

Other Signs and Symptoms
A. Unilateral or bilateral hearing loss
B. Hearing noises as "ringing," "buzzing," and so forth
C. Fullness in ear(s)

Subjective Data
A. Elicit the onset, duration, progression, and severity of symptoms. Note whether symptoms are bilateral or unilateral.
B. Obtain the patient's history of past or recent trauma.
C. Review the patient's occupational and recreational exposure to risk factors.
D. Review the patient's medical history and medications, including over-the-counter drugs and prescriptions.
E. Review the patient's history for recent URI or ear infections, especially for chronic ear infections.
F. Elicit data about any previous hearing loss, how it was treated, and how it affected daily activities. There is often a history of previous ear disease with conductive hearing loss.

G. Review the patient's other symptoms such as dizziness, fullness or pressure in the ears, and noises.

H. Review what causes difficulty with hearing, high tones versus low frequencies. Can patient hear people talking, the television at normal volume, doorbells ringing, telephone ringing, and watch ticking?

Physical Examination

A. Temperature.

B. Inspect
1. Examine both ears for comparison.
2. Externally inspect ears for discharge; note color and odor. Obstruction of the auditory canal by impacted cerumen, a foreign body, exostoses, external otitis, otitis media with effusion, or scarring or perforation of the eardrum due to chronic otitis may be present.
3. Conduct otoscopic examination to observe the auditory canal for cerumen impaction or foreign body.
4. Inspect tympanic membrane for color, landmarks, contour, perforation, and acute otitis media. A reddish mass visible through the intact tympanic membrane may indicate a high-riding jugular bulb, an aberrant internal carotid artery, or a glomus tumor.

C. Palpate: Palpate auricle and mastoid area for tenderness, swelling, or nodules. Check lymph nodes if infection is suspected.

D. Neurologic testing: Weber's and Rinne tests
1. In the Weber's test, the tuning fork is perceived more loudly in the conductively deaf ear.
2. The Rinne test shows that bone conduction is better than air conduction (normal is when air conduction is greater than bone conduction).

Diagnostic Tests

A. Audiogram in primary setting
B. Air insufflation for tympanic membrane mobility
C. Tympanometry brain stem–evoked response audiogram
D. CT scan or MRI after consultation with an otolaryngologist

Differential Diagnoses

A. Congenital hearing loss
B. Traumatic hearing loss
C. Ototoxicity
D. Presbycusis
E. Meniere's syndrome
F. Acoustic neuroma
G. Cholesteatoma
H. Infection
I. Cerumen impaction
J. Otitis externa
K. Foreign body in the ear
L. Tumors
M. Otosclerosis
N. Perforation of tympanic membrane
O. Serous otitis media
P. Hypothyroidism
Q. Paget's disease

Plan

A. General interventions: Treat any primary cause (i.e., remove impacted cerumen).

B. Patient teaching
1. Discuss avoiding loud noises, using earplugs, and so forth.
2. Instruct the patient not to insert small objects into the ear.

C. Pharmaceutical therapy: Treat primary condition if applicable.

Follow-up

A. If the primary cause of hearing loss is not identified, refer the patient to a physician.

Consultation/Referral

A. The patient should be referred to an otolaryngologist for an extensive workup when the primary cause cannot be identified.

Individual Considerations

A. Pediatrics
1. Most children are able to respond to a test of gross hearing using a small bell. To determine the patient's hearing ability, note if the child stops moving when the bell is rung and if the child turns his or her head toward the sound.
2. When examining children, pull the pinna back and slightly upward to straighten the canal.

B. Adults: The external auditory canal in the adult can best be exposed by pulling the earlobe upward and backward.

C. Geriatrics
1. Impaired hearing among the elderly is common and can impair the quality of life.
2. People with seriously impaired hearing often become withdrawn or appear confused.
3. Subtle hearing loss may go unrecognized.
4. Impacted cerumen is very common in the elderly.

OTITIS EXTERNA

Definition

A. Otitis externa is a common, acute, self-limiting inflammation or infection of the external auditory canal and auricle.

Incidence

A. Otitis externa is seen in patients of all ages. Incidence is higher during summer months. All varieties (with exception of necrotizing otitis externa) are common.

Pathogenesis

A. Acute diffuse otitis externa (swimmer's ear): *Pseudomonas* is the most common bacterial infection (67%), followed by *Staphylococcus* and *Streptococcus*. Infection can also be fungal (*Aspergillus,* 90%). Bacterial or fungal invasion is usually preceded by trauma to ear canal, aggressive cleaning of the naturally bactericidal cerumen, or frequent submersion in water (swimming).

B. Chronic otitis externa: condition generally results from a persistent, low-grade infection and inflammation with *Pseudomonas*.

C. Eczematous otitis externa: otitis externa associated with primary coexistent skin disorder such as atopic dermatitis, seborrheic dermatitis, and psoriasis.

D. Necrotizing or malignant otitis externa: invasive *Pseudomonas* infection results in skull base osteomyelitis. It is most commonly seen in the immunocompromised or diabetic geriatric patient.

Predisposing Factors

A. Ear trauma from scratching with a foreign object or fingernail, overly vigorous cleaning of cerumen from canal

B. Humid climate

C. Frequent swimming

D. Use of a hearing aid

E. Eczema (eczematous otitis externa)

F. Debilitating disease (necrotizing otitis externa)

Common Complaints

A. Otalgia

B. Itching

C. Erythematous and swollen canal

D. Purulent discharge

E. Hearing loss from edema and obstruction of canal with drainage

Other Signs and Symptoms

A. Plugged ear sensation (aural fullness)

B. Tenderness to palpation (tragus)

Subjective Data

A. Elicit onset, duration, and intensity of ear discomfort.

B. Inquire into the patient's history of previous ear infections.

C. Determine whether the patient notes any degree of hearing loss.

D. Question the patient about recent exposure to immersion in water (swimming).

E. Question the patient as to ear canal cleaning practices and any recent trauma to canal.

Physical Examination

A. Temperature.

B. Inspect
   1. Carefully examine the ear with otoscope due to extreme tenderness.
   2. Observe the ear for erythematous and edematous external canal; look for otorrhea and debris.
   3. Observe tympanic membrane, which may appear normal.
   4. Inspect nose and throat.

C. Auscultation: Auscultate heart and lungs.

D. Palpate
   1. Apply gentle pressure to tragus and manipulate pinna to assess for tenderness.
   2. Palpate cervical lymph nodes.

Diagnostic Tests

A. Examine ear canal scrapings and drainage under microscope for hyphae (if fungal infection is suspected from previous history or ineffective topical therapy).

B. Culture vesicular lesions for viruses.

Differential Diagnoses

A. Otitis externa.

B. Otitis media.

C. Foreign body.

D. Mastoiditis.

E. Hearing loss.

F. Wisdom tooth eruption.

G. Herpetic otitis externa (vesicular eruptions in the ear canal are associated with herpetic otitis externa).

H. Necrotizing or malignant otitis externa (life-threatening condition that occurs in diabetic or immunocompromised patients). Cranial nerve palsies (of the seventh, ninth, and twelfth cranial nerves) and periostitis of the skull base have been associated with necrotizing otitis externa.

Plan

A. General interventions
   1. When the patient's ear canal is sufficiently blocked by edema or drainage, preventing passage of ear drops, cautiously irrigate the canal and insert a cotton wick (approximately 1 in. long for adults) to allow passage of drops.
   2. Insert the wick by gently rotating it while inserting it into ear. The patient then places ear drops on the wick. The drops are absorbed through the wick, which allows medicine to reach the external canal. The wick may need to be changed daily or several times per week by the provider.

B. Patient teaching
   1. See the Section III Patient Teaching Guide for this chapter, "Otitis Externa."
   2. The patient should be advised to keep water out of the ear for 4–6 weeks. The patient should not swim until symptoms are completely resolved and the wick is removed.
   3. Bathing or showering is permitted with a cotton ball coated with petroleum jelly inserted into the ear to block water passage into the ear canal.

C. Pharmaceutical therapy
   1. For early, mild cases associated with swimming in which the primary symptom is pruritus, homemade preparations of 50% isopropyl alcohol and 50% vinegar can be used as a drying agent and to create an unsatisfactory environment for *Pseudomonas* growth.
   2. Vosol or Vosol HC may be prescribed with the same indication with instructions to instill 5 drops in the ear canal 3–4 times daily. (Vosol and Vosol HC are contraindicated with perforated eardrum; Vosol HC is contraindicated with viral otic infections.)
   3. For more moderate infections involving otalgia and edema, bacitracin zinc, neomycin sulfate, polymyxin B sulfate, and hydrocortisone (Cortisporin) otic suspension may be used. Adults apply 4 drops to canal four times daily for 7 days; children apply 3 drops to canal four times daily for 7 days. The suspension is recommended over the solution if the integrity of the tympanic membrane is in question. Nystatin 100,000 units/mL or clotrimazole topical solutions may be used for candidal or yeast infections.

4. Severe or resistant infections may require management with oral antibiotics and antifungals:
   a. Ciprofloxacin for pseudomonal infections; dicloxacillin or cephalexin for staphylococcal infections.
   b. Itraconazole (Sporanox) for treatment of otomycosis (fungal otitis externa).
5. For analgesia, use acetaminophen or ibuprofen. Short-term use of opiates may be necessary when acetaminophen and ibuprofen fail to control pain.

Follow-up
A. Usual follow-up is within 48 hours to assess improvement. Recheck in 2 weeks.
B. In severe cases requiring antibiotic drops instilled by means of a wick, follow-up may be required daily or several times per week to remove and replace wick.

Consultation/Referral
A Parenteral antibiotics are required for necrotizing otitis externa. These patients should be immediately referred to a physician.
B. Consult or refer the patient to a physician if osteomyelitis is suspected.

Individual Considerations
Geriatrics:

A. Persistent otitis externa in the geriatric patient (especially those who are immunocompromised or diabetic) may evolve into osteomyelitis of the skull base.
B. The external ear is painful and edematous, and a foul, green discharge is usually present.
C. Treatment may require parenteral gentamicin with a β-lactam agent. Surgery may be necessary.
D. Oral fluoroquinolones may be useful if infection has not progressed to osteomyelitis.

OTITIS MEDIA WITH EFFUSION

Definition
A. In patients with otitis media with effusion, asymptomatic middle ear fluid is present.

Incidence
A. Otitis media with effusion is seen in patients of all ages.
B. After the onset of acute otitis media (AOM), approximately 70% of children have fluid present at 2 weeks.
   1. 40% have fluid present at 1 month.
   2. 20% have fluid present at 2 months.
   3. 10% have an effusion at 3 months.

Pathogenesis
A. The effusion may be sterile fluid secondary to URI and eustachian tube dysfunction. It may be residual fluid after an episode of acute otitis media.

Predisposing Factors
A. Recent otitis media
B. Concurrent URI

Common Complaints
A. Ear pain
B. Increased pressure sensation in the ears
C. Recent hearing loss

Other Signs and Symptoms
A. The patient has a sense of fullness in the ears.

Subjective Data
A. Elicit onset and duration of symptoms.
B. Question the patient about recent history of otitis media or URI.
C. Question the patient about hearing loss.
D. Determine if the patient has a past history of frequent otitis media.

Physical Examination
A. Check temperature, pulse, respirations, and blood pressure.
B. Inspect
   1. Inspect ears, noting fluid level, serous middle fluid, and a translucent membrane with decreased mobility.
   2. Inspect nose, mouth, and throat.
C. Auscultation: Auscultate heart and lungs.
D. Palpate: Palpate head, neck, and lymph nodes.
E. Neurological examination: Weber's test and Rinne test with tuning fork.

Diagnostic Tests
A. Pneumatic otoscopy reveals decreased mobility. **Assessment with pneumatic otoscopy is strongly recommended.**
B. Negative pressure on tympanogram.

Differential Diagnoses
A. Otitis media with effusion
B. Cerumen impaction
C. Acute otitis media
D. Foreign body in the ear

Plan
A. General interventions: None is required.
B. Patient teaching: See the Section III Patient Teaching Guide for this chapter, "Otitis Media With Effusion."
C. Pharmaceutical therapy
   1. Persistent otitis media with effusion (lasting 6 weeks to 4 months) can be treated by observation alone or with antibiotic therapy.
   2. Consider antibiotic prophylaxis if effusion resolves and the patient has had more than three episodes in less than 6 months.
   3. Drug of choice: amoxicillin 40–50 mg/kg/day divided into three daily doses for 14–21 days.
   4. Trimethoprim with sulfamethoxazole 8 mg/kg/day of trimethoprim (40 mg/kg/day of sulfamethoxazole) divided into two daily doses for 14–21 days.
   5. Erythromycin and sulfisoxazole (Pediazole) 40 mg/kg/day of erythromycin (150 mg/kg/day of sulfisoxazole) divided into four daily doses for 14–21 days.
   6. Otitis media with effusion in adults and adolescents who have URI or allergies can be treated with decongestants, antihistamines, and nasal sprays.

Follow-up
A. Recheck the patient's ears after 4–6 weeks to evaluate effectiveness of treatment.

Consultation/Referral

A. Consult or refer the patient to a physician if treatment is not effective or if the patient has a persistent effusion (at least 3 months) along with a hearing loss of 20 dB or more.

B. Consider referring the patient to an otolaryngologist.

Individual Considerations

A. Pregnancy: Do not use sulfa medications (sulfonamides) in pregnant clients at term.

B. Geriatrics:
 1. Otitis media with effusion may be present in the elderly, usually unilaterally, and usually associated with an URI or allergies due to a blocked eustachian tube.
 2. If there is no accompanying URI, a nasopharyngeal mass must be ruled out.

TINNITUS

Definition

A. Tinnitus comes from the Latin word *tinnire,* which means "to ring." It refers to any sound heard in the ears or head.

Incidence

A. It is estimated that 6.4% of the adult population has experienced tinnitus at some point. More than 7 million people in the United States are thought to experience tinnitus.

Pathogenesis

A. Tinnitus is poorly understood. It is best described as a nonspecific manifestation of pathology of the inner ear, eighth cranial nerve, or the central auditory mechanism.

Predisposing Factors

A. Cerumen impaction.
B. Tympanic membrane perforation.
C. Fluid in the middle ear.
D. Acute otitis media.
E. Acoustic trauma.
F. Ototoxic drugs
 1. Sulfas
 2. Aminoglycosides
 3. Salicylate
 4. Indomethacin
 5. Propranolol
 6. Levodopa
 7. Carbamazepine.
G. Vascular aneurysm.
H. Jugular bulb anomaly. Compression of the ipsilateral jugular vein abolishes the objective tinnitus of a jugular megabulb anomaly.
I. Anemia.
J. Temporomandibular joint syndrome.
K. Hypertension.

Common Complaints

A. Ringing
B. Roaring
C. Buzzing
D. Clicking
E. Hissing
F. Hearing loss

Other Signs and Symptoms

A. "Muffled" hearing
B. Change in own voice, lower pitch

Subjective Data

A. Review the onset, duration, course, and type of symptoms; note whether they are bilateral or unilateral.
B. Determine the frequency and quality of sound; is the ringing constant, intermittent, or pulsating?
C. Review all medications, including over-the-counter drugs and prescriptions.
D. Determine whether the patient has experienced trauma (domestic violence, motor vehicle accident, and so forth).
E. Rule out a recent sinus, oral, or ear infection.
F. Review any previous occurrences. Ask: How was it treated?
G. Review work, hobbies, and music habits for noise levels (potential damage).
H. Assess the date of last hearing exam, and if there was any known hearing loss.
I. Review whether patient uses cotton-tipped swabs or other small objects for ear cleaning.

Physical Examination

A. Temperature if infectious cause is suspected.
B. Inspect
 1. Observe the external ear for discharge; note color and odor.
 2. Conduct otoscopic exam of the auditory canal for cerumen impaction or foreign body.
 3. Inspect tympanic membrane for color, landmarks, contour, perforation, and acute otitis media.
  a. The landmarks (umbo, handle of malleus, and the light reflex) should be visible on a normal exam.
  b. The tympanic membrane should be pearly gray in color and translucent.
  c. A bulging tympanic membrane is more conical, usually with a loss of bony landmarks and a distorted light reflex.
  d. A retracted tympanic membrane is more concave, usually with accentuated bony landmarks and a distorted light reflex (pathologic conditions in the middle ear may be reflected by characteristics of the tympanic membrane).
C. Auscultation: The skull should be auscultated for a bruit if the origin of the problem remains obscure.
D. Palpate
 1. Palpate auricle and mastoid area for tenderness, swelling, or nodules.
 2. Check lymph nodes if infection is suspected.
E. Visual Exam: Check for nystagmus if vertigo is reported.
F. Neurologic exam
 1. The eighth cranial nerve is tested by evaluating hearing.
 2. First evaluate how the patient responds to your questions.

3. Patients who speak in a monotone or with erratic volume may have hearing loss.
4. Check the patient's response to a soft whisper (should respond at least 50% of the time).
5. Rinne and Weber's testing: The Rinne test is performed by placing the struck tuning fork against the mastoid bone. Begin counting or timing the interval from the start to when the patient can no longer hear. Continue counting or timing the interval to determine the length of time sound is heard by air conduction. Air-conducted sound should be heard twice as long as bone-conducted sound after bone conduction stops.

Diagnostic Tests

A. Audiogram is performed in the primary care setting; other testing is performed by an otolaryngologist. Any association of the sound with respiration, drug use, vertigo, noise trauma, or ear infection should be checked. When the problem is present only at night, it suggests increased awareness of normal head sounds.
B. CT scan or MRI after referral to an otolaryngologist
C. Posterior fossa myelography

Differential Diagnoses

A. Tinnitus
B. Cerumen impaction
C. Foreign body in the ear
D. Acute otitis media
E. Otitis externa
F. Acoustic traumas
G. Vascular aneurysm
H. Temporomandibular joint syndrome
I. Otosclerosis
J. Ototoxicity
K. Meniere's syndrome
L. Presbycusis
M. Central nervous system lesion

Plan

A. Patient teaching
1. Stress the importance of not placing small objects in the ear and using cotton-tipped applicators to clean external ear only.
2. Suggest to the patient that keeping a radio on for background noise often facilitates sleep or work.
B. Pharmaceutical therapy:
1. No medication "cures" tinnitus.
2. Vasodilators, tranquilizers, antidepressants, and seizure medications have been shown to reduce symptoms.
3. Placebos are also of therapeutic value.

Follow-up

A. No specific follow-up is required for tinnitus unless a treatable problem is identified.

Consultation/Referral

A. Consult with an otolaryngologist as indicated.
B. Referral of an anxious patient to the otolaryngologist may be necessary to satisfy him or her that everything has been explored and that there is no serious or correctable underlying condition.
C. Any patient with a history of head trauma should be referred to a physician because tinnitus may be associated with an arteriovenous fistula or an aneurysm of the intrapetrous portion of the internal carotid artery.

REFERENCES

Behrman, R., & Vaughan, V. (1996). *Nelson text-book of pediatrics.* Philadelphia: W. B. Saunders.

Berman, S. (1995). Otitis media in children. *The New England Journal of Medicine, 332,* 1560–1565.

Bojrab, D. I., Bruderly, T., & Abdulrazzak, Y. (1996). Diseases of the external auditory canal: Otitis externa. *Otolaryngologic Clinics of North America, 29,* 761–781.

Dambro, M. R. (1997). *Griffith's five minute clinical consult.* Baltimore: Williams & Wilkins.

Fihn, S. D., & McGee, S. R. (1992). *Outpatient medicine.* Philadelphia: W. B. Saunders.

Freeman, R. (1995). Impacted cerumen: How to safely remove ear wax in an office visit. *Geriatrics, 50,* 52–53.

Goroll, A. H., May, L. A., & Mulley, A. G. (1995). *Primary care medicine: Office evaluation and management of the adult patient.* Philadelphia: J. B. Lippincott.

Harrison, C., & Belhorn, T. (1991). Antibiotic treatment failures in acute otitis media. *Pediatric Annals, 20,* 600–608.

Hay, W., Groothuis, J., Hayward, A., & Levin, M. (Eds.). (1995). *Current pediatric diagnosis and treatment.* Norwalk, CT: Appleton & Lange.

Kaleida, P. (1997). The COMPLETES exam for otitis. *Contemporary Pediatrics, 14,* 93–101.

Osguthorpe, J. D., & Nielsen, D. R. (2006). Otitis externa: Review and clinical update. *American Family Physician, 74,* 1510–1516.

Otitis Media Guideline Panel. (1994a). Managing otitis media with effusion. *Pediatrics, 84,* 766–775.

Otitis Media Guideline Panel. (1994b). Managing otitis media with effusion in young children. *Pediatrics, 94,* 766–773.

Sanders, R. (2001). Otitis externa: A practical guide to treatment and prevention. *American Family Physician, 64,* 927–936, 941–942.

Schmitt, B. D. (1996). Guide for parents: How to treat swimmer's ear. *Contemporary Pediatrics, 13,* 65–66.

Thibodeau, D., & Lo, B. (2008). Otitis externa: What you need to know. *Clinician Reviews/Convenient Care, 1*(3), 1–8.

Tierney, L., McPhee, S., & Papadakis, M. (Eds.). (1996). *Current medical diagnosis and treatment.* Stamford, CT: Appleton & Lange.

Valentino, R. L. (2009). Chronic dysfunction of the eustacian tube. *The Clinical Advisor, 12,* 21–25.

Weimert, T. A. (1992). Common ENT emergencies, part I: The acute ear. *Emergency Medicine, 24,* 134–148.

Zivic, R., & King, S. (1993). Cerumen-impaction management for clients of all ages. *Nurse Practitioner, 18,* 33–36, 39.

Nasal Guidelines

Jill C. Cash

CHAPTER 6

ALLERGIC RHINITIS

Definition
A. Allergic rhinitis is a chronic or recurrent condition characterized by nasal congestion, clear nasal discharge, sneezing, nasal itching, conjunctival itching, and periorbital edema. It usually occurs seasonally after exposure to allergens (same time every year, associated with pollen count), or it may be perennial (year-round, related to indoor inhalants, animal dander, and mold). "Allergic" suggests that a specific IgE antibody mediates the condition.

Incidence
A. Prevalence varies according to geographic region. Twenty to twenty-five percent of adults have allergic rhinitis.

Pathogenesis
A. This is an IgE-mediated inflammatory disease involving nasal mucosa; IgE antibodies bind to mast cells in the respiratory epithelium, and histamine is released. This results in immediate local vasodilatation, mucosal edema, and increased mucus production.

Predisposing Factors
A. Genetic predisposition to allergy
B. Exposure to allergic stimuli: pollens, molds, animal dander, dust mites, and indoor inhalants

Common Complaints
A. Nasal congestion
B. Sneezing
C. Clear rhinorrhea
D. Coughing from postnasal drip
E. Sore throat
F. Itchy, puffy eyes with tearing

Other Signs and Symptoms
A. Dry mouth from mouth breathing, snoring
B. Itchy nose
C. Loss of smell and taste
D. Eczema rash
E. Shortness of breath, difficulty breathing, and wheezing
F. Headache
G. Halitosis

Subjective Data
A. Ask about onset, course, and duration of symptoms.
B. Inquire about characteristics of nasal discharge.
C. Inquire about exposure to people with similar symptoms.
D. Ask about seasonal impact on symptoms.
E. Inquire about other diseases caused by allergens, such as asthma, eczema, and urticaria.
F. Rule out pregnancy.
G. Ask female patients about their birth control method, specifically birth control pills.
H. Review exposure to irritants.
I. Ask about any past or recent nasal trauma.

Physical Examination
A. Vital signs: temperature, blood pressure, pulse, and respirations.
B. Inspect
  1. Examine face. Note Dennie's lines (skin folds under eyes) and allergic salute (transverse crease on nose from chronic rubbing of nose).
  2. Examine eyes and conjunctivae.
    a. Tearing; red, swollen eyelids; and allergic shiners (dark circles under eye from venous congestion in maxillary sinuses) are seen with allergies.
    b. Palpebral conjunctiva pale and swollen, bulbar conjunctiva injected.
  3. Examine ears, nose, and throat.
    a. Red, dull, bulging, perforated tympanic membrane is seen with **otitis media**.
    b. Nasal redness, swelling, polyps, enlarged turbinates are seen with **upper respiratory infection**. Mucosa appears pale blue, boggy with clear discharge in chronic allergy.
    c. Cobblestone appearance in pharynx, tonsils, and adenoids seen in chronic allergies.
    d. Use otoscope light to transilluminate under superior orbital ridge of frontal sinus cavity and also

maxillary sinus cavity to assess for fluid in sinus cavity. Healthy sinuses contain air and light up symmetrically.

C. Palpate
   1. Palpate face and frontal maxillary sinuses for tenderness.
   2. Examine head and neck for enlarged lymph nodes.
D. Percuss
   1. Percuss sinus cavities and mastoid bone.
   2. Percuss chest for consolidation.
E. Auscultate: Auscultate lungs and heart.

Diagnostic Tests

Diagnosis may be made from history and physical. Other diagnostic tests include:

A. Wright's stain of nasal secretions: eosinophils present confirm allergy
B. Skin testing for allergies
C. RadioAllergoSorbent Test (RAST Test)
D. CBC with increased eosinophils (confirm allergy)

Differential Diagnoses

A. Allergic rhinitis
B. Upper respiratory infection
C. Medication-induced rhinitis
D. Sinusitis
E. Otitis media
F. Deviated septum
G. Nasal polyps
H. Endocrine conditions such as hypothyroidism
I. Influenza

Plan

A. General interventions
   1. Avoid allergens (most effective treatment).
   2. Keep bedroom as allergen-free as possible.
B. Patient teaching: See the Section III Patient Teaching Guide for this chapter, "Allergic Rhinitis."
C. Pharmaceutical therapy
   1. Antihistamines (H_1 receptor antagonists) are drugs of choice. Several may need to be tried before an effective one is found. Drugs may also need to be switched occasionally to prevent tolerance.
      a. Azelastine HCl (Astelin) metered nasal spray, 137 μg per metered dose.
         i. Children younger than 5 years: not recommended.
         ii. Children 5–11 years: 1 spray each nostril twice daily.
         iii. Adults: two sprays per nostril twice daily.
      b. Loratadine (Claritin) 10 mg by mouth daily (adults).
         i. Children younger than 2 years: not recommended.
         ii. Children 2–5 years: 5 mg daily.
         iii. Children 6 years and older: 10 mg daily.
      c. Fexofenadine HCl (Allegra) 60 mg capsules orally twice daily (adults) or 180 mg daily.
         i. Children younger than 6 years: not recommended.
         ii. Children 6–11 years: 30 mg twice daily.
      d. Cetirizine HCl (Zyrtec):
         i. Adults and children 12 years and older: 5–10 mg by mouth daily depending on symptom severity.
         ii. Zyrtec 5 mg daily for patients with renal or hepatic impairment.
         iii. Children 2–6 years: 2.5 mg daily.
         iv. Children 6–11 years: 5–10 mg (1–2 teaspoons) by mouth daily depending on symptom severity.
      e. Montelukast (Singulair): Not recommended for children younger than 6 months.
         i. Children 6–23 months: One 4 mg granule packet.
         ii. Children 2–5 years: one 4 mg chewable tab or granule packet.
         iii. Children 6–14 years: one 5 mg tab.
         iv. Children older than 15 years and adults: take one 10 mg tab daily.
      f. Levocetirizine dihydrochloride (xyzal):
         i. Children younger than 6 years: not recommended.
         ii. Children 6–11 years: max 2.5 mg once daily in PM.
         iii. Adults: 2.5–5 mg daily in PM. Precautions for renal impairment.
   2. Topical decongestants for significant congestion of the mucous membranes.
      These drugs may also stimulate the sympathetic nervous system and cause insomnia, nervousness, and palpitations. **Use no longer than 3–5 days. Discontinuing these drugs after 5 days may result in a rebound effect.**
      a. Oxymetazoline hydrochloride (Afrin) spray or drops:
         i. Adults and children 6 years and older: two to three drops or sprays of 0.05% solution in each nostril twice daily.
         ii. Children 2–6 years: two to three drops of 0.025% solution in each nostril twice daily.
      b. Phenylephrine (Neo-Synephrine) spray or drops:
         i. Adults and children 12 years and older: two to three drops or one to two sprays in each nostril, or small amount of jelly applied to nasal mucosa, every 4 hours as needed. Do not use for more than 3–5 days.
         ii. Children 6–12 years: two to three drops or one to two sprays of 0.25% solution in each nostril every 4 hours as needed. Do not use for more than 3–5 days.
         iii. Children younger than 6 years: two to three drops of 0.125% solution every 4 hours in each nostril as needed. Contact physician if symptoms persist beyond 3 days.
   3. Steroid sprays may be used to decrease nasal inflammation. Sprays do not cause significant systemic absorption in usual doses, but occasionally they may cause pharyngeal fungal infections.
      a. Beclomethasone dipropionate (Beconase, Vancenase): Adults and children older than 12 years: one

to two sprays in each nostril two or three times daily.

    b. Fluticasone propionate (Flonase): Adults and children 4 years and older: two sprays daily or one spray twice daily. Maintenance dosing: one spray in each nostril daily.

    c. Triamcinolone acetonide (Nasacort AQ): Adults and children 6 years and older: two sprays daily.

    d. Mometasone furoate (Nasonex): Adults: 2 sprays each nostril once daily. Children younger than 2 years: not recommended. Children 2–11 years: 1 spray each nostril daily.

    e. Fluticasone furoate (Veramyst):

      i. Adults: 2 sprays each nostril daily.

        (a). Maintenance: 1 spray each nostril daily.

      ii. Children younger than 2 years: not recommended.

      iii. Children 2–11 years: 1 spray each nostril daily. May increase to 2 sprays daily if needed.

        (a). Maintenance dose: 1 spray each nostril daily.

    f. Budesonide (Rhinocort): Adults and children 6 years and older: two sprays twice daily.

4. Saline spray

    a. Saline spray is effective in liquefying thick secretions and helps keep mucosa moist.

    b. Use Netty pot to cleanse inside of nasal mucosa, daily use suggested.

5. Petroleum jelly applied with Q-tip to inside mucosa of nares 3–4 times a day helps to provide lubrication and hold in moisture to prevent nasal dryness and bleeding.

Follow-up

A. Patient should return for follow-up visit in 2–3 weeks if necessary, earlier if symptoms worsen after 3 days of treatment.

Consultation/Referral

A. Refer the patient to an allergist if symptoms continue and interfere with daily activities.

B. Allergist may prescribe immunotherapy following identification of offending allergens.

Individual Considerations

A. Pregnancy:

    1. Over-the-counter antihistimines such as Diphenhydramine HCl (Benadryl) may be used for up to 5 days.

    2. Over-the-counter decongestants such as oxymetazoline HC1 (Afrin) may be used up to 3 days.

EPISTAXIS

Definition

A. Epistaxis is a nosebleed or hemorrhage from the nose.

Incidence

A. About 11% of Americans have had at least one nosebleed.

Pathogenesis

A. Epistaxis is caused by disruption of the nasal mucosa. More than 90% of nosebleeds are related to local irritation rather than underlying anatomic lesions and are self-limiting. Most start in the anterior nasal cavity (Kisselbach's plexus).

B. Posterior nasal bleeding usually originates from the turbinates or lateral nasal wall.

Predisposing Factors

A. Local trauma, usually from nose picking

B. Acute inflammation from an upper respiratory infection (e.g., common cold, acute sinusitis, and allergic rhinitis)

C. Vigorous nose blowing

D. Inhalation of chemical irritants

E. Drying and crusting of nasal septum

F. Trauma

G. Cocaine use

H. Pregnancy

I. Neoplasm

J. Systemic causes

    1. Bleeding disorders (most common)

    2. Hypertension

    3. Arteriosclerosis

    4. Renal disease

Common Complaints

A. Common complaint is unusually severe or frequent nosebleeds.

Other Signs and Symptoms

A. Anterior epistaxis

    1. Unilateral

    2. Continuous, moderate bleeding from septum of nose

B. Posterior epistaxis

    1. Brisk (arterial) bleeding

    2. Blood flowing into pharynx (indicates a more serious problem)

Subjective Data

A. Inquire about amount, duration, and frequency of bleeding.

B. Ask about use of oral anticoagulants, aspirin, or aspirin-containing compounds (e.g., Pepto-Bismol, aspirin, Excedrin).

C. Ask about recent or current upper respiratory infections (URIs), family history of abnormal bleeding, recent surgery, or trauma.

D. Ask the first day of female patient's last menstrual period (if appropriate). Determine if the patient is pregnant.

E. Ask about possible foreign body in the nose.

F. Ask about cocaine use or occupational exposure to irritants or chemicals.

G. If the patient has a history of nosebleeds, how did the patient treat previous nosebleeds?

H. Has the patient ever been evaluated for a blood clotting abnormality, such as thrombocytopenia or platelet dysfunction?

I. Does the patient complain of bruising easily, melena, or heavy menstrual periods?

J. Ask about family history of bleeding disorders, such as hemophilia or von Willebrand's disease.

Physical Examination

A. Temperature, blood pressure (check for orthostatic hypertension), pulse, and respirations. **If nasal packing is required, take precaution and monitor patient closely for vasovagal episode during insertion of nasal packing.**

B. Inspect
1. Check airway patency with patient sitting and leaning forward.
2. Observe skin, mucous membranes, and conjunctiva for rash, pallor, purpura, petechiae, and telangiectasias.
3. Perform full eye exam, noting pupillary response.
4. Examine nose for septal perforation and ulcerations, which indicates cocaine use. Collagen diseases (such as lupus) are occasionally responsible for ulceration. Epistaxis is rare in hemophiliacs without trauma, but is characteristic of von Willebrand's disease.
5. Examine nasal discharge: a unilateral foul discharge with blood indicates a foreign body in the nose.
6. After bleeding has stopped:
   a. Inspect nasal mucosa for color, discharge, masses, lesions, and swelling of turbinates.
   b. Inspect nasal septum for alignment, septal perforation, and crusting.

C. Auscultate: heart and lungs.

D. Palpate: Check for enlarged lymph nodes in the neck to rule out Sarcoidosis, tuberculosis, or malignancy.

E. Percuss: Percuss sinuses.

Diagnostic Tests

A. **None is required unless the patient has recurrent or severe blood loss.**

B. Drug screen, if indicated.

C. Hematocrit and hemoglobin if bleeding is severe.

D. CBC with differential.

E. Platelets, prothrombin time (PT), and partial thromboplastin time (PTT) if bleeding disorder is suspected.

F. Sinus films if recurrent sinus pain, tenderness, and bleeding.

Differential Diagnoses

A. Epistaxis
B. Foreign body
C. Septal deformity
D. Perforated nasal septum
E. Coagulation disorder (von Willebrand's disease)
F. Nasal tumors
G. Drug-induced coagulapathy
H. Hypertension
I. Pregnancy

Plan

A. General interventions: Main goal is to control episodes of bleeding.

B. Patient teaching: See the Section III Patient Teaching Guide for this chapter, "Nosebleeds."

C. Medical/surgical management
1. To control *anterior septal bleeding*:
   a. Have patient sit and lean forward, apply pressure to reduce venous pressure, and prevent swallowing of blood.
   b. Soak a cotton pledget in phenylephrine (Neo-Synephrine), oxymetazoline HCl (Afrin), or epinephrine 1:1000, and apply with pressure against bleeding site for 5–10 min.
   c. Remove and check for bleeding after 10 min.
   d. If this fails, anesthetize mucous membrane by applying cotton soaked with a vasoconstrictor, such as 4% lidocaine (Xylocaine), Cocaine 4%, or Phenylephrine 0.25% for 5 min.
   e. Then apply a silver nitrate stick to bleeding site and any prominent vessels. Warn the patient this is painful.
   f. If bleeding still doesn't stop (rare), repeat last two steps. Then place a small amount of oxidized regenerated cellulose (Surgicel) against bleeding artery, or pack a small petroleum gauze strip in nasal vestibule for 24 hours. Monitor thepatient for vasovagal episode during the insertion of packing.
2. To control *posterior epistaxis*:
   a. Have the patient sit and lean forward.
   b. Control bleeding: Spray nose with topical anesthetic and vasoconstrictor, and apply pressure to bleeding site.
   c. **Consult a physician. The patient needs emergency room care immediately because of rapid blood loss.**
   d. Take blood pressure and pulse; order hematocrit; blood type and cross-match may be needed.

D. Pharmaceutical therapy: Drugs used to control bleeding (noted above).

Follow-up

A. Anterior nosebleeds are self-limited and require no follow-up.

B. For posterior nosebleeds, follow-up after hospital discharge.

Consultation/Referral

A. Posterior epistaxis: Consult or refer the patient to a physician immediately.

Individual Considerations

A. Pregnancy:
1. Nosebleeds are common.
2. Suggest use of saline spray to keep mucous membranes moist and humidifier at bedtime.
3. Follow use of saline spray with Vaseline applied with Q-tip daily to prevent recurrent nosebleeds.

B. Pediatric
1. Most common cause of nosebleeds is trauma from nose picking or rubbing.
2. Advise keeping fingernails short.
3. Applying water-based lubricant on rims of nostrils to maintain mucosal moisture may cause lipoid pneumonia in infants and children.

C. Geriatrics
1. Spontaneous posterior hemorrhage is more common in elderly patients.
2. Epistaxis is classically associated with hypertension or arteriosclerosis.

3. Airway obstruction from posterior packing is especially risky in elderly.
4. Applying water-based lubricant on rims of nostrils to maintain mucosal moisture may cause lipoid pneumonia in elderly.

NONALLERGIC RHINITIS

Definition
A. Nonallergic rhinitis is an inflammation of nasal mucous membranes, usually accompanied by a nasal discharge and mucosal edema. Nonallergic rhinitis disorder has no correlation to specific allergen exposures. It is classified in several ways: vasomotor, perennial, atrophic, geriatric, drug-induced, or rhinitis of pregnancy.

Incidence
A. Chronic or recurrent nasal congestion occurs in about 15%–20% of the population.

Pathogenesis
A. Vasomotor and perennial nonallergic rhinitis results from hyperreactive nasal mucosa.
B. Atrophic and geriatric rhinitis results from progressive degeneration and atrophy of the mucus membranes and bones of the nose.
C. Overuse of topical nasal decongestants can worsen symptoms and cause severe rebound congestion.
D. Cocaine abuse also causes nasal congestion and discharge.
E. Rhinitis in pregnancy results from hormonal increase; congestion abates with delivery.

Predisposing Factors
A. Adulthood
B. Abrupt changes in temperature, odors, and emotional stress
C. Other predisposing factors depend on type

Common Complaints
A. Nasal congestion
B. Sneezing
C. Clear rhinorrhea
D. Coughing
E. Sore throat
F. Itchy, puffy eyes

Subjective Data
A. Ask about onset, duration, and course of symptoms.
B. Inquire about the color and other characteristics of nasal discharge.
C. Ask about other discomforts and exposure to people with similar symptoms.
D. Inquire about seasonal impact on symptoms, previous treatments, and results.
E. Rule out pregnancy. Ask female patients about birth control method, specifically contraceptives.
F. Ask about use of prescription drugs, over-the-counter drugs (especially aspirin), and illicit drugs (cocaine).
G. Review medical history for other respiratory problems, such as asthma, emphysema, or chronic bronchitis.
H. With children, investigate possibility of a foreign object in nostrils.

Physical Examination
A. Temperature and blood pressure
B. Inspect
   1. Observe general appearance.
   2. Inspect conjunctivae for "allergic shiners" (dark circles under eyes), tearing, and eyelid swelling.
   3. Examine ears for signs of otitis media (red, bulging, perforated tympanic membrane, and purulent drainage).
   4. Examine nose for redness, swelling, polyps (soft, pedunculated, nontender, pale-gray smooth structures), enlarged turbinates, foreign objects, septal deviation, septal perforation (sign of cocaine abuse), ischemia, mucosal injury, atrophy, and "cobblestoned" pharyngeal mucosa (sign of allergy).
C. Auscultate: Auscultate lungs and heart.
D. Percuss
   1. Percuss sinus cavities and mastoid process.
   2. Percuss chest for consolidation.
E. Palpate
   1. Palpate face for sinus tenderness.
   2. Palpate head and neck for enlarged lymph nodes.

Diagnostic Tests
A. Skin testing for allergies may be done.

Differential Diagnoses
A. Nonallergic rhinitis
B. Allergic rhinitis
C. Upper respiratory infection
D. Foreign body
E. Sinusitis
F. Otitis media
G. Deviated septum
H. Nasal polyps
I. Endocrine conditions such as hypothyroidism and pregnancy
J. Drug use: oral contraceptives, aspirin, α-adrenergic blockers, cocaine, and nasal decongestant overuse

Plan
A. General interventions
   1. Avoid changes in temperature, odors, and emotional stress.
   2. Identify triggers for condition and address alleviating triggers.
B. Pharmaceutical therapy
   1. Vasomotor rhinitis: Physiologic saline solution as nasal spray, thorough cleansing of nares, topical ipratropium bromide, or inhaled ipratropium bromide (Atrovent) 3–6 puffs every 4 hours, not to exceed 12 inhalations per day.
   2. Atrophic rhinitis: guaifenesin (Guiatuss) 200 mg/5 mL, 10 mL orally every 4 hours, and physiologic saline nasal spray.
   3. Encourage use of Netty pot daily to cleanse sinus cavity. Cleansing sinus cavity daily will help to remove foreign materials inhaled and will also help with tissue edema.

Follow-up
A. Have patient return in 2 to 3 weeks and for biannual exams and/or as needed.

Consultation/Referral

A. Consult with a physician if symptoms continue despite treatment.

B. If treatment fails, refer the patient to allergist for testing.

Individual Consideration

A. Pregnancy: Reassure pregnant patients that rhinitis is a common hormonal response. Nonallergic rhinitis is not contagious and cannot cross the placenta.

SINUSITIS

Definition

Sinusitis is inflammation of mucous membranes lining paranasal sinuses. It may be acute, subacute, or chronic.

A. Acute sinusitis: abrupt onset of infection with symptom resolution after therapy.

B. Subacute sinusitis: persistent purulent nasal discharge despite therapy.

C. Chronic sinusitis: episodes of prolonged (greater than 3 months) inflammation and/or repeated or inadequately treated acute infections.

Incidence

A. Sinusitis is very prevalent. However, true incidence is unknown because people with frontal headaches or congestion self-medicate with over-the-counter (OTC) decongestants and then request antibiotics if symptoms persist. Incidence increases in spring and fall (allergy seasons) and in winter (cold season).

Pathogenesis

A. One cause is obstruction of mucus flow due to edema of nasal mucosa from allergies and upper respiratory infections.

B. Another cause is anatomical abnormalities that interfere with normal mucocilliary clearance mechanism.

C. Exposure to pathogens following URI also causes sinusitis. Pathogens include *Staphylococcus aureus, Haemophilus influenzae*, pneumococci, streptococci, and bacteroides. Incubation period depends on pathogen.

D. Dental abscess is a cause in 10% of cases.

E. Fungi such as *Mucor, Rhizopus*, and *Aspergillus* can produce invasive sinusitis in poorly controlled diabetics or people with leukemia.

F. Common cold is a cause in 0.5%–5.0% of cases.

Predisposing Factors

A. Recent upper respiratory infection (URI)

B. Allergens (pollens, molds, smoking, occupational exposure such as coal mining, and animal dander)

C. Nicotine/smoke exposure (first- or secondhand smoke)

D. Air pollutants

E. Deviated septum

F. Adenoidal hypertrophy

G. Dental abscess

H. Diving and swimming

I. Neoplasms

J. Cystic fibrosis

K. Trauma

L. Medical disorders (diabetes, immune disorders, inflammatory disorders, mucosal disorders, cystic fibrosis, and asthma)

M. Flying or rapid changes in altitude

Common Complaints

A. Yellow or green nasal discharge

B. Fever

C. Sore throat

D. Facial pain, frontal pain, or pressure that worsens when patient bends forward

E. Headache

F. Toothache

Other Signs and Symptoms

A. Nasal congestion

B. Purulent yellow or green drainage, color does not indicate bacterial infection

C. Cough (worse when lying down); may be chronic

D. Periorbital edema (especially early morning)

E. Malaise or fatigue

F. Halitosis

G. Snoring, mouth breathing

H. Nasal sounding speech

I. Anosmia (loss of sense of smell)

Potential Complications to Consider
Immediate ENT Referral

A. Meningitis (symptoms are increased fever, stiff neck)

B. Subdural and epidural purulent drainage

C. Brain abscess

D. Cavernous sinus thrombosis (acute thrombophlebitis due to infection in area where veins drain into cavernous sinus)

E. Tender periorbital edema (orbital cellulitis)

Subjective Data

A. Elicit onset, duration, and course of symptoms.

B. Inquire whether seasons affect symptoms.

C. Ask the patient about recent URI and how it was treated.
   1. Did the patient receive antibiotics?
   2. Did the patient finish the full course of antibiotics?

D. Ask about allergies.

E. Inquire about recent dental problems, especially dental abscesses.

F. Find out what home therapies and OTC medications the patient tried before the office visit.

G. Ask if the patient took a trip recently, especially by airplane.

H. With a child, look for a foreign object up the nose.

I. Inquire whether the patient was swimming or diving recently.

J. Review the patient's medical history for cystic fibrosis, asthma, nasal abnormalities (e.g., deviated septum), and other respiratory problems.

Physical Examination

A. Temperature, blood pressure, pulse, and respirations.

B. Inspect
   1. Observe eyes for periorbital swelling, "allergic shiners" (dark circles under eyes), tearing, and signs of orbital

cellulitis (conjunctival edema, drooping lid, decreased extraocular motion, and vision loss).

   2. Examine ears.

   3. Inspect the nose for erythema, edema, discharge, lack of nostril patency, septal deviation and polyps, and presence of a foreign body.

   4. Transilluminate in a darkened room maxillary and frontal sinuses. Absence of light reflection is not definitive.

   5. Examine the mouth and pharynx for erythema and tonsillar enlargement, check teeth for uneven surfaces (sign of grinding), and check retropharynx for evidence of postnasal drip.

C. Auscultate: Auscultate heart and lungs.

D. Palpate
   1. Palpate neck for lymphadenopathy.
   2. Palpate sinuses, but do not press on eyes.
      a. Frontal sinusitis: pain and tenderness over lower forehead (worse when bending forward) and purulent drainage from middle meatus of nasal turbinates.
      b. Maxillary sinusitis: pain and tenderness over cheeks from inner canthus to teeth (referred pain), edematous hard palate (severe cases), and purulent drainage in middle meatus.
      c. Ethmoid sinusitis: frontal or orbital headache, tenderness and erythema over upper lateral aspect of nose, drainage from anterior ethmoid cells through middle meatus, drainage of posterior cells through superior meatus.
      d. Sphenoid sinusitis (uncommon): frontal or orbital headache or facial pain (headache referred to top of head and deep into eyes), purulent drainage from superior meatus.

E. Percuss
   1. Tap maxillary teeth to rule out dental cause.
   2. Percuss maxillary and frontal sinuses and do chest percussion, if indicated.
   3. Percuss over affected area exacerbates pain.

F. Neurologic exam:
   1. Evaluate for signs of meningeal irritation, assessing for Brudzinski's sign, Kernig's sign, and nuchal rigidity.

Diagnostic Tests

A. **Diagnosis is usually made through history and physical.**

B. Consider sinus X-ray films, which show air-fluid level and thickening of sinus mucous membranes with sinusitis for chronic or recurrent sinusitis or complicated cases.

C. CT of sinuses indications include chronic sinusitis, recurrent sinusisits, allergic fungal sinusisits, or osteomeatal complex occusion.

Differential Diagnoses

A. Sinusitis
B. Headache (cluster, migraine)
C. Rhinitis (allergic or vasomotor)
D. Nasal polyps
E. Tumor
F. URI
G. Trigeminal neuralgia

Plan

A. General interventions: See below.

B. Patient teaching: See the Section III Patient Teaching Guide for this chapter, "Sinusitis."

C. Pharmaceutical therapy
   1. Antibiotics for infection
      a. Drugs of choice for acute sinusitis:
         i. Adults: Amoxilicillin 1000 mg three times a day for 10 days.
         ii. Penicillin allergy: Trimethoprim-sulfamethoxazole 160/800 mg twice a day for 10 days.
         iii. Doxycycline 100 mg twice daily for 10 days.
         iv. Children: Amoxil 80–90 mg/kg/day every 8 hours for 10–14 days v. Augmentin 80–90 mg/kg/day amoxil/ 6.4 mg /kg clavulatnate per day daily for 10–14 days.
      b. Other antibiotics for acute sinusitis:
         i. Adults: amoxicillin/clavulanate acid (Augmentin) 875/125 orally twice daily for 10–14 days.
         ii. Cefuroxime axetil (Ceftin) 250–500 mg twice daily for 14 days.
         iii. Levofloxacin (Levoquin) 500 mg by mouth once daily for 10 days.
         iv. Ciprofloxacin HCl (Cipro) 500 mg twice daily for 10 days.
         v. Azithromycin (Zithromax) 500 mg day 1, then 250 mg daily days 2–5.
         vi. Clarithromycin XR 1000 mg daily for 14 days.
         vii. Moxifloxacin (Avelox) 400 mg daily for 10 days.
      c. Children:
         i. Trimethoprim-sulfamethoxazole 8–12 mg/kg/day every 12 hours for 10 days.
         ii. Azithromycin (Zithromax) 10 mg/kg/day on day one, then 5 mg/kg/day days 2–5.
         iii. Clarithromycin 15mg/kg/day twice a day.
         iv. Levofloxacin (Levoquin) not used for children under 18 years.
      d. The same antibiotics can be used for chronic sinusitis, but treatment should last 3–4 weeks.

D. Oral and topical decongestants to correct the underlying edematous mucosa (use cautiously with hypertension).
   1. Adults and children older than 6 years: pseudoephedrine sulfate (Afrin) 0.05% spray or drops, two to three drops or sprays per nostril twice daily. Maximum for 3–5 days.
   2. Children 2–6 years: pseu-doephedrine sulfate (Afrin) 0.025% solution two to three drops per nostril twice daily. Use no longer than 3–5 days.
   3. Adults and children older than 12 years: phenylephrine (Neo-Synephrine) spray or drops, two to three drops or one to two sprays of 0.25% solution per nostril, or small amount of jelly to nasal mucosa, every 4 hours as needed. Do not use for more than 3–5 days.
   4. Pseudoephedrin HCl 60 mg every 4–6 hours as needed for congestion for adults.
   5. Nasal saline to nares three times daily as needed for hydrating nasal mucosa 0.25% solution spray or

drops, two to three drops or one to two sprays per nostril every 4 hours as needed. Do not use for more than 3–5 days.

    6. Children younger than 6 years: phenylephrine (Neo-Synephrine) 0.125% solution two to three drops every 4 hours per nostril as needed.

E. Steroid sprays may be used to decrease nasal inflammation:

    1. Beclomethasone dipropionate (Beconase AQ, Vancenase AQ); fluticasone (Flonase).

      a. Adults: 2 sprays daily.

      b. Children 4–12 years: 1 spray daily.

    2. Mometasone furoate monohydrate (Nasonex):

      a. Adults: 2 sprays daily.

      b. Children: 6–12 years: 1 spray daily.

F. Antihistimines are recommended to block histimine production in response to the allergy triggers and prevent allergy symptoms.

    1. Loratadine (Claritan) 10 mg daily for children over 6 years.

    2. Fexofenadine (Allegra) 180 mg daily in adults.

    3. Levocetirizine HCl(Xyzal) 5 mg daily for adults.

    4. Leukotriene inhibitors (Singulair, Accolate) may also be used for severe allergies and/or asthma.

G. Pediatric doses available on all products.

Follow-up

A. Recheck the patient in 3–4 days if signs and symptoms are not improving with use of treatment prescribed.

B. Recommend treatment for 10 days. For patients not improving may consider resistant to antibiotics and consider switching to different antibiotic for 14 days.

Consultation/Referral

A. Admission to hospital is needed if the patient has fever with facial cellulitis and mental changes.

B. Refer chronic sinusitis patients to an otolaryngologist if they do not improve in 4 weeks. They may need aspiration or surgery.

C. Refer to a physician or ENT for suspected neoplasm, abscess, osteomyelitis, meningitis, or sinus thrombosis.

Individual Considerations

A. Pediatrics: Children who present with normal to low-grade temperature and green mucous from nose for longer than 2 weeks, consider sinusitis.

B. Geriatrics:

    1. Precautionary measures should be used for patients with long-term nasogastric tubes. These patients are at higher risk for development of occult sinusitis.

    2. Precautions should be used with patients currently prescribed warfarin (Coumadin).

    3. Avoid use of TMP-SMX with warfarin due to the increase effect on the medication that can cause a significant increase in prothrombin time/international normalized ratio (PT/INR).

    4. Macrolides can also cause similar effects.

REFERENCES

Ferguson, B. J., Anon, J., Poole, M. D., Hendrick, K., Gilson, M., & Seltzer, E. G. (2002). Short treatment durations for acute bacterial rhinosinusitis: Five days of gemifloxacin versus 7 days of gemifloxacin. *Otolaryngology Head Neck Surgery, 127,* 1–6.

Luterman, M., Tellier, G., Lasko, B., & Leroy, B. (2003). Efficacy and tolerability of telithromycin for 5 or 10 days vs amoxicilllin/clavulanic acid for 10 days in acute maxillary sinusitis. *Ear Nose Throat Journal, 82,* 576–580, 582–584, 586.

CHAPTER 7

Throat and Mouth Guidelines

Jill C. Cash

AVULSED TOOTH

Definition
A. A tooth that has been completely displaced from its alveolar socket.

Incidence
A. Avulsion accounts for 0.5%–16% of all dental injuries to the permanent teeth. It occurs predominantly in children between ages 7 and 10. The upper central incisor is the most frequent tooth that is avulsed.

Pathogenesis
A. Trauma causes a tooth to be completely displaced from its alveolar socket.

Predisposing Factors
A. Erupting teeth are most susceptible to avulsion due to immature periodontal ligaments.

Common Complaints
A. Tooth displaced
B. Pain
C. Bleeding

Subjective Data
A. Ascertain the patient's age, and note if avulsed tooth is primary or permanent.
B. Determine time span the tooth has been avulsed (minutes or hours?).
C. Ask the patient about underlying cause or trauma. Are there any other injuries that need assessment, such as lacerations or concussion?

Physical Examination
A. Check temperature, pulse, respirations, and blood pressure.
B. Inspect
   1. Observe general appearance.
      a. Check for signs secondary to traumatic etiology, as necessary.
      b. Check to be sure patient is not in respiratory distress from aspirated tooth.
   2. Inspect gums and avulsed tooth, noting poor dental hygiene. **Do not touch root surface.**

Differential Diagnoses
A. Avulsed tooth
B. Luxation injuries: concussion and subluxation

Plan
A. Patient teaching: Tell the patient not to let tooth air-dry; it may cause permanent destruction of periodontal cells. Have him or her transport tooth in tooth socket, milk, or physiologic saline.
B. Medical and surgical management: If possible, replace tooth in socket, cover with gauze, and have the patient bite down on gauze during transport and prior to dental evaluation.

Follow-up
A. Follow-up is done with the dentist until stabilization is complete.

Consultation/Referral
A. Immediately refer the patient to a dentist or emergency room. Teeth replanted within 30 min have best prognosis. Teeth avulsed longer than 2 hours have a poor prognosis.

Individual Considerations
A. Pediatrics: Primary teeth do not need to be replaced.

DENTAL ABSCESS

Definition
A. A dental abscess is a space infection of the gingival or periodontal tissues.

Incidence
A. Incidence is unknown.

Pathogenesis
A. An abscess occurs when bacteria gain access into the gingiva or periodontal tissues.

Predisposing Factors
A. Poor dental hygiene
B. Dental caries

Common Complaints

A. Constant, severe jaw pain
B. Swelling
C. Difficulty chewing on tooth due to pain

Other Signs and Symptoms

A. Fever
B. Warmth, redness
C. Loss of appetite
D. Heat and cold sensitivity
E. Halitosis

Potential Complications

Risk of complications increases with valvular disease. The following are complications:

A. Sepsis
B. Leukocytosis associated with facial cellulitis

Subjective Data

A. Elicit information from the patient regarding onset, duration, location, and quality of pain.
B. Note radiation of pain as well as alleviating or aggravating factors.
C. Note if pain is brought on by contact with hot, cold, or sweet substances; this may indicate periapical abscess or dental caries.
D. Ask if the patient has a fever. If so, how high and for how long?
E. Inquire about history of mitral valve prolapse or rheumatic fever.

Physical Examination

A. Check temperature, pulse, respirations, and blood pressure.
B. Inspect
   1. Inspect teeth for caries, mobility of teeth or protrusion from sockets, and gum disease.
   2. Examine teeth for erosion, enamel decalcification, diminished tooth size, discoloration, and sensitivity to temperature changes.
C. Palpate neck and submental area for enlarged, tender lymph nodes.
D. Percuss all teeth. Tenderness is diagnostic of an abscess.
E. Auscultate heart, if indicated.

Diagnostic Tests

A. None usually required.
B. WBC, if cellulitis is suspected.

Differential Diagnoses

A. Dental abscess
B. Periodontal disease
C. Cellulitis

Plan

A. General interventions: Advise patient to apply a heating pad to painful facial area for comfort. Advise soft diet until pain resolves.
B. Pharmaceutical therapy
   1. Drug of choice: penicillin V potassium (Pen-Vee-K) 250–500 mg orally every 6 hours while the patient awaits dental consultation.

2. Other medications:
   a. Cephalexin (Keflex) 500 mg every 6 hours until dental consultation.
   b. Clindamycin (Cleocin) 300 mg orally every 6 hours until dental consultation.
3. For discomfort and fever: ibuprofen (Advil) 400–600 mg orally every 6–8 hours, not to exceed 1,200 mg/day.

Follow-up

A. Follow up 2–3 days after dental exam to evaluate results.

Consultation/Referral

A. Advise the patient to see a dentist promptly, even if pain resolves.

Individual Considerations

A. Pregnancy
   1. Patients may safely have dental procedures during pregnancy.
   2. X-ray films may be taken with lead shield over patient's abdomen.
   3. Epinephrine and nitrous oxide should not be used during dental procedures.
   4. Tetracycline should not be used; it causes staining of fetal bones and teeth.

EPIGLOTTITIS

Definition

A. Epiglottitis is inflammation and swelling of the epiglottis and is a medical emergency.

Incidence

A. Epiglottitis usually occurs in children between ages 2–8 years, but it may also occur in adults. Incidence has decreased dramatically since the *Haemophilus influenzae* vaccine was introduced.

Pathogenesis

A. Epiglottitis is almost always caused by *H. influenzae,* although *Streptococcus pneumoniae* and *Streptococcus pyogenes* have also been implicated.

Predisposing Factors

A. Upper respiratory infection

Common Complaints

A. Sudden onset of fever
B. Sudden onset of dysphagia
C. Sudden onset of drooling
D. Sudden onset of muffled voice

Other Signs and Symptoms

A. Respiratory distress
B. Stridor
C. Very ill appearance

Subjective Data

A. Determine onset, duration, and course of illness.
B. Is child's breathing labored?

C. Are the child's breathing problems affecting his or her ability to eat or drink?

D. Has he or she had a fever?

E. Has he or she had trouble swallowing or talking?

Physical Examination

A. Temperature, pulse, respirations and blood pressure.

B. Inspect
   1. Observe overall appearance.
   2. Check nail beds and lips for cyanosis.
   3. Note drooling or difficulty swallowing.
   4. Note breathing pattern and rhythm.
   5. Do not examine throat—airway occlusion may result.

C. Auscultate: Auscultate heart and lungs.

Diagnostic Tests

A. Lateral neck radiograph confirms diagnosis. However, this test may delay establishment of airway.

Differential Diagnoses

A. Epiglottitis

B. Bacterial tracheitis (a pediatric emergency)

C. Viral croup

D. Foreign body aspiration

E. Retropharyngeal abscess

Plan

A. Medical/surgical management
   1. Immediate admission to hospital.
   2. While awaiting transport to hospital, establish patent airway, start oxygen, and assemble airway equipment. Move child as little as possible.
   3. Insert intravenous access for fluids and antibiotic administration.
   4. If respiratory arrest occurs, you may not be able to see the airway to intubate. An AMBU bag and mask may work temporarily, but nasogastric (NG) tube insertion may be necessary to prevent gastric distension.
   5. Prompt recognition and appropriate treatment usually results in rapid resolution of swelling and inflammation.

B. Pharmaceutical therapy
   1. IV fluids.
   2. Antibiotics; IV antibiotics after physician consultation.
   3. Obtain blood and epiglotis cultures prior to starting antibioitics.
   4. Drug of choice:
      a. Cefotaxime (Claforan) 100–200 mg/kg/day every 8 hours IV.
      b. Ceftriaxone (Rocephin) 50–100 mg/kg/day every 12 hours IV.
      c. Ampicillin-sulbactam (Unasyn) 150 mg/kg/day every 6 hours IV.
      d. Amoxicillin-clavulanate acid 100 mg/kg/day every 8 hours IV.
   5. May give Tylenol as needed.

Follow-up

A. Follow-up care occurs in the hospital.

B. An airway specialist should evaluate the patient in the operating room.

Consultation/Referral

A. If you suspect epiglottitis, refer the patient to a physician immediately.

ORAL CANCER, LEUKOPLAKIA

Definition

A. Oral cancer is cancer of the buccal mucosa, tongue, gingiva, hard palate, soft palate, or lips. White patches, known as leukoplakia, or red, velvety patches, known as erythroplakia, on the buccal mucosa may indicate premalignant lesions.

Incidence

A. Oral cancer is primarily seen in the elderly. Male-to-female predominance is 2:1.

B. There are 30,000 new cases each year and 8,000 deaths each year.

C. Oral cancer represents 3% of all newly diagnosed cancers and 2% of all cancer-related deaths.

D. Frequency of oral cancer of cheek and gum rises 50-fold among long-term users of smokeless tobacco.

Pathogenesis

Pathogenesis is unknown; 50% of oral cancers already have metastasized at time of diagnosis. The following factors are involved.

A. Use of tobacco in all its forms is highly correlated with risk of oral cancer.

B. Risk of oral cancer also is high with heavy alcohol consumption. Whether this is due to a direct effect of alcohol on the oral mucosa or to associated smoking or vitamin deficiency remains unclear.

C. Chronic iron deficiency leading to Plummer-Vinson syndrome is known to alter mucosal tissues, and this change may be related to increased oral cancer. Research has shown that a diet low in fruits and vegetables contributes to oral cancer.

D. Epstein-Barr virus and papillomavirus have been found in cells of the tongue manifesting oral hairy leukoplakia, a hyperplastic change found in AIDS patients. HPV is found in approximately 20%–30% of cases of oral cancer.

E. Occupational hazards also exist from sun exposure. It is estimated that 30% of those with oral cancer worked outdoors.

Predisposing Factors

A. Male gender

B. Age over 40 years for men, over 50 years for women

C. African American ancestry

D. Smoking or use of other tobacco products, including such smokeless products as snuff and dip

E. Alcohol consumption

F. Sun exposure

G. Poor diet, deficient in vitamins A, C, and E and high in salted or smoked meats, fats, and oils

H. Previous cancer

Common Complaints

A. Oral sores that do not heal; this is what most commonly leads patients to seek medical care

B. Poorly fitting dentures

C. Bleeding mucosa or gingiva without apparent cause

D. Difficulty swallowing, usually indicates more advanced disease

E. Altered sensations: burning or numbness, usually indicates more advanced disease

F. Leukoplakia or erythroplakia

Other Signs and Symptoms

A. No symptoms, possibly

B. Decreased appetite related to altered taste

C. Increased salivation

D. Sore throat

E. Foul breath odor

F. Neck mass

Subjective Data

A. Review onset, course, and duration of symptoms. Question the patient regarding altered taste, sensations, difficulty swallowing, and foul breath.

B. Evaluate for risk factors. See predisposing factors.

C. Ask the patient about previous history of cancer and treatments.

D. Review the patient's use of tobacco products, including age of onset, amount of daily use, and quit dates.

E. Evaluate amount of alcohol intake, including age of onset, amount of daily use, and quit dates.

F. Review the patient's general health history for other chronic conditions.

G. Review medication history, including prescription and OTC drug use, especially aspirin.

H. Take dental history, including previous gum surgery, how long ago dentures were fitted, and if they always fit well.

I. Establish usual weight. Is there any weight loss related to altered taste, and if so, how much and in what length of time?

Physical Examination

A. Check temperature, pulse, respirations, blood pressure, and weight.

B. Inspect
1. Observe general appearance.
2. Note quality of voice patterns.
3. Note odor of breath.
4. Inspect lips, gums, tongue, buccal mucosa for swelling, discoloration, bleeding, asymmetry, leukoplakia, and erythroplasia. Take out dentures first.
   a. Leukoplakia ranges from slightly raised, white, translucent areas to dense, white, opaque plaques, with or without adjacent ulceration. Normal intraoral mucosa is pinkish or salmon-colored.
   b. Mucosal erythroplasia is red, inflammatory, or erythroplastic mucosal changes. It appears smooth, granular, and minimally elevated, with or without leukoplakia, and it persists more than 14 days.
   c. Erythroplakia may mimic inflammatory lesions, but it can be differentiated by failure of the affected area to blanch with light pressure. **Erythroplakia is a malignant change seen as red, velvety, plaquelike lesion on mucous membrane.**

d. Other oral lesions appear black, blue, or brown.

e. Approximately 90% of cancers are squamous cell carcinomas, and most occur in sites accessible by clinical examination: tongue, oropharynx (soft palate, lingual aspect of retro-molar trigone, anterior tonsillar pillar), and floor of mouth.

f. Cancer of lip is a lesion that fails to heal.

g. Signs and symptoms of cancer of tongue are swelling, ulceration, areas of tenderness or bleeding, abnormal texture, and limited movement.

C. Palpate
1. Palpate mouth for masses. Try to remove or scrape patches.
2. Palpate lymph nodes: cervical (anterior/posterior chain), submandibular, sublingual, and submental, pre/postauricular; check nodes for size, firmness, and tenderness.

D. Auscultate lungs and heart. The lungs are the most frequently involved extranodal metastatic site.

Diagnostic Tests

A. HIV, if indicated.

B. Staining of oral lesion with toluidine blue: lesion stains dark blue after rinsing with acetic acid. Normal tissue does not absorb the stain.

C. Biopsy for persistent lesions (more than 2 weeks): essential to differentiate from blue-black lesion of malignant melanoma.

D. Chest radiography to rule out metastasis.

E. Consider CT, MRI, or bone scan to rule out metastasis.

Differential Diagnoses

A. Oral leukoplakia

B. Pulpitis

C. Periapical abscess

D. Gingivitis

E. Periodontitis

F. Lichen planus

G. Oral candidiasis

H. Discoid lupus

I. Pemphigus vulgaris

Plan

A. General interventions
1. Advise the patient to stop smoking and stop using oral tobacco products.
2. Advise the patient to decrease alcohol consumption.
3. Encourage routine dental care and exams.

B. Pharmaceutical therapy: Erythroplakia does not respond to antifungal therapy.

Follow-up

A. If immediate biopsy is not indicated, ask the patient to return for reevaluation in 2 weeks, after eliminating irritants and noxious agents.

Consultation/Referral

A. Refer the patient to an otolaryngologist and/or dentist for immediate biopsy for deeply ulcerative or fungating lesions. Follow-up treatment may include one or more of following: wide excision, radical neck dissection, radiation, and chemotherapy.

Individual Considerations

A. Pediatrics
   1. Currently, the highest rate is in smokeless tobacco use.
   2. Oral screening should be considered annually in adolescents who use tobacco and/or alcohol.
B. Adults: The American Cancer Society recommends that people between age 20 and 40 years undergo an oral cancer screening every 3 years, and that those over age 40 years be screened every year. Oral screening should be considered annually in adults who use tobacco and/or alcohol.

Patient Resources

Oral Cancer Foundation: http://oralcancerfoundation.org/
American Cancer Society: www.cancer.org
National Cancer Institute: www.cancer.gov
American Academy of Family Physicians: www.aafp.org

PHARYNGITIS

Definition

A. Pharyngitis is inflammation of the pharynx and surrounding lymph tissue.

Incidence

A. Pharyngitis is the fourth most common symptom seen in medical practice.

Pathogenesis

Pharyngitis may be due to viral, bacterial, and fungal agents, as well as other atypical agents.

A. Viral agents include coxsackievirus, ECHO viruses, and Epstein-Barr virus.
B. Bacterial agents include Group A β-hemolytic streptococcus, *Neisseria gonorrhoeae,* and *Corynebacterium diphtheriae.*
C. The fungal source is *Candida albicans.*
D. Atypical agent include *Mycoplasma pneumoniae* and *Chlamydia trachomatis* (rare).
E. Noninfectious causes include allergic rhinitis, postnasal drip, mouth breathing, and trauma.

Predisposing Factors

A. Cigarette smoking
B. Allergies
C. Upper respiratory infections
D. Oral sex
E. Drugs (antibiotics and immunosuppressants)
F. Debilitating illnesses (such as cancer) that can cause *Candida albicans* to proliferate

Common Complaints

A. Common complaints are sore and/or scratchy throat
B. Fever
C. Headache
D. Malaise

Other Signs and Symptoms

A. Oral vesicles
B. Exudate on throat
C. Lymphadenopathy
D. Fatigue
E. Dysphasia
F. Abdominal pain
G. Vomiting

Potential Complications

Without proper antimicrobial treatment, streptococcal pharyngitis can lead to serious complications such as the following:

A. Suppurative adenitis with tender, enlarged lymph nodes
B. Scarlet fever
C. Peritonsillar abscess
D. Glomerulonephritis
E. Rheumatic fever

Subjective Data

A. Ask the patient about onset, course, and duration of symptoms. Ask about dyspnea or dysphagia.
B. Inquire about mouth lesions, rhinorrhea, cough, drooling, and fever.
C. Ask about malaise, headache, fatigue, and fever; these are symptoms of mononucleosis.
D. Take a sexual history, if indicated. Ask if family members or sexual partners have the same signs and symptoms. Pharyngeal gonorrhea has no symptoms, so high-risk patients should be tested.
E. Ask whether symptoms have caused decreased intake of food and fluid.
F. Determine history of heart disease; previous strep pharyngitis; rheumatic fever; and other respiratory diseases, such as asthma, emphysema, and chronic allergies.
G. If rash is present, find out when it first occurred and if it has spread.
H. Ask about signs and symptoms of urinary tract infection and pyelonephritis.
I. Ask about a history of herpes, immunosuppressive disorders, and steroid use.
J. Review immunization history.

Physical Examination

A. Temperature and blood pressure, if indicated.
B. Inspect
   1. Observe general appearance.
   2. Examine the mouth, pharynx, tonsils, and hard and soft palate for vesicles and ulcers, candidal patches, erythema, hypertrophy, exudate, and stomatitis. Check gum and palate for petechiae and tongue for color and inflammation.
      a. Herpangina are small oral vesicles on the fauces and soft palate caused by the coxsackievirus.
      b. Herpes causes vesicles and small ulcers (stomatitis) of the buccal mucosa, tongue, and pharynx.
      c. Trench mouth (gingivitis) and necrotic tonsillar ulcers (Vincent's angina) cause foul breath, pain, pharyngeal exudate, and a gray membranous inflammation that bleeds easily.
      d. *Candida albicans* (thrush) may be painful and causes cheesy, white exudate.
      e. Oral candidiasis may be the first symptom of HIV.
      f. Peritonsillar cellulitis causes inflamed, edematous tonsils; grayish-white exudate, high fever, rigors, and leukocytosis. Peritonsillar abscess (palpable-mass) may also develop.

g. Mononucleosis causes tonsillar exudates in 50% of patients; 33% develop petechiae at junction of hard and soft palate.

h. *Corynebacterium diphtheriae* causes a whitish-blue pharyngeal exudate "pseudomembrane" that covers the pharynx and bleeds if removal is attempted.

3. Examine the ears, nose, and throat.

4. Inspect skin for rashes.

a. Pastia's lines are petechiae present in a linear pattern along major skin folds in axillae and antecubital fossa that are seen with group A strep.

b. Erythema marginatum, caused by group A streptococcus, is an evanescent, nonpruritic, pink rash mainly on the trunk and extremities. It may be brought out by heat application.

C. Auscultate: Auscultate heart and lungs.

D. Percuss
1. Percuss abdomen, especially spleen area.
2. Percuss chest.

E. Palpate
1. Palpate lymph nodes, especially of the anterior and posterior cervical chains, axilla, and groin.
2. Palpate abdomen for organomegaly and suprapubic tenderness.
3. Palpate back for costovertebral angle (CVA) tenderness.

F. Neurologic exam: Check for nuchal rigidity and meningeal irritation.

Diagnostic Tests

A. Rapid strep test; if negative, then perform throat culture and sensitivity. **Throat culture and sensitivity is gold standard for diagnosis.**

B. Monospot test

C. CBC with differential

D. Gonorrhea culture

E. Blood cultures if sepsis is suspected

F. Radiograph of neck if possible trauma

Differential Diagnoses

A. Pharyngitis
B. Stomatitis
C. Rhinitis
D. Sinusitis with postnasal drip
E. Epiglottis
F. Peritonsillar abscess
G. Mononucleosis
H. Herpes simplex
I. Coxsackie A virus
J. *Corynebacterium diphtheriae*
K. Trench mouth
L. Vincent's angina
M. *Candida albicans*
N. HIV

Plan

A. General interventions
1. Patients with a history of rheumatic fever and those who have a household member with a documented group A streptococcal infection need immediate treatment without prior testing or even an office visit.

2. Assess patency of airway if tonsils are enlarged.
3. Do not put instruments in airway if you suspect epiglottitis.

B. Patient teaching: See the Section III Patient Teaching Guide for this chapter, "Pharyngitis."

C. Pharmaceutical therapy
1. Drug of choice: prescribe one of the following penicillins for possible and diagnosed strep throat.
   a. Penicillin V potassium (Pen-Vee-K)
      i. Adults and children more than 60 pounds: 250–500 mg orally three or four times daily for 10 days.
      ii. Children less than 40 pounds: 25–50 mg/kg/day three times daily for 10 days.
   b. Penicillin G benzathine combined with penicillin G procaine (Bicillin C-R)
      i. Adults and children more than 60 pounds: 1.8–2.4 million units in one dose by IM injection.
      ii. Children less than 60 pounds: 600,000 units in one dose by IM injection.

2. If the patient is allergic to penicillin:
   a. Adults: erythromycin (E-Mycin) 250 mg orally every 6 hours for 10 days.
   b. Adults: cefadroxil (Duricef) 500 mg orally twice daily for 10 days.
   c. Children younger than 12 years: erythromycin (E-Mycin) 40 mg/kg/day in dividedoral doses four times daily for 10 days.
   d. Children more than 40 pounds: erythromycin ethylsuccinate (E.E.S.) 250 mg orally four times daily for 10 days.

3. For pharyngeal gonorrhea
   a. Adults: ceftriaxone (Rocephin) 500 mg–1 g by IM injection.
   b. Children: ceftriaxone (Rocephin) 50–75 mg/kg in one dose by IM injection.

4. For *Mycoplasma pneumoniae* and *Chlamydia trachomatis*: erythromycin (E-Mycin) 250 mg orally three to four times daily for 10 days.

5. For pharyngeal candidiasis in the immunocompromised patient:
   a. Oral nystatin suspension (100,000 U/mL) 15 mL by swish-and-swallow method four times a day.
   b. Clotrimazole troche 10 mg held in mouth 15 to 30 min three times daily.

Follow-up

A. If symptoms do not improve in 3–4 days, recheck patient.

B. Do throat culture after treatment to see if patients with streptococcal pharyngitis are cured.

C. Treat sexual partners of patients with pharyngeal gonorrhea.

Consultation/Referral

A. Consult physician if patient has severe dysphagia or dyspnea, signaling possible airway obstruction.

B. Refer the patient to an otolaryngologist if peritonsillar abscess is noted.

Individual Considerations
A. Pediatrics
   1. Rheumatic fever follows between 0.5%–3% of ineffectively treated cases of group A streptococcal URIs.
   2. Twenty percent of children aged 5–15 years who are diagnosed with rheumatic fever had pharyngitis in the preceding 3 months.

STOMATITIS, MINOR RECURRENT APHTHOUS STOMATITIS

Definition
A. Stomatitis is tender, round, discrete, oval, shallow, 1- to 5-mm ulcers in the oral cavity. The ulcers are gray-white or yellow, on nonkeratinized skin, and surrounded by erythematous halos. They typically involve the labial and buccal mucosa and tongue, and adjacent tissue appears healthy.
B. Major recurrent aphthous stomatitis (RAS) has larger, deeper ulcers; lasts a longer period of time; usually recurs up to four times a year; and frequently leaves scars. It can cause significant dysphagia.

Incidence
A. Stomatitis affects 20%–50% of the population. It is very common in North America.

Pathogenesis
A. Cause is poorly understood. Genetic, immunologic, viral, or nutritional causes are possible.

Predisposing Factors
A. Minor trauma
B. History of recurrent aphthous stomatitis
C. Possible nutritional deficiency of iron, folic acid, or zinc
D. Hormonal changes

Common Complaints
A. Painful sore in mouth

Other Signs and Symptoms
A. Burning sensation in mouth for 24–48 hours before lesions appear

Subjective Data
A. Elicit history of aphthous stomatitis.
B. Ask the patient about prodrome of burning or stinging in the mouth.
C. Illicit information regarding previous illness and trauma.

Physical Examination
A. Check temperature, pulse, respirations, and blood pressure.
B. Inspect
   1. Inspect mouth for ulcers.
   2. Inspect ears, nose, and throat.
   3. Inspect skin, especially palms and soles, for lesions; indicates hand-foot-and-mouth disease
C. Auscultate
   1. Auscultate heart.
   2. Auscultate lungs.

Differential Diagnoses
A. Aphthous stomatitis
B. Herpetic stomatitis
C. Behçet's disease
D. Crohn's disease
E. HIV
F. Kawasaki syndrome
G. Hand-foot-and-mouth disease

Plan
A. Patient teaching: See the Section III Patient Teaching Guide for this chapter, "Aphthous Stomatitis."
B. Dietary management
   1. Advise patient to avoid spicy, salty, and hot foods.
   2. Suggest the patient use a straw when drinking to decrease pain.
C. Pharmaceutical therapy
   1. Mouthwash made of diphenhydramine (Benadryl), with Kaopectate, or Maalox or sucralfate, and viscous lidocaine three to four times a day. Leave out lidocaine when using in children. Tell the patient not to swallow medication.
   2. Sucralfate (Carafate) suspension 1 tsp four times a day may be used to swish in mouth and spit out for oral comfort.
   3. Glucocorticoid gel such as fluocinonide gel (Lidex) 0.05% two to four times a day, one of which is always at bedtime.
   4. Orabase with or without triamcinolone acetonide (Kenalog).

Follow-up
A. Follow-up as needed for treatment of recurrences.

Consultation/Referral
A. Refer the patient to or consult with a physician if ulcers are deeper or larger than 1–5 mm, if Kawasaki disease is suspected, or if no improvement is seen with adequate treatment.
B. Any lesion lasting longer than 3 weeks should be evaluated by a dentist or oral surgeon to rule out cancer.

Individual Considerations
A. Pregnancy: Avoid use of fluocinonide and triamcinolone acetonide (Kenalog) in pregnant or nursing women.
B. Pediatrics
   1. Avoid use of fluocinonide and triamcinolone acetonide (Kenalog).
   2. Do not use viscous lidocaine.

THRUSH

Definition
A. Thrush is oral candidiasis—an infection of the oral cavity and/or the pharynx caused by *Candida*.

Incidence
A. Thrush mainly affects bottle-fed infants; occasionally, debilitated older children are affected. Breast-fed infants may also be affected.

Pathogenesis

A. *Candida albicans* is normally not invasive unless the mouth is abraded.

Predisposing Factors

A. Use of broad-spectrum antibiotics
B. Adults:
  1. Human immunodeficiency virus
  2. Prolonged steroid use (systemic or inhaled cortico-steroids)
  3. Cancer treatments (radiation/chemotherapy)
  4. Dentures
  5. Malnutrition
C. Children:
  1. Endocrine disorders (thyroid disease, diabetes mellitus, and Addison's disease)
  2. HIV
  3. Cancer

Common Complaints

A. Soreness, pain of the mouth

Other Signs and Symptoms

A. Irritability in infants
B. Refusal to eat in infants
C. White plaques coating buccal mucosa

Subjective Data

A. Determine onset, duration, and course of illness.
B. Ask if the child refuses to eat.
C. Has the patient used antibiotics or other medications in the previous weeks?
D. Does the patient use inhaled or systemic steroid on a daily basis?

Physical Examination

A. Check temperature, pulse, respirations, and blood pressure.
B. Inspect
  1. Inspect oral cavity for white, curdlike plaques that cannot be removed.
  2. Inspect ears, nose, and throat.
  3. Inspect genital area for red rash and satellite papular lesions.

Differential Diagnoses

A. Thrush
B. Milk deposits on tongue or buccal mucosa
C. Stomatitis
D. Aphthous ulcer
E. Hairy leukoplakia

Plan

A. General interventions
  1. If the patient is breast-feeding, instruct the mother to clean breasts and nipples well with warm water between feedings to prevent contamination. Consider prescribing antifungal cream to be applied to breasts; this should be washed off before feedings.
  2. If bottle feeding, boil all bottles, nipples, and pacifiers to kill the organism.
B. Patient teaching: See the Section III Patient Teaching Guide for this chapter, "Oral Thrush."
C. Dietary management
  1. Have caregiver feed infant temporarily with a cup and spoon.
  2. Tell caregiver to keep infant well-hydrated.
D. Medical management
  1. Instruct caregiver to attempt removal of large plaques with a moistened cotton-tipped applicator and/or small, moist gauze pad.
  2. If thrush is recurrent or resistant, consider checking the mother for candidial vaginitis.
  3. Instruct the patient/family on proper use and cleaning/rinsing of inhalers/dentures to prevent reoccurrence of thrush.
E. Pharmaceutical therapy
  1. Oral candidiasis: nystatin (Mycostatin) oral suspension 1 mL four times a day for 1 week. Place medication in front of mouth on each side. Rub directly on plaques with a cotton swab. Adults: pastilles: 200,000 units lozenge four times a day for 14 days, or swish-and-swallow 500,000 units four times a day for 14 days or two 500,000 unit tabs three times daily for 14 days.
  2. Clotrimazole troche (Mycelex) : 10 mg 5 times daily for 14 days, monitor for side effects.
  3. Fluconazole: Adults: 200 mg × 1, then 100 mg daily for 5–7 days. Children: 5 mg/kg by mouth every day for 5 days or 6–12 mg/kg on first day, then 3–6 mg/kg for 10 days.
  4. Genital candidal dermatitis: nystatin cream 3–4 times a day for 7–10 days. Have caregiver discontinue use of all baby wipes, lotions, powders, and creams.

Follow-up

A. Instruct caregiver to telephone the office if the child refuses to eat, if there is no improvement, if thrush lasts more than 10 days, or if there is unexplained fever.

Consultation/Referral

A. Consult a physician if thrush does not resolve with adequate antifungal treatment.

REFERENCES

American Academy of Pediatrics. (2010). *2009 Red Book Online: Report of the Committee on Infectious Diseases.* Elk Grove Village, IL: American Academy of Pediatrics.

Beischer, N. A., & Mackay, E. V. (1986). *Obstetrics and the newborn* (2nd ed.). Philadelphia: W. B. Saunders.

Hoyle, C. (2009). Make your strep diagnosis spot on. *The Nurse Practitioner, 34,* 46–52.

King, J. (2009). Infectious mononucleosis: Update and considerations. *The Nurse Practitioner, 34,* 42–45.

Respiratory Guidelines

Cheryl A. Glass

◖ ASTHMA

Definition

Asthma is chronic airway inflammation characterized by recurrent episodes of wheezing, breathlessness, chest tightness, and cough, particularly at night and in the early morning. Episodes are associated with widespread, variable, often reversible airflow obstruction and bronchial hyper-responsiveness when airways are exposed to various stimuli or triggers. Asthma is responsible for lost school days, lost productivity, and presenteeism.

Asthma is classified four ways:

A. *Step 1—Mild intermittent:* Symptoms less than or equal to two/week; asymptomatic with normal peak expiratory flow rate (PEFR) between attacks; nighttime symptoms less than or equal to two/month; PEFR greater than 80% predicted with variability less than 20%.
B. *Step 2—Mild persistent:* Symptoms greater than two/week but less than one/day; exacerbations may affect activity; nighttime symptoms greater than two/month; PEFR greater than or equal to 80% predicted with variability 20%–30%.
C. *Step 3—Moderate persistent:* Daily symptoms requiring β_2 agonist use; attacks affect activity; exacerbations greater than or equal to two/week; nighttime symptoms greater than one/week; PEFR greater than 60% and greater than 80% predicted with variability greater than 30%.
D. *Step 4—Severe persistent:* Continuous symptoms with limited physical activity; frequent exacerbations; frequent nighttime symptoms; PEFR less than or equal to 60% predicted with greater than 30% variability.

Incidence

A. Asthma affects 16.4 million people in the United States. It is the most common chronic disease of childhood, affecting about 4.8 million children.

Pathogenesis

A. Asthma arises from a complex cycle of processes initiated by airway inflammation resulting from physical, chemical, and pharmacologic agents (such as environmental irritants, allergens, furry animals, cockroaches, dust mites, pollens and mold, cold air, viral respiratory infections, and exercise). It progresses to airway hyper-responsiveness, bronchoconstriction, airway wall edema, chronic mucus plug formation, and chronic airway remodeling.

Predisposing Factors

A. In children:
 1. Allergy or family history of allergy
 2. Atopy
B. In adults:
 1. Family history
 2. Coexisting sinusitis, nasal polyps, and sensitivity to aspirin or other nonsteroidal anti-inflammatory drugs (NSAIDs)
 3. Exposure in workplace to wood dust, metals, and animal products
 4. Premenstrual asthma (PMA)
C. In all ages:
 1. Inhalation of irritants such as tobacco smoke
 2. Viral respiratory infections
 3. Gastroesophageal reflux

Common Complaints

A. Recurrent cough (worse at night and early morning)
B. Recurrent wheezing
C. Recurrent shortness of breath
D. Recurrent chest tightness (may worsen with moderate activity)

Other Signs and Symptoms

A. Nocturnal awakening from symptoms
B. Variation of symptoms with seasons or environment
C. Chest discomfort, tightness with moderate activity

Subjective Data

A. Ask about onset, duration, and course of symptoms.
B. Inquire about sudden severe episodes of coughing, wheezing, and shortness of breath and whether precipitating factors can be identified.
C. Ask whether the patient has chest colds that take more than 10 days to resolve.

D. Ask whether symptoms seem to occur during certain seasons or during exposure to environmental irritants (such as tobacco smoke, perfume, or household pets).

E. Find out how often coughing, wheezing, or shortness of breath awakens the patient.

F. Ask if symptoms are caused or exacerbated by moderate exercise or physical activity.

G. Determine the family history of asthma, allergies, and eczema.

H. Determine if the patient is pregnant or has other medical problems. If so, do not prescribe β_2 adrenergics and use NSAIDs cautiously. The safest medications are Cromolyn sodium and anticholinergic drugs.

I. Administer the Asthma Control Test for adults or the Childhood Asthma Control Test for children ages 4–11 years. Both tests are available online from www.asthma control.com.

Physical Examination

A. Temperature, blood pressure, pulse and respirations. Obtain weight if failure to thrive is suspected.

B. Inspect
1. Especially in children, observe for hyper-expansion of thorax and signs that accessory muscles are being used (retractions, nasal flaring) or stridor.
2. Note appearance of hunched shoulders and/or chest deformity.
3. In children, inspect the nose for a foreign body.
4. In all patients, inspect ears, nose, and throat. Evaluate the presence of enlarged tonsils and adenoids, and nasal polyps.
5. Inspect skin for eczema, dermatitis, or other irritation that might signal allergy.
6. Observe for allergic shiners and pebbled conjunctiva.
7. Observe for digital clubbing.

C. Auscultate
1. Auscultate lung sounds. Note wheezing during normal expiration and prolonged expiration, which is seen with asthma.
2. Listen to all lung fields for an asymmetric wheeze.
3. Auscultate heart rate.

D. Percuss: Percuss lung fields.

Diagnostic Tests

A. Forced vital capacity (FVC) and forced expiratory volume (FEV_1) before and after the patient inhales a short-acting bronchodilator.

B. Chest radiograph and complete blood count (CBC) to exclude other diagnoses and infection.

C. Allergy testing is recommended for children with persistent asthma.

D. PEFR after inhalation of short-acting β_2 agonist. Diagnosis is confirmed if:
1. There is a 15% increase in PEFR after 15–20 min.
2. PEFR varies more than 20% between arising and 12 hours later in patients taking bronchodilators (or 10% without bronchodilators).
3. There is a greater than 15% decrease in PEFR after 6 min of running or exercise.

E. Consider a bronchial provocation test with histamine or methacholine for nondiagnostic spirometry.

Differential Diagnoses

A. In infants and children:
1. Asthma
2. Pulmonary infections
   a. Pneumonia
   b. Respiratory syncytial virus (RSV)
   c. Viral bronchiolitis
   d. Tuberculosis
3. Allergic rhinitis and sinusitis
4. Foreign body in the nose
5. Gastroesophageal reflux disease (GERD)
6. Cystic fibrosis
7. Bronchopulmonary dysplasia
8. Vocal cord dysfunction
9. Enlarged lymph nodes or tumors

B. In adults:
1. Asthma
2. Chronic obstructive pulmonary disease (COPD)
3. Gastroesophageal reflux disease (GERD)
4. Congestive heart failure (CHF)
5. Cough secondary to medications such as Angiotensin converting enzyme (ACE) inhibitors or β-blockers
6. Pneumonia
7. Pulmonary embolism
8. Laryngeal dysfunction
9. Benign and malignant tumors
10. Vocal cord dysfunction

Plan

A. General interventions
1. Review proper medication dosages. Short- and long-term agents come in several formulations, nebulizer, metered-dose inhaler (MDI), and a dry powder inhaler (DPI). Young children should have medication via nebulizer using an appropriate size face mask. The use the "blow-by" technique is not an appropriate means of administering medication.
2. Demonstrate correct use of inhalers, spacers, and nebulizer. If the patient does not use correct technique when using these devices, medication does not get delivered to the bronchioles and therefore the patient may believe the medication does not work. Most often the medication works well when delivered to the bronchioles correctly. See the Section III Patient Teaching Guide for this chapter, "How to Use a Metered-Dose Inhaler."
3. Stress the importance of using a peak flow monitor at home to monitor progress of the disease. See Section III Patient Teaching Guide for this chapter, "Peak Flow Monitoring and Asthma Action Plan."
4. Short-acting β_2 agonists (SABA) are used for rescue from acute symptoms.
5. The use of a SABA more than twice a week for symptom relief indicates the patient has inadequate asthma control and needs an inhaled corticosteroid (ICS) as controller therapy.
6. Stress the need for an asthma action plan. See the Section III Patient Teaching Guide for this chapter, "Peak Flow Monitoring and Asthma Action Plan."

TABLE 8.1   Medications for Asthma and COPD (By Class/Alphabetical Order)

Brand	Generic	Drug Classification	Availability
(SABA) Short-acting beta agonist for rescue/fast-acting rescue			
Accuneb	Albuterol	Beta 2 agonist	Nebulizer
Albuterol	Albuterol sulfate	Beta 2 agonist	Inhal. solution Nebules Syrup
Combivent	Ipratropium + Albuterol	Combination anticholinergic + beta 2 agonist	MDI
Maxair Autohaler	Pirbuterol Acetate	Beta 2 agonist	MDI
ProAir HFA inhaler	Albuterol	Beta 2 agonist	MDI
Proventil HFA inhaler	Albuterol	Beta 2 agonist	MDI
Terbutaline sulfate	Brethine	Beta 2 agonist	Tablet
Ventolin HFA	Albuterol sustained release	Beta 2 agonist	MDI
Vospire ER	Albuterol	Beta 2 agonist	Extended release (ER) tablet
Xopenex	Levalbuterol Tartrate	Beta 2 agonist	HFA inhaler Concentrate solution for nebulizer
(LABA) Long-acting beta 2 agonist for maintenance/long-acting control			
Advair Diskus	Fluticasone + Salmeterol	Combination-steroid + long-acting beta 2 agonist (LABA)	Dry powder diskus MDI-HFA inhaler
Brovana	Arformoterol	Beta 2 agonist	Nebulizer
Foradil Aerolizer	Formoterol fumarate	Long-acting beta 2 agonist	Nebulizer Dry powder diskus
Perforomist	Formoterol solution	Beta 2 agonist	Nebulizer
Serevent Diskus	Salmeterol	Long-acting beta 2 agonist	Dry powder diskus
(ICS) Inhaled corticosteroid anti-inflammatory for maintenance or long-term control			
Aerobid & Aerobid M	Flunisolide	Inhaled corticosteroid	MDI MDI with menthol
Alvesco	Ciclesonide	Inhaled corticosteroid	MDI
Asmanex	Mometasone	Inhaled corticosteroid	Twisthaler dry powder
Beclovent	Beclomethasone Dipropionate	Inhaled corticosteroid	Dipro Powder Inhaler
Flovent HFA	Fluticasone	Inhaled corticosteroid	MDI
Pulmicort	Budesonide	Inhaled corticosteroid	Flexhaler & Respules
QVAR	Beclomethasone	Inhaled corticosteroid	MDI
Symbicort	Budesonide + Formoterol	Combination corticosteroid + long-acting beta 2 agonist	MDI
Leukotriene modifiers—Nonsteroidal anti-inflammatory			
Accolate	Zafirkalast	Leukotriene modifier	Tablet
Singulair	Montelukast	Leukotriene modifier	Chew tablet Tablet granules
Zyflo	Zileuton	Leukotriene modifier	Filmtab
Anticholinergics			
Atrovent HFA	Ipratropium	Antimuscarinic/antispasmodic	MDI and nebulized
DuoNeb	Ipratropium + Albuterol	Combination antimuscarinic/antispasmodic + beta 2 agonist	Nebulizer
Spiriva with HandiHaler	Tiotropium	Antimuscarinic/antispasmodic	Dry powder diskus

(continued)

TABLE 8.1 *(continued)*

Brand	Generic	Drug Classification	Availability
Mast cell stabilizer			
Intal	Cromolyn sodium	Mast cell stabilizer	MDI
Tilade	Nedocromil	Mast cell stabilizer	MDI
Methylxanthine			
Theo-24	Theophylline sustained-release	Methylxanthines respiratory smooth muscle relaxant	Tablet
Anti-IgE (IgE blocker) monoclonal antibody			
Xolair	Omalizmab	IgE blocker-immunomodulator	Subcutaneous injection
Systemic corticosteroids—used as a short-term "burst" for control			
Deltasone	Prednisone	Systemic corticosteroid	Tablet
Medrol	Methylprednisolone	Systemic corticosteroid	Tablet
Prelone	Prednisolone	Systemic corticosteroid	Tablet

MDI = Metered Dose Inhaler, HFA = Hydrofluoroalkanes

B. Patient teaching: See the Section III Patient Teaching Guide for this chapter, "Asthma."
C. Pharmaceutical therapy: Drugs are prescribed in a step-wise fashion for the type of asthma. The amount of medication used depends on the severity of asthma (Steps 1–6). **Prior to any medication/dosage changes, monitor the patient's compliance.** See Table 8.1.
   The following treatments are recommended for children 5 years old to adult:
   1. Mild intermittent asthma (Step 1)
      a. No long-term preventive medications are needed.
      b. Use short-acting beta agonists (SABAs) as rescue medication. May be used up to 4 times a day to treat exacerbation.
      c. Alternative medications include: Cromolyn, nedocromil, leukotriene modifier, or theophylline.
   2. Mild persistent asthma (Step 2)
      a. Low-dose inhaled corticosteroids (ICS) are used daily as a long-term preventive medication.
      b. Only Budesonide inhalation suspension is FDA approved for use in infants and children younger than 4 years.
      c. Alternative medications include: An ICS plus either a leukotriene modifier OR theophylline.
   3. Moderate persistent asthma (Step 3)
      a. Low-dose ICS plus a long-acting beta 2 agonist (LABA) OR a medium-dose ICS.
      b. ICS plus either a leukotriene modifier or theophylline or Zileuton.
   4. Severe persistent asthma (Step 4)
      a. Medium- to high-dose ICS plus either a LABA or Montelukast.
      b. Medium-dose ICS plus either a leukotriene modifier or theophylline.
      c. Second alternative: medium-dose ICS plus either leukotriene modifier, theophylline, or Zileuton.
      d. Consider Omalizumab for patients with allergies for severe persistent asthma.
   5. Step 5: preferred agents are high-dose ICS plus either LABA or Montelukast.
   6. Step 6: preferred agents are high-dose ICS plus either LABA or Montelukast and oral systemic corticosteroids.
   7. Mild-to-moderate asthma: Leukotriene modifiers are used to reduce the need for short-acting, inhaled β_2 agonists. They are also an alternative to low-dose, inhaled corticosteroids for patients with mild persistent asthma.
   8. Exercise-induced bronchospasm
      a. Short-acting inhaled β_2 agonist, two inhalations shortly before exercise is effective for 2–3 hours.
      b. Long-acting β_2 agonist, two inhalations is effective 10–12 hours.
   9. Hypertension and asthma: Drug of choice is a calcium channel blocker. Asthmatics also tolerate diuretics well.
   10. Theophylline can cause cardiac arrhythmias, therefore use it with caution and always follow-up with theophylline levels.
   11. Vaccinations
      a. Inhaled flu vaccine is not used in children with asthma. Inactivated influenza vaccine is safe, including children with severe asthma.
      b. Pneumococcal vaccine is recommended for children with asthma.

Follow-up

A. After acute episodes, follow-up within 1–2 hours or next day to monitor improvement until patient is stable.

B. For patients with mild intermittent or mild persistent asthma under control for at least 3 months, assess and follow-up at least every 6 months to provide education and reinforce positive behaviors. Gradually reduce medication dosage. If control is not achieved, consider increasing dosage after reviewing medication technique, compliance, and environmental control.

Consultation/Referral

A. Consider hospitalization for patients with acute episodes who do not completely respond to treatment within 1–2 hours.

B. If all therapies fail—including a short burst of Prednisone—refer patient to an asthma specialist.

C. Consult with a physician when the patient is pregnant or has other medical problems, or when standard treatment is ineffective.

Individual Considerations

A. Pregnancy
   1. Risks of uncontrolled asthma far outweigh risks to mother or fetus from drugs used to control the disease.
   2. Most drugs used to treat asthma and rhinitis, with the exception of brompheniramine, and epinephrine pose little increased risk to the fetus.
   3. Classes of drugs that do cause risk include decongestant, antibiotics (tetracycline, sulfonamides, and ciprofloxacin), live virus vaccines, immunotherapy (if doses are increased), and iodides. Always weigh benefits against risks, because adequate fetal oxygen supply is essential.
   4. If corticosteroids are necessary, recommend aerosolized forms due to their lower systemic effects. Prednisone or methylprednisolone are preferred and should be prescribed at minimum effective doses.
   5. Do not prescribe inhaled Triamcinolone because it is teratogenic.
   6. Drugs recommended during pregnancy
      a. A β_2 agonist, such as terbutaline, is preferred two inhalations every 4 hours as needed up to eight inhalations per day. Regular daily use suggests a need for additional medications.
      b. Cromolyn two inhalations four times daily as initial therapy for patients needing regular medication.
      c. Regular inhaled Beclomethasone if Cromolyn is not effective.
      d. Regular oral theophylline if Beclomethasone is not effective.
      e. Oral Prednisone if all other therapies fail, 1 week of 40 mg per day, followed by 1–2 weeks of tapering.

B. Geriatrics
   1. Half of elderly patients with asthma have first onset after age 65. Respiratory viruses are a common trigger.
   2. Recurrent episodes of shortness of breath may be primary symptom.
   3. Treatment is the same as with younger patients, with inhaled steroids the mainstay and oral steroids reserved for severe episodes. If oral steroids are prescribed, carefully monitor patient for complications and encourage measures to prevent bone loss.
   4. Inhaled anticholinergics and β_2 agonists are second-line treatment.
   5. Theophylline is rarely effective in the elderly. Asthma medications may have increased adverse effects in the elderly or may aggravate coexisting medical conditions, requiring medication adjustments. Also consider drug interactions and drug and disease interactions.

C. Pediatrics
   1. Spacing chambers are recommended for children to assist in proper delivery of medication.

Helpful Resources

Adult and Children Asthma Control tests: www.asthmacontrol.com

American Lung Association: http://www.lungusa.org/

Asthma & Allergy Foundation of America: http://www.aafa.org/

Global Initiative for Asthma (GINA) Instructions for Inhaler and Spacer Use: http://www.ginasthma.com/OtherResourcesItem.asp?l1=2&l2=3&intId=30

National Heart Lung and Blood Institute (NHLBI): http://www.nhilbi.nih.gov

BRONCHITIS, ACUTE

Definition

A. Acute bronchitis is inflammation of the tracheobronchial tree. Bronchitis is nearly always self-limited in the otherwise healthy individual. Generally, the clinical course of acute bronchitis lasts 10–14 days. The cause is usually infectious, but allergens and irritants may also produce a similar clinical profile. Asthma can be mistaken as acute bronchitis if the patient has no prior history of asthma.

Incidence

A. Bronchitis is more common in fall and winter in relation to the common cold or other respiratory illness. It occurs in both children (under 5 years of age) and adults and is diagnosed in women more frequently than men. Fewer than 5% of patients with bronchitis develop pneumonia.

Pathogenesis

A. Most attacks are caused by viral agents, such as adenovirus, influenza, parainfluenza viruses, and Respiratory syncytial virus (RSV).

B. Bacterial causes include *Bordetella pertussis, Mycobacterium tuberculosis, Corynebacterium diphtheriae, and Mycoplasma pneumoniae. Bordetella pertussis* should be considered in children who are incompletely vaccinated.

Predisposing Factors

A. Viral infection

B. Upper respiratory infection

C. Exposure to smoke

Common Complaints

A. The most common symptom initially is a dry, hacking or raspy sounding cough. The cough then loosens and becomes productive.

Other Signs and Symptoms

A. Sore throat
B. Rhinorrhea or nasal congestion
C. Rhonchi during respiration
D. Low-grade fever
E. Malaise
F. Retrosternal pain during deep breathing and coughing

Subjective Data

A. Ask about onset, duration, and course of symptoms.
B. Is cough productive?
C. Is there substernal discomfort?
D. Is there malaise or fatigue?
E. Has patient had a fever?
F. Does patient smoke? (Smoking aggravates bronchitis.)
G. A review of occupational history may be important in determining whether irritants play a role in symptoms.
H. Assess for symptoms of gastroesophageal reflux.

Physical Examination

A. Temperature and blood pressure. Consider pulse oximetry.
B. Inspect
   1. Observe overall appearance.
   2. Observe eyes, ears, nose, and throat (pharynx may be injected).
   3. Transilluminate sinuses.
C. Palpate: Palpate lymph nodes, maxillary and frontal sinuses.
D. Auscultate: Auscultate lungs for crackles, wheezing, and rhonchi.

Diagnostic Tests

A. Consider chest X-ray to exclude pneumonia.

Differential Diagnoses

A. Bronchitis
B. Upper respiratory infection
C. Asthma
D. Sinusitis
E. Cystic fibrosis
F. Aspiration
G. Respiratory tract anomalies
H. Foreign body aspiration
I. Pneumonia
J. Chronic obstructive pulmonary disease and emphysema
K. Pediatrics: Pertussis

Plan

A. General interventions—primarily supportive and should ensure the patient is adequately oxygenating.
   1. Tell the patient to increase fluid intake.
   2. Suggest trying humidity and mist therapy.
   3. Avoid irritants, such as smoke.
B. Patient teaching: See the Section III Patient Teaching Guide for this chapter, "Acute Bronchitis."
C. Pharmaceutical therapy.

1. Acetaminophen (Tylenol) for fever and malaise.
   a. Adults: 625–1,000 mg orally every 4 hours; not to exceed 4 g/day
   b. Pediatrics: For those younger than 12 years: 10–15 mg/kg/dose by mouth every 4–6 hours; not to exceed 2.6 g/day. For children older than 12 years: 325–650 mg by mouth every 4 hours; not to exceed 5 doses in 24 hours.
2. Expectorants such as guaifenesin with dextromethorphan (Robitussin DM, Humibid DM, Mytussin) to treat minor cough from bronchial/throat irritation.
   a. Adults and children older than 12 years: 10 ml by mouth every 4 hours
   b. Pediatrics: younger than 2 years: not recommended. For children 2–6 years: 2.5 mL by mouth every 4 hours and 6–12 years: 5 mL by mouth every 4 hours.
3. Among otherwise healthy individuals, antibiotics have not demonstrated benefit for acute bronchitis. However, consider oral antibiotics if symptoms persist 2 weeks with treatment (indicates bacterial infection).
   a. Erythromycin (EES, E-Mycin, Ery-Tab):
      i. Adults: 250–500 mg by mouth four times a day or 333 mg by mouth three times daily.
      ii. Pediatrics: 30–50 mg/kg/day by mouth divided four times a day
   b. Clarithromycin (Biaxin)
      i. Adults: 250–500 mg by mouth twice a day
      ii. Pediatrics: 7.5 mg/kg by mouth twice a day
   c. Azithromycin (Zithromax)
      i. Adults: day 1: 500 mg by mouth; then days 2–5: 250 mg by mouth
      ii. Pediatrics: 12 mg/kg by mouth every day. Do not exceed 500 mg/dose.
4. Albuterol (Ventolin) for patients with wheezes or rhonchi, or for patients with a history of bronchoconstriction.
   a. Adults: 2 puffs every 4–6 hours *or* 2–4 mg by mouth 3–4 times a day
   b. Pediatrics: 0.1–2 mg/kg by mouth three times daily

Follow-up

A. Follow-up if patient does not improve in 48 hours.

Consultation/Referral

A. In uncomplicated cases, mucus production decreases and cough disappears in 7–10 days. If symptoms persist, refer the patient to a physician.
B. Refer the patient if you note respiratory distress or if he or she appears ill and you suspect pneumonia.

Individual Considerations

A. Pediatrics:
   1. Children who have repeated episodes of bronchitis should be evaluated for congenital defects of the respiratory system.
   2. Instruct patients regarding the need for immunization against pertussis, diphtheria, and influenza, which reduces the risk of bronchitis.

B. Geriatrics: Monitor elderly patients for complications such as pneumonia. The elderly have a greater morbidity and mortality rate.

BRONCHITIS, CHRONIC

Definition
A. Chronic bronchitis is excessive mucus secretion with chronic or recurrent productive cough occurring 3 successive months a year for 2 consecutive years.
B. Others limit the definition to a productive cough that lasts more than 2 weeks despite therapy.
C. Patients with chronic bronchitis have more mucus than normal because of either increased production or decreased clearance. Coughing is the mechanism for clearing excess secretion.

Incidence
A. The incidence of chronic bronchitis is uncertain. There is a lack of definitive diagnostic criteria and considerable overlap with asthma. Visits for bronchitis is second only to otitis media and slightly more common than asthma.

Pathogenesis
A. Mucociliary clearance is delayed because of excess mucus production and loss of ciliated cells, leading to a productive cough. In children, chronic bronchitis follows either an endogenous response to an acute airway injury or continuous exposure to noxious environmental agents such as allergens or irritants.
B. Bacteria most often implicated are *Streptococcus pneumoniae, Haemophilus influenzae, Mycoplasma pneumoniae,* and *Moraxella catarrhalis.* The most common cause of chronic bronchitis in the pediatric population includes viral infections such as adenovirus, RSV, rhinovirus, and human bocavirus.

Predisposing Factors
A. Cigarette smoking
B. Cold weather
C. Acute viral infection
D. COPD/emphysema
E. Exposure to other airborne irritants
F. Chronic, recurrent aspiration or gastroesophageal reflux
G. Allergies

Common Complaints
A. Worsening cough: hacking, harsh, or raspy sounding.
B. Changes in color (yellow, white, or greenish), amount, and viscosity of sputum.
C. Children younger than 5 years rarely expectorate, sputum is usually seen in vomitus.
D. "Rattling" sound in chest.
E. Dyspnea/breathlessness.
F. Wheezing.

Other Signs and Symptoms
A. Difficulty breathing, retrosternal pain during a deep breath or cough
B. Rapid respirations
C. Fatigue
D. Headache
E. Loss of appetite
F. Fever
G. Myalgias
H. Arthralgias

Subjective Data
A. Determine the onset, course, and duration of illness.
B. Is the patient having trouble breathing?
C. Has there been a fever?
D. How is the patient's appetite? Is the patient drinking enough fluids?
E. Does the patient smoke or is exposed to secondhand smoke?
F. Review occupational history to evaluate exposure to irritants.

Physical Examination
A. Temperature and blood pressure.
B. Inspect
   1. Observe overall appearance.
   2. Inspect eyes, ears, nose, and throat. Conjunctivitis suggests adenovirus.
C. Auscultation
   1. Auscultate lungs in all fields. Lung sounds may sound normal to scattered, bilateral crackles, rhonchi, or large airway wheezing.
   2. Auscultate heart.
D. Percuss chest.
E. Palpate lymph.

Diagnostic Tests
A. **Patients with uncomplicated respiratory illness need little, if any, laboratory evaluation.**
B. Pulse oximetry.
C. Sputum culture to identify bacteria.
D. Chest radiography may help exclude other diseases or complications.
E. Pulmonary function studies may be indicated.
F. EKG and pulmonary function tests may be required for COPD patients.
G. Sweat test may be necessary to rule out cystic fibrosis.

Differential Diagnoses
A. Chronic bronchitis
B. Acute bronchitis
C. Asthma
D. Sinusitis
E. Cystic fibrosis
F. Bronchiectasis
G. Central airway obstruction
H. Pneumonia
I. Lung cancer
J. Aspiration syndrome
K. Gastroesophageal reflux
L. Tuberculosis

Plan
A. General interventions
   1. Rest during early phase of illness.
   2. Encourage stopping smoking and stay away from secondhand smoke.

3. Suggest exercise for patients with COPD.
4. The patient's goal is to improve symptoms, decrease cough and production of sputum.
5. Inform patients that increased sputum production may occur after smoking cessation and the patient may have airway reactivity (wheezing), especially seen in asthmatics.

B. Patient teaching: See the Section III Patient Teaching Guide for this chapter, "Chronic Bronchitis."

C. Dietary management
   1. Increase fluids.
   2. Eat nutritious food.

D. Pharmaceutical therapy
   1. Bronchodilators should be considered for bronchospasm.
      a. Albuterol sulfate (Proventil, Ventolin)
         i. Adults: MDI-2 actuations (90 mcg/actuation) inhaled every 4–6 hours
         ii. Pediatrics: MDI or nebulizer
            (a). Less than 1 year: 0.05–0.15 mg/kg dose every 4–6 hours
            (b). 1–5 years old: 1.25–2.5 mg/dose every 4–6 hours
            (c). 5–12 years old: 2.5 mg/dose every 4–6 hours
            (d). Over 12 years: 2.5–5 mg/dose every 6 hours
   2. Analgesics and antipyretics are used to control fever, myalgias, and arthralgias.
   3. Consider oral steroids to decrease inflammation.
      a. Adults: 5–60 mg/day by mouth
      b. Pediatrics: 1–2 mg/kg by mouth daily or in twice a day divided dosing. Do not exceed 80 mg/day.
      c. Tapering steroids is not necessary with short courses.
   4. Inhaled corticosteroids may be effective.
      a. Beclomethasone (Qvar) Available as a metered dose inhalant (MDI) that delivers 40 or 80 mcg/actuation.
         i. Adults MDI: 40–80 mcg inhaled by mouth twice a day, not to exceed 320 mcg twice a day.
         ii. Pediatrics MDI: 40 mcg inhaled by mouth twice a day, dose not to exceed 80 mcg twice a day.
      b. Fluticasone (Flovent HFA, Flovent Diskus). Available as MDI (44-mcg, 110-mcg, or 220-mcg per actuation) and Diskus power for inhalation (50-mcg, 100-mcg, or 250-mcg per actuation).
         i. Adult:
            (a). MDI: 88 mcg inhaled by mouth twice a day, not to exceed 440 mcg twice a day
            (b). Diskus: 100 mcg inhaled by mouth twice a day, not to exceed 500 mcg twice a day
         ii. Pediatrics:
            (a). MDI: Ages 4–11 years: 88 mcg inhaled by mouth twice a day; older than 11 years administer as adults.
            (b). Diskus: Ages 4–11 years: 50 mcg inhaled by mouth twice a day; older than 11 years administer as adults.

5. Antibiotics for bacterial infection.
   a. Erythromycin (EES, E-Mycin, Ery-Tab)
      i. Adults: 250–500 mg by mouth four times a day or 333 mg by mouth three times daily
      ii. Pediatrics: 30–50 mg/kg/d by mouth divided four times a day. Do not exceed 2 g/day.
   b. Clarithromycin (Biaxin)
      i. Adults: 250–500 mg by mouth twice a day
      ii. Pediatrics: 7.5 mg/kg by mouth twice a day
   c. Azithromycin (Zithromax)
      i. Adults: 500 mg by mouth on day 1, then 250 mg by mouth on days 2–5
      ii. Pediatrics: 10 mg/kg/day by mouth on day 1, then 5 mg/kg on days 2–5. Do not exceed adult dose.
   d. Amoxicillin-clavuanic acid (Augmentin)
      i. Adult: 250–500 mg by mouth every 8 hours
      ii. Pediatrics:
         (a). Less than 3 months old: 30 mg/kg/day by mouth divided to every 12 hours
         (b). 3 months or older: 40–80 mg/kg/day by mouth divided to every 12 hours.

Follow-up

Follow-up if there is no improvement in 3–4 days after starting therapy.

Consultation/Referral

A. Refer patients with respiratory distress to a physician. If respiratory failure occurs (rare), hospitalization may be needed.
B. Refer patients with COPD to a physician or pulmonary specialist.
C. Referral to a pediatric pulmonologist should be considered when symptoms persist and do not respond to initial therapy.

Individual Considerations

A. Pediatrics: Recurrent acute or chronic bronchitis should alert the clinician to the diagnosis of asthma. Recurrent episodes of acute or chronic bronchitis may also be associated with immunodefiencies.

BRONCHIOLITIS

Definition

A. Bronchiolitis is a narrowing and inflammation of the bronchioles, causing wheezing and mild to severe respiratory distress.

Incidence

A. Respiratory infection is seen in 25% of children younger than 12 months and 13% of children aged 1–2 years. Bronchiolitis occurs in infants and children. Infants are affected most often because of their small airways and insufficient collateral ventilation. It is one of the most common causes of acute hospitalizations in infants, especially during fall and winter.

Pathogenesis

The pathology results in obstruction of bronchioles from inflammation, edema, and debris, leading to hyperinflation of the lungs, increased airway resistance, atelectasis, and ventilation-perfusion mismatching.

A. Respiratory syncytial virus (RSV) is the most common cause. RSV bronchiolitis accounts for more than 90,000 pediatric hospitalizations and as many as 4,500 deaths annually.
B. Other causes include parainfluenza virus (10%–30%), adenovirus (5%–10%), influenza (10%–20%), *Chlamydia pneumoniae*, *Mycoplasma pneumoniae*, human bocavirus (HBoV), and human metapneumovirus (hMPV).

Predisposing Factors

A. Low birth weight, particularly premature infants
B. Chronic lung disease (CLD)
C. Parental smoking
D. Congenital heart disease
E. Chronic pulmonary disease (including bronchopulmonary dysplasia)
F. Immunodeficiency
G. Lower socioeconomic group
H. Crowded living conditions and day care
I. Gender: Bronchiolitis occurs in males 1.25 times more frequently than in females

Common Complaints

Clinical manifestations are initially subtle.

A. Infants become increasingly fussy.
B. Difficulty feeding during the 2–5 day incubation period.
C. Low-grade fever (usually less than 101.5°F).
D. Cough.
E. Tachypnea.
F. Wheezing.
G. Retractions.

Other Signs and Symptoms

A. Coryza
B. Irritability
C. Lethargy
D. Respiratory distress
E. Nasal flaring and grunting
F. Hypothermic (infants under 1 month)

Subjective Data

A. Determine onset, course, and duration of illness.
B. Are breathing problems affecting the ability to eat and drink?
C. Evaluate a history of fever, nausea, vomiting, or diarrhea.
D. Does the patient or any family members have asthma?

Physical Examination

A. Temperature and blood pressure.
B. Inspect
   1. Observe overall appearance.
   2. Note respiratory pattern.
   3. Check for tachypnea, which differentiates bronchiolitis from upper respiratory infections and bronchitis.
   4. Examine eyes, ears, and throat, noting other potential infections.
   5. Inspect nose for nasal flaring.
C. Auscultate
   1. Auscultate heart.
   2. Auscultate lungs. Note prolonged expiratory phase as seen with bronchiolitis.
D. Palpate liver and spleen.
E. Percuss: Percuss chest/lungs for hyperresonance.
F. Neurologic exam: Assess for irritability and lethargy.

Diagnostic Tests

A. **Diagnosis is made based on age and seasonal occurrence, tachypnea, and the presence of profuse coryza and fine rales, wheezes, or both upon auscultation.**
B. Pulse oximetry or arterial gases (ABGs) show hypoxemia.
C. Chest radiograph shows hyperexpansion, atelectasis, and infiltrates. Chest X-ray is also useful in excluding unexpected congenital anomalies.
D. White blood cell count (WBC) may be normal or show increased lymphocytes.
E. Viral isolation from nasopharyngeal secretions or rapid antigen detection (ELISA, immunofluorescence) for RSV can confirm diagnosis.

Differential Diagnoses

A. Bronchiolitis
B. Asthma
C. Viral or bacterial pneumonia
D. Aspiration syndromes
E. Pertussis
F. Cystic fibrosis
G. Cardiac disease
H. Reflux
I. Aspiration

Plan

A. General interventions
   1. Use a humidifier in the patient's bedroom.
   2. Clear stuffy nose with saline solution drops and suction out nares with bulb syringe.
   3. Infants should not be exposed to secondhand smoking.
   4. Monitor respiratory pattern.
B. Patient teaching: See the Section III Patient Teaching Guide for this chapter, "Bronchiolitis."
C. Dietary management
   1. Encourage fluids, such as juice and water. Dilute juice for younger infants.
   2. Offer small, frequent feedings.
D. Medical/surgical management
   1. Patients may only require supportive care. Patients with respiratory distress require hospitalization.
   2. Hypoxemic patients need oxygen therapy and possibly mechanical ventilation.
   3. Chest physiotherapy is not recommended.
E. Pharmaceutical therapy
   1. Bronchodilators should not be routinely used.
   2. Corticosteroids use is controversial.
   3. Antibacterials should be used only upon proven coexistence of a bacterial infection.
   4. Palivizumab (Synagis) prophylaxis should be administered to selective children.

Follow-up

A. Contact the patient within 12–24 hours for evaluation.

Consultation/Referral

A. Notify a doctor if the patient's breathing becomes labored, his or her wheezing becomes worse, and/or respiratory distress is suspected.

B. Refer patients with RSV to emergency room if moderate respiratory distress, dehydration, or hypoxemia occurs.

C. Younger patients in moderate to severe respiratory distress require hospitalization.

D. Infants under age 2 who have RSV often need to be hospitalized for supportive care, oxygen, and antiviral therapy.

E. Patients with pulmonary hypertension, bronchopulmonary dysplasia, or cystic fibrosis need hospitalization if their respiratory rate is greater than 60, their pulse oximetry is less than 92%, or they eat poorly.

Individual Considerations

A. Patients with pulmonary hypertension, bronchopulmonary dysplasia, or cystic fibrosis may have prolonged courses with high morbidity and mortality. Some may have reactive airway diseases in the future.

CHRONIC OBSTRUCTIVE PULMONARY DISEASE (COPD)

Definition

Chronic obstructive pulmonary disease is progressive, chronic, expiratory airway obstruction due to chronic bronchitis or emphysema. The relief of bronchoconstriction due to inflammation has some reversibility. Chronic bronchitis is a chronic productive cough for 3 months during 2 consecutive years. Emphysema is an abnormal, permanent enlargement (hyperinflation) of the air sacs, as well as the destruction of the elastic recoil. Many patients have both types of air restriction symptoms of chronic bronchitis and emphysematous destruction leading to chronic obstructive pulmonary disease (COPD). Patients with asthma whose airflow obstruction is completely reversible are not considered to have COPD. When an asthmatic patient does not have complete reversible airflow obstruction, they are considered to have COPD.

Irreversible airflow obstruction is a key factor in the patient's disability. The goal of COPD management is to improve daily quality of life (QOL) and the recurrence of exacerbations. Smoking cessation continues to be the most important therapeutic intervention.

The Global Initiative for Chronic Obstructive Lung Disease (GOLD) staging criteria are:

A. Stage I—Mild obstruction: FEV_1 greater than 80% of predicted value, some sputum and chronic cough

B. Stage II—Moderate obstruction: FEV_1 between 50% and 80% of predicted value, shortness of breath (SOB) on exertion, and chronic symptoms

C. Stage III—Severe obstruction: FEV_1 between 30% and 50% of predicted value, dyspnea, reduced exercise tolerance, exacerbations affecting quality of life

D. Stage IV—Very severe obstruction chronic respiratory failure: FEV1 less than 30% of predicted value or moderate obstruction FEV_1 less than 50% of the predicted value and chronic respiratory failure

Incidence

A. Approximately 12 million people in the United States have been diagnosed with COPD, however, another 12 million are considered undiagnosed. It is the fourth leading cause of death in the United States. COPD is most commonly seen in males (11.8%) versus females (8.5%). The exact worldwide prevalence is unknown.

Pathogenesis

A. Chronic bronchitis leads to the narrowing of the airway caliber and increase in airway resistance. Mucus gland enlargement is the histological hallmark of chronic bronchitis.

B. In emphysema the loss of the air sac's elastic recoil causes air limitation. Emphysema caused by smoking is the most severe in the upper lobes. Most patients with COPD have smoked 1 pack of cigarettes a day for 20 or more years before the symptomatic dyspnea, cough, and sputum.

Predisposing Factors

A. Cigarette smoking

B. Occupational, environmental, or atmospheric pollutants
1. Dust
2. Chemical fumes
3. Secondhand smoke
4. Air pollution

C. Genetic factor: α_1-antitrypsin deficiency (AAT)

D. Recurrent or chronic lower respiratory infections or disease

E. Age (most common in fifth decade of life)

Common Complaints

A. Chronic cough and colorless sputum, usually worse in morning

B. Dyspnea with exertion, progressing to dyspnea at rest

C. Wheezing

D. Difficulty speaking or performing tasks

E. Weight loss (decrease in fat-free mass)

Other Signs and Symptoms

A. Pursed-lip breathing
B. Use of accessory muscles
C. Tripod position
D. Barrel chest
E. Cyanosis (fingertips, tip of nose, around lips)
F. Tachypnea
G. Tachycardia
H. Difficulty speaking or performing tasks
I. Distended neck veins
J. Digital clubbing
K. Abnormal, diminished, or absent lung sounds
L. Mental status changes
M. Anxiety and depression
N. Pulmonary hypertension
O. Cor pulmonale
P. Left-sided heart failure

Subjective Data

A. Ask the patient about past respiratory problems and infections. Does he or she currently have fever, chills, or other signs of infection?

B. Ask about onset of cough and characteristics of sputum (amount, color, and presence of blood).

C. Determine cigar use and cigarette pack-year history (pack/day x number of years smoked).

D. Inquire about exposure to occupational or environmental irritants.

E. How far can the patient walk before becoming breathless? Is there more breathlessness walking on a slight incline?

F. Does the patient become breathless or tired when performing activities of daily living?

G. Ask about insomnia, anxiety, restlessness, edema, and weight change.

H. How many pillows does the patient sleep on? Does he or she have to sleep in a recliner or sitting up?

Physical Examination

A. Temperature, blood pressure, pulse, and respirations. The respiratory rate increases proportionally to disease severity. Height and weight to calculate the Body Mass Index (BMI). The patient may have a fairly normal examination early in the disease.

B. Inspect
  1. Observe general appearance: skin color, affect, posture, gait, amount of respiratory effort when walking; note increased anterior-posterior chest diameter.
  2. Examine sputum: frothy pink signals pulmonary edema. Hemoptysis as seen in tuberculosis.
  3. Examine fingers for clubbing; lips, fingertips, and nose for cyanosis.
  4. Observe the neck for distended veins and peripheral edema (advanced disease).
  5. Check for pursed-lip breathing and use of accessory muscles.

C. Auscultate
  1. Auscultate the heart.
  2. Auscultate lungs for wheezes, crackles, decreased breath sounds, and prolonged forced expiratory rate.
  3. Assess for vocal fremitus (vibration) and egophony (increased resonance and high-pitched bleating quality). Air trapping causes air pockets that don't transmit sound well. Absent ventricular lung sounds are a distinctive characteristic of COPD.
  4. Auscultate the carotids.

D. Percuss: Percuss chest for presence of hyper-resonance and for signs of consolidation.

E. Palpation
  1. Palpate the neck for lymphadenopathy.
  2. Palpate the chest.
  3. Evaluate abdomen for organomegaly.
  4. Evaluate pedal edema.

F. Mental status: Assess for decreased level of consciousness.

G. Six-minute walking distance (6MWD) testing to evaluate desaturation.

Diagnostic Tests

A. Spirometry is the gold standard for diagnosing COPD. Pulmonary Function Tests (PFTs) are used to diagnose, determine severity, and follow the disease progression of COPD. Spirometry before and after using bronchodilator.
  1. Forced expiratory volume in 1 second (FEV_1) is used as an index to airflow obstruction and evaluates the prognosis in emphysema.
  2. Forced vital capacity (FVC).
  3. FEV_1/FVC ratios less than 0.70.

B. Chest radiograph (not required to diagnose COPD but rules out other diagnoses).

C. CBC-evaluate polycythemia due to chronic hypoxia.

D. Sputum specimen for culture.

E. If the patient is younger than age 40 or has a family history of early onset of emphysema, measure α_1-antitrypsin levels.

F. Arterial blood gas.

G. EKG: note sinus tachycardia, atrial arrhythmias.

H. Two-diminsional echocardiogram is used to evaluate secondary pulmonary hypertension.

I. Chest CT is an alternative imaging study for emphysema, however, it is not required as a diagnostic tool.

J. Perform a PPD test if tuberculosis is suspected.

Differential Diagnoses

A. COPD

B. Heart failure

C. Pulmonary edema

D. Tuberculosis

E. α_1-antitrypsin deficiency (AAT)

F. Pneumonia

G. Pulmonary embolism

Plan

A. General interventions
  1. Educate and encourage active participation in the plan of care.
  2. Develop a smoking cessation plan; assess readiness to quit. Set a quit date, encourage a group smoking cessation program. Discuss smoking at every subsequent visit.
  3. Advise to stay away from secondhand smoke and limit exposure to other pulmonary irritants including extreme temperature changes.
  4. Advise exercise with physician approval.
  5. Educate and counsel patients regarding advance directives.
  6. Consider pulmonary rehabilitation if necessary.

B. Patient teaching: See the Section III Patient Teaching Guide for this chapter, "COPD."

C. Dietary management
  1. About 25% of COPD patients are malnourished because of coexisting medical conditions, depression, and the inability to shop for or prepare food.
  2. Suggest a low-carbohydrate diet. High carbohydrate intake may increase respiratory work by increasing CO_2 production.

D. Pharmaceutical therapy: Treatment guidelines are based on Spirometry.
  1. Stage I—The patient may be unaware he or she has COPD. Give influenza vaccine and use short-acting beta 2 agonist bronchodilators as needed.
  2. Stage II—Give influenza vaccine, plus short-acting beta 2 agonist bronchodilators as needed, plus

long-acting bronchodilator(s) plus cardiopulmonary rehabilitation.

3. Stage III—Give influenza vaccine, plus short-acting beta 2 agonist bronchodilators as needed, plus long-acting bronchodilator(s), plus cardiopulmonary rehabilitation, plus inhaled glucocorticoid steroids if patient has repeated exacerbations.

4. Stage IV—Give influenza vaccine, plus short-acting beta 2 agonist bronchodilator as needed, plus long-acting bronchodilator(s), plus cardiopulmonary rehabilitation, plus inhaled glucocorticoid steroids if repeated exacerbations plus long-term oxygen therapy (if the patient meet criteria for O2). Medicare guidelines require a patient's PaO_2 to be less than 55 mmHg or his or her resting oxygen saturation to be below 88% on room air.

5. Utilization of a spacer/holding chamber for inhalers should be encouraged.

6. Administer pneumonia vaccine for patients 65 years and older.

7. Prescribe pharmacologic agents/nicotine replacement therapy for smoking cessation.

8. Antibiotics are used empirically in COPD patients with acute exacerbation with symptoms of increased dyspnea, changes in cough, fever, or other evidence of an infection such as an infiltrate on CXR.

9. Mucolytic agents are not usually recommended.

Follow-up

A. For acute exacerbations, follow-up same day or following day.

B. Follow-up stable, chronic COPD every 1–2 months, depending on the patient's needs.

C. Monitor serum theophylline levels for toxicity.

D. Reevaluate patients on oxygen therapy in 1–3 months after starting oxygen.

E. Evaluate for osteoporosis; bone mineral density is lower in COPD patients and they are at risk for vertebral fractures.

Consultation/Referral

A. Consult with a physician if the patient has acute respiratory decompensation, severe cor pulmonale (distended neck veins, hepatomegaly, dependent peripheral edema, ascites, and pleural effusion).

B. Refer the patient to a pulmonary specialist for rehabilitation, if available.
1. Outpatient education for the patient and family
2. Exercise training
3. Breathing retraining, that is, purse-lip breathing, huff coughing
4. Correct administration of medications

C. Refer to a registered dietitian (RD) to provide Medical Nutrition Therapy (MNT). RDs focus on the prevention and treatment of weight loss associated with COPD and other comorbidities.

D. Send to a pulmonologist for evaluation for CPAP or BiPAP.

E. Send to a pulmonologist to evaluate for surgical intervention such as bullectomy, lung volume reduction surgery, or lung transplantation.

Individual Considerations

A. Pregnancy
1. COPD is rare except in α_1-antitrypsin deficiency.
2. Monitor drug treatment for potential teratogenic effects.

B. Geriatrics
1. Presentation may be atypical.
2. Patients should have annual flu vaccinations and Pneumococcal vaccination every 5 years.

COMMON COLD/UPPER RESPIRATORY INFECTION

Definition

A. The common cold is a self-limiting acute respiratory tract infection (ARTI) resulting from viral infection of the upper respiratory tract. It is also called acute nasopharyngitis. ARTI is characterized by mild coryzal symptoms, rhinorrhea, nasal obstruction, and sneezing.

Incidence

A. Upper respiratory tract infections are among the most frequent reasons for office visits. However, the true incidence is not known because patients treat themselves with over-the-counter and home remedies, as well as the seasonal and locational variability. Most children have six to eight colds a year; most adults have two to four.

Pathogenesis

A. Over 25%–80% of ARTIs are caused by a rhinovirus (greater than 100 antigenic serotypes). Other viral agents include coronavirus (10%–20%), respiratory syncytial virus, adenoviruses (5%), influenza viruses (10%–15%), and parainfluenza viruses. Incubation period is 1–5 days with viral shedding lasting up to 2 weeks.

B. Rhinoviral infections are chiefly limited to the upper respiratory tract but may cause otitis media and sinusitis.

Predisposing Factors

A. Exposure to airborne droplets.

B. Direct contact with virus by touching hands or skin of infected people, or by touching surfaces they touched, and then touching eyes or nose.

Common Complaints

A. Low-grade fever
B. Generalized malaise
C. Nasal congestion and discharge (initially clear, then yellow and thick)
D. Sneezing
E. Sore throat or hoarseness
F. Watery and/or inflamed eyes

Other Signs and Symptoms

A. Headache
B. Cough

Subjective Data

A. Elicit the onset, course, and duration of symptoms.

B. Inquire about color and other characteristics of nasal discharge and sputum. **Purulent nasal discharge after 14 days signals bacterial sinusitis.**

C. Inquire about other discomforts and exposure to people with similar symptoms.

D. Review allergens, seasonal problems, and exposure to irritants and smoke.

E. Review history for other respiratory problems, such as asthma, chronic bronchitis, and emphysema.

Physical Examination

A. Temperature and blood pressure.

B. Inspect
1. Observe general appearance.
2. Inspect eyes. **Note "allergic shiners," tearing, and eyelid swelling.**
3. Observe ears, throat, and mouth. **Otitis media is indicated by redness and bulging of tympanic membrane, or evidence of membrane perforation with drainage.**
4. Inspect nose for nasal redness, swelling, polyps, enlarged turbinates, septal deviation, and foreign bodies.
5. Transilluminate sinuses.
   a. Group A streptococci: tonsilar enlargement, exudate, petechiae.
   b. Allergies: "cobblestoned" pharyngeal mucosa.
   c. Mononucleosis: about half of patients with mononucleosis develop tonsillar exudates, and about one-third develop petechiae at the junction of the hard and soft palate, which is highly suggestive of the disease.

C. Auscultate:
1. Auscultate all lung fields.
2. Auscultate heart.

D. Percuss
1. Percuss sinus cavities and mastoid process of temporal bone to rule out otitis media.
2. Percuss chest for consolidation.

E. Palpate
1. Palpate face for sinus tenderness.
2. Examine head and neck for enlarged, tender lymph nodes.

Diagnostic Tests

A. Diagnosis may be made from history and physical. Because common cold manifestations are so prevalent, an aggressive workup is rarely necessary.

B. Consider rapid strep test if the patient has symptoms or was exposed to Group A streptococcus.

C. Consider throat culture if negative rapid strep and symptomatic.

Differential Diagnoses

A. Upper respiratory infection

B. Allergic rhinitis

C. Foreign body

D. Sinusitis

E. Influenza

F. Group A strep pharyngitis

G. Otitis media

H. Pneumonia

Plan

A. General interventions: No specific treatment.

B. Controlled trials reveal minimal therapeutic benefits of vitamin C for the treatment and prevention of colds. Zinc has no proven benefit. Echinacea has not shown any differences in rates of infection or severity of symptoms when compared with placebo. Validation and standardization of herbal products has not been completed.

C. Patient teaching: See the Section III Patient Teaching Guide for this chapter, "Common Cold."

D. Pharmaceutical therapy
1. **The American College of Chest Physicians released clinical practice guidelines in 2006 for the management of cough. Health care providers should refrain from recommending cough suppressants and over-the-counter (OTC) cough medicines for young children because of associated morbidity and mortality.**
2. **Antibiotics are ineffective in treating viral infection.**
3. Corticosteroids may actually increase viral replication and have no impact on cold symptoms.
4. Topical decongestants for rhinorrhea and nasal congestion
   a. Adults and children older than 6 years, pseudoephedrine (Afrin) nasal spray 0.05% two to three sprays per nostril twice daily, or phenylephrine (Neo-Synephrine) nasal spray 0.25%–1% two to three sprays per nostril every 4 hours as needed.
   b. Children younger than 6 years, saline nasal drops two to three drops per nostril 2–3 times daily. **Using nasal sprays longer than 2–3 days can result in rebound congestion and abuse of the drug.**
   c. As an alternative to pseudoephedrine and other nasal decongestants, consider clearing nasal congestion in infants with a rubber suction bulb; secretions can be softened with saline nose drops or a cool-mist humidifier.
5. Oral decongestants such as pseudoephedrine (Sudafed)
   a. Adults: pseudoephedrine (Sudafed) 60 mg every 4–6 hours or 120 mg every 12 hours.
   b. Children 2–6 years: pseudoephedrine (Sudafed) liquid 2.5 mL every 4–6 hours.
   c. Children older than 6 years: pseudoephedrine (Sudafed) liquid 5 mL every 4–6 hours, or pseudoephedrine (Sudafed) 30 mg every 4–6 hours.
6. Analgesics, such as acetaminophen (Tylenol) and ibuprofen (Advil), may be used for headache relief.
   a. Ibuprofen: Adult 200–400 mg by mouth while symptoms persist; not to exceed 3.2 g/day
   b. Ibuprofen: Pediatrics
      i. Less than 6 months: Not established
      ii. 6 months–12 years: 4–10 mg/kg/dose by mouth 3–4 times a day
      iii. Children older than 12 years: Administer as adults
7. Cough suppressants, if necessary: dextromethorphan (Benylin DM, Robitussin, Vicks Formula 44 pediatric formula).
   a. Adults and children older than 12 years: 10–20 mg orally every 4 hours, or 30 mg every 6–8 hours, or 60 mg extended-release liquid twice daily, to a maximum of 120 mg/day.

   b. Children 6–12 years: 5–10 mg every 4 hours.
   c. Children 2–6 years: 2.5–5 mg orally every 4–6 hours.
   d. Children under 2 years: Few data exist regarding the therapeutic or toxic levels of cough and cold medications in children younger than 2 years.
8. Colds have no allergic mechanism, so antihistamines are ineffective. The atropinelike drying effect from antihistamines may exacerbate congestion and obstruct the upper airway by impairing mucus flow.

Follow-up

A. None is recommended unless symptoms persist longer than 7 days from onset.

Consultation/Referral

A. Consult a physician if the patient has been reevaluated and given a new treatment plan but still has symptoms.
B. Refer the patient to an otolaryngologist if tonsillary abscess is suspected.

Individual Considerations

Pediatrics:

A. Oral decongestants are not recommended for children under 24 months of age.
B. The most common reported calls that involve OTC medications to poison control centers are for the ingestion of acetaminophen and cough and cold preparations.
   1. Accidental pediatric toxic ingestion is reported in children younger than 6 years and intentional toxic ingestion is more common is adolescents age 13–19 years.
   2. Adolescents have used Dextromethorphan as a recreational drug.

COUGH

Definition

A. Coughing is a mechanism that clears the airway of secretions and inhaled particles. The act of coughing has the potential to traumatize the upper airway (e.g., vocal cords). A chronic cough is one that lasts longer than 8 weeks.
B. Because coughing can be an affective behavior, psychological issues must be considered as a cause or effect of coughing.

Incidence

A. Data about the incidence of coughing is not available. However, most healthy people do not cough, and the main reason for coughing is airway clearance. A chronic cough is the most common presenting symptoms in adults who seek medical treatment in an ambulatory setting.

Pathogenesis

Stimulation of mucosal neural receptors in the nasopharynx, ears, larynx, trachea, and bronchi can produce a cough; so can acute inflammation and/or irritation of the respiratory tract. Cough is a reflex response that is mediated by the medulla but is subject to voluntary control. There is clear evidence that vagal afferent nerves regulate involuntary coughing. The "pathogenic triad of chronic cough" responsible for 92%–100% of chronic cough is:

A. Upper airway cough syndrome (UACS), previously referred to as postnasal drip syndrome.
B. Asthma
C. Gastroesophageal reflux disease (GERD)

Predisposing Factors

A. Pharyngeal irritants
B. Foreign body aspiration
C. Tuberculosis (persons in prisons and nursing homes and immigrants from endemic areas of TB)
D. Psychogenic factors (more common in children and with emotional stress)
E. Mediastinal or pulmonary masses
F. Congestive heart failure
G. Cystic fibrosis
H. Congenital malformations
I. Viral bronchitis
J. Asthma (sole symptom in 28%)
K. Mycoplasma infection
L. Upper airway cough syndrome (UACS), previously referred to as postnasal drip
M. Chronic sinusitis
N. Allergic rhinitis
O. Environmental irritants
P. Gastroesophageal reflux disease (GERD)
Q. Chronic bronchitis
R. Pulmonary edema
S. Medicating with angiotensin converting enzyme (ACE) inhibitors
T. Impacted cerumen and external otitis

Common Complaints

A. Common complaint is a cough that interferes with activities of daily living and sleeping leading to a decrease in a patient's quality of life.

Other Signs and Symptoms

A. Fatigue
B. Rhinitis
C. Epistaxis
D. Tickle in throat
E. Pharyngitis
F. Night sweats
G. Dyspnea
H. Fever
I. Sputum production
J. Hoarseness

Subjective Data

A. Elicit information about onset, duration, and course of the cough. Was onset recent or gradual? Does the cough occur at night? **Nocturnal cough may be caused by chronic interstitial pulmonary edema and may signal left-sided heart failure. Cough caused by asthma is also worse at night. Morning cough with sputum suggests bronchitis.**
B. Inquire about the cough's characteristics. For example, is it productive, dry, bronchospastic, brassy, wheezy, strong, or weak? If it is productive, is it bloody or mucoid? What

is the color, consistency, odor, and amount of sputum or mucus? Dry, irritative cough suggests viral respiratory infection. Severe or changing cough should be evaluated for bronchogenic carcinoma. Rusty-colored sputum suggests bacterial pneumonia. Green or very purulent sputum is due to degeneration of white cells. HIV cough also produces purulent sputum.

C. Inquire whether the cough is associated with eating and choking episodes. Wheezing or stridor with coughing may indicate a foreign body or aspiration.

D. Ask whether the cough is associated with postnasal drip, which produces a chronic cough, clear sputum, edematous nasal mucosa, and a "cobblestoned" pharyngeal mucosa.

E. Find out if the cough is associated with heartburn or a sour taste in the mouth, indicating GERD.

F. Ask about precipitating factors, such as exercise, cold air, or laughing. Also ask about alleviating factors. **Cough from asthma can be triggered or exacerbated by exposure to environmental irritants, allergens, cold, or exercise.**

G. Ask about current and previous work. Is the patient exposed to occupational and environmental irritants, such as dust, fumes, or gases? If so, what is the type, level, and duration of exposures?

H. Ask about family history of respiratory illness, such as cystic fibrosis or asthma.

I. Is the patient a smoker? If so, how much does he or she smoke, and how long has he or she smoked? Is he or she exposed to secondhand smoke? How much of the day? **Smoking is the main cause of chronic cough.**

J. Find out the date of the patient's last tuberculin skin test. Note recent exposure to TB.

K. Inquire about any exposure to the flu.

L. Does the patient have a history of heart problems?

M. Does the patient have a history of respiratory problems or other medical problems? Chronic bronchitis is a major cause of chronic cough and sputum production. Cough may also be an early sign of lung cancer; in late stages, cough occurs along with weight loss, anorexia, and dyspnea.

N. Review medications such as ACE inhibitors. Cough related to ACE inhibitors usually subsides within 2 weeks, but the median time is up to 26 days.

Physical Examination

A. Temperature and blood pressure, if indicated.

B. Inspect
1. Observe general appearance for cyanosis, difficulty breathing, use of axillary muscles, and finger clubbing.
2. Examine ears, nose, and throat.

C. Auscultate: Auscultate heart and lungs.

D. Percuss
1. Percuss sinus cavities and mastoid process.
2. Percuss chest and lungs for consolidation.

E. Palpate
1. Palpate face for sinus tenderness.
2. Examine head and neck for lymph nodes, masses, and jugular vein distension (JVD).

Diagnostic Tests

Testing can be held to a minimum by careful review of history and physical exam. Children with chronic cough should undergo, as a minimum, a chest X-ray and spirometry (if age appropriate).

A. WBC if infection suspected
B. HIV test if suspected
C. Sputum for Gram's stain, culture, and cytology
D. Mantoux test if indicated
E. Chest radiograph
F. Sweat chloride to rule out cystic fibrosis
G. Pulmonary function testing/spirometry
H. Methacholine challenge to rule out asthma
I. Esophageal pH monitoring to rule out GERD
J. CT scan if necessary

Differential Diagnoses

A. Environmental irritants
1. Cigarette, cigar, or pipe smoking
2. Pollutants (wood smoke, smog, burning leaves, and so on)
3. Dust
4. Lack of humidity

B. Lower respiratory tract problems
1. Lung cancer
2. Asthma
3. Chronic obstructive lung disease (includes bronchitis)
4. Interstitial lung disease
5. Congestive heart failure
6. Pneumonitis
7. Bronchiectasis

C. Upper respiratory tract problems
1. Chronic rhinitis
2. Chronic sinusitis
3. Disease of external auditory canal
4. Pharyngitis

D. Medication-induced cough from ACE inhibitors

E. Extrinsic compression lesions
1. Adenopathy
2. Malignancy
3. Aortic aneurysm

F. Psychogenic factors, more common in children and with emotional stress

G. Gastrointestinal problems such as reflux esophagitis

H. Genetic problems such as cystic fibrosis

Plan

A. General intervention: If sputum is purulent, obtain a sample for examination.

B. Patients with COPD and CF should be taught huffing as an adjunct to other methods of sputum clearance.

C. Patient teaching: See the Section III Patient Teaching Guide for this chapter, "Cough."

D. Pharmaceutical therapy
1. **The American College of Chest Physicians released clinical practice guidelines in 2006 for the management of cough. Health care providers should refrain from recommending cough suppressants and over-the-counter (OTC) cough medicines for young children because of associated morbidity and mortality.**

2. Therapy depends on various acute inflammatory and chronic irritating processes and on cause of cough. Refer to applicable sections of this chapter, such as "Asthma," "Tuberculosis," and see Chapter 10, "Gastrointestinal Guidelines."

Follow-up

A. The patient with a normal chest radiograph and no risk factors for lung cancer (e.g., smoking or occupational exposure) can be followed expectantly without further testing.

B. In patients whose cough resolves after the cessation of ACE inhibitors, and for whom there is a compelling reason to treat with these agents, a repeat trial of ACE inhibitors may be attempted.

C. See applicable sections for specific diagnoses.

Consultation/Referral

A. Consult a physician if symptoms persist after treatment. Reevaluate patient in 2 weeks if he or she is no better.

B. When a cough lasts for greater than 2 weeks without another apparent cause and it is accompanied by paroxysms of coughing, post-tussive vomiting, and/or inspiratory whooping sound, the diagnosis of a B *pertussis* infection should be made unless another diagnosis is proven.

C. Patients whose condition remains undiagnosed after a work-up and therapy may need referral to a cough specialist.

Individual Considerations

A. Pregnancy: Cough may be an early symptom of pulmonary edema. Watch intrapartum patients for signs of edema.

B. Pediatrics:
1. The most common reported calls that involve OTC medications to poison control centers are for the ingestion of acetaminophen and cough and cold preparations. Accidental pediatric toxic ingestion is reported in children younger than 6 years and intentional toxic ingestion is more common in adolescents age 13–19 years. Adolescents have used Dextromethorphan as a recreational drug.
2. Children with chronic productive purulent cough should always be investigated to document the presence or absence of bronchiectasis and to identify underlying and treatable causes such as cystic fibrosis and immune deficiency.

CROUP, VIRAL

Definition

A. Viral croup is an acute inflammatory disease of the larynx, also called laryngotracheobronchitis. Croup is the most common cause of stridor in febrile children. The uncomplicated disease usually wanes in 3–5 days but may persist up to 10 days. Croup is most often self-limited, but occasionally is severe and rarely, fatal. Lethargy, cyanosis, and decreasing retractions are indications of impending respiratory failure.

Incidence

A. The most common form of acute upper airway obstruction, croup generally affects children aged 3 months to 6 years. Croup has a peak incidence of 5 cases per 100 children per year during the second year of life. It is most prevalent in younger children in fall and early winter.

Pathogenesis

A. Parainfluenza 1 virus usually causes croup. The initial port of entry is the nose and nasopharynx. Other causes include parainfluenza virus types 2 and 3, respiratory syncytial virus, influenza virus, adenovirus, and *Mycoplasma pneumoniae*. Inflammation usually occurs in the entire airway, and edema formation in the subglottic space accounts for the predominant signs of upper airway obstruction.

Predisposing Factors

A. Upper respiratory tract infection
B. Male-to-female ratio is 2:1
C. Ages 3 months to 3 years (mean onset 18 months)

Common Complaints

A. Hoarseness
B. Cough progressing to a seal-like barking cough
C. Stridor, especially during sleep
D. Fever, usually absent or low-grade, but may be high
E. Runny nose

Subjective Data

A. Determine onset, duration, and course of illness.
B. Has the child been exposed to respiratory illness?
C. Is the child coughing? Having trouble breathing?
D. Has the child had fever, nausea, vomiting, or diarrhea?
E. Are immunizations up to date?

Physical Examination

Have the child sit upright in a parent's lap to perform the physical examination. Persistent crying increases oxygen demand and respiratory muscle fatigue.

A. Temperature and blood pressure.
B. Inspect
1. Observe overall appearance, noting respiratory pattern, retractions, nasal flaring, and air hunger. Children often sound terrible but don't look very ill.
2. Check nail beds and lips for cyanosis (ominous sign).
3. Assess skin and mucous membranes for signs of dehydration.
4. Observe for drooling or difficulty swallowing.
5. Inspect throat for foreign body. Inspect eyes, ears, nose, and throat for infection.
C. Auscultate
1. Auscultate heart. Tachycardia is out of proportion to fever.
2. Auscultate lungs for unequal breath sounds (signals foreign body aspiration). Stridor is an audible harsh, high-pitched musical sound that may be noted on inspiration or heard during both inspiration and expiration.
3. The Westley score is a way to quantify the severity of respiratory compromise. The severity of croup is evaluated by assessing inspiratory stridor, air entry, retractions, cyanosis, and level of consciousness. See Table 8.2.

TABLE 8.2 Westley Scoring for Croup

Symptom	Scoring
Inspiratory stridor	No inspiratory stridor = 0 points Stridor upon agitation = 1 points Stridor at rest = 2 points
Retractions	Mild = 1 points Moderate = 2 points Severe = 3 points
Air entry	Normal = 1 points Mild decrease = 1 point Marked decrease = 2 points
Cyanosis	None = 0 points Cyanosis upon agitation = 4 points Cyanosis at rest = 5 points
Level of consciousness	Normal = 0 points Depressed = 5 points

Mild disease = A score of less than 3 points. Occasional barking coughs, no stridor at rest, and mild to no suprasternal or subcostal retraction.
Moderate disease = A score of 3–6 points. Frequent cough, audible stridor at rest, visible retractions, but little distress or agitation.
Severe disease = A score greater than 6 points. Frequent cough, prominent inspiratory (occasional expiratory) stridor, obvious retraction, decreased air entry on auscultation, and significant distress and agitation.

Adapted from "Croup," by J. D. Cherry, 2008. *New England Journal of Medicine, 358,* 384–391.

D. Percuss: Percuss chest.
E. Palpate: Palpate neck to evaluate lymph nodes.
F. Neurologic exam: Assess level of alertness.

Diagnostic Tests

The diagnosis of croup is largely clinical, based on the presenting history and physical examination findings.

A. Pulse oximetry assesses respiratory status.
B. Laboratory testing is usually not needed for croup in a well-hydrated patient. However, a CBC may be indicated.
C. Imaging is not required in mild cases with a typical history that responds appropriately to treatment.
   1. Chest radiograph may show the "steeple or pencil sign."
   2. Anteroposterior (AP) soft tissue neck radiography may show subglottic narrowing.
D. Bronchoscopy or laryngoscopy may be required in unusual circumstances.
E. Arterial blood gases (ABGs) are unnecessary since they do not indicate hypoxia or hypercarbia unless respiratory fatigue is present.

Differential Diagnoses

A. Viral croup
B. Epiglottitis
C. Spasmodic croup
D. Membranous croup
E. Bacterial tracheitis
F. Retropharyngeal abscess
G. Diphtheria
H. Foreign bodies (Gastrointestinal or trachea)
I. Respiratory syncytial virus (RSV)
J. Measles
K. Varicella
L. Influenza A or B

Plan

A. General interventions
   1. Treatment is supportive for patients without stridor at rest.
   2. Stress rest and minimal activity.
   3. Cool mist therapy has not been shown to be clinically effective.
   4. Hot steam should be avoided due to the potential of scalding.
B. Patient teaching: See the Section III Patient Teaching Guide for this chapter, "Viral Croup."
C. Dietary management: Give plenty of fluids.
D. Medical/surgical management: If pulse oximetry shows desaturation, administer oxygen and monitor carefully.
E. Pharmaceutical therapy
   1. **Antibiotics are not indicated for the treatment of croup.**
   2. Acetaminophen (Tylenol) 5–15 mg/kg/dose for fever.
   3. In severe cases requiring hospitalization: nebulized racemic epinephrine (Asthmanefrin Solution) 0.5 mL of 2.25% solution in 2.5 mL sterile water may relieve airway obstruction up to 2 hours. Treatment may be repeated 3 times.
   4. Steroid use is controversial but may be considered if above therapy is ineffective. Steroids are used to decrease subglottic edema by suppressing local inflammatory process. Corticosteroids should not be given to children with untreated tuberculosis.
      a. Decadron (Dexamethasone) is the drug of choice. Pediatric dosing is 0.6 mg/kg every 6 hours orally or intramuscularly.

b. Budesonide (Pulmicort Respules inhalation suspension) has been shown to be equivalent to oral Dexamethasone. Pediatric dosing is 2 mg (2 mL of suspension) nebulized.

c. Prednisone (Deltasone) pediatric dosing is 1–2 mg/kg/day orally daily or in a divided dose twice a day for 5 days.

Follow-up

A. Call the parent in 12–24 hours to evaluate patient status.

Consultation/Referral

A. Consultation with an otolaryngologist and anesthesia prior to rapid sequence induction may be necessary if the patient is exhibiting rapid deterioration.

B. Refer the patient to a physician if he or she is a child who is severely ill with respiratory distress or dehydration.

C. Refer the patient to a physician if there is no improvement in 12–24 hours.

D. Patients with stridor at rest should be admitted to the hospital.

Individual Considerations

A. Most children improve within a few days.

B. Virus is most contagious during the first few days of fever.

C. Children may return to day care or school when temperature is normal and they feel better, even if cough lingers.

D. Children older than 5 years of age with recurrent croup should be referred to an otolaryngologist for evaluation.

EMPHYSEMA

Definition

A. Emphysema is an abnormal dilation and destruction of alveolar ducts and air spaces distal to the terminal bronchioles. Lung function slowly deteriorates over many years before the illness develops. Emphysema is one of the chronic obstructive pulmonary diseases (COPD)—a term that refers to conditions characterized by continued increased resistance to expiratory airflow. Chronic bronchitis, emphysema, and asthma comprise COPD. Chronic bronchitis and emphysema with airflow obstruction commonly occur together.

Incidence

A. Emphysema typically occurs in people older than age 50, with a peak occurrence between ages 65 and 75. Emphysema is more common in men (4%–6%) than in women (1%–3%).

Pathogenesis

A. Decreased gas exchange occurs due to focal destruction limited to the air spaces distal to the respiratory bronchioles causing airway obstruction, hyperinflation, loss of lung recoil, and destruction of alveolar-capillary interface.

Predisposing Factors

A. Long-term cigarette smoking

B. Occupational and environmental exposure to toxic agents

C. α_1-Protease inhibitor deficiency

D. Intravenous drug use secondary to pulmonary vascular damage from the insoluble fillers (e.g., cornstarch, cotton fibers, cellulose, talc)

E. Connective tissue disorders (e.g., Marfan syndrome and Ehlers-Danlos)

F. HIV

Common Complaints

A. Gradually progressing exertional dyspnea

B. Chronic cough

C. Wheezing

D. Fatigue

E. Weight loss

Other Signs and Symptoms

A. Cough with mild to moderate sputum production and clear-to-mucoid sputum

B. Early morning cough.

C. Shortness of breath.

D. Tachypnea.

E. Use of accessory muscles for breathing; pursed-lip breathing; *prolonged* expiration.

F. Barrel chest (increased anterior-to-posterior chest diameter).

G. Flushed skin.

H. Clubbed fingers.

I. Decreased libido.

J. Thin, wasted appearance.

K. Wheezing may occur particularly during exertion and exacerbations.

Subjective Data

A. Elicit information about onset, duration, and course of symptoms.

B. Determine if the patient is a smoker. If so, how much and for how long? Evaluate exposure to secondhand smoke. How much of the day?

C. Ask about current and previous work. Is the patient exposed to occupational and environmental irritants, such as dust, fumes, or gases? If so, what is the type, level, and duration of exposures?

D. Inquire about the cough's characteristics. Is it productive, dry, bronchospastic, brassy, wheezy, strong, or weak?

E. Question the patient about episodes of tachypnea, frequency of respiratory infections, and incidence of angina during exertion.

F. Does the patient have a hereditary disease (e.g., cystic fibrosis or α_1-antitrypsin deficiency), asthma, nasal abnormalities (e.g., deviated septum), or other respiratory problems (e.g., asthma)?

G. When was his or her last tuberculin skin test?

H. Find out the patient's usual weight, and assess how much weight loss has occurred and over what time period.

I. Evaluate current vaccination status for pneumonia and influenza.

Physical Examination

A. Temperature, blood pressure, and weight.

B. Inspect

1. Observe general appearance; note flushed skin color, use of accessory muscles, pallor around lips, pursed-lip

breathing, barrel chest (lung hyperinflation), and thinness.

2. Assess for peripheral edema
3. Dermal examination: Note finger clubbing and cyanosis.

C. Auscultate:
   1. Auscultate heart.
   2. Auscultate lungs: generally diffuse decreased breath sound.

D. Percuss: Percuss chest: hyper-resonance on percussion.

E. Palpate:
   1. Palpate abdomen.
   2. Evaluate pedal edema.

Diagnostic Tests

A. Pulse oximetry: blood gases if indicated.
B. α_1-Antitrypsin to rule out hereditary deficiency.
C. Tuberculin skin test.
D. **Pulmonary function tests reveal increased total lung capacity with poor respiratory expulsion and increased respiratory volume.**
E. EKG reveals sinus or supraventricular tachycardia.
F. Chest radiograph reveals hyperinflation, flat diaphragm, and enlarged heart.
G. Sputum evaluation and/or culture.

Differential Diagnoses

A. Emphysema
B. Chronic bronchitis
C. Chronic asthma
D. Bronchiectasis
E. Cystic fibrosis
F. Chronic asthmatic bronchitis
G. Tuberculosis
H. Alpha1-antitrypsin (AAT) deficiency
I. Congestive heart failure

Plan

A. Medical management: Supplemental oxygen therapy is indicated if the patient has a resting PaO_2 less than 55 mmHg or a PaO_2 less than 60 mmHg along with right heart failure or secondary polycythemia. Goals are to achieve a PaO_2 of greater than 55 mmHg (usually 1–3 L/min).
B. Patient teaching: See the Section III Patient Teaching Guide for this chapter, "Emphysema."
C. A smoking cessation plan is an essential part of a comprehensive treatment plan.
   1. Nicotine chewing gum produces better-quit rates than counseling alone.
   2. Transdermal nicotine patches have a long-term success rate of 22%–42%.
   3. The use of an antidepressant such as Zyban (150 mg twice a day) has been shown to be effective for smoking cessation and may be used in combination with nicotine replacement therapy.
   4. Chantix is a partial agonist selective for alpha4, beta 2 nicotinic acetylcholine receptors.
D. Pharmaceutical therapy
   1. Drugs of choice are inhaled beta 2 agonist. Beta 2 agonist are used primarily for relief of symptoms and in stable patients have an additive effect when used with an anticholinergic agent (e.g., ipratropium bromide). A spacer/chamber device should be used to improve delivery and reduce adverse effects. The following inhaled preparations have rapid action and fewer cardiac side effects:
      a. Ipratropium bromide (Atrovent) has bronchodilatory activity with minimum side effects.
         i. MDI: 2–4 puffs every 4–6 hours
         ii. Nebulizer: 250 mcg diluted with 2.5 mL normal saline every 4–6 hours
      b. Tiotropium (Spiriva) is a bronchodilator similar to Ipratropium. Available as a capsule form containing a dry powder or oral inhalation via HandiHaler inhalation device. Adults: 1 capsule (18 mcg) inhaled every day via the inhaler device.
      c. Metaproterenol sulfate (Alupent) is available as a liquid for nebulizer and metered-dose inhaler.
         i. MDI: 2 puffs every 3–4 hours
         ii. Nebulizer: 0.2–0.3 mL of 5% solution diluted to 2.5 mL with normal saline 3–4 times a day.
      d. Albuterol (Proventil, Ventolin) is available as a liquid for nebulizer, metered-dose inhaler (MDI) and dry powder inhaler.
         i. MDI: 1–4 puffs every 3–4 hours.
         ii. Nebulizer: 0.2–0.3 mL of 5% solution diluted to 2.5 mL with normal saline 3–4 times a day.
   2. If improvement is not satisfactory or tachyphylaxis occurs, give theophylline. Theophylline improves respiratory muscle function and stimulates the respiratory center as well as bronchodilates.
      a. Initial dose: 10 mg/kg/daily divided in oral doses every 8–12 hours
      b. Maintenance: 10 mg/kg/daily divided in oral doses every day or twice a day. Adjust doses in 25% increments to maintain serum theophylline level of 5–15 mcg/mL; not to exceed 800 mg/day.
   3. Oral steroids should be used to treat outpatients with acute exacerbations. Corticosteroids reduce mucosal edema, inhibit prostaglandins that cause bronchoconstriction, and increase responsiveness to bronchodilators. Taper dose as soon as bronchospasm is controlled. A minority of patients who respond to oral steroids can be maintained on long-term inhaled steroids.
   4. In patients with COPD, chronic infection or colonization of the lower airways is common. The goal of antibiotic therapy is not to eliminate organisms, but to treat acute exacerbations. If infection is present, give one of the following:
      a. Amoxicillin 500 mg orally three times daily.
      b. Clarithromycin 250–500 mg orally twice daily.
      c. Cefaclor (Ceclor) 250–500 mg orally every 8 hours. This drug is active against *Pneumococcus* and *H. influenzae*.
   5. Mucolytic agents in clinical practice are not recommended currently because of a lack of evidence for their benefit.
   6. Trivalent influenza vaccine is essential for all COPD patients. Give the patient the vaccine each October, at least 6 weeks before onset of flu season.

7. Pneumococcal vaccine is essential for COPD patients. Give as a single intramuscular injection of 0.5 mL.
8. α_1-Antitrypsin is needed for significant antitrypsin deficiency (less than 80 mg/dL). Patients get weekly or monthly infusions. Consult with a physician before therapy. A history of smoking rules out candidacy.

Follow-up

A. If the patient is acute, contact by phone in 24–48 hours and consider immediate referral.
B. Monitor the patient's body weight.
C. Serial pulmonary function tests may help guide therapy and offer prognostic information.
D. Monitor theophylline levels because of the drug's potential for toxicity. Adverse effects including nausea and nervousness are the most common. Other adverse effects include abdominal pain with cramps, anorexia, tremors, insomnia, cardiac arrhythmia, and seizures. Theophylline doses: 100–200 mg every 6–8 hours.

Consultation/Referral

A. If the patient's condition remains acute after 48 hours of treatment, consider immediate referral to a physician.
B. Refer the patient to a social worker for help in getting Meals on Wheels, handicapped parking, and finding other community resources.
C. A consultation with a pulmonary specialist is recommended.

Individual Considerations

A. Adults: Sexual dysfunction is common in patients with COPD; encourage other ways to display affection.
B. Geriatrics:
   1. Discuss course of disease, living wills, advanced directives, and resuscitation status early, before a crisis occurs.
   2. Theophylline is on the Beers list of drugs to use with caution in the geriatric population related to cardiovascular, renal, hepatic, insomnia, and peptic ulcers.

PNEUMONIA (BACTERIAL)

Definition

A. Pneumonia is inflammation and consolidation of lung tissue due to a bacterial pathogen. The causative agent and the anatomic location classify pneumonia. It is not uncommon to have acute viral and bacterial pneumonia concurrently.
B. Other types of pneumonia and pulmonary inflammation occur secondary to smoking, exposure to chemicals, fungi, near drowning, and from recurrent aspiration with gastroesophageal reflux.

Incidence

Pneumonia and other respiratory tract infections are the leading cause of death worldwide and account for 10–20 million hospitalizations per year.

A. Bacterial pneumonia is more prevalent in the very old and very young. Annual attack rate is 18:1,000.
B. Community-acquired pneumonia (CAP) in children younger than 5 years is approximately 0.026 episodes per child-year.

C. A higher mortality rate occurs in young infants, immunodeficiency, and adults with abnormal vital sign and certain pathogens.
D. The incident rate also varies by pathogens.

Pathogenesis

Pneumonia results from inflammation of the alveolar space. Lobar pneumonia has four stages:

A. Vascular congestion and alveolar edema within the first 24 hours of infection.
B. Red hepatization (2–3 days) is characterized by erythrocytes, neutrophils, and fibrin within the alveoli.
C. Gray hepatization (2–3 days) is characterized by a gray-brown to yellow color secondary to exudate.
D. Resorption and restoration of the pulmonary architecture. A rub may still be ascultated due to the fibrinous inflammation.

Bacterial causes include *Streptococcus pneumoniae* (most common pathogen), *Haemophilus influenzae* (second most common pathogen), *Staphylococcus aureus, Legionella, Chlamydia trachomatis, Chlamydia pneumoniae, Mycoplasma pneumoniae,* and *Pneumocystis carinii* pneumonia (PCP) in patients with HIV.

Predisposing Factors

A. Age extremes
B. COPD
C. Alcoholism
D. Cigarette smoking
E. Aspiration
F. Heart failure
G. Diabetes
H. Heart failure/heart disease
I. Crowded conditions (day care, dormitories)
J. Immunodeficiency
K. Congenital anomalies
L. Abnormal mucus clearance
M. Lack of immunization

Common Complaints

Acute onset of symptoms:

A. Fever
B. Shaking chills
C. Dyspnea, rapid, labored breathing
D. Cough
E. Rust-colored sputum

Other Signs and Symptoms

A. Increased respiratory rate (tachypnea)
B. Chest pain
C. URI symptoms such as pharyngitis
D. Headache
E. Nausea
F. Vomiting
G. Vague abdominal pain
H. Diarrhea
I. Myalgia
J. Arthralgias
K. Poor feeding
L. Lethargy in infants

Subjective Data

A. Determine the onset, duration, and course of illness.

B. Has the patient had fever or shaking chills?

C. Has there been breathing trouble? Are the breathing problems interfering with eating and drinking?

D. If a child, review the presence of acute onset of fever, cough, tachypnea, dyspnea, and grunting?

E. Is there a cough? Is the cough productive? What color is the sputum?

F. Are any other family members ill?

G. If a child, has he or she been hospitalized for pneumonia or respiratory distress before?

H. Review the history for any chronic diseases.

Physical Examination

A. Temperature, blood pressure, pulse and weight. Count respirations for a full minute.

B. Inspect
1. Observe overall appearance. Does the patient appear ill? Consider the clinical presentation, age of the person, and history.
2. Observe breathing pattern and the use of accessory muscles, grunting, retractions, and tachypnea.
3. Obtain a pulse oximetry to assess oxygen saturation.
4. Check nail beds and lips for cyanosis.
5. Examine the eyes, nose, ears, and throat.

C. Auscultate
1. Auscultate heart.
2. Auscultate lungs for the following (auscultate bases first in geriatric patients):
   a. Crackles (present in 80% of patients), wheezes, and decreased breath sounds.
   b. Whispered pectoriloquy (increased loudness of whisper during auscultation).
   c. Egophony (patient's "e" sounds like "a" during auscultation).
   d. Bronchophony (voice sounds louder than usual).

D. Percuss chest to identify areas of consolidation.

E. Palpate
1. Palpate chest for tactile fremitus (increased conduction when patient says "99").
2. Palpate lymph nodes for adenopathy.
3. Palpate sinuses for tenderness. Sinusitis is a sign of *Mycoplasma* infection.

Diagnostic Tests

A. Chest radiograph: Infiltrates confirm diagnosis. False negatives result from dehydration, evaluation in first 24 hours, and infection.

B. The World Health Organization (WHO) defines pneumonia solely on the basis of clinical finding observed by inspection and the timing of respirations.

C. Complete blood count.

D. Cultures
1. Blood cultures if critically ill, immunocompromised, or for persistent symptoms.
2. Sputum cultures are reserved for very ill patients for unusual presentations.

E. Consider rapid viral testing.

F. Consider skin testing for tuberculosis for high-risk exposure risk.

Differential Diagnoses

A. Pneumonia
1. Bacterial pneumonia
2. Viral pneumonia
3. Aspiration pneumonia
4. Chemical-induced pneumonia

B. Asthma

C. Bronchitis/bronchiolitis

D. Pertussis

E. Heart failure

F. Pulmonary embolus

G. Empyema and abscess

H. Aspiration of foreign body

Plan

A. General interventions:
1. Encourage rest during acute phase.
2. Encourage patients to avoid smoking/secondhand smoke.
3. A vaporizer may be used to increase humidity.
4. Encourage good hand washing or use of hand sanitizer.

B. Patient teaching: See the Section III Patient Teaching Guides for this chapter, "Bacterial Pneumonia: Adult" and "Bacterial Pneumonia: Child."

C. Dietary management: Encourage a nutritious diet with increased fluid intake.

D. Pharmaceutical therapy:
1. Treatment with antibiotics is empirical. Oral therapy should continue 7–10 days. See Table 8.3.
2. Acetaminophen (Tylenol) for fever.
3. Avoid cough suppressants.
4. Vaccines:
   a. Children: Heptavalent pneumonoccal vaccine is recommended for all children in the United States.
   b. Geriatrics: Pneumococcal vaccine

Follow-up

A. Patients/parents should know the signs of increasing respiratory distress and seek immediate medical attention.

B. Follow-up by telephone in 24 hours.

C. If there is no improvement after 48 hours on antibiotics, the patient is advised to call back.

D. Schedule a return visit in 2 weeks for evaluation.

E. Follow-up chest radiograph in 4–6 weeks for patients over 60 years and for those who smoke. However, if the patient is younger than 60 years, a nonsmoker, and feels well at 6-week follow-up, there is no need to follow-up with a chest radiograph.

Consultation/Referral

A. Patients who are immunocompromised or have signs of toxicity or hypoxia may need hospitalization. Refer them to a physician.

B. If the child is in moderate respiratory distress, dehydrated, or hypoxemic, consult with or refer the patient to a physician/hospital.

C. Poor prognostic signs that require referral are age older than 65 years, respiration rate greater than or equal to 30 breaths/minute, systolic BP less than 90 or diastolic

TABLE 8.3 Antibiotic Therapies for Pneumonia

Antibiotic	Adult Dosages	Pediatrics Dosages
Amoxicillin: oral (Amoxil, Trimox)	250 mg–500 mg TID Not exceed 1,500 mg/day	40 mg/kg/day divided TID 5–10 kg: 125 mg TID > 10 kg: 250 mg TID
Clarithromycin: oral (Biaxin)	250 mg–500 mg BID	15 mg/kg/day divided every 12 hours
Cefotaxime: intramuscular (Claforan)	> 50 kg: 1–2 gram IM every 6–8 hours. Not to exceed 12 g/day	< 50 kg: 100 mg–200 mg/dg/day IM divided doses every 6–8 hours
Doxycycline: oral (Doryx) Not recommended for children < 8 years	200 mg loading dose then 100 mg BID	> 8 yrs and < 100 lbs; 2 mg/lb divided in 2 doses for 2 day; then 1–2 mg/lb daily in 2 divided doses > 100 lbs: 100 mg orally every 12 hours
Azithromycin: oral (Zithromax)	500 mg loading dose then 250 mg daily on days 2–5	10 mg/kg initial dose (not to exceed 500 mg/day) then 5 mg/kg daily on days 2–5 (Not to exceed 250 mg/day)

Note: BID = twice a day. IM = Intramuscular. TID = three times daily.

BP less than 60, temperature greater than 101°F, altered mental status, extrapulmonary infection, WBC less than 4,000 or greater than 30,000.

D. Physician consultation is needed for suspected PCP.

Individual Considerations

E. Pregnancy
1. The annual U.S. rate of antepartum community-acquired pneumonia is 0.5–1.5 per 1,000 pregnancies.
2. Perinatal mortality may increase slightly due to associated increase in prematurity. Pneumonia puts older mothers at high risk of maternal death.
3. The symptoms of bacterial pneumonia are the same in pregnancy.
4. Chest radiographs are acceptable in pregnancy to diagnose pneumonia.

PNEUMONIA (VIRAL)

Definition

A. Viral pneumonia is inflammation and consolidation of lung tissue due to a viral pathogen.

Incidence

A. Viral pneumonia is the most common pediatric pulmonary infection. Viral agents account for only 2% up to 15% of pneumonia cases in adults. Viruses were documented in up to 45% of children. It is not uncommon to have concurrent viral and bacterial infections.

B. Children younger than 5 years and elderly persons have the highest rate of influenza-associated hospitalizations.

Pathogenesis

A. Pneumonia results from inflammation of the alveolar space and may compromise air exchange. Viral pneumonia is caused by influenza viruses, parainfluenza virus, and adenovirus and respiratory syncytial virus (RSV).

Predisposing Factors

A. Age extremes
B. Prematurity
C. Exposure to viral illness
D. Lack of immunization

Common Complaints

A. Fever
B. Cough
C. Dyspnea
D. Tachypnea

Other Signs and Symptoms

A. Upper respiratory prodrome
B. Poor appetite
C. Malaise/lethargy in pediatrics
D. Myalgia
E. Muscle aches
F. Headache
G. Fatigue
H. Chest pain/tightness

Subjective Data

A. Determine onset, duration, and course of illness.
B. Has the patient had fever, cough, and upper respiratory infection?
C. Have there been any flulike symptoms?
D. Has there been any labored breathing?
E. Has there been a cough? Is it a productive cough? What color is the sputum?
F. Are the breathing problems affecting the ability to eat or drink?
G. Has the child had nausea, vomiting, or diarrhea?

Physical Examination

A. Temperature, blood pressure, pulse, and respirations. Count respirations for a full minute.
B. Inspect

1. Observe overall appearance. Does the patient appear ill? Consider the clinical presentation, age of person, and history.
2. Observe respiratory pattern, grunting, nasal flaring, retractions, and use of accessory muscles.
3. Check pulse oximetry.
4. Check nail beds and lips for cyanosis.
5. Examine eyes, ears, nose, and throat.

C. Auscultate
1. Auscultate heart.
2. Auscultate lungs for the following (auscultate bases first in geriatric patients):
   a. Crackles, decreased breath sounds.
   b. Whispered pectoriloquy (patient's whispered sounds are louder than normal).
   c. Egophony (patient's "e" sounds like "a").
   d. Bronchophony (voice sounds louder than usual).

D. Percuss: Percuss chest for dull sound (consolidation).

E. Palpate
1. Palpate lymph nodes for swelling.
2. Palpate chest for tactile fremitus (increased conduction when patient says "99").
3. Palpate sinuses.

Diagnostic Tests
A. Chest radiograph reveals interstitial, perihilar, or diffuse infiltrates
B. CBC
C. Rapid viral tests per nasal swab
D. Sputum Gram's stain if indicated

Differential Diagnoses
A. Viral pneumonia
B. Bacterial pneumonia
C. Pertussis
D. Asthma
E. Bronchitis/bronchiolitis
F. Sinusitis
G. Foreign body obstruction
H. Aspiration

Plan
A. General interventions:
1. Tell the patient to rest during acute phase.
2. Avoid smoking or secondhand smoke.
3. Respiratory isolation; may use facial masks.
4. Encourage good hand washing or use of hand sanitizer.

B. Patient teaching: See the Section III Patient Teaching Guides for this chapter, "Viral Pneumonia: Adult" and "Viral Pneumonia: Child."

C. Dietary management: Encourage fluids and nutritious diet.

D. Pharmaceutical therapy: Antiviral agents:
1. Zanamivir (Relenza) is the recommended initial choice when influenza A infection or exposure is suspected. Zanamivir is administered by a metered-dose inhaler (MDI). The combination of Oseltamivir (Tamiflu) and Rimatadine, an adamantane, is considered a second-line alternative. Tamiflu resistance emerged in the United States during the 2008–2009 influenza season.
2. Acyclovir (Zovirax) for herpes viruses is administered as an IV infusion.
3. Ribavirin (Virazole) for RSV is administered as an aerosol.

E. Patients with viral pneumonia who are superinfected with bacterial organisms require antibiotic therapy.

F. Avoid cough suppressants.

G. Acetaminophen (Tylenol) for fever.

H. Immunizations
1. Recommend the influenza vaccine for prevention.
2. Consider RSV vaccine prophylaxis for pediatrics following the current American Academy of Pediatrics' recommendations.

Follow-up
Signs and symptoms may vary greatly according to the viral pathogen, severity of disease, and the patient's age.

A. Tell the patient to return to the clinic if no improvement is seen after 48 hours on antiviral agents.
B. Follow-up by phone in 24 hours.
C. Consider follow-up at 2 weeks if bronchoconstriction is noted on exam.

Consultation/Referral
A. Consult a physician if viral pneumonia is strongly suspected.
B. Consult a physician if the patient is pregnant.
C. Consult a physician or transfer to the hospital if in respiratory distress, dehydrated, or hypoxemic.
D. Hospitalization should be considered for infants younger than 2 months of age or premature with RSV, due to the risk of apnea.

Individual Considerations
A. Pregnancy: Ribavirin is contraindicated in pregnancy, class X drug.

◳ RESPIRATORY SYNCYTIAL VIRUS

Definition
A. Respiratory syncytial virus (RSV) is the most frequent cause of viral respiratory tract infection in infants. Most infants develop upper respiratory tract symptoms; 20%–30% develop lower respiratory tract disease with their first infection. Infection with RSV may produce minimal respiratory symptoms. Most previously healthy infants who develop RSV bronchiolitis do not require hospitalization. Preterm infants with respiratory symptoms with lethargy, irritability, and poor feeding may require admission for treatment.

Incidence
A. RSV is prevalent worldwide, with similar clinical manifestations and young age. Annual epidemics occur in fall, winter, and early spring, usually in temperate climates. Most infants are infected during the first year of life. Peak incidence of occurrence of severe RSV disease is observed at age 2–8 months. Virtually all children have been infected at least once by their third birthday. Reinfection with RSV throughout life is common.

B. The period of viral shedding usually is 3–8 days, but shedding may last longer. The incubation period ranges from 2–8 days.

Pathogenesis

A. RSV is an enveloped, nonsegmented, negative strand RNA virus of the *Paramyxoviridae* family. Two major strains (groups A and B) have been identified and strains of both often circulate concurrently.

B. Humans are the only source of infection. Transmission is by direct or close contact with contaminated secretions. RSV can persist on environmental surfaces for several hours and for a half-hour or more on hands.

Predisposing Factors

A. Prematurity
B. Congenital heart disease
C. Chronic pulmonary disease
D. Immunodeficiency

Common Complaints

A. Fever (< 101°F). 20% of patients have higher temperatures.
B. Decreased appetite.
C. Irritability.
D. Lethargy.
E. Rapid respirations.
F. Cough.
G. Coryza.

Other Signs and Symptoms

A. Tachypnea or apnea
B. Nasal flaring
C. Retractions
D. Crackles
E. Wheezes

Subjective Data

A. Ask about onset, duration, and course of illness.
B. Inquire whether the child is having trouble eating or drinking because of breathing problems.
C. Review other symptoms including fever, nausea, vomiting, or diarrhea.
D. Are there any labored breathing patterns?

Physical Examination

A. Temperature and blood pressure.
B. Inspect
   1. Observe general appearance.
   2. Note respiratory pattern, retractions, nasal flaring, grunting, and circumoral cyanosis.
   3. Inspect eyes, ears, nose, and throat. As many as 40% have an associated viral and/or bacterial otitis media.
   4. Assess hydration status: skin turgor, capillary refill, mucous membranes.
C. Auscultate
   1. Auscultate heart.
   2. Auscultate lungs for crackles and mild to moderate respiratory distress with scattered wheezes.
D. Percuss: Percuss chest.
E. Palpate
   1. Palpate lymph nodes for adenopathy.
   2. Palpate head and fontanelles (if applicable).

Diagnostic Tests

A. Rapid diagnostic assay of nasopharyngeal secretions are reliable in infants and young children.
B. Laboratory studies are frequently not indicated in the infant who is comfortable in room air, well hydrated, and feeding adequately. Nonspecific lab test may include CBC, serum electrolytes, and urinalysis.
C. Chest radiograph may show hyperexpansion, atelectasis, and/or infiltrates.
D. ABGs or pulse oximetry may show hypoxemia.

Differential Diagnoses

A. RSV
B. Viral or bacterial pneumonia
C. Asthma
D. Croup
E. Influenza
F. Neonatal sepsis

Plan

A. General interventions
   1. Most infants require only supportive care.
   2. Infants should never be exposed to cigarette smoke.
   3. Hydration is important.
   4. Contact precautions are recommended for the duration of RSV-associated illness among infants and young children. Adhere to appropriate hand hygiene practices.
   5. Prevention includes limiting, when feasible, exposure to contagious settings (e.g., childcare centers).
B. Patient teaching: See the Section III Patient Teaching Guide for this chapter, "Respiratory Syncytial Virus."
C. Dietary management
   1. Tell caregiver to offer juice, water, and other fluids frequently and to dilute juice for younger infants.
   2. Suggest offering small, frequent feedings.
D. Pharmacological therapy:
   1. Ribavirin is an antiviral drug that may be delivered by means of aerosol, but it is reserved for severely ill children or those at high risk.
   2. The use of bronchodilators and corticosteroids is controversial, but they may be indicated for hospitalized patients.
   3. Antibiotics are not indicated for RSV bronchiolitis or pneumonia unless there is a secondary bacterial infection.
   4. Respiratory Syncytial Virus Globulin Intravenous (RSV-IGIV) is no longer available.
   5. Palivizumab (Synagis) Immunoprophylaxis is extremely costly, however. the intervention may reduce hospitalizations of high-risk infants. Dosing: Palivizumab 15 mg/kg intramuscular every 30 days. Immunizations are given from 3–5 months depending on the gestational age, risk factors, and month that prophylaxis is started. The 2009 American Academy of Pediatrics eligibility criteria for Palivizumab prophylaxis criteria includes:
      a. Infants with chronic lung disease (CLD) younger than 24 months who receive supplemental oxygen,

bronchodilator, diuretic, or chronic corticosteroids. A maximum of 5 doses is recommended for this category.

   b. Infants born before 32 weeks' gestation (31 weeks, 6 days or less). A maximum of 5 monthly doses is recommended depending on gestational age and chronologic age at the start of RSV season.

   c. Infants born at 32 to less than 35 weeks' gestation (32 weeks + 0 days through 34 weeks + 6 days): Palivizumab prophylaxis should be limited to infants at greatest risk, younger than 3 months of age at the start of RSV season.

   d. Infants with congenital abnormalities of the airway or neuromuscular disease may be considered for immunoprophylaxis. A maximum of 5 doses of Palivizumab during the first year of life is recommended.

   e. Infants and children with congenital heart disease who are 24 months of age or younger with hemodynamically significant acyanotic congenital heart disease may benefit from immunoprophylaxis. The decision to treat should be based on the degree of physiologic cardiovascular compromise.

   f. Immunocompromised children with severe immunodeficiency or advanced acquired immunodeficiency syndromes (AIDS) may benefit from prophylaxis.

   g. There is insufficient data to determine the efficacy of Palivizumab with patients with cystic fibrosis.

Follow-up

A. Call the patient's caregiver in 12–24 hours to assess feeding and respiratory status.

Consultation/Referral

A. Refer the patient to a physician if the infant is in moderate respiratory distress, is dehydrated, or is hypoxemic.

B. Admit hypoxemic infants to the hospital for hydration; oxygen therapy; and, possibly, mechanical ventilation.

Individual Considerations

A. Pediatrics: All high-risk infants 6 months of age and older and their contacts should be administered the influenza vaccine as well as other recommended age-appropriate immunizations. Palivizumab does not interfere with response to vaccines.

B. Adults: Palivizumab (Synagis) is not approved for adults.

TUBERCULOSIS

Definition

A. Tuberculosis (TB) is an infectious disease. Tuberculosis is a granulomatous disease caused by *Mycobacterium tuberculosis, Mycobacterium bovis,* and other mycobacteria. Humans are the only reservoirs for *M tuberculosis.* Tuberculosis may involve multiple organs including the lungs, liver, spleen, kidney, brain, and bone.

B. In most immunocompetent individuals, macrophages are successful in containing the bacilli, and the infection is self-limited and often subclinical. As many as 60% of children and 5% of adults with primary TB are asymptomatic. When the pulmonary macrophages are unable to contain the bacilli, it leads to clinically apparent infection-progressive primary tuberculosis.

C. Postprimary (reactivation) tuberculosis is when the initial infection was successfully contained by the pulmonary macrophages, with bacilli remaining viable within the macrophages. Infection results when the host's immune status (T cells) is compromised.

Incidence

A. Tuberculosis is a worldwide infection and is considered a global public health emergency by the World Health Organization. TB can affect any age group. The lifetime risk of developing TB is 5%–10%, with increased risk and mortality noted with extremes of age. For patients with HIV infection, the risk of developing tuberculosis is 7%–10% per year.

B. Postprimary TB is a significant cause of worldwide morbidity and mortality. Pulmonary morbidity results from a chronic cough, hemoptysis, fibrosis, superinfection, bronchial stenosis, repeated pulmonary infections, or empyema. Morbidity also arises from chronic TB osteomyelitis, chronic renal insufficiency, and CNS TB.

Pathogenesis

A. Mycobacteria are non-spore-forming, slow-growing bacilli. Tuberculosis infection occurs by means of inhalation of airborne bacillus droplets from an infected host. The development of an infection depends on prolonged exposure (weeks) to an individual with active pulmonary tuberculosis. Bacilli travel through the pulmonary lymphatics or enter the vascular system and are disseminated to the brain, meninges, eyes, bones, joints, lymph nodes, kidneys, intestines, larynx, and skin. Incubation period from infection to positive skin test reaction is 2–10 weeks, although disease may not occur for many years or may never occur. The risk of disease is greatest within 2 years following infection.

Predisposing Factors

A. Exposure to someone with active disease.

B. High-risk groups: minorities, foreign-born people, prisoners, nursing home residents, indigents, migrant workers, and health care providers.

C. HIV infection is one of the most significant risk factors for TB.

D. Steroid therapy, cancer chemotherapy, and hematologic malignancies increase the risk of tuberculosis.

Common Complaints

A. Fever

B. Malaise

C. Weight loss/difficulty gaining weight

D. Cough

E. Night sweats

F. Chills

G. Occasional hemoptysis

Other Signs and Symptoms

A. Pulmonary TB: fatigue, irritability, undernutrition, with or without fever and cough

B. Glandular TB: chronic cervical adenitis
C. Meningeal TB: fever and meningeal signs, positive CSF
D. Failure to thrive
E. Anorexia

Subjective Data

A. Determine onset, duration, and course of illness.
B. Review symptom history: fever, night sweats, chills, or cough.
C. Review history of weight loss.
D. Review exposure history to someone that has TB.
E. What is the patient's living situation?
F. Review travel history to endemic areas with TB including China, Pakistan, Philippines, Thailand, Indonesia, Bangladesh, and the Democratic Republic of Congo.

Physical Examination

A complete physical examination is mandatory, including the following:

A. Temperature and blood pressure.
B. Inspect
   1. Observe overall appearance.
   2. Check skin for pallor.
   3. Inspect eyes, ears, nose, and throat.
C. Auscultate
   1. Auscultate heart.
   2. Auscultate lungs and chest for the following:
      a. Rales in upper posterior chest.
      b. Bronchophony (voice sounds louder than usual).
      c. Whispered pectoriloquy (patient's whispered sounds are louder than normal).
D. Percuss: Chest.
E. Palpate
   1. Palpate for lymphadenopathy, usually anterior or posterior cervical and supraclavicular nodes. Less commonly involved lymph nodes include submandibular, axillary, and inguinal lymph nodes.
   2. Palpate to evaluate hepatosplenomegaly.
F. Neurologic examination
   1. Evaluate the presence of nuchal rigidity.
   2. Deep tendon reflexes.

Diagnostic Tests

Diagnosis is based on a combination of tuberculin skin testing, purified protein derivative (PPD) testing, and sputum cultures. Bronchoscopy may be required to obtain specimens. Patients with primary TB may not undergo imaging; however, conventional chest radiography (CXR) may be preformed, and 15% of patients with primary TB have normal CXR findings.

Patients with progressive primary or postprimary TB may need a CT to evaluate parenchymal involvement, satellite lesions, bronchogenic spread, and miliary disease. Magnetic resonance imaging (MRI) may be ordered to evaluate complications, such as the extent of thoracic wall involvement with empyema.

A. Tuberculin skin test using the Mantoux test is the recommended method. The dosage of 0.1 mL or 5 tuberculin units (TU) of purified protein derivative (PPD) should be injected intradermally into the volar aspect of the forearm using a 27-gauge needle. A wheel should be raised and should measure approximately 6–10 mm in diameter. Skilled personnel should read the test in 48–72 hours after administration. Measure the amount of induration and not the erythema. Measure transverse to the long axis of the forearm. See Table 8.4.
B. Annual Mantoux tests for those at high risk. There is no need to repeat PPD once the patient has reacted and had a positive PPD.
C. Anteroposterior and lateral chest X-ray films: "snow-storm" appearance indicates miliary TB; segmental consolidation and hilar adenopathy are common; pleural effusion may be present.
D. CBC with differential.
E. Sputum culture with acid-fast smear. Nasopharyngeal secretions and saliva are not acceptable.

Differential Diagnoses

A. Tuberculosis
B. Bronchiectasis
C. Asthma
D. Histoplasmosis
E. Coccidioidomycosis
F. Blastomycosis
G. Malignancies
H. Other pulmonary infections
I. Aspiration pneumonia

Plan

A. General interventions:
   1. Report all suspected and confirmed cases of TB to the local health department.

TABLE 8.4 Interpretation of Mantoux Tuberculin Skin Test

Positive Reaction—Induration Size	Risk Factors
5 mm or more	Close contact with a known or suspected tuberculosis; immunosuppressive conditions (e.g., HIV); on immunosuppressive medications; or an abnormal chest X-ray—consistent with active TB, previously active TB, or clinical evidence of the disease.
10 mm or more	High-risk categories (i.e., homeless, HIV infected, users of illicit drugs, residents in nursing homes, incarcerated, or institutionalized); travel histories to high-prevalence areas of world; children who are at higher risk of dissemination of TB (i.e., younger than 5 years or immunosuppressed).
15 mm or more	Children aged 5 years or older without any risk factors for TB.

2. Directly observed therapy (DOT) is mandatory for the treatment of patients with coexistent HIV disease, those with multidrug-resistant (MDR) tuberculosis, and those who may be noncompliant.

3. Educate patients regarding compliance to therapy, adverse effect of medications, and follow-up care.

B. Pharmaceutical therapy

1. Contact public health authorities for up-to-date recommendations on medications. Medication protocols vary and include the following drugs: isoniazid (INH), rifampin (Rifadin), pyrazinamide (Tebrazid), and ethambutol (Etibi). See Table 8.5.

   a. Isoniazid (Laniazid, Nydrazid) dosing:

     i. Adults: 5–10 mg/kg by mouth (not to exceed 300 mg/day)

     ii. Pediatrics: 10–20 mg/kg by mouth every day; not to exceed 300 mg/day

   b. Rifampin (Rifadin) dosing:

     i. Adults: 600 mg by mouth every day

     ii. Pediatrics: 10–20 mg/kg by mouth every day; not to exceed 600 mg/day

   c. Pyrazinamide (Tebrazid) dosing

     i. Adults: 15–30 mg/kg by mouth every day; not to exceed 2 g/day

     ii. Pediatrics: Administer as in adults

   d. Ethambutol (Myambutol) dosing

     i. Adults with no previous anti-TB therapy: 15 mg/kg by mouth every day

     ii. Adults with previous therapy: 25 mg/kg by mouth every day

     iii. Pediatrics: For those older than 13 years administer as an adult; not recommended those younger than 13 years

2. Compliance with drug regimen is most important.

3. Drug resistance averages 5%–10% nationally and is increasing.

Follow-up

A. Regular follow-up every 4–8 weeks to ensure compliance and to monitor adverse effects and response of the medications.

B. Repeat chest radiograph may be performed after 2–3 months of therapy to observe the response to treatment for patients with pulmonary TB.

C. Consider monitoring liver enzymes monthly in the following patients:

1. Severe or disseminated TB

2. Concurrent or recent hepatic disease or hepatobiliary tract disease from other causes

3. Receiving high doses of INH (10 mg/kg/d) in combination with rifampin, pyrazinamide, or both drugs

4. Women who are pregnant or within the first 6 weeks postpartum

5. Clinical evidence of hepatotoxic effects

Consultation/Referral

A. An infectious diseases consultation may be helpful. The efficacy of vaccination with the bacilli Calmette-Guerin (BCG) vaccine is debated.

Individual Considerations

A. Pregnancy

1. Manage TB on a case-by-case basis with a physician.

2. Chemotherapy must be started immediately to protect both mother and fetus.

3. All pregnant women on INH therapy should receive pyridoxine.

4. The mother that has current disease but is noncontagious at delivery does not require separation of the infant and mother. The mothers can also breast-feed.

   a. Evaluation of the infant includes CXR and Mantoux test at age 4–6 weeks.

   b. If the Mantoux test is negative, a repeat test is warranted at age 3–4 months and at age 6 months.

   c. INH should be administered even if the Mantoux results and CXR do not suggest TB because sufficient cell-mediated immunity to prevent progressive disease may not develop until age 6 months.

5. The mother that has current disease and is contagious at delivery requires separation of the mother and infant until the mother is noncontagious. The management is the same as noted above.

B. Pediatrics

1. Most children and adolescents with positive skin tests are asymptomatic.

2. Mantoux tests are given at ages 1 year, between 4 and 6 years, between 11 and 16 years, and annually to children at risk.

TABLE 8.5 Treatment of Tuberculosis

Tuberculosis	Regimen	Duration
Pulmonary and cervical lymphadenopathy	Isoniazid (INH) + Rifampin	6 months
	*Supplement with pyrazinamide	*First 2 months only
Hilar adenopathy	Isoniazid + Rifampin daily	9 months
	OR	
	INH + Rifampin daily *then*	1 month
	INH + Rifampin twice a week	8 months
Bone and joint disease and miliary disease	INH + Rifampin + Pyrazinamide and streptomycin once a day *then*	2 months
	INH + Rifampin once a day	7–10 months
Tuberculosis in patients with HIV	Consult with a specialist	

REFERENCES

American Academy of Pediatrics. (2009). Respiratory syncytial virus. In L. K. Pickering (Ed.), *Red Book: 2009 Report of the Committee on Infectious Diseases* (26th ed., pp. 560–569). Elk Grove Village, IL: Author. Retrieved June 27, 2009, from http://aapredbook. aappublications.org.proxy.library.vanderbilt.edu/cgi/content/full/ 2009/1/3.110.

American Dietetic Association. (2009). American Dietetic Association chronic obstructive pulmonary disease (COPD) evidence-based nutrition practice guideline. Retrieved October 3, 2009, from http:// www.adaevidencelibrary.com/tmp/prn6D80E0CAFE734D8FC12 7FB5D0FBB7BEB.pdf.

Batra, V., & Ang, J. T. (2008, October 30). Tuberculosis. *emedicine.* Retrieved August 23, 2009, from http://emedicine.medscape.com/ article/969401-print.

Carolan, P. L., & Callahan, C. (2009, March 19). Bronchitis, acute and chronic. *emedicine.* Retrieved August 23, 2009, from http://emedi cine.medscape.com/article/1001332-print.

Catanzano, T. M., & Curtis, A. (2008, February 27). Lung, primary tuberculosis. *emedicine.* Retrieved August 23, 2009, from http:// emedicine.medscape.com/article/358610-print.

Centers for Disease Control and Prevention. (n.d.). Bronchitis (Chest cold). Retrieved August 23, 2009, from http://www.cdc.gov/gets mart/antibiotic-use/URI/bronchitis.html.

Centers for Disease Control and Prevention. (2007, January 12). Infants deaths associated with cough and cold medications: Two states, 2005. *MMWR, 56*(1), 1–4. Retrieved August 23, 2009, from http://www.cdc.gov/mmwr/preview/mmwrhtml/mm5601a1.htm.

Chen, H. H., & Jafek, B. W. (2008, February 1). Chronic cough. *emedicine.* Retrieved August 23, 2009, from http://emedicine.medscape. com/article/1048560-print.

Cherry, J. D. (2008). Croup. *The New England Journal of Medicine, 358,* 384–391.

DellaCroce, H. (2009). Guidelines for managing asthma. *The American Journal for Nurse Practitioners, 13,* 8–18.

DeNicola, L. K. (2008, September 18). Bronchiolitis. *emedicine.* Retrieved August 23, 2009, from http://emedicine.medscape.com/ article/961963-print.

Elder, M. A., & Mellon, M. (2008). Long-term inhaled corticosteroid therapy in children and adolescents with persistent asthma: Facilitating adherence to guidelines-based therapy. *The American Journal for Nurse Practitioners, 12,* 9–18.

Ellis, K. C. (2009). The differential diagnosis and management of asthma in the preschool-aged child. *Journal of the American Academy of Nurse Practitioners, 21,* 463–473.

Global Initiative for Chronic Obstructive Lung Disease. (2009). Pocket guide to COPD diagnosis, management, and prevention: A guide for health care professionals. Retrieved February 6, 2010, from http:// www.goldcopd.com/Guidelineitem.asp?l1=2&l2=1&intId=2002.

Harding, S. M. (2009, June 18). Gastroesophageal reflux and asthma. *UpToDate.* Retrieved September 20, 2009, from http://www.upto date.com/online/content/topic.do?topicKey=asthma/9465&selected Title=36-150&source=search_result.

Irwin, R. S., Bauman, M. H., Bolser, D. C., Boulet, L. P., Braman, S. S., Brightling, C. E., et al. (2006). Diagnosis and management of cough executive summary: ACCP evidence-based clinical practice guidelines. *Chest, 129,* 1S–23S.

Kamangar, N., & Nikhanj, N. S. (2009, August 14). Chronic obstructive pulmonary disease. *emedicine.* Retrieved August 23, 2009, from http://emedicine.medscape.com/article/297664-print.

King, L. (2009, August 11). Pediatrics, croup or laryngotracheobronchitis. *emedicine.* Retrieved August 23, 2009, from http://emedi cine.medscape.com/article/800866-print.

Krawczyk, J., Gharahbaghian, L., & Rutkowski, A. (2006, July 14). Toxicity, cough and cold preparation. *emedicine.* Retrieved August 23, 2009, from http://emedicine.medscape.com/article/1010513-print.

Krilov, L. R. (2009, July 27). Respiratory syncytial virus (RSV) infection. *emedicine.* Retrieved August 23, 2009, from http://emedicine. medscape.com/article/971488-print.

Lim, W. S., Baudouin, S. V., George, R. C., Hill, A. T., Jamieson, C., Leune, I. L., et al. (2009). British Thoracic Society guidelines for the management of community acquired pneumonia in adults: Update 2009. *Thorax, 64,* iii1–iii55.

Louden, M. (2009, June 23). Pediatrics, bronchiolitis. *emedicine.* Retrieved August 23, 2009, from http://emedicine.medscape.com/ article/800428-print.

Medscape Drug Reference. (n.d.). Theophylline oral. *Medscape.* Retrieved September 20, 2009, from http://www.medscape.com/ druginfo/dosage?drugid=3591&drugname=Theophylline+Oral& monotype=default.

MuÑiz, A., Molodow, R. E., & Defendi, G. L. (2008, November 21). Croup. *emedicine.* Retrieved August 23, 2009, from http://emedi cine.medscape.com/article/962972-overview.

Neuman, M. I. (2009, July 24). Pediatrics, pneumonia. *emedicine.* Retrieved August 27, 2009, from http://emedicine.medscape.com/ article/803364-print.

Newcomb, P. (2009). Safe control of pest and pet asthma triggers. *The American Journal for Nurse Practitioners, 5,* 571–578.

Nurse Practitioner Associates for Continuing Education. (2009, August). *COPD: Improving patient outcomes—You can made a difference.* Montvale, NJ: HayMarket Medical Education LP.

Ong, S. (2009, January 14). Bronchitis. *emedicine.* Retrieved August 23, 2009, from http://emedicine.medscape.com/article/807035-print.

Rajnik, M., & Murray, C. (2008, June 30). Rhinoviruses. *emedicine.* Retrieved September 7, 2009, from http://emedicine.medscape. com/article/227820-print.

Rennard, S. I. (2009, May 31). Chronic obstructive pulmonary disease: Definition, clinical manifestations, diagnosis, and staging. *UpToDate.* Retrieved September 20, 2009, from http://www.uptodate. com/online/content/topic.do?topicKey=copd/6333&view=print.

Rogers, N. F. (2008). Recognition and treatment of premenstrual asthma. *Women's Health Care: A Practical Journal for Nurse Practitioners, 7,* 18–23.

Sarver, N., & Murphy, K. (2009). Management of asthma: New approaches to establishing control. *Journal of the American Academy of Nurse Practitioners, 21,* 54–65.

Sharma, S. (2006, June 14). Emphysema. *emedicine.* Retrieved August 23, 2009, from http://emedicine.medscape.com/article/ 298283-print.

Sheffield, J. S., & Cunningham, F. G. (2009, October). Community-acquired pneumonia in pregnancy. *Obstetrics & Gynecology, 114,* 915–922.

Sherman, C. (2008). A larger role for PCPs in COPD management. *The Clinical Advisor, 11,* 67–73.

Vanhoose, K. J., & Wood, A. F. (2009). Current insight into childhood asthma: Implications for practice. *The American Journal for Nurse Practitioners, 13,* 10–18, 42.

Watts, B. (2009). Outpatient management of asthma in children age 5–11 years: Guidelines for practice. *Journal of the American Academy of Nurse Practitioners, 21,* 261–269.

Cardiovascular Guidelines

Christopher S. Shadowens

ACUTE MYOCARDIAL INFARCTION

Definition
A. Acute myocardial infarction (MI) is a prolonged lack of myocardial oxygenation leading to necrosis of a portion of the heart muscle. It is caused by atherosclerotic coronary artery disease that alone or in association with other factors causes complete blockage of one of the coronary arteries.

Incidence
A. Approximately 1.5 million Americans sustain an acute MI annually. Despite a marked decrease in incidence and mortality during the past three decades, MI continues to be the leading cause of death in this country, accounting for one-fourth of all fatalities. More women die from heart disease than men.

Pathogenesis
A. Abrupt coronary artery occlusion is the primary cause of most MIs. Occlusions can result from atherosclerotic plaque, intracoronary thrombus formation, or arterial spasm.

Predisposing Factors
A. Hypercholesterolemia: increased LDL, decreased HDL
B. Hypertriglyceridemia
C. Premature familial onset of coronary heart disease, or CHD, formerly called CAD, before age 55
D. Smoking
E. Hypertension
F. Obesity
G. Sedentary lifestyle
H. Diabetes mellitus
I. Aging
J. Stress

Common Complaints
A. Primary complaint: pain somewhere in chest, described as worst pain ever experienced
B. Nausea
C. Vomiting
D. Diaphoresis
E. Indigestion

Other Signs and Symptoms
A. Pain in abdomen, arm, back, jaw, and neck
B. Chest heaviness or tightness
C. Anxiety
D. Cough
E. Dyspnea
F. Hypertension or hypotension
G. Weakness, light-headedness, syncope
H. Pallor
I. Orthopnea

Potential Complications
A. Arrhythmias
B. Heart failure
C. Cardiogenic shock
D. Rupture of left ventricular papillary muscle
E. Ventricular septal rupture
F. Pericarditis or Dressler's syndrome
G. Ventricular aneurysm
H. Thromboembolism

Subjective Data
A. Ask the patient what activity brought about or preceded the episode.
B. Have the patient describe duration of pain and what time of day symptoms began.
C. Ask the patient to describe pain, for example, crushing, stabbing, or burning.
D. Ask the patient where sensation began and in what direction it radiates.
E. Have the patient rate pain on a scale of 1 to 10, with 1 being the least painful.
F. Ask the patient to list all medications currently being taken, particularly substances not prescribed and illicit drugs such as cocaine.

Physical Examination

Patients presenting with acute chest pain should be quickly assessed for the need to call emergency services/911 for immediate transport to the hospital.

A. Check temperature, pulse, respirations, and blood pressure.
B. Inspect.

1. Inspect general appearance, noting dyspnea and weakness.
2. Inspect skin for pallor and diaphoresis.
3. Inspect legs for edema.
4. Inspect chest wall for visible pulsations.
5. Inspect neck for jugular vein distension.
6. Observe nail beds for signs of cyanosis and note capillary filling time.

C. Palpate
1. Palpate abdomen for organomegaly.
2. Palpate peripheral pulses in legs.
3. Palpate femoral pulses.

D. Auscultate
1. Auscultate carotid arteries.
2. Auscultate abdomen.
3. Conduct a complete heart exam, checking for dysrhythmias.
4. Conduct a complete lung exam.

E. Mental status: Assess for confusion.

Diagnostic Tests

A. EKG: shows inverted T waves, ST segment elevation, and Q waves. One normal EKG initially does not always rule out MI; perform serial EKGs if MI suspected.
B. Cardiac enzymes: Creatinine kinase (CK) initially rises in 6–8 hours; isoenzyme (CK-MB) initially rises in 4–6 hours.
C. Cardiac troponin-I.
D. Chest radiography.
E. Cardiac catheterization.

Differential Diagnoses

A. Acute myocardial infarction
B. Unstable angina pectoris
C. Aortic dissection
D. Pulmonary embolism
E. Pericarditis
F. Esophageal spasm
G. Pancreatitis
H. Biliary tract disease

Plan

A. Patient teaching
1. Educate the patient about modifying controllable risk factors such as keeping diabetes and hypertension under control, diet, exercise, and stopping smoking.
2. If known CHD is present:
   a. Make sure the patient is aware of signs and symptoms of MI.
   b. Make sure the patient knows to seek medical attention or dial 911 if signs and symptoms occur.
   c. Encourage CPR training for family and/or close friends.
   d. The patient should carry nitroglycerin at all times and know how to use it.

B. Dietary management: Counsel the patient on nutrition and low-fat, low-cholesterol, low-sodium diet. Give diet handouts. See Appendix B for DASH diet.
C. Pharmaceutical therapy
1. When MI is suspected: aspirin 160–325 mg (four 81 mg baby aspirin) chewed or swallowed as soon as possible. Enteric coated aspirin delays absorption and therefore is not recommended.
2. Instruct the patient on how to take sublingual nitroglycerin tablets and other medications.
3. Oxygen therapy: 2–4 liters per nasal cannula.
4. Nitrates: Nitroglycerin sublingual 0.2–0.6 mg every 5 minutes for ischemic chest pain in the absence of hypotension.
5. If pain persists after three doses of nitroglycerin:
   a. Morphine sulfate IV; 2–4 mg IV, repeating every 5 minutes until pain resolves. Dose may be increased at 2–8 mg per dose as tolerated. Monitor side effects: nausea/vomiting, dizziness, hypotension, respiratory distress.
6. If no contraindications (bradycardia, heart failure, 2nd or 3rd degree heart block, asthma, shock), beta blockers may be started IV during the acute phase and changed to oral therapy during course of the treatment.
7. Fibrinolytic therapy may be used for patients with suspected MI with ST-Elevation Myocardial Infarction (STEMI) or Non-ST-Elevation Myocardial Infarction (NSTEMI) with left bundle brand block.

Follow-up

A. Follow-up is determined by patient's needs, severity of acute MI, and whether complications are present.

Consultation/Referral

If you suspect MI, refer patient for immediate hospitalization.

☐ ATHEROSCLEROSIS AND HYPERLIPIDEMIA

Definition

A. Atherosclerosis is a systemic disease characterized by lipid deposition and smooth muscle cell migration and proliferation in the intima of the larger arteries. Atheromatous changes lead to thrombotic stroke, peripheral vascular disease, CAD, and MI.
B. Hyperlipidemia is an elevation in serum lipoproteins and a major risk factor in the development of CHD. The two main lipids in blood are cholesterol and triglyceride. Cholesterol is a relatively insoluble lipid that is necessary for cell membrane formation, steroid and bile salt production, and the development of nerve sheaths. Cholesterol is composed of three clinically significant components: high-density lipoprotein (HDL), low-density lipoprotein (LDL), and very-low-density lipoprotein (VLDL). Triglyceride is found in VLDL particles, but its role in atherosclerosis is not clear.

Incidence

A. Incidence of atherosclerotic diseases increases with age. These diseases are by far the leading cause of death in the United States in people of all ages. Heart disease (CHD) accounted for more than 631,636 deaths in 2006, estimating that it caused 1 out of every 6 deaths in the United States in 2006. Coronary heart disease is the most common type of heart disease (Heron et al., 2009, 57-1-80). Based on the NHANES report 2003–2006 data, 17,600 American adults 20 years and older had CHD, with men being higher at 9% and women being 7%. CHD is the primary cause of morbidity and mortality in this country. In the United States, heart disease alone (medical services and lost time at work) will cost the country approximately $316.4 billion.

Pathogenesis

A. Atherosclerosis is in part attributed to the deposition of cholesterol and lipoproteins in arterial smooth muscle cells. Dietary factors, obesity, drugs, and genetic defects in lipoprotein particle metabolism influence lipid and lipoprotein concentrations in blood.

B. Primary hyperlipoproteinemias are either due to single-gene disorders transmitted by simple dominant or recessive mechanisms, or to multifactorial disorders with complicated inheritance patterns.

C. Secondary hyperlipoproteinemias (such as in thyroid disease and diabetes mellitus) occur as part of a constellation of abnormalities in certain metabolic pathways. The association between atherosclerosis, CHD, and hypercholesterolemia is well documented. HDL cholesterol comprises about one-fourth of the total serum cholesterol and acts as a scavenger, removing cholesterol from peripheral tissues and returning it to the liver, which produces a favorable cardioprotective effect. Elevated HDL levels are desirable. HDL levels over 60 mg/dL are a negative risk factor for CHD; those below 35 mg/dL are a major risk factor for CHD.

D. LDL cholesterol constitutes 70% of the total serum cholesterol. It is the most atherogenic cholesterol subgroup. LDL particles interact with platelets, damaged arterial endothelium, and smooth muscle cells in the process of plaque formation. LDL levels of 160 mg/dL or greater are associated with an increased number of cardiac events.

E. VLDL accounts for a small amount of total serum cholesterol and is responsible for carrying triglycerides from the liver. Its role in atherogenesis is uncertain, but an inverse relationship has been observed between VLDL and HDL.

Predisposing Factors

A. *High risk factors* for coronary heart disease (CHD) events (CHD risk equivalent):
 1. Clinical CHD
 2. Symptomatic carotid artery disease
 3. Peripheral arterial disease
 4. Abdominal aortic aneurysm

B. Presence of *major risk factors* (other than LDL):
 1. Age older than 45 years for men, or older than 55 years for women
 2. Cigarette smoking
 3. Low HDL cholesterol level, less than 40 mg/dL
 4. Family history of early CHD: MI or sudden cardiac death younger than 55 years in father or other male first-degree relative, before age 65 in mother or other female first-degree relative
 5. Hypertension (BP >140/90 mmHg or on antihypertensive medication).

HDL cholesterol of greater than 60 mg/dL is equal to "negative" risk factor and removes one risk factor from the total count.

Common Complaints

A. There are no complaints or symptoms associated with atherosclerosis and hyperlipidemia. Most lipid abnormalities are detected by routine laboratory testing or as part of a cardiovascular evaluation.

Subjective Data

A. Ask the patient if there is a history of cardiovascular disease.

B. Discuss his or her past medical history, including predisposing factors for cardiovascular disease.

C. Have the patient list current medications, including over-the-counter and herbal products.

D. Have the patient discuss his or her current diet and exercise routine.

E. Explore the patient's social habits, including use of alcohol and tobacco.

Physical Examination

A. Check temperature, pulse, respirations, blood pressure, height, and weight.

B. Inspect
 1. Funduscopic exam: Examine eyes for premature arcus cornealis, which is a gray opaque line around the cornea caused by lipoid degeneration, and for lipemia retinalis, or a pale retina with white blood vessels caused by excess serum lipids due to VLDL of more than 2,000 mg/dL or alcoholism.
 2. Inspect skin for xanthomas, which appear as red-brown or yellow papules, nodules, or plaque, caused by lipid deposits from high VLDL. Tendinous xanthomas are found on Achilles tendons, patellae, and hands.
 3. Inspect joints for Achilles tendonitis and arthritis.

C. Palpate
 1. Palpate abdomen for hepatomegaly or splenomegaly.
 2. Palpate neck and thyroid.

D. Auscultate
 1. Perform a complete heart exam.
 2. Perform a complete vascular exam.

Diagnostic Tests

A. Lipoprotein analysis, performed after patient fasts for 9–12 hours.
 1. Review ATP III Guidelines At-A-Glance Quick Desk Reference and perform steps 1–9 as recommended by the National Institutes of Health (see Table 9.1). Perform 10 year cardiovascular heart disease risk assessment.

B. Risk Screening Score and discuss results with the patient.

Differential Diagnoses

Assess patient for the following secondary causes of CHD and hyperlipidemia:

A. Athereroscerosis

B. Hyperlipidemia

C. Diabetes mellitus

D. Hypothyroidism

E. Nephrotic syndrome

TABLE 9.1 Step Therapy for Hyperlipidemia

STEP 1: Determine lipoprotein levels. Obtain complete lipoprotein profile after 9- to 12-hour fast.

ATP III Classification of LDL, Total, and HDL Cholesterol (mg/dL)

- **LDL Cholesterol—Primary Target of Therapy**

< 100	Optimal
100–129	Near optimal/above optimal
130–159	Borderline high
160–189	High
≥ 190	Very high

- **Total Cholesterol**

< 200	Desirable
200–239	Borderline high
≥ 240	High

- **HDL Cholesterol**

< 40	Low
≥ 60	High

STEP 2: Identify presence of clinical atherosclerotic disease that confers high risk for coronary heart disease (CHD) events (CHD risk equivalent):

- Clinical CHD
- Symptomatic carotid artery disease
- Peripheral arterial disease
- Abdominal aortic aneurysm.

STEP 3: Determine presence of major risk factors (other than LDL):

Major Risk Factors (Exclusive of LDL Cholesterol) That Modify LDL Goals

- Cigarette smoking
- Hypertension (BP 140/90 mmHg or on antihypertensive medication)
- Low HDL cholesterol (< 40 mg/dl)*
- Family history of premature CHD (CHD in male first-degree relative < 55 years; CHD in female first-degree relative < 65 years)
- Age (men 45 years; women 55 years)

*HDL cholesterol 60 mg/dL counts as a "negative" risk factor; its presence removes one risk factor from the total count.
Note: in ATP III, diabetes is regarded as a CHD risk equivalent.

STEP 4: If 2+ risk factors (other than LDL) are present without CHD or CHD risk equivalent, assess 10-year (short-term) CHD risk (see Framingham tables).

Three levels of 10-year risk:

- > 20%—CHD risk equivalent
- 10–20%
- < 10%

STEP 5: Determine risk category:

- Establish LDL goal of therapy.
- Determine need for therapeutic lifestyle changes (TLC).
- Determine level for drug consideration.

LDL Cholesterol Goals and Cutpoints for Therapeutic Lifestyle Changes (TLC) and Drug Therapy in Different Risk Categories.

Risk Category	LDL Goal	LDL Level at Which to Initiate Therapeutic Lifestyle Changes (TLC)	LDL Level at Which to Consider Drug Therapy
CHD or CHD risk equivalents (10-year risk > 20%)	< 100 mg/dL	≥ 100 mg/dL	≥ 130 mg/dL (100–129 mg/dL: drug optional)*

TABLE 9.1 *(continued)*

Risk Category	LDL Goal	LDL Level at Which to Initiate Therapeutic Lifestyle Changes (TLC)	LDL Level at Which to Consider Drug Therapy
2+ risk factors (10-year risk > 20%)	≥ 130 mg/dL	≥ 130 mg/dL	10-year risk 10–20%: ≥ 130 mg/dL 10-year risk < 10%: ≥ 160 mg/dL
0–1 risk factor**	≥ 160 mg/dL	≥ 160 mg/dL	≥ 190 mg/dL (160–189 mg/dL: LDL-lowering drug optional)

*Some authorities recommend use of LDL-lowering drugs in this category if an LDL cholesterol < 100 mg/dL cannot be achieved by therapeutic lifestyle changes. Others prefer use of drugs that primarily modify triglycerides and HDL, for example, nicotinic acid or fibrate. Clinical judgment also may call for deferring drug therapy in this subcategory.

**Almost all people with 0–1 risk factor have a 10-year risk < 10%, thus 10-year risk assessment in people with 0–1 risk factor is not necessary.

STEP 6: Initiate therapeutic lifestyle changes (TLC) if LDL is above goal.

TLC Features

- TLC diet:
  - o Saturated fat < 7% of calories, cholesterol < 200 mg/day.
  - o Consider increased viscous (soluble) fiber (10–25 g/day) and plant stanols/sterols (2g/day) as therapeutic options to enhance LDL lowering.
- Weight management
- Increased physical activity

STEP 7: Consider adding drug therapy if LDL exceeds levels shown in Step 5 table:

- Consider drug simultaneously with TLC for CHD and CHD equivalents.
- Consider adding drug to TLC after 3 months for other risk categories.

Drugs Affecting Lipoprotein Metabolism

Drug Class	Agents and Daily Doses	Lipid/Lipoprotein Effects	Side Effects	Contraindications
HMG CoA reductase inhibitors (statins)	Lovastatin (20–80 mg), Pravastatin (20–40 mg), Simvastatin (20–80 mg), Fluvastatin (20–80 mg), Atorvastatin (10–80 mg), Cerivastatin (0.4–0.8 mg)	LDL-C ↓18–55% HDL-C ↑5–15% TG ↓7–30%	Myopathy Increased liver enzymes	Absolute: • Active or chronic liver disease Relative: • Concomitant use of certain drugs*
Bile acid Sequestrants	Cholestyramine (4–16 g) Colestipol (5–20 g) Colesevelam (2.6–3.8 g)	LDL-C ↓15–30% HDL-C ↑3–5% TG No change or increase	Gastrointestinal distress Constipation Decreased absorption of other drugs	Absolute: • dysbeta-lipoproteinemia • TG > 400 mg/dL Relative: • TG > 200 mg/dL
Nicotinic acid	Immediate release (crystalline) nicotinic acid (1.5–3 gm), extended release nicotinic acid (Niaspan®) (1–2 g), sustained release nicotinic acid (1–2 g)	LDL-C ↓5–25% HDL-C ↑15–35% TG ↓20–50%	Flushing Hyperglycemia Hyperuricemia (or gout) Upper GI distress Hepatotoxicity	Absolute: • Chronic liver disease • Severe gout Relative: • Diabetes • Hyperuricemia • Peptic ulcer disease
Fibric acids	Gemfibrozil (600 mg BID) Fenofibrate (200 mg) Clofibrate (1,000 mg BID)	LDL-C ↓5–20% (may be increased in patients with high TG) HDL-C ↑10–20% TG ↓20–50%	Dyspepsia Gallstones Myopathy	Absolute: • Severe renal disease • Severe hepatic disease

*Cyclosporine, macrolide antibiotics, various antifungal agents, and cytochrome P-450 inhibitors (fibrates and niacin should be used with appropriate caution).

Note: BID = twice a day

(continued)

TABLE 9.1 *(continued)*

STEP 8: Identify metabolic syndrome and treat, if present, after 3 months of TLC.

Clinical Identification of the Metabolic Syndrome—Any 3 of the Following:

Risk Factor	Defining Level
Abdominal obesity* Men Women	Waist circumference** > 102 cm (> 40 in) > 88 cm (> 35 in)
Triglycerides	≥ 150 mg/dL
HDL cholesterol Men Women	< 40 mg/dl < 50 mg/dl
Blood pressure	≥ 130/ 85 mmHg
Fasting glucose	≥ 110 mg/dL

*Overweight and obesity are associated with insulin resistance and the metabolic syndrome. However, the presence of abdominal obesity is more highly correlated with the metabolic risk factors than is an elevated body mass index (BMI). Therefore, the simple measure of waist circumference is recommended to identify the body weight component of the metabolic syndrome.

**Some male patients can develop multiple metabolic risk factors when the waist circumference is only marginally increased, for example, 94–102 cm (37–39 in). Such patients may have a strong genetic contribution to insulin resistance. They should benefit from changes in life habits, similarly to men with categorical increases in waist circumference.

Treatment of the Metabolic Syndrome

- Treat underlying causes (overweight/obesity and physical inactivity):
  o Intensify weight management.
  o Increase physical activity.
- Treat lipid and nonlipid risk factors if they persist despite these lifestyle therapies:
  o Treat hypertension.
  o Use aspirin for CHD patients to reduce prothrombotic state.
  o Treat elevated triglycerides and/or low HDL (as shown in Step 9 below).

STEP 9: Treat elevated triglycerides.

ATP III Classification of Serum Triglycerides (mg/dL)

< 150	Normal
150–199	Borderline high
200–499	High
≥ 500	Very high

Treatment of Elevated Triglycerides (150 mg/dL)

- Primary aim of therapy is to reach LDL goal.
- Intensify weight management.
- Increase physical activity.
- If triglycerides are 200 mg/dL after LDL goal is reached, set secondary goal for non-HDL cholesterol (total HDL) 30 mg/dL higher than LDL goal.

Comparison of LDL Cholesterol and Non-HDL Cholesterol Goals for 3 Risk Categories

Risk Category	LDL Goal (mg/dL)	Non-HDL Goal (mg/dL)
CHD and CHD risk equivalent (10-year risk for CHD > 20%)	< 100	< 130
Multiple (2+) risk factors and 10-year risk 20%	< 130	< 160
0–1 risk factor	< 160	< 190

If triglycerides 200–499 mg/dL after LDL goal is reached, consider adding drug if needed to reach non-HDL goal:

- Intensify therapy with LDL-lowering drug, or
- Add nicotinic acid or fibrate to further lower VLDL.

TABLE 9.1 *(continued)*

If triglycerides 500 mg/dL, first lower triglycerides to prevent pancreatitis:

- Very low-fat diet (≤ 15% of calories from fat).
- Weight management and physical activity.
- Fibrate or nicotinic acid.
- When triglycerides < 500 mg/dL, turn to LDL-lowering therapy.

Treatment of Low HDL Cholesterol (<40 mg/dL)

- First reach LDL goal, then:
- Intensify weight management and increase physical activity.
- If triglycerides 200–499 mg/dL, achieve non-HDL goal.
- If triglycerides < 200 mg/dL (isolated low HDL) in CHD or CHD equivalent, consider nicotinic acid or fibrate.

Source: NIH Publication No. 01-3305

F. Porphyria
G. Obesity
H. Obstructive liver disease
I. Diuretic use

Plan

A. General interventions
   1. Encourage the patient to engage in physical activity to help raise HDL levels.
   2. Explain to the patient that walking vigorously for 30 min three times a week is associated with reduced coronary risks.
B. Patient teaching: See the Section III Patient Teaching Guide for this chapter, "Atherosclerosis and Hyperlipidemia."
C. Dietary management
   1. Advise the patient that diet modification is the first line of therapy for hyperlipidemia.
   2. Explain cholesterol-lowering diet. Give dietary recommendation sheets. See Appendix B for low fat/low cholesterol and DASH dietary approaches to stop hypertention.
   3. Explain that weight reduction in patients greater than 20% over ideal body weight can lower LDL and triglyceride levels.
D. Pharmaceutical therapy: Drug therapy is recommended for elevated LDL cholesterol levels despite diet therapy. Use clinical judgment when deciding potential benefits, possible side effects, and costs of drug treatment.
   1. Drug of choice: HMG-CoA reductase inhibitors (statins). These suppress activity of the key enzyme in cholesterol synthesis in liver; they are highly effective in lowering LDL but can cause liver toxicity, myositis, rhabdomyolysis, and low HDL. Monitor liver function tests before therapy begins, 4–6 weeks after starting drug therapy. Then check at 3–4 month intervals or more frequently, if necessary. Discontinue medications if abnormal lab values or adverse symptoms appear. Avoid concomitant drugs such as erythromycin, nicotine, azole antifungals, clofibrate, and gemfibrozil. Use caution with other medications.
   2. Bile acid sequestrants bind bile acids in GI tract; lower moderately elevated LDL by 20%; and may cause constipation, bloating, and poor absorption of other drugs.
   3. Nicotinic acid, or niacin: Mechanism of action is unknown. Discuss possibilities of flushing. Contraindicated with chronic liver disease and severe gout.
   4. Fibric acid derivatives: Highly effective in lowering triglycerides, and lowers VLDL, causes modest reduction in LDL, and raises HDL. May cause GI distress, rash, pain, blurred vision, anemia, and gallstones. May inhibit insulin and oral hypoglycemic absorption, and potentiates oral anticoagulants.

Follow-up

A. Measure patient's total cholesterol 4 weeks after initiation of **diet** and then at 3–4 month intervals.
B. If initiating medication therapy, obtain baseline blood work, including fasting lipid profile with liver function tests (LFTs) and a CBC. Recheck tests 4–6 weeks after starting drug therapy. Then check at 3–4 month intervals or more frequently, if necessary.

Individual Considerations

A. Patients with high cholesterol who are otherwise at low risk for CHD (particularly men over age 35 and premenopausal women) are candidates for primary prevention emphasizing diet modification and increased physical activity. It is recommended that drug therapy be used sparingly in these patients.
B. Lowering serum cholesterol reduces morbidity and mortality in patients with CHD, and it reduces the number of new cardiac events in those without known CHD.
C. Elevated triglycerides increase the risk of pancreatitis and diabetes.

CHEST PAIN

Definition
A. Chest pain is a localized sensation of distress or discomfort that may or may not be associated with actual tissue damage.

Incidence
A. Chest pain is one of the most common complaints of adult patients. Causes can range from minor disorders to life-threatening diseases, so every patient must be assessed carefully.

Pathogenesis
A. Cardiac etiology: ischemia, atherosclerosis, inflammation, or valvular problems due to angina, MI, pericarditis, endocarditis, dissecting aortic aneurysm, or mitral valve prolapse (MVP) (See Table 9.2)
B. Musculoskeletal etiology: muscle strain and inflammation due to costochondritis, chest wall syndrome, cervicodorsal arthritis, or intercostal myositis
C. Neurologic etiology: nerve inflammation and/or compression due to herpes zoster and nerve root compression
D. GI etiology: structural defects, inflammation, or infection due to GERD, hiatal hernia, esophageal spasm, pancreatitis, cholecystitis, or peptic ulcer disease (PUD)
E. Pleural etiology: inflammation, distension, or compression of pleural membranes due to pneumonia, pulmonary embolus, pulmonary hypertension, spontaneous pneumothorax, and lung and mediastinal tumors
F. Psychogenic etiology: stress due to anxiety, depression, or panic disorders

Predisposing Factors
A. These vary depending on etiology of pain.

Common Complaints
A. Primary complaint: pain somewhere in the chest
B. Fatigue
C. Cough
D. Indigestion

Other Signs and Symptoms
A. Pain may be typical of angina and MI.
B. Musculoskeletal pain may be relieved by position change, aggravated by body movement, reproducible, or caused by injury or trauma.
C. Neurologic pain is associated with skin lesion if herpes zoster is the causative agent.
D. GI pain may be associated with meals, certain positions, or an acid taste in mouth, or it may be referred to other sites.
E. Pleural pain is accompanied by cough, URI symptoms, or shortness of breath (SOB).
F. Psychogenic pain or pressure along with SOB and dizziness may be associated with a specific event or time.

Subjective Data
A. What precipitates and relieves the patient's chest pain?
B. Inquire about character of pain: location, radiation, quality, intensity, duration, and frequency.
C. Are other associated symptoms present?
D. Discuss any risk factors the patient may have for cardiac disease: smoking, hyperlipidemia, hypertension, sedentary lifestyle, and family history.
E. Review medical history as noted above.
F. Review all medications including prescription, over-the-counter, and herbal product.

Physical Examination
A. Check temperature, pulse, respirations, and blood pressure.
B. Inspect
   1. Inspect general appearance. Note patient position: sitting, lying, squatting. Relief of chest pain with recumbency suggests MVP; relief with squatting suggests hypertrophic cardiomyopathy. Noncardiac chest pain may be present along with cardiac chest pain.
   2. Inspect skin for jaundice, pallor, herpes zoster lesions, rash, or cyanosis.
   3. Inspect chest wall for herpes zoster lesions or signs of trauma.
   4. Inspect eyes by performing funduscopic exam.
   5. Inspect legs for signs of phlebitis: unilateral swelling, cyanosis, venous stasis, and diminished pulses.
   6. Inspect neck for enlarged thyroid and lymph nodes, midline trachea, and jugular venous distension.
C. Palpate
   1. Palpate chest wall for tenderness and swelling. Chest pain present in only one body position is usually not cardiac in origin.
   2. Palpate abdomen for masses, tenderness, bounding pulses, organomegaly, and ascites.
   3. Palpate femoral and distal pulses.
D. Auscultate
   1. Auscultate carotid arteries for bruits.
   2. Auscultate lungs for crackles, wheezes, equal breath sounds, and pleural rub.
   3. Auscultate abdomen for bruits and bowel sounds.
   4. Auscultate heart for murmurs, rubs, clicks, irregularities, or extra sounds.
E. Neurologic exam: Perform this if neurologic etiology is suspected.

Diagnostic Tests
A. Testing depends on information collected in exam. A normal physical exam, EKG, and/or lab test results in a patient with chest pain does not rule out CHD. Typical tests include the following:
   1. EKG
   2. Chest radiography, whenever diagnosis of chest pain is not clear
   3. Echocardiogram
   4. Stress test
   5. Cardiac catheterization
   6. Barium tests
   7. Endoscopy to rule out GI etiology
   8. Esophageal pH, low

Differential Diagnoses
A. Cardiac causes

TABLE 9.2 Comparison of Common Chest Pain Etiologies

Condition	Pain Findings	Associated Symptoms	Precipitating Factors	Relieving Factors	Physical Findings	Diagnostic Tests	Treatment Modalities
Cardiac-Stable Angina	Substernal, tight, dull pressure, usually last > 15 min		Exertion, cold, emotional stress	Rest, nitroglycerin Valsalva's maneuver	Sinus tach. bradycardia xanthomas, signs of HF	Resting EKG, stress EKG, cardiac enzymes, Echo angiogram	ASA BB Nitrate CCB
Prinzmetal's Angina (variant)	Substernal, achy, tight, dull pressure		Often occurs at rest; may awaken from sleep	Nitroglycerin	Same as stable angina	Resting EKG, angiogram	ASA Nitrates CCB
MI	Precordial, substernal, severe, crushing, squeezing, lasts > 15 min	Dyspnea, sweating, dizzy, radiation to neck/arm/jaw N&V, cough fever unstable V/S	Oxygen	Not relieved by nitroglycerin	S3 or S4 murmur, tachycardia, bradycardia pericardia friction rub, hyper/hypo tension	EKG, serial CK enzymes Echo, radionuclide studies	Analgesia, reperfusion, prevent and treatment complications limit infarcts Thrombolytic therapy for acute MI
MVP	Usually not substernal, often knife-like, may last 1–3 hr	Palpitations, fatigue, light-headed, arrhythmia, syncope		Recumbent position, BB, nitroglycerine	Midsytolic click and/or murmur, thin body status, SOB	Echo, EKG	Usually none, BB if palpitations or ventricular ectopy becomes disabling
Hypertrophic Cardiomegaly	Similar to angina	Dyspnea with exertion, arrhythmias, light-headed syncope	May be increased by nitroglycerin, exertion	BB, squatting	Systolic murmur, in creased upright position, Valsalva's maneuver, more forceful PMI	EKG, CXR, Echo, Doppler, Cardiac Cath	BB CCB Possible pacing and myomectomy, exercise restriction
Pericarditis	Retrosternal, sharp or dull, sudden onset, long duration, radiates to one side of the trapezius	Fever, myalgia, anorexia, anxiety, recent viral infection		Sitting up, leaning forward	Friction rub, SVT1, tachypnea, crackles, signs of cardiac tamponade	EKG, Echo CBC, ESR	Hospitalize r/o purulent process Analgesics
Endocarditis	Usually dull, retrosternal, may radiate to back	Fever, night sweats, joint pain, back pain, weight loss, headache, murmur			Systolic–diastolic murmur, petechiae, Osler's modes, Roth spots, neck vein distention, pleural or pericardia rub, pain in extremities, splenomegaly hematuria	CBC, ESR blood cultures, Echo	Hospitalize, for antibiotic therapy
GI-Esophageal spasm	May be identical to angina		Alcohol or cold liquids	May be relieved by nitroglycerin		Esophageal manometry	Nitroglycerin anti-cholinergics esophageal dilation

(continued)

TABLE 9.2 *(continued)*

Condition	Pain Findings	Associated Symptoms	Precipitating Factors	Relieving Factors	Physical Findings	Diagnostic Tests	Treatment Modalities
Esophagitis	Burning, tightness	Heartburn, water brash	Overeating, alcohol, recumbent position	Antacids	May have slight to moderate epigastric tenderness	Esophago-scophy	Lifestyle modification, Antacid, H2 blocker, PPI, Pro-motility agent
Musculosteletal Costochondritis	Sharp, sometimes pleuritic, parasternal costochondral pain		Sneezing, cough on deep inspiration, or twisting motions, reaching overhead		Erythema at sites of tenderness; positive pinpoint tenderness at costochondral junctions	CXR to r/o other causes	NSAIDS, ASA, Ibuprofen, Naproxen, heat application

1. CHD
   a. Acute MI: chest pain lasting more than 15 min
   b. Unstable angina pectoris
   c. Stable angina pectoris
   d. Prinzmetal's, or variant, angina
2. Valvular heart disease
   a. MVP
   b. Aortic stenosis
3. Hypertrophic cardiomyopathy
4. Pericarditis
5. Endocarditis
6. Aortic dissection
B. Noncardiac causes
   1. Pulmonary causes
      a. Pneumonia
      b. Pleurisy
      c. Pulmonary embolism
      d. Pulmonary hypertension
      e. Pneumothorax
      f. Tracheobronchitis
      g. Lung cancer
   2. GI causes
      a. GERD
      b. Esophageal spasm
      c. Peptic ulcer disease
      d. Pancreatitis
      e. Cholecystitis
      f. Flatulence
   3. Rheumatology causes
      a. Fibromyalgia
      b. Costochondritis
      c. Arthritis
   4. Chest wall causes
      a. Rib fracture
      b. Muscle strain
      c. Cervical or thoracic spine disease
      d. Metastatic bone disease
      e. Breast conditions
   5. Neurologic causes
      a. Herpes zoster

   b. Postherpetic pain syndrome
   c. Nerve root compression
   6. Psychogenic causes
      a. Panic disorder
      b. Generalized anxiety
      c. Depression
      d. Somatoform disorders

Plan
A. General interventions: Direct management toward primary disorder causing the symptom.
B. Patient teaching
   1. Teach the patient about medications.
   2. Encourage CPR training for the patient's family and/or close friends.
   3. Explain to the patient and family when and how to call 911 and the importance of going to ER immediately so that thrombolytic therapy can be considered. A positive response to nitroglycerin does not confirm the presence of CAD.
C. Pharmaceutical therapy
   1. Cardiac pain: nitroglycerin
   2. GI pain: H2 blocker, PPI
   3. Musculoskeletal pain: NSAIDS
   4. Psychogenic pain
      a. SSRIs
      b. Tricyclic antidepressants
      c. Benzodiazepines

Follow-up
A. Follow patients with CAD for an indefinite period of time to detect recurrence or progression of disease.
B. Other follow-up depends on etiology of chest pain.

Consultation/Referral
A. Consult a physician when chest pain is cardiac in origin. If cardiac origin is found in a pregnant patient, call for a cardiology consultation as soon as possible for comanagement.

Individual Considerations

A. Pregnancy: Evaluate chest pain in the same manner as in nonpregnant patients.
B. Pediatrics
  1. Chest pain usually does not represent serious cardiovascular disease.
  2. Pericarditis is one of the most frequent causes of chest pain associated with a febrile illness.
  3. Exercise-induced chest pain may be indicative of asthma.
  4. A chest wall syndrome like costochondritis is another frequent etiology.
C. Geriatrics
  1. Frail elderly patients usually do not present with "typical" symptom complex of chest pain. Often, the only symptoms of acute MI are lethargy, decreased level of consciousness (LOC), crackles, CHF, persistent cough, or hypotension.
  2. Prescribe medications for frail elderly patients in half the usual dosage and then slowly taper upward to the desired effect.

▣ CHRONIC VENOUS INSUFFICIENCY

Definition

A. Chronic venous insufficiency is a venous system impairment that inhibits normal return of blood to the heart. It is most commonly due to improper functioning of the valves in the vessels.

Incidence

A. It is estimated that 7 million Americans are affected by venous insufficiency. More than 500,000 have stasis ulcers. It is more common in women and the elderly, and it tends to be familial.

Pathogenesis

A. Valves in the thigh and deep venous system become incompetent, which impairs proper blood return to the heart.

Predisposing Factors

A. Defective valves in vessels and heart
B. Obesity
C. Increased pressure on pelvic veins due to obesity or pregnancy
D. Prolonged standing
E. Women
F. Increases with advanced maternal age
G. Familial tendency

Common Complaints

A. Early stages may be asymptomatic.
B. Achy lower extremities.
C. Lower extremity swelling.
D. Night cramps in lower extremities.

Subjective Data

A. Ask the patient when symptoms began, noting their frequency, timing, and duration.
B. Ask what relief measures have been used and what was the result.

C. Inquire whether the patient has a family history of venous insufficiency.
D. Inquire whether the patient notes pain with exercise. If so, is relief noted with rest?
E. Ask if the patient smokes. If so, how much per day?
F. Ask if the patient has noted lower extremity swelling. If so, ask how long there has been swelling and to describe it.
G. Ask the patient about any trauma to lower extremities.
H. Inquire about the patient's occupation.

Physical Examination

A. Check temperature, pulse, respirations, and blood pressure.
B. Inspect
  1. Inspect lower extremities for dilated veins.
  2. Inspect lower extremities for ulcers, which signal vascular disease, and measure size of ulcer. Ulcers are commonly seen on the malleoli. Lesions have irregular borders with brown to brownish-red discoloration. Ankle edema is commonly seen. Peripheral pulses may be normal.
  3. Inspect skin color on lower extremities or upper extremities; note signs of Raynaud's phenomenon.
  4. Note any clubbing or cyanosis of nail beds.
C. Palpate
  1. Palpate lower extremities for peripheral pulses. Absent peripheral pulses signal acute arterial occlusion. Pulses may be normal with leg ulcers.
  2. Palpate lower extremities for skin sensation.
  3. Palpate lower extremities for edema.
  4. Check for Homans' sign, which is discomfort behind knee and in calf area caused by forced dorsiflexion of foot. Positive sign may indicate calf vein thrombosis.

Diagnostic Tests

A. Culture and sensitivity, CBC, if secondary infection is present.
B. Trendelenburg's test: observe saphenofemoral junction.
C. Doppler ultrasonography.
D. Venogram.
E. Ankle brachial indices.
F. BNP (Brain natriuretic peptide).

Differential Diagnoses

A. Chronic venous insufficiency
B. Arterial insufficiency, signaled by muscle pain on exercise
C. Peripheral neuritis
D. Osteoarthritis
E. Lower extremity ulcers with secondary infection

Plan

A. General interventions
  1. Encourage weight loss for obese patients.
  2. Encourage frequent rest periods with elevation of lower extremities when possible.
  3. Tell the patient to avoid long periods of sitting or standing.
  4. Tell the patient not to cross the legs.

B. Patient teaching
   1. Teach proper foot and leg care to enhance recovery of ulcers.
   2. Teach the patient how to prevent or care for secondary infections.
C. Medical management:
   1. Prescribe supportive hose.
   2. Consider TED hose for advanced disease.
   3. Surgery may be required.

Follow-up
A. Reevaluate the patient in 1 month. If presenting symptoms worsen, see the patient as often as needed.

Consultation/Referral
A. Consider referring the patient to a specialist for ligation and stripping of saphenous veins and, if appropriate, injection therapy.

CONGESTIVE HEART FAILURE

Definition
Congestive heart failure (CHF) is failure of the heart to pump sufficient blood to meet the metabolic demands of the tissues. It may also be defined according to the primary dysfunction and clinical manifestations.

A. Systolic failure
   1. Primary hallmark is low ejection fractions (< 45%) due to weak, inefficient systolic contractions.
   2. S3 ventricular gallop rhythm commonly occurs.
   3. Systolic failure is often the result of CHD and/or ML.
   4. It can result from right- or left-sided failure, or both.
B. Diastolic failure: the primary hallmark is normal ejection fraction (> 45%) but poor compliance of ventricle, which impedes ventricular diastolic filling.
   1. S4 atrial gallop rhythm commonly occurs.
   2. Diastolic failure is often the result of hypertrophy due to hypertensive disease.
C. Left ventricular failure (LVF): the most common type.
   1. LVF results when the left ventricle is unable to pump its blood volume to tissues.
   2. LVF results in low cardiac output and backward pulmonary congestion.
   3. LVF is often the consequence of CHD, MI, valvular heart disease, cardiomyopathies, and hypertensive heart disease.
D. Right ventricular failure (RVF)
   1. RVF occurs when the right ventricle is unable to pump its venous return to left heart.
   2. RVF results in backward systemic congestion and low cardiac output from left ventricle.
   3. RVF is often the consequence of severe left ventricular failure, right ventricular infarction, COPD, and pulmonary hypertension.

Incidence
A. More than 3 million people in the United States have chronic heart failure. It is more common in men than women between the ages of 40 and 75. However, the incidence is equal after the age of 75. More than 30%–40% of patients are hospitalized yearly. CHF is the most frequent inpatient diagnosis for people over the age of 65.

Pathogenesis
A. Injuries to the myocardium may cause loss of functioning muscle. Compensatory mechanisms, including cardiac hypertrophy and neurohumoral processes, lead to adverse long-term effects. An inotropic insult results in incomplete emptying (systolic failure), and a compliance abnormality results in incomplete filling (diastolic failure). Most heart failure has some degree of both abnormalities.

Predisposing Factors
A. Atherosclerotic heart disease
B. MI
C. Rheumatic heart disease involving mitral and aortic valves
D. Cardiomyopathies
E. Hypertensive heart disease
F. Aortic stenosis or regurgitation
G. Thyrotoxicosis
H. Pregnancy-related disorders, such as multiple births with preexisting heart disease
I. Volume overload
J. β-Blockers or other cardiac depressants
K. Pulmonary embolism
L. Systemic infection
M. Arrhythmias
N. Renal disease

Common Complaints
Patients are assigned the New York Heart Association classifications by their tolerance of physical activity and shortness of breath. This classification may change according to their progression or regression of their cardiovascular disease (see Table 9.3).

A. Dyspnea on exertion
B. Hemoptysis
C. Fatigue
D. Cough
E. Orthopnea
F. Edema
G. Paroxysmal nocturnal dyspnea
H. Nausea
I. Right upper abdominal pain or fullness

Other Signs and Symptoms
A. **Left Ventricular Failure:**
   1. Hemoptysis
   2. Bibasilar crackles
   3. S3 gallop
   4. Murmurs
   5. Exercise intolerance
   6. Weakness
   7. Cough
   8. Orthopnea
   9. Nocturnal dyspnea
   10. Tachycardia
   11. Pallor
   12. Cyanosis

TABLE 9.3   New York Heart Association Functional Classification for Heart Failure

Functional Class	Activities	Objective Assessment
AHA Class I ACCF Stage A	**No limitation.** Ordinary activity does not cause undue fatigue, palpitation, dyspnea, or angina.	No objective evidence of CV disease
AHA Class II ACCF Stage B	**Slight limitations.** Fatigue, palpitation, SOB, angina with ordinary physical activity.	Objective evidence—minimal CV disease
AHA Class III ACCF Stage C	**Marked limitations.** No discomfort at rest. Fatigue, palpitation, SOB, and angina with less than usual activities.	Objective evidence—moderately severe CV disease
AHA Class IV ACCPF Stage D	**Inability to do physical activity without discomfort.** Symptoms are present at rest and become worse with activity.	Objective evidence—severe CV disease

Modified from American Heart Association (http://www.americanheart.org/) and includes staging by the American College of Cardiology Foundation (ACCF).

B. **Right Ventricular Failure:**
1. Anorexia
2. Constipation
3. Jugular venous distention (JVD)
4. Hepatomegaly
5. Hepatojugular reflux (HJR)
6. Murmurs
7. Exercise intolerance
8. Weakness
9. Nocturia
10. Tachycardia
11. Pallor or cyanosis

Subjective Data
A. Ask the patient if he or she has difficulty breathing.
B. Ask how many pillows he or she sleeps on. Does the patient need to sit up in a recliner to sleep?
C. Inquire about how often he or she wakes up at night with SOB.
D. Inquire about how far the patient can walk without getting SOB. Have the patient describe his or her routine activities of daily living and how well he or she tolerates each activity.
E. Discuss the patient's history of heart disease, heart attack hypertension, or hyperlipidemia.
F. Ask the patient about current medications, prescription, over-the-counter, and herbal products.
G. Question the patient regarding all symptoms found in the "Common Complaints" section.
H. Discuss drug history.
I. Has the patient ever been treated for cancer/chemotherapy and how long ago?

Physical Examination
A. Check temperature, pulse respirations, blood pressure, height and weight.
1. Check blood pressure sitting, standing, and lying down.
2. Be alert for abnormal vital signs: hypotension, narrow or wide pulse pressure, tachycardia, bradycardia, and tachypnea.
3. Calculate BMI.
4. On all subsequent visits note weight gain of more than 1 pound per day over 3 consecutive days or 3 pounds in 1 day.
B. Inspect
1. Inspect overall physical appearance. Is the patient in distress?
2. Inspect skin: note pallor, cyanosis, and temperature.
3. Inspect neck: check jugular veins for distension.
4. Inspect extremities: note edema, cyanosis, pallor, and ulcers.
C. Palpate
1. Palpate abdomen for hepatomegaly and hepatojugular reflux (HJR).
2. Palpate extremities for peripheral pulses.
3. Palpate chest wall for displaced point of maximal impulse (PMI), lifts, heaves, and thrills.
D. Auscultate
1. Auscultate heart for murmurs; tachycardia; S1, S3, or S4 gallops; and other abnormalities.
2. Auscultate lungs: note moderate-to-severe crackles, edema, and other abnormal sounds.
3. Auscultate neck and carotid arteries.
E. Mental status: Check mental status because confusion may occur, especially in the elderly.

Diagnostic Tests
Full initial and serial assessment recommended by the American College of Cardiology Foundation (ACCF) and the American Heart Association (AHA) 2009 Clinical guidelines are available at http://circ.ahajournals.org/cgi/content/full/119/14/1977#FIG1192064.

A. CBC, electrolytes, BUN, creatinine, LFTs, FBS/HgA1C
B. Thyroid profile, lipid profile
C. BNP (Brain natriuretic peptide) and NT-proBNP to stratify/staging
D. 2-D echo with Doppler-ejection fraction
E. EKG
F. Arteriography in the presence of angina
G. Exercise stress test
H. Holter monitoring for history of MI
I. Evaluation for sleep apnea (OSA)

Differential Diagnoses

A. CHF
   1. LVF.
   2. RVF.
B. Renal disease or nephrotic syndrome.
C. Liver disease.
D. Asthma.
E. COPD: to distinguish between progressing LVF and a COPD exacerbation when both conditions are present, the presence of weight gain and an S3 gallop indicates LVF, not COPD.

Plan

A. General interventions:
   1. Determine the etiology of the failure state and treat appropriately.
   2. The goals of therapy are to improve the patient's quality of life by reducing symptoms, decreasing morbidity, and prolonging survival.
B. Patient teaching
   1. Teach the patient to weigh daily at the same time, on the same scale, and in the same clothing. Tell the patient to call his or her health care provider if there are gains of more than 3 pounds in 1 day or more than 1 pound/day over a 3-day period.
   2. Encourage him or her to lose weight.
   3. Recommend regular, moderate exercise as long as dyspnea is not induced.
   4. Encourage smoking cessation if at all possible.
   5. Instruct the patient about all medications and possible side effects. Do not to use OTC medicines without consulting. NSAIDS are contraindicated in heart failure.
   6. Encourage exercise even though the patient may only tolerate a few minutes of walking to increase his or her endurance and strengthen muscles.
C. Dietary management:
   1. Read food labels for sodium content.
   2. Teach dietary modifications especially including salt restrictions.
   3. Abstention from alcohol.
   4. See Appendix B for the DASH diet (Tables B.3 and B.5).
   5. Other diet changes include low fat/low cholesterol and the use of
      a. Monounsaturated fats decrease cholesterol
         i. Canola oil
         ii. Olive oil
      b. Polyunsaturated fats decrease cholesterol but not as well as monounsaturated
         i. Vegetable and fish oils
         ii. Corn, safflower, peanut, and soybean oils
      c. Avoid saturated fats
         i. Animal fats and some plant fats
         ii. Butter and lard
         iii. Coconut oil and palm oil
D. Pharmaceutical therapy
   1. Therapy is based on extent of cardiac impairment and severity of symptoms.
   2. **Full therapy guidelines/algothrim recommended by the American College of Cardiology Foundation (ACCF)** and the American Heart Association (AHA) 2009 Clinical guidelines are available at: http://circ.ahajournals.org/cgi/content/full/119/14/1977 Treatment algothrim available at http://circ.ahajournals.org/cgi/content/full/119/14/1977#FIG1192064.
   3. Drug classifications for antihypertensive and cardiac medication are noted in Table 9.4.
E. Biventricular pacing or an implantable defibrillator may be necessary for advanced HF.
F. Discuss the need for compassionate care/hospice when heart failure does not respond despite maximal therapy.
G. Discuss the patient's desire for an evaluation as a heart transplant candidate.

Follow-up

A. Heart failure patients should be comanaged with a physician.
B. Close follow-up is essential if the patient is to be maintained as an outpatient.
C. Appointments every 1–2 weeks may be necessary with additional appointments depending on the patient's symptoms, such as increasing shortness of breath, inability to lie flat to sleep, nocturnal moist cough, and increase in daily weight.
D. Lab monitoring is required for electrolytes, BUN, creatinine, proteinuria, and digoxin level.

Consultation/Referral

A. Consult a physician when the patient requires the next level up in pharmacologic management.
B. Cardiology consultation for staging and hospital management.

Individual Considerations

A. Pregnancy
   1. CHF is uncommon in healthy women without coexisting heart disease.
   2. Pregnancy in a patient with heart disease is considered high risk.
B. Pediatrics: CHF is usually associated with congenital heart defects.
C. Adults
   1. The 5-year survival rate is 25% for men and 38% for women.
   2. Predictors of poor outcome include an ejection fraction (EF) of less than 25%, ischemic etiology, ventricular arrhythmias, serum sodium greater than 130 mEq/L, poor functional class, low cardiac index, and high filling pressures.
D. Geriatrics
   1. In very frail elderly patients or those in long-term care settings, the only sign may be increased agitation or acute change in LOC.

DYSRHYTHMIAS

Definition

Dysrhythmias are abnormal heart rhythms. Common types are the following:

A. Bradycardia: heart rate less than 60 beats/minute; impulse originates in SA node.

TABLE 9.4 Antihypertensive and Cardiac Medications (Sorted Alphabetically)

Drug	Brand Name	Drug Class
Accupril	Quinapril	ACE Inhibitor
Aceon	Perindopril erbumine	ACE Inhibitor
Adalat CC	Dihydropyridine/Nifedipine	Calcium Channel Blocker
Alavide	Irbesartan + HCTZ	Combination-ARB + Diuretic
Aldactazide	Spironolactone + HCTZ	Combination-K+ sparing + Thiazide
Aldactone	Spironolactone	Diuretic-K+ Sparing
Amiloride/HCTZ	Amiloride/HCTZ	Combination + Diureic
Altace	Ramipril	ACE Inhibitor
Atacand	Candesartan Cilexetil	Angiotensin II Receptor Blocker (ARB)
Atacand HCT	Candesartan + HCTZ	Combination-ARB + Diuretic
Avapro	Irbesartan	Angiotensin II Receptor Blocker (ARB)
Azor	Amlodipine +01mesartan	Calcium Channel Blocker + ARB
Benicar	Olmesartan medoxomil	Angiotensin II Receptor Blocker (ARB)
Benicar HCT	Olmesartan + HCTZ	Combination-ARB + Diuretic
Betapace	Sotalol	Beta Blocker/Class II and III Antiarrhythmic
Betapace AF	Sotalol	Class II and III Antiarrhythmics
Bidil	Isosorbide dinitrate + Hydralazine	Nitrate + Diuretic
Bumex	Butetanide	LOOP Diuretic
Bystolic	Nebivolol	Beta Blocker-cardioselective
Caduet	Amlodipine + atorvastatin	Calcium Channel Blocker/Amliodipline/Atorvasatin
Calan	Verapamil	Calcium Channel Blocker/Antianginal
Calan SR	Verapamil	Calcium Channel Blocker
Capoten	Captopril	ACE Inhibitor/CHF
Capozide	Captopril + HCTZ	Combination-Ace + Diuretic
Cardizem LA	Dilitiazem	Calcium Channel Blocker
Cardura	Doxazosin	Alpha 2 blocker AAB
Catapres	Clonidine	Central alpha agonist
Chlorothiazide	Various	Thiazide Diuretic
Cleviprex	Dihydropyridine	Calcium Channel Blocker
Cordarone	Amiodarone	Class II and III Antiarrhythmics
Coreg CR	Carvedolol	Beta Blocker-Non cardioselective/CHF
Corgard	Nadolol	Beta Blocker-Non cardioselective/Antianginal
Corzide	Nadolol + HCTZ	Combination-Beta blocker (non cardioselective) + Diuretic
Covera HS	Verapamil	Calcium Channel Blocker/Antianginal
Cozaar	Losartan	Angiotensin II Receptor Blocker (ARB)
Demadex	Torsemide	LOOP Diuretic
Digoxin	Digoxin	Cardiac gyloside/Antiarrythmic
Dilacor XR	Diltiazem	Calcium Channel Blocker/Antianginal
Dilatrate SR	Isosorbide dinitrate	Nitrate
Diovan	Valsartan	Angiotensin II Receptor Blocker (ARB)/CHF Class II-IV
Diovan HCT	Valsartain + HCTZ	Combination-ARB + Diuretic
Diuril	Chlorothiazide	Thiazide Diuretic
Dyazide	Triamterene + HCTZ	Combination-K+ sparing + Thiazide
Dynacirc CR	Isradipine Controlled release	Calcium Channel Blocker

(continued)

TABLE 9.4 *(continued)*

Drug	Brand Name	Drug Class
Edecrin	Ethacrynic acid	LOOP Diuretic
Exforge	Dihydropyridine+Amlodipine	Calcium Channel Blocker + ARB
HCTZ	Hydrochlorothiazide	Thiazide Diuretic
Hytrin	Terazosin	Alpha 1 blocker
Hyzaar	Losartan potassium + HCTZ	Combination-ARB + Diuretic
Imdur	Isosorbide dinitrate	Nitrate
Inderal	Propranolol	Beta Blocker-Non cardioselective/Antianginal/Antiarrythmic
Inderide	Propranolol + HCTZ	Combination-Beta blocker (non cardioselective) + Diuretic
Innopran XL	Propranolol HCL ext release	Beta Blocker-Non cardioselective
Inspra	Eplerenone	Aldosterone Receptor Blocker-mineralocorticoid selective/CHF
ISMO	Isosorbide dinitrate	Nitrate
Isoptin SR	Verapamil	Calcium Channel Blocker
Isosorbide dinitrate	Various	Nitrate
Kerlone	Betaxolol	Beta Blocker-Cardioselective
Lanoxin	Digoxin	Cardiac gyloside/Antiarrythmic
Lasix	Furosemide	LOOP Diuretic
Lopressor	Metoprolol tartrate	Beta Blocker-Cardioselective/Antianginal
Lopressor HCT	Metoprolol + HCTZ	Combination-Beta blocker (Cardioselective) + Diuretic
Lotensin	Benazepril	Ace Inhibitor
Lotensin HCT	Benazepril + HCTZ	Combination-Ace + Diuretic
Lotrel	Amlodipine + Benazepril	Combination-Calcium Channel Blocker + Ace Inhibitor
Mavik	Trandolapril	Ace Inhibitor/CHF
Maxide	Triamterene + HCTZ	Combination-K+ sparing + Thiazide
Micardis	Telmisartan	Angiotensin II Receptor Blocker (ARB)
Micardis HCT	Telmisartan + HCTZ	Combination-ARB + Diuretic
Microzide	Hydrochlorothiazide (HCTZ)	Diuretic
Minitran	Nitroglycerin	Nitrate
Monoket	Isosorbide dinitrate	Nitrate
Monopril	Fosinopril	Ace Inhibitor/CHF
Multaq	Dronedarone	Antiarrhythmic
Nicardipine	Various	Calcium Channel Blocker
Nitro-BID	Nitroglycerin	Nitrate
Nitro-Dur	Nitroglycerin	Nitrate
Nitrolingual	Nitroglycerin	Nitrate
Nitrostat	Nitroglycerin	Nitrate
Normodyne	Labetolol	Beta Blocker
Norpace	Disopyramide	Antiarrhythmics-Class 1-Ventricular
Norvasc	Amlodipine	Calcium Channel Blocker/Antianginal
Pindolol	Pindolol	Beta Blocker-Non cardioselective
Plendil	Felodipine	Calcium Channel Blocker
Prinivil	Lisinopril	Ace Inhibitor/CHF
Prinizide	Lisinopril + HCTZ	Combination-Ace Inhibitor + Thiazide Diuretic
Procanbid	Procainamide	Antiarrhythmics-Class 1a-Ventricular
Procardia XL	Nifedipine	Calcium Channel Blocker/Antianginal
Quinidine gluconate	Various	Antiarrhythmics-Class 1 Atrial and Ventricular

TABLE 9.4 *(continued)*

Drug	Brand Name	Drug Class
Quinidine sulfate	Various	Antiarrhythmics-Class 1 Atrial and Ventricular
Ranexa	Ranolazine	Antianginal
Rythmol	Propafenone	Antiarrhythmics-Class 1c-Ventricular
Sular	Nisoldipine	Calcium Channel Blocker
Tambocor	Flecainide	Antiarrhythmics-Class 1c-Ventricular
Tarka	Trandolapril + Verapamil	Combinaiton-Ace + Calcium Channel Blocker
Tekturna	Aliskiren	Direct renin inhibitor
Tekturna HCT	Aliskiren + HCTZ	Direct renin inhibitor + Thiazide diuretic
Tenex	Guanfacine	Central alpha agonist
Tenoretic	Atenolol + Chlorthalidone	Combination-Beta blocker (Cardioselective) + Diuretic
Tenormin	Atenolol	Beta Blocker-Cardioselective/Antianginal
Teventen	Eprosartan	Angiotensin II Receptor Blocker (ARB)
Teventen HCT	Eposartan + HCTZ	Combination-ARB + Diuretic
Tiazac	Diltiazem	Calcium Channel Blocker/Antianginal
Timolide	Timolol malate + HCTZ	Combination-Beta blocker (non cardioselective) + Diuretic
Tenormin	Atenolol	Beta Blocker-Cardioselective
Toprol XL	Metoprolol	Beta Blocker-Cardioselective/Antianginal/CHF Class II or III
Trandate	Labetolol	Beta Blocker-Non cardioselective
Twynsta	Telmisartan + Amlodipine	ARB + Calcium Channel Blocker
Uniretic	Moexipril + HCTZ	Combination-Ace + Diuretic
Univasc	Ameoxipril	Ace Inhibitor
Vaseretic	Enalapril + HCTZ	Combination-Ace + Diuretic
Vasotec	Enlapril	Ace Inhibitor/CHF with Digitalis an diuretics
Verelan PM	Verapamil	Calcium Channel Blocker
Zaroxolyn	Metolazone	Diuretic-Quinazoline
Zebeta	Bisoprolol	Beta Blocker-Cardioselective
Zestoretic	Lisinopril + HCTZ	Combination-Ace + Diuretic
Zestril	Lisinopril	Ace Inhibitor/CHF with Digitalis and diuretics
Ziac	Bisoprolol + HCTZ	Combination-Beta blocker (Cardioselective) + Diuretic

B. Tachycardia: heart rate greater than 100–160 beats/minute; impulse originates in SA node.
C. Supraventricular tachydysrhythmias (SVTs): heart rate greater than 100 beats/minute; originates
   1. Atrioventricular (AV) nodal reentrant tachycardia (AVNRT) is intranodal reentry by means of fast and slow conduction pathways within the AV junction.
   2. Orthodromic AV reentrant tachycardia (AVRT) is tachycardia across accessory pathways associated with preexcitation.
D. Atrial fibrillation: chaotic electrical activity caused by rapid discharges from numerous ectopic foci in atria. Atrial rate is difficult to count. Three types of atrial fibrillation:
   1. Paroxysmal atrial fibrillation occurs in patients who usually have normal sinus rhythm (NSR).
   2. Chronic atrial fibrillation occurs in patients who have a permanent fibrillation rather than brief episodes of symptoms.

3. Premature ventricular contractions (PVCs) are impulses that form within Purkinje network.

Incidence

A. SVTs are the most common cardiac arrhythmias presenting to health care providers.
B. AVNRTs account for 60%–70% of all SVTs.
C. AVRTs account for 30%–40%. Greater than 90% of younger children who present with SVTs are likely to have an AVRT, but once they reach adolescence, AVNRT is the primary cause of SVT in about one-third of these patients.
D. Atrial fibrillation is most common cardiac tachydysrhythmia, affecting approximately 2% of the general population. Prevalence increases with age to 5% of those over age 69. The presence of atrial fibrillation is associated with a fivefold increase in risk of morbidity, a twofold increase in mortality, and an increased incidence of embolic stroke.
E. PVCs are common, and their frequency increases with age.

Pathogenesis

A. Bradycardia: Dominance of the parasympathetic nervous system, with excessive vagal stimulation to the heart, causes a decreased heart rate of sinus node discharge.

B. Tachycardia: Dominant sympathetic nervous system stimulation of the heart or vagal inhibition results in positive chronotropic, dromotropic, and inotropic effects.

C. AVRT: The most classic form of this SVT is Wolff-Parkinson-White (WPW) syndrome. Reentry occurs in a loop using atrial myocardium, AV node-His-Purkinje system, ventricular myocardium, and an accessory AV connection. During sinus rhythm, antegrade conduction through the accessory connection depolarizes the myocardium earlier than would occur by conduction through the AV node-His-Purkinje system, preexcitation is present, and a delta wave (slurring of initial deflection of the QRS complex) is usually seen on the surface 12-lead EKG.

D. AVNRT: The most common form is antegrade conduction, which occurs through a pathway with a short effective refractory period (ERP) and a longer conduction time. This pathway is often referred to as the slow pathway.

E. Atrial fibrillation: Multiple, rapid impulses from many foci depolarize the atria in a totally disorganized manner. In the chaos, no P waves, no atrial contraction, loss of atrial kick, and a totally irregular ventricular response occur. The atria quiver, which leads to formation of mural thrombi and potential embolic events.

F. Premature PVCs: These originate in the ventricles as a result of increased irritability in those cells.

Predisposing Factors

A. Bradycardia
   1. Increased vagal tone
   2. Decreased sympathetic drive
   3. Ischemia to SA node
   4. Drugs: digitalis, propranolol, sedatives, PTU or Tapazole, aminophylline, caffeine, alcohol, nicotine, and sympathomimetics
   5. Normal variant in athletes
   6. Normal body response to insult
   7. Atrial enlargement
   8. Acute MI
   9. CHF
   10. Rheumatic heart disease
   11. Hypertensive heart disease
   12. Thyroid disease
   13. Hypothermia
   14. Electrolyte abnormality
   15. Acidosis
   16. Infection

B. Tachycardia
   1. Decreased vagal tone
   2. Increased sympathetic tone
   3. MI

C. SVT
   1. Digitalis toxicity
   2. Catecholamines

D. Atrial fibrillation

   1. Myocardial ischemia
   2. Thyrotoxicosis

E. PVC: stress

Common Complaints

A. Symptoms may not be present; however, patient may note irregular heartbeat.

B. Palpitations.

C. Chest discomfort.

D. SOB.

E. Dizziness.

F. Diaphoresis.

G. Weakness.

H. Syncope.

I. Nausea.

Subjective Data

A. Obtain an accurate health and medical history.

B. Explore precipitating factors, such as emotional stress, alcohol or drug use, hot tub or bath use.

C. Inquire about onset and duration of symptoms.

D. Explore whether the patient has had concomitant weight loss, mood changes, and tremor, which are often associated with hyperthyroidism.

E. Carefully determine the number of previous episodes of palpitations or symptoms and what treatment, if any, was initiated.

F. Review all medications including prescription, over-the-counter, and herbal products.

Physical Examination

A. Temperature, pulse, respirations, blood pressure, and weight
   1. Sinus bradycardia: pulse rate decreased
   2. EKG: normal
   3. Sinus tachycardia
      a. Pulse regular
      b. Systolic BP constant
   4. Atrial fibrillation
      a. Pulse irregular
      b. Systolic BP changing
   5. AVNRT
      a. Pulse regular; atrioventricular (AV) block usual
      b. Systolic BP constant; electrical alternans rare
   6. AVRT
      a. Pulse regular; AV block not present
      b. Systolic BP constant; electrical alternans common, especially at high heart rates
   7. PVC: pulse diminished or absent

B. Inspect
   1. General appearance
      a. Is the patient in respiratory distress?
      b. Does the patient look apathetic? This is a sign of a thyroid problem.
   2. Inspect the skin for flushing or pallor.
   3. Examine the eyes, noting lid lag.
   4. Assess the neck for carotid artery bruits, jugular vein distension, or thyromegaly.
      a. With sinus tachycardia, neck vein pulsation is normal.

b. With atrial fibrillation, neck vein pulsation is irregular; assess for thyromegaly.

c. AVNRT: Assess the neck veins for "frogsign," in which the atria contract against closed AV valves, producing rapid, regular, expansive venous pulsation in the neck, resembling rhythmic puffing motion of a frog.

d. AVRT: Assess for frog sign.

C. Auscultate for abnormal heart sounds. Heart rhythm may be regular or irregular, depending on type of dysrhythmia. Have the patient perform vagal maneuver (Valsalva's maneuver). If vagal maneuver responds to rapid heart rate and the cycle is broken, it is likely the patient has AVRT. If it does not respond, it is possible the patient has AVNRT.

1. Sinus bradycardia
   a. Rate less than 60 beats/minute.
   b. Rhythm regular.
2. Sinus tachycardia
   a. Rate = 160–200 beats/minute.
   b. Rhythm regular; gradual onset and cessation.
   c. Loudness of first heart sound is constant.
3. Atrial fibrillation
   a. Rate: atrial rate is nonmeasurable, ventricular rate is variable, usually rapid at onset.
   b. Rhythm: atrial and ventricular rhythms are irregular.
   c. Loudness of first heart sound changes.
4. AVNRT
   a. AV block present, usually.
   b. Loudness of first heart sound is constant.
5. AVRT
   a. AV block not present.
   b. Loudness of first heart sound is constant.
6. PVC
   a. Rate depends on underlying rhythm.
   b. Rhythm: prematurity interrupts regularity of rhythm.

Diagnostic Tests

A. EKG
B. Drug screen
   1. Digitalis
   2. Aminophylline
   3. Illicit drugs
C. Electrolytes
D. ABGs if indicated

Differential Diagnoses

A. Multifocal atrial tachycardia
B. Sinus tachycardia with multiple premature atrial contractions
C. Atrial flutter
D. Ventricular tachycardia
E. AV blocks

Plan

A. General interventions:
   1. Remove as many predisposing factors as possible.
   2. Stop smoking.
B. Patient teaching
   1. Teach relaxation techniques.

2. Teach the patient and his or her family signs of hemodynamic compromise, including rapid heart rate, unexplained weight gain, worsening dyspnea on exertion, and decreased exercise tolerance.
3. Teach and reassure the patient about long-term medication therapy and its side effects.
4. Discuss the need for a pacemaker/defibrillator or surgical ablation.

C. Pharmaceutical therapy
   1. Initial treatment usually is prescribed by a physician.
   2. Selection of treatment modality should be based on underlying pathophysiology.
   3. For reentrant cases (AVNRT, AVRT), agents that block the reentrant circuit are more effective:
      a. Digitalis
      b. β-Blockers
      c. Calcium channel blockers
   4. Episodes caused by increased automaticity are treated with the following:
      a. Quinidine gluconate (Quinaglute)
      b. Procainamide HCl (Procan SR)
      c. Disopyramide phosphate (Norpace CR)
   5. Chronic atrial fibrillation is treated with anticoagulants such as warfarin sodium (Coumadin).
      a. Start therapy as soon as possible if a history of underlying heart disease is present.
      b. Evaluate Prothrombin Time/International Normalized Ratio (PT/INR) on a regular basis to monitor for therapeutic response to warfarin sodium treatment.

Follow-up

A. Patients who have their first episode of atrial fibrillation should return to clinic within 24–48 hours for reevaluation.
B. Patients on antiarrhythmic agents should have liver enzymes measured during first 4–8 weeks of therapy.
C. Patients with risk factors for developing cardiac complications to therapy should have EKGs during first weeks of therapy and every 3–6 months thereafter.
D. Monitor patients on digoxin carefully for digitalis toxicity.
E. Patients on digitalis should be carefully monitored for signs of toxicity. Caution the patient regarding medication interactions with digitalis.

Consultation/Referral

A. Consult a physician when there are questions about the difference between a narrow and wide QRS complex.
B. Consult a physician if the patient has an abnormal EKG pattern, refractory atrial fibrillation, suspicion of WPW syndrome, or sick sinus syndrome.
C. Patients with hemodynamic instability should be referred to a hospital or 911 immediately.
D. Patients unable to tolerate their dysrhythmia should be hospitalized immediately.

Individual Considerations

A. Pregnancy: Digitalis is safe during pregnancy.
B. Pediatrics
   1. PSVT is probably the most common pediatric arrhythmia.

2. Instruct young adult patients without underlying heart disease to quit/avoid smoking, avoid sleep deprivation, and limit use of alcohol and stimulants.

HYPERTENSION

Definition

A. Hypertension is sustained elevated blood pressure (BP). The Joint National Committee released its seventh annual report in 2003 (JNC VII). The JNC-VIII is expected to be released fall 2011. The JNC VII defines hypertension in adults (see Table 9.5).

Incidence

A. Hypertension occurs in approximately 20%–25% of population, with approximately 70% of cases falling in Stage I category.

Pathogenesis

Over 90% of cases have no identifiable cause, thus constituting the category of primary or essential hypertension. The remaining 10% of cases have the following secondary causes:

A. Renal causes
   1. Glomerulonephritis
   2. Pyelonephritis
   3. Polycystic kidney disease
B. Endocrine causes
   1. Primary hyperaldosteronism
   2. Pheochromocytoma
   3. Hyperthyroidism
   4. Cushing's syndrome
C. Vascular causes
   1. Corarctation of aorta
   2. Renal artery stenosis
D. Chemical/medication induced
   1. Oral contraceptives
   2. NSAIDs
   3. Decongestants
   4. Antidepressants
   5. Sympathomimetics
   6. Corticosteroids
   7. Lithium
   8. Ergotamine alkaloids
   9. Cyclosporine
   10. Monoamine oxidase inhibitors (MAOIs), in combination with certain drugs or foods
   11. Appetite suppressants, in combination with certain drugs or foods
   12. Cocaine
   13. Amphetamines

Predisposing Factors

When making a diagnosis, consider not only the absolute BP reading, but also the presence or absence of other cardiovascular risk factors. Factors include the following:

A. Family history of hypertension
B. Obesity
C. Alcohol consumption
D. Stress
E. Sedentary lifestyle
F. African American ancestry
G. Male gender
H. Age over 30 years
I. Excessive salt intake
J. Medications
K. Drug use

Common Complaints

A. Hypertension is asymptomatic in the majority of patients.

Other Signs and Symptoms

A. Headaches
B. Advanced disease: organ-specific complaints with end-organ damage
C. Retinopathy

Potential Complications

A. CVA
B. MI
C. Renal failure

Subjective Data

A. Ask the patient about any family history of hypertension or cardiac or renal disease.
B. Ask if the patient has ever been diagnosed with hypertension or cardiac or renal disease.
C. Ask if the patient ever had any high BP readings.
D. Ask if the patient has ever been treated for any of the above problems.
E. Ask about other risk factors, like smoking, drinking, high fat intake, obesity, and/or diabetes.
F. Inquire about the patient's lifestyle, exercise regimen, work environment, and stress level.

TABLE 9.5 JNC VII Classification of Blood Pressure in Adults		
Blood Pressure Classification	**Systolic Blood Pressure mmHg**	**Diastolic Blood Pressure mmHg**
Normal	< 120	and < 80
Prehypertension	120–139	or 80–89
Stage 1 Hypertension	140–159	or 90–99
Stage 2 Hypertension	≥ 160	or ≥ 100

Seventh Report of the Joint National Committee (JNC VII) Prevention, Detection, Evaluation, and Treatment of High Blood Pressure, 2003: http://www.nhlbi.nih.gov/guidelines/hypertension/express.pdf.

G. Ask the patient about symptoms that suggest secondary etiology:
1. Palpitations, headache, diaphoresis (pheochromocytoma)
2. Anxiety, weight gain or loss (thyroid abnormality)
3. Muscle weakness, polyuria (primary aldosteronism)
H. Find out if the patient is taking drugs that elevate BP.
I. Ask if the patient feels nervous when having his or her blood pressure taken in the office ("white coat hypertension").
J. Review current medications including prescription, over-the-counter, and herbal products.
K. Review current recreational drug use.

Physical Examination

A. Check temperature, pulse, blood pressure, height, weight, waist circumference, and distribution of body fat. Calculate BMI.
1. Make diagnosis after averaging two or more elevated BP readings taken at least 6 hours apart.
2. When patient's SBP and DBP fall into two different categories, use higher category to classify his or her BP.
3. For accurate measurement, use correct size cuff for patient (adult, large adult, or thigh cuff).
B. Inspect
1. Observe overall appearance.
2. Conduct funduscopic exam; look for papilledema, exudates, AV nicking, anterior nicking.
3. Inspect the neck for jugular vein distension.
C. Palpate
1. Palpate the neck; check thyroid for enlargement.
2. Palpate the abdomen for masses or organomegaly.
3. Palpate the extremities; assess peripheral pulses and note edema.
4. Assess deep tendon reflexes (DTRs).
D. Auscultate
1. Auscultate heart, noting PMI.
2. Auscultate lungs; check for bronchospasm and rales.
3. Auscultate neck; assess carotid arteries for bruits.

Diagnostic Tests

A. CBC
B. Liver function tests (LDH, uric acid)
C. Chemistry profile
D. Lipid profile

TABLE 9.6 Modifiable and Nonmodifiable Risk for Control of Hypertension

Modifiable	Nonmodifiable
Sedentary lifestyle	Age
Smoking	Gender
Diet	Ethnicity
Lipid control	Diabetes
Sodium intake	Postmenopausal
Alcohol intake	Family history
Obesity	

E. Urinalysis for proteinura
F. EKG
G. If history, physical exam, or lab tests indicate the need, obtain the following:
1. Intravenous pyelography (IVP)
2. Renal arteriogram
3. Plasma renin
4. Catecholamines
5. Chest radiography
6. Aortogram
7. Ultrasonography
8. Sleep study

Differential Diagnoses

A. Primary hypertension
B. Secondary hypertension

Plan

A. General interventions (see Table 9.6):
1. Advise overweight patients to lose weight. Loss of as little as 10 pounds reduces BP in many patients.
2. Advise the patient to limit or discontinue alcohol intake.
3. Encourage the patient to stop smoking.
4. Suggest to the patient that he or she increase aerobic activity to 30–45 min, three to five times/week.
5. Encourage some form of relaxation technique.
B. Patient teaching
1. Stress asymptomatic nature of disease.
2. Stress importance of ongoing monitoring and treatment under the direction of a health care provider.
3. Review risk factors for cardiac, renal, and cerebrovascular disease and possible preventive measures.
C. Dietary management: Review specific dietary measures. Give dietary recommendation sheets. See Appendix B for low fat/low cholesterol and DASH dietary approaches to stop hypertension.
1. Diet alone will only make the lowest incremental change in blood pressure; therefore, it should be combined with lifestyle modification; stop smoking, weight loss, and exercise are essential.
2. It is essential for the patient/family to read labels for sodium, fat content, and serving sizes.
3. Other dietary changes include low fat–low cholesterol diets, which includes limiting fats.
   a. Use monounsaturated fats to decrease cholesterol
      i. Canola oil
      ii. Olive oil
   b. Use in limited quantities: polyunsaturated fats decrease cholesterol but not as well as monounsaturated
      i. Vegetable and fish oils
      ii. Corn, safflower, peanut, and soybean oils
   c. Limit saturated fats
      i. Animal fats and some plant fats
      ii. Butter and lard
      iii. Coconut oil and palm oil
D. Pharmaceutical therapy
1. If lifestyle changes alone are not adequate to control hypertension consider drug therapy. Medication doses

are dependent of age, ethnicity, and comorbid conditions. Most patients will require two or more medications to control their blood pressure. The blood pressure goal is less than 130/85 unless the patient is a diabetic, then the blood pressure should be less than 130/80 to protect renal function. Consider starting antihypertensive and/or diuretics. (see Table 9.4 for drugs and classifications). See Exhibit 9.1.
   a. Diuretics
   b. Beta blocker
   c. ACE inhibitors
   d. Calcium channel blockers
   e. Alpha-adrenergic blockers
   f. Arterial vasodilators

2. Antihypertensive/diuretics should be started low and increased if there is inadequate response to initial therapy and nonadherence is ruled out. Consider the following:
   a. Increasing drug dose
   b. Substituting another drug
   c. Adding a second drug from another class; a diuretic is recommended if not already being used.

3. If response is still inadequate, add a second or third drug or diuretic if not already tried.

4. Evaluate the patient for secondary causes if severe hypertension is resistant to therapy.

5. Inadequate response to drug therapy may be caused by the following:
   a. "White-coat" hypertension: have the patient begin to take and record his or her blood pressure at home and bring the values.
   b. Using regular BP cuff on obese patient.
   c. Nonadherence to therapy.
   d. Volume overload due to excessive salt intake, progressive renal damage, fluid retention from BP reduction, and inadequate diuretic therapy.
   e. Drug problems: dose too low, wrong type of diuretic, inappropriate combinations, rapid inactivation, drug actions and interactions.
   f. Associated conditions: smoking, obesity, sleep apnea, insulin resistance, ethanol intake of greater than 30 mL (1 oz) per day, panic attacks, chronic pain, and organic brain syndrome.

6. Treat with decongestants very cautiously. Pseudoephedrine HCl (Sudafed) has the least cardiovascular effect.

7. Diuretics may worsen gout and diabetes.

8. β-blockers are contraindicated in asthma, heart failure, and heart block.

9. Use diltiazem HCl (Cardizem) and verapamil HCl (Calan) cautiously in heart failure or block.

10. ACE inhibitors may cause coughing.

Follow-up

A. If drug therapy is initiated, see the patient again in 2–4 weeks for follow-up.
B. Once the patient is stable, see him or her every 3–6 months.
C. Evaluate the patient yearly, including uric acid, creatinine, and potassium.
D. Review and discuss drug therapy compliance, effectiveness, and adverse reactions (including effect on sexual activity) at each visit.

Consultation/Referral

A. If the patient is pregnant, consult a physician before prescribing medications. Many antihypertensive drugs are harmful to the fetus.
B. Consult a physician if the patient is having an acute hypertensive emergency: DBP greater than 130 mmHg.
C. Consult/comanage with a physician if the patient needs more than two drugs for therapy.

Individual Considerations

A. Pregnancy
   1. Hypertension may be either chronic or pregnancy-induced.
   2. Hypertension is considered chronic if it is present before pregnancy or diagnosed prior to the 20th week of gestation.
   3. Pregnancy-induced hypertension is diagnosed if SBP increases 30 mmHg or more, or DBP increases 15 mmHg or more, compared with BP readings before the 20th week of gestation. When BP readings are not known, a reading of 140/90 or higher is considered abnormal.
   4. Maternal as well as fetal mortality and morbidity improve with treatment.

B. Pediatrics
   1. Evaluate BP at every visit starting at age 3.
   2. Hypertension can occur in many acute illnesses, or it may be a chronic problem.
   3. Determine high BP by correlating height indexes with BP readings.

C. Geriatrics
   1. The general approach to drug therapy in the geriatric population is to start low and go slow.
   2. Check the Beers list for harmful drugs in the geriatric population. A Pharmacist's Letter reference copy is located on the Internet at http://www.fmda.org/beers.pdf.
   3. Evaluate side effects including dizziness and sedation.

MURMURS

Definition

A murmur is turbulent blood flow through the heart as a result of one or more of the following etiologies:

A. Narrow valve opening, stenosis
B. Incomplete valve closure, regurgitant or insufficient blood flow
C. Abnormal opening through chambers, atrial or ventricular septal defect
D. Rapid blood flow through normal valve structures; occurs during pregnancy, with increased physiologic demand states, and in children
E. No abnormality; occurs in patients with thin chest walls and in children

Incidence

A. Approximately 80% of children have a physiologic murmur at one time or another. Four percent of women studied in the Framingham study had a murmur related to mitral valve prolapse (MVP).

EXHIBIT 9.1 **Algorithm for Treatment of Hypertension**

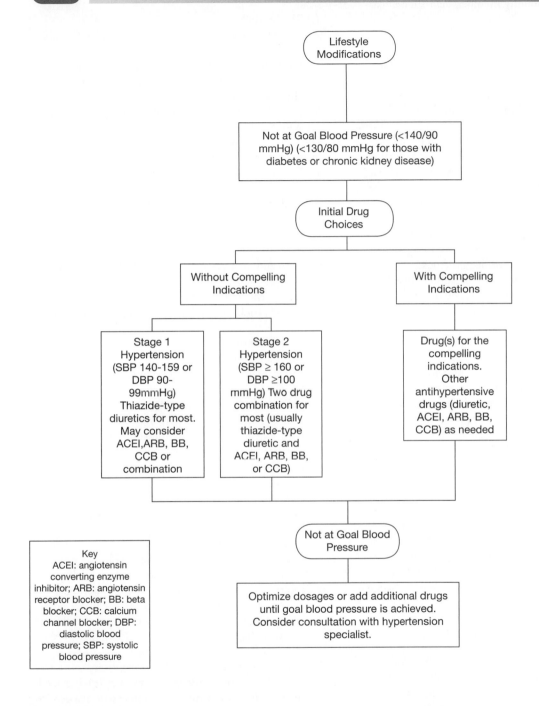

Pathogenesis

A. Pathogenesis depends on specific etiology, but rheumatic disease, calcific changes, ischemic insults, congenital abnormalities, and degenerative diseases are all contributors to the development of a murmur.

Common Complaints

A. Often no symptoms are present and murmur is found on routine examination.

B. Complaints with advanced valvular disease:
   1. Chest pain
   2. Dyspnea
   3. Palpitations
   4. SOB
   5. Exercise intolerance
   6. Postural light-headedness

Subjective Data

A. Has the patient ever been diagnosed with a murmur?

B. Did the patient have frequent strep infections as a child?

C. Ask the patient about any recent viral infections.

D. Question the patient about chest pain; SOB; palpitations; diaphoresis; light-headedness; or syncope, especially with exertion.

E. Ask the patient if any family members had sudden cardiac death before age 55.

Physical Examination

A. Check temperature, pulse, respirations, and blood pressure.

B. Inspect the chest for lifts and heaves.

C. Palpate the chest for lifts, heaves, and thrills.

D. Auscultate
   1. Auscultate heart for splitting of heart sounds, slicks, rubs, and murmurs; use bell and diaphragm of stethoscope to auscultate patient in left lateral, supine, standing, and squatting positions and after having patient run in place or do jumping jacks for 2–3 minutes.
      a. A new, systolic, regurgitant murmur in the setting of an acute MI may indicate a ruptured papillary muscle and possible cardiogenic shock.
      b. When a new murmur is audible, differentiate location, timing, quality, intensity, and duration. Note if radiation to neck, axilla, or back is present.
      c. Note location of murmur.
         i. Aortic: second right intercostal space (ICS) next to sternum
         ii. Pulmonic: second left ICS next to sternum
         iii. Tricuspid: fifth left ICS next to sternum
         iv. Mitral: fifth left ICS at midclavicular line
      d. If murmur is heard, have the patient squat, stand, and/or perform Valsalva maneuver. Squatting will increase the blood to the heart and increase the left ventricle blood volume and stroke volume that will increase the sound of the murmur. Standing and the Valsalva maneuver will provide the opposite, in which the venous return will drop and decrease the ventricle size and stroke volume and soften the sound of the murmur.
      e. If the sound of the murmur occurs in the opposite action, softer when squatting and louder when standing or during Valsalva maneuver, consider hypertrophic cardiomyopathy or mitral valve prolapse as the diagnosis.
   2. Auscultate the neck and axilla for radiation.

Diagnostic Tests

A. EKG

B. Echocardiogram

C. Chest radiography

Differential Diagnoses

Major differentiation should be in the description of murmur, as this aids in identification of the murmur.

A. Timing
   1. Identify when the murmur occurs in the cardiac cycle.
   2. Systolic murmurs may or may not be normal.
      a. Occurs between the "S1" lub and the "S2" dub.
   3. Diastolic murmurs are always abnormal.
      a. Occurs between the "S2" dub and the "S1" lub.

B. Quality: Is the sound harsh, blowing, musical, rumbling, vibratory, or soft?

C. Intensity: Murmurs are usually graded on a six-point scale:
   1. Barely audible
   2. Audible but soft
   3. Easily audible
   4. Easily audible, but a thrill is usually palpable
   5. Audible with only the rim of the stethoscope on the chest wall; thrill present
   6. Audible with the stethoscope barely off the chest wall; thrill present

D. Duration: Identify location and timing in the specific phase of cardiac cycle:
   1. Holosystolic: throughout systole
   2. Holodiastolic: throughout diastole
   3. Midsystolic: midway between S1 and S3
   4. Middiastolic: midway between S2 and S1
   5. Decrescendo: starts loud at the beginning, then tapers off
   6. Crescendo: Starts soft at the beginning, then gets louder

E. Radiation: Murmur can be heard in another place, such as the neck, back, left axilla, or across precordium. Sound usually radiates in the direction of blood flow.

F. Location: Identify location on chest wall.

G. Systolic murmurs:
   1. *Mitral regurgitation:* Holosystolic, blowing may be loud. Located at 5th intercostal space (ICS) and radiates to left axilla/back. Heard best left lateral position and sudden squatting, intensity decreases with Valsalva's maneuver and standing.
   2. *Physiologic:* Early to midsystolic, low-pitch normal S1–S2, located at left lower sternal edge at 3th–4th intercostal space (ICS). Heard best with bell and supine and disappears when sitting up or holding breath. Commonly seen in children, pregnancy, and infection.
   3. *Aortic stenosis:* Loud, hard crescendo-decrescendo at 2nd right ICS and radiates to neck. Heard best leaning forward, increases with leg raise and lying flat. Decreases with valsalva and handgrip standing.
   4. *Mitral valve prolapse:* Midsystolic click heard before late systolic murmur, heard best at 5th left ICS. Heard best with diaphragm; sitting or squatting may increase intensity.
   5. *Tricuspid regurgitation:* Holosystolic, heard left lower sternal border or apex when right ventricle is enlarged. Intensity increases with inspiration and decreases with expiration. Straight leg raises may increase intensity. May also see hepatojugular reflux.
   6. *Pulmonic stenosis:* Prolonged, loud S2 or crescendo-descrendo, usually greater than 3/6 at 2nd ICS and radiates to neck; increases with inspiration.
   7. *Hypertrophic cardiomyopathy (aortic outflow obstruction):* Peaks at midsystole; loud, harsh tone at left, lower sternal border that may radiate to neck. Increases with Valsalva maneuver and standing, decreases with sudden squatting. Note carotid upstroke brisk.
   8. Systolic murmurs are benign or pathologic.

H. Diastolic murmurs:
1. *Mitral stenosis:* Rumbling extends beyond middiastole at 5th ICS. Increases with left lateral position. May hear snap after S2.
2. *Aortic regurgitation:* High-pitch faint, decrescendo may start with S2, at 3rd left ICS and radiates down sternal edge. Heard best leaning forward, holding breath. Increases with sudden squatting or handgrip. May hear displaced point maximal intensity, S3, bounding pulse.
3. Diastolic murmurs are always pathologic.

Plan

A. General interventions
1. Major therapeutic goals are to preserve quality of life, increase life expectancy and exercise capacity, and reduce risk of complications.
2. Activity restriction is not necessary in patients with asymptomatic valvular disease.
B. Patient teaching: Reassure the patient regarding specific diagnosis. Counsel him or her regarding his or her specific condition. Teach the patient signs and symptoms to report to the health provider, including chest pain, SOB, difficulty breathing, and so forth.
C. Medical and surgical management: Patients who need progressive increases in medications to control symptoms may be candidates for valve replacement surgery.
D. Pharmaceutical therapy:
The 2007 American Heart Association Guidelines (AHA) do not recommend endocarditis antimicrobial prophylaxis treatment for common valvular lesions that include bicuspid aortic valve, acquired aortic or mitral valve disease (including mitral valve prolapse with regurgitation), and hypertrophic cardiomyopathy with latent or resting obstruction.
1. Endocarditis prophylaxis treatment: cardiac conditions It **is** recommended for high-risk cardiac condition abnormalities to have prophylactic treatment. These specific **cardiac conditions include:**
   a. Prosthetic cardiac valve or prosthetic material used for cardiac valve repair
   b. Previous infective endocarditis
   c. Congenital heart disease
   d. Postcardiac transplant valvulopathy
2. **Procedures for high-risk patients** mentioned above that require prophylaxis treatment include:
   a. All dental procedures with manipulation of gingival tissue or periapical region of teeth or perforation of oral mucosa
   b. Incision or biopsy of respiratory mucosa or any invasive procedure of the respiratory tract system
   c. Procedures that include infected skin or musculoskeletal tissue
3. Antibiotic prophylactic regimens include single dose 30–60 min prior to procedure:
   a. Amoxicillin 2 g by mouth, IM, or IV for adults or 50 mg/kg for children single dose
   b. Ampicillin 2g IM or IV or 50 mg/kg IM or IV ×1.
   c. Allergy to PCN: Cephelexin 2 g by mouth for adults or 50 mg/kg for children
   d. Azithromycin or clarithromycin 500 gm for adults or 15 mg/kg for children
   e. Allergic to above: consider Cefazolin or ceftriaxone 1 gm IM or IV for adults or 50 mg/kg IM or IV for children or clindamycin 600 mg IM or IV for adults or 20 mg/kg IM or IV children
4. Prophylaxis treatment is not recommended for treatment for gastrointestinal or genitourinary tract procedures (Gopalakrishnan, Shukla, & Tak, 2009).
5. Other pharmaceutical treatments depend on the specific valvular abnormality.
   a. Mitral stenosis: the mitral valve has narrowing that does not allow adequate blood to the left ventricle during diastole, usually due to rheumatic heart disease. Mitral heart disease is the most commonly seen valve affect with rheumatic heart disease.
   b. Diuretics such as furosemide (Lasix) or hydrochlorothiazide (HydroDiuril) are used to control edema.
   c. Digoxin (Lanoxin) or β-blockers are used to control atrial fibrillation and irregular heart rate.
   d. Warfarin (Coumadin) and the antiplatelet agent aspirin (Bayer) are used to prevent clotting.
   e. Mitral valve prolapse (MVP): the echocardiogram is the recommended test for diagnosis of MVP. Usually no medications are recommended unless symptomatic and required.
      i. Beta blockers (such as Atenolol) may be used for palpitations.
      ii. Diuretics should be avoided in patients who are volume reserved.
      iii. Oral contraceptives should be avoided in women who exhibit neurologic symptoms.
   f. Mitral regurgitation: diuretics, digitalis, and afterload reducing agents for CHF.
      i. Aortic stenosis.
      ii. Diuretics are used for CHF.
      iii. Avoid vasodilators; they may result in profound, irreversible hypotension.
      iv. Echocardiograms should be performed every 6–12 months to follow progression of narrowing of the left ventricle across the aortic valve.
   g. Aortic regurgitation: Afterload reducing agents, digitalis, and diuretics are recommended.

Follow-up

A. Most patients with valvular disease should be evaluated at least once a year.
B. Patients on oral anticoagulation drugs need monthly or as needed Prothrombin Time/International Normalized Ratio (PT/INRs).

Consultation/Referral

A. Consult a physician if the patient is diagnosed with a new murmur or exercise-induced symptoms during a sports physical.

B. Refer patients with newly diagnosed murmurs to a cardiologist after obtaining echocardiogram results. Drug therapy should be initiated according to diagnosis and symptoms.

C. Onset of atrial fibrillation with rapid ventricular response is an indication for immediate hospitalization.

D. Refer patients with systemic embolization to a physician for emergent anticoagulation therapy and chronic oral anticoagulant therapy. Discuss the possibility of valve replacement with a cardiologist.

E. If a new murmur is diagnosed in a pregnant patient with a history of cardiac disease, refer her to a physician immediately.

F. All diastolic murmurs in pediatric patients indicate pathology and need to be evaluated by a physician.

Individual Considerations

A. Pregnancy: The development of a new, "high-flow" murmur in a healthy woman is not uncommon due to physiologic changes occurring during pregnancy.

B. Pediatrics: Perform a thorough cardiac exam on patients from the time they are newborns through adolescence, so that if a murmur is detected, it can be compared.

C. Geriatrics: A systolic murmur heard best in the aortic area may indicate aortic sclerosis due to aging of the aortic valve, rather than true aortic stenosis.

PALPITATIONS

Definition

A. Palpitations are a feeling in the chest or an unpleasant awareness of the heartbeat.

Incidence

A. The incidence of palpitations may range from 1%–8% of patients in a general practice setting.

Pathogenesis

Palpitations may be caused by the following:

A. Increase in stroke volume or contractility
B. Sudden change in heart rate or rhythm
C. Unusual cardiac movement within thorax
D. Hyperkinetic states, which cause constant pounding
E. Valvular heart disease that produces large stroke volumes
F. Catecholamine release during anxiety or panic attacks

Predisposing Factors

A. Cardiac defects
B. Severe anemia
C. Hyperthyroidism
D. Pregnancy
E. Fever
F. Anxiety
G. Stimulants, such as caffeine and certain drugs
H. Emotions, such as fear
I. Exertion
J. Diabetes mellitus and insulin reaction

Common Complaints

A. Palpitations are often described as a turning over or flopping sensation in the chest, but symptoms vary enormously.

B. Most patients are free of palpitations at the time of the exam.

Other Signs and Symptoms

A. Fluttering in the chest
B. SOB
C. Pounding in the chest and neck
D. Diaphoresis
E. Light-headedness
F. Anxiety or fear

Subjective Data

A. Ask the patient when symptoms first presented and how they have changed.

B. Have the patient describe the characteristics of the palpitations, such as rapid, regular, irregular, or slow.

C. Ask the patient what precipitates the palpitations. Does anything terminate them, or do they go away on their own?

D. Inquire whether symptoms occur or change with exercise.

E. Ask the patient about other associated symptoms with the palpitations.

F. Ask how often the episodes occur and how long each lasts.

G. Discuss any previous treatments for this condition and the results.

H. Ask the patient about risk factors for CHD and prior cardiac history.

I. Question the patient's use of over-the-counter decongestants and diet pills. Obtain complete list of medications the patient is currently taking.

Physical Examination

A. Check temperature, pulse (count the pulse for 1 full minute), respirations, and blood pressure.

B. Inspect
   1. Inspect overall appearance.
   2. Inspect the skin for diaphoresis and pallor.
   3. Inspect the neck for thyromegaly or jugular vein distension.
   4. Inspect the legs for edema.

C. Palpate
   1. Palpate the skin for temperature and dryness.
   2. Palpate the lower extremities for edema and calf tenderness.
   3. Palpate the neck for thyroid enlargement.

D. Auscultate
   1. Auscultate the heart for abnormal rhythms.
   2. Auscultate the lungs.
   3. Auscultate the neck and carotid arteries for bruits.

E. Mental status: Does the patient appear light-headed, anxious, or fearful?

Diagnostic Tests

A. Hgb to rule out anemia, if suggestive on exam
B. TSH to rule out hyperthyroidism, if suggestive on exam
C. EKG during episode, if possible: most diagnostic
D. Ambulatory monitoring if symptoms continue, either 24-hour Holter monitor or patient-activated transtelephonic monitoring
E. Treadmill test if palpitations are provoked by exercise

Differential Diagnoses

A. Palpitations are secondary to the underlying problem, such as anxiety, medications, or cardiac or pulmonary origin.

Plan

A. General interventions: Provide reassurance if the palpitations result from a neurotic concern.
B. Patient teaching
   1. Caution the patient to avoid any factors that trigger episodes.
   2. Teach the patient the vagal maneuver, which is effective in halting palpitations.
C. Medical and surgical management: Correct any underlying problem (e.g., cardiac or pulmonary).
D. Pharmaceutical therapy: Discontinue all nonessential medications that could cause palpitations.

Follow-up

A. Depending on the etiology of palpitations and the existence of comorbid conditions, the prognosis in patients with no underlying cardiac disease is generally favorable.

Consultation/Referral

A. Consult a physician if the patient has a history of palpitations leading to syncope or near syncope, anginalike chest pain, or dyspnea. These patients are candidates for referral to a cardiologist and/or inpatient evaluation.
B. Hemodynamically compromised patients need prompt hospital admission.

⬢ PERIPHERAL ARTERIAL DISEASE

Definition

A. Peripheral arterial disease is lower limb ischemia that produces pain in the lower extremities. It is usually noted with exercise and is relieved with rest. Ischemia is caused by an accumulation of fatty deposits (atherosclerotic changes) on the lining of the arteries that impede the blood flow to the lower extremities.

Incidence

A. Lipid buildup on the lining of the arteries is commonly seen earlier in men than in women.

Pathogenesis

A. Atherosclerosis limits the perfusion of blood to the lower extremities, in which the oxygen supply does not meet the demand, producing pain in the lower extremities. Collateral circulation develops to compensate for obstructed vessels. As the disease progresses, collateral circulation deteriorates, and symptoms are observed.

Predisposing Factors

A. Metabolic syndrome
   1. Atherosclerosis
   2. Diabetes mellitus
   3. Hypertension
   4. Hyperlipidemia
B. Smoking
C. Middle age; usually seen after age 40
D. Male gender

Common Complaints

A. Pain in lower extremities with exercise, relieved with rest
B. Numbness and tingling sensation in lower extremities, usually unilateral

Other Signs and Symptoms

A. Asymptomatic at first
B. Disease progress:
   1. Pain in the buttocks, hips, and thighs with aortoiliac disease
   2. Calf pain with femoropopliteal disease
   3. Male impotence
C. Advanced disease:
   1. Pain in the lower extremities at rest
   2. Numbness or burning when extremities are dependent
   3. Ischemic ulcerations
   4. Hair loss
   5. Skin color changes in dependent and elevated positions

Subjective Data

A. Ask the patient when presenting complaints began.
B. Inquire if the pain increases with exercise and improves with rest. If so, what other measures relieve pain?
C. Note duration of the activity prior to symptoms. Is pain so intense it limits the patient's physical activity?
D. Has the patient noted other physical changes, such as changes in skin integrity or impotence?
E. Ask the patient if there is a family history of atherosclerosis.
F. Ask if the patient smokes. If so, note how much per day and for how many years.

Physical Examination

A. Check temperature, pulse, respirations, and blood pressure.
   1. BP should be evaluated in all extremities and should be equal.
   2. Ankle and brachial pressure ratio should be 1.0. If ratio is less than 1.0, consider arterial occlusive disease; if less than 0.5, consider severe ischemia.
B. Inspect
   1. Note color of the lower extremities in dependent and elevated positions.
   2. Note texture of skin, nails, hair on extremities. Thin, parchmentlike skin results from poor perfusion.
   3. Inspect the leg muscles for atrophy.
C. Palpate
   1. Palpate lower extremities for edema.
   2. Palpate peripheral pulses before and after exercise.
   3. Palpate Homans' sign: calf pain caused by forced dorsiflexion of foot.
D. Auscultate heart and lungs; auscultate carotid arteries and abdomen for bruits.

Diagnostic Tests

A. Doppler flow study
B. Ankle brachial index

Differential Diagnoses

A. Peripheral arterial disease
B. Acute arterial occlusion
C. Raynaud's phenomenon

Plan

A. General interventions
   1. Encourage daily exercise program and increased activity as tolerated.
B. Patient teaching: See the Section III Patient Teaching Guide for this chapter, "Peripheral Arterial Disease."
C. Dietary management: Encourage weight loss program for obese patients.
D. Medical and surgical management
   1. Encourage patient to wear appropriate stockings for supporting circulation in lower extremities. Also encourage patients to wear socks to bed.
   2. Have the patient monitor lower extremities for skin breakdown.
   3. Counsel patients with severe disease regarding possible surgical interventions.
E. Pharmaceutical therapy
   1. Hemorrheologic agents: pentoxifylline (Trental) 400 mg three times daily with meals.
   2. Anticoagulants may be used for long-term therapy for claudication.
   3. Vasodilators are also used for claudication.
   4. Aspirin therapy reduces risk of stroke and cardiovascular disease with severe disease.
   5. Aggressive therapy involves treating with lipid-lowering agents.

Follow-up

A. Recommend monthly follow-up to evaluate treatment modalities and responses.
B. Once the patient is stabilized, follow-up every 3 months or as necessary.

Consultation/Referral

A. Consult with a physician before prescribing long-term anticoagulation therapy or vasodilators.
B. Consult with or refer the patient to a physician if Doppler flow study is abnormal, or if claudication, ischemic pain at rest, gangrene, or ulceration with delayed healing occur.
C. Refer obese patients to a nutritionist. Medications should be prescribed by a physician.
D. Refer the patient to an exercise rehabilitation therapist to begin a walking exercise program.

Individual Considerations

A. Pediatrics
   1. Fatty lipid deposits are evident in children as young as age 10.
   2. Counsel parents regarding appropriate fat intake for children.
B. Geriatrics: Atherosclerosis is the leading cause of death for patients over age 65.

SYNCOPE

Definition

A. Syncope is a brief, sudden loss of consciousness and muscle tone secondary to cerebral ischemia, or inadequate oxygen or glucose delivery to brain tissue. Recovery is spontaneous.

Incidence

A. Syncope is a common problem in all age groups. An estimated 15% of children experience an episode by adulthood. Between 12%–48% of healthy young adults have lost consciousness (one-third following trauma), but most do not seek medical attention. Adults over age 75 in long-term care facilities have a 6% annual incidence of syncope, and 23% have had previous episodes. Syncopal episodes account for approximately 1%–6% of hospital admissions and 3% of emergency room visits.

Pathogenesis

The most common cause of syncope is inadequate cerebral perfusion caused by one of the following:

A. Vasomotor instability associated with a decrease in systemic vascular resistance and/or venous return. The following may cause syncope:
   1. Vasovagal episodes
   2. Situational syncope, from coughing, micturition, and defecation
   3. Medications
      a. Vasodilators
      b. Antiarrhythmics
      c. Diuretics
      d. Neurologic agents
      e. Glucose-regulating drugs
      f. Impotence therapy
B. Decrease in cardiac output caused by blood-flow obstruction within the heart or pulmonary circulation or by arrhythmias. This may be caused by the following:
   1. Aortic, pulmonic, and mitral stenosis
   2. Idiopathic hypertropic subaortic stenosis (IHSS)
   3. Pump failure
   4. Subclavian steal syndrome
   5. Seizures
C. Focal or generalized decrease in cerebral perfusion leading to transient ischemia due to cerebrovascular disease.
D. Metabolic abnormalities
   1. Hypoglycemia
   2. Hypocarbia and hypoxia usually do not result in syncope unless they are profound, although consciousness may be altered.
   3. Psychiatric illnesses associated with syncope include:
      a. Generalized anxiety
      b. Panic attacks
      c. Major depressive disorders

Predisposing Factors

A. Advanced age, caused by altered regulation of cerebral blood flow and/or systemic arterial pressure due to aging process and increased medication use
B. Other factors, depending on etiology
C. Medication use (noted above)

Common Complaints

A. Dizziness
B. Light-headedness
C. Fainting with no memory of events

Other Signs and Symptoms

A. Neuroautonomic regulations:
  1. Event triggered by changing position, turning head, wearing tight collars
  2. Nausea, warmth, diaphoresis, weakness 1 hour after eating
B. Cardiac causes: exercise-induced palpitations, chest pain, SOB with no warning prior to episode
C. Neurologic causes:
  1. Vertigo
  2. Diplopia
  3. Facial paresthesias
  4. Ataxia
  5. Auditory, visual, or vestibular disturbances
D. Metabolic or endocrine causes
  1. Restlessness
  2. Anxiety
  3. Confusion
  4. No recent food intake, low glucose level
E. Psychiatric: graceful fainting in presence of an audience

Subjective Data

A. Inquire if the patient ever experienced similar symptoms or episodes before.
B. Ask the patient or witness of episode to give a detailed description of loss of consciousness.
C. Question the patient regarding events leading up to the episode, noting prodromal symptoms.
D. Obtain a detailed account of symptoms after the episode, noting mental status.
E. Obtain a detailed medication history, addressing prescribed and OTC drugs, alcohol, and illicit preparations.
F. Review the patient's past medical history.

Physical Examination

A. Check temperature, pulse, respirations, and blood pressure.
  1. Measure BP and pulse in both arms and legs. Note BP differences between the arms.
  2. Measure BP several times during a 2-min period with the patient standing.
  3. Check for orthostatic hypotension, which is defined as a drop of 20 mmHg or more in SBP on standing:
    a. First, measure BP after the patient lies supine for 5–10 min.
    b. Then have the patient stand, and measure BP several times during a 2-min period.
B. Inspect the range of motion in the neck.
C. Palpate the abdomen, noting pulsatile expansion.
D. Auscultate
  1. Auscultate the heart with position changes. Note murmurs or extra heart sounds to rule out structural disease. Identify dysrhythmias such as bradycardia, supraventricular tachycardia, tachycardia, AV blocks, atrial fibrillation, bundle branch blocks, and sinus pauses or arrests.
  2. Auscultate the carotid arteries.
  3. Auscultate the abdomen for bruits.
E. Neurologic exam: Perform a complete exam, if indicated, including assessing 2nd–12th cranial nerves, Babinski's reflex, and gait.
F. Mental status: Assess mental health, if indicated.

Diagnostic Tests

The following tests are performed depending on history and physical exam results:

A. A 12-lead EKG, for essential baseline data. Identify acute and old EKG changes to rule out pathologic Q wave, ST segment elevation, and left ventricular hypertrophy.
B. Chest radiography, for essential baseline data. **Wide mediastinum signals aortic dissection.**
C. Echocardiogram.
D. Cardiac catheterization.
E. Lung scan.
F. Treadmill test.
G. Holter monitoring.
H. Tilt test.
I. Electrophysiologic studies.
J. EEG.
K. CT scan of head.
L. Cerebral flow studies.
M. Carotid Doppler ultrasonography.
N. Glucose tolerance test.
O. Chemistry profile, TSH, free T4, if hypoglycemia, hyponatremia, or hypothyroidism is suspected.

Differential Diagnoses

A. Irregular neuroautonomic regulations
  1. Neurocardiogenic causes
  2. Situational causes, such as coughing, defecation, diving, micturition, sneezing, swallowing, trumpet playing, vagal stimulation, weight lifting, postprandial state
  3. Orthostatic causes
    a. Hyperadrenergic state
    b. Hypoadrenergic state, primary or secondary autonomic insufficiency
    c. Carotid sinus syncope
    d. Cardioinhibitory state
    e. Vasodepressor stimulation
    f. Mixed
B. Cardiac causes
  1. Mechanical causes, such as aortic dissection, aortic stenosis, atrial myxoma, cardiac tamponade, global myocardial ischemia, hypertrophic cardiomyopathy, mitral stenosis, MI, prosthetic valve dysfunction, pulmonary embolism, pulmonary hypertension, pulmonary stenosis, and Takayasu's arteritis
  2. Electrical causes, such as AV block, long QT syndrome, pacemaker, sick sinus syndrome, supraventricular tachyarrhythmias, and ventricular tachyarrhythmias
C. Neurologic causes
  1. Neuralgias: glossopharyngeal, trigeminal
  2. Normal pressure hydrocephalus
  3. Subclavian steal
  4. Vertebrobasilar artery disease: compression, migraine, TIA
D. Metabolic or endocrine causes: hypoadrenalism, hypoglycemia, hyponatremia, hypothyroidism, and hypoxia
E. Psychiatric causes: anxiety, hysteria, major depression, panic disorder, somatization, and hyperventilation syndrome

Plan

A. General interventions: Management is directed at primary cause for the episode.
B. Patient teaching
1. If the patient has orthostatic hypotension, suggest that he or she wear elastic stockings, change positions slowly, sleep with the head of the bed elevated, and exercise legs before standing.
2. If syncope is induced by situations, warn the patient to avoid or alter his or her approach to such precipitating events.
3. If the patient has prodromal symptoms, such as nausea, light-headedness, pallor, sweating, or palpitations, advise him or her to lie down when they occur.
4. If the patient has hypersensitive carotid sinus reflex, recommend that he or she loosen his or her collar.
5. Tell patients to avoid prolonged standing. If they can't avoid it, they should contract their calf muscles to increase venous blood flow.
C. Dietary management: If not contraindicated, instruct patients with orthostatic hypotension to use salt liberally.
D. Pharmaceutical therapy: Therapy for neurocardiogenic syncope includes the following:
1. Drugs of choice are β-blockers.
2. Fludrocortisone acetate (Florinef Acetate), a corticosteroid, may be used alone or with β-blockers. Initial dosage is 0.1–0.2 mg/day; this may be increased gradually to 1.0–2.0 mg/day.
3. Other drugs include anticholinergic agents, disopyramide phosphate (Nor-pace), and selective serotonin-reuptake inhibitors.

Follow-up

A. Scheduling of return visits depends on etiology and severity of syncope and whether the patient has been placed on medications.

Consultation/Referral

A. Consult with or refer the patient to a physician when cardiac or neurologic involvement is suspected.
B. Consult or refer the patient to a physician if medication therapy is required.

Individual Considerations

A. Adults
1. In young adult athletes, be aware of symptoms of Marfan syndrome.
2. In older adults, coronary atherosclerosis may present along with syncope.
B. Geriatrics: Elderly patients may have multiple comorbid conditions, such as decreased cerebral blood flow and acute viral illness.

THROMBOPHLEBITIS

Definition

A. Superficial thrombophlebitis is inflammation of a vessel wall accompanied by blood stasis in varicose veins, which may also have clot formation.

B. Deep-vein thrombosis (DVT) is clot formation within a blood vessel, with inflammation of a vessel wall in the lower extremities. This can be life-threatening if embolization occurs in the lung.

Incidence

A. Varicose veins occur in approximately 10%–20% of adults, more frequently in women. The incidence of superficial thrombophlebitis is 50:100,000. With pregnancy, there is approximately a 49-fold increase of phlebitis. DVT is diagnosed in approximately 2 million people a year.

Pathogenesis

A. Superficial thrombosis is caused by infection, abuse of IV drugs, chemical irritation from overuse of IV route for diagnostic tests and drugs, and/or trauma. Several episodes can signal an underlying problem, such as carcinoma of the pancreas.
B. A common cause of varicose veins is blood flow stasis, basically due to valvular incompetence and/or dilation of the vessel lumen.
C. The cause of DVT is not always known; however, it is classically attributed to Virchow's triad: hypercoagulable state, vessel wall injury, and poor perfusion of blood supply.
D. Thrombi in the upper extremities commonly have iatrogenic causes, such as IV catheters.

Predisposing Factors

A. Hypercoagulablity states such as pregnancy
B. Oral contraceptive use
C. Blood disorders such as Factor XII deficiency
D. Malignancy
E. Lupus, positive anticardiolipin antibody
F. Sepsis
G. Surgery
H. Long bone trauma
I. Recent IV catheter access
J. Immobilization
K. Obesity
L. Varicose veins
M. Age older than 40
N. Stroke
O. MI
P. Family history of DVT

Common Complaints

These symptoms are common to superficial thrombophlebitis and DVT and occur along the course of a vein, usually in the lower extremities:

A. Swelling
B. Redness
C. Tenderness or pain

Other Signs and Symptoms

A. Superficial thrombophlebitis
1. Warm, tender, inflamed vessel with palpable cord
2. Fever or no fever
B. Varicose veins
1. Superficial dilated veins in lower extremities
2. Tiredness and heaviness in lower extremities

C. DVT
1. No symptoms may be present.
2. Symptoms may be unilateral, usually in lower extremities: extremity pain, swelling, and tenderness with palpation in affected extremity.
3. Erythema.
4. Warmth when touched.
5. Homans' sign, or pain in calf caused by forced dorsiflexion of foot, is commonly positive, but may be negative.

Potential Complications

A. Pulmonary embolism, especially if clots are in deep veins of thighs
B. Complete venous occlusion

Subjective Data

A. Query the patient regarding onset, duration, and intensity of symptoms.
B. Ask the patient about fever or other related symptoms.
C. Obtain a thorough medical history and account of recent physical activity.
D. Ask the patient if he or she has experienced any type of injury recently.
E. Inquire whether the patient has ever had similar symptoms or history of previous thrombophlebitis. If so, discuss treatment and therapy used and the results.
F. Review current medications: prescription, over-the-counter, and herbal. Ask specifically about oral contraceptives and hormone therapy.
G. Review the patient's occupation for sedentary lifestyle.
H. Review any recent plane travel.

Physical Examination

A. Check temperature, pulse, respirations, and blood pressure.
B. Inspect
1. Assess overall appearance. Evaluate for the presence of respiratory distress.
2. Inspect extremities, noting erythema and edema.
3. Measure circumference of each extremity.
C. Auscultate: Auscultate heart, lungs, and carotid arteries.
D. Palpate
1. Palpate extremities; check all pulses, including femoral, posttibial, pedal, and radial.
2. Palpate lower extremities for tenderness and palpable cord.
3. Test for Homans' sign in lower extremities bilaterally.

Diagnostic Tests

A. Contrast venography: definitive test
B. Doppler flow study of affected extremity
C. PT/PTT
D. Plethysmography

Differential Diagnoses

A. Thrombophlebitis
B. Varicose veins
C. Cellulitis
D. Strained muscle

Plan

A. General interventions
1. Advise all patients to stop smoking.
2. Tell the patient to avoid prolonged sitting or standing and not to cross or massage legs.
3. Advise the patient to avoid constrictive clothing such as knee-high hosiery.
4. Prescribe supportive hose.
5. Have the patient apply heat and elevate extremity for varicose veins or superficial thrombophlebitis.
6. Prescribe bed rest for superficial thrombophlebitis.
7. Tell patients with thrombophlebitis to discontinue oral contraceptives and hormone replacement.
8. DVT: Hospitalization is required.
B. Patient teaching: See the Section III Patient Teaching Guide for this chapter, "Deep Vein Thrombosis."
C. Pharmaceutical therapy for DVT: After hospitalization, anticoagulant therapy is prescribed by a physician.

Follow-up

A. Tell patients with varicose veins or superficial thrombophlebitis to return in 2 weeks or as needed.
B. Periodic follow-up is needed to monitor patients on anticoagulation therapy.
C. After acute problem is resolved, consider laboratory evaluation for hypercoagulation syndrome (protein C, protein S, and antithrombin III).

Consultation/Referral

A. If septic thrombophlebitis or DVT is diagnosed, refer the patient to a physician.
B. Hospitalization is required to initiate heparin therapy.

Individual Considerations

A. Pregnancy
1. Warfarin and NSAIDs are contraindicated.
2. Heparin is safe during pregnancy.
B. Geriatrics: Prognosis is poor for patients with septic thrombophlebitis.

REFERENCES

Abedin, Z., & Conner, R. (1989). *12 lead ECG Interpretation: The Self-Assessment Approach.* Philadelphia: W. B. Saunders.

Alpert, M., Hashimi, M. W., Concannon, M. D., Bikkina, M., & Mukerji, V. (1995). Pathogenesis, recognition, and management of common cardiac arrhythmias, Part II: Supraventricular premature beats and tachyarrhythmias. *Southern Medical Journal, 88,* 153–174.

American Heart Association 2009 Writing Group. (2009). 2009 Focused update: ACCF/AHA guidelines for the diagnosis and management of heart failure in adults. *Circulation, 119,* 1977–2016.

Arnstein, P., Buselli, E., & Rankin, S. (1996). Women and heart attacks: Prevention, diagnosis, and care. *Nurse Practitioner, 21,* 57–71.

Baer, M., & Goldschlager, N. (1995). Atrial fibrillation: An update on new management strategies. *Geriatrics, 50,* 22–28.

Barron, H., & Amidon, T. (1996). Options in antihypertensive drug therapy. *Postgraduate Medicine, 100,* 89–94.

Behrman, R., & Kliegman, R. (1994). *Nelson's essentials of pediatrics* (2nd ed.). Philadelphia: W. B. Saunders.

Berns, E. (1994). Nonpharmacologic therapy of tachyarrhythmias. *Comprehensive Therapy, 20,* 162–169.

Birdwell, B. G., Herberts, J. E., & Kroenke, K. (1993). Evaluating chest pain: The patient's presentation style alters the physician's diagnostic approach. *Archives of Internal Medicine, 325,* 1991.

Brugada, P., Gürsoy, S., Brugada, J., & Andries, E. (1993). Investigation of palpitations. *The Lancet, 341,* 1254–1258.

Burn, S., & Kaye, G. (1995). Identifying the causes of syncope and palpitations. *Practitioner, 239,* 666–669.

Cannon, Christopher P. (2008). Updated strategies and therapies for reducing ischemic and vascular events (STRIVE) ST-segment elevation myocardial infarction critical pathway toolkit. *Critical Pathways in Cardiology, 7,* 223–231.

Cannon, R. O. (1993). Chest pain with normal coronary angiograms. *New England Journal of Medicine, 328,* 1706.

Centers for Disease Control and Prevention. (2008). Disparities in adult awareness of heart attack warning signs and symptoms: 14 States, 2005. *MMWR, 57,* 175–179.

Champagne, M. A., Lamendola, C., & Miller, N. H. (2009). *National guidelines and tools for cardiovascular risk reduction.* New York: Philips Healthcare Communications.

Chobanian, A. V., Bakris, G. L., Black, H. R., Cushman, W. C., Green, L. A., Izzo, J. L., et al. (2003). Seventh report of the Joint National Committee on prevention, detection, evaluation, and treatment high blood pressure. *Hypertension, 42,* 1206–1252. Retrieved April 4, 2010, from http://hyper.ahajournals.org/cgi/content/full/42/6/1206

Choice of Lipid-Lowering Drugs. (1996). *The Medical Letter, 38,* 67–70.

Chun, H., & Sung, R. (1995). Supraventricular tachyarrhythmias. *Medical Clinics of North America, 79,* 1121–1134.

Cody, R. J. (1992). Management of refractory congestive heart failure. *American Journal of Cardiology, 69,* 141G–149G.

Coluccielo, S. (1994). Chest pain that isn't cardiac. *Emergency Medicine,* 71–79.

Conn, R. D., & O'Keefe, J. H. (2009). Cardiac physical diagnosis in the digital age: An important but increasingly neglected skill (from stethoscopes to microchips). *American Journal of Cardiology, 104,* 590–595.

Conover, M. (1992). *Understanding electrocardiography: Arrhythmias and the 12-lead ECG* (6th ed.). St. Louis: Mosby.

Dambo, M. (1995). *Griffith's 5 Minute Clinical Consult.* Baltimore: Williams & Wilkins.

Dubin, D. (1989). *Rapid interpretation of EKGs* (4th ed.). Tampa: Cover Publishing Company.

Epstein, M., & Bakris, G. (1996). Newer approaches to antihypertensive therapy. *Archives of Internal Medicine, 15,* 1969–1977.

Ewald, G., & McKenzie, C. (1995). *Manual of medical therapeutics: The Washington manual.* Boston: Little, Brown and Company.

Farrehi, P., Santingo, J., & Eage, K. (1995). Syncope: Diagnosis of cardiac and noncardiac causes. *Geriatrics, 50,* 24–30.

Fenstermacher, K., & Hudson, B. (1997). *Practice guidelines for family nurse practitioners.* Philadelphia: W. B. Saunders.

Fihn, S., & McGee, S. (1992). *Outpatient medicine.* Philadelphia: W. B. Saunders.

Freed, M. (1994). Advances in the diagnosis and therapy of syncope and palpitations in children. *Current Opinion in Pediatrics, 6,* 368–372.

Gandhi, S., & Santiesteban, H. (1996). Resistant hypertension. *Postgraduate Medicine, 100,* 97–107.

Giese, E. A., O'Connor, F. G., Depenbrock, P. J., & Oriscello, R. G. (2007). The athletic preparticipation evaluation: Cardiovascular assessment. *The American Family Physician.* Retrieved April 5, 2010, from http://www.aafp.org/afp/2007/0401/p1008.html

Gifford, R. (1997). What's new in the treatment of hypertension. *Cleveland Clinic Journal of Medicine, 64,* 143–149.

Gopalakrishnan, P. P., Shukla, S. K., & Tak, T. (2009). Infective endocarditis: Rationale for revised guidelines for antibiotic prophylaxis. *Clinical Medicine & Research, 7,* 63–66.

Goroll, A., May, L., & Mulley, A. (1995). *Primary care medicine office evaluation and management of the adult patient* (3rd ed.). Philadelphia: J. B. Lippincott.

Greene, H. (Ed.). (1996). *Clinical medicine* (2nd ed.). St. Louis: Mosby Year-Book.

Grossman, W. (1991). Diastolic dysfunction in congestive heart failure. *New England Journal of Medicine, 325,* 1557–1565.

Hanes, D., Weir, M., & Sowers, J. (1996). Gender considerations in hypertension pathophysiology and treatment. *The American Journal of Medicine, 101,* 3A-10s–3A-19s.

Hanifin, D. (2010). Cardiac auscultation 101: A basic science approach to diagnosing heart murmurs. *Journal of the American Academy of Physician Assistants.* Retrieved April, 6, 2010, from www.jaapa.com/cardiac-auscultation-101-a-basic-approach-to-diagnosing-heart-murmurs/article/167102/4

Hearns, P. (1994). Differentiating ischemia, injury, infarction: Expanding the 12-lead electrocardiogram. *Dimensions of Critical Care Nursing, 13,* 172–183.

Heron, M., Hoyert, D. L., Murphy, S. L., Xu, J., Kochanek, K. D., & Tejada-Vera, B. (2009). Deaths: Final data for 2006. National Vital Statistics Reports 57. Hyattsville, MD: National Center for Health Statistics. Retrieved April 3, 2010, from http://www.cdc.gov/nchs/data/nvsr/nvsr57/nvsr57_14.pdf

Hinson, J., Riordan, K., Hemphill, D., Randolph, C., & Fonseca, V. (1997). Hypertension education: An important and neglected part of the diabetes education curriculum? *The Diabetes Educator, 23,* 166–169.

Jamerson, K., & DeQuattro, V. (1996). The impact of ethnicity on response to antihypertensive therapy. *The American Journal of Medicine, 101,* 3A-22s–3A-30s.

Kapoor, W. (1994). Syncope in older adults. *Journal of the American Geriatrics Society, 42,* 426–436.

Kapoor, W. (1995). Workup and management of patients with syncope. *Medical Clinics of North America, 79,* l153–1168.

Koch, W. M. (1993). Swallowing disorders. *Medical Clinics of North America, 77,* 571–582.

Kugler, J., & Danford, D. (1996). Management of infants, children, and adolescents with paroxysmal supraventricular tachycardia. *Journal of Pediatrics, 129,* 324–338.

Lazarus, J., & Mauro, V. (1996). Syncope: Pathophysiology, diagnosis, and pharmacotherapy. *The Annals of Pharmacotherapy, 30,* 994–1003.

Lazzara, D., & Sellergren, C. (1996). Chest pain, making the right call. *Nursing, 96,* 2–51.

Lesh, M., Kalman, J., & Olgin, J. (1996). New approaches to treatment of atrial flutter and tachycardia. *Journal of Cardiovascular Electrophysiology, 7,* 368–381.

Linzer, M., Yang, E. H., Estes, N. A. 3rd, Wang, P., Vorperian, V. R., & Kapoor, W. N. (1997). Diagnosing syncope, Part 1: Value of history, physical examination, and electrocardiography. *Annals of Internal Medicine, 126,* 989–996.

Lloyd-Jones, D., Adams, R. J., Brown, T. M., Carnethon, M., Dais, S., De Simone, G., et al. (2010). Heart disease and stroke statistics—2010 update. A report from the American Heart Association Statistics Committee and Stroke Statistics Subcommittee. *Circulation, 121,* e1–e170.

Mukerji, B., Alper, M. A., & Mukerji, V. (1994). Musculoskeletal causes of chest pain. *Hospital Medicine, 30,* 26–39.

Ondrusek, R. (1996). Spotting an MI before it's an MI. *RN,* 26–30.

Paul, S. (1993). New pharmacologic agents for emergency management of supraventricular tachydys-rhythmias. *Critical Care Nursing Quarterly, l6,* 35-45.

Perez, A. (1996). Cardiac monitoring: Mastering the essentials. *RN,* 32–39.

Pharmacist's Letter/Prescriber's Letter. (2007, September). *Potentially harmful drugs in the elderly: Beers list and more.* 23: Detail document # 230907.

Rahman, M., Douglas, J., & Wright, J. (1997). Pathophysiology and treatment implications of hypertension in the African-American population. *Endocrinology and Metabolism Clinics of North America, 26,* 125–136.

Rakel, R. (1995). *Vonn's current therapy.* Philadelphia: W. B. Saunders.

Rakel, R. (1996). *Saunders manual of medical practice.* Philadelphia: W. B. Saunders.

Reynolds, E., & Baron, R. (1996). Hypertension in women and the elderly. *Postgraduate Medicine, 100,* 59–69.

Richter, J. E. (1991). Gastroesophageal reflux disease as a cause of chest pain. *Medical Clinics of North America, 75,* 1065–1080.

Robinson, A. (1996). Common varieties of supraventricular tachycardia: Differentiation and dangers. *Heart & Lung, 25,* 373–380.

Scheld, W. B., & Sands, M. A. (1990). Endocarditis and intravascular infections. In G. L. Mandel, R. G. Douglas, & K. E. Bennet (Eds.), *Principles and practices of infectious diseases.* New York: Churchill Livingstone.

Screening for High Blood Cholesterol and Other Lipid Abnormalities. (1996). *Guide to clinical preventive services: Report of U.S. Preventive Services Task Force* (2nd ed., pp. 15–32). Baltimore: Williams & Wilkins.

Seller, R. (1996). *Differential diagnosis for common complaints.* Philadelphia: W. B. Saunders.

Sexton, D. J. (2010, January). Antimicrobial prophylaxis for bacterial endocarditis. *UpToDate.* Retrieved April 6, 2010, from www.uptodate.com

Smith, T. W. (1993). Digoxin in heart failure. *New England Journal of Medicine, 329,* 51–58.

Spodick, D. (1996). Normal sinus heart rate: Appropriate thresholds for sinus tachycardia and bradycardia. *Southern Medical Journal, 89,* 666–667.

Spodick, D. H. (2010). Heart sounds: Important and neglected. *The American Journal of Cardiology, 105,* 1040.

Summary of the Second Report of the National Cholesterol Education Program (NCEP) Expert Panel on Detection, Evaluation, and Treatment of High Blood Cholesterol in Adults (Adult Treatment Panel II). (1993). *Journal of the American Medical Association, 269,* 3015–3023.

Taubert, K. A., & Dajaui, A. S. (1998, February). Preventing bacterial endocarditis: American Heart Association guidelines. Retrieved April 5, 2010, from http://www.aafp.org/afp/980201ap/taubert.html

Tierney, L., McPhee, S., & Papadakis, M. (Eds.). (1998). *Current medical diagnosis and treatment* (37th ed.). Stanford, CT: Appleton & Lange.

Tobin, L. (1999). Evaluating mild to moderate hypertension. *The Nurse Practitioner, 24,* 22–41.

U.S. Department of Health and Human Services. (2004). ATP III update 2004: Implications of recent clinical trials for the ATP III Guidelines. Retrieved April 5, 2010, from http://www.nhlbi.nih.gov/guidelines/cholesterol/atp3upd04.htm

U.S. Department of Health and Human Services. (2006). Your guide to lowering your blood pressure with DASH. NIH Publications No. 06–4082. Retrieved April 5, 2010, from http://www.nhlbi.nih.gov/health/public/heart/hbp/dash/new_dash.pdf

U.S. Department of Health and Human Services, National Institutes of Health. (2003). Seventh Report of the Joint National Committee (JNC VII) Prevention, Detection, Evaluation, and Treatment of High Blood Pressure. Retrieved April 4, 2010, from http://www.nhlbi.nih.gov/guidelines/hypertension/express.pdf

Weitz, H., & Weinstock, P. (1995). Approach to the patient with palpitations. *Medical Clinics of North America, 79,* 449–455.

Wellens, H., & Conover, M. (1992). *The ECG in emergency decision making.* Philadelphia: W. B. Saunders.

Williams, C., & Bernhardt, D. (1995). Syncope in athletes. *Sports Medicine, 19,* 223–234.

Wilson, W., Taubert K. A., Gewitz M., Lockhart, P. B., Baddour, L. M., Levison, M., et al. (2007). Prevention of infective endocarditis: Guidelines from the American Heart Association: A guideline from the American Heart Association Rheumatic Fever, Endocarditis, and Kawasaki Disease Committee, Council on Cardiovascular Disease in the Young, and the Council on Clinical Cardiology, Council on Cardiovascular Surgery and Anesthesia, and the Quality of Care and Outcomes Research Interdisciplinary Working Group. *Circulation, 116,* 1736–1754.

Young, J. (1995). The Fifth Report of the Joint National Committee on Detection, Evaluation, and Treatment of High Blood Pressure. *AAOHN Journal, 43,* 301–305.

Zellner, C., & Sudhir, K. (1995). Lifestyle modifications for hypertension. *Postgraduate Medicine, 100,* 75–79.

Zemel, M. B. (1997). Dietary pattern and hypertension: The DASH study. Dietary approaches to stop hypertension. *Nutrition Review, 55,* 303–305.

Gastrointestinal Guidelines

Cheryl A. Glass

ABDOMINAL PAIN

Definition

A. Abdominal pain is a common nonspecific complaint. The responsibility is for clinicians to determine which patients can be safely observed and treated symptomatically and which require further investigation or a specialist referral. Pain in the abdomen is secondary to problems relating to abdominal organs, and it is categorized as follows:

A. Acute pain: pain of less than a few days that has worsened progressively until presentation.

B. Chronic pain: interval of 12 weeks can be used to separate acute from chronic pain, that is, it has remained unchanged for months or years.

C. Emergent: pain that lasts 3 hours or longer, accompanied by a fever or vomiting.

Incidence

Abdominal pain is very common. Abdominal pain is present on questioning 75% of adolescent students and in about 50% of all adults. Gastroenteritis and irritable bowel syndrome are the most common cause of acute pain, and chronic stool retention is the most common cause of chronic pain. Other causes of abdominal pain include the following:

A. Acute appendicitis: occurs 10:100,000

B. Acute cholecystitis: varies according to age and ethnic origin

C. Intestinal obstruction, usually small intestines: accounts for 20% of acute abdominal conditions

D. Abdominal pain associated with pregnancy: ectopic pregnancy (1:200 pregnancies), miscarriage, and abruptio placenta

Pathogenesis

A. Pathogenesis depends on the origin of pain. Pain may result from inflammation, ischemia, distension, altered motility, obstruction, or ulceration.

Predisposing factors

A. Abdominal trauma

B. Motor vehicle accidents

C. Lactose intolerance

D. Pregnancy

E. Torsion

F. Psychogenic pain

G. Sickle cell disease

Common Complaints

Clinical presentation of abdominal pain is determined in part by the site of the involvement.

A. Acute or chronic onset of pain

B. Vomiting

C. Diarrhea

Other Signs and Symptoms

A. Bleeding.

B. Referred shoulder pain.

C. Fever.

D. Nausea or projectile vomiting.

E. Rigid abdomen.

F. Changes in vital signs.

G. Abdominal distension.

H. Constipation.

I. Guarding.

J. Rebound tenderness.

K. Biliary pain and right subcostal tenderness.

L. Anorexia.

M. Periumbilical discomfort; consider appendicitis if, within 2 to 12 hours, pain localizes in right lower quadrant (RLQ) at McBurney's point.

N. Dysuria.

O. Abdominal mass; do not overlook the possibility of pregnancy as the cause of a mass.

P. Melena (most common in peptic ulcer disease).

Subjective Data

Evaluate for a "surgical abdomen" defined as a rapidly worsening prognosis in the absence of surgical intervention. Patients should not eat or drink while a diagnosis of a surgical abdomen remains under consideration. Once a surgical abdomen has been excluded the remainder of the evaluation will be guided by the chronicity of symptoms along with the location of pain.

A. Review onset, duration, course, and quality of pain. Ask: Has this ever occurred before? What was the primary diagnosis? What was the previous treatment, and was it effective?

B. Determine pain rating on a 10-point scale, with 0 being no pain and 10 being equivalent to the worst pain the patient has ever felt. Review progression of pain.
C. Qualify the duration of pain in minutes, hours, days, weeks, or months. Does the pain interfere with sleep?
D. Review the pattern of pain.
   1. Review aggravating factors.
   2. Review alleviating factors
   3. Does the pain radiate?
E. If the patient is pregnant, determine her last missed menses (LMP). Has she had a previous hysterectomy or tubal ligation? Does she have a recent history of dyspareunia or dysmenorrhea that suggests pelvic pathology.
F. Review the patient's current medications and drug history, especially antibiotic, laxative, acetaminophen, aspirin, and NSAID use.
G. Rule out abdominal trauma from domestic violence, motor vehicle accidents, falls, or assaults.
H. Review bowel habits and note changes: constipation, diarrhea, anorexia, food intolerance, nausea, vomiting, or bloating.
I. Review the patient's history for sickle cell disease. Any African American presenting with leg or abdominal pain should be questioned regarding sickle cell disease or trait.
J. Review urinary function. Is there any urinary frequency, urgency, dysuria, flank pain, or back pain? If the patient is male, does he have any hesitancy, difficulty starting the urine stream, nocturia, low urinary volume, or any lower abdominal distension indicating urinary retention?
K. Review alcohol intake/history.

Physical Examination

A. Check temperature, pulse, respirations, and blood pressure; include orthostatic blood pressure.

Tachycardia or hypotension may be signs of a ruptured aortic aneurysm, septic shock, GI hemorrhage, or volume depletion.

B. Inspect
   1. Observe general appearance: facial expressions, walk, skin turgor; note grimace during exam.
   2. Perform eye and mouth exam to rule out iritis and aphthous ulcers of the mouth (extraintestinal manifestations of inflammatory bowel disease [IBD]).
   3. Examine the abdomen for the presence of a hernia at the umbilicus, groin, or near the site of prior surgical incisions.
   4. Examine the eyes and skin for jaundice.
C. Auscultate
   1. Auscultate for bowel sounds in all four quadrants of the abdomen.
   2. Evaluate heart and lungs.
   3. Check for bruits of aorta.
D. Percuss abdomen.
E. Palpate
   1. Palpate abdomen for masses, rebound tenderness, and peritoneal signs.
      a. Before palpating the abdomen, ask the patient to bend the knees to help with relaxation of the wall musculature.
      b. Elderly patients may lack classical peritoneal signs of rebound and guarding.

2. Check the abdomen for tender pulsatile mass at midline; it may indicate abdominal aortic aneurysm.
3. Palpate back; check for CVA tenderness.
4. Perform a bimanual examination in women regardless of whether the patient has had a hysterectomy or is postmenopausal.
   a. Evaluate the size and symmetry of the uterus.
   b. Evaluate the adnexal areas for presence of appropriately sized, mobile ovaries. A fixed, painful adnexal mass is suggestive of an endometriomoa or tubo-ovarian abscess.
   c. Endometriosis is suggested by localized tenderness in the cul-de-sac or uterosacral ligaments, palpable tender nodules, pain with uterine movement, tender, fixation of adnexal or uterus in a retroverted position.
5. Check for obturator sign, which is abdominal pain in response to passive internal rotation of the right hip from the 90° angle knee-hip flexion position.
6. Check for iliopsoas sign; perform this when an inflamed appendix is suspected. Positive psoas sign is the presence of lower quadrant pain noted as the supine patient raises his or her right leg from the hip while the examiner pushes downward against his or her lower thigh.
F. Perform a rectal exam including testing of stool for occult blood. **Failure to perform a rectal examination in patients with abdominal pain may be associated with an increased rate of misdiagnosis and should be considered a medicolegal pitfall.**

Diagnostic Tests
A. CBC with differential.
B. Electrolytes.
C. SMA 12.
D. Chemistry 20.
E. BUN.
F. Amylase.
G. Aminotransferases, alkaline phosphatase, and bilirubin.
H. Lipase.
I. Urinalysis; save sample for culture.
J. Serum HCG, if indicated.
K. Coproporphyrin, if lead poisoning is suspected.
L. Plain X-ray films of abdomen; consider CT of abdomen.
M. Abdominal ultrasonography.
N. GI series radiography.
O. Endoscopy; consider *Helicobacter pylori* testing.
P. Sigmoidoscopy.
Q. Barium enema: avoid with suspected obstruction.
R. Chest radiography.
S. Guaiac stool for occult blood.
T. Consider endoscopic retrograde cholangiopancreatography (ERCP) to visualize the distal common bile duct.
U. EKG to rule out cardiac pain.
V. Consider blood cultures for elderly that present with abdominal pain associated with either fever or hypothermia or when sepsis is suspected.

Differential Diagnoses
Location and duration of abdominal pain can often help significantly in narrowing the differential diagnosis.

A. Right upper quadrant (RUQ) pain
1. Acute cholecystitis and biliary colic
   a. Biliary tract: increased serum amylase.
   b. Ascending cholangitis presents with fever and jaundice in a patient with right upper quadrant pain.
   c. In acute cholecystitis, the typical pain is maximal in the RUQ or epigastrium, radiating to the scapular region, and is accompanied by nausea, vomiting, and fever without jaundice. *Murphy's sign,* or inspiratory arrest in response to upper quadrant palpation, may be seen with acute cholecystitis. RUQ tenderness to percussion or pressure of the gallbladder is also a suggestive finding.
   d. Ketoacidosis has been found to present with severe abdominal pain in 8% of instances and may be accompanied by emesis and an elevated white cell count. Acute intra-abdominal events such as cholecystitis may be the precipitant of ketoacidosis.
2. Acute hepatitis
3. Hepatic abscess
4. Hepatomegaly due to congestive heart failure
5. Perforated duodenal ulcer

A perforated ulcer is accompanied by an increased serum amylase.

6. Acute pancreatitis; bilateral pain

Pancreatitis is accompanied by an increased serum amylase.

7. Herpes zoster
8. Myocardial ischemia
9. Pleural or pulmonary pathology (e.g., pneumonia, pulmonary embolism, or empyema)
B. Right lower quadrant (RLQ) pain
1. Appendicitis often begins with symptoms of dull, steady, periumbilical pain and anorexia before localizing to the RLQ at McBurney's point.
2. Regional enteritis.
3. Leaking aneurysm.
4. Ruptured ectopic pregnancy.
5. Twisted ovarian cyst.
6. PID.
7. Ureteral calculi.
8. Incarcerated, strangulated inguinal hernia.
9. Endometriosis.
10. Meckel's diverticulitis.
11. Abdominal wall hematoma.
C. Left upper quadrant (LUQ) pain
1. Gastritis
2. Acute pancreatitis: epigastric pain that is relatively sudden and particularly when it radiates to the back and is associated with nausea, vomiting, and anorexia.
3. Splenic enlargement, rupture, infarction, aneurysm
4. Myocardial ischemia
5. Left lower lobe pneumonia
6. Acute pancreatitis; bilateral pain
D. Left lower quadrant (LLQ) pain

1. Sigmoid diverticulitis
2. Regional enteritis
3. Leaking aneurysm

Abdominal aortic aneurysm may present with a tender pulsatile mass at the abdominal midline. Vascular disorders such as acute arterial insufficiency, due to atherosclerosis or embolus, may present with severe abdominal pain, although mild, constant pain may be the only symptom for several days. Dissection or rupture of an abdominal aortic aneurysm produces severe acute abdominal pain and often radiates to the back or genitalia.

4. Ruptured ectopic pregnancy

Rupture of the fallopian tube generally causes sudden, acute, and localized abdominal pain. Internal hemorrhage causes syncope and referred shoulder pain, caused by phrenic nerve irritation. Diagnosis before tubal rupture may be difficult because symptoms and physical findings mimic other conditions such as appendicitis.

5. Twisted ovarian cyst
6. PID
7. Ureteral calculi
8. Incarcerated, strangulated inguinal hernia
E. Generalized abdominal pain
1. Trauma
   a. **Any person with a possible blow to the abdomen should have orthostatic blood pressure taken, careful palpation of the abdomen, serial abdominal circumferences measured, and be considered for abdominal imaging. Serial hemoglobin and hematocrit measurements should be obtained, if necessary.**
   b. In abdominal trauma, the spleen is the most commonly injured organ, especially in blunt abdominal trauma; the onset can be immediate or delayed.
   c. Nontraumatic splenic rupture is often associated with acute infectious mononucleosis.
2. Intestinal obstruction: Obstruction that develops slowly over weeks to months may be relatively subtle in presentation.

Acute obstruction presents with severe "colicky" pain or pain that is wavelike in nature; it makes the pain relentless.

3. Peritoneal irritation: Severe pain due to the rich innervation of the parietal peritoneum. Focal injury results in well-localized discomfort that is described as a sharp aching or burning.
4. Metabolic disturbances may mimic intra-abdominal etiologies.

Porphyria and lead poisoning sometimes simulate bowel obstruction, because they can cause cramping, abdominal pain, and hyperperistalsis.

5. Nonspecific dysfunctional abdominal pain and psychogenic abdominal pain are diagnoses of exclusion.

Plan
A. General interventions
1. If necessary, prepare the patient for emergency transport and hospitalization.
2. Management and follow-up of other causes of abdominal pain are variable and depend on diagnosis.

B. Patient teaching
  1. See the Section III Patient Teaching Guides for this chapter, "Abdominal Pain: Adults" and "Abdominal Pain: Children."
  2. Counsel the patient to keep a pain diary to include activity, foods, and other pain triggers; duration of pain; and what provides relief of symptoms.
C. Pharmaceutical therapy: Treatment depends on the findings from the history, physical, and testing and the clinical diagnosis.

Follow-up
A. Variable, depending on diagnosis.
B. Review pain diary.

Consultation/Referral
A. Consult the physician for the patient with acute abdominal pain and pain related to abdominal trauma.
B. For the obstetric patient, consult a physician for any bleeding or abdominal pain.

Individual Considerations
A. Pregnancy: There is no evidence that acute intra-abdominalsurgical emergencies are more common during pregnancy if ectopic pregnancy is excluded.
  1. The presence of peritoneal signs, rebound tenderness, and abdominal guarding is never normal in pregnancy.
  2. Bleeding complications include the following:
     a. First trimester: miscarriage and ectopic pregnancy
     b. Second and third trimester: abruptio placenta
  3. Physiologic changes of pregnancy may affect the presentation and evaluation of abdominal pain. The enlargement of the uterus can impede physical examination, affect the normal location of pelvic and abdominal organs, and mask or delay peritoneal signs.
  4. Severe preeclampsia: The clinical manifestations of liver involvement include right upper quadrant or midepigastric pain, elevated transaminases, and in severe cases, subcapsular hemorrhage or hepatic rupture.
B. Pediatrics
  1. The caregiver's lap makes the best examining surface; it is much better than having the child lie fixed and supine on a table.
  2. Observe the child's interaction and gait prior to examination. If able to stand, ask the child to hop as an assessment of peritoneal irritation. If the child is unwilling to stand, shaking the exam table or pelvis can also evaluate for peritoneal signs.
  3. An infant's abdomen should be examined during a time of relaxation and quiet, if possible. It is often best to do this at the start of the overall examination, especially before initiating any procedure that may cause distress.
  4. Allowing an infant to suck on a pacifier may help relax him or her.
  5. Tenderness or pain on palpation may be difficult to detect in an infant. However, pain and tenderness are assessed by such behaviors as change in the pitch of crying, facial grimacing, rejection of opportunity to suck, and drawing the knees to the abdomen with palpation.
  6. Urinary tract infections can cause abdominal pain, and often the child with a UTI does not complain of dysuria and frequency as adults typically do.
  7. Young children have inaccurate body perceptions and are inaccurate historians. The practitioner must rely on the caregiver and the examination for data. Consider psychosocial aspects of childcare and possible abuse.
  8. Appendicitis is the most common pediatric surgical emergency. The diagnosis can be difficult, because the classic symptoms are often not present.
  9. Intestinal malrotation must be considered when a healthy infant suddenly refuses to eat, vomits, becomes inconsolable, and develops abdominal distension.
  10. Intussusception presents as paroxysmal, colicky pain, and the infant often has currant jelly stools; a palpable right upper quadrant abdominal mass; and ultimately, distension.
  11. Young male patients may hesitate to report testicular pain.
C. Adults
  1. Obesity distorts the abdominal exam making organ palpation or pelvic examination difficult.
  2. With men older than age 40 and women older than age 50, suspect cardiac origin when presenting with epigastric pain. Consider obtaining EKG for patients in this age group.

While myocardial infarction "classically" presents with anterior chest pressure or pain, the patient may also have a gastritis or heartburn sensation, coupled with nausea and diaphoresis.

D. Geriatrics
  1. Elderly patients may have a vague or atypical presentation of pain, varying in location, severity, and presence of a fever or nonspecific findings on examination.
  2. Elderly patients have a diminished sensorium, allowing pathology to advance to a dangerous point prior to symptom development.
  3. In an older patient, a similar presentation to IBD with abdominal pain and a change in bowel habits can be the first sign of colon cancer.
  4. Abdominal aortic aneurysm (AAA) is observed almost exclusively in elderly patients. Maintain a high index of suspension in patients that present with a clinical picture suggestive of renal colic or musculoskeletal back pain.
  5. Elderly patients with urinary tract infections are less likely to have dysuria, frequency, or urgency.

⬛ APPENDICITIS

Definition
A. Appendicitis is acute inflammation of the appendix caused by the obstruction of the appendiceal lumen. Perforation is rare in the first 12 hours but the rate of perforation

increases after 72 hours. Prompt, early diagnosis, and operative intervention is the goal of treatment. The differential diagnoses for appendicitis include all abdominal sources of pain. Imaging studies appears to reduce the negative appendectomy rate to less than 10%.

Incidence

A. Acute appendicitis occurs at a rate of 10:100,000. It the most common condition in children (1%–8%) and during pregnancy (0.06%–0.1%) that requires emergency abdominal surgery. One in every 2,000 adults older than age 65 will develop appendicitis.

Pathogenesis

A. Foreign bodies, fecal material, tissue hypertrophy, strictures, or a bend or twist on the organ may cause obstruction of the appendix. The obstruction causes colicky pain. Bacterial invasion causes inflammation and leads to gangrene and perforation. The most common bacteria are *E. coli,* pseudomonas, *B. fragilis,* and *Peptostreptococcus* species.

Predisposing Factors

A. Pregnancy
B. Torsion
C. Abdominal trauma
D. Male gender, age 10–30

Common Complaints

A. Adults
1. Generalized or localized abdominal pain in the epigastric or periumbilical areas. Within 2–12 hours, pain localizes in right lower quadrant (RLQ) at McBurney's point, and intensity increases.
2. The location of the appendix is altered in pregnancy.
3. Pain typically develops before vomiting.
4. Nausea and/or vomiting (may be projectile).
5. Anorexia signals organic cause of abdominal pain.
B. Pediatrics
1. Children younger than 2 years:
a. Abdominal distention
b. Irritability
c. Lethargy
2. Children older than 2 years
a. Vomiting is often the first symptom.
b. Abdominal pain.
c. Fever.

Other Signs and Symptoms

A. Rigid abdomen
B. Changes in pulse (tachycardia), breathing, or skin temperature
C. Involuntary guarding
D. Rebound tenderness

Subjective Data

A. Review onset, duration, course, and quality of pain. Has pain ever occurred before? If so, what was the primary diagnosis? What was previous treatment, and was it effective?
B. Qualify the duration of pain in minutes, hours, days, weeks, or months. Does it interfere with sleep? Is there a pattern to the pain?
C. Have the patient rate the pain on a 10-point pain scale, with 0 being no pain and 10 being the worst pain the patient has ever felt.
D. Review aggravating or alleviating factors.
E. Determine last menstrual period to rule out pregnancy. Review sexual activity to help distinguish gynecological disorders.
F. Review current medications and drug history, especially antibiotic and laxative use.
G. Rule out abdominal trauma, motor vehicle accidents, falls, and assault.
H. Discuss bowel habits, including any changes, such as constipation or diarrhea; anorexia; food intolerance; nausea and vomiting; bloating.
I. Ask the patient about urinary frequency, urgency, dysuria, flank pain, and back pain. In males, ask about hesitancy, difficulty starting the urine stream, nocturia, low urinary volume, or lower abdominal distension (urinary retention).

Physical Examination

A. Check temperature, pulse, respirations, and blood pressure, including orthostatic BP.
B. Inspect
1. Observe general appearance: facial expressions (grimace during exam), walk, skin color and turgor, level of consciousness, and acuity level of pain.
2. Inspect abdomen for surgical scars.
C. Auscultate
1. Auscultate the abdomen for bowel sounds in all quadrants.
2. Auscultate heart and lungs.
D. Palpate: Note guarding with exam.
1. Palpate abdomen.
a. Ask the patient to bend his or her knees to help relax abdominal wall musculature. Note rebound tenderness. **Perform at end of exam** because positive response produces pain and muscle spasm that can interfere with subsequent exam.
b. Check for Murphy's sign, which is inspiratory arrest in response to right upper quadrant (RUQ) palpation, seen with acute cholecystitis.
2. Palpate back; note CVA tenderness.
3. Check for rebound tenderness.
4. Check for obturator sign, or abdominal pain in response to passive internal rotation of right hip from 90° angle hip-knee flexion position. A positive sign indicates pain secondary to irritation of obturator muscle with inflamed appendix.
5. Assess psoas sign or increased abdominal pain occurring when the patient attempts to raise his or her right thigh against the pressure of your hand placed over his or her right knee. Pain is caused by inflammation of the psoas muscle in acute appendicitis.
6. Check for the Apley rule, or the farther from the navel the pain, the more likely it is organic in origin.
7. Check for Rovsing's sign, or pain in the right lower quadrant (RLQ) on palpation of the left side.
8. The location of the appendix and pain is altered during pregnancy. See Figure 10.1.

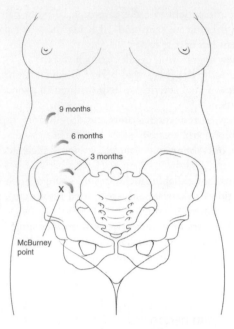

Figure 10.1 The position of the appendix alters during pregnancy and so must the site of incision to gain access.

E. Percuss abdomen.
F. Perform rectal exam, if indicated.

Diagnostic Tests
A. CBC with differential.
B. C reactive protein (CRP).
C. Urinalysis, to rule out urinary disorders.
D. HCG serum pregnancy test, if indicated.
E. Abdominal ultrasonography; any person with trauma to abdomen should have abdominal ultrasound.
F. CT scan.
G. MRI may be used as an alternative diagnostic test in pregnancy to avoid exposure to ionizing radiation.
H. Guaiac stool for occult blood.

Differential Diagnoses
Duration of pain can help significantly in narrowing differential diagnosis. Nonspecific dysfunctional abdominal pain and psychogenic abdominal pain are diagnoses of exclusion.

A. Appendicitis
B. Regional enteritis
C. Leaking aneurysm
D. Ruptured ectopic pregnancy
E. Twisted ovarian cyst
F. Pelvic inflammatory disease (PID)
G. Mittelschmerz, or ovulatory bleeding or pain
H. Endometriosis
I. Ureteral calculi
J. Incarcerated, strangulated groin hernia
K. Meckel's diverticulitis
L. Abdominal wall hematoma
M. Bowel obstruction
N. Intestinal malrotation
O. Intussesception
P. Testicular torsion

Plan
A. See the Section III Patient Teaching Guide for this chapter, "Abdominal Pain: Adults" and "Abdominal Pain: Children."
B. Medical and surgical management: appendectomy may need to be performed.
C. Pharmaceutical therapy: do not give antipyretics to mask fever, and do not administer cathartics because they may cause rupture.

Follow-up
A. Postoperative follow-up is with the surgeon.

Consultation/Referral
A. Physician consultation and possible emergency transport and hospitalization are often required.

Individual Considerations
A. Pregnancy
   1. Any abdominal pain or bleeding in the first 8 weeks after a missed menstrual period must be considered a symptom of possible **ectopic pregnancy.**
   2. The identification of intra-abdominal masses may be compromised by the enlarged uterus, but this problem may be partially obviated by examining the woman in the lateral position.
   3. The intestinal tract is progressively displaced upward, outward, and backward during pregnancy; bowel sounds are best heard lateral or superior to the uterus.
B. Pediatrics
   1. The caregiver's lap makes the best examining surface; it is much better than having the child lie fixed and supine on a table.
   2. If possible, examine the infant's abdomen during a time of relaxation and quiet. It is often best to do this at the start of the overall examination, especially before initiating any procedure that might cause distress. Allowing the infant to suck on a bottle or pacifier may help relax him or her.
   3. Tenderness or pain on palpation may be difficult to detect in the infant. However, pain and tenderness are assessed by such behaviors as change in the pitch of crying, facial grimacing, rejection of the opportunity to suck, and drawing knees to the abdomen with palpation.
   4. Intestinal malrotation must be considered when a healthy infant suddenly refuses to eat, vomits, becomes inconsolable, and develops abdominal distension.
   5. Young children have inaccurate body perceptions and are inaccurate historians, so rely on caregivers and examination for data, and consider psychosocial aspects such as childcare and child abuse.
   6. Intussusception presents as paroxysmal, colicky pain, and the infant often has currant jelly stools, a palpable RUQ, abdominal mass, and ultimately distension.

C. Adults
1. Obesity distorts abdominal exam, making organ palpation or pelvic exam difficult.
2. Immunocompromised patients are susceptive to infection. They may not exhibit the typical signs and symptoms of appendicitis; only mild tenderness on exam.
3. The CT exam is useful in the immunocompromised for diagnosis.
D. Geriatrics
1. The elderly tend to have a diminished inflammatory response, resulting in a less remarkable history and physical examination. Be aware of vague symptoms, such as milder pain, less pronounced fever, and leukocytosis with shift to left on differential.
2. A redundant sigmoid colon may also cause right-sided pain from sigmoid disease.
3. Prompt CT scanning is used for diagnosis and differential.

CELIAC DISEASE

Definition

A. Celiac disease (CD), previously known as celiac sprue, is an autoimmune disorder triggered by a well-defined environmental factor, gluten. CD is a permanent sensitivity to gluten, specifically; the people are unable to tolerate gliadin, the alcohol-soluble fraction of gluten. Three cereals contain gluten and are considered toxic for patients with celiac disease: wheat, rye, and barley. The disease primarily affects the small intestine. Onset of symptoms depends on the amount of gluten in the diet. Dietary nonadherence is the chief cause of persistent or recurrent symptoms. (See Appendix B: "Examples of Foods That Are Allowed or Avoided on a Gluten-Free Diet.")
B. Celiac disease is strongly associated with autoimmune conditions including type 1 diabetes, thyroiditis; as well as genetic syndromes including Down syndrome, Williams syndrome and Turner syndrome. The complications from CD include osteopenia, osteoporosis, infertility, short stature, delayed puberty, anemia, and gastrointestinal malignancies and lymphoma.

Incidence

A. Celiac disease can occur at any stage of life. The prevalence of CD in children is unknown. The prevalence of CD is approximately 1% of the general population in North America. The highest incidence (5%) is noted in the Sub-Saharan African population. The true incidence is undetermined due to asymptomatic disease and underdiagnosis.

Pathogenesis

A. Interactions between gluten and immune and genetic factors result in celiac disease. Gluten is poorly digested. The enzyme tissue transglutaminase (tTG) is the autoantigen against which abnormal immune response is directed. The immune responses promote an inflammatory reaction. Celiac disease primarily affects the mucosal layer of the small intestine. The classic celiac lesion is noted in the proximal small intestine.

B. The Marsh Classification is used to describe the progressive histological stages in CD. Marsh 1 and Marsh 2 may be seen in sow and cow's milk allergies.

Type 0: preinfiltrative stage (normal)
Type 1: infiltrative lesion (increased intraepithelial lymphocytes)
Type 2: hyperplastic lesion (type 1 plus hyperplastic crypts)
Type 3: destructive lesion (type 2 plus villous atrophy of progressively more severe degrees [termed 3a, 3b, and 3c])

Predisposing Factors

A. Female gender.
B. May be precipitated by an infectious diarrheal episode or other intestinal disease (e.g., rotavirus).
C. Genetic disorders
1. Down syndrome (8%–12%).
2. Type 1 diabetes (10%).
3. Turners syndrome (2%–10%).
4. Williams syndrome (8.2%).
D. Strong hereditary component (10% in first-degree relatives).
E. The introduction of gluten before 4 months of age is associated with an increased disease development.
F. Autoimmune thyroiditis.
G. Selective IgA deficiency.

Common Complaints

A. Asymptomatic
B. Chronic diarrhea or explosive watery diarrhea
C. Anorexia
D. Abdominal distention
E. Abdominal pain
F. Poor weight gain or weight loss
G. Vomiting
H. Steatorrhea (malabsorption of ingested fat)

Other Symptoms

A. Behavioral changes including irritability
B. Dehydration
C. Lethargy
D. Constipation
E. Failure to thrive
F. Short stature and delayed puberty
G. Dermatitis herpetiformis
H. Arthritis
I. Seizures
J. Weakness and fatigue
K. Dental enamel hypoplasia of permanent teeth
L. Iron-deficiency anemia unresponsive to treatment

Subjective Data

A. Review the onset, duration, course, and type of symptoms.
B. Review the patient's weight history.
C. Evaluate family history for celiac disease or members with similar histories.
D. Review current medications and drug history, especially antibiotic, laxative, and herbal products.
E. Review bowel habits and note changes: constipation, diarrhea, anorexia, and/or food intolerance.

Physical Examination

A. Vital signs including height and weight.
B. Inspect
  1. Observe general overall appearance.
  2. Oral examination to evaluate glossitis, dry mucosal membranes (dehydration), and the presence of oral aphthae.
  3. Examine the skin for the presence of dermatitis herpetiformis: a blistering rash involving the scalp, neck, elbows, knees, and buttocks.
  4. Evaluate the abdomen for the presence of bloating and protuberant "potbelly."
  5. Evaluate the patient's weight loss including muscle wasting.
C. Auscultate
  1. Auscultate for bowel sounds in all four quadrants of the abdomen.
D. Percuss abdomen.
E. Palpate
  1. Palpate the abdomen for masses, rebound tenderness, and peritoneal signs.
    a. Before palpating the abdomen, ask the patient to bend his or her knees to help with relaxation of the wall musculature.
  2. Perform a rectal examination including testing of stool for occult blood.

Diagnostic Tests

All testing should be performed while patients are following a gluten-rich diet.

A. Endoscopy for duodenal biopsies is the standard for diagnosing celiac disease.
B. IgA tissue transglutaminase antibody (IgA tTG) and EMA antibodies for symptomatic and asymptomatic patients.
C. Complete blood count (CBC) and electrolytes.
D. AST and ALT (liver enzymes normalize on a gluten-free diet).
E. Prothrombin time (PT) may be prolonged with malabsorption of vitamin K.
F. Stool culture, ova, and parasites.
G. Bone density (bone mineral density improves on gluten-free diet).
H. Human leukocyte antigen (HLA) haplotypes.
I. Colonoscopy if bloody stools or symptoms of colitis.
J. Radiograph including barium swallow study with a small bowel follow-through are usually nonspecific and are not indicated.
K. Sweat test to exclude cystic fibrosis (CF).
L. Other testing specific to nutritional deficiencies as needed.

Differential Diagnoses

A. Celiac disease
B. Failure to thrive
C. Food allergies
D. Inflammatory bowel disease (IBD)
  1. Crohn's disease
  2. Ulcerative colitis
E. Immunodeficiency disorders
F. Gastroenteritis (viral or bacterial)
G. Parasites
H. Fungal infection
I. Irritable bowel syndrome
J. Malabsorption
K. Lymphomas of the small intestine

Plan

A. Nutrition therapy is the only accepted treatment for celiac disease. Gluten-free dietary instructions should be given and reenforced. Consider a dietary consultation.
B. Monitor for iron and vitamin deficiencies because substitute flours are not fortified with B vitamins. Supplement with iron, folate, and vitamin B_{12} as needed.
C. Screen for osteoporosis.
D. Keep a food/symptom diary in order to eliminate trigger foods. See Appendix B: "Examples of Foods That Are Allowed or Avoided on a Gluten-Free Diet."
E. Gluten rechallenge is not generally recommended unless the diagnosis remains uncertain. The rechallenge is not mandatory for patients with good improvement of symptoms.
F. Pharmacology: Corticosteroids may be prescribed for rapid control of symptoms. Prednisone (Deltasone, Orasone, Sterapred)
  1. Adults: 30–40 mg per day, taper off completely in 6–8 weeks.
  2. Pediatrics: 1 mg/kg per day; not to exceed 30 mg/day. Taper off completely in 6–8 weeks. Children with celiac disease are rarely given steroids.

Follow-up

A. After the diagnosis of CD and a strict diet has been started, follow-up in 4–8 weeks or earlier if the patient has other comorbidities.
B. The Celiac Disease Guideline Committee recommends the measurement of tTGA after 6 months of a gluten-free diet.

Consultation/Referral

A. If the gluten-free diet fails, or the patient experiences new symptoms, a systematic evaluation is required.
B. Endocrine consultation for patients with Hashimoto thyroiditis and celiac disease.
C. Consultation with a pediatric gastroenterologist.

Individual Considerations

A. Pregnancy: Mothers with untreated celiac disease are at risk for preterm birth and low birth weight babies.
B. Pediatrics:
  1. Children may appear to have a "potbelly" with muscle wasting from malnutrition.
  2. Monitor growth and development. Utilize a growth chart to plot growth rates. As many as 10% of children with idiopathic short stature may have celiac disease.
  3. Breast-feeding has a protective role even if gluten is introduced while breast-feeding.

▣ CHOLECYSTITIS

Definition

A. Cholecystitis is acute or chronic inflammation of the gallbladder. Acute cholecystitis has associated stone formation (cholelithiasis) in 90% of all cases, causing obstruction and inflammation. Biliary sludge is a feature of chronic cholecystitis.

Incidence

A. Gallbladder disease afflicts more than 20 million Americans. The incidence in children is not known. Biliary sludge and/or gallstones are likely to form in 1 in 5 children with hemolytic anemia before their adolescent years. Most patients with an acute attack of cholecystitis have complete remission in 1–5 days; however, approximately 20% require surgical intervention. Mortality related to acute cholecystitis is 5%–10%, with the highest risk for patients older than age 60.

Pathogenesis

A. Cholecystitis occurs subsequent to bile stasis, bacterial infection, ischemia, or obstruction by a gallstone. Acute cholecystitis is related to the impaction of a calculus in the neck of the gallbladder in approximately 90% of cases. Spontaneous resolution may occur after the reestablishment of cystic duct patency.

B. *Escherichia coli* is the primary microorganism in 80% of cholecystitis infections.

C. Estrogen-induced alteration in bile salts may favor stone formation. Stones occur when cholesterol supersaturates the bile in the gallbladder and precipitates out of the bile. Cholesterol stones are the most common type of gallstones in the United States.

D. Pigment stones occur when free bilirubin combines with calcium. Pigment stones are found in patients with cirrhosis, hemolysis, and infections in the biliary tree.

E. Acalculous cholecystitis is associated with infection and local inflammation. Formation of gallstones is not necessary for the obstruction of the bile duct.

Predisposing Factors

A. Female gender.

B. Sudden starvation/prolonged fasting.

C. Medications
   1. Cholesterol-lowering drugs: stone formation increases in users of cholesterol-lowering drugs, which are known to increase biliary cholesterol saturation.
   2. Furosemide.
   3. Ceftriaxone.
   4. Cyclosporine.
   5. Opiate narcotic analgesics.
   6. Estrogen usage (oral contraceptives [OCP] and hormone replacement therapy [HRT]): stone formation increases in users of contraceptives and estrogens, which are known to increase biliary cholesterol saturation.

D. Bile acid malabsorption.

E. Genetic predisposition: Native Americans and those of Chinese or Japanese decent have a high incidence.

F. Parenteral nutrition (TPN).

G. Obesity.

H. Status postbariatric surgery.

I. Pregnancy secondary to elevated progesterone.

J. Increasing age.

K. Hemolytic anemia.

Common Complaints

A. Abrupt, severe abdominal pain lasting 24 hours

B. Constant aching pain in the right upper quadrant, right subcostal region, with radiation to the back and right shoulder

C. Nausea and vomiting

Other Signs and Symptoms

A. Anorexia.

B. Heartburn.

C. Upper abdominal fullness.

D. Biliary colic: sudden onset of severe pain in the epigastrium or right hypochondrium that subsides relatively slowly. Tenderness may remain for days.

E. Fat intolerance.

F. Fever, rarely.

G. Mild jaundice (20%).

H. Complicated disease such as an abscess or perforation symptoms include more severe localized persistent pain, tenderness, fever, chills, and leukocytosis.

Subjective Data

A. Review the onset, location, duration, course, and quality of pain.

B. Use a pain-rating scale, such as a 10-point pain scale with 0 being no pain and 10 being equivalent to the worst pain the patient has ever felt. Determine progression of the pain as well.

C. Review any alleviating factors, such as antacids, and any worsening factors, such as deep inspiration.

D. Review any pain radiating to the jaw, neck, shoulder, or arm.

E. Review onset of pain in relation to last meal and foods ingested.

F. Ask the patient about recurrent history of epigastric pain.

G. Obtain history and demographic data that may indicate the risk factors for biliary disease.

H. Review the date of the patient's last menstrual period (LMP), and if she is pregnant, establish gestational age.

Physical Examination

A. Check temperature, pulse, respirations, and blood pressure.

B. Inspect: Observe general appearance, facial expressions, walk, skin color (15% have jaundice) and turgor, and grimace during exam. Overall appearance is generally unremarkable between attacks; ill appearance occurs during acute attack.

C. Auscultate
   1. Heart.
   2. Lung fields.
   3. Abdomen for bowel sounds in all four quadrants.

D. Percuss abdomen.

E. Palpate
   1. Palpate abdomen; check for tenderness in the RUQ, especially with inspiration; assess for guarding and rebound tenderness.
   2. Check Murphy's sign. Positive Murphy's sign is inspiratory arrest secondary to extreme tenderness when subhepatic area is palpated during deep inspiration.

F. Perform rectal exam, if indicated.

Diagnostic Tests

A. Ultrasonography: study of choice
B. Amylase
C. CBC with differential
D. Alkaline phosphate
E. Bilirubin
F. Aspartate transaminase, or AST
G. Alanine transaminase, or ALT
H. Flat plate of abdomen (nonspecific; unable to differentiate between acute cholecystitis and biliary colic)
I. CT or MRI
J. Hepatobiliary (HIDA) scan
K. Endoscopic retrograde cholangiopancreatography (ERCP) and percutaneous transhepatic cholangiography (PTC)
L. EKG to rule out MI
M. Chest radiography to rule out pneumonia
N. Stool for occult blood to rule out bleeding
O. Urinalysis to rule out pyelonephritis and renal calculi
P. Pregnancy test if childbearing age

Differential Diagnoses

A. Acute cholecystitis
B. Acute pancreatitis
C. Peptic ulcer perforation
D. Acute hepatitis
E. Pneumonia or pleurisy
F. Myocardial infarction
G. Renal calculi
H. Gastric/peptic ulcer
I. Gastroesophageal reflux disease (GERD)
J. Pregnancy: urolithiasis, pyelonephritis

Plan

A. General interventions: Patients with a single episode of biliary colic are reasonable candidates for expectant management, as long as they continue to be free of recurrent pain.
B. Patient teaching
   1. No activity restriction is required.
   2. Treatment depends on acuteness of attack. Heat may be used as needed for pain. If pain continues to worsen, have the patient contact his or her health care provider. Hospitalization and/or surgery may be required depending on the severity of the attack.
C. Dietary management
   1. Counsel the patient to avoid fatty foods.
   2. Encourage the patient to avoid fasting and starvation diets, which make the bile even more lithogenic.
D. Surgical and medical management
   1. Stone dissolution, lithotripsy, may be used to break up the stone.
   2. Cholecystectomy may be recommended for symptomatic patients. The standard of care is the laparoscopic cholecystectomy. Conversion from a laparoscopic procedure to an open surgical procedure is approximately 5%.
E. Pharmaceutical therapy
   1. Acetaminophen (Tylenol) may be used as needed for pain.
   2. Anticholinergics are not helpful.
   3. Antibiotics, such as ampicillin or cefazolin (Ancef), flagyl, may be used for mild attacks.

Follow-up

A. See the patient at next pain attack to reevaluate.
B. Surgical follow-up in 2 weeks.

Consultation/Referral

A. For acute attack, consult a physician for possible surgical consultation referral.
B. Refer the patient for elective cholecystectomy when he or she has documented gallstones and recurrent biliary colic or a history of complication of gallstone disease such as pancreatitis.
C. Refer to a gastroenterologist for consideration of ERCP.

Individual Considerations

A. Pregnancy
   1. Right upper quadrant pain in pregnancy differential includes preeclampsia, pancreatitis, and appendicitis.
   2. In the absence of pancreatitis, maternal mortality should be rare, and fetal loss is generally estimated to be no more than 5%. However, if secondary pancreatitis is present, maternal mortality is 15%, and fetal loss is reported as high as 60%.
B. Pediatrics
   1. Patients with sickle cell disease are at higher risk for developing cholecystitis.
   2. Infants with cholecystitis may present with irritability, jaundice, and acholic (pale white) stools.
C. Geriatrics: Signs and symptoms may be nonspecific and vague. Localized tenderness may be the only presenting sign.

⬛ COLIC

Definition

A. Colic is a benign disorder characterized by abdominal spasms and rigidity that results in abdominal pain. Infants with colic exhibit persistent, unexplained, and inconsolable crying and move rapidly in and out of sleep. The infant is in good health, eats well, and gains weight appropriately, despite the daily crying episodes. Colic is self-limited.

Incidence

A. Between 8%–40% of all infants exhibit colic, regardless of ethnicity, gender, gestational age, breast- versus bottle-fed, or socioeconomic status.

Pathogenesis

A. Research has never conclusively identified a cause for colic, and many interventions are based on hypothesized causes, such as immature gastrointestinal function, milk allergy to casein or whey, and maternal anxiety. There has be a causal relationship between colic and family stress.

Predisposing Factors

A. Age: 2 weeks to 4 months; usually resolves by 6 months of age
B. Male gender: occurs more in males than females
C. First in birth order
D. Fruit juice intolerance (sorbitol-containing fruit juices)

Common Complaints

Crying characteristics:

A. Intense crying: louder, higher, and more variable in pitch.
B. The cry may sound like the baby is in pain or is screaming rather than crying.
C. Inconsolable.

Other Signs and Symptoms

A. Hands clenched
B. Abdominal distension
C. Legs flexed over abdomen
D. Short sleep cycles
E. Flatus
F. Fussiness
G. No disease process found on examination

Subjective Data

A. Review when the crying occurs and how long it lasts. What techniques help?
B. Review basic infant needs with caregivers, such as determining whether the infant is hungry or wet, has air bubbles, or is in an uncomfortable position.
C. Review feeding methods, technique, and burping. Crying that occurs directly after feeding may be associated with swallowing too much air or gastroesophageal reflux.
D. If the infant is breast-fed, review maternal diet for offending foods, including chocolate, pizza, spicy foods, cabbage, and so forth.
E. If the infant is breast-fed, review prescribed maternal drugs and any over-the-counter medications that she is taking, such as laxatives.
F. If the infant is bottle-fed, review preparation of formula and type of formula.
G. Review intake of fruit juices for possible carbohydrate intolerance to sorbitol.
H. Rule out the early introduction of solid foods.
I. Review any history of fever and high-pitched or shrill cry.
J. Have caregiver describe color, frequency, and softness of stools.
K. Review secondhand smoke exposure: there is an association between maternal smoking and colic.

Physical Examination

A. Check temperature, pulse, respirations, blood pressure, and weight.
B. Plot growth parameters: length, head circumference, and weight. **Note signs of failure to thrive (FTT). Failure to gain approximately 1 ounce per day may indicate FTT.**
C. Inspect
   1. Evaluate the skin for signs of abuse.
   2. Check fontanelles.
   3. Conduct ear, nose, and throat exam.
   4. Evaluate the skin and mucosa for signs of dehydration.
D. Auscultate: abdomen, heart, and lungs.
E. Percuss: Percuss the abdomen.
F. Palpate:
   1. Palpate abdomen for tenderness, masses, and distension.
   2. Feel anterior and posterior fontanelles.
   3. Testicular examination to evaluate torsion.

Diagnostic Tests

A. Colic is a diagnosis of exclusion and must be differentiated from identifiable causes of prolonged crying.
B. None is required if the infant is gaining weight and has a normal physical exam.
C. Consider urinalysis.
D. Stool for occult blood to rule out cow's milk allergy.

Differential Diagnoses

A. Colic
B. Infection
C. Obstruction
D. Injury
E. Abuse
F. Failure to thrive
G. Gastroesophageal reflux
H. Intussusception
I. Meningitis
J. Otitis media
K. Protein intolerance
L. Testicular torsion

Plan

A. Patient teaching
   1. Review feeding and burping techniques, making sure the baby is not over- or underfed.
   2. Reassure the family that the baby has no evidence of infant developmental problems and the problem is not related to poor parenting skills.
   3. Reassure families that colic does resolve over time.
   4. Encourage parents to take time away from the infant to rest and recoup the energy needed to deal with the demands of a crying baby.
   5. Empathize with parental frustration and provide coping techniques.

Physical abuse of the infant with colic may occur when crying is prolonged and parents have inadequate resources to cope.

   6. Consider a hypoallergenic diet (e.g., protein hydrolysate formula such as Alimentum, Nutramigen, or Pregestamil). The literature does not support the use of fiber-enriched formulas.
   7. See the Section III Patient Teaching Guide for this chapter, "Colic: Ways to Soothe a Fussy Baby."
   8. Teach caregivers to assess the child for signs of emergent abdominal problems such as fever, pallor, sweating, vomiting, diarrhea, and rigid and tender abdomen.
B. Dietary management
   1. Counsel the caregiver to consider changing formula from a milk-based to soy-based formula. If the infant is breast-fed, counsel caregiver not to switch to formula.
   2. Educate caregiver to avoid the use of homegrown mint teas for fussy babies. Fatalities have been reported secondary to ingestion of the pennyroyal form of mint, which produces toxic oil.
C. Pharmaceutical therapy
   1. Simethicone has little therapeutic benefit versus a placebo for treating colic by randomized controlled trials.

2. Antispasmodics have adverse effects including apnea, seizures, and coma. Dicyclomine is contraindicated in infants younger than 6 months of age and is not considered for the indication of colic by the manufacturer.
3. Lactase is not a therapeutic option for colic.
4. Probiotics lack evidence-based support for the treatment of colic.
5. Sedatives should not be used for the treatment of colic.
6. Herbal remedies are common in many cultures, but few herbal products have been evaluated for colic.

Follow-up

A. Reevaluate the child periodically to provide support and assess for other problems.
B. Review signs of emergent abdominal problems such as fever, pallor, sweating, vomiting, diarrhea, and rigid and tender abdomen.

Consultation/Referral

A. Consult a physician as necessary.
B. Consider a home-based nursing consultation.
C. Refer the breast-feeding mother for an observational feeding.

CONSTIPATION

Definition

Constipation is infrequent and difficult defecation of hard stools and a sensation of incomplete evacuation or straining. Constipation is a symptom, not a disease. The lower limit of normal stool frequency is 3 bowel movements a week. The Rome consensus criterion defines constipation as 2 or fewer stools weekly.

Three classifications of constipation are noted in the literature:

A. Functional constipation (slow-transit)
B. Irritable bowel syndrome
C. Outlet obstruction (sudden onset)

Incidence

A. The incidence of constipation is unknown due to frequent self-treatment. Constipation is commonly self-reported. Constipation occurs in more than 50% of patients with colorectal cancers; it is usually a symptom of advanced disease, but it may be the presenting complaint.

Pathogenesis

A. Constipation can be caused by an alteration of the filling of the rectum by colonic transportation and/or reflex defecation of stool.
B. Lack of exercise decreases propulsion of bowel contents.
C. During pregnancy, progesterone has a relaxing effect on the muscles of the gastrointestinal tract and causes a decrease in peristalsis. The compression of the intestines by the enlarging uterus causes constipation during pregnancy.
D. Habitual use of laxatives is associated with impaired motor activity and has the potential of producing hypokalemia.
E. Hypokalemia can produce a generalized ileus and is most often seen in patients who take diuretics.
F. Psychiatric disease and psychosocial distress have important roles. The exact mechanisms by which emotional difficulties lead to constipation remain unclear, but their contribution is widely recognized.
G. Drugs. See Table 10.1.

Predisposing Factors

A. Insufficient nutrition
   1. Low-fiber diet
   2. Low-fluid intake
B. Neurologic causes
   1. Spinal cord injury
   2. Parkinson's disease
   3. Multiple sclerosis
   4. Aganglionosis (Hirschsprung disease)
   5. Sacral nerve trauma/tumor
C. Sedentary lifestyle
D. Laxative abuse
E. Travel
F. Ignoring urge to defecate
G. Drug use (individual medications and polypharmacy)
H. Pregnancy, especially third trimester
I. Psychosocial problems
   1. Depression
   2. Sexual abuse
   3. Unusual attitudes to food and bowel function
J. Extremes of ages: infants and geriatrics
K. Hypothyroidism
L. Colorectal cancer
M. Irritable bowel syndrome
N. Pelvic floor disorders

TABLE 10.1 Drugs and Classifications That Cause and Increase Constipation

Anticholinergics (atropine, antidepressants, neuroleptics, anti-parkinsonian drugs)	Opiates
Antipsychotics	Cholestyramine (binds bile salts)
Anticonvulsants	Antacids (aluminum hydroxide and calcium carbonate)
Antihistamines	Iron supplements
Antihypertensives (calcium-channel blockers, clonidine, hydralazine, MAO inhibitors, methyldopa)	Nonsteroidal anti-inflammatory agents
Diuretics	Ganglionic blockers

1. Impaired function of the pelvic floor and/or external sphinchter
2. Pelvic floor obstruction
3. Rectal prolapse
4. Enterocele and/or rectocele
5. Rectal intussesception

Common Complaints
A. Hard infrequent stools
B. Straining
C. Inability to defecate when desired
D. Need for digital manipulation to facilitate evaculation

Other Signs and Symptoms
A. Hard, pebbly, rocklike stools
B. Painful defecation
C. Abdominal pain
D. Weight loss
E. Blood in stools

Potential Complications
A. A rectal prolapse of the mucosa is pink and looks like a doughnut or rosette. Complete prolapse involving the muscular wall is larger and red, and it has circular folds.

Subjective Data
A. Review the onset, duration, and course of symptoms.
  1. Is constipation a chronic or acute problem?
  2. If there has been a change in bowel habits, was it gradual or sudden?
  3. What feature does the patient rate most distressing?
B. Review bowel habits.
  1. Does the patient have a regular time for defecation?
  2. Review size, color, consistency, and frequency of stools.
  3. Is there any blood?
  4. Are there any periods of diarrhea?
  5. How often are laxatives being used and what doses?
  6. Are suppositories and enemas also required?
C. Review the patient's daily diet and fluid intake. Has there been any dietary change?
D. Review the patient's medication history: prescription and over-the-counter (refer to Table 10.1)
E. Review the patient's daily physical activity.
F. Review the patient's psychosocial history of stress, depression, anxiety, and coping mechanisms.
G. Review the patient's other health problems such as diabetes, depression, hypothyroidism, and hypercalcemia.
H. Review family history of constipation and colorectal cancer.

Physical Examination
A. Check temperature, pulse, respirations, blood pressure, and weight.
B. Inspect
  1. General overall assessment of nutritional status.
  2. Examine the skin, especially the rectum, for pallor and signs of dehydration and hypothyroidism.
  3. Evaluate for the presence of hernias.
  4. Anal inspection including the position, presence of perianal erythema, and skin tags.
C. Auscultate: Auscultate all four abdominal quadrants for bowel sounds. Bowel sounds may be high-pitched or absent.
D. Percuss: Percuss the abdomen.
E. Palpate
  1. Palpate the abdomen for masses, tenderness, distension, and fecal mass.
  2. Palpate the liver and spleen.
F. Digital rectal exam
  1. Examine the rectum for masses, hemorrhoid, fissures, fistula, prolapse, and inflammation.
  2. Evaluate for impaction, hard stool in ampulla.
  3. Perform an anal reflex test by a light pinprick or scratch.
  4. Evaluate sphincter tone.
    a. Disordered innervation of the anus is indicated by finding that the anal canal opens wide when the puborectalis muscle is pulled posteriorly.
    b. Evaluate the resting tone of the sphincter and squeezing effort.
    c. Instruct the patient to "expel the examination finger" to evaluate the force of expulsion.
G. Perform a neurologic examination for tone, strength, and reflexes to search for focal deficits and delayed relaxation phase of the ankle jerks, suggestive of hypothyroidism.
H. Pelvic examination to evaluate a prolapse or rectocele. Evaluate when the patient is at rest and with straining.
I. Perform mental status examination checking for signs of depression and somatization.

Diagnostic Studies
A. No tests are required for *common* constipation.
B. Tests to rule out differential diagnoses:
  1. CBC with differential.
  2. Thyroid studies.
  3. Potassium and calcium. **Patients taking diuretics should have serum potassium checked. Hypokalemia may reduce bowel contractility and produce an ileus.**
  4. Urinalysis.
  5. Serum glucose to rule out diabetes.
  6. Barium enema to evaluate megacolon and redundant sigmoid colon.
  7. Flexible sigmoid.
  8. Stool for occult blood.
  9. Anorectal function tests
    a. Manometry.
    b. Electromyography.

Differential Diagnoses
A. Constipation.
B. Intestinal obstruction: Acute onset of constipation requires ruling out an ileus, especially when accompanied by abdominal discomfort.
C. Hypothyroidism.
D. Psychosocial dysfunction.
E. Fecal impaction.
F. Neurologic disorders.
G. Multiple sclerosis.
H. Spinal cord injury.
I. Cancer.
J. Drug use.

K. Crohn's disease: Constipation is often the presenting complaint in Crohn's disease.
L. Diabetes (chronic dysmotility).

Plan

A. Patient teaching
   1. See the Section III Patient Teaching Guide for this chapter, "Tips to Relieve Constipation."
   2. Encourage the patient to exercise. Both exercise and dietary fiber stimulate the natural wavelike contraction of the colon that triggers the urge to defecate.
   3. Reassure the patient that recommended dietary changes and exercise help with constipation.
   4. Warn chronic laxative users that it may take 4–6 weeks before spontaneous bowel movements return.
   5. Teach the patient regarding potential complications of long-term constipation.
B. Dietary management: See Appendix B
C. Surgical and medical management
   1. Treatment of constipation is symptomatic and should begin with lifestyle and dietary changes.
   2. Evaluate and stop medications, if possible, that cause constipation.
   3. Fecal impaction may require a hypertonic enema (e.g., Fleet's) or manual removal to relieve the situation. Enemas should not be given routinely to treat constipation, because they disrupt normal defecation reflexes and the patient becomes dependent.
   4. Pelvic floor physiotherapy may be offered.
   5. Biofeedback has been effective for short-term treatment of intractable constipation.

TABLE 10.2 Laxatives

Bulk laxatives	Psyllium (Konsyl, Metamucil) Polycarbophil Methylcellulose (Citrucel)
Lubricating agents	Mineral oil[a]
Stimulant laxatives	Docusate Bile acids Bisacodyl[b] Castor oil Senna[b] Cascara Aloes Rhubarb
Osmotic agents	Magnesium and phosphate salts Lactulose (Kristalose)[a] Sorbitol[a] Polyethylene glycol (Colyte, Glycolax, Miralax)[b] Glycerin suppositories[a]
Selective 5-HT$_4$ receptor agonists	Prucalopride Tegaserod (Zelnorm) (HTF-919)

[a]Considered safe and effective in children.
[b]After a thorough evaluation, use in low doses for selected children when constipation is hard to manage.

6. Manual removal of fecal impaction can stimulate the vagus nerve and cause syncope and tachycardia. It is contraindicated in the following conditions:
   a. Pregnancy
   b. After genitourinary, rectal, perineal, abdominal, or gynecologic surgery
   c. Myocardial infarction, coronary insufficiency, pulmonary embolus, congestive heart failure, or heart block
   d. Gastrointestinal or vaginal bleeding
   e. Blood dyscrasias or bleeding disorders
   f. Hemorrhoids, fissures, and rectal polyps
D. Pharmaceutical therapy
   1. Bulk-forming agents decrease abdominal pain and improve stool consistency. They should be used if an increase in dietary fiber does not work. They act by causing retention of fluid and increasing fecal mass. They must be taken with plenty of fluids to prevent formation of an obstructing bolus. Flatulence and abdominal distension may occur, but long-term use is safe.
   2. Stimulant laxatives act by directly stimulating the colonic nerves. Suppositories are faster (20–60 min) versus oral laxatives (8–12 hours).
   3. Osmotic laxatives act by retaining fluid in the bowel by osmosis, changing the water distribution in the feces. Good hydration is important. See Table 10.2.
   4. Tegaserod (Zelnorm) is available by a restricted treatment investigational new drug (IND) for irritable bowel syndrome with constipation or chronic idiopathic constipation for women younger than 55 years. Specific guidelines must be met for prescribing.
   5. When severe depression requires the use of antidepressants, the least constipating agent should be selected (i.e., one with minimal anticholingeric activity).
   6. Treat other identified causes, for example, hypothyroidism.

Follow-up

A. Repeat assessment in 4 to 6 weeks.
B. If there is no evidence of obstruction, anemia, or occult blood loss, follow the patient expectantly for a few weeks on a conservative program that includes increased dietary fiber and increased exercise, and follow stool guaiac.
C. Failure to improve may indicate serious underlying cause and need for referral.

Consultation/Referral

A. Consider consultations with a gastroenterologist (adult or pediatric), pediatrician, gynecologist, surgeon, or psychologist/psychiatrist as indicated.

Individual Considerations

A. Pregnancy
   1. Constipation is very common in pregnancy secondary to progesterone and the enlarging uterus (see "Pathogenesis").

2. Constipation that results from iron supplementation can be avoided by increasing the intake of fluid and high-fiber foods, and increasing physical activity such as walking.
3. Bulking agents and lactulose will not enter breast milk. Senna, in large doses, will enter breast milk and may cause diarrhea and colic in infants.

B. Pediatrics
1. In infancy and childhood, most constipation is functional. Constipation can be associated with coercive toilet training, sexual abuse, excessive parental interventions, and toilet phobia.
2. If Hirschsprung disease is suspected, the patient should be evaluated by a pediatric gastroenterologist and a pediatric surgeon.
3. Reinforce that each infant has individual stool patterns. Formula-fed infants generally pass at least one stool each day, whereas breast-fed infants may pass a stool after every feeding or, occasionally, only one every 2–3 days.
4. Educate the parent about what constipation really is: dry, hard, and marblelike stools.
5. Infants may get red in the face and appear to be straining when having a bowel movement, but it is normal behavior and does not indicate constipation.
6. Rectal prolapse in children has been associated with cystic fibrosis.
7. Use a high-fiber diet and fluids first before other therapies.
8. Common times when constipation is likely to occur in the pediatric population are:
   a. Introduction of solid foods or cow's milk
      i. Recommended fiber intake is 20 grams/day.
      ii. Minimum fluid intake depends on the child's age.
      iii. Consumption of whole cow's milk should be limited to 24 ounces/day.
   b. Toilet training: a potty seat that provides appropriate foot support and leverage for elimination should be used.
   c. School entry.

C. Adults
1. The most common cause of chronic constipation in adults is failure to initiate defecation.
2. Diabetics should avoid stimulant laxatives such as lactulose and sorbitol. Their metabolites may influence blood glucose levels.

D. Geriatrics
1. Constipation in old people is not a result of aging, it is usually related to an increase in constipating factors such as chronic illnesses, immobility, dietary factors, medications, neurologic factors, and psychiatric conditions.
2. An important diagnostic concern in the elderly is the possibility of constipation being due to a colonic neoplasm. More than 25% of patients with colorectal carcinomas present with constipation.
3. Check for a fecal impaction, especially in elderly patients with a history of chronic constipation. Fecal impaction ranks as one of the major sources of anorectal discomfort among the elderly and bedridden. Chronic, incomplete evacuation leads to formation of an obstructing bolus of desiccated hard stool in the rectum.
4. Diarrhea rather than constipation is sometimes the only complaint, because of the collection of liquid stool distending the proximal colon and passing around the obstructing bolus.

CROHN'S DISEASE

Definition
A. Crohn's disease (CD) is a chronic inflammatory bowel disease (IBD) of the gastrointestinal tract that produces ulceration, fibrosis, and malabsorption. CD can involve any segment of the gastrointestinal (GI) tract from the mouth to the anus; the terminal ileum and colon are the most common sites. Pediatric patients are more likely to present with the disease limited to the small intestine.
B. The disease is chronic, relapsing, and incurable. Crohn's disease is characterized by episodes of remission and exacerbation. The most frequent cause of death in persons with IBD is the primary disease, followed by malignancy and thromboembolic disease. In most cases, symptoms do correspond well with the degree of inflammation present. The diagnosis is usually established with endoscopic finding in a patient with a compatible clinical history. Objective evidence for disease activity should be sought before administering medication with significant adverse effects.
C. More than 70% of patients with CD undergo surgery within 20 years of the diagnosis. Indications for surgery include stricture, intractable or fulminant disease, anorectal disease, and intra-abdominal abscess. The incidence of adenocarcinoma in CD is higher than in the general population. Lymphoma is also increased especially for patients with IBD treated with Azathioprine (6-MP).

Incidence
The incidence rate ranges from 5.8 cases per 100,000 to 7.3 cases per 100,000. An estimated 1–2 million people in the United States have ulcerative colitis or CD. The incidence of IBD has been reported to be highest in Jewish populations. The American Jewish population has one of the highest prevalences of IBD, 4–5 times that of the general population.

The peak incidence of CD is most common in late adolescence to the third decade of life. Children younger than 5 years and elderly persons are occasionally diagnosed.

Crohn's disease may involve the entire GI tract, note the incidence according to the location:

A. Eighty percent have small bowel involvement, usually in the distal ileum.
B. Fifty percent have ileocolitis (involves both the ileum and colon).
C. Twenty percent have disease limited to the colon with roughly one-half having sparing on the rectum.

D. A small percentage has predominant involvement of the mouth (aphthous ulcers) or gastroduodenal area; fewer have involvement of the esophagus (odynophagia and dysphagia) and proximal small bowel.

E. One-third has perianal disease (perianal pain, drainage from large skin tags, anal fissures, perirectal abscesses, and anorectal fistulae).

F. 15–20% have arthralgias. Arthritis is the most common complication.

Pathogenesis

Pathogenesis is unknown. The common end pathway is inflammation of the mucosal lining of the intestinal tract, causing ulceration, edema, bleeding, and fluid and electrolyte loss. Speculation for the pathogenesis includes:

A. Pathogenic organism (remains unidentified).
B. Immunologic response.
C. Autoimmune process.
D. Potential genes linked to IBD
  1. Chromosome 16 (*IBD1* gene).
  2. *CARD15* gene is noted to be a susceptibility gene for CD.
  3. Susceptibility genes on chromosomes 5 (5q31) and 6 (6p21 and 19p).

Predisposing Factors

A. Age between 15 and 35 years
B. Genetic predisposition/family history of Crohn's disease
  1. First-degree relatives 5- to 20-fold increased risk
  2. Children of a parent with IBD—5% risk
  3. 70% incidence in identical twins vs. 5%–10% in nonidentical twins
  4. Jewish populations
C. Smoking (increased risk for CD, but reduces risk in ulcerative colitis)

Common Complaints

The following cardinal symptoms occur in about 80% of patients:

A. Chronic diarrhea
B. Abdominal pain, the classic location is in right lower quadrant (appendicitislike)
C. Fatigue, commonly related to pain, inflammation, and anemia

Other Signs and Symptoms

Symptoms vary, depending on the location of the intestinal tract and extent of disease:

A. Constipation: early sign
B. Weight loss
C. Abdominal mass
D. Cramping with BM
E. Rectal bleeding or blood in stools
F. Perianal discomfort or soft or semiliquid irritating rectal discharge
G. Vomiting
H. Low-grade fever
I. Erythema nodosum (correlates well with the activity of disease)
J. Folate deficiency
K. Anorexia
L. Fissures and fistulas, sometimes extending to skin
M. Growth retardation—may be the only presenting sign in young patients

Subjective Data

A. Ask about onset, duration, and course of symptoms. Have any of the presenting symptoms occurred at any time in the past (flares of CD may have gone undiagnosed in the past)?
B. Review the patient's history and extent of diarrhea including frequency, consistency, color, quantity, and odor of stools. Evaluate if there are blood, mucus, pus, or food particles in the stools.
C. Inquire about recent travel to foreign countries.
D. Ask the patient if diarrhea represents a change in bowel habits. Is there nocturnal diarrhea?
E. Ask the patient what makes the diarrhea worse or better.
F. Inquire about previous GI surgery.
G. Review the patient's usual weight and any history of weight loss. If weight loss has occurred, how many pounds? How is patient's appetite?
H. Review family history of Crohn's disease, colon cancer, ulcerative colitis, and malabsorption syndrome.
I. How has the duration of current complaints affected the patient's work or usual social activities?
J. Review for duration and extraintestinal symptoms including:
  1. Urinary complications: renal calculi.
  2. Sclerosing cholangitis: fatigue and jaundice.
  3. Skin diseases
    a. Erythema nodosum: painful, tender, raised, purple lesion on the tibia.
    b. Pyoderma gangrenosum: inflamed patch of skin that has progressed to ulceration.
    c. Herpetic lesions related to immune suppression.
  4. Arthritic symptoms.
K. Review medications especially antibiotics and nonsteroidal anti-inflammatory drugs.
L. Review the patient's current tobacco/cigarette use.

Physical Examination

A. Check temperature, pulse, respirations, blood pressure, and weight.
B. Inspect
  1. Observe general appearance, noting pallor, wasting, apathetic appearance, ecchymosis, skin ulcerations, jaundice, and signs of Kaposi's sarcoma.
  2. Inspect the head and neck for aphthous ulcers, glossitis, stomatitis, and poor dentition.
  3. Inspect the abdomen for surgical scars.
  4. Eye examination for uveitis.
  5. Inspect joints for warmth and redness.
C. Auscultate the abdomen for bowel sounds in all quadrants for altered bowel sounds (obstruction).
D. Palpate
  1. Palpate the neck for goiter and lymphadenopathy.
  2. Palpate the abdomen for distension, ascites, tenderness rebound, guarding, and masses.

3. Palpate for hepatomegaly in RLQ.
4. Palpate the joints for tenderness.
E. Rectal exam
 1. Check anal sphincter for tags, control, and discharge.
 2. Palpate for masses, fissures, fistulas, and inflammation.
 3. Digital rectal examination to assess for anal strictures and rectal mass.
F. Neurologic exam: Assess for signs of vitamin B_{12} deficiency, including tingling sensation and numbness in hands or feet.

Diagnostic Tests
A Laboratory tests
 1. CBC with differential.
 2. Electrolytes and albumin.
 3. Erythrocyte sedimentation rate.
 4. Serum cobalamine (vitamin B_{12}).
 5. Serum iron studies.
 6. Folate.
 7. Liver enzymes and functioning tests (INR) and bilirubin.
 8. HIV.
 9. Celiac antibody testing should be considered.
B. Stool studies
 1. Guaiac
 2. Stool culture
 3. *C difficile* toxin assay
 4. Ova and parasites
C. Imaging
 1. Abdominal flat plate
 2. Barium enema
  a. Classic "string sign": narrow band of barium flowing through an inflamed or scarred area in terminal ileum; differentiates Crohn's disease from ulcerative colitis.
  b. "Rectal sparing": suggests CD in the presence of inflammatory changes in other parts of the colon.
  c. "Thumbprinting": indicates mucosal inflammation (may be seen on flat plate of abdomen).
  d. "Skip lesions": areas of inflammation with normal-appearing areas.
 3. Small bowel follow-through GI series.
 4. Fistulogram: used to guide the surgical correction.
 5. CT scan of the abdomen and pelvis (limited use in IBD but may detect fistulae).
D. Procedures with/without biopsy
 1. Colonoscopy: mucosa has characteristic cobblestone appearance.
 2. Flexible sigmoidoscopy with biopsy: reveals "skip areas" in colon, significant small bowel involvement, fistulas, and granulomas.
 3. Upper endoscopy: aphthous ulcerations occur in the stomach and duodenum in 5%–10%.
 4. Capsule enteroscopy: the major risk is the potential for the camera to become lodged at the point of stricture and require operative intervention.
 5. Skin biopsy.
E. Tuberculin purified protein derivative (PPD) skin test.

Differential Diagnoses
A. Crohn's disease
B. Ulcerative colitis
C. Appendicitis
D. Colon cancer
E. Irritable bowel syndrome
F. Anorexia nervosa
G. Perianal abscess
H. Intestinal protozoan and bacterial etiologies
I. Food poisoning
J. Cytomegalovirus
K. Intestinal TB

Plan
A. Patient teaching: See the Section III Patient Teaching Guide for this chapter, "Crohn's Disease."
B. Dietary management
 1. Adequate nutrition is critical to the promotion of healing. Sufficient protein and calories limit the stress on an inflamed and often strictured bowel.
 2. Patients with cramps and diarrhea should have the fiber content of their diets altered. Diet should include high fiber, low fat. (See Appendix B.)
 3. Those with steatorrhea benefit from decrease in fat intake to less than 80 g/day. Give the patient a copy of the Low Fat/Low Cholesterol Diet (see Appendix B).
 4. An empiric trial of restricting milk products may terminate diarrhea due to lactase deficiency.
 5. Patients with severe diarrhea may require partial bowel rest, which removes the stimulus that food has on bowel motility and secretion.
 6. Elemental diet preparations, such as Ensure, Sustacal, or Isocal, have been found to induce remission, improve symptoms, and decrease disease activity in patients with acute disease.
 7. Total parenteral nutrition (TPN) is used when the patient's oral intake is not adequate or surgery is indicated.
 8. Pretreatment screening for tuberculosis, using Mantoux (PPD) skin testing, is needed prior to initiation of immunomodulators and thiopurines.
 9. Immunization status
  a. Immunizations with inactivated vaccines should be brought up to date and rigorously maintained during treatment, including influenza, meningococcus, and pneumococcus.
  b. Check varicella titers prior to treatment with immunomodulators and re-immunize if titers are low.
  c. The risk of administering live vaccines (polio, rubella, and yellow fever) to patients on immunomodulators has not been established; however, most experts avoid live vaccines during treatment.
C. Medical and surgical management
 1. Surgery does not cure the patient and is reserved for intractable disease, perforation, obstruction, or severe bleeding.
 2. The objective of surgery is to remove grossly involved bowel and spare as much normal-appearing bowel as possible.

3. Postoperative recurrence rates are estimated at 30%–50% per decade and are inversely related to preoperative disease duration.

D. Pharmaceutical therapy: The medical management of CD can be divided into the treatment of an acute exacerbation and the maintenance of remission. In acute exacerbation, triggers such as underlying infection, fistula, perforation, and other pathology must be ruled out prior to the IV administration of glucocorticoids. The goal of chronic therapy is the remission of bowel inflammation. Therapies include:

1. Vitamin, mineral, and folic acid supplements are necessary for proper healing and avoidance of secondary complications, such as bone disease and anemia.
   a. Patient should take a multiple vitamin containing about five times the normal daily vitamin requirements.
   b. Folic acid supplementation is required for patients on sulfasalazine because it impairs folic acid absorption.
   c. Vitamin B_{12} replacement is required for patients who have ileal surgery.
   d. Vitamin D, 4,000 IU, is required for patients with steatorrhea.

2. Opiates provide symptomatic relief of diarrhea during acute phases of illness and chronic active colitis. Diphenoxylate and atropine (Lomotil), codeine, tincture of opium (Paregoric), and loperamide (Imodium A-D) all limit the number of BMs. Tincture of belladonna and other anticholinergics help control cramping.

3. Step-wise medication approach:
   a. Aminosalicylates (5-ASA) are a mainstay of therapy because of its anti-inflammatory activities and rapid absorption throughout the small intestines. Several formulations are available for targeting a specific region of the bowel.
      i. Sulfasalazine and Balsalazide are primarily released in the colon. Sulfasalazine (Azulfidine) for abdominal pain and diarrhea: begin with 500 mg four times daily with meals, then increase as tolerated over several days to 4 g/day. Continue for 2–4 weeks until symptoms abate, then decrease to the smallest dosage that controls symptoms (usually 2 g/day). Improvement typically occurs within 4–8 weeks. Chronic use does not maintain remissions.
      ii. Pentasa can be released in the duodenum to the distal colon. High doses 4 gram/day (16 pills a day) must be used to achieve modest effects. There are no pediatric studies to evaluate the efficacy of Pentasa.
      iii. Asacol is targeted for release in the distal ileum and colon; initial dosage is 800 mg three times/day for 6 weeks. Maintenance is 1.6 mg/day in divided doses.
      iv. Multi-matrix System (MMX) marketed as Lialda™ releases Mesalamine in the colon. Lialda is not recommend for pediatrics younger than 18 years. Dosage is 2.4 mg–4.8 mg once a day with meals, taken for 8 weeks.
      v. Rowasa is specific for the rectum and distal colon. Mesalamine (Rowasa) 800-mg tablets three times daily for total of 2.4 g/day for 6 weeks. Alternatively, 1 g control-release capsule four times daily for a total of 4 g/day for up to 8 weeks; or 4 g as a retention enema or suppository once daily, preferably at bedtime. Rectal form should be retained overnight, for about 8 hours. Usual course of therapy for rectal form is 3–6 weeks.

   b. Corticosteroids are used if IBD fails to respond to aminosalicylates. Corticosteroids should be tapered as rapidly as possible and do not have a role in maintaining remission.
      i. Budesonide is designed to be effective only in the treatment of disease involving the ileum and ascending colon. Budesonide is effective in the maintenance of short-term (3 months) but not long-term (1 year) remission.
         (a). Adults: Initial starting dose for an adolescent and adult is 9 mg/day, tapered by 3 mg increments.
         (b). Pediatrics: The optimal dosing in children is currently not defined. A respective study used oral budesonide in doses of 0.45 mg/kg/day (maximum dose of 9 mg/day).
      ii. Prednisone or Prednisolone:
         (a). Adults: For acute flare-ups: prednisone 60 mg/day initially. As acute disease subsides, steroid dosage is empirically tapered by 5–10 mg for 2 weeks to minimum necessary to control symptoms. Sometimes, alternate-day regimens control disease activity. Up to 4 months of steroids may be needed to treat an exacerbation.
         (b). Pediatrics: Prednisone or Prednisolone 1–2 mg/kg per day (maximum 60 mg/day) given orally or intravenously brings rapid improvement but should serve as a short-term induction therapy due to long-term side effects including growth failure, osteopenia, hirsutism, diabetes, psychosis, cataracts, and altered body shape and image.

   c. Immunomodulatory agents may be initiated for IBD refractory to corticosteroids or frequent flares that require steroids. These agents require monitoring of blood counts due to hematological toxicity. A 3% incidence of pancreatitis, allergic reactions, infections, and marrow toxicity is associated with their use. The main drawback to the use of Azathioprine and 6-MP is their slow onset. The effect of therapy is noted after 3–6 months of treatment. The Food and Drug Administration (FDA) recommends individuals should have thiopurine methyltransferase (TPMT) genotype or phenotype assessment before initiation of therapy with Azathioprine (AZA) or 6-MP to detect individuals who have low enzyme activity or who are homozygous deficient in TPMT.

   i. 6-mercaptopurine (6-MP)

     (a). Adults: Initially 50–75 mg per day titrated to 1.0–2.0 mg/kg/day.

     (b). Pediatrics: 1.0–2.0 mg/kg per day orally (maximum of 150 mg per day).

   ii. Azathioprine (AZA) (Imuran)

     (a). Adults: 1 mg/kg per day orally in 1–2 divided doses.

     (b). Pediatrics: 1.5–2.5 mg/kg per day orally (maximum 200 mg per day).

   iii. Methotrexate ([MTX] folic acid antagonist) has adverse effects including leukopenia, GI upset, and hypersensitivity pneumonitis.

     (a). Adults: Intramuscular or subcutaneous MTX given once a week is moderately effective in inducing and maintaining remission in adult patients with steroid-refractory or steroid dependent CD.

     (b). Pediatrics: Doses typically start at 15 mg/M2 per week and are advanced as tolerated to a maximum of 25 mg/M2 per week. Subcutaneously dosing for children is recommended to ensure absorption until the patient enters remission then switch to oral methotrexate.

     (c). Folic acid supplement (1 mg/daily) may reduce the likelihood of oral ulcers.

  d. Tumor necrosis factor (TNF)-alpha blocker

   i. Infliximab (Remicade®) is a chimeric monoclonal antibody to TNF factor alpha. Infliximab is effective for moderate to severe CD and for patients with fistulizing CD or resistant to steroids and conventional therapy. Infliximab can close perianal fistulas refractory to therapy with antibiotics and 6-MP. Currently used regimens involve the administration of three initial doses (0, 2, and 6/8 weeks) and follow up infusions at 8-week intervals if the patient responds. Infliximab has a half-life of approximately 10 dyas.

     (a). Adults: 5 mg/kg in a single IV dose. Patients that do not respond can sometimes respond to increasing the dosage to 10 mg/kg or increasing the frequency of infusions.

     (b). Pediatrics: Experience with Infliximab is growing; initial experience suggests a similar benefit to that observed in adults.

   ii. Certolizumab (Cimzia) is given subcutaneously in the abdomen or thigh.

     (a). Adults: 400 mg in two divided 200 mg injections on day 1, then at weeks 2 and 4. The maintenance dose is 400 mg subcutaneously every 4 weeks.

     (b). Pediatrics: Not recommended.

   iii. Adalimumab (Humira) is an antibody directed against TNF. It is also administered subcutaneously in the abdomen or thigh.

     (a). Adults (> 18 years of age) 160 mg administered in 4 injections in 1 day or divided over 2 days at week 1, then 80 mg subsequent at week 2. At week 4, start the maintenance dose of 40 mg every other week.

     (b). Pediatrics: Not recommended for those younger than 18 years.

  e. Natalizumab (Tysabri), a monocolonal antibody, is an effective induction agent for CD in adults. It is given as an IV infusion over 1 hour and requires a 1-hour observation period postinfusion.

   i. Adults (>18 years): 300 mg every 4 weeks. Discontinue after 12 weeks of induction therapy.

   ii. Pediatrics: Not recommended for those younger than18 years.

  f. Metronidazole or ciprofloxacin is utilized for perianal disease or inflammatory mass.

  g. Thalidomide, an inhibitor of both tumor necrosis factor and angiogenesis, has been used off-label to treat refractory inflammatory bowel disease.

Follow-up

A. Have the patient record his or her weight daily to monitor changes.

B. Assess frequency and consistency of stools to evaluate volume losses and effectiveness of therapy.

C. Instruct patients on self-medication to call the health provider's office if fever develops, diarrhea worsens, bleeding occurs, or abdominal pain becomes marked.

D. Monitoring patients on aminosalicylates should include CBC at least twice a year and urinalysis at least annually.

E. Monitoring patients on 6-MP requires frequent monitoring including CBC and aminotransferase levels (ALT and AST) before treatment, and again at 2, 3, 8, and 12 weeks after initiating therapy. When stable, monitor every 3 months thereafter, and 2–3 weeks after a change in dosage.

F. Monitoring patients on MTX includes a CBC and aminotransferases as with 6-MP/thiopurine therapies.

G. Periodic bone mineral density assessment is recommended for patients on long-term corticosteroid therapy (longer than 3 months). Osteopenia should be treated aggressively. The primary intervention includes dietary counseling and supplementation to ensure adequate intake of vitamin D and calcium.

H. Annual ophthalmologic examination are recommended for patients on long-term corticosteroids.

I. Patients who are using corticosteroids should be monitored for glucose intolerance and other metabolic abnormalities.

Consultation/Referral

A. Refer the patient to a gastroenterologist initially for evaluation. Treatment requires a multidisciplinary management with gastroenterologist and other subspecialists, including nutritionist, surgeon, rheumatologist, ophthalmologist, and social workers.

B. Promptly hospitalize for parenteral management patients who are toxic, bleeding heavily, in severe pain, or too sick to obtain adequate nutrition orally.

Individual Considerations

A. Pregnancy
   1. Active disease at time of conception is associated with increased incidence of miscarriage and postpartum exacerbation. It may also predispose the patient to other maternal and prenatal risks, such as premature labor, small-for-gestational-age babies, and stillbirth.
   2. Sulfasalazine and steroids are safe and effective during nursing or pregnancy.
   3. Women on Prednisone should receive supplementary steroids during labor and delivery as well as during other highly stressful times.
   4. Counsel women to attempt pregnancy only when the disease has been quiescent for several months.
   5. Withholding sulfasalazine for 2–3 days before delivery may be advisable to minimize neonatal jaundice due to bilirubin displacement.
B. Pediatrics
   1. Approximately 30% of children with CD are refractory to or dependent on steroids despite concomitant use of 6-MP. These patients may require conversion from thiopurine to methotrexate maintenance therapy, or treatment with a biologic agent.
   2. Sulfasalazine and olsalazine can be compounded into a suspension for young children to drink. It is recommended that other aminosalicylates be swallowed whole; however, Pentasa may be opened and administered by sprinkling the granules on soft food.
   3. Psychological counseling may be required in children secondary to the chronic relapsing nature of the illness, effects on body appearance and image such as short stature, and pubertal delay.
   4. Children with CD should undergo colonoscopy for cancer screening beginning 8–10 years after the diagnosis of their CD. The frequency of screening should be determined by the findings on the initial colonoscopy (around every 1–3 years).
C. Geriatrics: Elderly patients tend to have Crohn's disease confined to the distal colon, with only 40% having proctitis.

CYCLOSPORIASIS

Definition

A. Cyclosporiasis is a one-cell parasite that infects the upper small intestines. Causes of cyclosporiasis include drinking infected water or produce (fresh fruits, especially raspberries and vegetables) or exposure to the organism during travel to countries where it is endemic.
B. It manifests as protracted and relapsing gastroenteritis. The clinical syndrome consists of explosive watery diarrhea, nausea, anorexia, weight loss, fatigue, and abdominal cramps that may persist for 7 days to several weeks, with a waxing and waning course.
C. In an immunocompromised host, onset is insidious, and the condition becomes chronic with symptoms, and the shedding of oocysts continues indefinitely.

Incidence

A. The incidence of infection is unknown, although it is common around the world. It may be more common in spring and summer in the United States and Canada. It affects all ages.

Pathogenesis

A. Infection is caused by an 8- to 10-μm, spore-forming coccidian protozoan called *Cyclospora cayetanesis*. Transmission of oocysts is by oral-fecal route. Incubation period is days to weeks after excretion, depending on temperature and humidity.

Predisposing Factors

A. Incompetent or compromised immune system (e.g., infection with AIDS)
B. Travel to underdeveloped or tropical countries
C. Ingestion of contaminated food or water
D. Contact with animals that carry the parasite

Common Complaints

A. Abrupt, profuse, malodorous, watery diarrhea
B. Nausea
C. Vomiting
D. Anorexia
E. Substantial weight loss
F. Flulike symptoms
G. Abdominal cramps and bloating

Other Signs and Symptoms

A. Asymptomatic
B. Low-grade fever
C. Nausea and vomiting
D. Anorexia
E. Profound fatigue
F. Yellow-to-khaki-green stools
G. Bloating
H. Flatus
I. Dehydration

Subjective Data

A. Review onset, duration, and course of symptoms. Is diarrhea acute or chronic?
B. Question the patient about travel to areas known for cyclospora, such as Haiti, Puerto Rico, Pakistan, India, Mexico, Nepal, New Guinea, and Peru. It has also been seen in Chicago, Los Angeles, New York, Florida, and Massachusetts.
C. Review the patient's intake of medications and other substances that can cause diarrhea, especially antibiotics, laxatives, quinidine, magnesium-containing antacids, digitalis, loop diuretics, antihypertensives, alcohol, caffeine, herbal teas, and sorbitol-containing (sugar-free) gum and mints.
D. Ask about the nature of the patient's BMs, including frequency; consistency; volume; and presence of blood, pus, or mucus.

E. Review associated symptoms that need evaluation: fever, abdominal pain, and anorexia.

F. Ask the patient if other family members or sexual contacts are also ill.

G. Establish the patient's normal weight and any recent weight loss. How much weight was lost and over what period of time?

Physical Examination

A. Check temperature, pulse, respirations, blood pressure, and weight (vital signs are normal in most cases).

B. Inspect
   1. Inspect general appearance for signs of illness and dehydration.
      a. Inspect mucous membranes.
      b. Inspect infants' fontanelles.
      c. Decreased skin tugor.

C. Auscultate the abdomen for bowel sounds in all quadrants.

D. Palpate
   1. Palpate the abdomen for masses, rebound tenderness, guarding; may exhibit right upper quadrant pain (biliary disease).
   2. Palpate lymph nodes for enlargement.

E. Perform rectal exam.

Diagnostic Tests

Identification may be made by microscopic examination under ultraviolet light, by modified acid-fast staining, or by review of wet mounts of stool by experienced microscopists. Finding large numbers of white cells suggests an inflammatory or invasive diarrhea. The following tests are done:

A. Acid-fast Ziehl-Neelsen stained slide of stool.

B. Stool culture for ova and parasites: Parasites are passed intermittently, so three or more stools on alternating days should be examined.

C. Endoscopy with small bowel biopsy.

Differential Diagnoses

A. Cyclospora infection.

B. Giardiasis.

C. Malabsorption.

D. *E. coli* infection: *E. coli* causes diarrhea within hours of ingesting contaminated food. Confirm by checking if others were affected.

E. Irritable bowel syndrome: Leukocyte-free mucus is the hallmark of irritable bowel syndrome.

F. Viral diarrhea.

G. Lactose intolerance.

H. Other bacterial infections, for example, *Shigella, Salmonella, and Campylobacter.*

I. Cholera.

J. Crohn's disease.

Plan

A. General interventions
   1. Advise the patient to tell household members and sexual contacts to seek medical examination and treatment.

   2. Children and caregivers with diarrhea should be excluded from childcare centers until they become asymptomatic.

B. Patient teaching: See the Section III Patient Teaching Guides for this chapter, "Diarrhea (Adults and Children)."
   1. Discuss safe sexual practices.
   2. Teach contact precautions to those caring for diapered and/or incontinent children.

C. Dietary management
   1. Tell the patient to increase fluids. Fluid replacement is the basic approach to prevent dehydration from diarrhea.
   2. Tell the patient to restrict milk products to rule out lactose intolerance.
   3. Give the a patient a copy of Nausea and Vomiting Diet (Children and Adults)

D. Pharmaceutical therapy
   1. Drugs of choice are trimethoprim with sulfamethoxazole (TMP-SMZ). They can reduce shedding and stops diarrhea within 2 days.
      a. Adults
         i. Immunocompetent host: TMP 160 mg/SMZ 800 mg tablet orally twice a day for 7–10 days.
         ii. Immunocompromised host: TMP 160 mg/SMZ 800 mg tablet orally four times a day for 10 days, followed by prophylaxis with TMP 160 mg/SMZ 800 mg orally 3 times per week.
      b. Children
         i. For those younger than 2 months, do not prescribe TMP/SMZ.
         ii. For those older than 2 months: TMP 8 mg/kg, SMZ 40 mg/kg orally twice a day for 7 days for acute infections.
   2. Ciprofloxacin (Cipro) is the alternative treatment for patients with allergies to sulfamethoxazole.
      a. Adults: Cipro 500 mg orally twice a day for 10 days for acute infection.
      b. Adults: Prophylaxis in HIV: Cipro 500 mg orally 3 times a week.
      c. Pediatrics: For those younger than 18 years: not recommended.

Follow-up

A. See the patient in 1 week to verify continuing clinical improvement.

B. If diarrhea persists 2 weeks or more, a second evaluation is indicated.

C. Retest stools for blood and leukocytes; do a stool culture for ova and parasites.

D. Report cases of cyclosporiasis to the health department.

Consultation/Referral

A. Consult an infectious disease specialist and/or gastroenterologist if the patient has no symptom relief after completing therapies or has a prolonged or severe case.

Individual Considerations

A. Pregnancy: Treat during pregnancy.

DIARRHEA

Definition
A. Diarrhea is an abnormally high fluid content in the stool. Generally diarrhea also involves an increase in the frequency of bowel movements, which can range from 4–5 to more than 20 times a day. Diarrhea may be an acute onset or chronic/persistent diarrhea.
B. Acute diarrhea is usually self-limited; the most common complication of diarrhea is dehydration.
C. Chronic diarrhea is defined as lasting longer than 14 days.

Incidence
A. The incidence of diarrhea is unknown; however: it is responsible for 20% of pediatric referrals in children younger than 2 years and for 10% in children younger than 3 years of age. Morbidity has decreased because of the use of oral rehydration solutions; however, the global rate of mortality from acute diarrhea is 18% of children younger than age 5.
B. The incidence of *C difficile* infection is approximately 7% and 28% of patients who were hospitalized have positive cultures for the organism. *C difficile* associated diarrhea has a mortality rate as high as 25% in the frail elderly.

Pathogenesis
A. The increased water content in diarrhea stools is due to an imbalance in the physiology of the small and large intestinal processes. A bacterial infection is usually the cause of acute diarrhea in children. Other causes of diarrhea in children include malabsorption syndrome. See Table 10.3.

Predisposing Factors
A. Enteric infections.
B. Females have a higher incidence of *Campylobacter* species infections.

TABLE 10.3   Organisms That Cause Diarrhea

Viral organisms	Rotavirus
	Norovirus
	Adenovirus
	Calicivirus
	Astrovirus
Invasive bacteria	*Escherichia Coli*
	Klebsiella
	Clostridium difficile
	Clostridium perfringens
	Shigella
	Salmonella
	Campylobacter
	Cholera
	Yersinia
	Plesiomonas
	Aeromonas
Parasites	*Giardia*
	Entamoeba organisms
	Crytosporidium
	Glamblia

C. Young children.
D. Institutional: day care and skilled nursing facilities.
E. Food: raw or contaminated food.
F. Contaminated water or inadequate chlorinated water supply.
G. Travel.
H. Chemotherapy- or radiation-induced.
I. Vitamin deficiencies (Niacin and folate).
J. Vitamin toxicity (C, Niacin, and vitamin B_3).
K. Ingestion of heavy metals (copper, tin, or zinc) or toxins.
L. Ingestion of plants, mistletoe, or mushrooms.

Common Complaints
A. Frequent watery stool
B. Foul-smelling stools (fat malabsorption)
C. Flatulence
D. Abdominal cramping

Other Signs and Symptoms
A. Lethargy
B. Fever
C. Nausea and vomiting
D. Currant jelly stool (blood and mucus)
E. Anorexia

Subjective Data
A. Review the onset of diarrhea stools. What is the normal stool pattern?
B. Review the consistency, color, volume, and frequency of the stools.
C. Review dietary intake of raw foods, contaminated food, and nonabsorbable sugars including lactulose or lactose in lactose malabsorbers.
D. Review any contact with others that may have the same symptoms.
E. Have any of the stools contained blood?
F. Review travel history, including camping vacations.
G. Review any exposure to turtles or young dogs or cats.
H. Review medication history including antibiotics, vitamins, herbal production, laxatives, antacids that contain magnesium, opiate withdrawal, Olestra, and Methylxanthines (caffeine, theobromine, and theophylline).
I. Review any food allergies and history of lactose intolerance.
J. Evaluate the presence of other symptoms such as fever and abdominal pain.

Physical Examination
A. Temperature, pulse, respirations, blood pressure (standing and sitting) and weight.
B. Inspect
   1. Observe the patient's general overall appearance, the presence of lethargy or depressed consciousness, or grimace during exam.
   2. Evaluate muscle tone, skin turgor, reduced muscle, and fat mass.
   3. Exam mouth, lips, and mucus membranes for signs, symptoms, and severity of dehydration.
   4. Perianal examination for skin breakdown, erythema, and fissures.

C. Auscultation
   1. Assess heart and lungs.
   2. Auscultate the abdomen in all four quadrants.
   3. Assess the presence of borborygmi (significant increase in peristaltic action that may be audible and/or palpable).
D. Percuss abdomen.
E. Palpate
   1. Palpate the abdomen for masses, guarding, rebound tenderness, and peritoneal signs.
   2. For a newborn, palpate fontanels.
   3. Palpate for lymphadenopathy.
   4. Perform a rectal examination including testing of stool for occult blood.

Diagnostic Tests

A. Stool specimens for the evaluation of:
   1. Fecal leukocytes.
   2. Blood.
   3. Culture.
   4. Ova and parasites.
   5. Fecal alpha-1 antitrypsin levels.
   6. Viral antigen testing.
B. CBC-WBC may be elevated.
C. Albumin.
D. Electrolytes.
E. A colonoscopy for intestinal biopsy for chronic or protracted diarrhea or patients with AIDS should be done. A sigmoidoscopy alone may not reveal any abnormality.
F. Abdominal ultrasound to identify intussusception.
G. Abdominal CT.

Differential Diagnoses

A. Diarrhea: infectious etiology
B. Inflammatory bowel disease
   1. Crohn's disease
   2. Ulcerative colitis
C. Cystic fibrosis
D. Giardiasis
E. Protozan
F. Malabsorption syndromes
G. Intussusception
H. Stool impaction
I. Irritable bowel syndrome
J. Meckel diverticulum
K. Intolerance to lactose, carbohydrates, and protein
L. Antibiotic-associated diarrhea
M. Pseudomembranous colitis
N. Toxic megacolon
O. Appendicitis

Plan

A. See the Section III Patient Teaching Guide for this chapter, "Diarrhea (Adults and Children)."
B. Examination of stools for ova and parasites should be done every other day or every three days.
C. Rehydration with oral fluids for each diarrhea stool. Administer small amounts at frequent intervals.
D. Hold foods until hydration is completed. No evidence shows that bananas, rice, applesauce, and toast (BRAT) is useful and is not currently recommended.

E. Use antibiotics (or the discontinuation of antibiotics in the case of *C difficile*) or use antiparasitics agents depending on the etiology.
F. The use of probiotics, *Lactobacillus GG* (I, A) and *S boulardii* (II, B), has been found to be effective and may reduce the spread of rotavirus.
G. Encourage proper hygiene and food preparation to prevent spread and future infections.
H. Water should be boiled for at least 1 minute if contamination is suspected.

Follow-up

A. Follow-up depends on the severity of diarrhea and the age of the patient. Neonates require strict follow-up within a few days of illness.
B. Monitor children who require labor-intensive oral hydration. Hospitalization for IV hydration may be required.
C. Rotavirus vaccine is available for the prevention of rotavirus gastroenteritis. Rota Teq is administered in a 3-dose series for children aged 6–12 weeks and completing before 32 weeks. OR Rotarix oral vaccine is available in a 2-dose administration to patients aged 6–24 weeks.

Consultation/Referral

A. Evaluate the need for a surgical consultation (fulminant colitis, peritonitis, and toxic megacolon) or one with an infectious-disease specialist or a gastroenterologist.

Individual Considerations

A. Pediatrics
   1. Stool patterns vary widely. Breast-fed children may have up to 5–6 stools per day. Breast-fed infants with acute diarrhea should continue on breast milk.
   2. The younger the child, the higher the risk for severe, life-threatening dehydration and nutrient malabsorption.
B. Geriatrics: Review any hospitalizations within the last 72 hours as a cause of diarrhea.

DIVERTICULOSIS AND DIVERTICULITIS

Definition

A. Diverticulum is saclike protrusions of mucosa through the muscular colonic wall. Protrusions can occur in weakened areas of the bowel wall and blood vessels can penetrate. Diverticulosis is the presence of diverticula, but it does not imply a pathologic condition. Diverticulitis occurs when the diverticula become plugged and inflamed. Surgery is often the treatment of choice for young symptomatic patients. Diverticular disease is one of the most common causes of lower GI hemorrhage and a leading consideration in patients who present with brisk rectal bleeding.
B. There is no evidence of a relationship between the development of diverticula and smoking, caffeine, and alcohol consumption. However, an increased risk of developing diverticular disease is associated with a diet that is high in red meat and total fat content. This risk can be reduced by a diet high in fiber content, especially with fruits and vegetables (cellulose). (See Appendix B, Table B.7: Fiber Recommendations by Age.)

Incidence

Diverticulosis is very common and increases by age and gender.

A. Prevalence by age:
1. Age 40: 5%
2. Age 60: 30%
3. Age 80: 65%
B. Prevalence by gender:
1. Age younger than 50 years: more common in males
2. Age 50–70 years: slight predominance in women
3. Age older than 70 years: more common in women

Diverticulosis is symptomatic in 70% of cases. It leads to diverticulitis in 5%–25%; and is associated with bleeding in 5%-15%. The sigmoid colon is commonly affected. There are two types of diverticular disease and diverticulitis:

A. Simple, with no complications
B. Complicated, with abscesses, fistula, obstruction, perforation, and peritonitis leading to sepsis

Pathogenesis

A. The present theory that fiber is a protective agent against the development of diverticula and subsequent diverticulitis holds that insoluble fiber causes the formation of more bulky stool, which leads to decreased effectiveness in colonic segmentation. The overall result is that intracolonic pressure remains close to the normal range during colonic peristalsis. Diverticular sac can become inflamed when undigested food residues and bacteria get trapped in the thin-walled sacs. If this occurs, blood supply is mechanically compromised and bacterial invasion ensues.

Predisposing Factors

A. Advanced age
B. Obesity (84%–96%)
C. Low-residue diet
D. Complicated diverticular disease is increased with:
1. Patients who smoke
2. Use of nonsteroidal anti-inflammatory drugs (NSAIDS)
3. Acetaminophen use (especially paracetamol)

Common Complaints

A. Diverticulosis is usually asymptomatic.
B. Painless rectal bleeding is the hallmark of diverticular bleeding, with intermittent passage of maroon or bright red blood.
C. Common diverticulitis symptoms:
1. Left lower quadrant pain
2. Constipation

Other Signs and Symptoms

A. Back pain
B. Flatulence
C. Periodic abdominal distension
D. Borborygmi, or loud, prolonged gurgles caused by hyperactive intestinal peristalsis
E. Diarrhea
F. Nausea or vomiting
G. Dysuria
H. Tenderness on palpation, possible guarding
I. Fever, low-grade

Subjective Data

A. Review onset, duration, and course of symptoms, including size, color, consistency, and frequency of stools.
B. Ask the patient if constipation is a chronic or acute problem, and if it alternates with diarrhea.
C. Review the patient's daily diet and fluid intake.
D. Ask the patient about medication use, including iron supplements, NSAIDS, and acetaminophen.
E. Inquire about color, amount, and frequency of rectal bleeding. Does the patient strain when having a BM?
F. Review the patient's history of pain with defecation.

Physical Examination

A. Check temperature, pulse, respirations, blood pressure, and weight.
B. The physical examination may be relatively unremarkable, but most commonly reveals abdominal tenderness or a mass.
C. Inspection:
1. Observe the general overall appearance for signs of pain.
2. Inspect the abdomen in detail, assessing for distension.
D. Auscultate all four quadrants of the abdomen. Absent bowel sounds suggests peritoneal inflammation.
E. Percuss the abdomen.
F. Palpate
1. Palpate the abdomen for rebound tenderness or masses signaling possible abscess and tenderness.
2. Palpate beneath right costal arch, checking for Murphy's sign, or pain on deep inspiration.
G. Rectal exam: Evaluate for hemorrhoids, masses, fissures, fistulas, inflammation, and stool in ampulla.

Diagnostic Tests

A. The diagnosis of diverticular colitis is made endoscopically and histologically.
B. CT scan is becoming the optimal method of investigation for suspected acute diverticulitis.
C. CBC with differential: WBC may show leukocytosis with a shift to the left; hemoglobin and hematocrit may be low with chronic or acute bleeding.
D. Radiography: flat plate and upright films of abdomen to evaluate ileus or obstruction, free air, and perforation.
E. Abdominal ultrasonography to evaluate masses or abscess.
F. Proctosigmoidoscopy.
G. Barium enema (BE) after infection subsides. Caution a BE during acute phase may increase intraluminal pressure and cause bowel perforation.
H. Hemacult: stool.

Differential Diagnoses

A. Diverticulitis
B. Diverticulosis
C. Acute appendicitis
D. Bowel obstruction
E. Ischemic colitis

F. Colon cancer
G. Hemorrhoids
H. Constipation or impaction
I. Inflammatory bowel disease
J. Urologic disorder: pyelonephritis
K. Pelvic inflammatory disease (PID)

Plan

A. Stress importance of strict adherence to diet.
B. Dietary management
  1. NPO status for acute treatment.
  2. Full-liquid diet or low-fiber diet if not on bowel rest.
  3. Long-term dietary management:
    a. High-fiber diet including bran, beans, fruits and vegetables.
    b. Bulk agents if unable to tolerate bran.
    c. Note foods to avoid such as nuts.
C. Medical and surgical management: Acute treatment has not been well defined in diverticular disease.
  1. Acute treatment may include the following:
    a. NG tube placement.
    b. IV fluids.
  2. Surgical intervention is required for abscess, peritonitis, obstruction, fistula, and failure to improve after several days of medical management, or recurrence after successful medical management.
D. Pharmaceutical therapy: Optimal treatment has not been defined.
  1. Conservative management of diverticulosis: psyllium (Metamucil) 1–3 teaspoons in 8 oz liquid three times a day.
  2. Diverticulitis initial attack: Ciprofloxacin (Cipro) 500 mg orally twice daily and Metronidazole (Flagyl) 250 mg orally three times a day for 7–14 days. Amoxicillin/clavulanic or Sufamethoxazole-tipethoprim may also be used with Metronidazole.
  3. Aminosalicylates may be added if there is a lack of response.
  4. Relapse: May repeat with the same antibiotic regimen for 1 month.
  5. Chronic disease: Utilize long-term ciprofloxacin but not Metronidazole.
  6. Avoid laxatives, enemas, and opiates.

Follow-up

A. Follow up in 1 to 2 weeks. Continue conservative management if the patient has no signs of complications.

Consultation/Referral

A. Consult a physician if the patient has mild diverticulitis: temperature less than 101°F; WBC less than 13,000 to 15,000.
B. Arrange for prompt hospitalization and surgical consultation if the patient's temperature rises above 101.0°F, his or her pain worsens, peritoneal signs develop, or WBC continues to rise. Surgery consultation is required for abscess, peritonitis, obstruction, fistula, or failure to improve after several days of medical management.

ELEVATED LIVER ENZYMES

Definition

Liver function tests (LFTs) used to determine the health of the liver are not direct measures of its function. The liver has excretory, metabolic, protective, detoxication, hematologic, and circulatory functions. Liver function tests may be abnormal even in patients with a healthy liver. Normal laboratory chemistry values may vary according to age, gender, ethnicity, blood group, and postprandial state as well as other factors such as exercise and pregnancy. Common liver chemistry tests (see Table 10.4) include:

A. Differential diagnosis of the different types of jaundice.
B. Assess the severity of hepatocellular injury.
C. Follow the trend of the disease.
D. Diagnosis of the presence of latent liver disease (i.e., differential diagnosis of ascites or hematemesis).
E. Screening the suspected case during outbreaks of infective hepatitis.
F. Screening the persons exposed to hepatotoxic drugs.
G. Evaluate cholestatic problems.

Incidence

A. The incidence of elevated liver enzymes is undetermined. Abnormal elevations of serum liver chemistries may occur in 1%–4% of the asymptomatic population.

Pathogenesis

A. Pathogenesis varies by diagnosis.

Predisposing Factors

A. Predisposing factors are dependent on the suspected or known medical diagnosis.

Common Complaints

A. Asymptomatic
B. Pruritus
C. Jaundice
D. Ascites
E. Fatigue
F. Weight loss
G. Change in the color of urine (dark) or stools (clay-colored)

Subjective Data

A complete medical history is the single most important part of the evaluation of the patient with elevated LFTs.

A. Review medications including prescription, over-the-counter medications, as well as herbal therapies.
B. Determine the duration of LFT abnormalities (if known).
C. Review the presence of accompanying symptoms including arthralgias, myalgias, rash, abdominal pain, fever, pruritus, and changes in the color of urine or stool.
D. Has the patient experienced any anorexia, or weight loss? Over what period of time did weight loss occur?
E. Review parenteral exposures including transfusions, intravenous and intranasal drug use, tattoos, and sexual history.
F. Review the patient's recent travel history and possible exposure to contaminated foods.

TABLE 10.4 Liver Chemistry Tests and Implications

Liver Chemistry Test	Clinical Implication of Abnormality
Alanine aminotransferase (ALT)	Hepatocellular damage
Aspartate aminotransferase (AST)	Hepatocellular damage
Alkaline phosphatase (ALP)	Cholestasis, infiltrative disease, or biliary obstruction
Albumin	Synthetic function
Alpha-Fetoprotein	Cancer marker when elevated
Bile acids: Urine bile salts, bile pigments, and urobilinogen	Cholestasis or biliary obstruction, impaired hepatic update or secretion, or portal-systemic shunting
Bilirubin: Serum total, direct and indirect bilirubin	Cholestasis, impaired conjugation, or biliary obstruction
Cholesterol, serum triglycerides	Lipoprotein production and metabolism, chronic cholestasis
Fibrinogen	Liver damage/cirrhosis, acute liver insufficiency, poisoning
Gamma-GT (GGT)	Cholestasis or biliary obstruction, malignant involvement in hepatocellular disease, more sensitive than other enzymes in alcoholism
Hepatitis surface antigen, IGM, antibody, RNA, genotype, viral load	Differentiation of type of hepatitis
Lactate dehydrogenase	Hepatocellular damage not specific for hepatic disease
Total proteins, albumin globulin, (A/C ratio)	Hepatitis, advanced liver disease
Prothrombin time (PT)	Synthesis function in hepatocellular disease, fulminate hepatitis
Plasma ammonia	CNS dysfunction/toxicity or end-stage liver disease
5'-Nucleotidase	Cholestasis or biliary obstruction
Urea	End-stage liver disease

G. Review exposure to people with jaundice.

H. Review the patient's occupational history and exposure to hepatotoxins.

I. Review the patient's history of alcohol consumption.

Physical Examination

A. Temperature, pulse, respirations and blood pressure.

B. Observation:
1. Observe for temporal and proximal muscle wasting.
2. Eye and mouth (mucous membranes) examination for icterus.
3. Dermal examination for icterus, spider nevi, palmar erythema, presence of caput medusae (the presence of dilated veins seen on the abdomen; noted with cirrhosis of the liver and portal hypertension).
4. Evaluate the presence of gynecomastia.
5. Observe for the presence of jugular venous distention (JVD), a sign of right-sided heart failure that suggests hepatic congestion.

C. Auscultate: heart and lungs.

D. Percuss abdomen.

E. Palpate
1. Abdominal examination:
   a. Evaluate the presence of hepatomegaly; focus on the size and consistency of the liver.
   b. Evaluate the presence of splenomegaly; focus on the size of the spleen. An enlarged spleen is most easily appreciated with the patient in the right lateral decubitus position.
   c. Assess for ascites: presence of a fluid wave or shifting dullness.
   d. Assess for an abdominal mass.
2. Lymph nodes: evaluate lymphadenopathy.
3. Testicular examination for testicular atrophy (increased estrogen/reduced testosterone).

Diagnostic Tests

A. The particular LFT tests ordered are related to the suspected or identified medical diagnosis. Table 10.5 shows common serologic tests for viral hepatitis.

Differential Diagnoses

A. Table 10.6 shows differential diagnoses with elevated liver enzymes.

Plan

A. **The clinical significance of any liver chemistry test abnormality must be interpreted in the context of the clinical situation.** The plan of care is dependent upon the suspected or identified medical diagnosis. Lifestyle modifications, including discontinuance of medications and alcohol, weight loss, and dietary changes can be recommended as appropriate.

B. Patients with marked abnormalities of liver tests, or with signs and symptoms of chronic liver disease or hepatic decompensation (i.e., ascites, encephalopathy, coagulapathy, or portal hypertension), should be evaluated and treated in a more expeditious manner than asymptomatic patients.

TABLE 10.5 Serologic Tests for Hepatitis

Virologic Test	Usual Clinical Implication of a Positive Test
Hepatitis A-IgM	Positive in acute hepatitis A
Hepatitis A-IgG	Positive in response to previous hepatitis A infection or vaccination
Hepatitis B surface antigen	Positive during active hepatitis B infection
Hepatitis B surface antibody	Positive in response to previous hepatitis B infection or vaccination
Hepatitis B core antibody-IgM	Positive during active hepatitis B infection
Hepatitis B core antibody-IgG	Positive in response to current or prior hepatitis B infection
HBV-DNA	Positive during active hepatitis B infection
Hepatitis B e antigen	Positive test indicates replicative state of wild-type hepatitis B infection
Hepatitis B e antibody	Positive after replicative state of wild-type hepatitis B infection
HBV viral load	Assess hepatitis B virology
HCV-antibody enzyme-linked immunosorbent assay (ELISA)	Positive during or after hepatitis C infection
HCV-RIBA	Positive during or after hepatitis C infection
HCV-RNA	Positive during hepatitis C infection
HCV viral load	Assess hepatitis C virology
HCV genotype	Genotyping is used for evaluation of the length of therapy

TABLE 10.6 Differential Diagnosis With Elevated Liver Enzymes

Infiltrating diseases of the liver

- Sarcoidosis
- Tuberculosis
- Fungal infection
- Amyloidosis
- Lymphoma
- Metastatic malignancy
- Hepatocellular carcinoma

Acute viral hepatitis (A-E, EBV, CMV, herpes)	Wilson's disease (genetic disorder of biliary copper excretion)
Cholestatis disease	Acute bile duct obstruction
Chronic hepatitis B, C	Hemolysis
Steatosis/nonalcoholic steatohepatitis (NASH)	Myopathy
Hereditary hemochromatosis (HH)	Thyroid disorders
Medication/herbal-induced	Strenuous exercise-induced changes
alpha-1-antitrypsin deficiency	Pregnancy—HELLP syndrome
Cirrhosis	Toxin(s) exposure
Celiac disease	Acute Budd-Chiari syndrome
Alcohol-related liver injury	Anorexia nervosa

Follow-up

A. Follow-up testing for elevated liver function tests, including abdominal/liver ultrasonography, CT, MRI, and liver biopsy, is dependent on the risk factors for disease, symptoms and history, and physical finding of the suspected or identified medical diagnosis. A liver chemistry test that is normal does not ensure that the patient is free of liver disease. If a laboratory error is suspected, the laboratory test should be repeated.

Consultation/Referral

A. Consider a consultation or referral to a hepatologist, gastroenterologist, or infectious disease specialist.

Individual Considerations

Pregnancy: Hemolysis, elevated liver enzymes, and low platelets (HELLP syndrome) is a severe form of pregnancy-induced hypertension (PIH or preeclampsia). It may occur anywhere from the mid second trimester to immediate postpartum. HELLP syndrome occurs in 0.2%–0.6% of pregnancies. The etiology is unknown. The presence of laboratory abnormalities confirms the diagnosis. The treatment of HELLP syndrome will not be covered. However, the laboratory abnormalities that are noted include:

A. Hemolytic anemia
B. Proteinuria
C. Serum aspartate aminotransferase (AST) level (>70 IU/L)
D. Low platelet count (<10,000 cells/mL)
E. Serum lactate dehydrogenase (LDH) level (>600 IU/L)
F. Total bilirubin level (>1.2 mg/dL)

▣ GASTROENTERITIS, BACTERIAL AND VIRAL

Definition
A. Bacterial and viral gastroenteritis is an acute inflammation of the GI mucosa of the middle or lower intestine. It is primarily an acute, self-limited illness. Immunocompromised patients can develop unremitting or fatal symptoms from gastroenteritis.

Incidence
A. Gastroenteritis is very common, occurring in all age groups. Epidemic outbreaks of bacterial gastroenteritis occur in groups who have ingested contaminated food. Viral excretion can begin before symptoms. Gastroenteritis is responsible for an estimated 8 million health care visits and 250,000 hospitalization a year.

Pathogenesis
A. Gastroenteritis is commonly due to infectious agents—viruses, bacteria, and parasites (see Table 10.7). There are four viral agents: rotavirus, Norovirus, enteric adenovirus, and Astrovirus. Exotoxins produced by some organisms induce hypersecretion or increased peristalsis resulting in diarrhea or vomiting. Bacteria such as *E. coli* and *Salmonella* penetrate and invade the gastric mucosa and lead to diarrhea accompanied by fever and fecal

TABLE 10.7	Infectious Agents Causing Gastroenteritis
Causative Agent	**Incubation Period**
Noroviruses	12 hours–2 days
E. coli	24–72 hours
Campylobacter	2–5 days
Staphylococcus	1–6 hours
Shigella	8–24 hours
Botulism	12–36 hours
Giardia lamblia	7–21 days
Salmonella	6–72 hours
Rotaviruses	1–3 days
Adenovirus	5–8 days
Clostridium perfringes	10–12 hours
C. difficile	Variable
Listeria species	20 hours

leukocytes. Viruses destroy enterocytes of the upper jejunal villi, often producing secondary lactose intolerance.

Predisposing Factors
A. Travel to areas where cholera or *Giardia* is epidemic:
1. Ingestion of raw or undercooked seafood or drinks containing cholera-contaminated ice or water.
2. Ingestion of *Giardia*-contaminated water supplies.
B. Ingestion of food contaminated with *Salmonella* or *Shigella*. Foods that are often implicated are domestic fowl and eggs, custard-filled pastries, processed meats, foods warmed on steam tables, poultry, red meat, raw seafood, raw milk, rice, and bean sprouts due to the following:
1. Inadequate cooking time and temperatures
2. Poor hygiene, lack of hand washing
3. Improper storage of food
4. Ingestion of fruits and vegetables contaminated by an infected person or by animal products
C. Infection by person-to-person spread:
1. Day care centers: Rotavirus can be found on toys and hard surfaces.
2. Overcrowded environment, inadequate health care or education.
D. Contact with *Salmonella*-infected turtles, iguanas, and other reptiles.

Common Complaints
A. Abrupt onset of nausea and vomiting
B. Abrupt onset of diarrhea
C. Fever, sometimes

Other Signs and Symptoms
A. Explosive flatulence
B. Cramping abdominal pain
C. Abdominal tenderness
D. Frequent watery diarrhea
E. Myalgia
F. Headache
G. Weakness
H. Malaise

Subjective Data
A. Review onset, duration, and course of symptoms, including presence of abdominal pain and frequency of BMs. Ask the patient if anyone else in the family has the same symptoms.
B. Ask the patient about travel history, including travel to foreign countries and camping with ingestion of water from streams, springs, or untreated wells.
C. Ask the patient about crowded or unsanitary living conditions, use of day care centers, and institutional living.
D. Take a 24-hour diet history, including ingestion of prunes or beans.
E. Review diarrhea history:
1. How many stools?
2. How frequent are the diarrhea stools?
3. What color is the stool?
4. Does the stool contain mucus?
F. Inquire about other symptoms, such as fever or respiratory problems.

G. If the patient is an infant, ask caregiver about activity level, irritability, sleep pattern, fluid intake, and number of wet diapers.

H. If the patient is a child, ask about activity level and dietary and fluid intake.

I. Review drug history intake, including laxatives, antacids, antibiotics, quinine, or anticancer medications.

Physical Examination

A. Check temperature, pulse, respirations, blood pressure, and weight.
   1. Bacterial infections: temperatures between 101° and 102°F.
   2. Viral infections: temperatures of 103°F and above.
   3. Note hypotension and tachycardia.

B. Inspect
   1. Inspect general appearance; note if the patient is very ill.
   2. Assess hydration status. Signs of dehydration:
      a. Mild: slightly dry buccal mucous membranes, increased thirst, decreased urine output
      b. Moderate: sunken eyes, sunken fontanelle in infants, loss of skin turgor, dry buccal mucous membranes, decreased urine output
      c. Severe: signs of moderate dehydration and one or more of the following: rapid thready pulse, tachypnea, lethargy, and postural hypotension
   3. Assess activity level and behavior in infant or child.

C. Auscultate the abdomen in all quadrants for bowel sounds; note hyperactive bowel sounds, absent or hypoactive bowel sounds (common with botulism), and borborygmi.

D. Palpate the abdomen for diffuse tenderness, slight distension, masses, rebound tenderness, and spasm.

E. Rectal exam: Check for masses, fissures, inflammation, perianal erythema, or stool in ampulla.

F. Neurologic exam
   1. Check for dizziness, difficulty swallowing, and other neurologic signs.
   2. Neurologic signs and symptoms indicate botulism and require emergency intervention.

Diagnostic Tests

A. No immediate lab tests are required if dehydration is absent or mild and the patient feels well except for frequent diarrhea.

B. CBC with differential: serologic studies can detect viral pathogens.

C. Sedimentation rate: elevated with infections or inflammation.

D. Electrolytes, sodium, chlorides, potassium, and BUN.

E. Blood gases to assess acid-base balance, if indicated.

F. Blood cultures, if indicated.

G. Stool for guaiac, leukocytes, ova, and parasites; test specimens three times, every other day. Stool guaiac is usually negative in viral infections, positive in invasive bacterial infections. Large numbers of white cells in stool suggest inflammatory or invasive diarrhea, such as occurs with *Shigella, Salmonella, Campylobacter,* invasive *E. coli,* or *Entamoeba.* Mononuclear cells in stool are characteristic of salmonellosis.

H. Stool culture if blood or mucus, fever more than 24 hours, or leukocytes are present.

I. Special cultures for *Campylobacter* and cholera are required.

J. Urinalysis: excludes UTI as cause of nonspecific diarrhea; urine specific gravity to assess dehydration.

K. Sigmoidoscopy: skip bowel prep with gross blood, large numbers of leukocytes in stool, or severe illness.

L. Culture of food from suspected foci for *Salmonella.*

Differential Diagnoses

A. Gastroenteritis, bacterial and viral
B. Acute viral hepatitis
C. Acute appendicitis
D. Cholecystitis
E. Inflammatory bowel disease
F. PID
G. Intussusception
H. Bowel obstruction for other causes

Plan

A. General interventions
   1. Advise the patient to begin bed rest with progression to regular activities.
   2. If the patient is diapered and/or incontinent, tell the patient or caregiver to adhere strictly to contact precautions. Hand washing may decrease the spread.
   3. Diaper changing areas should be separate from food preparation areas.
   4. Chlorine-based disinfectants inactivate Rotavirus and may prevent disease transmission from contact with environmental surfaces.

B. Patient teaching: See the Section III Patient Teaching Guide for this chapter, "Diarrhea (Adults and Children)."

C. Dietary management:
   1. Patients should remain NPO and then slowly add clear liquids to maintain hydration.
   2. Hydration is one of the most important factors in prevention of complications.
   3. Recommend the BRAT diet (bananas, rice, applesauce, and toast) until the patient is able to tolerate other solids. (See Appendix B for "Nausea and Vomiting Diet Suggestions (Children and Adults)")

D. Pharmaceutical therapy
   1. The primary treatment for viral gastroenteritis is fluid replacement. There are not specific antiviral pharmaceutical therapies.
   2. Antibiotics may or may not be prescribed according to the bacterial source. Antimicrobial therapy is not indicated for uncomplicated (noninvasive) gastroenteritis because therapy does not shorten duration of the disease and can prolong duration of excretion of *Salmonella* organisms.
   3. Antidiarrheal therapy delays transit time, can reduce the severity and duration of abdominal cramping; however, it may prolong the course of some bacterial diarrhea such as *Shigella* and *E. coli.* Bismuth subsalicylate (Pepto-Bismol) (OTC) is not recommended for young children with gastroenteritis due to the potential toxicity from salicylate absorption.

4. Stop other medications that may be triggering diarrhea.
5. Vaccinate children with Rotavirus live vaccine:
   a. Rotavirus vaccine (RV) is administered for children between ages 6 weeks and 0 days to 14 weeks and 6 days of age. It should not be administered to infants older than 15 weeks.
   b. Repeat doses are given at 4 weeks apart. The maximum number of RV vaccine is a 3-dose series.
   c. If doses are administered at 2 and 4 months, a third dose at 6 months of age is not indicated.
   d. The final dose of RV should be administered by 8 months and 0 days of age.

Follow-up

A. Tell the patient to return if the condition worsens or if signs and symptoms have not abated in 48–72 hours. However, diarrhea due to *Salmonella* may be expected to persist for up to 2 weeks.
B. If diarrhea persists for 2 weeks or more, see the patient for a secondary evaluation.
C. Check with your local health department about outbreak notification of gastroenteritis.

Consultation/Referral

A. Refer patients to a physician immediately if they have dehydration, rebound tenderness, severe abdominal pain, neurologic symptoms, and intussesception.
B. Immediately refer infants under age 2 years with paroxysmal, severe abdominal pain and vomiting followed by currant jelly stool; they need immediate evaluation for intussesception.
C. Refer any patient with diarrhea longer than 7 days that has had no response to usual treatment.
D. Refer an immunocompromised patient.

Individual Considerations

A. Pediatrics
   1. Very young children are at a higher risk of mortality.
   2. Affected children may exhibit chronic diarrhea, or more than five watery or loose stools a day, but they develop normally and show no signs of malnutrition.
   3. Rotavirus is the most common cause of nosocomial diarrhea in children and an important cause of acute gastroenteritis in day care centers. Children whose stool cannot be contained by diapers or toilet use should be excluded from day care until diarrhea stops.
   4. Breast-feeding can continue during diarrhea.
B. Adults: Those with concomitant chronic debilitating disease are at a higher risk of mortality.
C. Geriatrics:
   1. Elderly are at a higher risk of mortality secondary to dehydration.
   2. Diminished thirst mechanism and decreased body water exacerbate dehydration.

GASTROESOPHAGEAL REFLUX DISEASE (GERD)

Definition

A. Gastroesophageal reflux (GER) is considered a normal physiologic process in healthy infants, children, and adults. Most episodes last less than 3 min, and most often occur 30–60 min after meals and with reclining positions. GERD is present when the symptoms, more than twice a week, cause troublesome symptoms or complications.
B. A very large population of patients will present after self-medicating with antacids, bicarbonate soda, and over-the-counter medications. The management of GERD should be tailored to the frequency, severity, and duration of symptoms.

Incidence

A. GERD is very common. Daily heartburn typically occurring postprandially has been estimated to affect 17%–65% of the normal adult population. Reflux esophagitis affects over 50% of women at some time during pregnancy. It is estimated that 30%–90% of asthmatics have GERD. Barrett's esophagus, which affects fewer than 1% of adults, is commonly associated with GERD.

Pathogenesis

A. Gastroesophageal reflux disease (GERD) is relaxation or incompetence of the lower esophagus persisting beyond the newborn period. Relaxation of the lower esophageal sphincter (LES) allows reflux of gastric acid and pepsin into the distal esophagus. Heartburn occurs when reverse peristaltic waves cause regurgitation of acidic stomach contents into the esophagus. Anatomical abnormalities such as a hiatal hernia predispose persons to GERD. Improper diet and nervous tension are also precipitating factors.
B. Gastroesophageal (GE) reflux has been identified as a trigger for asthma possibly by the activation of vagal reflexes and/or microaspiration. Asthma may promote GERD, and GERD may provoke asthma. Some asthma medications may reduce LES tone, further complicating the picture. Conversely, a patient with GERD may experience pulmonary disease as a response to the esophageal acid exposure.

Predisposing Factors

A. Obesity
B. Consuming large meals
C. Pregnancy
D. Immature, weak sphincter in newborns
E. Emotional stress
F. Increased abdominal pressure from tight clothes, straining to lift or defecate, or swallowing air
G. Ingesting drugs and foods that promote LES relaxation:
   1. Nonsteroidal anti-inflammatory agents (NSAIDS)
   2. Benzodiazepines
   3. Calcium channel blockers
   4. Theophylline
   5. Nitrates

6. Anticholinergics
7. Alcohol
8. Chocolate and peppermint
H. Smoking: increases stomach acid and LES pressure
I. Ingestion of caustic agents such as lye
J. Infection by agents, such as *Candida,* herpes simplex, or CMV, which directly attack the esophageal mucosa
K. Compromised immunity, from AIDS, diabetes, or chemotherapy
L. Asthma

Common Complaints
A. Heartburn
B. Regurgitation of fluid or food

Alarm Symptoms
A. Dysphagia (difficulty swallowing)
B. Unintentional weight loss
C. Predominant upper abdominal pain
D. Hematemesis (vomiting blood)
E. Melena (black feces/blood stool)
F. Odynophagia (painful swallowing)
G. Severe symptoms

Other Signs and Symptoms
A. Retrosternal aching or burning
B. Nocturnal aspiration, water or "acid" brash
C. Chronic cough, especially at bedtime
D. Hoarseness
E. Globus sensation
F. Nausea
G. Dental erosion
H. Infants: failure to thrive, vomiting

Subjective Data
A. Review onset, duration, and course of heartburn or other symptoms.
B. Review medication history including over-the-counter (OTC) medication and herbals. Specifically review the use of NSAIDS.
   1. Has the patient been taking OTC antacids, H_2 blockers, or OTC PPIs?
   2. How long has the patient been using these OTCs?
C. Ask the patient about alleviating and aggravating factors.
D. Review the patient's habits, including smoking and alcohol intake.
E. Inquire about other symptoms, such as weight loss, dysphagia, blood loss, regurgitation, and diarrhea.
F. Establish the patient's usual weight to determine extent of problem.
G. Ask the patient about any history of asthma and Crohn's disease.
H. Rule out ingestion of caustic agents especially in the pediatric population.
I. Review the patient's dietary history for bulimia.

Physical Examination
A. Check temperature, pulse, respirations, blood pressure, and weight.
B. General observation of respiratory distress including stridor.

C. Inspect:
   1. Throat examination and mouth evaluation for dental erosion.
   2. Assess swallowing ability.
D. Auscultate:
   1. Lungs: evaluate the presence of wheezing.
   2. Auscultate the heart.
   3. Evaluate the abdomen in all four quadrants.
E. Palpate:
   1. Abdomen for the presence of hepatosplenomegaly and masses.
   2. Assess the abdomen for tenderness or distention.
F. Perform rectal exam (if indicated for any history of hematemesis).

Diagnostic Tests
A. Clinical and history alone usually confirm the diagnosis in the vast majority of reflux sufferers.
B. Endoscopy with biopsy is usually first diagnostic tool in cases of caustic ingestion or suspected infectious etiology.
C. Ambulatory 24-hour pH monitoring: prolonged monitoring is the best clinical tool for diagnosing GERD in asthmatics. However, it is very expensive and not universally available.
D. Upper GI series or barium contrast radiography is not used to diagnose GERD but rules out anatomic abnormalities of the upper digestive tract.
E. Esophageal manometry: used to evaluate patients who have failed to respond to an empiric trial of proton pump inhibitors (PPI).
F. Guaiac test for occult blood. Bleeding may accompany reflux esophagitis and be slow and chronic, resulting in iron-deficiency anemia, or brisk, resulting in hematemesis. GERD may not be obvious to the clinician when obtaining a patient history, especially in an asthma patient with confounding respiratory symptoms.
G. Consider *H. pylori* testing.

Differential Diagnoses
A. GERD
B. MI/angina
C. Esophageal spasm
D. Gallbladder disease
E. Cancer-gastric or esophageal
F. Infections: CMV, herpes simplex virus, and *Candida*
G. Peptic ulcer
H. Ingestion of caustic substance
I. Self-induced vomiting/bulimia
J. Pyloric stenosis
K. Food allergy

Plan
A. General interventions: Management depends on cause and severity of symptoms.
B. Patient teaching: See the Section III Patient Teaching Guide for this chapter, "Gastroesophageal Reflux Disease (GERD)."
C. Dietary management: Weight loss is advised for overweight or obese patients with GERD symptoms. At the

present there is not supporting data for special dietary precautions.

D. Medical and surgical management
1. Surgery may be indicated for patients who do not respond to other approaches.
2. The Nissen fundoplication is a surgical procedure used to treat GERD in asthmatics. It improves the antireflux barrier and provides a lasting solution. Because it is not always successful, it is reserved for severe cases. The Nissen operation is often performed as a laparoscopic procedure.
3. Patients on nonsteroidal anti-inflammatory (NSAIDS) who experience upper gastric pain including reflux need to be referred for endoscopy as soon as possible.

E. Pharmaceutical therapy
1. The potential adverse effects of acid suppression include the increased risk of community-acquired pneumonia and GI infections.
2. Long-term use of acid suppression therapy without a diagnosis is not advised.
3. The target of pharmaceutical therapy is improvement in quality of life by the reduction/relief of symptoms and healing of erosive esophagitis (EE).
4. Histamine-2 receptor antagonists (H_2 blockers) are effective in managing milder, infrequent GI symptoms. Tolerance occurs with chronic use of H_2 blockers. Several H_2 blockers are currently available as prescription and over-the-counter (OTC): Nizatidine (Axid), Famotidine (Pepcid), Cimetidine (Tagamet), and Ranitidine (Zantac).
5. Proton pump inhibitors (PPIs) are used for both GERD and erosive esophagitis and are considered the "gold standard" of treatment. Dosages are age- and weight-based. Patients may experience a relapse in their GER symptoms after discontinuance and therefore may need to be tapered off or use a step-down approach with an antacid or an H_2 blocker. No PPI is approved for use in infants younger than

1 year. PPIs are currently available by prescription and OTC. See Table 10.8.

On-demand or self-directed therapy has been shown to be effective.

Follow-up
A. Empiric treatment with a PPI may be attempted for a short period except for patients presenting with any alarm symptoms. Schedule a return visit in 1–2 weeks to evaluate the relief of symptoms.
B. Patients have been having frequent relapses; failure to adequately respond or long-term OTC H_2 blockers and PPI use should have an endoscopic evaluation.
C. The need for prescribed long-term PPI treatment or the presence of alarm symptoms requires a gastroenterology consultation.
D. Patients that present with chest pain should be further evaluated/referred prior to prescribing medications for GERD.

Consultations
A. GERD diagnosis should not be made without a full evaluation in infants with vomiting or poor weight gain; refer to a pediatric gastroenterologist for evaluation.
B. Referral is necessary if the patients fails to improve after trying two different medications, or if the patient has dysphagia, recent weight loss, or blood loss.

Individual Considerations
A. Pregnancy
1. Underlying causes in pregnancy are diminished gastric motility and displacement of stomach by enlarging uterus.
2. To rule out pregnancy-induced hypertension (PIH), evaluate the patient immediately for signs and symptoms of sudden onset discomfort with no relief from antacids (PIH or HELLP syndrome).
B. Pediatrics
1. Some regurgitation is normal in neonates because the cardiac sphincter is immature and weak.

TABLE 10.8 Proton Pump Inhibitors

PPI	Available Dosages	Over the Counter
Omeprazole (Prilosec)	Capsules 10 mg, 20 mg, and 40 mg	Tablet 20 mg
Lansoprazole (Prevacid)	Capsules 15 mg and 30 mg Oral suspension and Solutab 15 mg and 30 mg IV (30 mg)	Capsule 15 mg
Rabeprazole (Aciphex)	Capsules 20 mg	Not available
Pantroprazole (Protonix)	Capsules 20 mg and 40 mg Oral suspension 30 mg IV 40 mg	Not available
Esomeprazole (Nexium)	Capsules 20 mg and 40 mg Oral suspension 20 mg and 40 mg IV 20 mg and 40 mg	Not available
Dexlansoprazole (Kapidex)	Capsules 30 mg and 60 mg	Not available
Omeprazole + sodium bicarbonate (Zegerid)	Capsules Omeprazole 20 mg and 20 mg plus 300 mg Na^+ Oral suspension Omeprazole 20 mg and 40 mg plus 460 mg Na^+	Not available

However, vomiting is an abnormal sign associated with overfeeding, sepsis, metabolic disorders such as galactosemia, increased intracranial pressure, and intestinal atresia and stenosis. Regurgitation and vomiting must be differentiated:

  a. Regurgitation most frequently occurs within the first hour after feeding in conjunction with burping or spontaneous eructation of air.
  b. Infants may exhibit refusal to eat, irritability, or arching on their back during or immediately after feeding.
  c. Vomiting, often projectile in nature, can occur at any time and results in the loss of significant amounts of body fluids and electrolytes.

2. Milk protein sensitivity should be ruled out.
3. There is no evidence to eliminate specific foods in children and adolescents to manage GERD.
4. The major agents used in children are gastric-acid buffering agents, mucosal surface barriers, and gastric antisecretory agents.

C. Geriatrics
1. GERD prevalence increases with age and may be associated with a hiatal hernia.
2. Prolonged reflux results in esophagitis and may lead to stricture development. Chronic recurrence may develop into Barrett's syndrome.
3. Treatment of GERD is the same as for general adults; however, do diagnostic testing in short-time sequence secondary to stricture and cancer in the elderly.

GIARDIA INTESTINALIS

Definition

A. *Giardiasis intestinalis* (formerly *Giardia lambia*) is the leading parasitic cause of diarrhea. Infestation can lead to malabsorption by coating large areas of the small bowel, particularly the lower duodenum and upper jejunum. Most people infected with *G intestinalis* remain asymptomatic, and most infections are self-limited.

Incidence

A. Giardiasis has a worldwide distribution and is especially prevalent in the United States and overseas. It is common in areas where water supplies are contaminated by human sewage. The age-specific prevalence of giardiasis is highest in childhood and adolescence and begins to decline thereafter.

Pathogenesis

A. *Giardiasis intestinalis* is a flagellated protozoan. Infective form is the cyst. Humans are the principal reservoir of infection, but *Giardia* can infect dogs, cats, beavers, and other animals that can contaminate water with feces containing cysts.
B. People become infected either directly, by hand-to-mouth transfer of cysts from feces of an infected person (e.g., childcare), or indirectly, by ingestion of fecal-contaminated water or food. Most community-wide epidemics result from contaminated water supplies.
C. Incubation period is 1–4 weeks, with an average of 7–10 days. The infective form is the cyst with infection limited to the small intestine and the biliary tract. Disease is communicable for as long as the infected person excretes cysts.

Predisposing Factors

A. Travel to endemic areas.
B. Subjection to unsanitary food handling.
C. Exposure to contaminated water supplies.
D. Association with day care centers.
E. Association with institutions for mentally retarded.
F. Male homosexuality.
G. Cystic fibrosis.
H. Immunocompromised individuals are at high risk.

Common Complaints

Acute complaints:

A. Explosive, foul-smelling diarrhea
B. Mucus in stools, bulky stools
C. Upper abdominal pain or discomfort
D. Flatulence
E. Nausea
F. Anorexia
G. Weight loss

Other Signs and Symptoms

Chronic complaints:

A. Intermittent loose stools (but not diarrhea)
B. Steatorrhea
C. Increased flatulence or distension
D. Vague abdominal discomfort
E. Fatigue related to anemia
F. Profound weight loss (10%–20% of body weight)
G. Malabsorption
H. Urticaria

Subjective Data

A. Review onset, duration, and course of symptoms. Is diarrhea acute or chronic?
B. Ask the patient about travel to areas known for giardiasis.
C. Review the patient's intake of medications and other substances that can cause diarrhea, especially antibiotics, laxatives, quinidine, magnesium-containing antacids, excess alcohol, caffeine, herbal teas, digitalis, loop diuretics, antihypertensive agents, and sorbitol-containing (sugar-free) gums and mints.
D. Review the nature of the patient's bowel movements, including frequency; consistency; volume; and presence of blood, pus, or mucus.
E. Does diarrhea have any relationship to meals: onset of diarrhea within hours of ingesting a potentially contaminated food is suggestive of bacterial infection such as *E. coli*; this is confirmed by checking if others were similarly affected.
F. Ask the patient about associated symptoms that need evaluation, such as fever, abdominal pain, or rash.
G. Ask the patient if other family members or sexual contacts are also ill.
H. Establish the patient's normal weight, and if any weight has recently been lost, review amount and over what period of time.

Physical Examination

The physical examination may reveal no specific finding.

A. Check temperature, pulse, respirations, blood pressure, and weight.
B. Inspect: general appearance for signs of dehydration; include evaluation of mucous membranes and infants' fontanelles.
C. Auscultate: abdomen for bowel sounds in all quadrants.
D. Palpate
   1. Palpate the abdomen for masses, tenderness, guarding, and rebound. Patients with periumbilical or right lower quadrant pain and copious volumes of watery stool are likely to have a small bowel etiology.
   2. Palpate lymph nodes for enlargement.
E. Perform rectal exam.

Diagnostic Tests

A. Stool bacteria culture and sensitivity.
B. Mucus stool for leukocytes: mucus free of leukocytes is the hallmark of irritable bowel syndrome (IBS); a large number of white cells suggests inflammatory or invasive diarrhea.
C. Stool for ova and parasites; test three times on alternate days. **Parasites are passed intermittently, so examine stools on alternating days.**
D. Stool for occult blood.
E. Endoscopy to identify cyst in duodenal fluid or small bowel tissue.

Differential Diagnoses

A. Giardiasis
B. Malabsorption
C. *E. coli* infection
D. Irritable bowel syndrome (IBS)
E. Viral diarrhea
F. Lactose intolerance
G. Other bacterial infections, such as *Shigella*, *Salmonella*, and *Campylobacter*
H. Crohn's disease
I. Sprue

Plan

A. General interventions
   1. Advise children and adult workers with diarrhea to stay away from day care centers until they become asymptomatic.
   2. Advise the patient's household and sexual contacts to seek medical examination and treatment.
B. Patient teaching
   1. See the Section III Patient Teaching Guide for this chapter, "Diarrhea (Adult and Children)."
   2. Discuss safe sexual practices. Avoiding oral-anal and oral-genital sex can decrease venereal transmission.
   3. Recommend contact precautions for duration of illness for diapered and/or incontinent children.
C. Dietary management
   1. Tell the patient or caregiver to prevent dehydration from diarrhea by increasing fluids.
   2. Advise restricting milk products to rule out lactose intolerance.

   3. Tell backpackers, campers, and people likely to be exposed to contaminated water to avoid drinking directly from streams. Boiling water kills infective cysts.
D. Pharmaceutical therapy
   1. Treatment of asymptomatic carriers is not generally recommended.
   2. Treat children with acute or chronic diarrhea who manifest failure to thrive, malabsorption, or other GI tract symptoms when *Giardia* has been identified.
   3. Metronidazole (Flagyl) is not FDA approved for the treatment of giardiasis; however, it is the principal agent used to treat giardiasis in the United States.
      a. Adults: 250 mg orally three times daily for 5 days.
      b. Pediatric: 15 mg/kg/day orally divided in three times daily dosing for 5 days; not to exceed 750 mg/day.
   4. Furazolidone (Furoxone) is only 80% effective, but is the only drug available in liquid suspension, so it is often more acceptable to children.
      a. Adult: 100 mg tablet or suspension orally for 7–10 days.
      b. Children:
         i. younger than 1 month old: not recommended.
         ii. older than 1 month: 5–8.8 mg/kg/day in 4 divided doses for 10 days; do not exceed 400 mg/day.
   5. Paromomycin (Humatin), a nonabsorbable aminoglycoside, is 50%–70% effective.
      a. Paromomycin is recommended for treatment of symptomatic infection in pregnant women.
      b. Adults and children: 25–35 mg/kg three times daily with meals for 7 days.

Follow-up

A. Relapses after treatment are common especially in immunocompromised patients.
B. Schedule follow-ups at 6 weeks and 6 months after treatment, as indicated.
C. If diarrhea persists for 2 weeks or more, secondary evaluation is indicated. Stools should be examined again for blood, leukocytes, and parasites.
D. Patients who remain undiagnosed after an extensive evaluation and trial of metronidazole (Flagyl) often turn out to have irritable bowel syndrome or surreptitious laxative abuse.

Consultation/Referral

A. Consult a physician if the patient has no relief of symptoms after completion of therapies.
B. Consultations with a pediatric infectious disease specialist and pediatric gastroenterologist are recommended.

Individual Considerations

A. Pregnancy:
   1. Treatment of patients during pregnancy is recommended. Giardiasis in pregnancy is associated with dehydration, malabsorption, or severe symptoms.
   2. Malabsorptive symptoms may persist since regeneration of functioning intestinal mucosa requires time.
   3. Breast-feeding appears to protect infants from *Giardia intestinalis*.

B. Pediatrics:
1. When an outbreak is suspected in a childcare setting, the local health department should be notified to investigate.
2. Children who are carriers do not have to be excluded from childcare; however, personal hygiene/universal precautions should be followed.

HEMORRHOIDS

Definition
A. Hemorrhoids are varicosities and stretched mucosal or submucosal tissue protruding into the anal canal. Internal hemorrhoids are above the anorectal line and covered by rectal mucosa. Internal hemorrhoids are graded by severity (see Table 10.9).
B. External hemorrhoids are below the anorectal line, covered by anal skin, and appear as painless, flaccid skin tags. See Figure 10.2.
C. When blood within the hemorrhoid becomes clotted due to obstruction, the hemorrhoids are referred to as thrombosed and appear as blue, shiny masses.

Incidence
A. The incidence of hemorrhoids is unknown. Patients tend to present after utilizing and failure of over-the-counter treatments. Hemorrhoids are common in people between 20 and 50 years of age. They are uncommon in people under age 20 years except secondary to pregnancy.

Pathogenesis
A. Mechanism is unknown. Prolapse may be initiated by shearing force from passage of large firm stool, an increase in venous pressure from heart failure (HF) or pregnancy, or by straining that occurs with lifting or defecation.

Predisposing Factors
A. Pressure associated with constipation
B. Pelvic congestion
C. Poor pelvic musculature
D. Pregnancy
E. Constipation or straining with stool
F. Portal hypertension, cirrhosis
G. Low-fiber diet
H. Sedentary jobs, such as driving trucks, piloting planes
I. Loss of muscle tone due to advanced age
J. Anal intercourse

Common Complaints
A. Cardinal features:
1. Bleeding: painless, bright red bleeding with defecation (internal)
2. Anal pruritus
3. Prolapse
4. Pain related to thrombosis

Other Signs and Symptoms
A. Visible prolapsed mass
B. Incomplete defecation
C. Leakage of feces (internal hemorrhoids)
D. Excessive moisture
E. Weakness or fatigue, with anemia

Subjective Data
A. Review onset and duration of symptoms, especially the history of rectal bleeding.
B. Review the patient's history of hemorrhoids and treatments, including surgery.

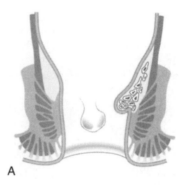

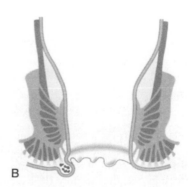

Figure 10.2 Internal and external hemorrhoids. A. Internal hemorrhoid: Covered by a thin sheet of tissue called mucous membrane, an internal hemorrhoid bulges into the rectal opening and may sink a bit during bowel movements. B. External hemorrhoid: Covered by skin, an external hemorrhoid protrudes from the rectum.

Grade	Severity
TABLE 10.9	**Severity of Hemorrhoids Used to Guide Treatment Options**
I	The hemorrhoids do not prolapse.
II	The hemorrhoids prolapse upon defecation but reduce spontaneously.
III	The hemorrhoids prolapse upon defecation and must be reduced manually.
IV	The hemorrhoids are prolapsed and cannot be reduced manually.

C. Ask the patient about recent pregnancy, liver disease, and constipation.

D. Inquire about the patient's job and level of daily activity.

E. Review the patient's sexual practices for anal intercourse.

F. Review the patient's dietary history for fluid intake and sources/amount of fiber.

Physical Examination

A. Check temperature, pulse, respirations, blood pressure, and weight.

B. Inspection
   1. Observation of rectal area for skin tags, prolapse, irritation, fissures, and condyloma.
      a. Internal hemorrhoids are usually not visible unless prolapsed.
      b. External hemorrhoids protrude with straining or standing.
   2. Using anoscopy: visualize internal rectum for hemorrhoids, fissures, or masses.

C. Palpate:
   1. Palpate abdomen for masses.
   2. Internal hemorrhoids are usually not palpable unless thrombosed.
   3. Digital rectal examination.

Diagnostic Tests

A. Hematocrit and hemoglobin, if bleeding present

B. Anoscopy: reveals internal hemorrhoids as bright red to purplish bulges

C. Sigmoidoscopy or colonoscopy (geriatric population)

D. Stool for guaiac testing

E. Air-contrast barium enema for atypical bleeding

Differential Diagnoses

A. Hemorrhoids

B. Condyloma acuminata

C. Rectal prolapse

D. Rectal bleeding due to one of the following:
   1. Colorectal cancer
   2. Polyps
   3. Anal fissure
   4. Fistula
   5. Abscess
   6. IBS
   7. Diverticulitis
   8. Pelvic tumor

Plan

A. General interventions: No treatment is necessary if the patient is asymptomatic except for maintaining regular bowel habits and performing comfort measures.

B. Patient teaching: See the Section III Patient Teaching Guide for this chapter, "Hemorrhoids."

C. Dietary management: High-fiber diet and an adequate fluid intake should be continued indefinitely. (See Appendix B, Table B.7: Fiber Recommendations by Age.)

D. Medical and surgical management

1. Use warm sitz baths up to 3 times a day for irritation and pruritus.

2. Conservative treatment for thrombosed hemorrhoid includes lying prone and applying ice pack to area.

3. Incision and evacuation of thrombosis or clot may be performed under local anesthesia. Other treatments for thrombosed hemorrhoids noted in clinical trials have included:
   a. Nitroglycerin 0.5% topical ointment for temporary analgesia. The most common side effect was headache.
   b. Topical nifedipine.
   c. In a small study, one intrasphincter injection of botulinum toxin relieved pain within 24 hours.

4. Symptomatic Grade I, Grade II and some Grade III hemorrhoids may be treated by:
   a. Rubber band ligation (most widely used and is associated with fewer complications than surgery)
   b. Bipolar, infrared, and laser coagulation (may require more than 1 treatment).
   c. Sclerotherapy

5. External hemorrhoids usually do not require surgical therapy unless in cases of thrombosis. For selective Grade III and Grade IV internal and strangulated hemorrhoids that fail medical and nonoperative therapies, surgical treatment is required. **Hemorrhoidectomy is treatment of last choice because it requires hospitalization and extended recovery period, and it risks compromising competence of anal sphincter.** Hemorrhoidectomy complications include:
   a. Urinary retention
   b. Urinary tract infection
   c. Fecal impaction
   d. Pain
   e. Hemorrhage
   f. Stricture formation (1%) or sphincter damage (rare)

E. Pharmaceutical therapy
   1. Drug of choice: bulk-forming agents such as psyllium seed (Metamucil), methylcellulose (Citrucel), or calcium polycarbophil (Fibercon), 1–3 tsp in 8 oz liquid three times a day. Maintenance dose is 1–3 tsp after dinner.
   2. Stool softener: docusate sodium (Colace) or docusate calcium (Doxidan) 100 mg three times daily.
   3. For irritation and pruritis, topical creams and anesthetics are found in OTC products such as Anusol, pramoxine HCl (Tronolane Cream), Preparation H, and topical hydrocortisone preparations.
   4. An oral analgesic such as codeine may be prescribed for thrombosed hemorrhoids. However, codeine causes constipation.

Follow-up

A. None is necessary if resolution occurs and the patient is asymptomatic.

B. Reevaluate the patient in 2 weeks for further treatment if symptoms persist.

C. Evaluate the patient with an intervention in 7–10 days.

Consultation/Referral

A. Refer the patient with acute thrombosis of external hemorrhoids to a physician.

B. Refer the patient to a surgeon if hemorrhoids bleed repeatedly, prolapse, produce intractable pain, or are thrombosed, and if 3–5 consecutive days of treatment do not provide relief.

Individual Considerations

A. Pregnancy: Labor, which results in pressure on the pelvic floor by the presenting part of the fetus and the expulsive efforts of the woman, may aggravate hemorrhoids, causing protrusion and inflammation during the puerperium. Hemorrhoids may be pushed back after delivery to prevent them from becoming swollen and painful.

B. Pediatrics: Rectal prolapse in children is associated with cystic fibrosis.

Prolapse looks like a pink doughnut or rosette; complete prolapse involving the muscular wall is larger and red, and it has circular folds.

C. Geriatrics:
1. Prolapse of rectal mucosa is more common in the elderly.
2. Colonoscopy is recommended in the geriatric population to exclude malignancy or other underlying disease.

HEPATITIS A

Definition

A. Hepatitis A is an acute self-limited illness with inflammation of the liver caused by a viral infection. Hepatitis A virus (HAV) is spread by viral shedding. All cases of hepatitis A are reportable to the public health department.

B. The highest titers of HAV in the stool of infected patients occur 1–2 weeks before onset of illness (jaundice or elevation of liver enzymes), during which time patients are most likely to transmit infection. Risk subsequently diminishes and is minimal in the week after onset of jaundice. Few children younger than 6 years old have concomitant jaundice, whereas up to 70% of older children and adults will have jaundice. Fulminant hepatitis is rare, and chronic infectious and carrier states do not occur.

C. Duration of HAV infection is typically 8 weeks, but prolonged disease, as long as 6 months, can occur in 10%–15% of symptomatic patients especially in neonates and young children.

D. The major methods of prevention include improved sanitation of water sources, improved hygiene practice prior to food preparation and diaper changes, immunization with the hepatitis A vaccine, and administration of immune globulin (IG).

Incidence

A. From 30% to 35% of acute hepatitis cases in the United States are due to hepatitis A virus (HAV). In developing countries, where infection is endemic, most people are infected during the first decade of life. In United States the incidence of HAV has declined since 1995 due to the administration of the HAV vaccine.

B. Outbreak in custodial institutions accounts for about 10%–15% of reported HAV in the United States. No appreciable seasonal variation in incidence has been noted.

C. The incidence of mortality from HAV is 0%–1%. The single most important determinant of illness severity is age; a direct correlation between increasing age and the likelihood of adverse events is present.

Pathogenesis

A. HAV is a small, RNA enterovirus classified as a member of the picornavirus group. Viral replication depends on hepatocyte uptake and synthesis, and assembly occurs exclusively in liver cells. Transmission of HAV is person-to-person primarily by the fecal-oral route and parenterally. Incubation period is 15–50 days, with an average of 25–30 days.

B. Common-source food- and water-borne epidemics have occurred, including several caused by shellfish contaminated with human sewage. Nosocomial outbreaks have occurred as a result of shedding of HAV virus from infected, asymptomatic neonates, children, or adults.

Predisposing Factors

A. Ingestion of infected water, food, and shellfish

B. Close personal contact with an HAV-infected person
1. Contact with a child who attends a childcare center
2. Male homosexual activity
3. Vertical transmission from mother to fetus (limited)

C. Poor sanitation or personal hygiene

D. Crowded living conditions

E. Recent travel in developing countries where HAV is endemic

F. IV drug abuse

Common Complaints

A. Malaise

B. Anorexia

C. Nausea

D. Low-grade fever

Other Signs and Symptoms

A. Infants and children: mild, nonspecific, flulike symptoms without jaundice.

B. Adults: severe, prolonged course with fatigue, headache, vomiting, and symptoms noted above.

C. Icteric phase: tea-colored urine, clay-colored stool, jaundice, abdominal pain, pruritus, and enlarged liver.

D. Relapsing hepatitis A is more common in the elderly. There generally has been a protracted course of symptoms and a relapse of symptoms following an apparent resolution.

Subjective Data

A. Review duration, onset, and severity of symptoms, including specifics about urine or stool color changes.

B. Ask the patient about family members and sexual contacts with similar symptoms.

C. Review the patient's history of blood transfusions, IV drug use, and alcohol abuse.
D. Inquire about occupational exposure.
E. Ask the patient about recent international travel.
F. Review immunization status.
G. Review medications for a possible Tylenol overdose or Ecstasy use as a cause for acute drug-induced liver injury.

Physical Examination

A. Check temperature, pulse, respirations, blood pressure, and weight.
B. Inspect
  1. Note general appearance.
  2. Inspect the skin for slight jaundice or rash.
  3. Inspect mucus membranes and nail beds.
  4. Inspect eyes for yellow sclera.
C. Auscultate lung fields, all quadrants of the abdomen, and the heart.
D. Percuss the abdomen.
E. Palpate
  1. Palpate all quadrants of the abdomen for masses, liver tenderness, and hepatosplenomegaly (about 10% of cases).

Diagnostic Tests

A. Viral serology for typing HAV, IgG, and IgM. **Serum IgM presents at onset of illness and disappears within 4 months, generally indicating current or recent infection. However, it may persist for 6 months or longer. Presence of IgG anti-HAV antibodies without virus-specific IgM indicates past infection and immunity.**
B. Liver function studies, including ALT, AST, LDH, and alkaline phosphatase.
C. Bilirubin, direct and indirect.
D. CBC.
E. Prothrombin time.
F. Urinalysis: reveals proteinuria and bilirubinuria.
G. Imaging studies are usually not indicated for hepatitis A infection. An ultrasound may be used to exclude other pathology.

Differential Diagnoses

A. HAV
B. Mononucleosis
C. Cancer
D. Obstructive jaundice
E. Alcoholic hepatitis or cirrhosis
F. Hepatotoxic drug use
  1. Drug-induced liver injury (e.g., Tylenol, Ecstasy)
  2. Drug-induced hypersensitivity reaction (e.g., Sulfasalazine hypersensitivity)
G. Food poisoning
H. Exclusion of other hepatitis types
I. Cytomegalovirus
J. Acute HIV infection

Plan

A. General interventions
  1. Contact precautions are recommended for diapered and/or incontinent patients for 1 week after onset of symptoms.

2. Children and adults with acute HAV infection should be excluded from school, work, and childcare centers for 1 week after onset of illness.
3. Hepatitis is self-limiting and does not require therapy. Treatment is supportive.
   a. Limit activities secondary to malaise.
   b. Oral contraceptives and hormone replacement therapy should be stopped to avoid cholestasis.
   c. Alcohol consumption is not advised.
4. Encourage strict hand washing.
B. Patient teaching
1. See the Section III Patient Teaching Guide for this chapter, "Jaundice and Hepatitis."
2. Teach the patient that major methods for prevention are improved sanitation (e.g., of water sources and in food preparation) and personal hygiene.
3. Food and travel precautions include:
   a. Avoid uncontrolled water resources: use bottled water, boil water, or add iodine to inactivate the virus.
   b. Avoid raw shellfish.
   c. Avoid uncooked foods.
   d. All fruit should be washed and peeled.
C. Dietary management: Encourage optimum nutrition.
D. Pharmaceutical therapy
1. Immune globulin (IG) (Gammar): Preexposure administration is 0.02 mL/kg × 2 doses intramuscularly. HAV vaccine preexposure is preferred in all populations unless contraindicated.
2. Postexposure IG administration given intramuscularly within 2 weeks of HAV exposure is 80%–90% effective in preventing symptomatic infection.
   a. Time of exposure—2 weeks or less
      i. Younger than 12 months: 0.02 mL/kg of IG given IM into a large muscle. No more than 3 mL in one site should be given to small children and infants.
      ii. 12 months–40 years: Hepatitis A vaccine.
      iii. 41 years and older: 0.02 mL/kg IG given IM into a large muscle. No more than 5 mL should be administered into one site for an adult or large child.
   b. Postexposure prophylaxis with IG is recommended for the following:
      i. Household and sexual contacts of infected persons.
      ii. Newborn infants of HAV-infected mothers.
      iii. Childcare center staff, children, and their household contacts.
      iv. Students when transmission within school is documented.
      v. Staff in institutions and hospitals.
      vi. People who ingested HAV-contaminated food or water, within 2 weeks of last exposure.
3. Vaccines
   a. Two inactivated HAV vaccines, Havrix and Vaqta, are available in the United States.
   b. Twinrix is combination hepatitis A (Havrix) and hepatitis B (Engerix-B) vaccine available in the United States for ages 18 years or older. See Table 10.10.

4. HAV vaccine is recommended for the following:
   a. Children 2 years and older in defined and circumscribed communities with high endemic rates and/or periodic outbreaks of HAV infection.
   b. Patients with chronic liver disease.
   c. Homosexual and bisexual men.
   d. Users of injections and illicit drugs.
   e. Those with occupational risk of exposure, such as handlers of nonhuman primates and persons working with HAV in a laboratory setting.
   f. Travelers who need preexposure immunoprophylaxis.
   g. Patients with clotting-factor disorders such as hemophilia.
5. HAV vaccine is potentially indicated for the following:
   a. Childcare center staff and children.
   b. Patients and staff in custodial care institutions.
   c. Hospital personnel.
   d. Food handlers.
   e. Patients with hemophilia.

6. HAV vaccine may be administered simultaneously with other vaccines, but it should be given in a separate syringe and at a separate site.
7. The need for an additional hepatitis A booster beyond the 2-dose primary immunizations has not been established.
8. Immune response in immunocompromised patients such as HIV may be suboptimal. The vaccine is inactivated; therefore, no special precautions are needed when vaccinating immunocompromised patients.
9. Nausea and vomiting are treated by antiemetics.
10. Tylenol may be administered for fever and arthralgia but is strictly limited to a maximum dose of 3–4 g/day in adults.

Follow-up
A. Dehydration may require hospital admission.
B. Follow-up in 2 weeks for reevaluation.
C. Check for hepatitis B immunity and vaccinate.
D. Hepatitis A is reportable to the public health department.

TABLE 10.10 Dosages and Schedules for Hepatitis A Vaccines

A. HAVIRIX®

Licensed dosages and schedules for HAVRIX®[1]				
Age	Dose (ELISA units)[2]	Volume (mL)	No. of doses	Schedule (mos)[3]
12 mos–18 yrs	720	0.5	2	0, 6–12
≥ 19 years	1,440	1.0	2	0, 6–12

[1]Hepatitis A vaccine, inactivated, GlaxoSmithKline.
[2]Enzyme-linked immunosorbent assay units.
[3]0 months represents timing of the initial dose; subsequent numbers represent months after the initial dose.

B. VAQTA®

Licensed dosages and schedules for VAQTA®[1]				
Age	Dose (U.)[2]	Volume (mL)	No. of doses	Schedule (mos)[3]
12 mos–18 yrs	25	0.5	2	0, 6–18
≥ 19 years	50	1.0	2	0, 6–18

[1]Hepatitis A vaccine, inactivated, Merck & Co., Inc.
[2]Units.
[3]0 months represents timing of the initial dose; subsequent numbers represent months after the initial dose.

C. TWINRIX®

Licensed dosages and schedules for TWINRIX®[1]				
Age	Dose (ELISA units)[2]	Volume (mL)	No. of doses	Schedule[3]
≥ 18 yrs	720	1.0	3	0, 1, 6 mos
≥ 18 yrs	720	1.0	4	0, 7, 21–30 days + 12 mos[3]

[1]Combined hepatitis A and hepatitis B vaccine, inactivated, GlaxoSmithKline.
[2]Enzyme-linked immunosorbent assay units.
[3]This 4-dose schedule enables patients to receive 3 doses in 21 days; this schedule is used prior to planned exposure with short notice and requires a fourth dose at 12 months.

From Centers for Disease Control and Prevention: http://www.cdc.gov/hepatitis/HAV/HAVfaq.htm.

Consultation/Referral

A. Consult a physician if necessary.

Individual Considerations

A. Pregnancy
1. Pregnant women recently exposed to HAV should receive prophylactic gamma globulin.
2. HAV is an inactivated vaccine and is considered safe during pregnancy.
3. HAV infection during pregnancy is associated with increased risk of premature labor and delivery.

B. Pediatrics
1. In the United States, the highest rates for symptomatic HAV infection occur in children 5–14 years of age, and the lowest rates occur in children from birth to 4 years.
2. Children who have received HAV vaccine rarely have detectable anti-HAV IgM titers.
3. Risk of outbreak in childcare centers increases with the number of children under age 2 who wear diapers.

C. Adults: In the United States, the lowest rate of HAV infection is in people older than 40.

D. Geriatrics
1. The elderly have greater numbers of HAV antibodies, resulting in fewer cases.
2. Symptoms are usually vague. Fatigue; pruritus; and the classic symptoms of jaundice, hepatomegaly, and liver tenderness are commonly absent in the elderly.
3. Diagnostic test results in the elderly include elevated bilirubin, lower or normal transaminase and alkaline phosphatase, and normal ultrasonography.
4. Treatment is supportive. Corticosteroids may relieve symptoms but prolong the disease state due to prolonged viral replication.

HEPATITIS B

Definition

A. Hepatitis B is inflammation of the liver caused by hepatitis B virus (HBV). Acute HBV infection cannot be distinguished from other forms of acute viral hepatitis on the basis of clinical signs and symptoms or nonspecific laboratory findings. Acutely infected patients may be asymptomatic or symptomatic. The likelihood of developing symptoms of acute hepatitis is age dependent.

B. Chronic HBV infection is defined as the presence of hepatitis B surface antigen (HBsAg) in serum for at least 6 months or by the presence of HBsAg in a person who tests negative for antibody of the immunoglobulin (Ig) M subclass to hepatitis B core antigen (IgM anti-HBc).

C. HBV is the main cause of cirrhosis and hepatocellular carcinoma (HCC) worldwide. For selected candidates, liver transplantation currently seems to be the only viable treatment for the latest stages of hepatitis B.

D. Antiviral treatment may be effective in approximately one-third of the patients who receive it. Eight different genotypes (A through H) have been identified. The progression of the disease seems to be more accelerated, and the response to treatment with antiviral agents is less favorable for patients infected by genotype C compared with those infected by genotype B. Genotypes A or B have a better response to interferon (IFN) treatment compared with patients infected by genotype C or D.

Incidence

A. An estimated one-third of the global population has been infected with HBV. Approximately 350 million people are lifelong carriers, and only 2% spontaneously seroconvert annually. Of chronically infected patients, 15%–40% will develop cirrhosis, progressing to liver failure and/or HCC.

B. Acute hepatitis B occurs in 1–2 out of every 1,000 pregnancies in the United States, and chronic infection occurs in 5–15 out of every 1,000 pregnancies. The course of maternal HBV infections does not seem to be affected by coexistent pregnancy. However, premature labor and delivery is increased.

C. Chronic HBV infections with persistence of hepatitis B surface antigen (HBsAg) occur in as many as 90% of infants infected by perinatal transmission; in 30% of children 1–5 years old infected after birth; and in 5%–10% of older children, adolescents, and adults with HBV infection.

Pathogenesis

A. HBV is a hepadnavirus. HBV-related liver injury is largely caused by immune-mediated mechanisms mediated via cytotoxic T-lymphocyte lysis of infected hepatocytes. The virus is transmitted through blood or body fluids, such as wound exudates, semen, cervical secretions, and saliva that are HBsAg positive. It is not transmitted by the fecal-oral route or by water. Blood and serum contain the highest concentration of virus; saliva contains the lowest.

B. Incubation period is 45–160 days (2–5 months), with an average of 120 days. An infected person can infect others 4–6 weeks before symptoms appear and for an unpredictable time thereafter.

C. The production of antibodies against HBsAg confers protective immunity and can be detected in patients who have recovered from HBV or in those patients that have been vaccinated. The immunoglobulin M (IgM) subtype indicates an acute infection or reactivation. IgG subtype indicates chronic infection.

Predisposing Factors

A. Higher prevalence in blacks and other populations.
1. Hispanic origin
2. Asian origin
3. Alaskan Eskimos
4. Asian Pacific islanders
5. Australian aborigines

B. Sexual contact is the major mode of transmission.
1. High number of sexual partners
2. An early age of first intercourse
3. Homosexuality/bisexuality

C. IV drug use, sharing needles.

D. Work in health care profession.

E. Household exposure.

F. Perinatal exposure, by vertical infection.
G. Receiving blood transfusions or blood products, for hemophilia and hemodialysis.
H. Breast-feeding, by transmission in breast milk.
I. Staffing or residing in institutions.
J. International travel.
K. Incarceration in long-term correction facilities.
L. Percutaneous contact with inanimate objects contaminated with HBV; virus can survive 1 week or longer.

Common Complaints

A. The following symptoms occur in the acute phase of HBV.
   1. Anicteric hepatitis: asymptomatic (majority of patients)
   2. Icteric hepatitis: associated with a prodromal period
      a. Anorexia
      b. Nausea and vomiting
      c. Low-grade fever
      d. Myalgia
      e. Fatigue
      f. Aversion to food and cigarettes
      g. Intermittent, mild to moderate right upper quadrant and epigastric pain
   3. Hyperacute, acute, and subacute hepatitis symptoms
      a. Hepatic encephalopathy
      b. Somnolence
      c. Disturbances in sleep pattern
      d. Mental confusion
      e. Coma
B. The following symptoms occur in the chronic phase of HBV:
   1. Asymptomatic: may be healthy carriers without any evidence of active disease
   2. During the replicative state common symptoms are:
      a. Fatigue
      b. Anorexia
      c. Nausea
      d. Mild upper quadrant pain or discomfort
      e. Hepatic decompensation

Other Signs and Symptoms

A. In young children
   1. Jaundice and other symptoms may not be present.
   2. Symptoms may be prolonged and insidious compared with HAV.
B. Icteric phase (10 days after the appearance of constitutional symptoms and lasts for 1–3 months)
   1. Jaundice of sclera and skin
   2. Tea-colored urine
   3. Clay-colored stools, often precede jaundice
   4. Right upper quadrant tenderness
   5. Enlarged liver

Subjective Data

A. Review onset, duration, course, and severity of symptoms. Ask the patient for specifics about urine and stool color.
B. Ask the patient about other family members and sexual contacts with similar symptoms.
C. Discuss the patient's history of blood transfusions, IV drug use, and alcohol abuse.
D. Review the patient's occupational exposure.
E. Inquire about recent international travel.
F. Establish the patient's usual weight; note amount of any weight lost and over what length of time.
G. Review for a history of variceal bleeding.

Physical Examination

A. Check temperature, pulse, respirations, blood pressure, and weight.
B. Inspect
   1. Observe general appearance, muscle wasting, ascites, and peripheral edema.
   2. Inspect the skin for jaundice, palmar erythema, rash, spider nevi, spider angioma, and dehydration.
   3. Inspect the eyes for yellow sclera.
   4. Inspect the mucous membranes and nail beds.
   5. Evaluate for the presence of gynecomastia.
C. Auscultate
   1. Auscultate lung fields and the heart.
   2. Auscultate all quadrants of the abdomen.
D. Percuss abdomen.
E. Palpate
   1. Palpate all quadrants of the abdomen for masses, liver enlargement or tenderness, hepatomegaly and splenomegaly.
   2. Palpate the lymph nodes for lymphadenopathy.
   3. Palpate for testicular atrophy.

Diagnostic Tests

A. Diagnostic test for HBV antigens and antibodies (see Table 10.11).
B. CBC with differential.
C. Complete liver panel:
   1. AST/ALT
   2. Bilirubin
   3. Prothrombin time (PT)
   4. Albumin
D. Other viral infection markers: HCV and HDV.
E. Alkaline phosphatase.
F. Serum iron levels.
G. Gamma-glutamyl transpeptidase (GGT).
H. HBV genotype.
I. HBV DNA viral load.
J. Imaging:
   1. Abdominal ultrasound
   2. CT or MRI to help exclude biliary obstruction
K. Liver biopsy to assess the severity of disease.
L. Pregnancy testing for antiviral therapy.
M. Before oral antiviral therapy is introduced, all patients should be screened for HIV.

Differential Diagnoses

A. Hepatitis B
B. Exclusion of other types of hepatitis (A, C, D, E, viral or autoimmune hepatitis)
C. Infectious mononucleosis
D. Hepatotoxic drug ingestion, for example, chloramphenicol, acetaminophen, or methyldopa

TABLE 10.11 Diagnostic Tests for HBV Antigens and Antibodies

Factors to Be Tested	HBV Antigen or Antibody	Indication
HBsAg	Hepatitis B surface antigen	Detects acutely or chronically infected; antigen used in hepatitis B vaccine
Anti-HBs	Antibody to HBsAg	Identifies resolved HBV infections; determines immunity after immunization
HBeAg	Hepatitis B e antigen	Identifies at-risk of transmitting HBV
Anti-HBe	Antibody to HBeAg	Identifies lower-risk of transmitting HBV
Anti-HBc	Antibody to hepatitis B core antigen; IgM (HBcAg)	Identifies acute, resolved, or chronic HBV infection. Anti-HBc is not present after immunization.
IgM anti HBc	IgM antibody to HBcAg	Identifies acute or recent HBV infections (includes HBsAg-negative during the window phase of infection)

E. Carcinoma

F. Alcoholic cirrhosis

G. Hemochromatosis

H. Wilson's disease

Plan

A. General interventions:
   1. No specific therapy for acute HBV infection is available.
   2. Before any form of HBV therapy is started, and optimally at the first presentation, the patient needs to be provided with information about the natural history of chronic hepatitis B infection and the fact that most infections remain entirely without symptoms even in those with severe disease, so that there is a need for regular lifelong monitoring.

B. Patient teaching
   1. See the Section III Patient Teaching Guide for this chapter, "Jaundice and Hepatitis."
   2. Tell the patient to avoid sexual activity until he or she is free of HBsAg.
   3. History of anaphylactic reaction to common baker's yeast is a contraindication to HBV vaccination.
   4. There are no dietary restrictions with acute and chronic hepatitis (without cirrhosis). Decompensated cirrhosis, portal hypertension, or encephalopathy are prescribed:
      a. Low-sodium diet (1.5 g/day)
      b. High-protein diet (white-meat protein, e.g., pork, turkey, and fish)
      c. Fluid restriction of 1.5 L/day in the presence of hyponatremia

C. Pharmaceutical therapy
   1. Primary prevention includes vaccination of high-risk individuals including teens. Vaccination is up to 95% effective.
   2. HBV vaccine is recommended preexposure for the following groups:
      a. All infants: All major authorities recommend that all children receive a complete series of HBV immunizations during the first 18 months of life. Infants born to HbsAg-positive mothers

should begin receiving immunizations at birth (HBIG).
      b. Children at risk of acquiring HBV by person-to-person (horizontal) transmission.
      c. All adolescents.
      d. IV drug users.
      e. Sexually active heterosexuals with more than one sex partner in the previous 6 months or who have an STI.
      f. Health care workers and others at occupational risk.
      g. Residents and staff of institutions for developmentally disabled persons.
      h. Staff of nonresidential childcare centers.
      i. Patients undergoing hemodialysis.
      j. Patients with bleeding disorders who receive clotting factor concentrates.
      k. Household contacts and sexual partners of HBV carriers.
      l. Members of households with adoptees who are HBsAg positive.
      m. International travelers to areas of high or intermediate endemicity.
      n. Inmates of long-term correctional facilities.
   3. Hepatitis B vaccine can be given concurrently with other vaccines.
   4. Early prophylaxis is paramount after an HBsAg needle stick (see Table 10.12). H-BIG should be administered immediately, no later than 48 hours, after exposure. Postexposure prophylaxis HBV vaccine is recommended.
   5. Currently, interferon alfa-2b (Intron A) or alfa-2a (Roferon-A), pegylated IFN alfa-2a (Pegasys), lamivudine (Epivir), telbivudine (Tyzeka), adefovir dipivoxil (Hepsera), entecavir (Baraclude), and tenofovir (Viread) are the main treatment drugs approved globally (see Table 10.13).
      a. Lamivudine and telbivudine are not recommended as first-line agents in the treatment of HBV.
      b. Antivirals may be given as monotherapy or in combination during clinical trials.
      c. Many of the antivirals do not have pediatric dosages established.

d. All antivirals require close monitoring due to side effect profiles.

e. Dose adjustment is required in the presence of renal impairment, dialysis, and used in caution in patients with a history of pancreatitis.

D. Orthotopic liver transplantation (OLT) is the treatment of choice for patients with fulminant hepatic failure who do not recover and for patients with end-stage liver disease.

Follow-up

A. Laboratory monitoring:
1. Monitor liver function (ALT) every 3–6 months for active disease.
2. Monitor HBeAg every 3–6 months dependent on ALT levels.
3. Monitor CBC and creatinine every month (1–2 days prior to treatment).
4. Monitor HBV DNA every 3–6 months when the patient is on treatment in the reactivation phase.

B. Risk of exposure to HBsAg ceases when antigen disappears from bloodstream, usually within 6–8 weeks of infection. Repeated serum determinations of HBsAg can help define when precautions may be relaxed.

C. Laboratory, physical examination, and psychosocial evaluation is required for antiviral therapy.

D. The American Association for the Study of Liver Disease (AASLD) recommends HCC surveillance using ultrasound in the following types of patients with chronic HBV.
1. Asian men over the age of 40 and Asian women over the age of 50
2. All patients with cirrhosis, regardless of age
3. Patients with a family history of HCC; any age
4. Africans over the age of 20
5. Any individual with HBV/HIV coinfection

Consultation/Referral

A. Patients with persistently elevated serum transaminase concentrations (exceeding twice the upper limits of normal), as well as those with elevated serum alpha-fetoprotein concentrations or abnormal ultrasounds, should be referred to a gastroenterologist for further management.

TABLE 10.12 Postexposure Hepatitis B Prophylaxis After Percutaneous Exposure

Exposed Person	HBsAg Negative	Unknown or Not Tested	Treatment When Source Is HBsAg Positive
Unimmunized	Initiate hepatitis B vaccine series	Initiate hepatitis B vaccine series	Administer 1 dose of HBIG 0.06 mL/kg IM; then initiate hepatitis B vaccine series
Previously immunized: known responder	No treatment	No treatment	No treatment
Previously immunized: known nonresponder	No treatment	If known high-risk source, treat as if source was HBsAg positive	Administer 1 dose of HBIG 0.06 mL/kg IM; then initiate reimmunization or HBIG (2 doses) hepatitis B vaccine series
Previously immunized: response unknown	No treatment	Test exposed person for anti-HBs. If adequate, no treatment. If inadequate, administer vaccine booster	Test exposed person for anti-HBs and administer vaccine booster dose. 2 additional doses should be administered to complete a 3-dose reimmunization series

---

TABLE 10.13 Comparisons of Approved Treatments for Chronic Hepatitis B

	HBeAg Positive Normal ALT	HBeAg Negative Positive Chronic Hepatitis	HBeAg Negative Chronic Hepatitis
IFN or peginterferon alfa	No therapy	Indicated	Indicated
Lamivudine	No therapy	Indicated: high rate of resistance	Indicated: high rate of resistance
Adefovir	No therapy	Indicated	Indicated
Entecavir	No therapy	Indicated	Indicated
Telbivudine	No therapy	Indicated: high rate of resistance	Indicated: high rate of resistance
Tenofovir	No therapy	Indicated	Indicated

Individual Considerations

A. Pregnancy
1. No adverse effect on developing fetus has been observed when pregnant women are vaccinated against HBV.
2. Many antivirals are pregnancy Category X drugs.
3. Pregnancy and lactation are not a contraindication to vaccination.
4. Prenatal HBsAg testing of all pregnant women is recommended to identify newborns who require immediate postexposure prophylaxis.
5. Breast-feeding by an HBsAg-positive mother poses no additional risk for acquisition of HBV infection by infant.

B. Pediatrics
1. Infants born to HBsAg-positive mothers need no special care other than removal of maternal blood by a gloved attendant and standard universal precautions.
2. All infants, including those who are premature, born to HbsAg-positive mothers need HBIG within 12 hours of birth.
3. More than 90% of infants infected perinatally will develop chronic HBV infection.
4. Adoptees from countries where HBV infection is endemic should be screened for HBsAg. If child is HBsAg positive, previously unimmunized family members and other household contacts should be vaccinated, preferably before adoption.
5. Persons infected as infants or young children are at higher risk of death due to liver disease than those infected as adults.
6. Interferon-α has limited effectiveness in chronic infections acquired during early childhood.

C. Adults
1. Most HBV infections are acquired in adolescence or adulthood, largely as a result of IV drug use, sexual contact, or occupational or household exposure. HBV infection is associated with other sexually transmitted diseases, including syphilis.
2. Patients who have received a blood transfusion should refrain from blood donation for 6 months, the incubation period for HBV. Blood should never be donated if the patient is a hepatitis B carrier or was infected with hepatitis C.

D. Geriatrics
1. The elderly have fewer cases of HBV due to diminished immune response; however, they tend to be asymptomatic HBV carriers.
2. Those who do develop the disease have a greater tendency to deteriorate into chronic liver failure or chronic hepatitis.

Resources

American Association for the Study of Liver Diseases: www.aasld.org
American Liver Foundation: www.liverfoundation.org
Centers for Disease Control and Prevention: www.cdc.gov/hepatitis
Hepatitis and HIV: www.hivandhepatitis.com
Hepatitis B Foundation: www.hepb.org
Hepatitis Foundation International: www.hepfi.org
Immunization Action Coalition: www.immunize.org

National Institute of Diabetes and Digestive and Kidney Diseases: www2.niddk.nih.gov
United Network for Organ Sharing: www.unos.org

HEPATITIS C

Definition

A. Hepatitis C is an inflammation of the liver caused by the hepatitis C virus. Hepatitis C virus (HCV) has signs and symptoms often undistinguishable from those of hepatitis A (HAV) or hepatitis B (HBV). The disease tends to be asymptomatic to mild and has an insidious onset. Acute fulminate infection is rare. The major feature of HCV is its propensity to become chronic. Persistent infection occurs in at least 70%–80% of patients, even in the absence of biochemical evidence of liver disease. Approximately 65%–70% of patients develop chronic hepatitis, and 20% develop cirrhosis.

B. Multiple (6) HCV genotypes and subtypes exist. The genotype is a major factor in the effectiveness of the patient's response to therapy. Approximately 50% of patients infected with genotype 1 and approximately 80% of patients with genotypes 2 and 3 achieve a SVR. Combination therapy with pegylated interferon-alfa and ribavirin results in sustained virologic response (SVR). SVR is defined as undetectable HCV RNA 12 months or more after treatment cessation.

C. The development of chronic hepatitis and its complications increase with several factors including older age at acquisition, HIV infection, excessive alcohol consumption, and male gender. Among children, live disease progression appears to be accelerated with comorbid conditions including cancer, iron overload, thalassemia, or coinfection with HIV.

D. HCV is the leading cause of nonalcoholic hepatic failure and cirrhosis, and the cause of 90% of post-transfusion hepatitis. Primary hepatocellular carcinoma also occurs in these patients.

Incidence

A. In 2005, the prevalence of acute symptomatic HCV infection in the United States is estimated at 0.2 per 100,000. Approximately 1.3% of the general U.S. population has chronic HCV. The virus occurs in all age groups. Seroprevalence rates among individuals vary according to their associated risk factors. The highest rates, between 60% and 90%, occur in persons with large or repeated direct percutaneous exposure to blood or blood products, such as IV drug users and patients with hemophilia who have received multiple blood transfusions.

B. Seroprevalence among pregnant women in the United States has been estimated at 1%–2%. Maternal-fetal (vertical) transmission is only 5% from women who are HCV RNA positive at the time of delivery. Maternal coinfection with HIV has been associated with increased risk of perinatal transmission of HCV RNA.

C. Serum anti-HCV antibody and HCV RNA have been detected in colostrum. However, although only a limited number of patients have been studied, the rate of transmission among breast-fed infants is the same as among bottle-fed infants.

D. More than 20% of adults with chronic infection progresses to cirrhosis an average of 20 years after their initial infection. Patients with cirrhosis have a secondary risk of portal hypertension, liver failure, and other complications. HCV is the leading indication for liver transplantation among adults in the United States.

E. Hepatocellular carcinoma (HCC) is diagnosed an average of 30 years after initial HCV infection in 1%–5% of patients, most of whom have underlying cirrhosis.

Pathogenesis

A. HCV is a small, single-stranded RNA virus with a lipid envelope and is a member of the Flavivirus family. Infection is spread primarily by parenteral exposure to blood and blood products from HCV-infected persons. In the United States, the current risk of HCV infection following blood transfusion is estimated at 0.1% or less because of exclusion of high-risk individuals from the pool of blood donors and screening for HCV. Sexual transmission of HCV is uncommon except with high-risk behavior.

B. The incubation period averages 6–7 weeks, with a range of 2 weeks to 6 months. The time from exposure to the development of viremia generally is 1–2 weeks.

Predisposing Factors

All people with HCV-RNA in their blood are considered to be infectious. The following groups are at high risk for HCV infection and should be tested:

A. IV drug users who have shared needles.

B. Intranasal cocaine users, presumably resulting from epistaxis and shared equipment.

C. Hemophiliacs, hemodialysis patients, and those who received blood transfusions before 1992.

D. Health care workers with percutaneous exposures.

E. Individuals with multiple sexual partners.

F. Transmission among contacts living with infected persons may occur with percutaneous or mucosal exposure to blood.

G. Infants of infected mothers, by vertical transmission.

H. HCV is more common in males than females.

I. Tattooing, body piercing, and acupuncture with unsterile equipment.

Common Complaints

A. Malaise

B. Anorexia

C. Nausea

D. Myalgia

Other Signs and Symptoms

A. Jaundice is rare in acute phase (25%).

B. Hepatomegaly is present in one-third of patients with an acute infection.

C. Ascites.

D. Spider nevi.

Subjective Data

A. Review duration, onset, and severity of symptoms.

B. Ask the patient about other family members and sexual contacts with similar symptoms.

C. Review the patient's history of blood transfusions, IV drug use, and alcohol abuse.

D. Ask the patient about occupational exposure.

E. Ask about high-risk sexual practices.

Physical Examination

A. Check temperature, pulse, respirations, blood pressure, and weight.

B. Inspect
   1. Observe general appearance, muscle wasting, edema, and demeanor. Administer a depression self-assessment tool at each visit when on HCV therapy.
   2. Inspect the skin for jaundice, rash, dehydration, palmar erythema, excoriations, spider nevi, and tattoos/piercings.
   3. Inspect the eyes for yellow sclera.
   4. Inspect mucous membranes and nail beds for clubbing and cyanosis.
   5. Inspect for gynecomastia and small testes.

C. Auscultate
   1. Auscultate lung fields and heart.
   2. Auscultate all quadrants of the abdomen and evaluate for abdominal bruit.

D. Percuss the abdomen.

E. Palpate
   1. Palpate all quadrants of the abdomen for masses; liver enlargement or tenderness; characteristics of cirrhosis; and hepatosplenomegaly, which occurs in about 10% of cases.
   2. Palpate the lymph nodes for lymphadenopathy and enlarged parotid.

Diagnostic Tests

A. Laboratory tests:
   1. Immunoglobulin (Ig) G antibody enzyme immunoassays for HCV and NAA tests to detect HCV RNA
   2. HCV genotyping
   3. HCV viral load: quantitative assay used as a prognostic indicator for patients undergoing antiviral therapy
   4. ALT and AST
   5. Hepatitis A IgM and IgG
   6. Hepatitis B surface antigen and antibody, core antibody
   7. CMV IgM and IgG (and/or CMV in urine culture)
   8. Epstein-Barr virus IgM and IgG
   9. HIV IgG enzyme-linked immunoassay (ELISA)
   10. Alpha-fetoprotein

B. Ultrasonography is used for monitoring HCV-related complications.

C. Liver biopsy is the most accurate method of evaluating the extent of HCV-related liver disease. Liver biopsy is the gold standard for determining histologic grade and stage of fibrosis/cirrhosis. The *absolute* requirement for a liver biopsy prior to the institution of medication therapy is currently under discussion. For patients with genotypes 2 and 3, the likelihood of response to therapy is so high that the benefits of treatment may outweigh the risk of biopsy and histological considerations.

D. Prior to the institution/during antiviral therapy perform the following tests:

1. CBC with platelets.
2. Viral load.
3. Liver function (ALT/AST).
4. Pregnancy test.
5. Thyroid profile.
6. Blood glucose/A1C.
7. Consider a dilated retinal examination.
8. Consider a stress test.
9. Screen for alcohol abuse, drug abuse, and/or depression.

Differential Diagnoses

A. Hepatitis C
B. Hepatitis A
C. Hepatitis B
D. Alcoholic liver disease
E. Drug toxicities
F. Opportunistic infections associated with HIV infection

Plan

A. Patient teaching
   1. See the Section III Patient Teaching Guide for this chapter, "Jaundice and Hepatitis."
   2. Warn the patient of the possibility of transmission to others, and tell the patient to refrain from donating blood, organs, tissues, or semen and from sharing toothbrushes and razors.
   3. All patients with chronic HCV should be immunized against Hepatitis A and Hepatitis B.
   4. Counsel the patient to avoid hepatotoxic medications and alcohol.
   5. Immunoprophylaxis for postexposure prophylaxis with immune globulin is not recommended.
   6. Patients and their spouses should be counseled to not become pregnant while on therapy and for 6 months after the completion of treatment.
B. Pharmaceutical therapy is aimed at inhibiting HCV replication and eradicating infection. Response to treatment varies depending on the HCV genotype. All treatment regimens are associated with adverse events including flulike symptoms, hematologic abnormalities, and neuropsychiatric symptoms.

   The FDA approves alpha Interferon (IFN) or pegylated IFN *alone* or peginterferon-alfa *in combination* with ribavirin for the treatment of chronic HCV in adults. IFN stimulates the production of another protein that inhibits viral replication. Improvements are not typically sustained after monotherapy is discontinued. The use of ribavirin in combination with IFN is more effective than either drug alone and provides a sustained response.
   1. Interferon alfa-2b (Intron A)
      a. Adults: 3 million IU subcutaneous 3 times a week for 12 months.
      b. The FDA has approved the use of non-pegylated interferon-alfa-2b in combination with ribavirin for treatment of HCV infection in children 3–17 years of age. Pediatrics: 3 million IU/m^2 subcutaneous/week administered with ribavirin (Rebetol, Copegus). Rebetron is a kit that contains ribavirin and IFN alpha-2b.
   2. Interferon alfa-2a (Roferon)

      a. Adults: 3 million IU subcutaneous 3 times a week.
      b. Pediatric dose has not been established.
   3. Interferon alfacon-1 (Infergens)
      a. Adults: 9 mcg subcutaneous 3 times a week.
      b. Pediatric dose has not been established.
   4. Pegylated interferon alfa-2a (Pegasys) and alfa-2b (PEG-Intron). Pegasys uses a standard dosage regardless of the patient's weight, whereas PEG-Intron uses weight-based dosing. Pediatric dosages have not been established for either pegylated IFN.
      a. Adults: Pegasys 180 mcg subcutaneous every week for monotherapy or combined with ribavirin.
      b. PEG-Intron monotherapy: 1.5 mcg/kg/wk subcutaneous for 1 year.
      c. PEG-Intron in combination with oral ribavirin: 1.5 mg/kg/wk subcutaneous for 1 year.
   5. Refer Table 10.14 for Ribavirin dosing.
   6. Manage side effects with therapeutic agents related to symptoms. For management of neutropenia dose reduction of Ribavirin is required.

Follow-up

A. Test the patient within 5–6 weeks after onset of hepatitis; 80% of patients are positive for serum anti-HCV antibody.
B. Persons with chronic HCV infections should be vaccinated against hepatitis A and B, unless they previously have been demonstrated to be nonsusceptible.
C. Children with chronic infection should be screened periodically for chronic hepatitis with serum liver function tests because of their potential long-term risk for chronic liver disease. Definitive recommendations on frequency have not been established.
D. Monitor for mental dysfunction related to IFN including depression, psychosis, aggressive behavior, hallucinations, violent behavior, suicidal ideation, suicide attempt, and homicidal ideation (rare) even without previous history of psychiatric illness.
E. Monitor for side effects related to IFN and Ribavirin (see Table 10.15).

Consultation/Referral

A. Referrals include gastroenterologist, psychiatrist, endocrinologist, neurologist, hematologist, dietician, and social workers.
B. Patients that are coinfected with HBV or HIV or have end-stage renal disease should be referred out for treatment.
C. Children with severe disease or histologically advanced pathology (bridging necrosis or active cirrhosis) should be referred to a specialist in the management of chronic HCV infection.
D. Children with persistently elevated serum transaminase concentrations, or those exceeding twice the upper limits of normal, should be referred to a gastroenterologist for further management.

Individual Considerations

A. Pregnancy
   1. No data currently exist to support counseling a woman against pregnancy.

TABLE 10.14 Ribavirin Dosing for Pediatrics and Adults

Dose/Age	Weight	Dosage Information Based on Genotype
Rebetol administered with IFN alfa-2b < 3 years	N/A	Dosage not established
Rebetol administered with IFN alfa-2b ≥ to 3 years	≤ 25 kg and unable to swallow capsules	15 mg/kg/dose po divided bid with meals. Treatment duration is 24 wk for Genotype 2/3 or 48 wk for Genotype 1
Rebetol administered with IFN alfa-2b ≥ to 3 years	25–36 kg	200 mg po bid with meals. Treatment duration is 24 wk for Genotype 2/3 or 48 wk for Genotype 1
Rebetol administered with IFN alfa-2b ≥ to 3 years	37–49 kg	200 mg po every AM and 400 mg po every PM Treatment duration is 24 wk for Genotype 2/3 or 48 wk for Genotype 1
Rebetol administered with IFN alfa-2b ≥ to 3 years	50–61 kg	400 mg po bid. Treatment duration is 24 wk for Genotype 2/3 or 48 wk for Genotype 1
Rebetol administered with IFN alfa-2b ≥ to 3 years	> 62 kg	Administer as in adults. Treatment duration is 24 wk for Genotype 2/3 or 48 wk for Genotype 1
Rebetol administered with IFN alfa-2b Adults	< 75 kg	400 mg po every AM and 600 mg po every PM Treatment duration is 24 wk for Genotype 2/3 or 48 wk for Genotype 1
Rebetol administered with IFN alfa-2b Adults	> 75 kg	600 mg po bid. Treatment duration is 24 wk for Genotype 2/3 or 48 wk for Genotype 1
Copegus administered with peginterferon alfa-2a	≤ 75 kg	1,000 mg/day po divided bid with meals for 48 wk based on Genotype 1/4
Copegus administered with peginterferon alfa-2a	> 75 kg	1,200 mg/day po divided bid with meals for 48 wk based on Genotype 1/4
Copegus administered with peginterferon alfa-2a	Weight not defined	800 mg/day po divided bid with meals for 24 wk based on Genotype 2/3

Note. po = by mouth; bid = twice a day.

TABLE 10.15 Side Effects to IFN and Ribavirin Therapies

Side Effects Related to IFN	Side Effects Related to Ribavirin
Flulike symptoms	Hemolytic anemia (dose related)
Marrow suppression (especially leukopenia and thrombocytopenia)	Chest congestion
Autoimmune disorders especially thyroiditis	Dry cough
Hair loss	Dyspnea
Rash	Rash
Diarrhea	Diarrhea
Sleep disorders	Pruritus
Visual disorders including retinal hemorrhages	Gout
Weight loss	Nausea
Seizures	Sinus disorders
Hearing loss	Teratogenicity
Pancreatitis	
Interstitial pneumonitis	
Injection site reactions	

2. Routine serologic testing of pregnant women for HCV infection is not recommended.

3. According to current guidelines of the U.S. Public Health Service, maternal HCV infection is not a contraindication to breast-feeding. HCV-positive mothers should consider abstaining from breast-feeding if their nipples are cracked or bleeding.

4. Ribavirin is a pregnancy Class X drug with abortifacients protential.

5. IFN is a pregnancy Class C drug and should be used only if the benefits outweigh the risk to the fetus. IFN is a pregnancy Category X when combined with Ribavirin.

B. Pediatrics

1. Serologic testing for anti-HCV antibodies in children born to women previously identified to be HCV infected is recommended because approximately 5% acquire the infection. Duration of passive maternal antibody in infants is unknown. Testing for anti-HCV antibodies should not be performed until after 12 months of age.

2. Exclusion of children with HCV infections from out-of-home childcare centers is not indicated.

3. The FDA does not approve interferon-α for children under age 18.

4. The need for testing for alpha-fetoprotein concentration and for abdominal ultrasonography in children has not been determined.

5. Routine serologic testing of adoptees, either domestic or international, is not recommended.

C. Adults

1. Infected persons with steady partners do not need to change their sexual practices. However, they should be informed of the possible risk of transmission and of what precautions to use to prevent transmission.

2. Persons with multiple partners should be advised to reduce the number of partners and to use condoms to prevent transmission.

3. The best means of limiting transfusion-associated HCV is to rely exclusively on volunteer rather than commercial blood donors and to screen donors for anti-HCV antibodies.

D. Geriatrics: There are fewer cases of HCV in the elderly than in other age groups. However, they tend to develop chronic hepatitis or hepatic failure.

Resources

American Association for the Study of Liver Diseases: www.aasld.org

American Liver Foundation: www.liverfoundation.org

Centers for Disease Control and Prevention: www.cdc.gov/hepatitis

Hepatitis and HIV: www.hivandhepatitis.com

Hepatitis Foundation International: www.hepfi.org

Immunization Action Coalition: www.immunize.org

National Institute of Diabetes and Digestive and Kidney Diseases: www2.niddk.nih.gov

United Network for Organ Sharing: www.unos.org

HERNIAS, ABDOMINAL

Definition

A hernia is the protrusion of a peritoneum-lined sac through some defect in the abdominal wall. Abdominal wall hernias are the most common surgical procedure. Hernias are a leading cause of disability and work loss. Types include the following:

A. Umbilical hernia: occurs when the intestinal muscles fail to close around the umbilicus, allowing the omentum and/or intestines to protrude into the weaker area.

B. Incisional hernia: caused by a defect in the abdominal musculature that develops after a surgical incision.

C. Epigastric hernia: protrusion of fat or omentum through the linea alba between the umbilicus and the xiphoid. Epigastric hernias are generally less than 2 cm in diameter.

D. Diastasis recti: acquired hernia most often due to pregnancy and obesity. The right and left rectus muscles separate, but there is no facial defect.

Incidence

A. Umbilical hernias are more common in African American infants, women, and the elderly. This type of hernia has a higher risk of incarceration and strangulation and therefore a greater mortality because the large bowel is frequently entrapped.

B. Epigastric hernias are most common in men 20–50 years old.

C. Incisional hernias typically are noted in the early postoperative period; however, there is an increase in incisional hernias during pregnancy. In addition to hernias, separation of the recti abdominis muscles (diastasis recti) is often caused by pregnancy or obesity.

Pathogenesis

A. Incisional hernias are due to failure of fascial tissues to heal and close.

B. Epigastric hernias are defects in the abdominal midline between the umbilicus and the xyphoid process. They are usually related to a congenital weakness, increased intra-abdominal pressure, surrounding muscle weakness, or chronic abdominal wall strain.

C. An umbilical hernia is caused by failure of the umbilical ring to obliterate after birth. In the infant, the umbilical ring often closes spontaneously within the first 1–2 years of life. Increased abdominal pressure or congenital defects cause abdominal hernias that allow abdominal contents to protrude through the opening defect.

Predisposing Factors

A. Congenital predisposition

B. Female gender

C. Obesity

D. Multiparity

E. Cirrhosis and ascites

F. Trauma or straining

G. African American ancestry and infancy

H. Chronic cough; can precipitate or worsen herniation

I. Previous abdominal surgery

J. Straining, coughing, and sneezing in infancy

K. Straining with chronic constipation

L. Incisional hernia factors
1. Smoking
2. Connective tissue disorder
3. Infection
4. Malnutrition
5. Immunosuppressive medications

Common Complaints
A. Bulge of abdomen or of a previous scar
B. Symptoms aggravated by cough and straining
C. Varying degrees of discomfort

Other Signs and Symptoms
A. Incisional: bulge through incision wall (may be intermittent).
B. Epigastric: small, usually painless subcutaneous mass.
C. Umbilical
   1. Adult: vague, intermittent pain; palpable mass.
   2. Infant: vomiting and irritability.
D. Reducible or irreducible: Signs and symptoms are related to the degree of pressure of their contents rather than to size. Most patients are asymptomatic or complain of only mild pain.
E. Strangulated: colicky abdominal pain, nausea, vomiting, abdominal distension, hyper-peristalsis

Subjective Data
A. Review onset, duration, and course of symptoms.
B. Ask the patient about previous abdominal surgeries, wound infection, and pregnancies.
C. Review history of straining, trauma, or physical labor.
D. Determine if the patient has signs and symptoms of strangulation of entrapped bowel: pain, nausea, vomiting, distension, and fever.
E. Determine if the patient can reduce hernia.
F. Ask the patient whether the hernia is enlarging and uncomfortable.
G. Review the patient's bowel history, specifically constipation.
H. Review the patient's history for chronic obstructive pulmonary disease/chronic cough.
I. Review the patient's history for symptoms of obstructive uropathy.
J. Review how the hernia affects the patient's activities of daily living (ADLs).

Physical Examination
Examination is the same for all types of abdominal hernias. Perform exam while the patient is standing and supine. History and physical examination are the best means of diagnosing hernias.

A. Check temperature, pulse, respirations, and blood pressure.
B. Inspect
   1. Inspect contour and symmetry of the abdomen for bulges or masses. The bulge may be asymmetric.
   2. Inspect irreducible hernias for discoloration, edema, and ascites.
   3. Assess for hernia:
      a. Have the patient perform Valsalva's maneuver while standing.
      b. Have the patient lie supine, lift head from exam table, and then bear down to tense abdomen.
C. Auscultate all quadrants of the abdomen for bowel sounds.
D. Percuss liver, spleen, and abdomen.
E. Palpate
   1. Palpate the entire abdomen for masses, hepatomegaly, and ascites. Umbilical hernias may be obscured by subcutaneous fat.
   2. Palpate the groin.
   3. Palpate the hernia, to try to gently reduce it.

Diagnostic Tests
A. None is required if the hernia is easily reducible (depending on the type of hernia).
B. CBC: WBC increased, HCT increased.
C. Electrolytes: Na⁺ increased or decreased.
D. Abdominal radiography: reveals abnormally high levels of gas in bowel.
E. Ultrasonography, if strangulation is suspected.
F. CT scan of the abdomen and pelvic may be indicated.

Differential Diagnoses
A. Abdominal hernia
B. Diastasis recti
C. Ascites
D. Abdominal wall tumor or cyst

Plan
A. Patient teaching
   1. Discuss the hernia and available options for treatment.
   2. Teach the patient signs and symptoms of strangulation.
   3. Instruct the patient to refrain from heavy lifting.
   4. Advise the patient to wear a support garment.
B. Medical and surgical management
   1. Try to reduce hernia unless strangulated. See the Section II Procedure, "Hernia Reduction (Inguinal/Groin)."
      a. Easily reducible: abdominal contents can be easily returned to their original compartment. Allows symptomatic relief.
      b. Incarcerated: cannot be returned to its original compartment. The incarcerated tissue may be bowel, omentum, or other abdominal contents.
      c. Strangulated: surgical emergency—blood supply to the herniated tissue is compromised.
   2. Do not try to reduce strangulated hernias, because reduction can cause gangrenous bowel to enter peritoneal cavity.
   3. A truss fits snugly over a hernia to prevent abdominal contents from entering the hernial sac. It does not cure a hernia and is used only when the patient is not a surgical candidate.
   4. Umbilical hernia repair is best performed under general anesthesia in children.
   5. Surgery may be done laparoscopically or through an open procedure and by sutured or mesh repair depending on the age of the person, type and size of the hernia, and the presence of strangulation.

Follow-up
A. Instruct the patient to call the office if fever or severe pain occur. Otherwise, no follow-up is required unless for postoperative repair. Postoperative follow-up is with the physician who performed the surgery.

Consultation/Referral
Consult a physician if the patient has abdominal tenderness, discoloration, or edema at the site; fever; or signs of bowel obstruction.

A. Pregnancy
   1. Incisional hernias are more common during pregnancy because of increased intra-abdominal pressure.
   2. Bowel obstruction secondary to previous scarring may also be seen and is most common when the uterus emerges from the pelvis early in the second trimester, when the uterus is maximally distended at term, and in immediate puerperium when the uterus promptly decreases in size.
B. Pediatrics
   1. Infants with umbilical hernias require no special treatment because the majority of these hernias close by the fifth year.
   2. The infant's abdomen should be soft. Masses may be due to enlargement of tumors or liver. Liver is normally felt 1–3 cm below right costal margin.
   3. Tell caregivers that the umbilicus normally everts when a baby cries. However, they should report if the lump becomes large or irreducible, particularly if the baby is vomiting. These signs indicate strangulation and the need for urgent surgery.

HERNIAS, PELVIC

Definition

A hernia is the protrusion of a peritoneum-lined sac through some defect from one anatomical space to another. As shown in Figure 10.3, there are three types of pelvic (inguinal) hernias distinguished by presentation:

A. Indirect: protrudes through internal inguinal ring; can remain in canal, exit external ring, or pass into scrotum; unilateral or bilateral
B. Direct: protrudes through external inguinal ring; located in region of Hesselbach's triangle; rarely enters scrotum
C. Femoral: protrudes through femoral ring, femoral canal, and fossa ovalis

Incidence

A. Indirect inguinal hernias are the most common type of hernia. They affect both sexes, but most often are seen in children and young males (7:1 male-to-female ratio). Incidence increases with age.
B. Direct inguinal hernias are less common than indirect inguinal hernias. They occur more often in males and are more common over age 40.
C. Femoral hernias are the least common type of hernia. They are rarely seen in children and occur more often in females (1.8:1 female-to-male ratio). Right-side presentation is more common than left.
D. Among inguinal hernias, a sliding component is found in 3%; they are overwhelmingly on the left side (left-to-right ratio, 4.5:1). Sliding hernias are much more common in men than in women, and the predominance increases with age. Female infants have a high incidence of sliding tub, ovary, or broad ligament hernias.
E. Primary perineal hernias occur most often in elderly multiparous women.

Pathogenesis

Pelvic hernias occur because there is a potential space for protrusion—commonly of the bowel, but occasionally of the omentum.

A. Indirect and direct hernias arise along the course that the testicle travels as it exits the abdomen and enters the scrotum during intrauterine life. Indirect hernias may be due to a congenital defect in which the processus vaginalis remains patent.
B. Femoral hernias occur at the fossa ovalis, where the femoral artery exits the abdomen.

Predisposing Factors

A. Pregnancy
B. Straining
C. Age
D. Obesity
E. Gender
F. Repetitive stress/hard physical labor
G. Congenital defect

Common Complaints

A. Bulging or swelling localized in the groin or scrotum
B. Dull ache in lower abdomen or groin
C. Swelling of labia majora in women

Other Signs and Symptoms

A. Ability to reduce hernia
B. Exacerbation on standing, straining, or coughing
C. Strangulation:
   1. Colicky abdominal pain
   2. Nausea or vomiting
   3. Hyperperistalsis
   4. Fever
   5. Edema
   6. Discoloration
   7. Tenderness
D. Infants:
   1. Distress
   2. Vomiting
   3. Poor feeding

Subjective Data

A. Review time of onset, duration, and course of hernia, and swelling.
B. Review any symptoms and quality of pain. Outright pain with hernias is unusual, and its presence should raise the possibility of incarceration or strangulation.
C. Ask the patient about history of straining, trauma, physical labor, and pregnancy.
D. Inquire about symptoms of obstruction or strangulation of entrapped bowel: pain, nausea, and vomiting. Groin pain and tenderness are generally absent in strangulated femoral hernias.
E. Determine if the patient can reduce the hernia.
F. Review irritating (e.g., exercise, straining, cough) and alleviating factors.
G. Review bowel habits, particularly constipation.
H. Evaluate history of COPD and cough.

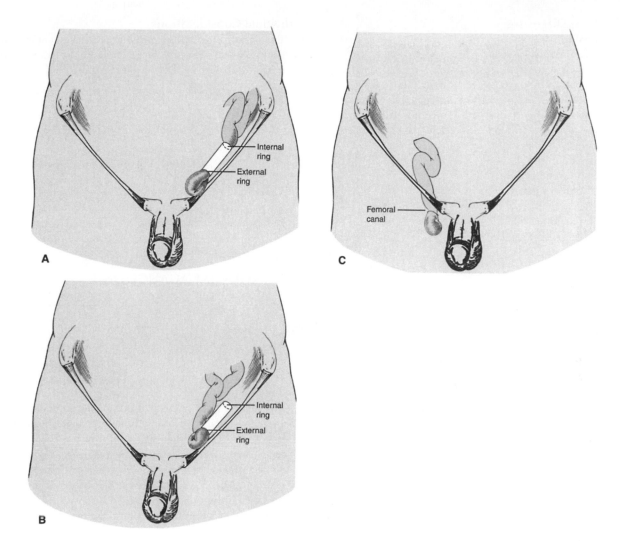

Figure 10.3 Pelvic hernias. A. Indirect hernia comes down canal and touches the fingertip on exam. B. Direct hernia bulges anteriorly, pushes against the side of the finger on exam. C. Femoral hernia protrudes through femoral ring, femoral canal, and fossa ovalis, so the inguinal canal is empty on exam.

Physical Examination

Physical examination is same for all types of hernias and is directed at determining the type of hernia and whether it is reducible, incarcerated, or strangulated. Perform the exam while the patient is standing and supine. Palpation is best done with the patient standing.

A. Check temperature, pulse, respirations, and blood pressure.
B. Inspect
  1. Inspect for discoloration and edema of the herniated area.
  2. Inspect for visible hernia. Instruct the patient to perform Valsalva's maneuver to increase intra-abdominal pressure.
  3. Transillumination of the scrotum to evaluate any bowel contents.
  4. Inspect for the presence of ascites.
C. Auscultate abdomen for bowel sounds.
D. Palpate
  1. Palpate the groin for lymphadenopathy, masses, and tenderness.

  a. Males: Using the second or third finger, invaginate the scrotal skin, with and without cough and strain. There will be some degree of pressure with this maneuver, but a true hernia can typically be felt as a "silky" impulse tapping against the finger. Palpate the scrotum: scrotal lump is either soft or unusually firm.
  b. Females: Visually examine for a bulge, and then place two or three fingers across the inguinal canal and ask the patient to bear down or cough to elicit the characteristic bulge or impulse. Palpate the labia for swelling: either soft or unusually firm.

Diagnostic Tests

A. History and physical examination remain the best means of diagnosing hernias.
B. Ultrasonography for abdominal masses and strangulation.
C. MRI appears to be able to differentiate inguinal and femoral hernias with a high sensitivity.
D. Sigmoidoscopy is not recommended as a screening test.

Differential Diagnoses

A. Inguinal or pelvic hernia
B. Acute conditions include:
1. Testicular torsion causes sudden, excruciating pain in or around the testicle, which may spread to the lower abdomen; the pain may get worse with standing. Other signs and symptoms include swelling, rising of the affected testicle, nausea, vomiting, fever, and fainting or light-headedness.
2. Epididymitis
C. Nonacute conditions include:
1. Testicular tumor
2. Muscle strain
3. Hip arthritis
4. Undescended testicle
5. Hydrocele
6. Varicocele
7. Spermatocele

Plan

A. Patient teaching
1. Tell the patient to call the office right away if he finds a lump or swelling in the scrotum, even if it is small or painless. Testicular tumors are usually painless.
2. Discuss condition and treatment options with the patient.
   a. Surgery is the only effective treatment.
   b. Watchful waiting rather than surgical repair is an option if the patient is asymptomatic as long as he is aware of the risk and understands the need for prompt attention should symptoms of complication occur.
   c. Nonsurgical therapy for groin hernias is the use of a truss. There is insufficient data to determine the efficacy of trusses in controlling symptoms. A truss has the potential risks of bowel constriction; prolonged use of a truss can lead to atrophy of the spermatic corn or fusion to the hernial sac.
3. Teach the patient signs of strangulation.
4. Instruct the patient to avoid heavy lifting.
B. Medical and surgical management: Gently reduce a groin hernia while the patient lies supine with hips slightly flexed to relax the abdominal muscles.

Follow-up

A. Tell the patient to return to the office if fever, severe pain, or strangulation occurs.
B. Postoperative evaluation for hernia recurrences as needed:
1. Immediately from repair
2. Greater than 6 months and up to 5 years from repair
3. Late recurrences beyond 5 years from the repair

Consultation/Referral

A. Refer patients with femoral hernias to a physician. These hernias need to be repaired as soon as possible because of increased risk of incarceration and strangulation.
B. Strangulated hernias are nonreducible and blood supply to protruded tissue is compromised. Refer patients for immediate surgical intervention.

Individual Considerations

A. Pregnancy: Preexisting groin hernias may become more symptomatic during the first trimester of pregnancy. The symptoms must be differentiated from round ligament pain.
B. Pediatrics:
1. A high incidence (16%–25%) of inguinal hernias occurs in premature infants. The incidence is inversely related to weight.
2. In infants, the only symptom of a hernia may be increased irritability.
C. Geriatrics: Signs and symptoms of prostatism are frequently present in men with hernias and may require relief before herniorrhaphy.

HIRSCHSPRUNG DISEASE, OR CONGENITAL AGANGLIONIC MEGACOLON

Definition

A. Hirschsprung disease (HD) is the major cause of intestinal obstruction in newborns. HD is a motor disorder of the gut. The aganglionic segment is aperistaltic and remains in a state of contraction causing a functional obstruction. The majority of HD patients are diagnosed in the neonatal period. Although infants appear normal at birth, more than half do not pass meconium for more than 48 hours. Absence of peristalsis causes feces to accumulate proximal to the defect and leads to intestinal obstruction. Bacterial enterocolitis is the most severe complication of untreated Hirschsprung's disease, and mortality from the complications may be as great as 25%–30%.

Incidence

A. Hirschsprung disease occurs in 1 in every 3,000–7,000 live births. It is uncommon in premature infants.
B. Occurrence is more often in males; however, long-segment disease increases in females.
C. About 10%–50% of cases have familial incidence. Around eight genetic mutations have been identified.
D. Hirschsprung is associated with other chromosomal abnormalities and syndromes:
1. Trisomy 21 (Down syndrome)
2. Cardiac disease (septal defects)
3. Bardet-Biedl syndrome (BBS)
4. Congenial central hypoventilation syndrome (CCHS)
5. Waardenburg syndrome
6. Smith-Lemli-Opitz syndrome
E. Approximately 80% of affected patients have the disorder limited to the rectum or rectosigmoid region.
F. From 3%–5% of affected patients have aganglionosis of the entire colon.
G. The disease is three times more common in people of European ancestry.
H. Around 25% of HD patients have associated congenital anomalies of the kidney and urinary tract (hydronephrosis and renal hypoplasia).

Pathogenesis

A. The disorder is due to congenital absence of ganglion cells in both Meissner's (submucosal) and Auerbach's (myenteric) plexus. It occurs secondary to the failure of migration of ganglia from the neural crest, which normally occurs before the 12th week of gestation. The disorder starts in the distal rectum and extends proximally to involve a varying amount of the bowel.

Predisposing Factors

A. Full-term infant of normal weight
B. European ancestry
C. Male gender
D. Family history of disorder
E. Down syndrome

Common Complaints

A. Newborns: failure to pass meconium for more than 48 hours
B. Blast sign: explosive expulsion of gas and stool after the use of a digital rectal examination
C. Children: failure to grow
D. Constipation
E. Abdominal distension

Other Signs and Symptoms

A. Newborns:
   1. Overflow-type diarrhea
   2. Bile- or feces-stained vomitus
   3. Failure to thrive
   4. Anorexia due to early satiety, abdominal discomfort, and distention
   5. Temporary relief with enema
B. Older infants and children (nearly all children with HD are diagnosed during the first 2 years of life):
   1. Constipation since birth; may have a history of requiring a daily enema
   2. Intestinal obstruction
   3. Progressive abdominal distension with visible peristaltic activity
   4. Temporary relief with enema
   5. Ribbonlike, fluidlike, or pellet stools
   6. Failure to thrive
   7. Anemia

Subjective Data

A. In newborns, review onset, duration, and course of symptoms, including number of bowel movements, passage of first stool, and expulsion of flatus.
B. Ask the patient or caregiver about family history of Hirschsprung disease.
C. Review the infant's weight and growth parameters.
D. Inquire about other symptoms of bowel obstruction, such as vomiting and diarrhea.
E. Ask about other complications such as blood in stool.
F. Review history of bowel movements and feeding habits, including onset of constipation, character of stools (ribbonlike or fluid-filled), frequency of bowel movements, and use of enemas.

Physical Examination

A. Check temperature, pulse, respirations, blood pressure, weight, and growth parameters, including length, and head circumference.
B. Inspect
   1. Note general appearance, level of activity, abdominal distention, and signs of malnutrition.
   2. Inspect fontanelles for signs of dehydration.
C. Auscultate the abdomen for bowel sounds in all quadrants.
D. Percuss the abdomen for organomegaly.
E. Palpate the abdomen for distension and masses.
F. Rectal exam
   1. Check for "tight" anal sphincter and absence of stool in rectal ampulla.
   2. Many infants have relief of symptoms and pass large amounts of stool and flatus after exam (Blast sign).

Diagnostic Tests

A. Rectal biopsy is considered the gold standard for diagnosis of HD. The biopsy is obtained by mucosal suction.
B. Contrast barium enema: 25% of cases appear normal.
C. Anorectal manometry.
D. Ultrasonography.
E. Chemistry panel to evaluate fluid and electrolyte management.

Differential Diagnoses

A. Hirschsprung disease
B. Meconium peritonitis
C. Meconium plug syndrome
D. Meconium ileus
E. Intestinal obstruction
F. Enterocolitis
G. Megacolon
H. Hypothyroidism

Plan

A. Patient teaching
   1. Prepare caregivers or the patient for referral or consultation.
   2. Teach caregivers or the patient about Hirschsprung disease and treatment therapy.
B. Medical and surgical management
   1. Treatment consists of colostomy performed proximal to aganglionic segment with biopsies taken at the time of surgery to identify level of involvement. Definitive repair can then be performed when the infant is 6–12 months old.
   2. The mainstay of treatment is surgery; however, in older children when symptoms are chronic, but not severe, treatment may consist of isotonic enemas, stool softeners, and low-residue diet.

Follow-up

A. Pediatric surgeons and gastroenterologists should generally care for children with Hirschsprung disease.

Consultation/Referral

A. Consult or refer the patient to a physician if Hirschsprung disease is suspected in an infant.
B. Consider genetic testing.

Individual Considerations

Pediatrics:

A. Recurrence risk is proportional to the length of aganglionic segment of the colon.

B. Infants who have symptom relief after rectal examination and pass large amounts of stool and gas (Blast sign) can have recurrence of symptoms, often fail to grow normally, can have constipation or diarrhea, and may have protein loss in their stool.

HOOKWORM, ANCYLOSTOMA DUODENALE AND NECATOR AMERICANUS DEFINITIONS

A. Hookworm is a chronic, debilitating parasitic disease with vague symptoms that vary in proportion to the degree of iron-deficiency anemia and hypoproteinemia of the host. The adult hookworm attach to the intestinal wall and ingests the host's blood and nutrients. Chronic infection in children may lead to physical growth delay, deficits cognition, and developmental delay. Anemia and hypoproteinemia are produced by the blood-clotting activity of adult nematodes in the intestines.

Incidence

A. Incidence in the United States is unknown. Globally about 740 million are infected with hookworms.

Pathogenesis

A. Disease is caused by infection with *Ancylostoma duodenale, A. ceylonicum,* and *Necator americanus* intestinal parasites. Mixed infections are common. Humans are the major reservoir. *A. duodenale* may be ingested. Eggs of nematode hatch into larvae that penetrate soles of feet and palms of hands from contact with contaminated soil. Contact for 5–10 min results in skin penetration. Larvae are carried by circulation to lungs and eventually to their final habitat, the small intestines. Eggs are passed in stools of infected persons. Although hookworms are not transmitted from person to person, infected persons can contaminate soil by defecation as long as they are untreated.

B. Incubation period, or the time from exposure to eggs excreted in stool to the development of noncutaneous symptoms, is 4–12 weeks. The appearance of parasites in the blood is 4–6 weeks. Adult worms or larvae are rarely seen.

Predisposing Factors

A. Living in or traveling to rural, tropic, or subtropics where soil contamination with human feces is common.

B. Exposure to loose, sandy, moist, shady, well-aerated, warm soil where larvae and eggs thrive.

C. Agricultural workers are at high risk.

D. Tourists with bare feet or open footwear that exposes skin to contaminated soil.

E. Military troops in endemic areas.

F. Children.

Common Complaints

A. Intense stinging or burning at penetration site, followed by pruritus and papulovesicular rash that persists for 1–2 weeks

B. Fatigue

C. Weight loss

D. Vague abdominal discomfort

E. Loss of appetite

Other Signs and Symptoms

A. Pharyngeal itching, after oral ingestion.

B. Hoarseness.

C. Nausea or vomiting.

D. Cough or wheeze, from pulmonary infiltration due to heavy infestation.

E. Colicky abdominal pain or diarrhea: late sign, occurring with marked eosinophilia 29–38 days after exposure.

F. Anemia is the principal manifestation of hookworm infestation; it occurs secondary to blood loss.

G. Edema.

H. Diarrhea.

Subjective Data

A. Review onset, duration, and course of symptoms, including recent episodes of intense itching of feet, palms of hands, or buttocks.

B. Establish patient's normal weight and amount of any weight lost, over what length of time.

C. Inquire about abdominal symptoms, including onset and intensity.

D. Review other GI symptoms such as diarrhea.

E. Review any transitory chest symptoms, such as cough or wheezing. Is there a history of asthma?

F. Ask the patient if any other family members are exhibiting the same symptoms.

Physical Examination

A. Check temperature, pulse, respirations, blood pressure, and weight.

B. Inspect skin on the entire body especially the soles of both feet. Erythematous, papular vesicular lesions may be excoriated from scratching. Rash persists for 1–2 weeks.

C. Palpate the abdomen for masses and tenderness.

D. Auscultate the abdomen and lungs.

Diagnostic Tests

A. Identification of hookworm eggs in feces is diagnostic. Fecal egg excretion does not become detectable until around 2 months after dermal exposure. Repeated stool samples may be needed for diagnosis.

B. Hgb and HCT for anemia.

C. CBC with differential: may have mild eosinophilia.

D. Beaver direct smear, Stoll egg-counting, or Kato-Katz techniques quantify infection.

E. Endoscopic examination may reveal the adult worms.

Differential Diagnoses

A. Hookworm

B. Asthma

C. Poor nutrition

D. Giardiasis

Plan

A. Patient teaching
1. Discuss the dangers of going barefoot outdoors with the patient.
2. Explain that good hand washing is critical, especially after defecation.
3. There is no direct person-to-person transmission.
4. Use good sanitary practices to prevent soil contamination.

B. Dietary management: Teach the patient how to correct anemia through good nutrition.

C. Pharmaceutical therapy
1. Mebendazole (Vermox) 100 mg orally twice a day for 3 days OR a one-time single dose of 500 mg.
2. Pyrantel pamoate (Pyrantel) 11 mg/kg per day for 3 days; do not exceed 1 g/day.
3. Albendazole (Albenza) 400 mg one-time dose.
4. Iron therapy helps correct anemia.
5. At the present time, there is no hookworm vaccine.
6. Ivermectin (Stromectol) is ineffective against hookworms.

Follow-up

A. Stool should be examined again 2 weeks after therapy is completed. If results are positive, repeating therapy is indicated.

Consultation/Referral

A. Refer pregnant patients to a physician.

B. Refer children to a physician if hemoglobin is less than 6 g/dL. Cardiac decompensation occasionally develops in children with hemoglobin concentrations of less than 6 g/dL.

Individual Considerations

A. Pregnancy
1. Anthelmintics are in Pregnancy Category C; however, risks versus benefits should be considered.
2. Adequate protein and iron nutrition should be maintained throughout pregnancy.
3. Consider delaying treatment until after delivery if necessary.

B. Pediatrics
1. All medications are advised for children 2 years of age and older.
2. Severely affected children may require a blood transfusion.

IRRITABLE BOWEL SYNDROME (IBS)

Definition

Irritable bowel syndrome (IBS) is the most common of the GI motility disorders. IBS is responsible for significant direct and indirect health care costs. It is a relapsing functional disturbance of intestinal motility marked by a common symptom complex that includes bloating and abdominal pain or discomfort associated with defecation. Bladder dysfunction has been identified in 50% of patients with IBS. Patients commonly transition between subgroups.

IBS is defined by symptom-based diagnostic criteria, in the absence of detectable organic causes. Rome III criteria for IBS is related to stool characteristics.

A. IBS with diarrhea predominant (IBS-D): Loose stools (small volume, pasty/mushy or watery) more than 25% of the time and hard stools less than 25% of the time.

B. IBS with constipation (small, hard, pelletlike stools) predominant (IBS-C): Hard stools more than 25% of the time and loose stools less than 25% of the time.

C. IBS with alternating bouts of constipation and diarrhea, mixed or cyclic pattern (IBS-M): Both hard and soft stools more than 25% of the time.

D. On clinical grounds other subclassifications are used:
1. Based on symptoms
   a. IBS with predominant bowel dysfunction
   b. IBS with predominant pain
   c. IBS with predominant bloating
2. Based on precipitating factors:
   a. Postinfectious (PI-IBS)
   b. Food-induced (meal-induced)
   c. Stress-related

Incidence

A. IBS is common, accounting for about 50% of GI complaints seen by health care professionals, and is a major cause of morbidity in the United States. Studies suggest nearly 20% of all adults suffer from some form of the condition; however, only a fraction seeks medical help. IBS is recognized in children; symptoms consistent with IBS are reported in 16% of students aged 11–17. IBS is not described in preschool-aged children.

Pathogenesis

A. IBS has an absence of detectable pathology and laboratory tests are unrevealing. The understanding of IBS has evolved from a disturbance in bowel motor activity to a more integrated understanding of visceral hypersensitivity and brain-gut interaction. It is thought to be both a normal response to severe stress and a learned visceral response to stress leading to the following:

A. Nonpropulsive colonic contractions lead to constipation-predominant IBS.

B. Increased contraction in the small bowel and proximal colon with diminished activity in the distal colon, leading to diarrhea-predominant IBS.

C. Most patients with functional disorders appear to have inappropriate perception of physiologic events and altered reflex responses in different gut regions.

D. The brain-gut transmitters act at different sites in the brain and gut and lead to varied effects on gastrointestinal motility, pain control, emotional behavior, and immunity. Serotonin plays a critical role in the regulation of GI motility, secretion, and sensation. Studies have shown that IBS may be related to an imbalance in mucosal serotonin (5-hydroxytryptamine) and 5-HT availability caused by defects in 5-HT production, serotonin receptors, or serotonin transport.

Predisposing Factors

A. Age
   1. 50% of IBS occurs prior to age 35.
   2. 40% of IBS occurs between ages 35–50.
B. Gender
   1. Women are 2–3 times more likely to have IBS.
   2. In pediatrics, both sexes are equally affected.
C. Emotional factors and situational stress.
D. Prior GI infection–induced IBS.
E. Genetics is considered a factor.
F. Carbohydrate intolerance may produce significant symptoms.

Common Complaints

A. Chronic relapsing stool pattern:
   1. Diarrhea over three loose stools per day OR
   2. Alternation of diarrhea with constipation. Diarrhea is typically small in volume, has visible mucous, and may follow a hard movement by a few hours. OR
   3. Constipation: less than three BMs per week.
B. Feeling of incomplete evacuation.
C. Abdominal distention and bloating.
D. Straining with bowel movements.
E. Aching or cramps in periumbilical or lower abdominal region.
F. Pain relief with BM.

Other Signs and Symptoms

A. Change in bowel function.
B. Clear mucous stool.
C. Pain may be precipitated by meals.
D. Pain radiating to left chest or arm, from gas in splenic flexure. Nocturnal pain is unusual and is considered a warning sign.
E. Flatulence.
F. Nausea.
G. Anxiety.
H. Depression.
I. Preoccupation with bowel symptoms.
J. Extraintestinal symptoms
   1. Dysmenorrhea.
   2. Urinary frequency, urgency, and incomplete bladder emptying.

EXHIBIT 10.1 **Red Flag Symptoms That Require Additional Tests or Examination**

Onset of symptoms after age 50

Unintended weight loss

Nocturnal symptoms

Blood in stools

Abdominal/rectal masses

Fever

---

   3. Impaired sexual function and dyspareunia.
   4. Fibromyalgia.
K. Menses may exacerbate IBS symptoms
L. **Red-flag symptoms (see Exhibit 10.1).**

Subjective Data

A. Review pattern of main symptoms, including onset, duration, and usual course.
B. Ask the patient what are the predominant symptoms—abdominal pain, diarrhea, or constipation.
C. Review the patient's history for stress factors, and ask if recurrent symptoms occur in relation to them.
D. Ask what other symptoms occur with the pain, diarrhea, or constipation, such as bloating, blood in stool, or nighttime bowel movements. **Bleeding, weight loss, and nocturnal diarrhea are not characteristic of IBS. IBS symptoms disappear during sleep.**
E. Establish patient's normal weight history, and determine amount of weight loss, if any, over what time period.
F. Review the patient's diet including
   1. Response to milk or lactose products
   2. Artificial sweetners
   3. Alcohol intake
   4. Irregular or inadequate meals
   5. Insufficient fluid intake
   6. Excessive fiber intake
   7. Obsession with dietary hygiene
G. Inquire about the patient's prescription, herbal, and OTC medications. Ask specifically about the use of laxatives.
H. Review travel and food history for dominant history of diarrhea.
I. Ask the patient if there is a family history of colon cancer, ulcerative colitis, Crohn's disease, or malabsorption.
J. Is there any fever accompanying lower abdominal pain?
K. What is the relation of symptoms to menstruation?

Physical Examination

A. Check temperature, pulse, respirations, blood pressure, and weight.
B. Inspect
   1. Observe general appearance. Does the patient appear anxious or depressed?
   2. Inspect abdominal contour for masses and bulges.
C. Auscultate all quadrants of the abdomen for bowel sounds; note whether they are normal or mildly hyperactive.
D. Percuss the abdomen for tympany or dullness.
E. Palpate the abdomen
   1. Evaluate the abdomen for mild tenderness, rigidity, guarding, and masses.
   2. Evaluate for hepatosplenomegaly.
   3. Evaluate for lymphadenopathy.
F. Rectal exam
   1. Check for masses and tenderness.
   2. Obtain stool for diagnostic tests.
   3. Rectal exam is normal with IBS.

Diagnostic Tests

A. Diagnosis of IBS is usually suspected on the basis of the patient's history and physical examination without additional tests. See Table 10.16.
B. CBC.
C. Sedimentation rate or C-reactive protein.
D. Serum potassium, if the patient is on diuretics; hypokalemia may reduce bowel contractility and produce an ileus.
E. Blood glucose, if diarrhea predominates; rule out diabetes mellitus, which may present as diarrhea due to diabetic gastroenteropathy.
F. Thyroid function study.
G. Stool specimen: culture for leukocytes and fat, ova and parasites and occult blood. Leukocyte-free mucous is a hallmark of IBS.
H. Stool cultures for *Clostridium difficile* toxin assay, if clinically indicated.
I. Barium enema and/or proctosigmoidoscopy for severe signs and symptoms, after consultation or referral.
J. Celiac serology, if appropriate.

Differential Diagnoses

A. IBS
B. Inflammatory bowel disease (Crohn's/ulcerative colitis)
C. Viral or bacterial gastroenteritis
D. GI neoplasm
E. Acute diarrhea due to protozoa or bacteria
F. Lactose insufficiency/deficiency
G. Laxative abuse
H. Drug side effect
I. Diabetes
J. Celiac spruce/gluten etiology
K. Diverticulitis
L. Failure to thrive in children
M. Endometriosis/PID
N. Zollinger-Ellison syndrome

Plan

A. General interventions
   1. Advise the patient to keep a diary of events of BMs and precipitating factors.
   2. Encourage the patient to quit smoking because nicotine may aggravate symptoms.
   3. Recommend daily exercise to reduce stress.

TABLE 10.16 Rome III Diagnostic Criteria for IBS

Onset of symptoms at least 6 months before diagnosis

Recurrent abdominal pain or discomfort for > 3 days per month during the past three months

At least 2 of the following features:

A. Improvement with defecation
B. Association with a change in frequency of stool
C. Association with a change in stool form

---

   4. Stress management should be encouraged, including counseling, tapes, meditation, and yoga.
B. Patient teaching: See the Section III Patient Teaching Guide for this chapter, "Irritable Bowel Syndrome."
C. Dietary management
   1. Prescribe a high-fiber diet.
   2. Tell the patient to avoid foods that aggravate the bowel. Tell him or her to avoid gas-producing foods, such as broccoli, beans, onions, garlic, and so forth. When diarrhea predominates, dietary review is essential for clues of intolerance to lactose or sorbitol.
D. Pharmaceutical therapy
   1. Tell the patient to stop all nonessential medications that may affect bowel function, especially irritant laxatives. Avoid narcotics, depressants, and other long-term drug use if possible.
   2. Recommend eliminating sorbitol-containing candy and restricting lactose-containing milk products.
   3. Drug of choice: psyllium hydrophilic mucilloid (Metamucil) 1 tbs per day in 8 oz juice or water, followed with another 8 oz of liquid. This treats both diarrhea and constipation.
   4. Pain relief:
      a. Opiates should be avoided due to the risk of dependence and addiction in chronic conditions.
      b. NSAIDs have an undesirable side effect on the gastrointestinal tract.
      c. Antispasmodics and anticholinergic agents (IBS-D predominant)
         i. Hyoscyamine (Levsin, Levbid)
            (a). Levsin 0.125–0.25 mg (1–2 tablets) orally or sublingual every 4 hours; not to exceed 12 tablets a day.
            (b). Levbid 0.375–0.75 mg orally twice a day.
            (c). Pediatric doses are dependant on age and weight.
         ii. Dicyclomine (Bentyl) 20–40 mg four times a day; discontinue if not effective within 2 weeks or if 80 mg daily is associated with adverse effects.
      d. Tricyclic antidepressants for diarrhea-predominant IBS. Tricyclics should be avoided for constipated patients.
         i. Amitriptyline (Elavil) 10 mg every bedtime initially, titrate up slowly to 75 mg/day at bedtime as needed.
         ii. Desipramine (Norpramin) 10 mg every bedtime initially, titrate up slowly up to 75 mg/day.
         iii. Imipramine (Tofranil) 10–50 mg orally every bedtime.
   5. Selective serotonin reuptake inhibitors (SSRIs):
      a. Paroxetine (Paxil) 10–60 mg/day.
      b. Citalopram (Celexa) 5–60 mg/day.
   6. Antidiarrheals
      a. Opiate-derived are reserved for very severe cases secondary to the potential for abuse.
      b. Loperamide (Imodium)

i. Adults: 2–12 mg orally in divided twice a day/three times daily doses; doses differ greatly among individuals.

ii. Pediatrics older than 2 years: 0.08 mg–0.24 mg/kg/d orally divided in twice a day/three times daily doses; not to exceed 2 mg/dose.

c. Alosetron (Lotronex), a 5 hydroxytryptamine-3 (5-HT$_3$) receptor antagonist, is indicated for women with severe diarrhea-predominant IBS.

7. Laxatives and stool softeners (IBS-C predominant)

a. Mineral oil 15–45 mL orally daily or in divided three times daily dosing.

b. Stimulant laxatives may be necessary intermittently for short periods, but prolonged use of stimulant laxatives should be avoided.

8. Lubiprostone (Amitiza), a selective C-2 chloride-channel activator is indicated for women 18 years and over with constipation-predominant IBS. 8-μ doses twice a day with food and water.

9. Probiotics.

Follow-up

A. Reevaluate the effectiveness of treatment in 2 weeks. Treatment may be challenging for symptom management and numerous tests that are inconclusive, but rule out pathology.

B. If symptoms persist without relief, have the patient return as needed.

C. Return if diarrhea lasts more than 2 weeks.

Consultation/Referral

A. Refer to a gastroenterologist for red-flag symptoms.

B. Refer to a pediatric gastroenterologist if findings from the patient's history, physical examination, or screening laboratory tests are suggestive of organic disease.

C. Alosetron (Lotronex) is prescribed under a restricted distribution program through a gastroenterologist.

D. Consult a physician if all treatment options fail.

E. Consider a psychiatric consultation, if indicated for anxiety, depression, somatization, and symptom-related fears.

Individual Considerations

A. Pediatrics:

1. Irritable bowel syndrome is recognized in children, and many patients trace the onset of symptoms to childhood.

2. Children who have a history of recurrent abdominal pain are at increased risk of IBS during adolescence and young adulthood.

3. The recommended daily intake of fiber (in grams) for children is estimated by adding 4 to their age in years.

B. Adults:

1. Annual rectal examination and sigmoidoscopy are recommended after age 40.

2. When constipation predominates, rule out malignancy, particularly in patients over age 40 who have weight loss or a family history of colon cancer.

JAUNDICE

Definition

A. Jaundice is a yellow tinge of the skin or mucous membranes. It is a symptom, not a disease. The diagnostic approach begins with gathering a comprehensive history, physical examination, and screening labs. The differential diagnosis is formulated and further testing may be warranted. The onset of jaundice usually prompts the patient or family to seek medical attention.

Incidence

A. Incidence is variable according to pathogenesis, age, and population.

Pathogenesis

The mechanism responsible for jaundice includes excess bilirubin production, decreased hepatic uptake, impaired conjugation, intrahepatic cholestasis, extrahepatic obstruction, and hepatocellular injury. See Table 10.17.

However, it is important to recognize that more than one mechanism can be operating in a given case (i.e., sickle cell anemia and HIV).

A. Excess bilirubin production results from accelerated red cell destruction. The excessive amounts of hemoglobin and resultant bilirubin released into the bloodstream overwhelm the liver's normal capacity for uptake, and an unconjugated hyperbilirubinemia ensues.

B. With decreased uptake and conjugation, there is often a concurrent, acquired illness such as infection, cardiac disease, or cancer. Hereditary conditions, such as Gilbert and Crigler-Najjar syndromes, are responsible.

C. Intrahepatic cholestasis may occur at a number of levels: intracellularly (e.g., hepatitis), at the canalicular level (when estrogen-induced), at the ductule (phenothiazine exposure), at the septal ducts (primary biliary cirrhosis), and at the intralobular ducts (cholangiocarcinoma).

D. Extrahepatic obstruction occurs when stone, stricture, or tumor blocks the flow of bile within the extrahepatic bil-

TABLE 10.17 **Classification of Jaundice According to Bile Pigment and by Mechanism**

Unconjugated Hyperbilirubinemia	Conjugated Hyperbilirubinemia
Increased/overproduction of bilirubin	Hepatocellular injury/disease
Impaired/decreased hepatic uptake of bilirubin	Intrahepatic cholestasis
Impaired/decreased conjugation	Extrahepatic cholestasis (biliary obstruction)

iary tree. A history of gallstones, biliary tract surgery, or malignancy may be elicited.

Predisposing Factors

A. Previous blood transfusion
B. Travel to an area endemic for hepatitis
C. Raw shellfish consumption
D. IV drug abuse
E. High-risk sexual practices
F. Family history of episodic jaundice
G. History of gallstones
H. Previous biliary tract surgery
I. Alcoholism
J. Chemical exposure
K. Working in the health care profession

Common Complaints

A. Pruritus
B. Dark, tea-colored urine, from conjugated bilirubinuria
C. Light, clay-colored stools, from absence of bile
D. Fatigue

Other Signs and Symptoms

A. Enlarged liver
B. Splenomegaly
C. Fever
D. Chills
E. GI: appetite loss, weight loss, abdominal pain, nausea or vomiting
F. Ascites
G. Shortness of breath
H. Palpitations
I. Ecchymosis
J. Steatorrhea, severe
K. Asterixis

Subjective Data

A. Review onset, duration, and course of symptoms.
B. Review medication history for drugs/herbals that may induce jaundice (see Table 10.18).
C. Inquire about recent blood transfusions. Are there any known blood disorders in the patient's family history?
D. Ask about contact with a person who has an infection, such as infectious hepatitis.
E. Ask about unprotected sexual activity/HIV status.
F. Review ingestion of potentially contaminated food or water, including *Amanita* mushrooms, milk, or shellfish.
G. Ask about the patient's exposure to any toxic chemicals, such as carbon tetrachloride, chloroform, phosphorus, arsenic, ethanol, or halothane (Fluothane).
H. Review the patient's history of nonsterile needle punctures.
I. Review the patient's medical/surgical history for gallstones, hepatitis, tumor, pancreatitis, Wilson's disease, Budd-Chiari syndrome, liver surgery, or transplantation. Is there a family history of gallstones?
J. Ask how much alcohol the patient has ingested over the years.
K. Ask about dark urine or white or clay-colored stool.

TABLE 10.18   Drugs and Herbals Associated With Jaundice

Acetaminophen (Tylenol)

Alkylated steroids

Aminobenzoic acid

Antidiabetic drugs

Arsenic

Chlorpromazine

Ethinyl estradiol/oral contraceptives/hormone replacement

Herbal medications (e.g., Jamaican bush tea)

Isoniazid (INH)

Mercaptopurine (Purinethol)

Methyldopa (Aldomet)

Monoamine oxidase inhibitors

Perphenazine (Trilafon)

Phenothiazine derivatives

Propylthiouracil (PTU)

Rifampin

Sulfonamides

Total parenteral nutrition

L. Inquire about dyspepsia, anorexia, nausea, vomiting, RUQ or epigastric pain, or pain radiating to back or shoulder blade. Ask: What is the relationship of pain to eating?
M. Inquire about fever, fatigue, malaise, loss of vigor and strength, easy bruising, and weight loss.
N. Review travel history.

Physical Examination

A. Check temperature, pulse, respirations, blood pressure, and weight. Marked weight loss accompanied by jaundice suggests carcinoma of the head of the pancreas or metastatic disease obstructing the common duct.
B. Inspect
 1. Inspect skin, mouth, palms, and sclera for yellow tinge. Severe jaundice may cause greenish tinge from oxidation of bilirubin to biliverdin.
   a. In fair-skinned people, discoloration is most evident on the face, trunk, and sclera (sclera icterus).
   b. In dark-skinned people, discoloration is most evident in sclera and roof of mouth.
   c. In newborns, jaundice first appears over face or upper body, then progresses over larger areas; it can also be seen in conjunctivae of the eyes.
   d. Jaundice is most noticeable in natural sunlight. In artificial or poor light, it may be hard to detect.
 2. Inspect the skin for spider angiomata, rashes or scratches from severe itching due to pruritus and for bruising or petechiae.
 3. Inspect the palms for erythema or overt bleeding.

4. Inspect the chest for gynecomastia.

C. Palpate the abdomen for tenderness, masses, liver enlargement in RUQ, and ascites.

1. Extrahepatic obstruction and intrahepatic cholestasis may be identical in presentation.

2. Tenderness is minimal unless cholangitis or rapid distension occur.

3. Splenomegaly is unlikely except in primary biliary cirrhosis.

4. Gallbladder may be palpable (Courvoisier sign) when there is gradual development of the biliary tree. Sudden onset of pain results from passage of stone that becomes wedged into common duct; fever and sepsis shortly thereafter indicates cholangitis.

5. Malignancy usually presents as a rock-hard mass.

6. Absence of abdominal pain does not rule out obstruction, especially when it develops slowly from tumor growth or primary biliary cirrhosis.

7. Advanced hepatocellular disease is indicated by a small liver, signs of portal hypertension (ascites, splenomegaly, prominent abdominal venous pattern), asterixis, peripheral edema (from hypoalbuminemia), spider angiomata, gynecomastia, palmar erythema, and testicular atrophy.

D. Percuss the abdomen.

E. Auscultate the heart, lungs, and abdomen for bowel sounds.

F. Neurologic exam

1. Note level of consciousness.

2. Note asterixis, or flapping tremor elicited when arms are extended and wrists dorsiflexed.

G. Rectal exam: Check for masses.

Diagnostic Tests

A. Initial laboratory tests:

1. Serum bilirubin: direct, indirect (unconjugated), and total; clinically, jaundice becomes noticeable when levels reach 2.0–2.5 mg/dL.

   a. Intrahepatic cholestasis and extrahepatic obstruction: elevated conjugated bilirubin, elevated serum alkaline phosphatase, mild to moderate rise in transaminase.

   b. Gilbert syndrome is the most common cause of decreased uptake and unconjugated hyperbilirubinemia. It is a benign disorder that produces recurrent self-limited episodes of mild jaundice. Typically, the unconjugated fraction rises to no more than 1.5–3.0 mg/100 mL. In Gilbert syndrome, fasting and minor illness can precipitate jaundice.

2. Alkaline phosphatase

3. Aspartate transaminase (AST)/Alanine transaminase (ALT)

   a. Elevation of ALT and AST may indicate liver cell damage or may be caused by opiates and aspirin.

   b. Aspirin may also decrease AST and ALT.

4. Prothrombin time (PT)

   a. PT may be prolonged due to malabsorption, but it is reversible by vitamin K injection.

   b. Prolonged PT unresponsive to parenteral vitamin K strongly suggests hepatocellular failure.

   c. Cholestasis and obstruction may also produce prolongation of PT but can be reversed by vitamin K.

   d. Phenazopyridine (Pyridium) may cause a false-positive bilirubin result.

B. Other laboratory testing as needed:

1. Total serum protein.

2. Serum albumin and globulin

   a. Albumin decreases with cirrhosis and chronic hepatitis.

   b. Globulin increases with cirrhosis, chronic obstructive jaundice, and viral hepatitis.

   c. To interpret albumin level, consider dietary intake and sources of possible protein loss.

3. Cholesterol.

4. Lactate dehydrogenase (LDH).

5. Gamma-Glutamyltransferase (GGT).

6. Serum ammonia.

7. Bile acids radioimmunoassay: elevated levels indicate hepatic disease.

8. Serologic tests for viral hepatitis.

9. Serum iron, transferrin, and ferritin to evaluate hemochromatosis.

10. Serum ceruloplasmin levels to evaluate Wilson's disease.

11. Alpha-1 antitrypsin activity to evaluate alpha-1 antitrypsin deficiency.

12. Urine for bilirubin-bilirubinuria may be an early sign of liver disease.

    a. Collect specimens over a 2-hour period after lunch.

    b. Place specimen in a dark brown container and send to lab immediately to prevent decomposition.

C. Abdominal ultrasound is considered the screening procedure of choice. More selective imaging procedures are ordered based on clinical evaluation.

D. Other imaging procedures:

1. Endoscopic ultrasound.

2. Hepatobiliary scan (HIDA scan): uses radioactive isotopes.

3. Oral cholecystography.

4. Endoscopic retrograde cholangiopancreatography (ERCP).

5. Percutaneous transhepatic cholangiography (PTC).

6. Helical CT.

7. Magnetic resonance cholangiopancreatography (MRCP) is an alternative to ERCP.

8. Liver biopsy may be indicated for definitive diagnosis.

Differential Diagnoses

A. Jaundice is a symptom, not a diagnosis.

B. Cancer of pancreas.

C. Obstruction of biliary tract.

D. Icteric phase of hepatitis.

E. Cirrhosis.

F. Right-sided heart failure.

G. Chronic hemolysis from prosthetic heart valve.

Plan
A. Management depends on primary diagnosis. Most patients can be managed on an ambulatory basis, unless they are unable to maintain hydration or begin to show evidence of severe hepatocellular failure.

Follow-up
A. See the patient 2–4 weeks after initial diagnosis and referral.
B. Subsequent routine evaluations are related to primary diagnosis.

Consultation/Referral
A. Consult with a gastroenterologist familiar with liver disease and needle biopsy techniques when hepatocellular disease is suspected; when there is evidence of hepatic failure, portal hypertension, or encephalopathy; or when jaundice persists longer than 3 months.
B. Consultation with a gastroenterologist, surgeon, or radiologist experienced in evaluation of jaundice can be very useful when there is clinical suspicion of extrahepatic obstruction.
C. Admission is mandatory when jaundice is complicated by a fever and peritoneal signs indicative of cholangitis. IV antibiotics and prompt surgical consultation are required.

Individual Considerations
A. Pregnancy
1. Viral hepatitis is the most frequent cause of jaundice in pregnancy.
2. Intrahepatic cholestasis in pregnancy is associated with modest maternal risks, including increased risk of peripartum bleeding and increased likelihood of subsequent cholelithiasis.
3. Cholestyramine resin, generally 4 g every 4–6 hours, has been reported to afford some relief of pruritus in 50% of affected women, presumably by removing a portion of the bile acids by irreversible binding in the gut.
4. Pregnant women who take cholestyramine are at increased risk for depletion of vitamin K-dependent coagulation factors and should be followed with serial PT times. Such women should also receive prophylactic vitamin K supplementation. If PT becomes prolonged, medication should be discontinued.
B. Pediatrics
1. Hepatitis predominates as cause of jaundice.
2. Neonatal jaundice is more common when the mother is an insulin-dependent diabetic, probably resulting from a higher hematocrit developed in utero, especially if oxygen availability is decreased. Newborn jaundice due to liver immaturity is common. It begins on day 2, peaks at 1 week, and disappears in 2–3 weeks. About half of all full-term newborns and 90% of premature newborns have some degree of jaundice. Jaundice is usually mild and can be treated with hydration and ultraviolet lamp exposure.
3. Intense, persistent jaundice suggests liver disease or severe, overwhelming infection.

4. In Rh isoimmunization infants without appropriate treatment (exchange transfusion), progressive jaundice leads to brain damage (kernicterus), death, or severe handicap (deafness, spasticity, and choreoathetosis).
C. Geriatrics: Stones and tumors are often responsible for jaundice.

MALABSORPTION

Definition
A. Malabsorption syndrome is a group of signs and symptoms occurring as a result of digestive problems and absorption of nutrients. There may be a resultant decrease in absorption of fat-soluble vitamins A, D, E, and K. Poor absorption of carbohydrates, minerals, and proteins may also occur.
B. The presentation of malabsorption varies from severe overt symptoms with weight loss to discrete oligosymptomatic changes in hematological/laboratory tests that are found incidentally. Malabsorption can result from congenital defects or from acquired defects, such as bariatric surgery, and may be either global or partial. The degree of nutrient malabsorption from bariatric surgery is dependent on the type of bariatric procedure.

Incidence
A. Incidence is unknown.

Pathogenesis
A. Deficiency of intestinal enzymes: lactase deficiency
B. Inadequate digestion caused by disease of the pancreas (such as cystic fibrosis), gallbladder, or liver
C. Change in bacteria that normally live in the intestinal tract
D. Disease of intestinal walls, such as helminthes (worms) or parasites, tropical sprue, and celiac disease
E. Surgery that reduces the intestinal tract, decreasing the area for absorption such as bariatric surgery
F. Intolerance to gluten, or celiac sprue

Predisposing Factors
A. Lactose deficiency
1. Incidence is increased in African Americans, Indians, and Asians.
2. Jews typically have onset in adulthood.
B. Family history of malabsorption or cystic fibrosis
C. Use of drugs, such as mineral oil or other laxatives
D. Excess alcohol consumption
E. Travel to foreign countries
F. Intestinal surgery, especially bariatric procedures

Common Complaints
A. Diarrhea, stools pale, greasy, and copious
B. Foul-smelling stools, frequently with mucus
C. Weight loss despite adequate food intake
D. Gas or vague abdominal discomfort
E. Anorexia

Other Signs and Symptoms
A. Early malabsorption:

1. Minimal weight loss
2. Softer, more frequent stools
3. Steatorrhea; stools "float" because of increased trapped gas
4. Abdominal discomfort
5. Bloating

B. Later signs: Above symptoms plus the following:
1. Marked weight loss
2. Foul-smelling, bulky, greasy stools

C. Malabsorption of fats and carbohydrates: Previous symptoms plus the following:
1. Foul-smelling, bulky, greasy, "sticky" stools that may be difficult to flush down the toilet
2. Ecchymosis
3. Bone pain
4. Glossitis
5. Muscle tenderness
6. Cramping in lower abdomen after BM

D. Malabsorption of lactose:
1. Nausea and bloating
2. Cramps
3. Diarrhea after ingesting more than customary intake of milk products
4. Absent or mild weight loss and steatorrhea
5. Good appetite

E. Edema: with severe protein depletion

F. Ecchymosis and bleeding disorders secondary to vitamin K malabsorption

Subjective Data

A. Review onset, duration, and course of symptoms. Are there any other family members with the same history/symptoms?

B. Ask the patient about dietary intake history.

C. Review any changes in bowel movements and stool characteristics.

D. Inquire about recent travel to areas known for giardiasis or other parasites.

E. Document weight loss, how much, and over what period of time.

F. Review previous GI surgery including the bariatric procedures and reversals, small bowel resections, and partial or total resection of the pancreas.

G. Ask the patient about signs and symptoms of inflammatory bowel disease, such as easy bruising, paresthesia, and sore tongue.

H. Ask about any irradiation treatment.

Physical Examination

A. Check temperature, pulse, respirations, blood pressure (may have orthostatic hypotension), and weight.

B. Inspect
1. Observe general appearance, noting wasting and apathetic appearance.
2. If the patient experiences a bowel movement after the examination, observe the stool for volume, appearance, presence of blood, mucus, and the presence of gross worms/parasites.
3. Inspect the skin for ecchymosis, jaundice, pallor, surgical scars, stigmata of hyperthyroidism or

hepatocellular failure, or signs of Kaposi's sarcoma. Alopecia or seborrheic dermatitis may be present.
4. Inspect the ears, nose, and throat for glossitis, stomatitis, aphthous ulcers, poor dentition, and goiter.

C. Auscultate
1. Auscultate the heart for tachycardia.
2. Auscultate the abdomen in all four quadrants for bowel sounds noting borborygmi.

D. Palpate
1. Palpate all lymph nodes; look for lymphadenopathy.
2. Palpate the abdomen for organomegaly, focal tenderness, masses, distension, and ascites.

E. Neurologic exam: Assess for signs of vitamin B_{12} deficiency including motor weakness, peripheral neuropathy, or ataxia.

F. Rectal exam: Note tenderness, discharge, blood, and stool.

Diagnostic Tests

A. Assessment of stool fat: qualitative assessment on a single specimen.

B. Quantitative assessment of a 72-hour stool collection while the patient is following a 100 gm fat/day diet.

C. Increased fecal fat: test for celiac disease.

D. Abdominal ultrasound.

E. Colonoscopy to evaluate and obtain biopsies.

F. Endoscopy to evaluate and obtain biopsies.

G. Barium studies.

H. Consider CT of the abdomen.

I. Endoscopic retrograde cholangiopancreatogram (ERCP) helps to document malabsorption due to pancreatic or biliary-related disorders.

J. Breath tests for carbohydrate malabsorption.

K. CBC and electrolytes.

L. Serum iron, vitamin $B_{12,}$ and folate concentrations.

M. Prothrombin time (PT): may be prolonged due to vitamin K deficiency.

N. Vitamin levels: vitamins A, D, E, and K may be decreased.

O. Total protein: may be decreased.

P. Albumin: may be decreased.

Q. Serum amylase.

R. Stool for ova and parasites; obtain on alternate days for three or more specimens because parasites are passed intermittently.

Differential Diagnoses

A. Malabsorption
B. AIDS
C. Alcoholism
D. Worms or parasites
E. Cystic fibrosis
F. Failure to thrive
G. Celiac disease
H. Tropical sprue
I. Side effect from bariatric surgery
J. Disaccharidase deficiencies (lactase)
K. Fructose intolerance
L. Milk or protein allergy
M. Whipple disease
N. Zollinger-Ellison syndrome

Plan

A. General interventions: Treatment depends on underlying cause.

B. Patient teaching: See the Section III Patient Teaching Guide for this chapter, "Lactose Intolerance and Malabsorption."

C. Dietary management: In most patients, diet modification or dietary supplements restore health.

D. Pharmaceutical therapy
   1. Vitamin supplements: Fat-soluble vitamins A, D, and K are most likely to be depleted. Supplements help prevent malnutrition, even though caloric intake may be replenished.
      a. Vitamin A: 25,000–50,000 U/day orally.
      b. Vitamin D: 30,000 U/day orally.
      c. Vitamin K: 4–12 mg/day orally.
      d. Vitamin B_{12}: 1,000 g/month by IM injection.
   2. Enzyme replacements: These replace endogenous exocrine pancreatic enzymes and aid in digestion of starches, fat, and proteins. Pancreatic supplements are typically expressed in USP units. One IU is equivalent to approximately 2–3 USP units.
      a. Pancreatin, adults and children: Doses vary with the condition being treated. Oral doses are given before or with meals or each snack. It may also be given in divided doses at 1- to 2-hour intervals throughout the day.
      b. Pancrelipase (Creon, Pancrease, Ultrase, Viokase): This must be given with each meal or snack:
         i. Adults: 1–3 capsules or tablets orally with meals; titrate dose to desired clinical response.
         ii. Children: 500 to 2,000 U of lipase/kg/meal orally, dosage should be individualized to the patient's response. Adjust dose according to stool fat and nitrogen content.
   3. Antispasmodics
      a. Anticholinergic agents are used to reduce the cholinergic stimulation of colonic activity that occurs in response to a meal.
      b. Drug of choice: dicyclomine hydrochloride (Antispas), 10–20 mg orally before meals.
   4. Iron and folic acid supplementation are usually required for celiac disease.
   5. Calcium and magnesium supplementation are required after extensive small intestinal resection.

Follow-up

A. If exam is normal, observe the patient for 1 month and have the patient keep a diary of food intake and weight.

B. For persistent malabsorption monitor for osteoporosis/bone mass with a DEXA scan.

Consultation/Referral

A. Any patient with weight loss of 15 kg is likely to have a life-threatening condition and requires prompt consultation and hospitalization.

B. Consult a gastroenterologist when malabsorption is documented by 72-hour stool fat assessment.

C. Consider a dietary consultation.

D. Refer back to the bariatric surgeon/center depending on surgical complications from bariatric surgery.

E. Consider a referral for allergy testing to milk and proteins.

Individual Considerations

Geriatrics

A. To identify impediments to adequate food intake, question the patient about social isolation, depression, bereavement, physical impairment, poor dentition, and poverty.

B. Loss of taste is sometimes responsible for poor intake and should be checked.

NAUSEA AND VOMITING

Definition

Nausea and vomiting are common symptoms for many conditions and diseases and include several terms to describe the symptoms (see Table 10.19).

A. Hyperemesis gravidarum is a condition of persistent, uncontrollable vomiting that begins in the first weeks of pregnancy and may continue throughout pregnancy.

B. Chronic nausea and vomiting is defined as at least 1 month in duration.

C. Complications of nausea and vomiting include fluid depletion, hypokalemia, and metabolic alkalosis.

Incidence

A. Nausea and vomiting are very common and the etiology is dependent on the disease/condition. During pregnancy, 70%–85% of women experience nausea and/or vomiting; 50% have both nausea and vomiting. Onset after the initial nine weeks of pregnancy should direct especially careful evaluation for another cause within the differential diagnoses of nausea and vomiting in nonpregnant patients. Hyperemesis gravidarum occurs in 1 in every 0.5%–2% of pregnancies.

Pathogenesis

A. Protective mechanisms are activated by numerous gastrointestinal (GI) and non-GI causes. Normal function of the upper GI tract involves an interaction between the gut and the central nervous system. Nausea and vomiting in pregnancy are related to increased hormones, including human chorionic gonadotropin (HCG), estrogen, and progesterone, as well as decreased gastric motility and relative hypoglycemia that results from a night-long fast.

Predisposing Factors

A. Acute nausea and vomiting
   1. Medications: digitalis toxicity, opiate use, chemotherapy agents, drug withdrawal, nicotine/nicotine patches, antibiotics, hormones, and antivirals
   2. Ketoacidosis
   3. Pregnancy or hormones
   4. Binge drinking
   5. Hepatitis

B. Recurrent or chronic nausea and vomiting
   1. Psychogenic vomiting
   2. Metabolic disturbances
   3. Gastric retention

TABLE 10.19	Definitions of Terminology Used to Describe Nausea and Vomiting
Vomiting	Forceful oral expulsion of gastric contents associated with contraction of the abdominal and chest wall musculature
Nausea	The unpleasant sensation of the imminent need to vomit, usually referred to the throat or epigastrium; a sensation that may or may not ultimately lead to vomiting
Regurgitation	The act by which food is brought back into the mouth without the abdominal and diaphragmatic muscular activity that characterizes vomiting
Anorexia	Loss of desire to eat; a true loss of appetite
Sitophobia	Fear of eating because of subsequent or associated discomfort
Early satiety	Fear of being full after eating an unusually small quantity of food
Retching	Spasmodic respiratory movements against a closed glottis with contraction of the abdominal musculature without expulsion of any gastric contents, referred to as "dry heaves"
Rumination	Chewing and swallowing of regurgitated food that has come back into the mouth through voluntary increase in abdominal pressure within minutes of eating or during eating; rumination may be accompanied by weight loss and bulimia

4. Bile reflux
5. Pregnancy
C. Nausea and vomiting with abdominal pain
  1. Viral gastroenteritis
  2. Acute gastritis
  3. Food poisoning
  4. Peptic ulcer disease
  5. Acute pancreatitis
  6. Small bowel obstruction
  7. Acute appendicitis
  8. Acute cholecystitis
  9. Acute cholangitis
  10. Acute pyelonephritis
  11. Inferior MI
D. Nausea and vomiting with neurologic symptoms
  1. Increased intracranial pressure
  2. Midline cerebellar hemorrhage
  3. Vestibular disturbances
  4. Migraine headaches
  5. Autonomic dysfunction

Common Complaints
A. Food aversion
B. Inability to retain food or liquids

Other Signs and Symptoms
A. Increased salivation
B. Bitter taste, "acid brash": indicates ulcer or small bowel obstruction
C. Weight loss
D. Dehydration
E. Sweating
F. Fast pulse
G. Pale skin
H. Rapid breathing

Subjective Data
A. Review onset, duration (acute or chronic problem?), and course of symptoms, including the quality (projectile?) and quantity of emesis. What was the color, taste, and consistency of the emesis? Was there blood present?
  1. Vomiting bright red blood indicates a hemorrhage—**peptic ulcer.**
  2. Dark red blood indicates a hemorrhage—**esophageal or gastric varices.**
  3. Coffee grounds material is indicative of digested blood from a slowly bleeding gastric or duodenal ulcer.
  4. Vomiting fecal material is a sign of distal **small-bowel obstruction** and blind-loop syndrome.
B. Ask the patient about other symptoms, including pain, fever, diarrhea, and headache.
C. Inquire if other family members are also ill and what are their symptoms.
D. Review the timing of vomiting in relation to meals, time of day, odors, and activity. Does vomiting occur before or after food intake?
E. Ask the patient about medication intake such as antibiotics, chemotherapy, herbals, digitalis, opiates, and birth control pills.
F. Ask about self-image, binge eating, and self-induced emesis.
G. Review any exposure to hepatitis or travel to places with poor sanitation and outbreaks of cholera.
H. Review the patient's medical history for vertigo, head injury, jaundice, diabetes, hypertension, and pregnancy.
I. Inquire about first day of last period and birth control method used.
J. Establish usual weight. Has there been any recent weight change, how many pounds, and over what period of time?
K. Ask about the patient's history of diabetes, gallbladder disease, ulcer disease, or cancer.

Physical Examination
A. Check temperature, pulse, respirations, blood pressure, and weight.
B. Inspect
  1. Observe general overall appearance of skin for pallor and signs of dehydration. Tenting of skin when it is

rolled between your thumb and index finger may indicate dehydration.
2. Inspect for signs of autonomic insufficiency. Postural hypotension, lack of sweat, or blunted pulse and blood pressure responses to Valsalva's maneuver suggest autonomic dysfunction and a bowel motility problem as the underlying etiology of nausea and vomiting. Postural hypotension indicates marked volume depletion or circulatory collapse.
3. Oral exam: Inspect mouth, teeth, and gums.
4. Inspect fontanelles in infants.
C. Palpate
1. Palpate the abdomen for masses, distension, tenderness, signs of peritonitis, and organomegaly.
2. Palpate the back; note CVA tenderness.
D. Percuss the abdomen.
E. Auscultate
1. Auscultate the abdomen for bowel sounds in all quadrants.
2. Auscultate the heart and lungs.
F. Perform rectal exam.

Diagnostic Tests
A. Urine: urinalysis, pregnancy test, culture and sensitivity, if indicated
B. Serum labs: multiple chemistry profile, including amylase, electrolytes, BUN, creatinine, glucose, and transaminase
C. Drug screen
D. Upper GI
E. Ultrasonography, to rule out molar pregnancy if persistent nausea and vomiting, especially after 16 weeks' gestation
F. Stool for occult blood
G. Endoscopy
H. Head CT scan, if indicated
I. Gastric scintigraphy, to rule out gastroparesis if indicated
J. EKG if chest pain/myocardial infarction is suspected

Differential Diagnoses
A. See Predisposing Factors.

Plan
A. General interventions: Assess hydration status. Proceed to IV hydration and antiemetics until ketones clear.
B. Patient teaching: See Patient Teaching Sheet: "Nausea and Vomiting Diet Suggestions (Children and Adults)"
C. Dietary management: see Appendix B "Nausea and Vomiting Diet Suggestions (Children and Adults)"
D. Pharmaceutical therapy (not an exhaustive list)
1. Antiemetics
a. Emetrol; available OTC:
i. Adults: 15–30 mL by mouth at 15-min intervals.
ii. Children older than 2 years: 5–10 mL by mouth at 15-min intervals.
iii. Children younger than 2 years or less than 30 lb: dose is not available.
iv. Tell the patient not to dilute the drug or take fluids 15 min before or after taking the medication.

b. Promethazine (Phenergan):
i. Drug of choice for gastroenteritis.
ii. Adults: 25–50 mg by mouth or per rectum every 4–6 hours.
iii. Children older than 2 years: 12.5–25 mg by mouth every 12 hours.
iv. Children younger than 2 years or less than 30 lb: not recommended.
c. Trimethobenzamide (Tigan):
i. Used for gastroenteritis and motion sickness.
ii. Adults: 250 mg three or four times daily.
iii. Children older than 2 years, 30–90 lb: 100–200 mg by mouth three to four times daily.
iv. Children younger than 2 years: 100-mg rectal suppository, three to four times in 1 day.
d. Prochlorperazine (Compazine):
i. Adults: 5–10 mg three or four times daily; spanules 10 mg every 12 hours; suppositories 25 mg twice daily.
ii. Children 40–85 lb: 5 mg twice daily, up to a maximum of 15 mg/day.
iii. Children younger than 2 years, 20–39 lb: 2.5 mg one to two times a day, up to maximum of 7.5 mg/day.
iv. Children younger than 2 years or less than 20 lb: not recommended.
2. Outpatient IV hydration in pregnancy: 1 liter lactated Ringer's solution to correct dehydration and restore electrolyte balance. Check urine ketones after first liter to determine if additional liter is necessary to clear ketones.
3. 5-HT3 antagonists
a. Ondansetron (Zofran)
i. Adults: 8–24 mg as directed for nausea related to chemotherapy or other diagnoses.
ii. Children ages 4–11: 4 mg as directed for nausea from chemotherapy or other diagnoses.
b. Granisetron (Sancuso): Transdermal patch for patients on chemotherapy. Transdermal patches should not be cut.
i. Adults: 1 patch on the outer arm 24–48 hours before chemotherapy; may wear up to 7 days.
ii. Children: not recommended for those younger than 18 years of age.

Follow-up
A. Tell the patient to call or visit the office in 24 hours to check response and nutritional intake.
B. Tell parents that are giving simple treatment at home to call the office promptly if projectile or prolonged vomiting occur.

Consultation/Referral
A. Hyperemesis gravidarum may require hospitalization to correct fluid and electrolyte imbalance.
B. Consult a physician and hospitalize the patient promptly if there is evidence of bowel obstruction; increased intracranial pressure (ICP); or another GI, neurologic, or metabolic emergency. **First priority is to rule out acute surgical etiology such as bowel obstruction and peritonitis.**

C. Call for a pediatric consultation immediately for vomiting lasting more than 24 hours, projectile vomiting, vomiting after a fall or head injury, or prolonged vomiting coupled with diarrhea.

D. Call for a psychiatric consultation for suspected psychogenic nausea and vomiting.

E. If postural hypotension occurs, especially in elderly patients, hospital admission for parenteral fluid and electrolyte replacement is indicated.

Individual Considerations

A. Pregnancy
1. Determine whether the woman is ingesting nonfood substances, such as starch, clay, or toothpaste, which would indicate pica.
2. Intractable nausea and vomiting require ultrasonography to rule out hydatidiform mole.
3. Emetrol, promethazine (Phenergan), and prochlorperazine (Compazine) may be used during pregnancy.
4. Uncorrected hyperemesis gravidarum can result in severe electrolyte imbalance and possible hepatic and renal damage. The major concern for fetal well-being is uncorrected ketosis, which may result in fetal abnormalities or death in early pregnancy.
5. Tell the patient to eat toast or a dry cracker before arising; to eat small, frequent meals and snacks; to drink fluids separately from meals; and to avoid fatty, fried, greasy, or spicy foods and foods with strong odors.

B. Pediatrics
1. The differential diagnosis of vomiting is age-dependent.
2. For neonates and young infants, the most frequent diagnostic consideration are:
   a. GERD
   b. Excessive feeding volume
   c. Increased intracranial pressure/meningitis
   d. Food allergy
   e. Intestinal obstruction
      i. Malrotation without volvulus
      ii. Hirschsprung disease
      iii. Intussesception
      iv. Intestinal atresia
      v. Pyloric stenosis
3. Older infants and children differential diagnoses include:
   a. Gastroenteritis
   b. GERD
   c. Gastroparesis
   d. Mechanical obstruction
   e. Munchausen syndrome by proxy
4. Adolescents disorders include the disorders affecting children as well as:
   a. Appendicitis
   b. Inflammatory bowel disease
   c. Pregnancy
   d. Bulimia or psychogenic vomiting
5. Question caregivers regarding the infant's feeding, activity level, irritability, lethargy, and number of wet diapers.

6. Otitis media, pharyngitis, and UTIs may present with nausea and/or vomiting in the pediatric population.
7. Rumination syndrome is a behavioral disorder that is most commonly identified among mentally disadvantaged children and adolescents of normal mental capacity. The behavior consists of daily, effortless regurgitation of undigested food within minutes of starting or completing ingestion of a meal.

▢ PEPTIC ULCER DISEASE

Definition

A. Peptic ulcer disease (PUD) is circumscribed ulceration of the GI mucosa occurring in areas exposed to acid and pepsin. The patient's prior ulcer history tends to predict future behavior and risk of future complications. Complications include bleeding ulcer, perforation, and obstruction.

B. The stomach is divided on the basis of its physiologic functions into two main portions. The proximal two thirds, the fundic gland area, acts as a receptable for ingested food and secretes acid and pepsin. The distal third, the pyloric gland area, mixes and propels food into the duodenum and produces the hormone gastrin. "Peptic" lesions may occur in the esophagus (esophagitis), stomach (gastritis), or duodenum (duodenitis). See Figure 10.4.

C. There is often no correlation between the presence of an active ulcer, noted by endoscopy, and symptoms. And the disappearance of symptoms does not guarantee ulcer healing.

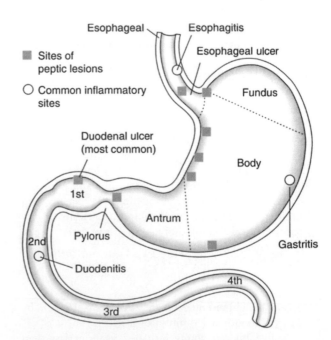

Figure 10.4 Location of ulcers.
From *The Lippincott Manual of Nursing Practice, 9th ed.,* by S. Nettina, 2010. Philadelphia: Wolters Kluwer Health/ Lippincott Williams & Wilkins.

Incidence

A. The annual incidence of peptic ulcer is estimated to range from 0.1%–1.8%. The ulcer incidence in H. pylori-infected individuals is about 1% per year. The recurrence rate is 50%–80% during the 6–12 months following the initial ulcer healing, although relapses are not always symptomatic. Some peptic ulcers heal spontaneously and 2–20 of patients have multiple simultaneous ulcers.

B. From 16%–31% of ulcers are caused by nonsteroidal anti-inflammatory drugs (NSAIDs). Epidemiologic studies show that risks of peptic ulcer and death are three to six times higher among people who take NSAIDs. Cigarette smokers are twice as likely to develop ulcers as nonsmokers.

Pathogenesis

A. Although the precise mechanisms of ulcer formation remain incompletely understood, the process appears to involve the interplay of acid production, pepsin secretion, bacterial infection, and mucosal defense mechanisms. Excess acid production is the hallmark of duodenal ulcer disease. Pepsin secretion is also elevated in duodenal ulcer (DU) disease.

B. The relation of aspirin and other NSAIDs to ulcer disease is due largely to the drugs' potent inhibition of gastric mucosal prostaglandin synthesis. In addition to prostaglandin inhibition, many NSAID preparations produce acute diffuse mucosal injury by means of a direct erosive effect.

Predisposing Factors

A. Use of NSAIDs, especially aspirin
B. Smoking
C. Genetic factors
D. Male gender
  1. Peak prevalence of duodenal ulcer occurs between ages 45 and 54.
  2. Peak prevalence of gastric ulcer occurs between ages 55 and 64.
E. Excessive alcohol consumption, which stimulates acid secretion
F. Improper diet, irregular meals, and skipped meals
G. Helicobacter pylori (H. pylori) infection; prevalence increases with age
H. Severe physiologic stress
  1. Burns
  2. CNS trauma
  3. Surgery
  4. Severe medical illness
    a. Cirrhosis
    b. COPD
    c. Renal failure
    d. Organ transplantation
I. Other causes
  1. Radiation-induced ulcer
  2. Chemotherapy-induced ulcer
  3. Vascular insufficiency
  4. Duodenal obstruction

Common Complaints

A. Pain described as aching, boring, gnawing, or burning feeling
B. Epigastric pain, in upper right and left upper quadrants of the abdomen or occasionally below breast
C. Pain that awakens the patient at night or in early morning

Other Signs and Symptoms

A. Asymptomatic
B. GI distress 1–3 hours after a meal, on an empty stomach
C. Pain relieved by food, antacids, or vomiting
D. Nausea and vomiting
E. Hematemesis
F. Chest discomfort
G. Blood in stools, "grape jelly" or maroon-colored stools
H. Loss of appetite or weight
I. Weight gain; with duodenal ulcer may eat more to ease pain
J. Anemia

Signs and Symptoms of Bleeding

A. Massive bleeding
  1. Acute, bright red hematemesis or large amount of melena with clots in the stool, or "grape jelly" stool
  2. Rapid pulse, drop in blood pressure, hypovolemia, and shock
B. Subacute bleeding
  1. Intermittent melena or coffee-ground emesis
  2. Hypotension
  3. Weakness and dizziness
C. Chronic bleeding
  1. Intermittent appearance of blood
  2. Increased weakness, paleness, or shortness of breath
  3. Occult blood

Subjective Data

A. Ask the patient to describe onset, duration, type, and location of pain. Does it occur at any special time, for example, before meals, after meals, or during the night?
B. Has the patient had a previous ulcer? What was the treatment; if oral treatment was prescribed, did the patient complete the therapy?
C. Have the patient describe what alleviates pain, such as taking antacids, and what worsens pain, such as use of aspirin, oral steroids, or NSAIDs.
D. Review associated symptoms, such as nausea, vomiting, and heartburn.
E. Ask the patient if any first-degree relatives have ulcers.
F. Inquire whether the patient is a smoker. If so, how much and for how long?
G. Ask the patient about alcohol consumption: how much and for how long?
H. Inquire whether any blood has ever been vomited or passed in stool. If so, have the patient describe it.
I. Take the patient's dietary history, including time of meals, frequency of skipped meals, weight loss, and so forth.
J. Obtain past medical history of associated diseases, such as cirrhosis, pancreatitis, arthritis, COPD, and, hyperparathyroidism.
K. If the patient suspects blood in stool, ask if there has been a change in bowel pattern, presence of abdominal pain or tenderness, and what kind of food, such as red beets, the patient recently ingested.

Physical Examination

A. Check temperature, pulse, respirations, blood pressure, and weight.

B. Palpate the abdomen for tenderness, rigidity, masses, and liver or spleen enlargement.

C. Percuss the abdomen for hepatosplenomegaly.

D. Auscultate the abdomen for bowel sounds in all quadrants.

E. Rectal exam
   1. Check for tenderness and masses.
   2. Take stool specimen.

Diagnostic Tests

A. CBC.

B. Stool for occult blood.

C. Coagulation studies.

D. Testing for *H. pylori*
   1. Urea breath test (UBT).
   2. Serum test for *H. pylori* antibodies.
   3. Stool *H. pylori* antigen testing.
   4. Endoscopic biopsy testing.

E. Radiography with barium meal.

F. Endoscopy with biopsy, after GI consultation; test is expensive and requires sedation.

G. Mucosal biopsy, after GI consultation, to rule out cancer.

H. Measurement of acid secretion is not useful in the routine evaluation of PUD.

Differential Diagnoses

A. Peptic ulcer disease

B. Gastroesophageal reflux disease (GERD)

C. Zollinger-Ellison syndrome: fasting serum gastrin level 500 pg/mL in presence of acid hypersecretion is diagnostic

D. Cancer
   1. Gastric lymphoma
   2. Gastric cancer
   3. Pancreatic cancer

E. Pancreatitis (acute or chronic)

F. Myocardial ischemia

G. Diverticulitis

H. Drug-induced dyspepsia
   1. Theophylline
   2. Digitalis

I. Crohn's disease involving the stomach or duodenum

J. Gastric infections

Plan

A. General interventions: Goals are to alleviate pain, promote healing, limit complications, and prevent recurrences while minimizing costs and side effects of treatment.
   1. Encourage the patient to stop taking NSAIDs, unless medically indicated.
      a. If NSAID use in unavoidable, the lowest possible dose and duration and cotherapy with a PPI or Misoprostol are recommended.
   2. Smoking cessation should be highly encouraged at each visit.

B. Patient teaching: See the Section III Patient Teaching Guide for this chapter, "Management of Ulcers."

C. Dietary management: Advise the patient to avoid alcohol, coffee, including decaffeinated, and other caffeine-containing beverages because they stimulate acid secretion. (See Appendix B, Table B.9: Bland Foods With Limited Odors.)

D. Medical and surgical management
   1. Diagnostic evaluation of the ulcer is by means of endoscopy.
   2. Test for *H. pylori*.
      a. A single negative *H. pylori* test should be interpreted cautiously, especially in the face of active bleeding. Blood in the stomach can alter the pH indicator in the rapid urease test. False negatives are likely and additional testing for *H. pylori* is essential.
      b. Concurrent use of a proton pump inhibitor (PPI), antibiotics, or bismuth will cause a false negative test.
   3. Surgery remains an option for treatment of refractory disease and complications. The most serious indications for surgery include brisk bleeding of 6–8 units of blood in 24 hours, recurrent bleeding episodes, perforation, gastric outlet obstruction refractory to medical therapy, and failure of a benign gastric ulcer to heal after 15 weeks. Emergency intervention may be required, such as NPO status, IV, NG tube, oxygen therapy, or blood transfusion. If life-threatening bleeding occurs, treat shock.

E. Pharmaceutical therapy:
   1. The treatment of peptic ulcer begins with the eradication of *H. pylori* in infected individuals. Empiric therapy for the infection is reasonable for uncomplicated cases in the absence of NSAID use. Documenting infection, even in patients with known ulcers, is an essential step prior to initiating antimicrobial therapy.
      a. Anti-*H. pylori* regimen given orally four times a day for 14 days
         i. Metronidazole (Flagyl) 300 mg
         ii. Amoxicillin 500 mg
         iii. Clarithromycin 250 mg
         iv. Plus an antacid for symptom control
      b. Helidac therapy (sold in a combination pack) oral doses four times a day for 14 days
         i. Choose an H_2 receptor antagonist
         ii. Metronidazole (Flagyl) 250 mg four times daily
         iii. Tetracycline 500 mg four times daily
         iv. Bismuth subsalicylate 2 chew tablets four times a daily
   2. Antisecretory therapy is the mainstay of therapy in uninfected patients and is used for maintenance therapy in selected cases. Full doses of H_2 receptor antagonist provide effective initial therapy; however, PPIs are more effective.

      Patients with uncomplicated, small (<1 cm) DU or GU who have received adequate treatment for *H. pylori* probably are asymptomatic and do not need any further therapy directed at ulcer healing. Maintenance acid suppression following *H. pyloric* eradication is recommended for patients with a complicated DU.

If the ulcer is giant (>2 cm), densely fibrosed ulcer beds, or a high-risk patient with a protracted prior history, then the patient should be kept on a PPI until a follow-up endoscopy.

a. H₂ receptor antagonists: split dose, evening, and nighttime therapy are all effective. In the United States cimetidine, ranitidine, and famotidine are approved for GU healing.
   i. Cimetidine (Tagamet) 400 mg orally twice a day or 800 mg at bedtime for 6–8 weeks
   ii. Ranitidine (Zantac) 150 mg orally twice a day or 300 mg at bedtime
   iii. Famotidine (Pepsid) 20 mg orally twice a day or 40 mg at bedtime
   iv. Nizatidine (Axid) 150 mg orally twice a day or 300 mg at bedtime
b. Proton pump inhibitors are effective in inducing ulcer healing. The PPIs are the most potent inhibitors of gastric acid secretion. Once-daily dosing is generally sufficient for acid inhibition; however, a second dose may be necessary and should be given before the evening meal. Once-daily PPI dosing inhibits acid output by 66% after 5 days. Optimal dosing is immediately before breakfast.
   i. Omeprazole (Prilosec/Zegerid) 20–40 mg every morning for 4 weeks
   ii. Esomeprazole (Nexium) 20–40 mg every morning for 4–8 weeks
   iii. Lansoprazole (Prevacid) 15–30 mg every morning for 4 weeks
   iv. Dexlansoprazole (Kapidex) 30–60 mg every morning for 4–8 weeks
   v. Pantoprazole (Protonix) 20–40 mg every morning for 4 weeks
   vi. Rabeprazole (Aciphex) 20 mg every morning for 4 weeks

   PPIs should not be given concomitantly with prostaglandins, or other antisecretory agents because of the marked reduction in their effects.

   An H₂ antagonist can be used with a PPI if given after a sufficient interval between their administrations; the minimal times have not been established. The H₂ antagonist could be given at bedtime for breakthrough symptoms after a morning dose of a PPI.
3. Sucralfate (Carafate) 1 g orally four times daily, 1 hour before meals and at bedtime; maintenance therapy is 1 g twice daily. Sucralfate is not recommended for *H. pylori* or NSAID ulcers.
4. Misoprostol (Cytotec, a prostaglandin analogue) is effective for peptic ulcers due to NSAID use; PUs respond well to Misoprostol 100–200 mcg orally four times a day.

Follow-up
A. Therapeutic trial of lifestyle changes combined with an H₂ receptor antagonist, sucralfate, or omeprazole for 1–2 weeks should provide relief. Reevaluate the patient after 2 weeks, and if symptoms are improved, prescribe a full course of 6–8 weeks.
B. Reevaluate the patient again at 8 weeks, after the full course of therapy is completed.
C. Consider repeating breath test to confirm eradication of *H. pylori*.
D. Some authorities advocate routine endoscopic or radiological documentation of healing. However, there are no studies showing this to be cost-effective in uncomplicated cases in which symptoms resolve within 4–6 weeks and do not recur.
E. For refractory gastric ulcer, that is, persistent pain after 8 weeks despite a full medical regimen or unresponsive to treatment for *H. pylori*, endoscopic examination and biopsy are needed, especially in patients over age 40 who are at increased risk of gastric cancer. Barium study is not sufficient, because even malignant ulcers may shrink in size in response to therapy.
F. Evaluate refractory cases for Zollinger-Ellison syndrome, especially when there are multiple ulcers, occurrences in unusual places, marked abdominal pain, or a secretory diarrhea.

Consultation/Referral
A. Consult both a surgeon and a gastroenterologist and admit the patient to a hospital when symptoms of hemorrhage, penetration, perforation, or gastric outlet obstruction are present.
B. Refer patients with recurrences or refractory disease to a physician for evaluation for *H. pylori* infection by endoscopy or breath test. If present, eradicate with a 2-week course of triple therapy.

Individual Considerations
A. Pregnancy: The drugs Misoprostol and Ranitidine are abortifacients. They cross the placental barrier and are excreted in breast milk and are contraindicated in pregnancy or suspected pregnancy. Use in sexually active women of childbearing age should be done with proper warning and detailed patient education.
B. Adults
   1. Duodenal ulcers are more common in people between ages 45 and 54; gastric ulcers, between 55 and 64 years.
   2. Patients over age 40 are at greater risk of gastric cancer and should undergo either an upper GI series or endoscopy to document the nature and location of lesions when there is strong clinical suspicion of ulcer disease.
   3. Gastritis not associated with reflux is present in 75% of people over age 50.
C. Geriatrics
   1. Silent disease is particularly common among the elderly and those using NSAIDs.
   2. Lethargy, confusion, slurred speech, agitation, and visual hallucinations have been reported with Cimetidine, particularly in the elderly.

3. In the elderly, duodenal ulcer symptoms remain classic with early morning awakening to pain, then quick relief by food or antacids. Gastric ulcer symptoms are less obvious, with burning or gnawing pain experienced in less than 50% of elderly patients.

4. Anemia may be the only symptom of gastric cancer. Cancer must always be considered and confirmed by endoscopy with biopsy.

PINWORM, ENTEROBIASIS VERMICULARIS

Definition
A. Pinworm, *Enterobiasis vermicularis,* is the most common helminth infection. It is characterized by a white, thread-like worm infestation.

Incidence
A. Pinworm is very common. *Enterobiasis* occurs worldwide and commonly occurs in family clusters. It has a high incidence of re-infection. Exact data are not available because helminth infestations are not CDC reportable.

Pathogenesis
A. The *Enterobius vermicularis* adult nematode, or round-worm, lives in the human rectum or colon and emerges onto the perianal skin to lay eggs. It is transmissible by direct transfer of infective eggs to mouth, or indirectly through clothing, bedding, food, or other articles contaminated with eggs of the parasite. Period of communicability is as long as female nematodes are discharging eggs on perianal skin. Eggs remain infective in an indoor environment, usually 2–3 weeks. Humans are the only known hosts; dogs and cats do not harbor *E. vermicularis.*

B. Incubation period is 1–2 months or longer, from ingestion of an egg until an adult gravid female migrates to the perianal region.

Predisposing Factors
A. Preschool and school age
B. Member of a family of an infected person
C. Institutional residence
D. Overcrowded living conditions

Common Complaints
A. Intense, nighttime anal pruritus
B. Irritability in infants and children

Other Signs and Symptoms
A. Disturbed sleep or insomnia
B. Pruritus vulvae
C. Urethritis
D. Vaginitis
E. Local irritation
F. Secondary infections from scratching
G. Loss of appetite or weight loss
H. Grinding teeth at night
I. Enuresis

Subjective Data
A. Review onset, duration, course, and time of symptoms, especially anal itching.

B. Ask the patient about symptoms in other family members.
C. Inquire about genital irritation symptoms in female children.

Physical Examination
A. Check temperature, pulse, respirations, blood pressure, and weight.
B. Inspect anus and female genitals for irritation and skin abrasions.

Diagnostic Tests
A. Press sticky side of transparent (not translucent) cellulose tape against perianal folds, and then press tape on glass slide. Eggs are most likely to be present on awakening and before the person bathes or uses the toilet.
B. Urinalysis to rule out UTI.
C. Stool specimen for ova and parasite; adult worms in feces are diagnostic.

Differential Diagnoses
A. Pinworms
B. UTI
C. Poor hygiene
D. Chemical irritants, soaps, and bubble baths

Plan
A. Patient teaching
   1. See the Section III Patient Teaching Guide for this chapter, "Roundworms and Pinworms."
   2. Teach the mother how to obtain a specimen from a child.
   3. Infected people should bathe in the morning to remove eggs.
   4. Use good hand washing before eating or preparing food.
   5. Keep fingernails short and avoid nail biting.
   6. All household members should be treated as a group when there are multiple instances.
B. Pharmaceutical therapy
   1. Mebendazole (Vermox) 100 mg orally twice a day for 3 days OR a one-time single dose of 500 mg.
   2. Pyrantel pamoate (Pyrantel) 11 mg/kg per day for 3 days; do not exceed 1 g/day.
   3. Albendazole (Albenza) 400 mg one-time dose.

Follow-up
A. If single-dose therapy is not effective, a second course of medication is advised in 3 weeks.

Consultation/Referral
A. Consult a physician if the patient is pregnant.

Individual Considerations
A. Pregnancy: Anthelmintics are in Pregnancy Class C; however, the risks versus benefits should be considered.
B. Pediatrics
   1. All medications are advised for children 2 years of age and older.
   2. Pinworms may predispose children to developing UTIs.
   3. No unusual cleansing other than basic hygiene measures should be undertaken. Excessive zeal in this regard can induce guilt and is counterproductive.

4. The best time to examine a child is 2–3 hours after he or she falls asleep.

C. Adults have the lowest incidence of pinworms.

POST-BARIATRIC SURGERY MANAGEMENT

Definition

A. The optimal management of overweight and obesity starts with a combination of diet, exercise, and behavior modification. Some patients eventually require bariatric surgery. Bariatric surgery is a therapeutic option for the management of carefully selected patients with severe obesity (BMI >40 or >35 with two significant comorbidities). There are several types of bariatric procedures that help promote weight loss by restricting food intake by limiting the amount of food that can be ingested and/or by decreasing the absorption of nutrients from the gut. See Table 10.20.

B. Restrictive procedures limit caloric intake by downsizing the stomach's reservoir capacity leaving the absorptive function of the small intestine intact. The primary mechanism of malabsorptive procedures is to decrease the effectiveness of nutrient absorption by shortening the length of functional small intestine. Some procedures have both a restrictive and malabsorptive component. The Roux-en-Y (RYGB), for example, is primarily a restrictive operation in which a small gastric pouch limits oral intake. See Figure 10.5.

Incidence

A. The Centers for Disease Control and Prevention (CDC) notes that more than one-third of the U.S. adult population and 16% of U.S. children are obese. Approximately 25% of bariatric surgery patients have surgical complications. Currently the most commonly performed gastric bypass procedure is the laparoscopic Roux-en-Y, representing 70%–75% of the procedures.

Pathogenesis

The pathogenesis of obesity is reviewed under "Obesity" in Chapter 19, "Endocrine Guidelines." The incidences of complications vary by surgical procedure and whether the surgery was performed laparoscopically or by an open surgical procedure. Post-operative complications may occur immediately or may occur long-term after surgery.

A. The laparoscopic adjustable gastric banding (LAGB), although simpler in comparison to malabsorptive procedures, tends to produce more gradual weight loss and patients may experience band slippage. Deficiency of fat-soluble vitamins, thiamine, and folate has been observed, especially if the patient develops frequent vomiting.

B. Profound weight loss can be achieved by the malabsorption operations (e.g., BPD, Sleeve procedure, or BPD-DS), depending on the effective length of the functional small bowel segment. The benefit of superior weight loss is often offset by the significant metabolic complications such as protein caloric malnutrition and various micronutrient deficiencies. See Figure 10.6.

C. The small bowel reconfiguration of the Roux-en-Y (RYGB) provides additional mechanisms favoring weight loss but includes side effects such as dumping physiology and malabsorption. Deficiency of iron, vitamin B_{12}, folate, calcium, and Vitamin D has been frequently observed after Roux-en-Y (RYGB) gastric bypass surgery.

Common Complaints

A. Metabolic alteration
1. Vitamin deficiencies
   a. Vitamin B_1 (Thiamine): loss of appetite, nausea, and vomiting. Neurologic symptoms include mental confusion, abnormal eye movement, hearing loss, weakness, and paraesthesia may occur if left unidentified.
   b. Vitamin B_{12}: pernious anemia, fatigue, sore tongue, anorexia, paraesthesia, impaired sense of smell, positive Babinski's sign, loss of deep tendon reflexes, and unsteady gait.
   c. Fat-soluble vitamins (A, D, E, and K): night blindness, delayed healing, gait disturbance, and petechiae.
2. Iron deficiency: fatigue, pallor, and picas.
3. Calcium deficiency: osteoporosis.
4. Protein deficiency: hair loss.

B. Surgical complications
1. Gastrointestinal bleeding.
2. Dumping syndrome occurs in approximately 50% of patients after RYGB. Dumping syndrome is characterized by symptoms of nausea, shaking, diaphoresis, and diarrhea shortly after eating foods containing high amounts of refined sugars.
3. Gastric leakage.
4. Bowel obstruction.
5. Bowel stricture.

TABLE 10.20 Bariatric Surgeries and Mechanism of Action

Restrictive Procedures	Malabsorptive Procedures	Restrictive and Malabsorptive Combination Procedure
1. Vertical Banded Gastroplasty (VBG)—not commonly performed	1. Biliopancreatic Diversion (BPD)	1. Roux-en-Y (RYGB)
2. Laparoscopic Adjustable Gastric Banding (LAGB)	2. Duodenal Switch (DS)	
3. Gastric Sleeve (GS)	3. Bilopancreatic Diversion & Duodenal Switch (BPD-DS)	

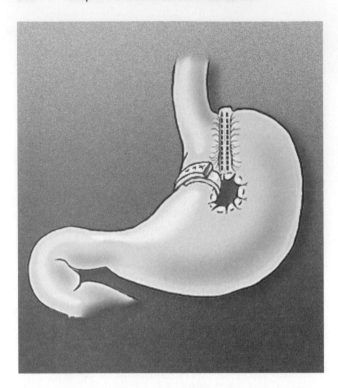

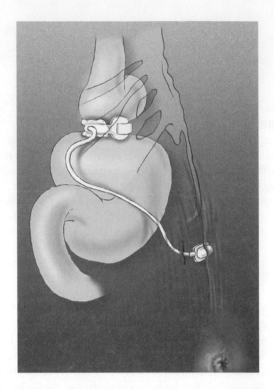

Figure 10.5a Gastric bypass procedures: Vertical banded gastroplasty.
Reprinted with permission of American Society of Metabolic and Bariatric Surgery, copyright 2009, all rights reserved.

Figure 10.5b Gastric bypass procedure: Laparoscopic adjustable gastric band.
Reprinted with permission of American Society of Metabolic and Bariatric Surgery, copyright 2009, all rights reserved.

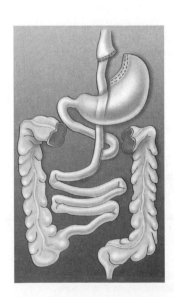

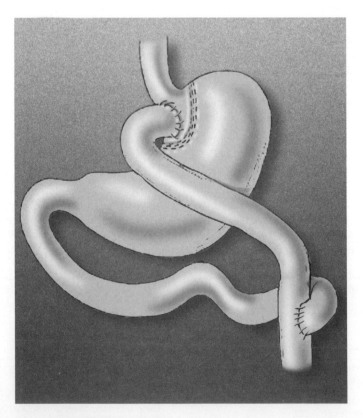

Figure 10.5c Gastric bypass procedures: Roux-en-y gastric bypass (RYGB).
Reprinted with permission of American Society of Metabolic and Bariatric Surgery, copyright 2009, all rights reserved.

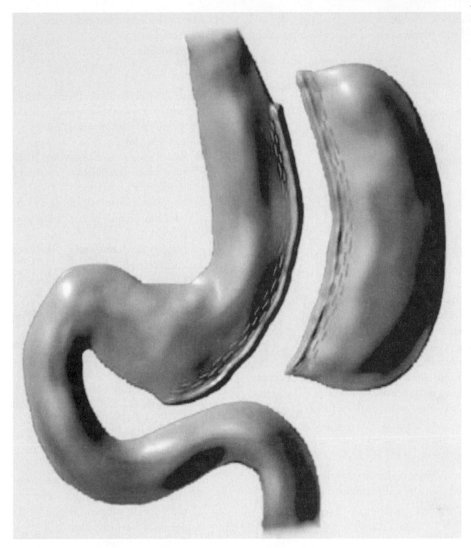

Figure 10.6 Sleeve bypass procedure with stomach resection.
Reprinted with permission from "Surgical Approaches to the Treatment of Obesity: Bariatric Surgery," by B. R. Smith, P. Schauer, & N. T. Nguyen, 2008, *Endocrinology and Metabolism Clinic of North America, 37, 949.*

6. Band slippage leading to gastric prolapse.
7. Infection.
8. Deep vein thrombus (DVT).
9. Ulcers.

Other Signs and Symptoms

A. Excessive nausea and vomiting after a laparoscopic adjustable gastric band (LAGB) may require band adjustment, relieving the tension of the gastric band to reduce or resolve the symptoms.
B. The postsurgical gastric bypass patient may express disappointment and depression if he or she does not loose weight fast enough, or as expected.
 1. Weight loss from the Roux gastric bypass generally levels off in 1–2 years. A weight regain of up to 20 lb from the weight loss nadir to a long-term plateau is common.
 2. Weight loss after the LAGB is about 50% of the excess body weight and about 25% of the BMI at 2 years postsurgery.

3. Weight loss after the Sleeve procedure is between 6.7%–130% of excessive weight. Patients that experience less than 25% loss of excess weight are considered failures and may be revised to a Roux gastric bypass or biliopancreatic diversion with duodenal switch (BP-DS).
4. Weight loss from the BPD or duodenal switch is about 66.3%–73.9% of the excess body weight. Significant weight loss is primarily due to malabsorption and therefore the patients experience more complications because of decreased absorption of food, vitamins, minerals, and protein deficiency.

Subjective Data

A. Review onset and duration of symptoms.
B. Elicit the date of the gastric bypass surgical procedure and any history of reoperations for band slippages, failure to loose weight, or surgical reversals.
C. Elicit a history of any surgical complications.
D. Ask the patient about other symptoms depending on the type of surgical procedure.

E. Evaluate the location level of pain/discomfort.
F. Evaluate the overall psychosocial changes since surgery.

Physical Examination

A. Check height, weight, waist and hip circumference. Calculate BMI, pulse, respirations, and blood pressure. Check temperature if infection is suspected.
B. Inspect
   1. Examine the skin, evaluate surgical site(s), evaluate redness and tenderness.
   2. Oral/dental examination.
   3. Evaluate for dehydration.
   4. Eye examination: evaluate eye movement (thiamine deficiency).
   5. Evaluate gait.
   6. General overview of personal presence and affect.
   7. Check for positive Homan's sign (dorsiflex the foot).
C. Auscultate
   1. Auscultate the heart and lungs.
   2. Auscultate the abdomen for bowel sounds.
D. Palpate abdomen
   1. Evaluate the presence of tenderness.
   2. Evaluate for masses.
E. Neurological examination: Perform neurological exam, including checking deep tendon reflexes (DTRs), sense of smell, and checking for Babinski reflex (vitamin B_{12} deficiency).

Diagnostic Tests

A. Monitor HgA1c and blood glucose closely since diabetes has been resolved postsurgical procedures.
B. CBC with differential.
C. Reticulocyte count.
D. Serum vitamin B_{12} level.
E. Abdominal ultrasound.
F. CT scan.
G. Doppler ultrasound of limb for suspected deep vein thrombus.
H. Pulmonary ventilation/perfusion scan for suspected pulmonary embolus.
I. Dexa Scan.
J. Endoscopy.

Differential Diagnoses

A. Postoperative surgical complication(s)
   1. Infection
   2. Abdominal pain
   3. Fascial dehiscence
   4. Deep vein thrombosis
   5. Bowel obstruction
   6. Band slippage
   7. Anastomosis leakage
   8. Stomal stenosis/stricture
B. Cholecystitis
C. Dumping syndrome
D. Food intolerance
E. Gastric ulcer
F. Gastroenteritis
G. Vitamin deficiency
H. Malnutrition/protein deficiency
I. Incisional hernia
J. Osteoporosis

Plan

A. General interventions: Post-bariatric surgery requires a lifelong follow-up to evaluate micronutritional deficiencies as well as psychosocial changes.
B. Patient teaching
   1. Avoid foods, such as sweets, that provoke dumping syndrome. The patient may need to keep a food diary to identify all triggers.
   2. Supplemental of vitamins and iron (if indicated) is a lifelong requirement. Take iron supplements with food.
   3. Surgery does not replace the need for a balance diet and exercise.
   4. Diabetics may need to check their blood glucose more frequently.
   5. Consume food slowly and avoid liquids when eating.
   6. Lifelong follow-up is required.
C. Pharmaceutical therapy
   1. Evaluate the need for adjustment of antidiabetic and antihypertensive medications.
   2. Vitamin B_{12} 1,000 mcg intramuscular every month for life or take Vitamin B_{12} 1,000–2,000 mcg sublingual daily. The dose may be reduced if long-term monitoring shows elevated vitamin B_{12} levels.
   3. The patient needs one daily multiple vitamin containing B vitamins and vitamin C and fat-soluble vitamins and minerals. Some patients require a liquid vitamin preparation because the stomach pouch does not tolerate pills.
   4. Prenatal vitamins are useful for those at risk for iron deficiency or whose diets put them at risk for folic acid deficiency.
   5. Vitamin D 800 IU daily. Most multivitamin supplements contain 400 IU of vitamin D. Additional supplementation is recommended by taking a second multivitamin, or by ingesting a second supplement containing calcium and Vitamin D.
   6. Vitamin A 30,000 IU daily for 1 week.
   7. Calcium 1,200–1,500 mg daily. Calcium citrate may be better absorbed than calcium carbonate after gastric bypass.
   8. Osteopenia and metabolic bone disease after RYGB have been reported. Calcium 1,200–1,500 mg with Vitamin D 800 IU will avoid metabolic bone disease.
   9. Iron supplementation of 640 mg/day especially for menstruating women, those patients intolerant to iron-containing foods, and those who develop iron deficiency anemia. Iron absorption is improved when iron is administered with Vitamin C.
   10. Patients with persistent vomiting or other cause of inadequate nutrient intake should receive thiamin 50 mg daily.
   11. Long-term anticoagulation may be required for DVT/PE.

Follow-up

A. Reevaluation depends on the complication and side effect profiles.

B. If no surgical complications, reevaluate on a schedule:
1. Every 3 months: CBC, glucose, and creatinine.
2. Every 6 months: protein and albumin, liver functions, iron, ferritin, total iron binding capacity (TIBC), B_{12}, folic acid, and calcium.
3. Annually: CBC, glucose, protein and albumin, creatinine, liver functions, B_{12}, folic acid, calcium, and iron, ferritin, and TIBC.
4. Consider Dexa Scan to evaluate osteopenia/osteoporosis.

Consultation/Referral

A. Physician referrals as indicated:
1. Gastroenterology consultation
2. Bariatric surgeon for surgical complications and revisions
3. Surgeon for cholecystectomy or panniculectomy
4. Nutrition consultation
5. Psychologist consultation

ROUNDWORM, ASCARIS LUMBRICOIDES

Definition

A. Roundworm, *Ascaris lumbricoides,* is a helminthic parasitic infection of the lumen of the small intestines and sometimes the lungs. Most infections with *A. lumbricoides* are asymptomatic. Roundworms are brownish, are the size and shape of earthworms, and can be seen easily without a microscope. The majority of worms are noted in the jejunum but can be noted from the esophagus to the rectum. Ova can survive for prolonged periods, up to 10 years. The eggs are resistant to normal water purification but can be removed by boiling and water filtration.

Incidence

A. *A. lumbricoides* are very common, approximately 25% of the world's population, more than 1 billion people, are infected with these human intestinal nematodes. It is the third most frequent helminth infection, only the hookworm and whipworm exceed it. It occurs worldwide, especially in tropical and warm climates. It affects people of all ages but is most common in young children.

B. Individuals can be asymptomatic and continue to shed eggs for years. The parasitic eggs are extremely durable in various environments and each produces a high number of eggs. Bowel obstruction occurs in 1 in 500 children and is the most common cause of acute abdominal surgery in endemic areas.

Pathogenesis

A. *Ascaris lumbricoides* is a large roundworm that infects humans. It is contracted by ingesting eggs in contaminated soil through eating the soil (pica), children playing in contaminated soil, eating unwashed fruits and raw vegetables, and by drinking water contaminated with feces, or touching food with soil-contaminated hands. Occasionally, transplacental migration of larvae has been reported.

B. The life cycle of *A. lumbricoides* is 4–8 weeks, and feces contain eggs about 2 months after ingestion of embryonated eggs. Female roundworms produce 200,000 eggs per day, which are excreted in stool and must incubate in soil for 2–3 weeks for the embryo to form and become infectious (second-stage larvae). The interval between ingestion of egg and development of egg-laying adults is approximately 8 weeks. If infection is untreated, adult worms can live 10–24 months, resulting in daily excretion of large numbers of ova.

C. The ingested ova hatch in the small intestine (jejunum or ileum) and release larvae. They then may migrate via blood or via the lymphatic system to the heart, lungs, the biliary tree, and occasionally the kidney or brain. It takes approximately 4 days for the larvae to reach the lungs, after maturation they are passed through the bronchi and the trachea and are subsequently swallowed.

Predisposing Factors

A. Crowded or unsanitary living conditions
B. Tropical or warm climates, including the southern United States
C. Preschool or early school age (2–10 years)
D. Tend to cluster in families
E. Residence in areas where human feces are used as fertilizer
F. Travelers to endemic areas (Asia, Africa, and South America)

Common Complaints

A. Asymptomatic
B. Restlessness at night
C. Colicky abdominal pain
D. Frequent fatigue
E. Worms found in bowel movements or in bed

Other Signs and Symptoms

A. Transient respiratory symptoms during migration
B. Nausea and vomiting
C. Anorexia and erratic or poor appetite
D. Fever
E. Irritability
F. Diarrhea or constipation
G. Weight loss or gain
H. Dry cough or wheezing, from larvae in lungs
I. Parasites regurgitated or passed through nares of febrile patients
J. Acute transient pneumonitis
K. Acute obstructive jaundice
L. Appendicitis
M. Urticaria
N. Impaired absorption of protein, lactose, and vitamin A
O. Burning chest pain

Subjective Data

A. Review onset, duration, and course of symptoms.
B. Ask about any problems with pica.
C. Inquire about worms in stool or emesis.
D. Review history of pets treated for worms.
E. Establish normal weight for evaluation.

Physical Examination

A. Check temperature, pulse, respirations, blood pressure, and weight. Plot the child's height and weight on a growth curve.
B. Inspect the skin to rule out jaundice and evaluate uticaria.
C. Auscultate
   1. Auscultate the lungs to evaluate the presence of rales, wheezes, and tachypnea.
   2. Auscultate the heart.
   3. Auscultate the abdomen.
D. Palpate the abdomen for distention, tenderness, and masses (worm bolus). Upper right quadrant, lower right quadrant, or hypogastrium tenderness may suggest complications of ascariasis.
E. Percuss the abdomen: dullness may be noted.

Diagnostic Tests

A. None, if the worm is visualized; they are occasionally passed from the rectum, nose, and seen in vomitus.
B. Stool for occult blood, ova and parasites, and culture.
C. CBC: eosinophilia may be noted particularly during the migration of larvae through the lungs.
D. Plain abdominal radiograph.
E. Ultrasound/CT to diagnose hepatobiliary or pancreatic ascariasis. ERCP is used for diagnosis and removal.
F. Chest radiography; rarely needed.
G. Microscopic wet prep of sputum may be helpful with respiratory symptoms.

Differential Diagnoses

A. Roundworm
B. Asthma
C. Pneumonia
D. Poor nutrition
E. Giardiasis
F. Pancreatitis from other causes

Plan

A. Patient teaching
   1. See the Section III Patient Teaching Guide for this chapter, "Roundworms and Pinworms."
   2. Stress the importance of maintaining a clean play area for children.
   3. Stress sanitary disposal of feces stops transmission.
   4. Explain that household bleach is ineffective in killing eggs or worms.
   5. All family members must be treated with medication.
   6. There is no direct person-to-person transmission.
B. Pharmaceutical therapy
   1. Treatment of symptomatic and asymptomatic infections may be achieved by a single dose of the following agents:
      a. Pyrantel pamoate (Antiminth) 11 mg/kg up to a maximum of 1 g given in a single dose. The single dose is 90% effective.
      b. Mebendazole (Vermox) 100 mg twice daily for 3 days or 500 mg as a single dose. Both the single and 3-day treatment are about 95% effective.
         i. The World Health Organization recommends for children 1-year old be given half

of the dose (50 mg) as for older children and adults.
      c. Anthelminth therapy is not usually given at the time of pulmonary symptoms. Dying larvae may increase complications over migrating larvae.
   2. Administer the drug to all family members to decrease risk of spreading infection.
   3. Consider Vitamin A supplement if growth is retarded.

Follow-up

A. Reexamine a stool specimen in 2 weeks to determine if the therapy was successful in elimination of the worms. If the patient is not cured give a second course of medication.
B. Therapy is effective for adult worms only. Reevaluate in 2–3 months for detectable eggs.
C. Endoscopy or laparoscopic extraction of worms may be required with hepatobiliary infestations.

Consultation/Referral

A. Consult with a physician if the patient is pregnant or is considered a surgical risk.

Individual Considerations

A. Pregnancy: Anthelmintics are Pregnancy Class C; however, risks versus benefits should be considered.
B. Pediatrics
   1. All medications are advised for children 2 years of age and older.
   2. Children are more prone to acute intestinal obstruction because they have smaller diameters of the intestinal lumen and often have large numbers of worms.
C. Adults: Acute intestinal obstruction may develop with heavy infestation.

ULCERATIVE COLITIS

Definition

Ulcerative colitis (UC) is one of the two inflammatory bowel diseases, along with Crohn's disease. UC is limited to the colon; it extends proximally from the anal verge in an uninterrupted pattern to part or the entire colon. Neither ulcerative colitis nor Crohn's disease should be confused with irritable bowel syndrome (IBS), which affects the motility of the colon. Smoking is negatively associated with UC; the relationship is reversed in Crohn's disease (CD). The general course of UC is intermittent exacerbations and remissions. In severe cases, surgery may result in a cure.

Histologically, most of the pathology of UC is limited to the mucosa and submucosal. The extent of ulcerative colitis is defined by the following:

A. Pan-ulcerative (total colitis): extensive disease with evidence of UC proximal to the splenic flexure. Massive dilation of the colon (toxic megacolon) may lead to bowel perforation.
B. Left-sided disease: continuous UC that is present from the rectum, the descending colon up to, but not proximal to, the splenic flexure.

C. Proctosigmoiditis: the disease is limited to the rectum with or without sigmoid involvement.

Incidence

A. The annual incidence of UC is 1–3 per 100,000 depending on the country.

Pathogenesis

A. UC may be considered an autoimmune disease. Persons with UC often have p-antineutrophil cytoplasmic antibodies. Abnormalities of humoral and cell-mediated immunity and/or generalized enhanced reactivity against intestinal bacterial antigen may also be causes of UC.

Predisposing Factors

A. Caucasian
B. Jewish descent
C. 30% more females than males
D. Genetic susceptibility (chromosomes 12 and 16)

Common Complaints

A. Frequent small-volume diarrhea
B. Bloody diarrhea with or without mucus
C. Severe bowel urgency
D. Abdominal cramps and pain with bowel movement
E. Constipation
F. Anorexia

Other Signs and Symptoms

A. Tenesmus
B. Abdominal tenderness
C. Arthralgias
D. Fatigue secondary to anemia
E. Failure to thrive in children
F. Severe UC
   1. Fever
   2. Tachycardia
   3. Significant abdominal tenderness
   4. Signs of volume depletion

Subjective Data

A. Review the onset, duration, signs, and symptoms.
B. Review the patient's recent travel history or camping for the presence of intestinal infection.
C. Review the patient's medication history including antibiotics and nonsteroidal anti-inflammatory drugs (NSAIDs).
D. Review family history for IBD, celiac disease, and colorectal cancer.
E. Review the patient's history or contact related to tuberculosis.

Physical Examination

A. Temperature, pulse, blood pressure and weight.
B. Inspection
   1. Observe the general overall appearance for nutritional status, cachexia, and pallor.
   2. Observe the perianal region for the presence of tags, fissures, fistulas, and abscess.
   3. Observe the abdomen for distention and presence of surgical scars.
C. Auscultation
   1. Auscultate the heart and lungs.
   2. Auscultate all four quadrants of the abdomen.

D. Palpation
   1. Palpate all four quadrants of the abdomen, observing for tenderness, rebound, and guarding.
   2. Evaluate the presence of hepatomegaly.
   3. Digital rectal examination to assess for anal strictures and rectal masses.

Diagnostic Tests

A. Laboratory tests
   1. CBC with electrolytes.
   2. Platelet count.
   3. Sedimentation rate.
   4. C-reactive protein.
   5. Cytomegalovirus (chronic immunosuppressive steroids).
   6. HIV.
B. Stool testing
   1. Evaluate bacterial, viral, or parasitic causes of diarrhea.
   2. Occult blood.
   3. Fecal leukocytes.
C. Colonoscopy with biopsy.
D. Plain abdominal radiograph.
E. CT scan.
F. Celiac antibody testing should be considered.
G. Intestinal TB testing should be considered.

Differential Diagnoses

A. Ulcerative colitis
B. Ischemic colitis (especially in the elderly)
C. Toxic megacolon
D. Colon cancer
E. Adenocarcinoma
F. Rectal cancer
G. Radiation colitis
H. Intestinal infections
I. Intestinal lymphoma
J. Chronic diverticulitis

Plan

A. Dietary considerations:
   1. Many patients with UC have concurrent lactose intolerance. (See Appendix for Lactose Intolerance dietary recommendations)
   2. Decrease dietary fiber during increased disease activity.
   3. Low-residue diet may decrease the frequency of bowel movements.
   4. High-residue diet may be helpful in ulcerative proctitis when constipation is the dominant symptom. (See Appendix B, Table B.7: Fiber Recommendations by Age.)
B. Stress reduction and stress management may improve symptoms.
C. Pharmacologic treatment:
   1. Aminosalicylates (5-ASA) class of anti-inflammatory drugs:
      a. Sulfasalazine (Azulfidine) for mild to moderate UC and remission maintenance.
         i. Induction: 4–6 grams/day orally in divided doses
         ii. Maintenance: 2–4 grams/day orally in divided doses

b. Balsalazide (Colazal) for mild to moderate UC and remission maintenance.
i. Induction: 6.75 grams/day, given three times daily, dosing
ii. Maintenance: 3–6 grams/day, given twice a day, dosing
c. Mesalamine (Asacol, Pentasa, Rowasa) for mild to moderate UC and remission maintenance.
i. Asacol: 2.4–4.8 grams/day orally in three times daily dosing
ii. Pentasa: 2–4 grams/day orally in four times a day dosing
iii. Rowasa enema: 4 grams/60 mL rectally at bedtime
2. Corticosteroids suppress the immune system and are used for moderate to severe UC: Prednisone (Deltasone, Orasone).
a. Induction: 40–60 mg/day by mouth for 7–14 days followed by gradual taper by 5 mg/week
b. Maintenance: 2.5–5 mg/week
3. Immune modifiers are used to decrease corticosteroids dosage.
a. Azathioprine (Imuran) 2–3 mg/kg/day orally
b. 6-Mercaptopurine (Purinethol) 1–1.5 mg/kg/day orally
4. Antibiotics
a. Cyclosoporine (Neoral, Sandimmune)
i. IV infusion: 2–4 mg/kg/day
ii. Can be switched to a doubled oral dose for outpatient therapy
b. Ciprofloxacin (Cipro) 500 mg orally twice a day
5. Biologic therapy for moderate to severe UC: Infliximab (Remicade) infusion therapy
a. Induction therapy: 5 mg/kg at 0, 2, and 6 weeks.
b. Maintenance: 5 mg/kg every 8 weeks.
c. Tuberculin skin test is recommended prior to therapy.
D. Indications for the consideration of a total colectomy
1. Failed medical therapy: refractory UC
2. Severe hemorrhage
3. Fulminate colitis not responsive to treatment
4. Toxic megacolon
5. Obstruction or stricture
6. Failure to thrive in children

Follow-up

A. Screening colonoscopy is recommended for all patients with UC for 8–10 years after the onset of symptoms due to the increase in colonic neoplasia.
B. Patients with extensive UC or left-sided colitis with negative findings on the screening colonoscopy should begin surveillance colonoscopy in 1–2 years.
C. Patients that require long-term steroids are at increased risk of osteoporosis.

Consultation/Referral

A. Gastroenterologist for confirmatory diagnosis with a colonoscopy.
B. Consultation with a surgeon for severe or fulminant colitis. Toxic megacolon is a life-threatening complication and requires urgent surgical intervention.

RESOURCES

Crohn's and Colitis Foundation of America (CCFA): http://www.ccfa.org

REFERENCES

Aberra, F. N., Gronczewski, C. A., & Katz, J. P. (2009, August 4). Clostridium difficile colitis. *emedicine*. Retrieved August, 23, 2009, from http://emedicine.medscape.com/article/186458-print.

American Academy of Pediatrics. (2009a). *Ascaris lumbricoides* infections. In L. K. Pickering (Ed.), *Red Book: 2009 Report of the Committee on Infectious Diseases* (26th ed., pp. 221–222). Elk Grove Village, IL: Author. Retrieved October 22, 2009, from http://aapredbook.aappublications.org.proxy.library.vanderbilt.edu/cgi/content/full/2009/1/3.8.

American Academy of Pediatrics. (2009b). Cyclosporiasis. In L. K. Pickering (Ed.), *Red Book: 2009 Report of the Committee on Infectious Diseases* (26th ed., pp. 274–275). Elk Grove Village, IL: Author. Retrieved October 22, 2009, from http://aapredbook.aappublications.org.proxy.library.vanderbilt.edu/cgi/content/full/2009/1/3.34.

American Academy of Pediatrics. (2009c). *Giardia intestinalis* infections. In L. K. Pickering (Ed.), *Red Book: 2009 Report of the Committee on Infectious Diseases* (26th ed., pp. 303–305). Elk Grove Village, IL: Author. Retrieved October 22, 2009, from http://aapredbook.aappublications.org.proxy.library.vanderbilt.edu/cgi/content/full/2009/1/3.44.

American Academy of Pediatrics. (2009d). Hepatitis A. In L. K. Pickering (Ed.), *Red Book: 2009 Report of the Committee on Infectious Diseases* (26th ed., pp. 329–337). Elk Grove Village, IL: Author. Retrieved June 27, 2009, from http://aapredbook.aappublications.org.proxy.library.vanderbilt.edu/cgi/content/full/2009/1/2.9.1.

American Academy of Pediatrics. (2009e). Hepatitis B. In L. K. Pickering (Ed.), *Red Book: 2009 Report of the Committee on Infectious Diseases* (26th ed., pp. 337–356). Elk Grove Village, IL: Author. Retrieved June 27, 2009, from http://aapredbook.aappublications.org.proxy.library.vanderbilt.edu/cgi/content/full/2009/1/3.53.

American Academy of Pediatrics. (2009f). Hepatitis C. In L. K. Pickering (Ed.), *Red Book: 2009 Report of the Committee on Infectious Diseases* (26th ed., pp. 357–360). Elk Grove Village, IL: Author. Retrieved June 27, 2009, from http://aapredbook.aappublications.org.proxy.library.vanderbilt.edu/cgi/content/full/2009/1/3.54.

American Academy of Pediatrics. (2009g). Hookworm infections (Ancylostoma duodenale and necator americanus). In L. K. Pickering (Ed.), *Red Book: 2009 Report of the Committee on Infectious Diseases* (26th ed., pp. 375–376). Elk Grove Village, IL: Author. Retrieved June 27, 2009, from http://aapredbook.aappublications.org.proxy.library.vanderbilt.edu/cgi/content/full/2009/1/3.59.

American Academy of Pediatrics. (2009h). Pinworm infection (Enterobius vermicularis). In L. K. Pickering (Ed.), *Red Book: 2009 Report of the Committee on Infectious Diseases* (26th ed., pp. 519–520). Elk Grove Village, IL: Author. Retrieved June 27, 2009, from http://aapredbook.aappublications.org.proxy.library.vanderbilt.edu/cgi/content/full/2009/1/3.99.

American Academy of Pediatrics. (2009i). Shigellai infections. In L. K. Pickering (Ed.), *Red Book: 2009 Report of the Committee on Infectious Diseases* (26th ed., pp. 593–596). Elk Grove Village, IL: Author. Retrieved June 27, 2009, from http://aapredbook.aappublications.org.proxy.library.vanderbilt.edu/cgi/content/full/2009/1/3.120.

American Gastroenterological Association. (2001). AGA technical review on nausea and vomiting. *Gastroenterology, 120*, 263–286.

American Gastroenterological Association. (2004). American Gastroenterological Association Institute medical position statement: Diagnosis and treatment of hemorrhoids. *Gastroenterology, 126*, 1461–1462.

American Gastroenterological Association. (2006a). American Gastroenterological Association Institute medical position statement on corticosteroids, immunomodulators, and Infliximab in inflammatory bowel disease. *Gastroenterology, 130*, 935–939.

American Gastroenterological Association. (2006b). American Gastroenterological Association Institute medical position statement on the diagnosis and management of celiac disease. *Gastroenterology, 131,* 1977–1980.

American Gastroenterological Association. (2006c). American Gastroenterological Association Institute medical position statement on the management of hepatitis C. *Gastroenterology, 130,* 225–230.

American Gastroenterological Association. (2008). American Gastroenterological Association Institute medical position statement on the management of gastroesophageal reflux disease. *Gastroenterology, 135,* 1383–1391.

American Gastroenterological Association Clinical Practice Committee. (2002). AGA technical review on the evaluation of liver chemistry tests. *Gastroenterology, 123,* 1367–1384.

Barth, W. H., & Goldberg, J. E. (2009, June 2). Appendicitis in pregnancy. *UpToDate.* Retrieved September 20, 2009, from http://www.uptodate.com/online/content/topic.do?topicKey=maternal/7304&view=print.

Basson, M. D. (2008, August 13). Constipation. *emedicine.* Retrieved August 23, 2009, from http://emedicine.medscape.com/article/184704-print.

Bennett, N. J., Domachowske, J., & Strickland, D. K. (2008, August 12). Hepatitis C. *emedicine.* Retrieved August 23, 2009, from http://emedicine.medscape.com/article/964761-overview.

Blacklow, N. R. (2009, January). Prevention and treatment of viral gastroenteritis in adults. *UpToDate.* Retrieved September 20, 2009, from http://www.uptodate.com/online/content/topic.do?topicKey=gi_infec/12064&view=print.

Bleday, R. (2009, May 1). Patient information: Hemorrhoids. *UptoDate.* Retrieved September 20, 2009, from http://www.uptodate.com/online/content/topic.do?topicKey=digestiv/8271&view=print.

Bleday, R., & Breen, E. (2009, May 1). Treatment of hemorrhoids. *UpToDate.* Retrieved September 20, 2009, from http://www.uptodate.com/online/content/topic.do?topicKey=colosurg/6160&view=print.

Boan, J., & Mun, E. C. (2009). Management of patients after bariatric surgery. *UpToDate.* Retrieved January 22, 2009, from http://www.uptodate.com.

Bonheur, J. L., Arya, M., Frye, R. E., & Tamer, M. A. (2009, February 19). Gastroenteritis, bacterial. *emedicine.* Retrieved January 27, 2010, from http://emedicine.medscape.com/article/176400-print.

Bousvaros, A., & Leichtner A. (2009, June 17). Overview of the management of Crohn's disease in children and adolescents. *UpToDate.* Retrieved September 20, 2009, from http://www.uptodate.com/online/content/topic.do?topicKey=pedigast/12773&view=print.

Brooks, D. C. (2009, January 6). Classification and diagnosis of groin hernias. *UpToDate.* Retrieved October 17, 2009, from http://www.uptodate.com/online/content/topic.do?topicKey=hernsurg/2279&selectedTitle=1~150&source=search_result.

Brooks, D. C. (2009, April 2). Abdominal wall hernias. *UpToDate.* Retrieved October 17, 2009, from http://www.uptodate.com/online/content/topic.do?topicKey=hernsurg/2830&selectedTitle=2~150&source=search_result.

Brooks, D. C. (2009, April 16). Treatment of groin hernias. *UpToDate.* Retrieved October 17, 2009, from http://www.uptodate.com/online/content/topic.do?topicKey=hernsurg/2541&selectedTitle=3~150&source=search_result.

Buchwald, H. (2005). Consensus conference statement on bariatric surgery for morbid obesity: Health implications for patients, health professionals, and third-party payers. *Surgery for Obesity and Related Diseases, 1,* 371–381.

Buchwald, H., Avidor, Y., Braunwald, Y., Jensen, E., Pories, W., Fahrback, K., et al. (2004). Bariatric surgery: A systematic review and meta-analysis. *Journal of the American Medical Association, 292,* 1724–1737.

Budd, G. M., & Falkenstein, K. (2009). Bariatric surgery: Putting the squeeze on obesity. *The Nurse Practitioner, 34,* 39–45.

Chowdhury, N. R., & Chowdhury, J. R. (2009, May 1). Diagnostic approach to the patient with jaundice or asymptomatic hyperbilirubinemia. *UpToDate.* Retrieved on October 17, 2009, from http://www.uptodate.com/online/content/topic.do?topicKey=hep_dis/8241&view=print

Ciclitira, P. J. (2009, May 1). Management of celiac disease in adults. *UpToDate.* Retrieved September 20, 2009, from http://www.uptodate.com/online/content/topic.do?topicKey=mal_synd/5722&view=print

Crohn's & Colitis Foundation of America. (2008, July 25). About ulcerative colitis & proctitis. Retrieved November 21, 2009, from http://www.ccfa.org/info/about/ucp

Deshpande, P. G. (2009, October 7). Colic. *emedicine.* Retrieved October 15, 2009, from http://emedicine.medscape.com/article/927760-print

Felberbauer, F. X., Langer, F., Shakeri-Manesch, S., Schmaldienst, E., Kees, M., Kriwanek, S., et al. (2008). Laparoscopic sleeve gastrectomy as an isolated bariatric procedure: Intermediate-term results from a large series in three Austrian centers. *Obesity Surgery, 18,* 814–818.

Gladden, D., Migala, A. F., Beverly, C. S., & Wolff, J. (2008, August 4). Cholecystitis. *emedicine.* Retrieved August 23, 2009, from http://emedicine.medscape.com/article/171886-print

Green, P. H. R., & Cellier, C. (2007). Celiac disease medical progress. *The New England Journal of Medicine, 357*(17), 1731–1744.

Guandalini, S., & Vallee, P. A. (2009, April 29). Celiac disease. *emedicine.* Retrieved August 23, 2009, from http://emedicine.medscape.com/article/932104-print

Haburchak, D. R. (2008, September 12). Ascariasis. *emedicine.* Retrieved on October 13, 2009, from http://emedicine.medscape.com/article/212510-overview

Hebra, A., & Miller, M. (2008, November 18). Cholecystitis. *emedicine.* Retrieved August 23, 2009, from http://emedicine.medscape.com/article/927340-print

Hill, I. D. (2009, May 1). Management of celiac disease in children. *UpToDate.* Retrieved September 20, 2009, from http://www.uptodate.com/online/content/topic.do?topicKey=pedigast/9506&view=print

Hokelek, M., & Nissen, M. D. (2008, December 17). Giardiasis. *emedicine.* Retrieved October 22, 2009, from http://emedicine.medscape.com/article/998168-print

Hvas, A. M., & Nexo, E. (2006). Diagnosis and treatment of vitamin B12 deficiency. An update. *Haematologica/The Hematology Journal, 91,* 1506–1512.

Iannelli, A., Dainesc, R., Piche, T., Facchiano, E., & Gugenheim, J. (2008). Laparoscopic sleeve gastrectomy for morbid obesity. *World Journal of Gastroenterology, 14,* 821–827.

Kahn, A. N., MacDonald, S., Patankar, T. A., Krishna, L. R., Chandramohan, H., Sherlock, R. D., et al. (2009, February 4). Cholecystitis, acute. *emedicine.* Retrieved August 23, 2009, from http://emedicine.medscape.com/article/365698-overview

Kaplan, M. M. (2009a, May 1). Approach to the patient with abnormal liver function tests. *UpToDate.* Retrieved September 27, 2009, from http://www.uptodate.com/online/content/topic.do?topicKey=hep_dis/14684&view=print

Kaplan, M. M. (2009b, May 1). Clinical aspect of serum bilirubin determination. *UpToDate.* Retrieved October 17, 2009, from http://www.uptodate.com/online/content/topic.do?topicKey=hep_dis/12335&view=print

Kelly, C. P. (2009, May 1). Diagnosis of celiac disease. *UpToDate.* Retrieved September 20, 2009, from http://www.uptodate.com/online/content/topic.do?topicKey=mal_synd/2879&selectedTitle=3~150&source=search_result

Klapproth, J. M., & Yang, V. W. (2008a, August 14). Celiac sprue. *emedicine.* Retrieved August 23, 2009, from http://emedicine.medscape.com/article/171805-print

Klapproth, J. M. A., & Yang, V. W. (2008b, August 14). Malabsorption. *emedicine.* Retrieved August 23, 2009, from http://emedicine.medscape.com/article/180785-overview

Le, T. H. (2008, August 7). Ulcerative colitis. *emedicine.* Retrieved August 23, 2009, from http://emedicine.medscape.com/article/183084-overview

Leder, K., & Weller, P. F. (2009a, May 1). Ascariasis. *UpToDate.* Retrieved September 20, 2009, from http://www.uptodate.com/online/content/topic.do?topicKey=parasite/11831&view=print

Leder, K., & Weller, P. F. (2009b, May 1). Epidemiology, clinical manifestations, and diagnosis of giardiasis. *UpToDate.* Retrieved

October 22, 2009, from http://www.uptodate.com/online/content/topic.do?topicKey=parasite/7013&view=print

Leder, K., & Weller, P. F. (2009c, May 1). Treatment and prevention of giardiasis in adults. *UpToDate*. Retrieved October 22, 2009, from http://www.uptodate.com/online/content/topic.do?topicKey=parasite/18011&view=print

Lee, S. L., & Shekherdimain, S. (2008, November 24). Hirschsprung disease. *emedicine*. Retrieved October 17, 2009, from http://emedicine.medscape.com/article/178493-print

Madoff, R. D., & Fleshman, J. W. (2004). American Gastroenterological Association technical review on the diagnosis and treatment of hemorrhoids. *Gastroenterology, 126*(5), 1463–1473.

Maggard, M. A., Shugarman, L. R., Suttorp, M., Maglione, M., Sugerman, H. J., Livingston, E. H., et al. (2005). Meta-analysis: Surgical treatment of obesity. *Annals of Internal Medicine, 142*, 547–559.

Mason, J. B., & Milovic, V. (2009, May 1). Overview of the treatment of malabsorption. *UpToDate*. Retrieved September 20, 2009, from http://www.uptodate.com/online/content/topic.do?topicKey=mal_synd/7320&view=print

Milovic, V., & Mason, J. B. (2009, May 1). Clinical features and diagnosis of malabsorption. *UpToDate*. Retrieved September 20, 2009, from http://www.uptodate.com/online/content/topic.do?topicKey=mal_synd/6513&view=print

Mun, E. C., & Tavakkolizadeh, A. (2009, February 9). Surgical management of severe obesity. *UpToDate*. Retrieved April 21, 2009, from http://www.uptodate.com

Nettina, S. (2010). *The Lippincott manual of nursing practice* (9th ed.). Philadelphia: Wolters Kluwer Health/Lippincott Williams & Wilkins.

Neville, H. L. (2008, November 17). Hirschsprung disease. *emedicine*. Retrieved October 17, 2009, from http://emedicine.medscape.com/article/929733-print

North American Society for Pediatric Gastroenterology, Hepatology and Nutrition. (2005). Guideline for the diagnosis and treatment of celiac disease in children: Recommendation of the North American Society for Pediatric Gastroenterology, Hepatology and Nutrition. *Journal of Pediatric Gastroenterology and Nutrition, 40*(1), 1–19.

Orzano, A. J., & Scott, J. G. (2004). Diagnosis and treatment of obesity in adults: An applied evidence-based review. *Journal American Board Family Practice, 17*, 359–369.

Reddy, S. (2009). An evidence-based review of obesity and bariatric surgery. *The Journal for Nurse Practitioners, 5*, 22–28.

Ren, C. J., & Fielding, G. A. (2003). Laparoscopic adjustable gastric banding: Surgical technique. *Journal of Laparoendoscopic & Advanced Surgical Techniques, 13*, 257–263.

Rowe, W. A. (2008, April 28). Inflammatory bowel disease. *emedicine*. Retrieved November 21, 2009, from http://emedicine.medscape.com/article/179037-print

Roy, P. K., Choudhary, A., Bradley, A. G., Othman, M., Bragg, J., Dehadrai, G., et al. (2009, August 19). Liver disease and pregnancy. *emedicine*. Retrieved August 23, 2009, from http://emedicine.medscape.com/article/188143-print

Shah, M., Simha, V., & Garg, A. (2006). Review: Long-term impact of bariatric surgery on body weight, comorbidities, and nutritional status. *The Journal of Clinical Endocrinology & Metabolism, 91*, 4223–4231.

Sharma, G. D. (2008, October 17). Cystic fibrosis. *emedicine*. Retrieved October 21, 2009, from http://emedicine.medscape.com/article/1001602-print

Shoff, W. H., Behrman, A. J., & Shepherd, S. (2007, July 5). Cyclospora. *emedicine*. Retrieved October 24, 2009, from http://emedicine.medscape.com/article/236105-print

Shoff, W. H., Moore, S., & Greenberg, M. E. (2008, June 11). Ascariasis. *emedicine*. Retrieved October 13, 2009, from http://emedicine.medscape.com/article/996482-overview

Singhal, V., Schwenk, W. F., & Kumar, S. (2007). Evaluation and management of childhood and adolescent obesity. *Mayo Clinic Proceedings, 82*, 1258–1264.

Smith, B. R., Schauer, P., & Nguyen, N. T. (2008). Surgical approaches to the treatment of obesity: Bariatric surgery. *Endocrinology & Metabolism Clinic of North America, 37*, 943–964.

The University of Chicago Celiac Disease Center. (n.d.). Gluten free diet. Retrieved October 3, 2009, from http://www.celiacdisease.net/gluten-free-diet

Tolan, R. W., & Schroeder, C. J. (2009, January 21). Cyclosporiasis. *emedicine*. Retrieved October 24, 2009, from http://emedicine.medscape.com/article/996978-print

Turner, T. L., & Palamountain, S. (2009a, May 1). Clinical features and etiology of colic. *UpToDate*. Retrieved September 20, 2009, from http://www.uptodate.com/online/content/topic.do?topicKey=behavior/2155&view=print

Turner, T. L., & Palamountain, S. (2009b, May 1). Evaluation and management of colic. *UpToDate*. Retrieved September 20, 2009, from http://www.uptodate.com/online/content/topic.do?topicKey=behavior/4542&view=print

Tyler-Evans, M. E., & Meyer, B. (2009). Post-bariatric surgery: Management considerations for NPs. *The American Journal for Nurse Practitioners, 13*, 29–33.

Utah Library of Medicine. (n.d.). Hepatitic pathology: Caput medusae. Retrieved September 20, 2009, from http://library.med.utah.edu/WebPath/LIVEHTML/LIVER061.html

Weller, P. F. (2009, May 1). Anthelminthic therapies. *UpToDate*. Retrieved September 20, 2009, from http://www.uptodate.com/online/content/topic.do?topicKey=antibiot/7691&view=print

Weller, P. F, & Leder, K. (2009, May 1). Hookworm infection. *UpToDate*. Retrieved September 20, 2009, from http://www.uptodate.com/online/content/topic.do?topicKey=parasite/6485&view=print

Wesson, D. E. (2009, May 1). Congenital aganglionic megacolon (Hirschsprung disease). *UpToDate*. Retrieved September 20, 2009, from http://www.uptodate.com/online/content/topic.do?topicKey=pedigast/7877&view=print

World Gastroenterology Organisation. (n.d.). WGO practice guideline: Malabsorption. Retrieved October 18, 2009, from http://www.worldgastroenterology.org/assets/downloads/en/pdf/guidelines/13_malabsorption_en.pdf

World Gastroenterology Organisation Global Guidelines. (2009, June). Inflammatory bowel disease: A global perspective. Retrieved November 21, 2009, from http://www.worldgastroenterology.org/assets/downloads/en/pdf/guidelines/21_inflammatory_bowel_disease.pdf

Yitzhak, A., Mizrahi, S., & Aninoach, E. (2006). Laparoscopic gastric banding in Adolescents. *Obesity Surgery, 16*, 1318–1322.

CHAPTER 11

Genitourinary Guidelines

Cheryl A. Glass

BENIGN PROSTATIC HYPERTROPHY

Definition
A. Benign prostatic hypertrophy (BPH) is enlargement of the prostate gland that constricts the urethra, causing urinary symptoms. BPH is not believed to be a risk factor for prostate cancer. BPH occurs primarily in the central or transitional zone of the prostate, while prostate cancer originates primarily in the peripheral part of the prostate.

Incidence
A. BPH increases progressively with age. The prevalence of prostatic hyperplasia increases from 8% in men aged 31–40 years to 40%–50% in men aged 51–60 years to over 80% in men older than 80 years.

Pathogenesis
A. Exact cause is unknown; BPH may be a response to the androgen hormone. The process of aging and the presence of circulating androgens are required for the development of BPH. Hyperplasia, in which the normally thin and fibrous outer capsule of the prostate becomes spongy and thick, and the contraction of muscle fibers cause pressure on the urethra. This requires the bladder musculature to work harder to empty urine.

Predisposing Factors
A. Advancing age.
B. Race: African American men younger than 65 years old may need treatment more often than Caucasian men.
C. Genetic predisposition: Increases with a positive family history of BPH having moderate to severe lower urinary tract symptoms.

Common Complaints
The clinical manifestations of BPH are lower urinary tract symptoms that typically appear slowly and progress gradually over a period of years.

A. Difficulty starting urine flow.
B. Dribbling.
C. Bladder does not feel like it completely empties.
D. Frequency of urination.

Other Signs and Symptoms
A. Obstructive symptoms
   1. Hesitancy
   2. Diminution in size and force of urinary stream
   3. Stream interruption (double voiding)
   4. Urinary retention
B. Irritative voiding symptoms
   1. Urgency
   2. Frequency
   3. Nocturia
   4. Painless hematuria: an early symptom; may also indicate malignancy
C. Severe late symptoms with untreated BPH:
   1. Acute urinary retention
   2. Recurrent urinary tract infections
   3. Hydronephrosis
   4. Loss of renal concentrating ability
   5. Systemic acidosis and renal failure

Subjective Data
A. Have the patient complete the American Urologic Association symptom score (AUASS) assessment tool at each visit to track symptoms. The AUA symptom score (see Table 11.1) is used to assess the severity of symptoms of BPH.
B. Review the onset, duration, and course of symptoms. The AUASS assessment tool can be used to quantitatively assess BPH symptoms over time.
C. Does the patient have signs of a urinary tract infection?
D. Is there any blood in the urine or pain in the bladder region (evaluate bladder tumor or calculi)?
E. Does the patient have new symptoms such as bone or back pain, loss of appetite, or weight loss (rules out cancer)?
F. Review the patient's history for medical illness, including diabetes and neurologic problems.
G. Review previous urinary problems, surgeries, infections, treatments, success of treatments, and testing.
H. Review the patient's history of sexual dysfunction and any new sexual partners (sexually transmitted infections).
I. Review the patient's history of urethral trauma, urethritis, or urethral instrumentation that could have led to urethral stricture.

TABLE 11.1 American Urologic Association Symptom Score

AUA SYMPTOM SCORE (AUASS)

PATIENT NAME: _____ TODAY'S DATE: _____

(Circle One Number on Each Line)	Not at All	Less Than 1 Time in 5	Less Than Half the Time	About Half the Time	More Than Half the Time	Almost Always
Over the past month or so, how often have you had a sensation of not emptying your bladder completely after you finished urinating?	0	1	2	3	4	5
During the past month or so, how often have you had to urinate again less than two hours after you finished urinating?	0	1	2	3	4	5
During the past month or so, how often have you found you stopped and started again several times when you urinated?	0	1	2	3	4	5
During the past month or so, how often have you found it difficult to postpone urination?	0	1	2	3	4	5
During the past month or so, how often have you had a weak urinary stream?	0	1	2	3	4	5
During the past month or so, how often have you had to push or strain to begin urination?	0	1	2	3	4	5
	None	1 Time	2 Times	3 Times	4 Times	5 or More Times
Over the past month, how many times per night did you most typically get up to urinate from the time you went to bed at night until the time you got up in the morning?	0	1	2	3	4	5

Add the score for each number above and write the total in the space to the right. **TOTAL:** _____

SYMPTOM SCORE: 1–7 (Mild) 8–19 (Moderate) 20–35 (Severe)

QUALITY OF LIFE (QOL)

	Delighted	Pleased	Mostly Satisfied	Mixed	Mostly Dissatisfied	Unhappy	Terrible
How would you feel if you had to live with your urinary condition the way it is now, no better, no worse, for the rest of your life?	0	1	2	3	4	5	6

Used with permission from Associates in Urology, West Orange, NJ: www.njurology.com.

J. Review medications, both prescription and over-the-counter drugs including sinus or cold products, anticholinergic drugs (impair bladder function), and sympathomimetic drugs (increase outflow resistance).

K. Review family history of BPH and prostate cancer.

Physical Examination

A. Temperature, blood pressure, and weight (if indicated).

B. Inspect
1. General appearance for discomfort or acute discomfort with urinary retention.
2. Consider having the patient void: Normal urination for a man is the ability to empty the bladder of 300 mL of urine in 12–15 seconds.
3. Examine the urethral meatus for discharge.
4. Retract foreskin (if present) and assess for hygiene and smegma.
5. Check the shaft of the penis, glans, and prepuce for lesions.
6. Check inguinal and femoral areas for bulges or hernias; have the patient bear down and cough, and re-examine him.
7. Perform a neurological examination.

C. Palpate
1. Palpate the abdomen for masses or bladder distension.
2. Palpate lymph nodes in the groin for enlargement.
3. Check costovertebral angle (CVA) tenderness.
4. Palpate the testes and epididymides for inflammation, tenderness, and masses.
5. Palpate the scrotum for hydrocele or varicocele.

D. Digital rectal exam (DRE)
1. Note sphincter tone, nodules or masses, and tenderness.
2. Palpate the two lateral lobes of the prostate gland and its median sulcus for irregularities, nodules, induration, swelling, or tenderness just above the prostate anteriorly; determine whether the rectum lies adjacent to the peritoneal cavity. If possible, palpate this region for peritoneal masses and tenderness.

Diagnostic Tests

A. Urinalysis: evaluate for infection and hematuria.

B. Urine culture if indicated (patients with BPH are more susceptible to urinary tract infections).

C. Serum creatinine concentration: an ultrasound of the bladder, ureters, and kidneys is indicated if the serum creatinine concentration is high.

D. Optional studies
1. Prostate-specific antigen (PSA): reference ranges vary by age and ethnicity and may be elevated with BPH.
2. Urodynamic testing including maximal urinary flow rate.
3. Postvoid residual (as shown by in-out catheterization, radiography, or ultrasound).
4. Cystourethroscopy (assists in planning for surgical therapy).

Differential Diagnoses

A. Benign prostatic hypertrophy: classifications of BPH from the score of the AUA symptom assessment tool:

1. Mild = total AUA symptom score 1–7
2. Moderate = total AUA symptom score 8–19
3. Severe = total AUA symptom score 20–35

B. Other obstructive causes: prostate cancer, urethral obstruction, urethral stricture, and vesical neck obstruction

C. Neurogenic bladder

D. Cystitis

E. Prostatitis

F. Bladder calculi

Plan

A. General interventions
1. Have the patient complete a 24-hour voiding chart with assessment of frequency and volume.
2. Any patient with other than mild symptoms needs referral to a urologist to discuss treatment options (surgery or drugs).
3. Monitor the patient with mild symptoms every 3–6 months to determine the progression of symptoms. Imaging studies are not routinely necessary in typical cases of BPH unless there is hematuria, an elevated creatinine, or another indication.
4. Treat concurrent UTI and sexually transmitted infections (STIs).

B. Patient teaching
1. See the Section III Patient Teaching Guide for this chapter, "Benign Prostatic Hypertrophy."
2. Patients should be instructed about the hyptotensive effect, asthenia, nasal congestion, and effect on ejaculation of the long-acting alpha-1-antagonists. The hypotensive effects can be potentiated by concomitant use of phosphodiesterase-5 (PDE-5) inhibitors sildenafil (Viagra), tadalafil (Cialis), or vardenafil (Levitra).
3. Alpha-1-antagonists have been associated with intraoperative floppy iris syndrome. Patients need to discuss using these meds with their ophthalmologist prior to eye surgery.

C. Pharmaceutical therapy
1. Five long-acting alpha-1-antagonists are FDA approved for treatment of BPH.
   a. Terazosin (Hytrin): increases hypotensive effect with PDE-5 inhibitor.
   b. Doxazosin (Cardura): increases hypotensive effect with PDE-5 inhibitor.
   c. Tamsulosin (Flomax) decreases ejaculate volume.
   d. Alfuzosin (Uroxatral) generally does not cause ejaculation problems.
   e. Silodosin (Rapaflo) may produce retrograde ejaculation.
2. Prazosin (Minipress), a short-acting alpha-1-antagonist, is occasionally used but other medications are preferred.
3. Two 5-alpha-reductase inhibitors are FDA approved for BPH. The major side effects of these drugs are decreased libido and ejaculatory or erectile dysfunction.
   a. Finastride (Proscar)
   b. Dutasteride (Avodart)
4. There are no herbal supplements that have been approved by the FDA for the treatment of BPH; however, patients may report taking saw palmetto.

Follow-up

A. See the patient in 2–3 weeks to monitor symptoms after specialty referral.
B. PSA testing: baseline testing should begin at age 40.
C. Prostate-specific antigen (PSA) is an amino acid glycoprotein specific to prostate disease, but not exclusive to prostate cancer. **Once the patient has exhibited an elevated PSA level, repeat the test yearly. Patients who have undergone treatment for prostate cancer are monitored for recurrence by the PSA levels.**
D. Surgical procedures: Transurethral resection of the prostate (TURP). Sexual dysfunction may occur after a TURP, including decreased libido, impotence, and ejaculatory difficulties. Balloon dilation may be used to reduce symptoms; however, relapse is common.

Individual Considerations

A. Geriatrics: Elderly men require special attention because their symptoms may be poorly expressed or confusing.

CHRONIC KIDNEY DISEASE IN ADULTS (CKD) *by Debbie Croley*

Definition

Chronic kidney disease (CKD) is specifically defined as:

A. The persistent and usually progressive reduction in glomerular filtration rate (GFR) less than 60 mL/min/1.73 m², and/or
B. Albuminuria more than 30 mg of urinary albumin per gram of urinary creatinine.

CKD is a disorder that leads to progressive kidney damage from a variety of causes including diabetes, hypertension, cardiovascular disease, urinary obstructions, prolonged use of nephrotoxic medications, and inherited diseases such as polycystic kidney disease. Associated comorbidities of CKD include renal osteodystrophy, anemia, metabolic acidosis, and malnutrition. Early recognition of CKD as well as treatment of complications can improve long-term outcomes.

Stages of CKD

A. Stage 1 disease is defined by a normal GFR (greater than 90 mL/min per 1.73m²) and persistent albuminuria.
B. Stage 2 disease is a GFR between 60 and 89 mL/min per 1.73 m² and persistent albuminuria.
C. Stage 3 disease is a GFR between 30 and 59 mL/min per 1.73 m².
D. Stage 4 disease is a GFR between 15 and 29 mL/min per 1.73 m².
E. Stage 5 disease is a GFR of less than 15mL/min per 1.73 m² or end-stage renal disease.

Incidence

A. Kidney disease is the ninth leading cause of death in the United States. It is estimated that 80,000 new cases of non-dialysis-dependent CKD are diagnosed annually and the incidence of CKD and end-stage renal disease (ESRD) has doubled every decade since 1980. The 2006 National Health and Nutrition Examination Survey (NHANES) estimated the prevalence of CKD for adults older than 20 years in the United States was 16.8%.
B. By age group, CKD was more prevalent among older persons aged above 60 (39.4%) than among younger persons aged 40–59 (12.6%) or ages 20–39 (8.5%). CKD prevalence was greater among persons with diabetes than among those without diabetes (40.2% vs. 15.4%), and among persons with cardiovascular disease than among those without cardiovascular disease (28.2% vs. 15.4%). CKD is higher among persons with hypertension than among those without hypertension (24.6% vs. 12.5%). In addition, CKD prevalence was greater among non-Hispanic blacks (19.9%) and Mexican Americans (18.7%) than among non-Hispanic whites (16.1%).

Pathogenesis

Blood from the renal arteries and their subdivisions is delivered to the glomeruli. The glomeruli form an ultrafiltrate, nearly free of protein and blood elements, which subsequently flows into the renal tubules. The tubules reabsorb and secrete solute and/or water from the ultrafiltrate. The final tubular fluid, the urine, leaves the kidney, draining sequentially into the renal pelvis, ureter, and bladder, from which it is excreted through the urethra. The causes of chronic kidney disease are traditionally classified by which portion of the renal anatomy is most affected by the disorder.

A. Vascular disease: Vascular disorders of the kidneys may involve partial or complete occlusion of large, medium, or small renal vessels. Examples of macro vascular or large renal vessel disease are renal artery stenosis, and atherosclerotic disease. Benign hypertensive arteriolar nephrosclerosis results when chronic hypertension damages small blood vessels, glomeruli, renal tubules, and interstitial tissues. Glomerulosclerosis is a severe micro vascular or small vessel kidney disease caused by diabetes and uncontrolled hypertension in which glomerular function of blood filtration is lost as fibrous scar tissue replaces the glomeruli. Loss of glomerular function leads to proteinuria, hematuria, hypertension, and nephrosis, with variable progression to end-stage renal disease. Proteinuria occurs because of changes to capillary endothelial cells, the glomerular basement membrane (GBM), or podocytes, which normally filter serum protein selectively by size and charge.
B. Tubular and interstitial disease: As with vascular disease, chronic tubulointerstitial nephritis (CTIN) can be primary or secondary to glomerular damage and renovascular vascular disease. CTIN arises when chronic tubular insults cause gradual interstitial infiltration and fibrosis, tubular atrophy and dysfunction, and a gradual deterioration of renal function usually over years. Causes of CTIN are immune disorders, infections, reflux or obstructive nephropathy, and drugs. Analgesic abuse nephropathy (AAN) is a type of CTIN caused by cumulative lifetime use of large amounts of certain analgesics such as nonsteroidal anti-inflammatory drugs (NSAIDs).

Predisposing Factors

A. Diabetes
B. Hypertension

C. Cardiovascular disease

D. Chronic use of analgesics such as NSAIDs

E. Autoimmune disorder

F. Polycystic kidney disease

G. Urinary tract obstructions such as benign prostatic hyperplasia (BPH) or kidney stones

H. Recurrent urinary tract infections

I. Age over 60

J. African American, Native American, or Hispanic ethnicity

K. Smoking

L. Exposure to toxins

M. Family history of kidney disease

Common Complaints

A. For CKD Stage 1 and 2 there are usually no presenting complaints; however, hypertension (HTN) is usually present. CKD is usually identified through routine screening of kidney function and urine tests for micro albumin.

Signs and Symptoms

In CKD Stage 3, the person will develop CKD complications but still will not usually have identifiable signs/symptoms:

A. Hypertension

B. Decreased dietary calcium absorption

C. Reduced renal phosphate excretion

D. Elevation of parathyroid hormone

E. Altered lipoprotein metabolism

F. Reduced spontaneous protein intake

G. Anemia

H. Left ventricular hypertrophy

I. Salt and water retention

J. Decreased renal potassium excretion

These complications gradually worsen as the person moves to Stage 4 CKD. The person will begin to display signs and symptoms of complications such as:

A. Changes in bone density

B. Fatigue and pallor related to anemia

C. Edema

D. Decreases in muscle mass

As the CKD progresses to Stage 5, in addition to gradual worsening of the signs/symptoms noted in Stages 3 and 4, the person will experience symptoms indicating chronic uremia:

A. Impaired sleep

B. Nocturia

C. Fatigue

D. Anorexia, nausea, vomiting, and weight change

E. Decreased mental acuity

F. Pruritis

G. Edema

H. Respiratory symptoms including orthopnea and dyspnea

I. Muscle cramps, twitching, and restless legs

J. Peripheral neuropathy

Subjective Data

A. Review the patient's medical history to identify risk factors for CKD (previously noted in predisposing factors).

B. Elicit information about how well risk factors such as DM and HTN are controlled.

C. Review onset and duration of signs/symptoms of CKD complications and uremia.

D. Review all medications—including all over-the-counter (OTC) medications, especially NSAIDs, and supplements. Obtain specific information about dosing and length of time drug was used.

E. Elicit smoking history.

Physical Exam

A. Observe general demeanor, attentiveness, and signs of fatigue.

B. Measure
   1. Height, weight, and body mass index.
   2. Vital signs, including orthostatic blood pressure and pulse.

C. Inspect
   1. Inspect skin for color, moisture, turgor, and signs of scratching due to chronic pruritis.
   2. Inspect the neck for jugular venous distention.
   3. Inspect the abdomen for distention.
   4. Inspect the extremities for edema, muscle mass, and signs of pain disorders such as arthritis.

D. Auscultate
   1. Auscultate the lungs for rales.
   2. Auscultate the heart for cardiac heave, gallop, or rub.
   3. Auscultate for abdominal or femoral bruit.

E. Palpate abdomen for masses, distention, palpable bladder, or flank tenderness.

F. Neurological exam for sensation and vibratory sense on both feet.

Diagnostic Tests

Laboratory testing is critical in ascertaining the stage, course, chronicity, and complications (and associated comorbid conditions) of CKD.

A. Routine kidney function tests:
   1. Serum creatinine
   2. BUN
   3. Urinalysis
   4. Measuring glomerular filtration rate: The severity of CKD should be classified based on the level of the estimated glomerular filtration rate (eGFR). Serum creatinine alone should *not* be used as a measure of kidney function. Kidney function in patients with CKD should be assessed by formula-based estimation of GFR (eGFR), preferably using the 4-variable Modification of Diet in Renal Disease (MDRD) equation. Clinicians who do not have access to an automated tool may use a Web-based tool at http://www.nkdep.nih.gov/professionals/gfr_calculators/index.htm.

   Calculate eGFRs using the actual MDRD equation:

$$eGFR = 186 \times [SCr]{-}1.154 \times [age]{-}0.203 \times [0.742 \text{ if female}] \times [1.210 \text{ if black}]$$

   Key: GFR = glomerular filtration rate; MDRD = Modification of Diet in Renal Disease; SCr = Serum creatinine concentration

B. Assessing proteinuria

1. When screening adults at increased risk for chronic kidney disease, albumin in the urine should be measured in a spot urine sample using either:
   a. Albumin-specific dipstick.
   b. Albumin-to-creatinine ratio.
   c. It is usually not necessary to obtain a timed urine collection (overnight or 24-hour).
   d. First morning specimens are preferred, but random specimens are acceptable if first morning specimens are not available.
   e. In most cases, screening with urine dipsticks is acceptable for detecting proteinuria:
   f. Standard urine dipsticks are acceptable for detecting increased total urine protein.
   g. Albumin-specific dipsticks are acceptable for detecting albuminuria.
2. Patients with a positive dipstick test (1_ or greater) should undergo confirmation of proteinuria by a quantitative measurement (protein-to-creatinine ratio or albumin-to-creatinine ratio) within 3 months.
3. Patients with two or more positive quantitative tests spaced apart by 1–2 weeks should be diagnosed as having persistent proteinuria and undergo further evaluation and management for chronic kidney disease.

Other Lab Tests: To Determine CKD Complications

A. CBC
B. If hemoglobin (Hgb) level is less than 12 g/dL in females, and Hgb levels of less than 13.5 g/dL in adult males, also do blood cell indices, absolute reticulocyte count, serum iron, total iron binding capacity, percent transferrin saturation, serum ferritin, white blood cell count and differential, platelet count, and testing for blood in stool.
C. Lipid profile and triglycerides
D. Total protein, serum albumin, pre-albumin
E. Sodium
F. Potassium
G. Chloride
H. Bicarbonate
I. Calcium
J. Phosphorus
K. Parathyroid hormone

Differential Diagnosis

A. Evaluation is meant to determine whether kidney disease is acute or chronic and to determine prerenal or post-renal causation.

Plan

The treatment plan will focus on patients in earlier stages of CKD—Stage 1, 2, and 3. Persons with Stage 4 and 5 CKD need specialized interventions provided by nephrologists and should be referred immediately.

A. General interventions for the patient with Stage 1–5 renal failure
   1. Provide support to the patient.
   2. Initiate appropriate referrals for a nephrologist, patient education, and social and financial support as soon as possible.

3. For Stage 4 or 5 CKD, access devices for hemodialysis such as a primary Arterio Venous (AV) Fistula or graft require months to mature and should be in place for 6 months prior to the start of dialysis.

B. Patient teaching
   1. Instruct the patient in how kidneys work and how their body is affected by the CKD.
   2. Emphasize the importance of following instructions to prevent further kidney damage:
      a. Follow medication management instructions as carefully as possible.
      b. No OTC medications should be taken that are not approved by the provider.
      c. Keeping diabetes and hypertension under good control is crucial to maintaining kidney function.
      d. Preventing cardiovascular complications by lowering cholesterol and BP is more important when you have CKD.
      e. Smoking cessation is an important way to prevent worsening kidney function.
      f. Routine follow-ups with provider are necessary to monitor kidney function. Patients should be educated and encouraged to keep all appointments.
      g. Follow dietary instructions regarding protein, fats, sodium, and minerals.
      h. Dietary intake of protein is usually restricted to 0.8–1.0 g/kg per day of high biologic value protein.
      i. Dietary sodium should be restricted to no more than 2 grams daily.
      j. Potassium should be restricted to 40–70 meq/day.
      k. Calories should be restricted to 35 kcal/kg/day; if the body weight is greater than 120 percent of normal or the patient is older than 60 years of age a lower amount may be prescribed.
      l. Fat intake should be about 30%–40% of total daily caloric intake.
      m. Phosphorus should be restricted to 600–800 mg/day.
      n. Calcium should be restricted to 1,400–1,600 mg/day.
      o. Magnesium should be restricted to 200–300 mg/day.
   3. Instruct when to notify the provider with urgent signs/symptoms or changes in kidney function.
      a. Changes in urine volume
      b. Anorexia, nausea, and vomiting
      c. Increased edema
      d. Shortness of breath (SOB)
      e. Increased fatigue
      f. Difficulty concentrating
      g. Muscle weakness, cramping, or twitching
      h. Fever
      i. Chest pain
C. Pharmaceutical therapy in CKD is used to prevent progression of CKD and to manage symptoms of complications of CKD. General Principles:
   1. Always prescribe the smallest effective dose of any medication.

2. Start with a low dose and gradually increase. Dosage intervals may need to be extended.

3. Monitor the effect of any new medication on kidney function with appropriate follow-ups.

4. Provide education to the patient of signs/symptoms to report to the provider immediately regarding drug therapy.

5. Avoid use of nephrotoxic drugs such as radiographic contrast materials, aminoglycoside antibiotics, and NSAIDs.

6. *Immunizations:* Some vaccines in usual doses provide protection, while other vaccines require more frequent dosing, or larger doses to achieve and maintain protective antibodies. Protective antibody titers may fall and booster doses should be given if appropriate. In general the recommendations are:
   a. Annual influenza vaccination
   b. Pneumococcal vaccine with a single booster dose 5 years after the initial dose
   c. Hepatitis B vaccine series for patients prior to starting dialysis

7. *Hypertension control and kidney protection:* It is recommended that hypertension therapy achieve a goal of blood pressure of 130/80 or less. Use of an Angiotensin converting enzyme (ACE) inhibitor or Angiotensin II receptor blocker (ARB) therapy in early stages of CKD with persons who have proteinuria can preserve kidney function. The clinician should monitor serum potassium upon initiation of the therapy. It is common for the serum potassium to initially rise then return to normal levels in 2–3 months. Follow-up serum potassium levels are recommended. In the early stages of CKD, with no proteinuria, the ACE inhibitors and ARBs have not been shown to be effective in protecting kidney function. Hypertension control can still be achieved with the ACE/ARB drugs but other antihypertensive drugs can be used as well.

8. *Fluid overload:* The combination of sodium restrictions and a loop diuretic such as furosemide (Lasix) can lower intraglomerular pressure and provide some kidney protection.

9. *Hyperkalemia:* Hyperkalemia is managed with a low potassium diet in combination with prescribing a loop diuretic such as furosemide. If a patient is on an ACE or ARB, the addition of the loop diuretic will compensate for the elevation of serum potassium related to the ACE/ARB treatment.

10. *Metabolic acidosis:* Build-up of hydrogen ions causes bicarbonate levels to fall below acceptable levels. Sodium bicarbonate in a daily dose of 0.5–1 meq/kg per day is often given. This prevents the symptoms of metabolic acidosis, which can increase muscle mass loss and worsen bone disease.

11. *Renal osteodystrophy:* The development of renal osteodystrophy is caused by hyperphosphatemia and hypocalcemia that are secondary to the decreased kidney function. In order to compensate, the patient will develop secondary hyperparathyroidism. Dietary restriction of phosphate to 800 mg/day is recommended. In Stage 3 CKD, the patient will usually require an oral phosphate binder like calcium carbonate or calcium acetate to prevent hyperphosphatemia. Oral phosphate binders must be taken with meals to be effective. It is imperative to avoid phosphate binders that contain aluminum or magnesium. To suppress parathyroid hormone secretion, the patient is given Calcitriol, a vitamin D analog.

12. *Anemia:* Use of elemental iron 200 mg such as ferrous sulfate 325 mg three times daily (65 mg elemental iron per dose) is recommended to maintain the percent transferrin saturation greater than 20%, and the serum ferritin level to be greater than 100 ng/mL.

    Although primarily used in patients with end-stage renal disease, erythropoietic agents (EPO), such as Epoetin Alfa (Procrit), Epogen, and darbepoietin alfa (Aranesp), are also used to correct the anemia in those with chronic kidney disease who do not yet require dialysis. Dosages of the EPO agents should be prescribed in order to maintain Hgb levels in the range of 11–12 g/dL in predialysis patients with CKD.

13. *Dyslipidemia:* Management of dyslipidemia has been shown to slow progression of CKD. Statins and fibrates are commonly prescribed to lower total cholesterol and LDL, and triglycerides. The incidence of untoward side effects with statins and fibrates is increased in persons with CKD; therefore, lower dosages and careful monitoring is required.

Follow-up

A. Regular, consistent follow-up appointments to monitor progression of CKD, management of complications of CKD, and management of comorbidities such as DM and HTN are recommended.

Consultation/Referral

A. Early referral to a nephrologist is recommended for anyone who has CKD. Referral to a nephrologist must be done as quickly as possible for symptomatic patients with Stage 4 or 5. Consultation with an endocrinologist or hypertension specialist may be helpful in cases where DM and HTN continue to be poorly controlled.

B. Counseling on renal transplantation should be completed by a nephrologist after the patient is evaluated as a candidate for kidney transplantation on what types of transplant are available and how the transplant process works.

C. Referral to a dietician for nutritional counseling and education to assist the patient to understand and follow complex dietary instructions is recommended.

D. Patients with Stage 4 or 5 CKD need counseling regarding the psychosocial and financial impact of progressive renal disease. Referral to a renal social worker or case manager can help the patient understand his or her health insurance benefits, how the transition to Medicare occurs after the health insurance benefit changes, and to help the patient deal with concerns about work or family life.

E. Patients should be referred to educational and support organizations for further education regarding CKD.

F. Web sites:
1. National Kidney Foundation: www.kidney.org
2. National Kidney Disease Education Program: www.nkdep.nih.gov

Individual Considerations

A. Although renal replacement therapy is widely available, some patients, especially the more debilitated elderly or those who have a terminal illness, may request end-of-life counseling including advanced directives.

EPIDIDYMITIS

Definition

A. Epididymitis is acute infection of the epididymis, the coiled segment of the spermatic duct that connects the efferent duct from the posterior aspect of the testicle to the vas deferens. Epididymitis is commonly found to develop during strenuous exertion in conjunction with a full bladder. It is important to differentiate epididymitis from testicular torsion, a true urologic emergency.

Incidence

A. Epididymitis is the fifth most common urologic diagnosis in men aged 18–50 years. There are approximately 600,000 medical visits per year related to epididymitis. An estimated 1 in 1,000 men develops epididymitis annually. Chronic epididymitis may account for up to 80% of scrotal pain noted in the outpatient setting.

Pathogenesis

A. The exact pathophysiology is unclear. The cause may be the retrograde passage of infected urine from the prostatic urethra to the epididymis from the ejaculatory ducts and vas deferens. Reflux may be induced by having the patient perform Valsalva or may be from strenuous exertion. Pathogens include *Chlamydia trachomatis*, *Neisseria gonorrhea*, *E. coli*, *Proteus* species, *Klebsiella* species, *Pseudomonas*, *Mycoplasma* species, and *Treponema pallidum*.

Predisposing Factors

A. Age
1. Age younger than 40: generally associated with urethritis, chlamydia, or gonorrhea
2. Age older than 40: generally associated with urinary tract infections (UTIs), prostatitis, reflux of infected urine, coliform bacteria, or *Pseudomonas*
B. Urinary tract infections
C. Tuberculosis (occasional)
D. Vasectomy
E. Indwelling urethral catheter
F. Urethral stricture
G. Amiodarone-high drug concentrations (dose-dependent)
H. Anal intercourse (coliform bacteria)

Common Complaints

A. Swelling and tenderness of the scrotum (usually located on one side)

B. Fever
C. Chronic epididymitis:
1. Epididymal pain and inflammation that last more than 6 weeks
2. May be accompanied by scrotal induration

Other Signs and Symptoms

A. Gradual onset of localized, unilateral testicular pain. The patient may get relief with elevation of scrotum, which *is* positive **Prehn's sign.**
B. Urethral discharge.
C. Dysuria.
D. Fever and chills.

Subjective Data

A. Elicit the onset, duration, and course of the patient's symptoms.
B. Review the patient's history for vasectomy or trauma to the groin.
C. Are there any other symptoms, including fever, dysuria, or discharge?
D. What makes the pain better? Ask about elevating the scrotum.
E. Does the patient's sexual partner(s) have any symptoms or discharge?
F. Has there been any recent instrumentation or catheterization?
G. Is the pain unilateral or bilateral?
H. Review medication history for Amiodarone.

Physical Examination

A. Temperature and blood pressure.
B. Inspection
1. Examine the patient generally for discomfort before and during examination.
2. Check the urethral meatus for discharge. Retract foreskin (if present) and assess for hygiene and smegma. Check the shaft of the penis, glans, and prepuce for lesions.
3. Check the inguinal and femoral areas for bulges and hernias; have the patient bear down and cough, and reexamine him.
C. Palpate
1. Palpate testes and epididymides for inflammation, tenderness, and masses. In chronic cases, epididymis feels firm and lumpy. Vas deferens may be beaded.
2. Check Prehn's sign by elevating the affected hemiscrotum. This action relieves the pain of epididymitis but exacerbates the pain of torsion.
3. Elicit a cremasteric reflex. Stroking inner thigh should result in rise of the testicle and scrotum on the affected side. A normal cremasteric reflex indicates that testicular torsion is less likely.
4. Palpate scrotum for hydrocele or varicocele.
5. Check for costovertebral angle (CVA) tenderness.
6. Examine the abdomen for masses, urinary distension, tenderness, and organomegaly.
7. Palpate lymph nodes in the groin.
D. Rectal exam: Check for symmetry, swelling, tenderness, and enlarged prostate.

Diagnostic Tests
A. WBC
B. Urinalysis and urine cultures
C. Urethra swab (before void, after prostate massage) for gonorrhea and Chlamydia culture
D. In patients older than 40: express prostatic secretions
E. TB skin test to rule out tuberculosis

Differential Diagnoses
A. Epididymitis
B. Testicular torsion
C. Testicular tumor
D. Prostatitis
E. Incarcerated inguinal hernia
F. Orchitis (occurs with parotitis)
G. Trauma
H. Vasectomy side effect
I. Folliculitis
J. Herpes outbreak

Plan
A. Patient teaching: See the Section III Patient Teaching Guide for this chapter, "Epididymitis."
B. Pharmaceutical therapy
   1. Nonsteroidal anti-inflammatory drugs (NSAIDs) for pain management.
   2. Antitubercular triple therapy consists of rifampin, isoniazid, and pyrazinamide for 6 months.
      a. Rifampin (Rifadin) 450 mg orally every day for 2 months; then 900 mg orally every day for an additional 4 months.
      b. Isoniazid (Laniazid) 300 mg orally every day for 2 months; then 600 mg orally every day for an additional 4 months.
      c. Pyrazinamide 25 mg/kg/day orally for 2 months only.
   3. Amiodarone epididymitis usually responds to a dosage reduction or discontinuation.
   4. Antibiotic therapy for STI or UTI based on cultures. Both sexual partners must be treated with an STI.
      a. Gonorrhea: Ceftriaxone (Rocephin) 250 mg × 1 dose intramuscularly.
         i. Fluoroquinolones are no longer recommended to treat gonococcal infection because of the high rate of resistant organisms.
      b. Chlamydia: Doxycycline (Vibramycin) 100 mg orally, twice a day for 10 days.
      c. Azithromycin 1 gram orally as a single dose for chlamydia and gonococcal infections: 2 grams orally as a single dose.
      d. Ofloxacin (Floxin) 400 mg orally twice a day for 14 days.
      e. Trimethoprim and sulfamethoxazole (Bactrim, Bactrim DS, Septra, Septra DS) 160 mg and 800 mg, respectively, one tablet twice a day for 14 days.

Follow-up
A. See the patient in 2–10 days depending on severity of infection. Inadequate treatment can result in abscess formation and decreased fertility.

B. Culture urine at the end of treatment (test of cure).
C. Failure to recognize and treat both partners for STIs is a potential legal pitfall.
D. Consider testing for HIV.

Consultation/Referral
A. Obtain an immediate consultation with a urologist if testicular torsion or failed medical treatment is suspected.
B. Consult physician for the following:
   1. Intravenous pyelography (IVP)
   2. Doppler ultrasonography
   3. Scrotal ultrasonography
   4. Radionuclide scrotal imaging
C. Refer for evaluation of pediatric patients for an underlying congenital anomaly.

Individual Considerations
A. Partner: Treat sexual partners for STI. Consider testing for HIV.
B. Pediatric: Epididymitis is rare prepubertal, and testicular torsion is more common in this age group.

HEMATURIA

Definition
A. Hematuria is blood in the urine. Microscopic hematuria is defined as three or more red blood cells (RBCs) per high-power microscope field (HPF) in urinary sediment from 2 of 3 properly collected, clean-catch midstream urine specimens.
B. Asymptomatic microscopic hematuria can range from minor findings that do not require treatment to highly significant, life-threatening lesions. Microscopic hematuria is an incidental finding. The American Urologic Association (AUA) recommends an appropriate renal or urologic evaluation with asymptomatic microscopic hematuria for patients who are at risk for urologic disease or primary renal disease.
C. If the excretion rate exceeds 1 million RBCs, macroscopic or gross hematuria is noted. Gross hematuria (macroscopic) is suspected when red or brown urine is present. Glomerulonephritis is associated with brown urine while bleeding from the lower urinary tract is suggested by pink or red urine. Gross hematuria with passage of clots almost always indicates a lower urinary tract source.

Incidence
A. The prevalence of asymptomatic hematuria is from 0.19%–21% of the general population. Less than 3% excrete 10 RBC/HPF. Every disease of the genitourinary tract can produce hematuria.

Pathogenesis
A. Prerenal pathology
   1. Coagulopathy: hemophilia or idiopathic thrombocytopenia purpura (ITP)
   2. Drugs: anticoagulants, aspirin
   3. Sickle cell disease or trait
   4. Collagen vascular disease; lupus
   5. Wilms' tumor

B. Renal pathology
  1. Nonglomerular pathology
    a. Pyelonephritis
    b. Polycystic kidney disease
    c. Granulomatous disease; TB
    d. Malignant neoplasm
    e. Congenital and vascular anomalies
  2. Glomerular pathology
    a. Glomerulonephritis
    b. Berger's disease
    c. Lupus nephritis
    d. Benign familial hematuria
    e. Vascular abnormalities; vasculitis
    f. Alport's syndrome; familial nephritis
C. Postrenal pathology
  1. Renal calculi
  2. Ureteritis
  3. Cystitis
  4. Prostatitis
  5. Benign prostatic hyperplasia
  6. Epididymitis
  7. Urethritis
  8. Malignant neoplasm
D. False hematuria
  1. Vaginal bleeding
  2. Recent circumcision
  3. Pigmentation
    a. Food: beets, blackberries
    b. Medications: quinine sulfate, phenazopyridine, and rifampin
E. Other causes
  1. Trauma
  2. Strenuous exercise (marathons)
  3. Fever

Predisposing Factors
A. See pathogenesis.

Common Complaints
A. Pink or red urine (clots may be present) or brown cola-colored urine on toilet tissue is the common complaint.

Other Signs and Symptoms
A. Pain may or may not be present. Colicky flank pain radiating to the groin suggests a kidney stone. Significant flank pain of renal colic is usually secondary to renal calculi but may occasionally be associated with passage of clots.
B. Frequency, dysuria, urgency, and suprapubic pain occur with cystitis and inflammatory lesions of the lower urinary tract.
C. Dull flank pain with fever and chills may accompany pyelonephritis.
D. Hesitancy and dribbling of the urine suggest benign prostatic hypertrophy.

Subjective Data
A. Elicit onset, duration, and occurrence (beginning, ending, or during voiding) of hematuria. Describe the color and amount: is it "pink on tissue" or bright red in the toilet and tissue?

B. Question the patient regarding past medical history of renal disease, systemic disease such as lupus, or sickle cell disease.
C. Review medications: aspirin, warfarin (Coumadin), and laxatives containing phenolphthalein. Rifampin and phenazopyridine HC1 (Pyridium) can change the color of urine to orange or red.
D. Review other symptoms, such as dysuria, fever, chills, pain, and hesitancy with voiding.
E. Establish whether the blood was urinary, from the vagina (after intercourse or during menstruation), or rectal (from hemorrhoids or strain with BM). Is the patient postpartum?
F. Does the patient bruise easily? Does the patient have bleeding noted when flossing teeth or with brushing?
G. Has the patient had a recent bout of pharyngitis with a rash, hematuria, edema, or hypertension (glomerulonephritis)?
H. Has he or she had any recent trauma, car accident, or strenuous exercise (i.e., marathon)?
I. Does the patient know if he or she has had any exposure to tuberculosis?
J. Is there any family history of kidney disease, stones, and familial nephritis?
K. Does the patient have any current outbreaks of herpes or other sexually transmitted infection (STI)?
L. Review the patient's smoking history.
M. Review occupation exposure to chemicals or dyes (benzenes or aromatic amines).
N. Review food intake of foods such as beets and blackberries.

Physical Examination
A. Temperature, blood pressure, and weight in the presence of recent weight gain or edema.
B. **Male or female patients**
  1. Inspect
    a. Inspect mouth: check tonsils for enlargement and gums for petechiae.
    b. Examine skin for signs of bleeding or bruises and pallor.
    c. Examine for edema.
  2. Palpate
    a. Check the back and abdomen for CVA tenderness.
    b. Check the abdomen for masses, urinary distension, tenderness, and organomegaly.
    c. Palpate groin lymph nodes for enlargement.
  3. Auscultate
    a. Auscultate the heart and lungs
    b. Auscultate for abdominal bruits.
C. **Female patients**
  1. Inspect
    a. Direct visualization of the external genitalia for inflammation, ulcerations, nodules, lesions, and hemorrhoids.
    b. Ask the patient to bear down to check for cystocele and rectocele.
    c. Speculum exam: Observe for atrophic vaginitis, torn tissue, discharge, and friable cervix.

2. Palpate
   a. Milk urethra for discharge.
   b. Bimanual exam: Check for cervical motion tenderness and adnexal masses.

D. **Male patients**
1. Inspect
   a. Direct visualization of the genital; check the urethral meatus for discharge.
   b. Retract the foreskin (if present) and assess for hygiene and smegma. Check the shaft of the penis, glans, and prepuce for lesions or urethral meatal erosion.
2. Palpate
   a. Palpate the testes and epididymides for inflammation, tenderness, and masses; palpate the scrotum for hydrocele or varicocele.
   b. Check the inguinal and femoral areas for bulges and hernias; have the patient bear down and cough, and reexamine him.
   c. Rectal exam: Check for swollen or tender prostate.

Diagnostic Tests

A. Urinalysis:
1. Centrifuge the urine specimen to see if the red or brown color is in the urine sediment or supernatant.
2. If the supernatant is red to brown test for heme (hemoglobin or myoglobin) with a urine dipstick. Semen is in urine after ejaculation and may cause a positive heme reaction on the dipstick.
3. A positive dipstick must always be confirmed with a microscopic examination.
4. Urine culture and sensitivity
5. Urine cytology

B. After the physical exam and consultation, consider the following:
1. CBC with differential.
2. BUN.
3. Creatinine.
4. PT, PTT, platelet count, and bleeding time (if indicated).
5. Sickle cell testing (if indicated).
6. Four-glass urine test for male patient (See the Section II Procedure, "Expressed Prostatic Secretions").
7. Collect 24-hour urine for calcium, uric acid, protein, and creatinine. Follow with a 24-hour urine collection for creatinine and protein to assess renal function and quantitatively assess the degree of proteinuria.
8. Culture for GC and chlamydia.
9. Urine culture for acid-fast bacillus.
10. TB skin testing.
11. IVP or renal ultrasonography.
12. Voiding cystourethrography.
13. A CT scan of the abdomen or pelvis should be considered with a history of trauma to determine the source of blood.

C. Based on history, consider the following tests:
1. Strep testing to detect poststreptococcal glomerulonephritis.
2. Antinuclear antibody to detect lupus nephritis.

D. Urological referral testing includes:
1. Cystoscopy or ureteroscopy.
2. CT or MRI if mass is suspected. CT is considered the best imaging modality for the evaluation of urinary stones, renal and perirenal infections, and associated complications.
3. Renal biopsy.

Differential Diagnoses

A. See pathogenesis for differential diagnoses.

Plan

A. General interventions
1. Investigate and diagnose cause(s). Only a limited workup (electrolytes, CBC) is needed in patients younger than 50 years old with normal physical exam. Patients older than 50 years need detailed investigation and referral.
2. Repeat urinalysis in 2 weeks.

B. Pharmaceutical therapy: None is recommended for hematuria unless an infection is diagnosed.

Follow-up

A. If no cause is obvious at first visit, recheck urine for blood in 2–5 days. Otherwise, follow up as recommended for cause.

B. Culture urine for acid-fast bacillus if sterile pyuria and hematuria persist.

Consultation/Referral

A. The presence of significant proteinuria (excretion of > 1,000 mg per 24 hours), red cell cast or renal insufficiency, or a predominance of dysmorphic RBCs in the urine should prompt an evaluation for renal parenchymal disease by a nephrologist. Red cell casts are considered virtually pathognomonic for glomerular bleeding.

Individual Considerations

A. Women:
1. Nonpregnant: rule out menstruation and sexual activity.
2. Pregnancy: rule out vaginal bleeding such as threaten abortion, abruption, or placenta previa.
3. Ultrasound can be used to evaluate the pregnant woman. CT should not be used secondary to the radiation exposure.

B. Pediatrics:
1. Urinary tract infection is the most common cause for hematuria in children. Irritation or ulceration of the perineum or urethral meatus is the next most common cause, followed by trauma.
2. The majority of children who present with gross hematuria have an easily recognizable and apparent cause. The underlying etiology is generally easy to establish by a complete history, physical examination, and urinalysis.
3. Renal ultrasound is the preferred modality for evaluation in children.
4. Cystoscopy is rarely indicated for hematuria in children. It usually is reserved for the child with a bladder mass noted on ultrasound and the child with urethral abnormalities due to trauma.

C. Geriatrics: The risk of malignancy increases among older individuals with a significant history of smoking or analgesic abuse.

HYDROCELE

Definition
A. Hydrocele is collection of fluid between layers of the processus vaginalis producing swelling in the scrotum or inguinal area. Cystic masses containing fluid or sperm often develop spontaneously. Inguinal hernia and hydrocele share similar etiology and pathophysiology and may coexist.

Incidence
A. Incidence is unknown; hydrocele occurs in 10% of the male pediatric population at birth or in the neonatal period. It occurs infrequently in adulthood.

Pathogenesis
A. Congenital: patent processus vaginalis (PPV).
B. Reactive: inflammatory condition in the scrotum (e.g., trauma, torsion, infection).
C. Idiopathic: arise over a long period of time (most common).
D. Hydroceles are believed to arise from an imbalance of secretion and reabsorption of fluid from the tunica vaginalis.

Predisposing Factors
A. Males; most commonly seen in childhood.

Common Complaints
A. Swollen scrotum is the common indication.

Other Signs and Symptoms
A. Painless swollen scrotum; pain increases with the size of the mass.
B. Rarely does a hydrocele become infected and cause pain.

Subjective Data
A. Elicit onset, duration, and course of swelling: is scrotal sac full all day, or does the patient have a flat scrotum in the morning and a gradual increase in fluid during the day?
B. How old is the patient? Has this ever occurred before? If so, what happened and how was it treated?
C. Review the patient's history for injury to the scrotum.
D. Is there any pain or other symptoms related to hernia with the swelling?
E. Review other symptoms such as discharge, dysuria, fever, or backaches.
F. Review birth control method (vasectomy).

Physical Examination
A. Temperature and blood pressure.
B. Inspect—Careful exam is necessary to rule out masses and tumor.
   1. Examine in the supine and standing positions.
   2. Genital exam: Note amount of swelling, symmetry, lesions, discharge, hernias, varices, and color of scrotum.
   3. Transilluminate scrotum to determine if the lesion is cystic, solid, or a varicocele. In a dark room, transillumination light appears as a red glow with serous fluid. If normal, blood and tissue do not transilluminate; however, the bowel may transilluminate.
C. Auscultate: Auscultate the scrotum for bowel sounds to rule out hernia.
D. Palpate
   1. Check warmth, tenderness, swelling, and any nodularity; if mass is present, check if it has solid versus cystic feel.
   2. Palpate lymph nodes: supraclavicular, chest, abdomen, and groin.
   3. Check for inguinal hernia.
   4. Palpate the abdomen for masses, rebound, and tenderness.

Diagnostic Tests
A. Laboratory evaluate is not required for the evaluation of hydroceles.
B. Scrotal ultrasonography.

Differential Diagnoses
A. Hydrocele: nontender, smooth, and firm. Palpation should reveal confinement to the scrotum unless hydrocele has been present for a long time. Hydrocele transilluminates.
B. Varicocele: feels like a "bag of worms."
C. Hernia: herniated bowel makes gurgling sounds upon auscultation of the scrotum.
D. Testicular tumors tend to occur in young men and are the most common tumor in males from ages 15–30. Consider tumor if the onset is acute. Tumors feel firm, nontender, and fixed and do not transilluminate. Inguinal lymphadenopathy may also be seen. The patient may complain of heaviness with a tumor.
E. Testicular torsion.
F. Orchitis: rare except with mumps. Orchitis is usually unilateral and is associated with fever, swelling, pain, and tenderness. On occasion, parotitis is absent.
G. Epididymitis: inflammation is often concurrent with a urinary tract infection. Epididymis is very tender; scrotal elevating may relieve the pain.
H. Spermatocele: cystic swelling of the epididymis. It is not as large as a hydrocele, but it also transilluminates.

Plan
A. General interventions: Monitor children every 3 months until resolution or until a decision is made to refer to a specialist for evaluation.
B. Factors that indicate surgical repair:
   1. Failure to resolve by age 2
   2. Continued discomfort
   3. Enlargement or waxing and waning in volume
   4. Unsightly appearance
   5. Secondary infection
C. Pharmaceutical therapy: None is recommended.

Follow-up
A. Monitor every 3 months.

Consultation/Referral
A. Refer to a urologist for evaluation, as needed.

Individual Considerations
A. Pediatrics: An infant testicle usually measures 1 cm. Parent may notice a hydrocele that fluctuates slightly in size and usually resolves on its own by 6 months of age.
B. Adults: If an adult experiences a hydrocele, he should be instructed to return for evaluation if the hydrocele becomes larger or uncomfortable, or if it interferes with sexual intercourse.

⬤ INTERSTITIAL CYSTITIS

Definition
A. Interstitial cystitis (IC) is a chronic condition that results in recurring discomfort or suprapubic pain, pressure in the bladder, and surrounding pelvic region related to bladder filling. IC is also commonly known as painful bladder syndrome (PBS). IC/PBS includes all cases of urinary pain with persistent urge to void or urinary frequency that cannot be attributed to other causes (i.e., infection, stones, or other pathology).
B. The persistent urge to void helps to distinguish the symptoms of IC/PBS from those of overactive bladder (OAB). IC/PBS affects quality of life related to social activities, lost work productivity, sleep deprivation due to urinary frequency, fatigue, and even depression.

Incidence
A. Actual prevalence is unknown because of the variability of diagnostic criteria. It is not uncommon for patients to experience a lag time of 5–7 years before diagnosis. It is estimated that in the United States, IC/PBS affects 700,000 to 1 million people. The majority of the affected persons are women.

Pathogenesis
A. The pathophysiology of IC/PBS remains unclear. It is not established whether IC/PBS is a localized condition just involving the bladder or whether it is a systemic disease that affects the bladder.

Predisposing Factors
A. In both genders with a higher prevalence in females
B. Mean age of diagnosis is 42–45 years
C. Urinary tract infection
D. Prostatitis
E. Chronic yeast infections
F. Posthysterectomy or other pelvic surgery
G. Medications
   1. Calcium channel blockers
   2. Cardiac glycosides

Common Complaints
A. Persistent urge to void/frequency
B. Mild discomfort to intense pain with bladder filling and/ or emptying
C. Frequency
D. Urgency
E. Nocturia

Other Signs and Symptoms
A. Combination of urgency and frequency
B. Pressure
C. Increase in symptoms during menstruation
D. Pain during vaginal intercourse
E. Low back pain with bladder filling

Subjective Data
A. Review onset, frequency, duration, and severity of symptoms.
B. Evaluate if the pain of bladder filling is partially or completely relieved by voiding.
C. Does the patient void frequently in order to maintain a low bladder volume and avoid discomfort versus voiding frequently to avoid urge incontinence (overactive bladder)?
D. Are there any foods or drinks (e.g., citrus, beer, coffee) that exacerbate symptoms?
E. Are symptoms increased after stress, exercise, intercourse, being seated for long periods of time, or during the menstrual cycle?
F. How much do the symptoms affect the patient's quality of life (e.g., sleep disturbance, loss of work, avoiding activities)?
G. Does the patient have any other chronic pain syndromes such as IBS, chronic fatigue, dyspareunia, or fibromyalgia?
H. Review the patient's surgical history and history of genitourinary cancers.
I. Has there been any trauma or falls onto the coccyx?
J. Review the patient's history of urinary tract infections, urinary retention, and urinary tract stones.

Physical Examination
A. Temperature and blood pressure.
B. Inspection
   1. Note general appearance for signs of depression and discomfort before and during examination.
   2. Inspect the male external genitalia for redness, edema, lesions, and discharge.
   3. Inspect female genitalia for discharge, lesions, fissures; inspect cervix for cervicitis.
C. Auscultate:
   1. Auscultate the heart and lungs.
   2. Auscultate bowel sounds in all four quadrants.
D. Palpate
   1. Palpate back; note costovertebral angle (CVA) tenderness.
   2. Palpate the abdomen for suprapubic tenderness, rebound masses, or pain.
   3. Perform bimanual exam to rule out other infections and pelvic inflammatory disease (tenderness of the cervix, uterus, and adnexal should be absent).
   4. Males: Complete palpation of external genitalia, prostate, and rectal exam.
E. Percuss: Percuss the bladder and costovertebral angles for tenderness.

Diagnostic Tests
A. Urinalysis with microscopy to exclude hematuria.
B. Urine culture and sensitivity.

C. Postvoid residual volume by straight catheter or ultrasound.
D. Urodynamic testing is not currently considered to have a role in the diagnosis of IC/PBS.
E. Cystoscopy usually reserved for gross or microscopic hematuria.
F. Hydrodistention is not required for diagnosis or treatment.
G. Bladder biopsy is not required for diagnosis; however, it is used for exclusion of other disorders.
H. The potassium sensitivity test is not recommended for routine use since results are nonspecific for IC/PBS.

Differential Diagnoses

A. Interstitial cystitis
B. Urinary tract infection
C. Endometriosis
D. Vulvodynia
E. Irritable bowel syndrome

Plan

A. Behavioral modifications
 1. Restrict fluids to 64 ounces/day, divided into 16 ounces per meal and 8 ounces between meals.
 2. Progressive timed voiding on a 2–3 hour schedule. If the patient is unable to hold urine for this interval, progressively increase urine storage time between void by 15 min per week until the goal of 2–3 hour interval is reached.
 3. Kegel exercises: perform 15 pelvic muscle Kegel contractions twice a day.
 4. Psychosocial support is an integral part of chronic pain disorders.
 5. Several foods have been identified as bladder irritants including foods rich in potassium. Patients may try the elimination of foods/drinks and reintroduce them one at a time to identify any items that make their symptoms worse. Examples include:
  a Alcohol
  b. Tomatoes
  c. Spices
  d. Chocolate
  e. Caffeinated and citrus beverages
  d. Artificial sweeteners
B. Pharmacological therapies
 1. Pentosan polysulfate sodium (Elmiron) is the only oral medication approved by the Food and Drug Administration (FDA) for the treatment of IC.
  a. Dosage: 100 mg orally three times daily
 2. Amitriptyline (Elavil) is used in the treatment of other pain syndromes including IC. May utilize a self-titration dose of 25 mg orally every night and increase in increments of 25 mg every week to a maximum dose of 100 mg orally a day.
 3. Intravesical dimethyl solfoxide (DMSO) (Rimso-50) is the only drug approved by the FDA for bladder instillation.
 4. Treat any comorbid depression.
 5. Treat any comorbid infections (e.g., urinary tract infections, sexually transmitted infections), inflammatory bowel disease, or endometriosis.
 6. Other medications that have been used for symptomatic relief are:
  a. Hydroxyzine hydrochloride 25–75 mg orally at bedtime.
  b. Gabapentin 300 mg up to 2,400 mg in divided doses. Gabapentin requires careful dose titration due to sedation.
  c. Macrodantin 100 mg/day.
  d. Urised 4 tablets/day.

Follow-up

A. Allodynia, the perception of nonnoxious stimuli such as touch as being noxious or painful, may be present; therefore, an adequate pelvic examination may not be possible. Consider empiric treatment and have the patient return for a pelvic examination to finish evaluation.

Consultation/Referral

A. Refer to a urologist for more through workup and testing.
B. Refer to a pain management specialist if indicated.
C. Electrical stimulation therapy may be considered. The implanted sacral neuromodulation device is FDA approved for the treatment of urinary urgency and frequency, but not specifically for the treatment of IC/PBS.

Resources

International Painful Bladder Foundation: http://www.painful-bladder.org/
Interstitial Cystitis Association: http://www.ichelp.org/
Interstitial Cystitis Network: http://www.ic-network.com/

⬡ PROSTATITIS

Definition

Prostatitis is acute or chronic infection of the prostate gland. Prostatitis is the most important cause of urinary infection in men. There are four types of prostatitis:

A. I Acute bacterial prostatitis (least common)
B. II Chronic bacterial prostatitis
C. III Chronic prostatitis/chronic pelvic pain syndrome (common in men of any age)
 1. IIIA. Inflammatory (presence of white cells in the semen expressed prostatic secretions, or voided bladder urine postprostatic massage)
 2. IIIB. Noninflammatory (absence of white cells)
D. IV Asymptomatic inflammatory prostatitis

Incidence

A. Approximately 8.2% of men have prostatitis sometime during their lives. Prostatitis constitutes about 2 million outpatient visits a year of office visits to a urologist, and primary care providers. Chronic prostatitis/chronic pelvic pain constitutes 90%–95% of cases.

Predisposing Factors

A. More common in younger and middle-aged men
B. Sexual transmission of bacteria
C. Neuromuscular dysfunction
D. Structural voiding dysfunction

Pathogenesis

A. Nonbacterial prostatitis is an inflammatory condition with an unknown etiology. Infection results in prostatitis in four ways:
   1. Ascending infection of urethra.
   2. Reflux of infected urine into the prostate through ejaculatory and prostatic ducts that empty into the prostatic urethra.
   3. Hematogenous spread causes bacterial prostatitis.
   4. Invasion by rectal bacteria by direct extension or lymph system spread.
B. Causative organisms: *E. coli, Pseudomonas, Enterococci, Ureaplasma, Gardnerella vaginalis, Trichomonas vaginalis, Chlamydia trachomatis, Chlamydia, Mycoplasma,* or *Neisseria gonorrhoeae. Cytomegalovirus (CMV), Mycobacterium turberculosis,* and fungi have been associated with prostatitis in HIV-infected patients.
C. Incubation period depends on pathogen.

Common Complaints

A. Dysuria
B. Perineal, rectal, or suprapubic pain (chronic pain syndrome)
C. Less urine flow
D. Spiking fever
E. Back pain
F. Sexual dysfunction

Other Signs and Symptoms

A. Acute bacterial prostatitis
   1. Fever and chills, malaise
   2. Acute onset of dysuria
   3. Hesitancy
   4. Urinary frequency and low back pain
   5. Pain with intercourse and with defecation
   6. Initial or terminal hematuria and edema with acute urinary retention
   7. Arthralgia or myalgia
   8. Nocturia
B. Chronic bacterial prostatitis
   1. Usually presents with recurrent UTI.
   2. May be asymptomatic between acute episodes; some men have large fluctuation in the symptom severity.
   3. Perineal, inguinal, or suprapubic pain, or irritative symptoms on voiding such as frequency and urgency.
   4. Hematuria, hematospermia, or painful ejaculations.
   5. Prostatic calculi.
C. Nonbacterial prostatitis (most common)
   1. Pain: prostatic, lower back, perineum, groin, scrotum, or suprapubic pain; ejaculatory pain
   2. Dysuria, urinary frequency, urgency, hesitancy, and decreased urine flow
   3. Penile discharge
D. Asymptomatic inflammatory prostatitis is found when looking for causes of infertility and testing for prostate cancer.

Subjective Data

A. Ask the patient to complete the NIH Chronic Prostatitis Symptom Index (NIH-CPSI) self-evaluation form (see Table 11.2). The assessment tool evaluates pain, urinary symptoms, and the impact on quality of life.
   1. Mild = 0–14 total score
   2. Moderate = 15–29 total score
   3. Severe = 30–43 total score
   An online NIH symptom index that self-scores is available at http://www.prostateinstitute.org/pro_nih.htm.
B. Review the onset, duration, and course of symptoms.
C. Are there any other symptoms such as discharge, pain, hematuria, hesitancy, back pain, or weight loss?
D. Has the patient ever had the same symptoms? If so, how were they treated?
E. Does any sexual partner(s) have any symptoms, lesions, or known STIs?
F. Has the patient noted any impaired urinary flow?
G. Has the patient required any recent urethral catheterization or instrumentation?

Physical Examination

A. Temperature and blood pressure.
B. Inspect
   1. Examine the patient generally for discomfort before and during examination.
   2. Check the urethral meatus for discharge.
   3. Retract foreskin (if present) and assess for hygiene and smegma.
   4. Check the shaft of the penis, glans, and prepuce for lesions.
C. Palpate
   1. Palpate testes and epididymides for inflammation, tenderness, and masses; palpate scrotum for hydrocele or varicocele.
   2. Check back for CVA tenderness.
   3. Evaluate for an enlarged tender bladder due to urinary retention.
   4. Palpate the abdomen for masses, urinary distension, suprapubic tenderness, and organomegaly.
   5. Palpate inguinal lymph nodes; check the inguinal and femoral areas for bulges and hernias; have the patient bear down and cough, and reexamine him.
   6. Rectal exam
      a. Check for symmetry, swelling, tenderness, and enlarged prostate.
      b. In acute prostatitis, rectal examination reveals the prostate gland to be exquisitely tender and boggy.
      c. A fluctuant prostatic mass suggests an abscess that may require surgical intervention.
      d. Perform prostate massage for postmassage urine sample.

Diagnostic Tests

A. Acute infection
   1. CBC with differential.
   2. Urinalysis, urine culture, and sensitivity (if indicated).
   3. Gram's stain, culture of expressed prostatic secretions (EPS); see the Section II Procedure, "Expressed Prostatic Secretions."
      a. **Avoid vigorous massage when obtaining specimen because of the risk of inducing bacteremia.**

TABLE 11.2 NIH Chronic Prostatitis Symptoms Index (NIH-CPSI)

Pain or Discomfort

1. In the last week, have you experienced any pain or discomfort in the following areas?

	Yes	No
a. Area between rectum and testicles (perineum)	$\square_1$	$\square_0$
b. Testicles	$\square_1$	$\square_0$
c. Tip of the penis (not related tourination)	$\square_1$	$\square_0$
d. Below your waist, in your pubic or bladder area	$\square_1$	$\square_0$

2. In the last week, have you experienced:

	Yes	No
a. Pain or burning during urination?	$\square_1$	$\square_0$
b. Pain or discomfort during or after sexual climax (ejaculation)?	$\square_1$	$\square_0$

3. How often have you had pain or discomfort in any of these areas over the last week?

- $\square_0$ Never
- $\square_1$ Rarely
- $\square_2$ Sometimes
- $\square_3$ Often
- $\square_4$ Usually
- $\square_5$ Always

4. Which number best describes your AVERAGE pain or discomfort on the days that you had it, over the last week?

$\square$ $\square$ $\square$ $\square$ $\square$ $\square$ $\square$ $\square$ $\square$ $\square$ $\square$
0   1   2   3   4   5   6   7   8   9   10
NO   PAIN AS
PAIN   BAD AS
                                     YOU CAN
                                     IMAGINE

Urination

5. How often have you had a sensation of not emptying your bladder completely afer you finished urinating, over the las week?

- $\square_0$ Not at all
- $\square_1$ Less than 1 time in 5
- $\square_2$ Less than half the time
- $\square_3$ About half the time
- $\square_4$ More than half the time
- $\square_5$ Almost always

6. How often have you had to urinate again less than two hours after you finished urinating, over the last week?

- $\square_0$ Not at all
- $\square_1$ Less than 1 time in 5
- $\square_2$ Less than half the time
- $\square_3$ About half the time
- $\square_4$ More than half the time
- $\square_5$ Almost always

Impact of Symptoms

7. How much have your symptoms kept you from doing the kinds of things you would usually do, over the last week?

- $\square_0$ None
- $\square_1$ Only a little
- $\square_2$ Some
- $\square_3$ A lot

8. How much did you think about your symptoms, over the last week?

- $\square_0$ None
- $\square_1$ Only a little
- $\square_2$ Som
- $\square_3$ A lot

Quality of Life

9. If you were to spend the rest of your life with your symptoms just the way they have been during the last week, how would you feel about that?

- $\square_0$ Delighted
- $\square_1$ Pleased
- $\square_2$ Mostly satisfied
- $\square_3$ Mixed (about equally satisfied and dissatisfied)
- $\square_4$ Mostly dissatisfied
- $\square_5$ Unhappy
- $\square_6$ Terrible

Scoring the NIH-Chronic Prostatitis Svmptom Index Domains

Pain: Total of items 1a, 1b, 1c, 1d, 2a, 2b, 3, and 4 = _____

Urinary Symptoms: Total of items 5 and 6 = _____

Quality of Life Impact: Total of items 7, 8, and 9 = _____

b. Gram's stain of EPS demonstrates infectious organisms or WBC typical of an immune response (>10 WBC/HPF is abnormal). Patients with abnormal WBC but no bacterial growth may have chlamydial or *Ureaplasma* infection and need to be tested or treated empirically.

B. Chronic infection
   1. BUN
   2. CBC with differential
   3. Creatinine

C. Chronic bacterial prostatitis
   1. If recurrent infections are confirmed; evaluate for structural or functional abnormality with CT scan.
   2. Measure residual urine after voiding.
   3. If no urologic abnormalities are found and repeated cultures indicate the same bacterial strain, chronic bacterial prostatitis is likely.

D. Other tests such as ultrasound, MRI, and biopsies as required to rule out other pathology.

Differential Diagnoses

A. Prostatitis
   1. Acute: readily evident by clinical presentation and exam.
   2. Chronic: more difficult to diagnose. The hallmark symptom is recurrent urinary tract infection. It often resembles prostatic hypertrophy, strictures, and prostatic carcinoma.
   3. Chronic pelvic pain syndrome.

B. Pyelonephritis.

C. Epididymitis.

D. Anal fistulas and fissures.

E. Benign prostatic hypertrophy (BPH) causes urinary retention due to obstruction.

F. Urethral stricture or stone.

G. Chronic pain syndromes/back pain.

Plan

A. General interventions
   1. Patients with acute prostatitis may need hospitalization and IV therapy for severe infection (high fever, increased WBC, dehydration). Less toxic patients may be treated on an outpatient basis.
   2. Older men without evidence of infection with lower tract symptoms should have urine cytology to rule out malignancy.

B. Patient teaching
   1. See the Section III Patient Teaching Guide for this chapter, "Prostatitis."
   2. Having the patient self-massage to reduce symptoms is questionable; the massage of an acutely infected gland is contraindicated because of the risk of bacteremia.
   3. Recommend sitz baths 2–3 times daily.

C. Dietary management
   1. Increase fluid intake.
   2. Decrease caffeine and alcohol, which can irritate the urethra.

D. Pharmaceutical therapy
   1. Analgesics (NSAIDs) and stool softeners may be needed.

2. Discontinue or reduce the dosage (if possible) of the patient's anticholinergics, sedatives, and antidepressants because they may impair bladder function.

3. Inpatient: Ampicillin and Gentamicin by IV infusion until the patient is afebrile for 24 hours, then switch to oral therapy.

4. Acute outpatient therapy: the usual course of treatment is 4 weeks based on the high response rate in clinical trials. Choose one of the following oral treatments depending on the causative organism:
   a. Trimethoprim and sulfamethoxazole (or co-trimoxazole, Bactrim DS) 160 mg and 800 mg, respectively, one tablet twice daily for 4 weeks.
   b. Cephalexin 500 mg four times a day for 4 weeks.
   c. Ciprofloxacin 500 mg twice daily for 4 weeks.
   d. Amoxicillin 500 mg three times daily for 4 weeks.
   e. Doxycycline 100 mg twice daily for 4 weeks.

5. Low-dose suppressive therapy with an agent that has shown to be effective may be considered.

6. There are no formal guidelines for the management of chronic bacterial prostatitis or chronic pelvic pain syndrome. Strategies are currently focused on symptomatic relief. Alpha-blockers may be used to control symptoms.

Follow-up

A. See the patient in 2–10 days depending on the patient's symptoms and course.

B. Culture urine at completion of drug therapy. Test of cure for antibiotics requires elimination of bacteria from prostatic fluid to prevent chronic flares. Some patients may not achieve cure even after 6–12 weeks of therapy.

C. Patients that achieve a partial response may be given a second course of antibiotics. Those failing to demonstrate an organism may benefit from a course of doxycycline or erythromycin for *Chlamydia* and/or *Ureaplasma* coverage.

D. Notify the health department for reportable sexually transmitted infections (STIs).

Consultation/Referral

A. Obtain a referral to a urologist for recurrent acute bacterial prostatic infections or infections that persist. Cystoscopy may be required to rule out interstitial cystitis.

PROTEINURIA

Definition

Proteinuria is excess protein (albumin) in urine. The measurement of protein excretion is used to establish the diagnosis and to follow the course of glomerular disease. There are three types of abnormal proteinuria:

A. Glomerular proteinuria (albuminuria): due to increased filtration of macromolecules across the glomerular capillary wall. The standard urine dipstick is able to detect glomerular proteinuria.

B. Tubular proteinuria: related to interference with proximal tubular reabsorption. A urinary dipstick is unable to detect tubular proteinuria.

C. Overflow proteinuria: increased excretion secondary to an overproduction of a particular protein. A urinary dipstick is unable to detect overflow protein.

The normal rate of albumin excretion is less than 20 mg/day; the rate is about 4–7 mg/day in healthy young adults and increases with age and an increase in body weight. Persistent albumin excretion between 30 and 300 mg/day is called microalbuminuria. Values of 300 mg/day of protein are considered overt proteinuria or macroalbuminuria.

In patients with diabetes, microalbuminuria usually indicates incipient diabetic nephropathy. In nondiabetics, the presence of microalbuminuria is associated with cardiovascular disease. Protein is a cardinal sign of pregnancy-induced hypertension (PIH).

Incidence

A. Incidence is unknown. Proteinuria may be a symptom of functional etiologies (due to fever, exercise, or orthostatic proteinuria), or it may be a symptom of a serious condition such as glomerulonephritis with rapidly deteriorating renal function.

Pathogenesis

A. Pathogenesis depends on the underlying etiology. An alteration in glomerular filtration that increases excretion (filtration) of plasma proteins occurs. Increased glomerular permeability, increased production of abnormal proteins (Bence Jones protein), decreased tubular reabsorption, surgical traumas, and infections may increase urinary protein. Urinary protein may also be affected by dietary protein intake.

Predisposing Factors

A. Fever
B. Increased exercise
C. Urinary tract infection
D. Medications
   1. Penicillamine
   2. NSAIDs
   3. Angiotensin converting enzyme (ACE) inhibitors
E. Heavy metal exposure
   1. Gold
   2. Cadmium
   3. Mercury
F. Allergens
G. Family history of proteinuria or pyelonephritis
H. Hypertension
I. Renal disease
J. Congestive heart failure (CHF) or endocarditis
K. Diabetes
L. Lupus
M. HIV and syphilis
N. Hepatitis B
O. Malignancy
   1. Lymphoma
   2. Hodgkin's disease
   3. Breast tumor
   4. Lung tumor
   5. Colon tumor
P. Heroin use
Q. Pregnancy-induced hypertension

Common Complaints

A. No complaints
B. Increased weight
C. Decreased urine output

Other Signs and Symptoms

A. Proteinuria may be an incidental finding and have no symptoms. The use of urine dipstick for screening is acceptable for first detecting proteinuria; however, the dipstick should not be used to quantify the amount of urinary protein. Protein concentration is a function of urine volume as well as the quantity of protein present.
B. Edema: slight to pitting.
C. Nephrotic syndrome: hypercholesterolemia and hypertriglyceridemia
D. Protein malnutrition: anorexia and vomiting

Subjective Data

A. Review the onset, course, and duration of presenting complaints.
B. Question the patient concerning urinary output, thirst or fluid intake, edema, increase in weight. Establish usual weight history.
C. If a woman, establish the first day of the patient's last period. Is she pregnant? If so, what is the fetus' gestational age? Is there edema, hypertension, headache, visual changes (scotoma), hyperreflexia, and/or right upper quadrant pain?
D. Review the patient's past medical history for renal disease, diabetes, congestive heart failure, and substance abuse.
E. Does the patient have signs or symptoms of a urinary tract infection or pyelonephritis?
F. Review the patient's recent history for exertion, emotional stress, surgical trauma, fever, and any acute illness.
G. When was the patient's last evaluation for cholesterol? Is he or she on any special diet?
H. Review medication list including prescribed and over-the-counter medications.

Physical Examination

A. Temperature, blood pressure, pulse, respirations and weight.
B. Inspect
   1. Inspect overall general appearance for edema (pedal, hand, facial, or periorbital edema) or ascites.
   2. Evaluate for protein wasting.
   3. Evaluate for jugular vein distension.
   4. Funduscopic exam: evaluate for retinopathy.
C. Auscultate: Auscultate the heart and lungs.
D. Palpate
   1. Examine the abdomen; evaluate bladder distension, suprapubic tenderness, masses, or abdominal tenderness.
   2. Palpate for CVA tenderness.
   3. Check deep tendon reflexes especially in pregnant women.

Diagnostic Tests

A. The gold standard for measurement of protein excretion is a 24-hour urine collection.

B. Protein to creatinine ratio on a random urine specimen.
C. Albumin and creatinine.
D. Lipid profile.
E. BUN: serves as an index of renal excretory capacity. Urea is the nitrogenous end product of protein metabolism.
F. Urinalysis, urine culture, and sensitivity (if indicated).
G. Other testing related to physical finding.
H. Renal biopsy is required to establish the diagnosis in most cases.

Differential Diagnoses
A. See predisposing factors.

Plan
A. Patients with hematuria and proteinuria need a 24-hour urine collection for protein and creatinine clearance.
B. Once significant proteinuria is established, the evaluation turns to establishing whether the patient is asymptomatic or symptomatic, and if asymptomatic, whether the proteinuria is transient or persistent.
   1. Asymptomatic: Reevaluate urine specimens for sediment, 24-hour protein, orthostatic or exercise-induced proteinuria, and so on. Invasive procedures and extensive workup are not necessary.
   2. Symptomatic: Reevaluate by focusing on the risk factors, potential systemic disease; refer the patient to a specialist if significant disease is suspected.
C. Management for nephrotic syndrome includes diet with sodium and protein restriction, loop and distal-acting diuretics, control of cholesterol (low-saturated-fat, low-cholesterol diet), lipid-lowering agents, administering pneumococcal and influenza vaccines to prevent infections, and use of steroids and immunosuppressive agent as necessary.
D. Patient teaching
   1. Encourage low-fat/low-cholesterol diet if hyperlipidemia is present.
   2. Encourage sodium- and protein-restricted diet for nephrotic syndrome.
E. Pharmaceutical therapy: There is no specific drug therapy for excess protein. Use drug therapy appropriate to the underlying medical disease causing proteinuria. In patients with chronic kidney disease, the administration of Angiotension converting enzyme (ACE) inhibitors and/or Angiotensin II receptor blockers (ARBs) is aimed at reducing the degree of proteinuria.

Follow-up
A. Recheck urine in 1–3 weeks if benign or functional proteinuria is suspected. Assess for vasculitic skin changes, rashes, retinopathy, lymphadenopathy, signs of heart failure, abdominal masses, organomegaly, guaiac stools, prostatic enlargement, and joint inflammation.

Consultation/Referral
A. Consider patient referral if kidney damage is progressing from medical disease (systemic lupus erythematosus, hypertension [HTN], diabetes).
B. Refer the patient as necessary; hypertension is a poor prognostic sign for significant renal impairment.
C. Consultation for diagnostic tests to be considered: kidney, ureter, and bladder (KUB); IVP; renal ultrasonography; renal biopsy.

Individual Considerations
A. Pregnancy:
   1. Protein excretion is considered abnormal in pregnancy when it exceeds 300 mg/24 hours or greater than 0.2 grams of protein per gram of creatinine in a random urine specimen.
   2. Abnormal protein may indicate onset of pregnancy-induced hypertension. The distinction between renal disease that predates conception and PIH is important because it affects clinical management.
   3. Monitor urine protein and BP at each prenatal visit and refer the patient if urinary protein remains elevated.
B. Pediatrics: Proteinuria may be seen in school-aged children during routine sports or school exams. It is most likely due to orthostatic proteinuria. However, reevaluate urine in 2–3 weeks. Obtain clean catch urine, using the first voided urine in the morning.
C. Geriatrics: Renal function deteriorates in the elderly who may also have coexisting medical conditions (HTN, diabetes) that may cause nephropathy.

PYELONEPHRITIS

Definition
A. Pyelonephritis is an acute infection and inflammatory disease of the upper urinary tract (renal pelvis, tubules, and interstitial tissue) of one or both kidneys. Acute pyelonephritis is a urinary tract infection that has progressed from the lower urinary tract.
B. Fever has been strongly correlated with the diagnosis of acute pyelonephritis; therefore, patients with clinical symptoms of pyelonephritis in the absence of fever should be evaluated for alternative diagnoses.
C. Acute pyelonephritis characteristically causes some scarring to the kidney and may lead to significant damage, kidney failure, abscess formation, and sepsis.

Incidence
A. Thirty percent of the female population has at least one urinary tract infection in their lifetime. The incidence of pyelonephritis in pregnancy is 1%–2%. Most cases develop as a consequence of undiagnosed or inadequately treated lower urinary tract infection (UTI).
B. Upper tract infections are less common and more serious than lower tract infections. After puberty, the prevalence of UTIs increases slightly in females, but remains low in males. After age 65, UTIs are more common with an equal incidence in both sexes.

Pathogenesis
A. Pyelonephritis is due to ascending infection from the bladder usually caused by gram-negative bacteria in 80%–90% of cases (*E. coli, Proteus mirabilis, Klebsiella*

pneumoniae, Enterobacter, Pseudomonas). Gram-positive causative agents are less common; 10%–15% of cases are due to *Staphylococcus saprophyticus.*

B. In women, the short urethra in close proximity to the perirectal area makes colonization possible. In pregnancy, the increased nutrient content of urine and urinary stasis facilitate bacterial growth.

Predisposing Factors

A. Previous urinary tract infection, cystitis, and pyelonephritis
B. Sickle cell disease
C. Diabetes
D. Urinary catheterization
E. Obstruction: calculi, tumors, and urethral strictures
F. Neurogenic bladder disease: strokes, multiple sclerosis, and spinal cord injuries
G. Urinary reflux
H. HIV
I. Trauma
J. Gender
1. Females
a. Increased sexual activity, failure to void after intercourse, diaphragms, and spermicides
b. Pregnancy
2. Males
a. Homosexuality
b. Uncircumcised penis
c. Sexual partner with colonization
d. Obstruction: prostatic hypertrophy

Common Complaints

A. Shaking, chills, and fever
B. Flank pain or tenderness
C. Urinary frequency or urgency
D. Blood in urine

Other Signs and Symptoms

A. Adults (particularly the elderly): may be asymptomatic with cystitis
B. Children: nausea and vomiting
C. Fever, palpitations, and dizziness
D. Costovertebral angle (CVA) tenderness
E. Headache
F. Urinary frequency, nocturia, hematuria, and dysuria (not always present in upper tract infections)
G. Abdominal pain and suprapubic heaviness
H. Pregnancy: uterine contractions
I. Shortness of breath

Subjective Data

A. Review the onset, course, and duration of symptoms.
B. Are there any problems with voiding? Frequency, urgency, and dysuria distinguishes lower urinary tract infection from pyelonephritis.
C. Review the patient's history of fever and any treatment.
D. Are there any other symptoms, odor, and nausea?
E. Have the patient point to the area of the backache. Is it unilateral or bilateral? What makes the backache better?

F. In women, rule out pregnancy; review first day of last menses.
G. Rule out sickle cell disease, diabetes, and multiple sclerosis.
H. Review the patient's previous history of genitourinary tract problems, stones, UTIs, previous pyelonephritis, any previous testing, and any previous anomalies.
I. Review the strength and character of the urinary stream, especially in older men.
J. Review the patient's history for active herpes lesion. Does urine flow hurt when urine stream begins? Or is the pain noted when urine passes over the lesion?
K. Review drug allergies.

Physical Examination

A. Temperature, pulse, and blood pressure; note orthostatic hypotension. Tachycardia may or may not be present, depending on associated fever, dehydration, and sepsis.
B. Inspect
1. Note general appearance for respiratory distress and dehydration.
2. Inspect the male external genitalia for redness, edema, lesions, and discharge.
3. Inspect the female genitalia for discharge, lesions, and fissures; inspect cervix for cervicitis.
C. Palpate
1. Palpate the back; check CVA tenderness (usually unilateral over the involved kidney).
2. Palpate the abdomen for suprapubic tenderness, rebound masses, or pain.
3. Perform a pelvic examination to rule out other infections and pelvic inflammatory disease (tenderness of the cervix, uterus, and adnexal should be absent).
D. Auscultate: Auscultate the lungs and heart.
E. Pregnancy
1. Check fetal heart rate; fetal tachycardia may be present with fever.
2. Palpate for uterine tenderness and contractions.
3. Pelvic examination for cervical dilation, if indicated for increased risk of preterm labor.
F. Males: Complete palpation of external genitalia, prostate, and rectal exam.

Diagnostic Tests

A. Urine: Urinalysis
1. Leukocyte esterase on dipstick detects pyuria or WBCs.
2. Significant pyuria is greater than 2–5 leukocytes per high power field (HPF).
3. Urine may need to be obtained from straight in-and-out catheterization if the patient is incontinent or has dementia.
B. CBC with differential or WBC, especially with systemic symptoms.
C. Blood culture, if indicated.
D. ABGs, if indicated.
E. Consider sedimentation rate, especially with severe illness and in the elderly.
F. Urine culture and sensitivity.

G. Culture for gonorrhea and chlamydia, if symptoms associated with sexually transmitted infection (STI).
H. Wet prep, if symptoms associated with STI.
I. Imaging studies are not routinely required for the diagnosis of acute pyelonephritis but can be helpful.
   1. Renal ultrasonography.
   2. IVP, if indicated.
   3. Voiding cystourethrogram; if abnormal, consider IVP or renal ultrasonography.

Differential Diagnoses
A. Pyelonephritis
B. Appendicitis
C. Cholecystitis
D. Pancreatitis
E. Diverticulitis
F. Pneumonia
G. Prostatitis
H. Epididymitis
I. Pelvic inflammatory disease (PID)

Plan
A. General interventions: Many severe infections (increased WBC, dehydration or vomiting, high fever) may need hospital admission for IV therapy. Risk factors include older adult, coexisting illness, pregnancy, and uncontrolled vomiting.
B. Give instruction on early recognition of UTIs. See the Section III Patient Teaching Guide for "Urinary Tract Infection (Acute Cystitis)."
C. Dietary management
   1. Increase fluids; have the patient drink at least one large glass of water every hour while awake.
   2. Encourage the patient to drink cranberry juice to help fight and prevent urinary tract infections. If the taste is objectionable, he or she may mix cranberry juice 1:1 with another juice such as grape juice.
D. Pharmaceutical therapy
   1. Acetaminophen (Tylenol) for fever.
   2. Antibiotics: Empiric antibiotic selection should be guided by culture results. Patients with delayed response to therapy should also receive a longer course of antibiotics of 14–21 days.
      a. Adults
         i. Trimethoprim and sulfamethoxazole (TMP-SMX) (Septra DS, Bactrim DS) 160 mg and 800 mg, respectively, one tablet twice daily for 7–14 days.
         ii. Ciprofloxacin (Cipro) 250–500 mg twice daily for 7–14 days. **Shorter antibiotic treatments are not recommended for males.**
         iii. Levofloxacin (Levaquin) 750 mg once daily for 5–7 days (FDA approval for uncomplicated pyelonephritis only; this dosage is not appropriate for complicated pyelonephritis). May be extended for a total of 14 days.
      b. Children less than 2 years old are usually treated for 10 days, children older than 2 years who are afebrile and without abnormalities of the urinary tract or have previous episodes of UTIs are usually treated for 5 days.
         i. Cefixime (Suprax) 16 mg/kg per day in two divided doses on the first day, followed by 8 mg/kg once a day.
         ii. Cefdinir (Omnicef) 14mg/kg per day in two divided doses.
         iii. Ceftibuten (Cedax) 9 mg/kg once a day.
         iv. The use of Ciprofloxacin in children is reserved for complicated UTIs and complicated pyelonephritis; it is not a first-line agent.
      c. Nitrofurantoin (Macrodantin) should not be used to treat UTI/pyelonephritis in adults or children; it is excreted in the urine but does not achieve therapeutic serum levels.

Follow-up
A. Follow up with the patient in 12–24 hours by phone or office visit. Patients with persistent fever or clinical symptoms after 48–72 hours of appropriate antibiotic therapy should undergo radiological evaluation.
B. Culture urine after antibiotic is completed (2 weeks) and again in 3 months for patients with recurrent symptoms.
C. Women with recurrence of pyelonephritis need further urologic investigation.

Consultation/Referral
A. Consult physician and consider hospitalization for infants with both lower and upper infections, children with pyelonephritis, and children with recurrent infections.
B. Consult or refer the patient to a physician if he or she requires IVP, cystoscopy, or renal biopsy.
C. IV therapy and hospitalization is needed in all cases suggestive of bacteremia in children who are vomiting, children younger than 2 years, and children with documented parenchymal damage.
D. Males with persistent bladder infections need a urologic consultation.
E. Pyelonephritis in men suggests structural problems and needs hospitalization and further evaluation (IVP).

Individual Considerations
A. Pregnancy: Based upon the higher risk of complications in pregnancy, pyelonephritis has traditionally been treated with hospitalization and intravenous antibiotics until the woman is afebrile for 24 hours and symptoms improve.
B. Pediatrics
   1. Always order a urine culture and sensitivity on children suspected of UTI.
   2. Suprapubic aspiration of the bladder should be considered in young infants.
   3. Voiding cystogram should be considered in all children less than 16 years with a documented UTI.
   4. Indications for hospitalization include:
      a. Age younger than 2 months
      b. Clinical urosepsis or potential bacteremia

c. Immunocompromised patient
d. Vomiting or inability to tolerate oral medication
e. Lack of adequate outpatient follow-up (e.g., no phone, live far from hospital)
f. Failure to respond to outpatient therapy

C. Males
1. Consider ordering renal function tests (BUN and creatinine).
2. Men over 50 years of age: consider urologic consultation and IVP.

D. Geriatrics
1. Patients may need hospitalization for IV antibiotics and hydration.
2. Bladder or kidney infections may be common in patients with long-term urinary catheters and can lead to septicemia if untreated or unrecognized.

RENAL CALCULI, OR KIDNEY STONES (NEPHROLITHIASIS)

Definition

A. Renal calculi, or kidney stones, are due to the formation of crystals in the urinary system from the kidneys to the bladder. Nephrolithiasis refers to renal stone disease; urolithiasis refers to the presence of stones in the urinary system. The majority of stones (80%) consist of calcium usually as calcium oxalate, but they can contain uric acid, struvite (magnesium, ammonium, and phosphate), oxalic acid, phosphate salts, or the amino acid cystine. Spontaneous passage of a stone is related to the stone size and location. Approximately one-half of symptomatic patients require intervention for stone removal.

Incidence

A. Renal calculi are very common with a higher incidence noted in males. At lease 12% of men and 5% of women have at least one symptomatic stone by age 70. Initial cases typically occur between ages 30 and 40 and the prevalence increases with age. Idiopathic nephrolithiasis is common in males, whereas primary hyperparathyroidism is more common in females.

B. Most kidney stones pass spontaneously; however, 10%–30% do not pass and can cause continuing pain, infection, or obstruction.

Pathogenesis

A. The formation of uric acid stones requires continued and excessive oversaturation of urine with stone-forming constituents, uric acid, calcium, and oxalate. Dehydration, hyperuricosuria, and significantly acidic urine contribute to uric acid supersaturation and stone formation. Struvite stones form only when the urinary tract is infected with urea-splitting organisms such as *Proteus* species.

B. Hydroureteronephrosis is the most significant renal alteration in pregnancy. Dilatation is greater on the right side than the left because of pressure due to physiological engorgement of the right ovarian vein and dextrorotation of the uterus.

Predisposing Factors

A. Male
B. Dehydration (poor intake and immobility)
C. Chronic obstruction with stasis of urine
D. Hypercalcemia caused by hyperparathyroidism; renal tubular acidosis; multiple myeloma; or excessive intake of vitamin D, milk, and alkali
E. Diet high in purines and abnormal purine metabolism (gout)
F. Pregnancy (1 per 1,500)
G. Chronic infections
H. Foreign bodies
I. Excessive oxalate absorption in inflammatory bowel disease, bowel resection, or ileostomy
J. Previous stone formation
K. Family history of nephrolithiasis
L. Medications
1. Vitamins A, C, and D
2. Loop diuretics
3. Acetazolamide
4. Ammonium chloride
5. Calcium-containing medications including alkali and antacids
6. Indinavir
7. Sulfadiazine
M. Obesity
N. Diabetes

Common Complaints

A. Severe flank and groin pain
B. Blood in urine
C. Asymptomatic

Other Signs and Symptoms

A. Unilateral flank pain that radiates to the groin.
B. Sudden onset of colicky pain.
C. Hematuria.

The timing and appearance of hematuria is important. Hematuria seen at the beginning of the urine stream may indicate bleeding in the urethra. Terminal hematuria, or blood in the end of the urine stream, denotes bladder neck or the prostate as the source. Lastly, blood throughout the entire urination suggests a lesion.

D. Nausea and vomiting.
E. Restlessness.
F. Symptoms common with cystitis or inflammatory lesions of the lower tract are usually absent: frequency, dysuria, urgency, and suprapubic pain.

Subjective Data

A. Review the onset, duration, and course of symptoms.
B. Review other signs and symptoms of urinary tract infection or pyelonephritis: frequency, dysuria, and fever.
C. Have the patient describe pain (colicky); note intensity (use a 1- to 10-point scale, 10 being the worst pain) and the characteristics of pain (constant, intermittent).
D. Has the patient ever had a stone before? How was it treated? What tests were performed? Has the patient ever seen a urologist?

E. Review dietary intake of high animal protein in the diet, milk, and other calcium-containing products for excessive intake.
F. Review the patient's medication history including excessive vitamin C or D supplements, antacids that contain calcium, and other medications noted in the predisposing factors.
G. Ask the patient to describe any hematuria or blood clots passed.
H. Ask about recent trauma to the back or abdomen.
I. Is there a family history of stone formation?
J. Is the patient pregnant?

Physical Examination

A. Temperature and blood pressure. Children: growth measurements to evaluate poor weight gain and/or failure to thrive (congenital and chronic conditions).
B. Inspect
   1. Inspect general appearance for discomfort before and during exam. Patients with renal colic are extremely restless and exhibit active movement on presentation.
   2. During the examination evaluate voluntary guarding of the abdominal musculature.
   3. Inspect external genitalia (male or female) for lesions, discharge, inflammation, and ulcerations.
   4. Assess for peripheral edema.
C. Auscultate
   1. Auscultate the abdomen, noting bruits if present.
   2. Auscultate bowel sounds.
D. Palpate
   1. "Milk" the urethra for discharge.
   2. Palpate the abdomen for masses and tenderness, organomegaly, and suprapubic tenderness.
   3. Palpate the groin; check lymph nodes.
   4. Palpate the back and abdomen.
   5. Check for the presence of costovertebral angle (CVA) tenderness.
E. Perform pelvic or bimanual exam, if indicated, to rule out pelvic inflammatory disease (PID).

Diagnostic Tests

A. Serum BUN, creatinine, calcium, and uric acid.
B. Stone for analysis.
C. Urinalysis.
   1. pH determination (pH > 7.5 is compatible with infection lithiasis, and a pH of < 5.5 favors uric acid lithiasis).
   2. Red cell casts strongly suggest glomerulonephritis.
   3. Evaluate urine sediment for crystalluria.
D. Urine culture, if indicated.
E. 24-hour urine for creatinine, calcium, uric acid, oxalate, pH, and sodium measurement.
   1. Patient should be on his or her usual diet before taking 24-hour specimen.
   2. Collection should be 1–2 months after any interventions including shock-wave, lithotripsy, uretoscopy, or percutaneous stone removal.
F. KUB or renal ultrasonography.
G. Serum electrolytes; consider fasting serum calcium and phosphorus and parathyroid hormone.

H. Consider CT since it is more sensitive and can identify anatomic abnormalities; however, CT is more costly.
I. Intravenous pyelogram (IVP) should rarely be used.
J. Pregnancy test (if indicated) to rule out and ectopic pregnancy.

Differential Diagnoses

A. Kidney stone(s): associated with colicky flank pain radiating to the groin. Significant flank pain of renal colic is usually secondary to renal calculi but may occasionally be associated with passage of clots.
B. Urinary tract infection: Passage of large, bulky blood clots implicates the bladder as the source, whereas long, shoestring-shaped specks or thin, stringy clots suggest an upper urinary tract or ureteral origin.
C. Acute abdomen/appendicitis.
D. Cholecystitis.
E. Pyelonephritis: associated with dull flank pain with fever and chills. In evaluating urine sediment, the presence of white cells and bacteria favors a diagnosis of pyelonephritis or interstitial nephritis.
F. PID.
G. Inflammatory bowel disease.
H. Urinary tract obstruction.
I. Constipation.

Plan

A. General interventions
   1. Increase fluids to allow passage of stone. Strain all urine to recover stone for analysis.
   2. Reduce possibility of recurrence with dietary modifications.
   3. Patient is usually referred for imaging after evaluation of creatinine.
   4. Patients can be managed on an outpatient basis with close follow-up if stones are small (< 6 mm).
B. Dietary management
   1. Force fluids to maintain a daily output of 2–3 liters of urine. Fluid intake that increases urinary production of at least 2 liters of urine per day increases the flow rate and lowers the urine solute concentration.
   2. Dietary consultation may be needed secondary to stone analysis.
C. Pharmaceutical therapy
   1. Pain medication (narcotic and nonnarcotic) is a priority.
   2. Antibiotics should be given for infection.
   3. Other medical/pharmaceutical management depends upon the etiology of the stone.

Follow-up

A. Reevaluate the patient in 24 hours by phone or in the clinic.
B. Evaluate sooner if pain increases, due to potential to progress to complete obstruction.
C. Recurrent stone formation is a manifestation of a systemic disease; evaluate for the management of the metabolic abnormality.

Consultation/Referral

A. Patients with severe pain, nausea, and vomiting need hospitalization for IV hydration and pain control. Consult with a physician.

B. Patients with severe symptoms and persistent obstruction beyond 3–4 days should be referred for urologic evaluation.

C. Refer for surgical interventions: Lithotripsy, urethroscope interventions, extracorporeal shock wave lithotripsy, and percutaneous ultra sonic lithotripsy may be indicated. Treatment varies based upon the location and size of the stone. Laparscopy may be indicated for the removal of a large or severely impacted ureteral calculi.

Individual Considerations

A. Pregnancy
1. Urolithiasis is the most common cause of nonobstetrical abdominal pain that requires hospitalization in pregnancy.
2. 80%–90% are diagnosed in the first trimester.
3. Renal ultrasound is the first-line screening test for pregnant patients. CT is reserved for complex cases.
4. Conservative treatment is used: bed rest, hydration, and analgesia.
5. Invasive measures include stent placement, ureteroscopy, and percutaneous nephrostomy.
6. Upon presentation, rule out:
   a. Ectopic pregnancy
   b. Abruptio placenta
   c. Preterm labor

B. Pediatrics
1. Young children generally do not present with the classic acute onset of flank pain; instead they may present with abdominal pain. Stone detection may be when abdominal imaging is performed.
2. Hematuria can present as the sole symptom or in conjunction with abdominal pain.
3. Ten percent of children present with symptoms of dysuria and urgency.

TESTICULAR TORSION

Definition

A. Testicular torsion is twisting of the testicle around the vas deferens, with compromise in the blood supply and possible necrosis to the testicles. Testicular torsion is a urologic emergency and is the most frequent cause of testicle loss in the adolescent male population. Approximately 40% of all cases of acute scrotal pain and swelling are diagnosed with testicular torsion. There is often a history of recurrent episodes of testicular pain before torsion.

Incidence

A. Incidence in males younger than 25 years old is approximately 1 in 4,000. Although torsion can occur at any age, the largest number of cases occur during adolescence.

B. The bell clapper congenital anomaly is present in approximately 12% of males, and 40% have the abnormality in the contralateral testicle.

Pathogenesis

A. Testicular torsion and torsion of the spermatic cord is due to abnormal fixation of the testicle to the scrotum, allowing free rotation. The bell clapper deformity allows the testicle to twist spontaneously on the spermatic cord. Venous occlusion and engorgement cause arterial ischemia and infarction of the testicle.

Predisposing Factors

A. Trauma to testicle
B. Spontaneous occurrence
C. Congenital bell clapper anomaly
D. Exercise
E. Undescended testicle
F. Active cremasteric reflex

Common Complaints

A. Sudden onset of severe unilateral scrotal pain
B. Swelling of scrotal sac

Other Signs and Symptoms

A. Sudden onset of testicular pain, may radiate to groin
B. Possible edema
C. Abdominal pain (20%–30%)
D. Nausea and vomiting (50% of cases)
E. Fever (16%)
F. Urinary frequency (4%)

Subjective Data

A. Review the onset, duration, and course of symptoms.
B. Review for a history of prior episodes on intermittent testicular pain that resolved spontaneously.
C. Review abdominal symptoms such as pain, nausea and vomiting, and fever.
D. Review urethral discharge (possible STI) and dysuria.
E. Review the patient's history for trauma to the scrotum or testicle.

Physical Examination

A. Temperature, blood pressure, pulse and respirations.
B. Inspect
1. Observe the patient generally for pain before and during examination.
2. Visualize the scrotal sac for edema, symmetry, lesions, discharge, color (especially for blue dot superior to the affected testicle). Testis is located high in the scrotum as a result of shortening of the cord by twisting.
3. Check the inguinal and femoral areas for bulges and hernias.
C. Auscultate
1. Auscultate all four quadrants of the abdomen; note bowel sounds.
2. Assess the scrotum for bowel noise.
D. Palpate
1. Palpate the abdomen for masses, rebound, and tenderness or guarding.
2. Palpate the groin; check the lymph nodes.
3. Examine for an inguinal hernia.
4. Genital exam

a. Check warmth, tenderness, swelling, and any nodularity; if a mass is present, check if it is solid or cystic. The testes should be sensitive to gentle compression but not tender. They should feel smooth, rubbery, and free of nodules.

b. Elicit a cremasteric reflex by stroking the inner thigh with a blunt object (reflex hammer or ink pen). The testicle and scrotum should rise on the stroked side. Cremasteric reflex is usually absent in testicular torsion.

c. Elevate the scrotum; there is usually no relief in pain with torsion. Elevation of the scrotum may improve the pain of epididymitis (Prehn's sign).

Diagnostic Tests

A. Urinalysis: normal in 90% of cases of testicular torsion
B. Doppler ultrasonography for blood flow and scrotal ultrasonography

Differential Diagnoses

A. **Testicular torsion: Firm, tender mass of acute onset in an afebrile young man with a history of prior episodes must be considered to represent torsion until proven otherwise.**
B. Epididymitis
C. Orchitis
D. Hydrocele
E. Testicular tumor: usually a hard, enlarged, painless testicle
F. Acute appendicitis
G. Scrotal/testicular trauma
H. Varicocele

Plan

A. Testicular torsion is a urologic emergency requiring surgery.
B. Immediately refer the patient to a urologist.
C. Symptoms **over 6 hours** can indicate testicular necrosis.
D. The opposite testicle is usually stabilized at the same surgery.

Pharmaceutical Therapy

A. None

Follow-up

A. Patient should follow up with the urologist as directed.

Consultation/Referral

A. All patients with suspected testicular torsion need to be immediately evaluated by a physician and referred to a urologist.

Individual Considerations

A. Pediatrics: Neonatal testicular torsion is rare. The exact mechanism is unknown. The torsion may occur prenatal (at or within 24 hours of delivery) or postnatal (within first 30 days of delivery). On physical examination a hardened, fixed nontender scrotal mass with a discolored scrotum is noted. Management is controversial due to the lack of data whether the testis can be salvaged and the risk for concomitant or subsequent torsion of the contralateral side.
B. Geriatrics: In older males, rule out epididymitis especially with new sexual partners or with symptoms of dysuria and urethral discharge.

UNDESCENDED TESTES, OR CRYPTORCHIDISM

Definition

A. Undescended testicle(s) or cryptorchidism is a testicle that is not within the scrotum and cannot be manipulated from the inguinal canal into the scrotum or is absent. Spontaneous descent of testes usually happens at the end of the first year. Bilaterally absent testicles is anorchia.

Incidence

A. Approximately 10% of males have bilateral cryptorchidism.
B. In unilateral cases, the left-side predominance is noted.
C. Between 2%–5% of full-term and 30% of premature male infants are born with an undescended testicle.
D. Twenty percent of boys have at least one nonpalpable testis.

Pathogenesis

A. An absent testicle may be due to agenesis or to an intrauterine vascular problem such as torsion. It may also be related to the lack of gonadotropic and androgenic hormones during fetal development. Most undescended testes are a result of a mechanical factor, a hernia sac, or a shortened spermatic artery that impedes the testes' descent into the scrotum.

Predisposing Factors

A. Prematurity, the testes descend into the scrotum at approximately 36 weeks' gestation. Most testicles will complete their descent within the first few months of life.
B. Twinning
C. Congenital disorder of testosterone secretion or testosterone action
   1. Kallmann syndrome
   2. Abdominal wall defects
   3. Neural tube defects
   4. Cerebral palsy
   5. Genetic syndromes:
      a. Trisomy 18
      b. Trisomy 13
      c. Noonan syndrome
      d. Prader-Willi syndrome

Common Complaints

A. Empty scrotum
B. Small, flat, undeveloped scrotum
C. Inguinal hernia

Other Signs and Symptoms

A. Absence of testicle noted on newborn examination or by parents during a bath or diaper change

Subjective Data

A. Review the course, duration, and symptoms. Has the testis ever been noticed in the scrotum during a bath or while the baby has been relaxed?
B. Note gestational age and birth weight at delivery (term versus preterm).
C. Has any health care provider ever noted that the testis was not descended or was absent upon examination?

D. Review the maternal history for evidence of an endocrine disturbance during pregnancy.

E. Review family history of congenital abnormalities, genital anomalies, and abnormal pubertal development.

F. Review if the patient has undergone prior inguinal surgery.

Physical Examination

A. Temperature, blood pressure, pulse and respirations.

B. Inspect
  1. Check the scrotum for size, shape, rugae, and any anomaly particularly hypospadias.
  2. Look for a bulge in the inguinal area.
  3. Transilluminate the scrotum to look for testes, and note fluid (if present).

To locate the testis, darken the room and shine a bright light from behind the scrotum. In a normal male, the testis stands out as the darker area.

C. Palpate
  1. Before you palpate the scrotum, place the thumb and index finger of one hand over the inguinal canals at the upper part of the scrotal sac. This maneuver helps prevent retraction of the testes into the inguinal canal or abdomen.
  2. Check each side of scrotum to detect the presence of the testes and other masses. If either of the testicles is not palpable, place a finger over the upper inguinal ring and gently push toward the scrotum. You may feel a soft mass in the inguinal canal. Try to push it toward the scrotum and palpate it with your thumb and index finger. The testicle of a newborn is approximately 1 cm in diameter.
  3. When any mass other than the testicle or spermatic cord is palpated in the scrotum, determine if it is filled with fluid, gas, or solid material. It is most likely to be a hernia or hydrocele. If it is reducible, then transilluminate to differentiate a hydrocele from a hernia.
  4. Check the cremasteric reflex: Scrotal sac retracts in response to cold hands and/or abrupt handling (yo-yo reflex).
  5. Bimanual digital rectal examination maybe used to evaluate the nonpalpable testis.

Diagnostic Tests

A. For unilateral undescended testis without hypospadias, no laboratory studies are needed.

B. Hormone levels (testosterone) may be obtained if both testes are nonpalpable.

C. Karyotype to rule out chromosomal abnormalities.

D. Ultrasonography of the abdomen.

E. Possible CT of the abdomen.

Differential Diagnoses

A. Undescended testis, one or both

B. Anorchia (complete absence)

C. Retractile testis

D. Ectopic testis

E. Ambiguous genitalia: In male-appearing genitals, at least one testis must be palpated; if not, ambiguous genitalia cannot be eliminated. A deep cleft in the scrotum (bifid scrotum) is usually associated with other genitourinary anomalies or ambiguous genitalia.

F. Tumor: A hard, enlarged, painless testicle may indicate a tumor.

Plan

A. General interventions
  1. Refer all children with cryptorchidism by 1 year of age to a surgeon for evaluation.
  2. Surgery (orchiopexy) is usually indicated before 18 months, and no later than 3 years of age, secondary to the increased risks of malignancy, infertility, testicular torsion, trauma, and hernia. After orchiopexy, the rate of fertility in these children is about 80%–90%.

B. Pharmaceutical therapy: Hormonal therapy is carried out by a specialist.

Follow-up

A. Monitor the patient's testicles at each well-child visit.

B. Males who have undescended testicles may have an increased risk of developing breast cancer and developing testicular germ cell cancers.

C. Testicular cancer screening should be done during and after puberty.

D. Men with a history of undescended testes have an increased incidence of infertility (lower sperm counts, sperm of lower quality, and low fertility rates).

E. Testicular torsion is 10 times higher in undescended testes. Torsion of an intra-abdominal testis can present as an acute abdomen.

Consultation/Referral

A. **A mass that does not transilluminate or reduce with gentle pressure is likely to be an incarcerated hernia. This is a surgical emergency.**

B. Refer the patient for urologic recommendations regarding surgery.

Individual Considerations

Pediatrics

A. Examine a child in the tailor's position or with the child sitting on a chair or examination table with legs in "frog position," kneeling or standing. *Note:* If the child sits cross-legged, it abolishes the reflex of the cremaster muscle.

B. Examine adolescents while standing and straining.

C. Examination of an adolescent includes evaluation of maturation described by Tanner.

URINARY INCONTINENCE

Definition

A. Urinary incontinence (UI) is the involuntary loss of urine severe enough to have unpleasant social or hygienic consequences. Urinary incontinence is diagnosed primarily on history; inquire about UI at every interview. UI is a symptom of an underlying disease process in most cases; some cases are reversible with appropriate treatment.

B. UI can be divided into the following categories: functional, urge, overflow, stress, and mixed. Each category has a unique etiology, pathophysiology, symptoms, and management.

Incidence

A. The exact incidence of IU is unknown. In a survey, only 45% of women and 22% of men reported UI occurring at least once a week ever sought care for their symptoms. Urinary incontinence has been estimated to affect at least 10 million adults in America. In the elderly incontinence affects 15%–30% community-dwelling and 50% of the nursing home residents. The cost of incontinence has been approximated at $10.3 billion annually. The elderly are more frequently affected; however, incontinence is not a consequence of normal aging.

Pathogenesis

Urinary incontinence (UI) can be caused by pathologic, anatomic, or physiologic factors and differs by the type of incontinence:

A. Functional incontinence: loss of urine due to the inability to get to the bathroom, either due to problems of mobility or cognition.
B. Urge incontinence: inability to delay voiding after the sensation of fullness is perceived. Common causes are detrusor hyperactivity or hyperreflexia associated with disorders of the lower urinary tract, tumors, stones, uterine prolapse, cystitis, urethritis, impaired bladder contractility. Central nervous system disorders such as stroke, dementia, parkinsonism, or spinal cord injury can also be causative factors.
C. Overflow incontinence: loss of urine associated with an overdistension of the bladder. Common causes are anatomic obstruction by an enlarged prostate, a prolapsed cystocele, acontractile bladder due to diabetes, spinal cord injury, multiple sclerosis, or suprasactal cord lesions.
D. Stress incontinence: involuntary loss of urine during coughing, sneezing, laughing, bending over, or other physical activity that increases intra-abdominal pressure.

Predisposing Factors

A. Age over 60 years
B. Female: 85% of cases are in women
C. Increased parity
D. Previous GU surgeries, including prostate surgery
E. Restricted mobility
F. Menopause
G. Infections
H. Chronic illnesses (e.g., diabetes)
I. Fecal impactions
J. Excessive urinary output
K. Delirium
L. Dementia
M. Neurologic or psychiatric disorders
N. Variety of medications

Common Complaints

A. Urgency: sudden and compelling desire to pass urine.
B. Urge incontinence: involuntary leakage accompanied by urgency. Precipitating factors:
   1. Hearing running water
   2. Placing hands in water
   3. Trying to unlock the door when returning home
C. Stress incontinence: involuntary leakage with the following precipitating factors:
   1. Exertion
   2. Sneezing/coughing
   3. May experience leakage with little or no activity
D. Overactive bladder (OAB): symptoms may occur with or without urge incontinence.
   1. Urgency
   2. Frequency
   3. Nocturia

Other Signs and Symptoms

A. Mixed incontinence: urge and stress leakage
B. Experiencing leakage with little or no activity
C. Continuous leakage (i.e., dribbling)
D. Daytime frequency
E. Nocturia: up one or more times a night to void
F. Slow urine stream, intermittent stream, or hesitancy
G. Need to strain to start, maintain, or improve voiding
H. Incomplete emptying sensation

Subjective Data

A. Question the patient regarding onset, duration, and severity of the incontinence.
   1. Do you ever leak urine/water when you don't want to?
   2. Do you ever leak urine when you cough, laugh, or exercise?
   3. Do you ever leak urine on the way to the bathroom (urgency)?
   4. Do you ever use pads, tissue, or cloth in your underwear to catch urine?
B. Elicit situations when UI is worse, when it is improved, what stimuli are associated with increasing UI (high fluid intake, high caffeine intake, agitation).
C. Review whether the female patient is pre- or postmenopause.
D. Review other lower urinary tract symptoms such as nocturia.
E. Review the patient's history of bowel function (i.e., fecal incontinence). If constipation is a problem, abdominal pressure from a large retained stool can cause symptoms including retention.
F. Review medications including over-the-counter drugs and herbals.
G. Preview previous continence therapy including surgical treatments.
H. Review the impact of incontinence on quality of life including work impairment, sexual dysfunction, activities of daily living, sleep, recreation activity, and social interaction, and depression.
I. Assess whether the elderly patient has incontinence despite toileting.
J. Review sexual function.

Physical Examination

A. Both *sexes*
   1. Temperature, pulse, blood pressure, and respirations.
   2. Inspection for evidence of cardiac overload: pedal edema.
   3. Auscultate the lungs for evidence of fluid overload: rales.

4. Perform neurologic examination to determine the presence of sensation.
5. Palpate the abdomen for masses, fullness over bladder, and tenderness.
6. Assess cognitive and functional status including mobility, transfers, manual dexterity, and ability to toilet in the elderly.
7. Screen for depression.

B. Females
1. Inspect perineal skin for irritation, thinning, vaginal atrophy, and vaginal discharge.
2. Remove the top blade of the speculum and evaluate the vaginal wall support.
3. Ask the woman to cough to reevaluate the vaginal wall support.
4. Palpate
   a. Perform a bimanual pelvic exam for prolapse, masses, or tenderness.
   b. Perform rectal exam for sphincter tone, masses, and fecal impaction.

C. Males
1. Inspection
   a. Inspect the glans penis for abnormalities in urethral meatus.
   b. Uncircumcised men should be evaluated for phimosis and balanitis.
2. Palpate: Perform rectal exam for sphincter tone, masses, fecal impaction, prostate size and contour.

Diagnostic Tests

The history, physical examination, and urinalysis are sufficient to guide initial therapy. Other tests include:

A. Urine culture and sensitivity if infection is suspected.
B. Urine cytology if hematuria or pelvic pain.
C. Cystometry. See the Section II Procedure, "Bedside Cystometry."
D. Postvoid residual (PVR) by catheterization or ultrasound. A PVR of less than 50 mL is considered adequate emptying and greater than 200 mL is considered inadequate and suggests either detrusor weakness or obstruction. Indications for PVR:
1. Men with mild to moderate lower urinary symptoms
2. Men with overactive bladder (urgency)
3. Persons with spinal cord injury or Parkinson's disease
4. Persons with prior episodes of urinary retention
5. Person with severe constipation

Differential Diagnoses

Eight reversible causes of transient incontinence can be remembered by using the mnemonic DIAPPERS:

Delirium
Infection (urinary)
Atrophic urethritis and vaginitis
Pharmaceuticals
Psychologic disorders, especially depression
Excessive urine output
Restricted mobility
Stool impaction

Plan

A. Functional UI: Therapy is directed at the cause of the condition, such as overdiuresis, inability to go to the toilet, or poor access to toilet facilities.
B. Behavioral interventions
1. A bladder diary (see Table 11.3) may provide information on usual timing and circumstances of urinary incontinence.
2. Timed scheduled voiding and/or prompted caregiver scheduled toileting.
3. Bladder training by systematic ability to delay voiding through the use of urge of inhibition.
4. Stress incontinence: Kegel perineal exercises may improve UI by 30%–90%. Exercises using graduated vaginal cones or weights induce pelvic muscle tone and strength, reducing UI.
5. Overflow UI: the use of Crede's method for expressing the bladder, by applying pressure with the hands placed in the suprapubic area after voiding to assist in emptying.
6. Intermittent catheterization is an option frequently utilized after other measures have failed or overflow UI.
C. Patient education: See the Section III Patient Teaching Guide for this chapter, "Urinary Incontinence: Women."
D. Surgical treatment is based on the cause of incontinence.
E. Continence pessaries may benefit women with stress urinary incontinence.
F. Electrical stimulation may be prescribed to inhibit bladder instability and improve striated and levator contractility and efficiency.
G. Treatment of concomitant constipation is an important step in the treatment of incontinence.
H. Treatment of vaginal atrophy another important step in the treatment of incontinence.
I. Pharmaceutical therapy
1. Use of anticholinergic and antispasmodic drugs to decrease reflex bladder contractions and increase bladder capacity **(contraindicated in angle-closure glaucoma and with gastric retention).**
   a. Oxybutynin (Ditropan): oral and transdermal formulation:
      i. Immediate release (IR): initial oral dose is 2.5 mg 2–3 times/day followed by titration as needed to 20 mg/day in divided doses.
      ii. Extended release (ER): 5 mg orally once/day and titrated up to 20–30 mg once a day.
      iii. Transdermal formulation: 3.8 mg, the patch should be changed twice a week.
   b. Tolterodine (Detrol)
      i. Immediate release (IR): 1–2 mg orally twice a day.
      ii. Extended release (ER): 2–4 mg orally per day.
   c. Fesoterodine (Toviaz): 4–8 mg orally daily.
   d. Trospium (Sanctura): must be taken on an empty stomach.
      i. Immediate release (IR): 20 mg orally twice a day.
      ii. Extended release (ER): 60 mg orally every morning.

TABLE 11.3 Bladder Control Diary

Your Daily Bladder Diary

This diary will help you and your health care team figure out the causes of your bladder control trouble. The "sample" line shows you how to use the diary. Use this sheet as a master for making copies that you can use as a bladder diary for as many days as you need.

Your name: _____

Date: _____

Time	Drinks		Trips to the Bathroom		Accidental Leaks	Did you feel a strong urge to go?	What were you doing at the time?
	What kind?	How much?	How many times?	How Much urine? (circle one)	How much? (circle one)	Circle one	Sneezing, exercising, having sex, lifting, etc.
Sample	Coffee	2 cups	✓✓	⊙ ○ ○ sm med lg	○ ⊙ ○ sm med lg	Yes (No)	Running
6–7 a.m.				○ ○ ○	○ ○ ○	Yes No	
7–8 a.m.				○ ○ ○	○ ○ ○	Yes No	
8–9 a.m.				○ ○ ○	○ ○ ○	Yes No	
9–10 a.m.				○ ○ ○	○ ○ ○	Yes No	
10–11 a.m.				○ ○ ○	○ ○ ○	Yes No	
11–12 noon				○ ○ ○	○ ○ ○	Yes No	
12–1 p.m.				○ ○ ○	○ ○ ○	Yes No	
1–2 p.m.				○ ○ ○	○ ○ ○	Yes No	
2–3 p.m.				○ ○ ○	○ ○ ○	Yes No	
3–4 p.m.				○ ○ ○	○ ○ ○	Yes No	
4–5 p.m				○ ○ ○	○ ○ ○	Yes No	
5–6 p.m.				○ ○ ○	○ ○ ○	Yes No	
6–7 p.m.				○ ○ ○	○ ○ ○	Yes No	
7–8 p.m.				○ ○ ○	○ ○ ○	Yes No	
8–9 p.m.				○ ○ ○	○ ○ ○	Yes No	
9–10 p.m.				○ ○ ○	○ ○ ○	Yes No	
10–11 p.m.				○ ○ ○	○ ○ ○	Yes No	
11–12 midnight				○ ○ ○	○ ○ ○	Yes No	
12–1 a.m.				○ ○ ○	○ ○ ○	Yes No	
1–2 a.m.				○ ○ ○	○ ○ ○	Yes No	
2–3 a.m.				○ ○ ○	○ ○ ○	Yes No	
3–4 a.m.				○ ○ ○	○ ○ ○	Yes No	
4–5 a.m.				○ ○ ○	○ ○ ○	Yes No	
5–6 a.m.				○ ○ ○	○ ○ ○	Yes No	

(continued)

TABLE 11.3 *(continued)*

I used _____ pads today. I used _____ diapers today (write number).

Questions to ask my health care team: _____

_____

_____

_____

_____

Let's Talk About Bladder Control for Women is a public health awareness campaign conducted by the National Kidney and Urologic Diseases Information Clearinghouse (NKUDIC), an information dissemination service of the National Institute of Diabetes and Digestive and Kidney Diseases (NIDDK), National Institutes of Health.

From National Kidney and Urologic Diseases Information Clearinghouse (NKUDIC), National Institutes of Health (NIH). http://kidney.niddk.nih.gov/kudiseases/pubs/bcw_ez/insertB.htm

Please see Section III "Patient Teaching Guides for Chapter 11: Genitourinary Disorders" for a copy of this table to hand out to patients.

    e. Darifenacin (Enablex): 7.5–15 mg orally daily.

    f. Solifenacin (Vesicare): 5 mg orally daily initially; may increase to 10 mg daily.

2. α-Adrenergic antagonists stimulate urethral smooth muscle contraction.

    a. Imipramine (Tofranil): used for childhood enuresis.

      i. Children younger than 6 years: not recommended.

      ii. Children older than 6 years: 25 mg initially one hour before bedtime.

      iii. Children 6–12 years: 25 mg initially one hour before bedtime; increase up to 50 mg after 1 week.

      vi. Children older than 12 years: 25 mg initially one hour before bedtime; may increase up to 75 mg as needed.

3. For postmenopausal women, estrogen may restore urethral mucosal; use the same type, dosage, and the patient selection criteria as with estrogen therapy (ET).

Follow-up

A. Follow-up is based on the type and cause of UI.

Consultation/Referral

A. When to consult a physician for UI depends on the type and cause of UI. Urinary incontinence is a problem that can be successfully treated.

B. Refer to a specialist for incontinence with abdominal and/or pelvic pain or hematuria in the absence of a UTI, or when surgical treatment is desired.

C. Refer for urodynamic testing, which is considered the gold standard. Testing requires special equipment and training.

D. Refer to a gynecologist or urology clinic experienced in fitting a continence pessary.

Individual Considerations

A. Pregnancy: Stress incontinence is frequently associated with pregnancy and is treated with pelvic exercises.

B. Pediatrics: Most often experienced as enuresis. UI in previously bladder-controlled children requires a thorough workup and referral to a pediatrician.

C. Geriatrics

1. Incontinence in the elderly is a risk factor for falls. Many falls occur en route to the bathroom, especially at night.

2. Incontinence increases social isolation and depression.

3. Functional incontinence is common with older adults with arthritis, Parkinson's, or Alzheimer's diseases. Patients are unable to hold their urine until they reach the bathroom and undress. A toileting program usually assists in this situation.

URINARY TRACT INFECTION (ACUTE CYSTITIS)

Definition

A. Urinary tract infection (UTI) is an infection of the urinary bladder. UTI is defined as the presence of at least 100,000 organisms per mL of urine in an asymptomatic patient or more than 100 organisms per mL of urine with accompanying pyuria (> 7 white blood cells/mL) in a symptomatic patient. Asymptomatic bacteriuria (ASB) when left untreated is a risk factor for acute cystitis (40%) and pyelonephritis in 25%–30% in pregnancy.

B. UTIs can be divided anatomically into upper and lower tract (cystitis) infections. For a discussion of upper tract infection, see the section, "Pyelonephritis."

Incidence

A. Incidence depends on age and gender. The prevalence of UTI in males varies according to age. Young men rarely develop a UTI; however, the incidence in geriatric males may be as high as in geriatric females (up to 15%). In children, it occurs in 1% of males and 1%–5% of females.

B. Prevalence for females increases by 1% per decade and 2%–4% throughout childbearing years. The incidence of UTIs in pregnancy ranges from 4%–7%. By age 30, approximately 25% of women have experienced symptoms of a urinary tract infection. In pregnancy, the increased incidence is related to both hormonal influence and anatomic changes that increase the risk of urinary stasis and vesicoureteral reflux.

Pathogenesis

A. Bacteria ascend from the perineum through the urethra. The greater susceptibility of younger women and girls is related to a shorter urethra. In older women, it is related to estrogen-mediated dilation of the urethra.

B. The normal male urinary tract has many natural defenses to infection. The greater susceptibility of elderly males is related to problems with the prostate and other urologic disease and can be linked to the instrumentation required for therapy.

C. Gram-negative bacilli are the most common pathogens; 80%–90% of cases are related to coliform bacteria *(E. coli)*. It originates from fecal floras that colonize the periurethral area.

D. Other gram-negative bacteria include *Klebsiella pneumonia* or *Proteus mirabilis. Staphylococcus saprophyticus* (gram-positive coccus) accounts for about 10%–15% of urinary tract infections.

E. Other pathogens include *Enterobacter, Pseudomonas, Enterococci,* and *Staphylococci.* The incubation period depends on the pathogen.

Predisposing Factors

A. Female (until elderly, then equal frequency)
B. Pregnancy
C. Poor hygiene
D. Trauma
E. Instrumentation
F. Sexual intercourse
G. Oral contraceptive or diaphragm use
H. Diabetic female (there is no increased risk for diabetic males)
I. Anomalies of the genitourinary tract
J. Neurologic factors
K. Vesicourethral reflux
L. Obstruction: stones
M. Foreign bodies
N. Bubble baths and hot tubs
O. Douching
P. Anal intercourse
Q. HIV
R. Uncircumcised penis
S. Catheterization
T. Nosocomial infection

Common Complaints

A. Burning on urination
B. Frequency
C. Cloudy or bloody urine
D. Urgency

Other Signs and Symptoms

A. Asymptomatic
B. Frequency, dysuria, bladder spasms, suprapubic discomfort, urgency, and nocturia

C. Suprapubic pain
D. Fever
E. Costovertebral angle tenderness

Subjective Data

A. Review the onset, course, and duration of symptoms.
B. Does the patient have a fever and chills or back or flank pain (unilateral or bilateral)?
C. Are there any other genital problems such as herpes lesions or vaginal discharge?
D. Review the associated factors: sexual intercourse, douching, or bubble bath.
E. Ask female patients if they use appropriate hygiene practices after urination and bowel movements.
F. Is the patient pregnant? If not, what type of birth control does she use?
G. Is there any history of previous infections? How often, and how were they treated? Were any tests performed in a workup? Has the patient ever seen a urologist?
H. How much liquid or water does the patient drink every day? Note the amount of caffeine.
I. In older men, review the strength of the urinary flow, dribbling, hesitancy, and so forth.
J. Is there any history of other medical diseases including diabetes?

Physical Examination

A. Temperature, blood pressure, pulse, and respirations.
B. General observation of general appearance for discomfort before and during examination.
C. Auscultation of the heart and all lung fields.
D. Palpate
  1. Palpate the abdomen: kidneys, masses; assess for suprapubic tenderness.
  2. Palpate the back; note costovertebral angle (CVA) tenderness.
  3. Check for inguinal lymph node enlargement.
  4. Palpate the suprapubic area.
E. Percuss: Percuss over bladder and costovertebral angles for tenderness.
F. Females
  1. Inspect external genitalia for lesions, Bartholin's glands cysts, irritation, and discharge.
  2. Milk urethra for discharge.
  3. Assess rectal area.
  4. Speculum exam: Evaluate vaginal vault for discharge, cervicitis, and inflammation; evaluate for atrophic vaginal changes and torn tissue.
  5. Bimanual exam: Check for cervical motion, tenderness, and masses.
G. Males
  1. Inspect the penis/urinary meatus for lesions, signs of inflammation, and discharge. Retract the foreskin (if present) and assess for hygiene and smegma.
  2. Palpate the testes and epididymides for inflammation, tenderness, and masses.
  3. Rectal examination is mandatory: Check for swollen and tender prostate. In patients with suspected acute bacterial prostatitis, palpation should be very gentle due to the potential for bacteremia.

Diagnostic Tests

A. Urinalysis
   1. Appearance: should be clear. Cloudy urine may indicate presence of pyuria, pus, blood, cells, phosphate, or lymph fluid.
   2. Odor: usually faint aromatic odor; ammonia odor indicates *Proteus,* related to food changes; offensive odor indicates bacterial infection.
   3. pH: normal is around 6 (acid); may normally vary from 4.6–7.5.
   4. Specific gravity: reflects the kidney's ability to concentrate urine and the body's hydration or dehydration status. Normal is 1.005–1.025.
   5. Color: shows concentration; usually yellow or amber.
      a. Straw color = dilute urine
      b. Dark color = concentrated (dehydrated)
      c. Red or red-brown to blood = transfusion reaction, drugs, and bleeding lesions
      d. Yellow brown = bile duct disease, jaundice
      e. Dark brown or black = melanoma or leukemia
B. Cystitis: positive results
   1. Urinalysis dipstick findings: pH greater than 7.0, positive for leukocyte esterase and positive for nitrites.
   2. Microscopic exam of urine findings: WBC greater than 2–5, WBC/HPF, bacteria, positive Gram's stain for cocci or rods, yeast, and blood.
   3. Urine culture and sensitivity
      a. Positive culture standard 10^5 colony-forming units; symptomatic female 10^2; symptomatic males 10^3.
      b. Screening for asymptomatic bacteria is recommended for patients in pregnancy, for elderly males with documented prostatic or urologic abnormalities, for patients with a recent catheterization, and for patients with known stones or documented structural abnormalities.
      c. Clean catch urinalysis: catheterization or suprapubic aspiration may be necessary depending on patient's age and condition. Catheterization should be reserved for patients with an obstruction or for those that cannot cooperate or collect a clean catch urine specimen. The percutaneous bladder aspiration is used for young children and infants.
      d. Culture for STIs if suspected.
      e. Wet prep for female, if indicated.
C. Consider intravenous pyelogram (IVP) if ureteral obstruction is suspected, renal ultrasound, and CT scan.

Differential Diagnoses

A. Urinary tract infection: watch for systemic symptoms of pyelonephritis.
B. Vaginal or pelvic infection.
C. Prostatitis or epididymitis: tender, enlarged prostate; tender testicle or scrotum.
D. Bladder tumor.
E. Interstitial cystitis.
F. Urinary calculi.
G. Benign prostatic hypertrophy: changes in urinary stream and nocturia.

H. Urge incontinence.
I. Consider the possibility that chronic, asymptomatic infections are a potential source of disseminated infection, such as endocarditis. This is particularly likely in the male patient with prostate disease and infection requiring instrumentation.

Plan

A. Patient education: See the Section III Patient Teaching Guide for this chapter, "Urinary Tract Infection (Acute Cystitis)."
B. Dietary management
   1. Instruct the patient to increase fluids and drink at least one large glass of liquid every hour.
   2. Instruct the patient to avoid foods that irritate the bladder: caffeine, alcohol, and spicy foods.
   3. Encourage the patient to drink cranberry juice to help fight bladder infections. If the patient dislikes the taste of plain cranberry juice, have him or her mix it 1:1 with another juice, such as orange juice.
C. Pharmacologic therapy
   1. Antibiotics: 3-day course may be efficacious and is less expensive than the traditional 7- to 10-day course of therapy for uncomplicated infections.
   2. The antibiotic of choice depends on the specific bacteria found upon culture. Empiric antimicrobial therapy should cover all likely pathogens.
   3. Trimethoprim and sulfamethoxazole (Bactrim DS) 160 mg and 800 mg, respectively, one tablet twice daily for 3–10 days.
      a. Give above dosage for 1–3 days for uncomplicated cystitis in female.
      b. Give above dosage for 7–10 days to patients who are male, are elderly, or have recurrent UTI, or for complicated cases.
   4. Other antibiotics
      a. Trimethoprim (Trimpex) 100 mg twice daily for 10 days.
      b. Nitrofurantoin macrocrystals (Macrodantin) 100 mg four times daily for 7 days.
      c. Nitrofurantoin (Macrobid) 100 mg tablet: one tablet twice daily for 7 days.
      d. Lomefloxacin hydrochloride (Maxaquin) 400 mg every day for 3 days uncomplicated; 10–14 days for complicated.
      e. Amoxicillin (Amoxil) 500 mg three times daily for 7 days.
   5. Urinary analgesic if needed: phenazopyridine HCl (Pyridium) 100–200 mg three times daily for 1–2 days only. Educate the patient that this drug turns urine orange.
   6. Drug of choice for UTI or pyelonephritis in pregnancy:
      a. Nitrofurantoin (Macrobid) 100 mg: one tablet orally every 12 hours for 7–10 days.
      b. Nitrofurantoin macrocrystals (Macrodantin) 100 mg orally every 6 hours for 7–10 days. Generally prescribed if cost of Macrobid is a prohibitive factor.

c. If dysuria is present: phenazopyridine HCl (Pyridium) 200 mg orally three times daily for 3 days.
d. Alternative medications
    i. Ampicillin 500 mg orally four times daily for 10 days.
    ii. Cephalexin (Keflex) 500 mg orally four times daily for 10 days.
7. Consider prophylactic therapy for patients with chronic conditions (pregnancy, sickle cell disease) who have recurrent infections.

Follow-up
A. Have the patient return in 2 to 4 days for follow-up urinalysis after therapy. If urinalysis is abnormal, obtain urine culture.

Consultation/Referral
A. Refer all children with more than one urinary tract infection to a physician.
B. Young men do not have urinary tract infections very often; a urologic workup may be needed if etiology such as a sexually transmitted infection (STI) cannot be determined.
C. Patients with bacteriuria are also more likely to have identifiable abnormalities on an IVP, including small kidneys, delayed excretion, caliceal dilation and blunting, ureteral reflux, stones, and obstructive lesions.
D. Consult with a urologist is essential in all forms of prostatitis or in all but the most clear-cut cases of acute scrotum.

Individual Considerations
A. Women
    1. Recurrent infections are common in females.
    2. Repeat urine cultures and sensitivity after antibiotic course is complete (approximately 2–4 weeks after therapy is completed).
    3. If the patient is perimenopausal and has two or fewer UTIs a year, consider patient-initiated therapy to start when symptomatic. Consider topical estradiol cream for atrophic vaginitis. If the patient has three UTIs a year, prescribe a prophylactic single-dose regimen after intercourse. If infections are not related to intercourse, consider urine cultures every 2 months, with extended antibiotic therapy:
        a. Macrobid: one tablet at bedtime.
        b. Sulfamethoxazole 800 mg/trimethoprim 160 mg (Bactrim DS): one tablet at bedtime.
        c. Cephalexin (Keflex): 250 mg at bedtime.
B. Pregnancy
    1. The incidence of pyelonephritis in pregnancy is 1%–2%. Most cases develop as a consequence of undiagnosed or inadequately treated lower urinary tract infection.
    2. Approximately 75%–80% of pyelonephritis cases occur on the right side, with a 10%–15% incidence on the left side. A small percentage of cases are bilateral.
    3. GBS (group B *Streptococcus*) colonization has important implications during pregnancy. Intrapartum transmission may lead to neonatal GBS infection. Current guidelines recommend universal vaginal and rectal screening in all pregnant women at 35–37 weeks' gestation rather than be treated based on risk factors.
    4. A urine culture screening is recommended for all pregnant women at their first prenatal visit.
    5. Suppressive antibiotic therapy should be instituted in pregnant patients who develop acute cystitis, recurrent or persistent ASB, or pyelonephritis.
    6. Patients with sickle cell hemoglobinopathies are at increased risk for UTI and should be screened more aggressively and may benefit from antibiotic prophylaxis.
    7. Antibiotics that should not be used during pregnancy include:
        a. Tetracyclines (adverse on fetal teeth/bones and congenital defects)
        b. Quinolones (congenital defects)
        c. Trimethoprim in the first trimester (facial defects and cardiac abnormalities)
        d. Sulfonamides in the last trimester (kernicterus)
C. Pediatrics: Symptoms may include incontinence and abdominal pain.
D. Geriatrics: Patients may not have classic symptoms. Consider urinary tract infection if the patient presents with increased urinary incontinence, fever, and mental confusion.

VARICOCELE

Definition
A. Varicocele is engorgement of the internal spermatic veins above the testes. This vascular abnormality is a cause of decreased testicular function. Some varicoceles are easy to identify and may be surgically corrected. The presence of a varicocele does not mean that surgical correction is a necessity.

Incidence
A. Varicocele may occur in 15%–20% of normal males; 80%–90% of cases occur on the left side. Up to 35%–40% of men with a palpable left-sided varicocele may actually have bilateral varicoceles that are identified upon physical examination.
B. Right-sided varicocele is uncommon and can indicate retroperitoneal malignancy. Varicocele is the leading known cause of male infertility (40%). Decreased sperm counts, infertility, and testicular atrophy occur in 65%–75% of varicocele cases. There is no correlation between size of the varicocele and the degree of infertility.

Pathogenesis
A. The exact pathophysiologic mechanisms for varicocele are not fully identified. Varicocele may be due to valvular incompetence or elevated hydrostatic pressure in the spermatic veins. Testicular temperature elevation also appears to play a role in varicocele-induced dysfunction. **New varicocele in older men may be secondary to renal tumors.**

Predisposing Factors
A. Varicoceles generally manifest at the time of puberty.

Common Complaints
A. Asymptomatic
B. Infertility
C. Pain or discomfort in the scrotum

Other Signs and Symptoms
A. Pain or aching and heaviness in the scrotum.
B. Feels like "worms"; scrotum may have bluish discoloration.

Subjective Data
A. Note the onset, course, and duration of symptoms. When was the varicocele first noted?
B. Has the scrotum enlarged? If there is enlargement, over what time span? Does it collapse with lying or sitting down?
C. Is there any pain or discomfort?
D. Has there been any history of infertility?

Physical Examination
A. Vital signs, temperature as indicated.
B. Inspect
   1. The examination should be one when the patient is lying or standing in a warm room. Warm temperature promotes relaxation of the scrotum.
   2. Examine the general appearance of the penis; note scrotal size, shape, and rugae. Varicocele tends to collapse with the patient sitting or supine.
   3. Transilluminate the scrotum to visualize the varicocele.
C. Palpate
   1. Palpate each side of the scrotum for testicular size, presence of varicocele (Valsalva's maneuver performed while the patient stands helps to reveal a small varicocele), and absence of vas deferens.
   2. Palpate the spermatic cord between the thumb and forefingers while the patient performs a Valsalva maneuver.
      a. Varicocele should significantly diminish in size when the patient assumes the supine position.
   3. Evaluate whether the varicocele can be reduced while the patient is supine.
   4. Palpate the abdomen for hernias, masses, and tenderness.
   5. Rectal exam: Palpate the prostate and seminal vesicles for tenderness and other signs of infection.
D. Auscultate: Listen over the scrotum to assess bowel sounds to rule out hernia.

Diagnostic Tests
A. Scrotal ultrasound with high-resolution color-flow Doppler is the diagnostic method of choice when clinical exams are equivocal, but are not indicated for standard evaluation.
B. Semen analysis times 2, if indicated.
C. CT to evaluate retroperitoneal pathology (e.g., renal cell carcinoma) for the following:
   1. Sudden onset of varicocele
   2. Single right-sided varicocele

3. Any varicocele that is not reducible in the supine position

Differential Diagnoses
A. Varicocele is classifications:
   1. Grade I (small): palpable only on Valsalva maneuver, which increases intra-abdominal pressure and therefore impedes drainage and increases the varicocele size.
   2. Grade II (medium): palpable when standing and bearing down (Valsalva maneuver)
   3. Grade III (large): visible on inspection alone
   4. Subclinical: not palpable, vein larger than 3 mm on ultrasound; Doppler reflux on Valsalva maneuver
B. Hernia
C. Epididymitis
D. Hydrocele
E. Testicular tumor **Consider retroperitoneal tumor, especially if presenting symptoms have a sudden onset.**

Plan
A. Urologic consultation for diagnosis and possible surgery. Surgery should be considered when all of the following conditions are met:
   1. Palpable varicocele upon physical examination.
   2. Couple with known infertility.
   3. Female has normal fertility or potential treatable cause of infertility.
   4. Male partner has abnormal semen parameters or abnormal results from sperm function tests.
B. Athletic supporter for comfort.
C. Patient teaching
D. Pharmaceutical therapy: none is recommended.

Follow-up
A. After surgery, no follow-up is necessary if the patient is taught scrotal self-exam.
B. If no surgery is performed, the patient should be taught self-exam and instructed to return for pain or change in size and shape.
C. Adolescents with varicoceles should be followed with annual objective measurements of testis size and/or semen analyses in order to detect the earliest sign of varicocele-related testicular injury.

Consultation/Referral
A. Refer the patient to a urologist for surgical evaluation. Varicocelectomy is recommended in cases of pain and infertility, and it may be offered in the preadolescent to ensure proper testicular development.

REFERENCES
American Urological Association. (2009). Prostate-specific antigen best practice: 2009 update. Retrieved October 31, 2009, from http://www.auanet.org/content/guidelines-and-quality-care/clinical-guidelines/main-reports/psa09.pdf

Arias, E., Anderson, R. N., Kung, H. C., Murphy, S. L., & Kochanek, K. D. (2003, September18). Deaths: Final data for 2001. *National Vital Statistic Report, 52,* 1.

Associates in Urology. (n.d.). Patient questionnaire: AUA symptom score. Retrieved November 1, 2009, from http://www.njurology.com/_forms/auass.pdf

Clemens, J. Q., Calhoun, E. A., Litwin, M. S., McNaughton-Collins, M., Dunn, R. L., Crowley, E. M., et al. (2009). Rescoring the NIH Chronic Prostatitis Symptom Index (NIH-CPSI): Nothing new. *Prostate Cancer Prostatitis Diseases, 12,* 285–287.

Consensus Group. (2007). A multidisciplinary consensus meeting on IC/PBS. *Reviews in Urology, 9,* 81–83.

Cooper, C. S., & Docimo, S. G. (2009, May 1). Undescended testes (cryptorchidism). *UpToDate.* Retrieved October 17, 2009, from http://www.uptodate.com/online/content/topic.do?topicKey=gen_pedi/16379&view=print

Cornell University. (n.d.). *Male infertility.* James Buchanan Brady Foundation Department of Urology. Retrieved October 31, 2009, from http://www.cornellurology.com/infertility/gi/varicocele.shtml

Cunha, B. A. (2009, October 19). Urinary tract infection, males. *emedicine.* Retrieved November 1, 2009, from http://emedicine.medscape.com/article/231574-print

Cunningham, G. R., & Kadmon, D. (2009, May 1a). Clinical manifestations and diagnosis of benign prostatic hyperplasia. *UpToDate.* Retrieved October 17, 2009, from http://www.uptodate.com/online/content/topic.do?topicKey=primneph/8919&selectedTitle=3-150&source=search_result

Cunningham, G. R., & Kadmon, D. (2009, May 1b). Epidemiology and pathogenesis of benign prostatic hyperplasia. *UpToDate.* Retrieved October 17, 2009, from http://www.uptodate.com/online/content/topic.do?topicKey=primneph/9298&selectedTitle=4-150&source=search_result

Cunningham, G. R., & Kadmon, D. (2009, May 1c). Medical treatment of benign prostatic hyperplasia. *UpToDate.* Retrieved October 17, 2009, from http://www.uptodate.com/online/content/topic.do?topicKey=primneph/9599&selectedTitle=1-150&source=search_result

Department of Veterans Affairs, Department of Defense. (2008). *The VA/DoD clinical practice guideline for management of chronic kidney disease in primary care.* Retrieved September 4, 2009, from http://www.healthquality.va.gov/ckd/ckd_v478_sums.pdf-115

DuBeau, C. E. (2009, May 1a). Clinical presentation and diagnosis of urinary incontinence. *UpToDate.* Retrieved October 31, 2009, from http://www.uptodate.com/online/content/topic.do?topicKey=primneph/2274&selectedTitle=1-150&source=search_result

DuBeau, C. E. (2009, May 1b). Treatment of urinary incontinence. *UpToDate.* Retrieved October 31, 2009, from http://www.uptodate.com/online/content/topic.do?topicKey=primneph/6500&view=print

Evans, R. J. (2002). Treatment approaches for interstitial cystitis: Multimodality therapy. *Reviews in Urology, 4,* S16–S20.

Eyre, R. C. (2009, May 1). Evaluation of nonacute scrotal pathology in adult men. *UpToDate.* Retrieved October 31, 2009, from http://www.uptodate.com/online/content/topic.do?topicKey=primneph/10158&view=print

Fitzgerald, M. P. (2009, May 1a). Clinical features and diagnosis of painful bladder syndrome/interstitial cystitis. *UpToDate.* Retrieved October 17, 2009, from http://www.uptodate.com/online/content/topic.do?topicKey=urogynec/8671&view=print

Fitzgerald, M. P. (2009, May 1b). Treatment of painful bladder syndrome/interstitial cystitis. *UpToDate.* Retrieved October 17, 2009, from http://www.uptodate.com/online/content/topic.do?topicKey=urogynec/9272&view=print

Gagnadoux, M. F. (2009, May 1). Evaluation of gross hematuria in children. *UpToDate.* Retrieved October 17, 2009, from http://www.uptodate.com/online/content/topic.do?topicKey=pedineph/18271&selectedTitle=1-150&source=search_result

Grossfeld, G. D., Wolf, J. S., Litwin, M. S., et al. (2001). Asymptomatic microscopic hematuria in adults: Summary of the AUA best practice policy recommendations. *American Family Physician, 63,* 1145–1154.

Hanley, R. S., Stoffel, J. T., Zagha, R. M., et al. (2009). Multimodal therapy for painful bladder syndrome/interstitial cystitis: Pilot study combining behavioral, pharmacologic, and endoscopic therapies. *International Brazil Journal of Urology, 35,* 467–474.

Hayslett, J. P. (2009, May 1). Evaluation of proteinuria in pregnant women. *UpToDate.* Retrieved October 17, 2009, from http://www.uptodate.com/online/content/topic.do?topicKey=maternal/8748&view=print

Hedayati, T., & Keegan, M. (2009, July 29). Prostatitis. *emedicine.* Retrieved November 1, 2009, from http://emedicine.medscape.com/article/785418-print

Hittelman, A. (2009, May 1). Neonatal testicular torsion. *UpToDate.* Retrieved October 17, 2009, from http://www.uptodate.com/online/content/topic.do?topicKey=pediatri/5304&view=print

Hooton, T. M., & Stamm, W. E. (2009, May 1a). Clinical manifestations, diagnosis, and treatment of acute pyelonephritis. *UpToDate.* Retrieved October 17, 2009, from http://www.uptodate.com/online/content/topic.do?topicKey=uti_infe/6922&view=print

Hooton, T. M., & Stamm, W. E. (2009, May 1b). Urinary tract infections and asymptomatic bacteriuria in pregnancy. *UpToDate.* Retrieved October 17, 2009, from http://www.uptodate.com/online/content/topic.do?topicKey=uti_infe/7516&view=print

Jones, L. A., Woodman, P. J., & Ruiz, H. E. (2008, October 9). Urinary tract infections in pregnancy. *emedicine.* Retrieved November 1, 2009, from http://emedicine.medscape.com/article/452604-print

Kausz, A. T., & Gilbertson, D. T. (2006). Overview of vaccination in chronic kidney disease. *Advances in Chronic Kidney Disease, 13,* 209–214.

Kelepouris, E., & Agus, Z. S. (2009, May 1). Overview of heavy proteinuria and the nephrotic syndromes. *UpToDate.* Retrieved October 17, 2009, from http://www.uptodate.com/online/content/topic.do?topicKey=glom_dis/26669&view=print

Komaroff, A. L. (2009, May 1). Dysuria in adult women. *UpToDate.* Retrieved October 17, 2009, from http://www.uptodate.com/online/content/topic.do?topicKey=primneph/7408&view=print

Meyrier, A., & Fekete, T. (2009, May 1). Acute and chronic bacterial prostatitis. *UpToDate.* Retrieved November 1, 2009, from http://www.uptodate.com/online/content/topic.do?topicKey=uti_infe/6581&view=print

Minevich, E., & Tackett, L. (2007, February 9). Testicular torsion. *emedicine.* Retrieved October 25, 2009, from http://emedicine.medscape.com/article/438817-print

National Kidney Disease Education Program. (n.d.). *GFR calculators.* Retrieved September 4, 2009, from http://www.nkdep.nih.gov/professionals/gfr_calculators/index.htm

National Kidney Foundation. (2002). KDOQI clinical practice guidelines for chronic kidney disease: Evaluation, classification, and stratification. *American Journal of Kidney Disease, 39,* S1–S266.

Nettina, S. M. (1996). *The Lippincott manual of nursing practice* (6th ed.). Philadelphia: Lippincott-Raven Publishers.

Ortenberg, J., Collins, S., & Roth, C. C. (2009, September 21). Hydrocele and hernia in children. *emedicine.* Retrieved October 17, 2009, from http://emedicine.medscape.com/article/1015147-print

Post, T. W., & Rose, B. D. (2008, August 27). Diagnostic approach to the patient with acute or chronic kidney disease. *UpToDate Online 17.1.* Retrieved June 8, 2009, from http://www.uptodate.com/online/content/topic.do?topicKey=renldis/19906&view=print

Post, T. W., & Rose, B. D. (2009, January 29). Overview of the management of chronic kidney disease in adults. *UpToDate Online 17.1.* Retrieved June 8 2009, from http://www.uptodate.com/online/content/topic.do?topicKey=renldis/11615&view=print

The Practice Committee of the American Society for Reproductive Medicine. (2008). Report on varicocele and infertility. *Fertility and Sterility, 90,* S247–S249.

Preminger, G. M. (2009, May 1). Management of ureteral calculi. *UpToDate.* Retrieved October 17, 2009, from http://www.uptodate.com/online/content/topic.do?topicKey=renal_ur/8506&view=print

Preminger, G. M., & Curhan, G. C. (2009, May 1). The first kidney stone and asymptomatic nephrolithiasis in adults. *UpToDate.* Retrieved October 17, 2009, from http://www.uptodate.com/online/content/topic.do?topicKey=renal_ur/8506&view=print

The Prostate Institute. (2000). *NIH symptom index.* Retrieved November 7, 2009, from http://www.prostateinstitute.org/pro_nih.htm

Rose, B. D., & Fletcher, R. H. (2009, May 1). Evaluation of hematuria in adults. *UpToDate.* Retrieved October 17, 2009, from http://www.uptodate.com/online/content/topic.do?topicKey=renldis/7627&selectedTitle=1-150&source=search_result

Rose, B. D., & Post, T. W. (2009, May 1). Measurement of urinary protein excretion. *UpToDate*. Retrieved October 17, 2009, from http://www.uptodate.com/online/content/topic.do?topicKey=glom_dis/5359&view=print

Rosenberg, M. T., Newman, D. K., & Page, S. A. (2007). Interstitial cystitis/painful bladder syndrome: Symptom recognition is key to early identification, treatment. *Cleveland Clinic Journal of Medicine, 74*, S54–S62.

Rupp, T. J., & Zwanger, M. (2008, November 26). Testicular torsion. *emedicine*. Retrieved October 25, 2009, from http://emedicine.medscape.com/article/778086-print

Sabanegh, E. S., Konety, B. R., & Ching, C. B. (2008, June 12). Epididymitis. *emedicine*. Retrieved October 25, 2009, from http://emedicine.medscape.com/article/436154-print

Schaefer, A. J. (2006). Chronic prostatitis and the chronic pelvic pain syndrome. *The New England Journal of Medicine, 355*, 1690–1701.

Shaikh, N., & Hoberman, A. (2009, May 1). Acute management, imaging, and prognosis of urinary tract infections in children. *UpToDate*. Retrieved October 17, 2009, from http://www.uptodate.com/online/content/topic.do?topicKey=pedi_id/19627&view=print

Shoff, W. H., Green-McKenzie, J., Edwards, C., et al. (2009, January 7). Pyelonephritis, acute. *emedicine*. Retrieved November 11, 2009, from http://emedicine.medscape.com/article/245559-print

Smith, D. A., Chini, E., & Buntin, F. (2009). Incontinence in older adults: Options for realistic, effective treatment. *Advance for Nurse Practitioners, 71*, 41–44.

Smith, J., & Stapleton, F. B. (2009, May 1). Clinical features and diagnosis of nephrolithiasis in children. *UpToDate*. Retrieved October 17, 2009, from http://www.uptodate.com/online/content/topic.do?topicKey=pedineph/4407&view=print

Sumfest, J. M., Kolon, T. F., & Rukstalis, D. B. (2009, January 2). Cryptorchidism. *emedicine*. Retrieved October 31, 2009, from http://emedicine.medscape.com/article/438378-print

Swygard, H., Cohen, M. S., & Sena, A. C. (2009, May 1). Infectious causes of dysuria in adult men. *UpToDate*. Retrieved October 17, 2009, from http://www.uptodate.com/online/content/topic.do?topicKey=stds/9500&selectedTitle=4-59&source=search_result

The Testicular Cancer Resource Center. (2009, March 16). *How to do a testicular self examination*. Retrieved October 25, 2009, from http://tcrc.acor.org/tcexam.html

U.S. Department of Health and Human Services, National Institutes of Health. (2007). National Kidney and Urological Diseases Information Clearinghouse: *Urinary incontinence in women*. (NIH Publication No. 08–4132). Retrieved November 3, 2009, from http://kidney.niddk.nih.gov/kudiseases/pubs/pdf/UI-Women.pdf

U.S. Department of Health and Human Services, National Institutes of Health. (2008, April). National Kidney and Urological Disease Information Clearinghouse: *Interstitial cystitis/painful bladder syndrome*. (NIH Publication No. 08–3220). Retrieved November 2, 2009, from http://kidney.niddk.nih.gov/kudiseases/pubs/pdf/interstitialcystitis.pdf

U.S. Department of Health and Human Services, National Institutes of Health. (2008). National Kidney and Urological Diseases Information Clearinghouse: *Prostatitis: Disorders of the prostate*. (NIH Publication No. 08–4553). Retrieved November 3, 2009, from http://kidney.niddk.nih.gov/Kudiseases/pubs/pdf/Prostatitis.pdf

U.S. Department of Health and Human Services, National Institutes of Health. (n.d.). National Kidney and Urological Diseases Information Clearinghouse: *Bladder control diary*. Retrieved November 3, 2009, from http://kidney.niddk.nih.gov/kudiseases/pubs/bladdercontrol/index.htm

United States Renal Data System (USRDS). (2008). *USRDS 2008 Annual data report: Atlas of chronic kidney disease and end-stage renal disease in the United States*. National Institutes of Health, National Institute of Diabetes and Digestive and Kidney Diseases. Bethesda, MD. Retrieved September 4, 2009, from http://www.usrds.org/adr.htm

Wayment, R. O., & Schwartz, B. F. (2009, March 19). Pregnancy and urolithiasis. *emedicine*. Retrieved November 11, 2009, from http://emedicine.medscape.com/article/455830-print.

WebMD. (2009). Testicular self-exam. *emedicinehealth*. Retrieved October 25, 2009, from http://www.emedicinehealth.com/testicular_self-exam/page7_em.htm#Physician%20Treatment

White, W. M., & Kim, E. D. (2009, July 28). Varicocele. *emedicine*. Retrieved October 25, 2009, from http://emedicine.medscape.com/article/438591-print

Wolfe, J. S. (2009, September 28). Nephrolithiasis. *emedicine*. Retrieved November 11, 2009, from http://emedicine.medscape.com/article/437096-print

CHAPTER 12

Obstetrics Guidelines

Jill C. Cash

PRECONCEPTION COUNSELING: IDENTIFYING PATIENTS AT RISK

A woman's health before conception influences her ability not only to conceive, but also to maintain pregnancy and to achieve a healthy outcome. Some women are unaware that their medical conditions, medications, occupational exposure, or social practices may have negative consequences in the earliest weeks of pregnancy, before the pregnancy test is positive. They don't know that organogenesis begins around 17 days after fertilization. Steps to provide the ideal environment for the developing fetus are most likely to be effective if they precede the traditional initiation of prenatal care.

The goal of preconceptional care is to reduce perinatal mortality and morbidity. Targeting only self-referred women who are planning their next conception or women referred with risk factors can result in a significant number of missed opportunities for primary prevention. Nurses working with women of childbearing age and their families have a responsibility to promote reproductive health during every health encounter. Even among married women in the United States, the unintended pregnancy rate is nearly 40%; 85% of teen pregnancies are unintended.

The preconception interview is the time to review primary care health issues. Is the woman current on immunizations, determination of hepatitis status, rubella immunity, Pap smears, cultures for sexually transmitted diseases, and mammography (if appropriate)?

When discussing preconception plans, the patient's history as well as that of her partner should be evaluated for poor health habits (alcohol, smoking, drug use), exposure to toxic substances (radiation and chemicals), multiple sexual partners (risk of HIV, hepatitis, and STIs), and racial or ethnic origin. Preconceptional evaluation should include the following:

A. Maternal age: Pregnancy-induced hypertension (PIH) occurs at the extreme of ages, insulin-dependent diabetes increases with maternal age, and the risks of Down syndrome and other chromosomal abnormalities increase with age. Advanced maternal age is defined as 35 years of age at delivery. The American College of Obstetrics and Gynecology (ACOG) requires counseling on genetic testing options for women of advanced maternal age.

B. Racial or ethnic considerations: Inquire and test patients, if indicated, for **Tay-Sachs disease:** Eastern European Jewish or French Canadian ancestry; **thalassemia:** Mediterranean, Southeast Asian, Indian, Pakistani, or African ancestry; **sickle cell anemia:** African, Mediterranean, Middle Eastern, Caribbean, Latin American, or Indian ancestry; and **cystic fibrosis:** positive family history of cystic fibrosis.

C. Social issues: Screen every woman for physical and sexual abuse. There is an increased incidence of physical abuse in pregnancy. This assessment should be done only if the partner is not present. Information should be given to the patient concerning the available community, social, and legal resources, as well as an assessment of her immediate danger and an escape plan.

D. Financial: Discuss insurance, maternity benefits, work leave policy, and contingency plans for lost wages due to pregnancy complications with the patient.

E. Environmental and occupational considerations: Routine assessment of hobbies and home and employment environments may identify exposures that have been associated with adverse reproductive consequences that can be minimized in the preconceptual period.

F. Fetal effects are dependent on dose(s) and gestational age at exposure related to the following:
    1. Radiation: Fetal effects include microcephaly, mental retardation, eye anomalies, intrauterine growth retardation (IUGR), and visceral malformations. Lead aprons should be used to protect the patient for any radiation exposures.
    2. Heavy metals: Mercury exposure is related to brain damage and neuromuscular defects. Lead exposure is related to increased spontaneous abortion, low birth weight, brain damage, and increased premature rupture of membranes. Cadmium is retained by the fetal liver and kidney and is also associated with fetal craniofacial defects. Nickel is associated with neonatal deaths.

3. Pesticides: Occupations at risk for pesticide exposure include, but are not limited to, the following: ranch and farm workers (including migrant workers); gardeners (home and professional); grounds keepers; florists; structural pest control workers; hunting and fishing guides; health care workers who deal with contamination; and people employed in pesticide production, mixing, and application. Dioxin is associated with an increased rate of spontaneous abortion, myelomeningocele, and limb defects. The pesticides DDT and DDE are associated with increased abortion, prematurity, low birth weight, and PIH.

4. Other: Carbon monoxide is associated with increased stillbirths, neurologic deficits, seizures, spasticity, and retarded psychomotor development. Ozone is associated with increased spontaneous abortion and increased structural defects. Anesthetic gases are associated with increased abortion, birth defects, low birth weight, and infertility.

G. Infectious diseases: See Chapter 14, "Sexually Transmitted Infections Guidelines" and Chapter 15, "Infectious Disease Guidelines."

H. Medications: Assess and minimize the risk of exposure to medications by reviewing the patient's use of prescription and nonprescription drugs. Provide the patient with information on the safest choices and avoiding drugs associated with fetal risks. Phenytoin (Dilantin) taken by the father increases the congenital defect risk to the fetus by 8.3%. Defects include cleft lip and palate, congenital heart disease, microcephaly, caudal dysplasia, and caudal regression syndrome.

I. Medical problems: Health assessment of potential risk not only to the fetus but also to the woman, should she become pregnant, should be discussed. Care must be taken to identify and counsel all women whose life expectancy could be markedly reduced by pregnancy or whose fetus would have a high likelihood of complications. For example, women with known cardiac problems, epilepsy, transplanted organs, or uncontrolled diabetes and hypertension should be told of the risks associated with pregnancy.

J. Diabetes: Researchers have demonstrated a dose-related response between glycosylated hemoglobin (Hgb A1c) during the first trimester of pregnancy and the incidence of congenital defects: the better the glycemic control, the lower the risk for birth defects. The preconceptional plan for diabetes includes the following:

1. Change all patients on oral agents to insulin therapy before pregnancy is attempted.
   a. Achieve strict plasma glucose control.
   b. Reduce the Hgb A1c to 7% or less.
   c. Assess the patient for vasculopathy, neuropathy, nephropathy, and retinopathy.
   d. Provide or refer the patient for genetic and nutritional counseling.
   e. Enhance the woman's knowledge of diabetes during pregnancy.

K. Nutrition: Dietary evaluation and recommendations of alternatives that may benefit the fetus' development are important components of preconceptional counseling.

Evaluation of nutritional status should include assessment of the appropriate weight for the patient's height as well as a discussion of eating habits such as vegetarianism, fasting for religious or personal reasons, eating disorders, and the use of mega vitamins.

L. Obstetric considerations: Preconceptional reproductive history is an important tool for identifying factors that may be amenable to intervention. Review term, preterm, aborted (elective, spontaneous, and therapeutic) pregnancies, as well as a short history on living children. Review the gestational age at delivery of each neonate and any pregnancy and delivery complications. Preterm labor has a 30% recurrence risk, and PIH has a 25%–35% recurrence rate in subsequent pregnancies. In some instances, after preconceptual and genetic counseling, the couple may decide to forgo pregnancy or to use assisted reproductive technologies such as donor eggs and/or sperm.

M. Recurrent loss: The workup and counseling for recurrent losses include the evaluation for a uterine defect (septal or bicornate uterus or uterus didelphys), endocrine problem (luteal phase defect or hypothyroidism), chromosomal defect, or the presence of antiphospholipid syndrome. Antiphospholipid syndrome is defined as the presence of maternal anticardiolipin antibodies and/or lupus anticoagulant in association with recurrent pregnancy loss, thrombotic events, and/or thrombocytopenia. Approximately 10% of women with unexplained recurrent pregnancy loss test positive for anticardiolipin antibodies and/or lupus anticoagulant. In the nonpregnant patient, thrombosis of a single vessel is the most common complication associated with antiphospholipid syndrome.

N. Lifestyle: Queries regarding a woman's social lifestyle history should seek to identify behaviors and exposures that may compromise reproductive outcome. While environmental exposures are a frequent concern of couples considering pregnancy, women should be informed that, in general, maternal use of alcohol, tobacco, and other mood-altering drugs is more hazardous for a fetus than most other lifestyle choices.

1. Alcohol: Alcohol is a known teratogen. Research indicates that as many as 73% of 12- to 34-year-old women expose their fetuses to alcohol at some time during pregnancy. Fetal alcohol syndrome is associated with IUGR, reduction in the width of palpebral fissures, microcephaly, mental retardation and developmental delay, and maxillary hypoplasia.

2. Smoking: Fetal affects of smoking are also related to the dose-response effect. Smoking is associated with an increase in bleeding in pregnancy (abruption and placenta previa), IUGR, preterm birth, stillbirth, respiratory distress in the neonate, and sudden infant death syndrome. Counsel the patient on smoking cessation. Suggestions of ways to quit include nicotine fading (tapering and brand switching to lower tar and nicotine), monitoring smoking behavior, setting a contract to quit smoking, identifying social support or a buddy, and restricting area(s) as No Smoking Zone. Give the patient positive reinforcement for decreases and quitting.

3. Substance use: If substance exposure is complicated by addiction, structured recovery programs are usually needed to effect behavioral change.

O. Exercise: Exercise and recreational activities should be reviewed and discussed relative to safety, including the use of bike helmets, avoiding strenuous exercise, and hyperthermia. ACOG recommends that maternal heart rate (for pregnant women) not exceed 140 bpm. If the woman is not currently exercising, walking and swimming can be suggested. Heat exposure appears to be teratogenic. Use of saunas or hot tubs and high fevers in the first trimester have been associated with an increased risk of neural tube defects.

Preconception counseling helps to identify high-risk patients who need intensive care during pregnancy and delivery, and it identifies women that need referral for medical management, nutritional counseling, genetic counseling, or behavior modification. Prescribe a prenatal vitamin daily for any woman considering pregnancy.

ROUTINE PRENATAL CARE

Initial Prenatal Visit

The initial prenatal visit is a very important visit. A comprehensive health history is obtained; blood is drawn for baseline prenatal laboratory values to be established; and depending on the time, the physical examination may also be performed. Many practitioners have the patient return in 2 weeks to perform the physical exam due to the amount of time taken for the history and collecting blood for laboratory tests. Another variation is to obtain the baseline lab tests (except blood type and Rh factor) after the first trimester (to avoid unnecessary testing in the event the patient should have a miscarriage).

There are several prenatal flow sheets available. Most of the flow sheets are complete and cover the most important aspects of the history and exam. The American College of Obstetricians and Gynecologists has a standard form. Important information to cover is the patient's medical and surgical history (including previous obstetric history), family genetic history, psychiatric disorders, contraception history, medications taken since the last menstrual period, menstrual history, social habits (smoking, substance abuse, alcohol), environmental exposures (job, hobbies, and so on), exposure to abuse (mental, physical, sexual), and sources of social support and health promotion (immunizations up-to-date, etc.).

Laboratory tests that are ordered at the initial exam include the following: CBC, rubella titer, HIV (with the patient's consent), syphilis (RPR or VDRL), hepatitis B surface antigen, blood type and Rh factor, antibody screen, tuberculosis testing, urine culture and sensitivity, and bacterial vaginosis screen.

Optional tests include hemoglobin A1c, sickle cell screening, thyroid profile, and hepatitis C. Other tests performed with the physical examination include Pap smear and cultures for chlamydia and gonorrhea. Additional tests may be ordered throughout the pregnancy:

A. 15–20 weeks gestation: maternal serum multiple marker screening (optional test per patient wishes and father of baby and other family history).

B. 18–20 weeks gestation: obstetric ultrasonography.

C. 24–28 weeks gestation: one-hour glucola; if the results are greater than 129 mg/dL, order 3-hour glucose tolerance test. Also perform first trimester diabetes testing for advanced maternal age or patient history of gestational diabetes.

D. 35–37 weeks gestation: vaginal culture for group B *Streptococcus* infection.

E. American Academy of Pediatrics recommends universal screening for group B *Streptococcus* infection at 36 weeks' gestation.

Special tests: Even with the best preconceptional plan and modifications, about 2%–3% of all babies have a major congenital malformation.

1. In about 90% of the cases, neural tube defects are not expected on the basis of past history. Neural tube defects (NTD) are associated with multifactorial causes, including environmental factors, undernutrition (lack of folic acid), chromosomal defects, maternal hyperthermia, diabetes, clomiphene citrate (Clomid) induction, and maternal obesity.

2. In 1996, the Food and Drug Administration (FDA) approved a population-based strategy, effective January 1998, to fortify grain food sources with folic acid. The recurrence risk of NTD is 15% without the use of preconceptional doses of folic acid. Even with the FDA strategy, folic acid supplement of 4 mg per day at least 1 month before conception and during the first trimester of pregnancy is recommended.

One example is genetic testing. If the mother is 35 years or older at the time of delivery, or if she has a family history of any abnormal genetic disorders, such as Down syndrome, in the family she should be offered genetic counseling and/or testing. The parents choose whether they would like to have genetic testing performed to evaluate the fetus for abnormal chromosomes. The following tests can be performed for genetic screening:

A. 10–12 weeks gestation: chorionic villus sampling.

B. 15–18 weeks gestation: amniocentesis.

C. Amniocentesis can also detect elevated protein levels (alpha-fetoprotein and the presence of acetylcholinesterase) in the amniotic fluid. Therefore, if the amniocentesis is performed, both genetic information and spinal cord defects can be evaluated.

The initial visit is also a time for teaching the pregnant patient (see Exhibit 12.1). Literature and brochures on health promotion (i.e., breast self-exam and smoking cessation) and information regarding the normal changes, discomforts, and concerns during pregnancy should be provided, along with the practice after hours contact telephone number. Reassure the patient that as the pregnancy progresses you can answer questions she may have; however, these resources may provide the information she is looking for. Encourage the patient to enroll in childbirth education, sibling classes (if applicable), breast-feeding classes, and any other classes of interest to her and her partner.

After the initial prenatal visit is completed, the other visits go fairly quickly with routine evaluation of vital signs, urine evaluation for glucose and protein, and fetal assessment.

EXHIBIT 12.1 **Routine Prenatal Patient Education Topics**

TOPIC	DATES
Prenatal care in your practice	_____
(Office visits, blood tests) prenatal handouts	_____
Diet/nutrition/weight gain	_____
Enrolled in WIC	_____
Substance use (alcohol, smoking, drugs)	_____
Domestic violence (history, type of injuries)	_____
OTC medication use	_____
Activity: work and exercise	_____
Travel	_____
Clothing	_____
Personal hygiene	_____
Cats	_____
Sexual activity	_____
Physiologic changes during pregnancy	_____
Fetal development	_____
Father's role during pregnancy	_____
Common discomforts/treatments	_____
Symptoms to report immediately	_____
Fetal kick counts	_____
Prenatal classes	_____
Breast-feeding/bottle feeding	_____
Circumcision	_____
Infant supply preparation	_____
Safety/car safety	_____
Preparing for delivery	_____
When to come to the hospital	_____
Labor and delivery expectations	_____
Postpartum care	_____
First days with baby	_____
Postpartum birth control	_____

TESTS

Triple or quad screen	_____
One-hour glucola screen	_____
Ultrasonography	_____
Glucose tolerance test if applicable	_____
Amniocentesis/CVS if applicable	_____
Group B strep	_____

Fetal monitoring: kick counts: _____

NST: _____ BPP: _____

(Content discussed can be found in patient handout provided to patient at first prenatal visit.)

The routine schedule of appointments includes a visit every 4 weeks until 28 weeks' gestation, every 2 weeks until 36 weeks' gestation, then weekly until delivered.

A. Each visit should include documentation of the following:
   1. Weight
   2. Blood pressure
   3. Fundal height, fetal heart tones, and fetal movement
   4. Urine: protein and glucose

Each visit should evaluate and discuss possible problems of pregnancy, such as preterm labor, vaginal bleeding, and so on. A few questions to ask at each visit include:

   1. Have you had any blurred vision, spots before your eyes, or epigastric pain?
   2. Have you had any headaches? If so, evaluate and note source of relief.
   3. Have you had any nausea or vomiting? If so, note source of relief.
   4. Have you had any abdominal pain, contractions, backache, pelvic pressure, or other pain?
   5. Have you had any vaginal bleeding, discharge, or leakage of fluid?
   6. Evaluate fetal movement, noting when movement was first felt (quickening) and the daily fetal movement.
   7. Evaluate social support at home and in the work environment.
   8. If the patient smokes, ask about current habits. Teach the patient the effects of smoking on herself and the fetus (bleeding, intrauterine growth retardation, increased risk of miscarriage), and encourage her at each visit to cut down or quit.
   9. Discuss the effects of weight gain related to nutritional intake as opposed to complications of pregnancy-induced hypertension.

ANEMIA, IRON DEFICIENCY

Definition
A. Anemia in pregnancy results from decreased serum iron. The iron-binding capacity is increased. Red blood cells are microcytic and hypochromic. The Centers for Disease Control and the American College of Obstetricians and Gyencologists defines first trimester anemia as a hemoglobin of <11.0 g/dL/hematocrit of <33%, second trimester as a hemoglobin of <10.5 g/dL/hematocrit of <32%, and third trimester as a hemoglobin of <11.0 g/dL/hematocrit of <33%.

Incidence
A. Anemia is a common medical complication of pregnancy. Iron deficiency anemia constitutes 75%–95% of pregnancy-related anemias.

Pathogenesis
A. Increased demand for iron during pregnancy occurs because of increased maternal blood volume. Hemoglobin and hematocrit decrease during first and second trimester and usually increase during third trimester.

B. Another 0.5–1.0 mg/day of iron is needed for lactation. During most pregnancies, diet alone does not provide the necessary iron.

Predisposing Factors
A. Failure to take oral iron; often due to inability to tolerate oral iron supplements.
B. Multiple gestation; increases iron requirement and may contribute to increased blood loss at delivery.
C. Diet high in phosphorous or foods such as tea, coffee, milk, or soy.
D. Low iron and protein diet, eating nonfood items (pica).
E. Not eating foods that help with absorption of iron (orange juice, broccoli, strawberries).
F. History of gastrointestinal surgery may cause iron malabsorption (i.e., gastrectomy).
G. Chronic bleeding during pregnancy (i.e., placenta previa, marginal sinus separation of placenta, hemorrhoidal bleeding).
H. Short intervals between pregnancies.
I. Race: Non-Hispanic black females.
J. Age: Teenage girls.

Common Complaints
A. Tiredness
B. Inability to take prenatal vitamins because of nausea
C. Bleeding problems (see "Predisposing Factors")
D. Pica

Other Signs and Symptoms
A. Fatigue
B. Pale mucous membranes and skin
C. Tachycardia

Subjective Data
A. Elicit the onset, duration, and course of presenting symptoms.
B. Elicit information about the patient's "typical" dietary intake for meals and snacks, and review pica (eating clay, starch, ice, and other nonnutritive substances).
C. Review the patient's intake of prenatal vitamins and supplemental iron. How often does she take iron? Elicit the reason for skipping the supplemental iron (nausea, constipation), if applicable.
D. Review the patient's history of gastrointestinal surgeries, irritable bowel syndrome (IBS), and Crohn's disease.
E. Review the patient's history for any type of anemia and previous treatment including blood transfusions.
F. Review pregnancy history for closely spaced pregnancies (two in a calendar year) and multiple gestation.
G. Review the patient's intake of medications for the use of aspirin and other nonsteroidal anti-inflammatory drugs (NSAIDs).

Physical Examination
A. Pulse and blood pressure: note postural hypotension and tachycardia.
B. Inspect: General appearance
   1. Inspect the skin, mucous membranes, and conjunctivae for pallor.

2. Observe the mouth and tongue: note atrophy of papillae and smooth, beefy red appearance of tongue with anemia.
3. Note dryness of skin. Inspect texture of nails (brittle, spoon-shaped, concave); inspect the hair for brittleness.

C. Palpate: Palpate the abdomen for masses; assess fundal height.
D. Auscultate: Auscultate the heart for systolic flow murmurs; auscultate lungs.

Diagnostic Tests

A. Hematocrit (HCT) and hemoglobin (Hgb):
   1. First trimester: less than 11g/dL Hgb or less than 33% Hct.
   2. Second trimester: less than 10.5 g/dL Hgb or less than 32% Hct.
   3. Third trimester: less than 11 g/dL Hgb or less than 33% Hct.
B. Peripheral blood smear: note microcytic and hypochromic RBCs on peripheral smear.
C. Sickle cell screen, if applicable.
D. Serum iron: low with anemia.
E. Iron-binding capacity: high iron-binding capacity with anemia.
F. Transferrin: saturation less than 15%.
G. Stool for occult blood, if applicable.
H. Emesis for presence of blood, if applicable.

Differential Diagnoses

A. Iron deficiency anemia.
B. Normal physiologic anemia of pregnancy: During normal pregnancy, concentrations of erythrocytes and hemoglobin usually fall because of the greater increase in plasma volume (increased by 45%) relative to the increase in erythrocyte volume (increased by 25%).
C. Megaloblastic anemia: This is commonly associated with iron deficiency anemia and is rarely seen alone.
D. Hemolytic anemia: sickle cell anemia, thalassemia, hereditary spherocytosis, and erythrocyte enzyme deficiency.
E. Aplastic anemia: bone marrow failure.
F. Hematologic malignancies: leukemia and lymphoma.
G. Clotting factor or other hemostatic deficiencies: hemophilia, von Willebrand's disease, ITP, and DIC.

Plan

A. Do initial evaluation of Hgb and HCT at first prenatal visit; repeat at 24–28 week blood draw with diabetes testing.
B. Diet counseling and nutrition consultation: The patient may be eligible for the WIC program (Women, Infants, and Children) that provides supplemental foods for pregnant women and young children. Ask your local health department for information available in your community.
   1. Advise the patient to take supplemental iron in addition to prenatal vitamins. If she is unable to tolerate prenatal vitamins, suggest a children's chewable vitamin, two tablets daily.

2. Encourage the patient to continue iron supplementation through the first month postpartum and throughout breast-feeding.
C. Patient teaching: See the Section III Patient Teaching Guide for this chapter, "Iron Deficiency Anemia (Pregnancy)."
D. Pharmaceutical therapy
   1. Prophylaxis: Oral iron supplements are recommended for all gestations with usual dose of 60 mg/day elemental iron, or 325 mg/day ferrous sulfate. Time-released tablets may help but are more expensive.
   2. Most prenatal vitamins contain supplemental iron. Therefore, if the woman is taking one vitamin daily, she may only need to take two iron tablets. Nausea and vomiting occur in 20%–25% of patients. These side effects are dose-related. Have the patient alter times of administration of the iron supplement to determine when the iron is best tolerated.
   3. Treatment: With iron deficiency anemia, three times the prophylactic dose of iron should be given, or 325 mg ferrous sulfate three times daily.
   4. Intramuscular or intravenous iron may be ordered for the small proportion of patients who do not tolerate oral iron due to gastrointestinal complaints, malabsorption syndrome, or noncompliance with the oral iron regimen.

Follow-up

A. Carry out routine prenatal and postpartum follow-up care. When the patient begins taking the recommended dose of supplemental iron, the RBC response can be measured in 2 weeks by an elevation in her reticulocyte count.
B. Repeat HCT after 4–6 weeks of therapy.
C. If no improvement is seen in reticulocyte count or HCT after 4 weeks of therapy and the patient has been compliant, another cause of anemia should be investigated.

Consultation/Referral

A. Consider consult with a physician if Hgb is less than 9 g/dL or HCT is less than or equal to 27% and does not improve with the above treatments.

PREGNANCY-INDUCED HYPERTENSION, OR PREECLAMPSIA

Definition

Pregnancy-induced hypertension (PIH; antiquated term *toxemia*) is hypertension with proteinuria and/or edema that develops during pregnancy and lasts or develops up to 6 weeks postpartum. Hypertension is defined as the following:

A. Increase of 30 mmHg systolic or 15 mmHg diastolic pressure over the baseline blood pressure, or BP, at first prenatal visit.
B. BP greater than or equal to 140/90 after 20 weeks' gestation if prior blood pressure is unknown. The values must be elevated on at least two separate occasions at least 6 hours apart. **Severity of hypertension is not necessarily associated with the severity of PIH.**
C. Eclampsia, or the occurrence of convulsions in a patient with preeclampsia.

D. Chronic hypertension in pregnancy is often complicated by superimposed PIH.

Incidence

A. Hypertensive disorders are the most common medical complication of pregnancy, with a reported incidence of between 5% and 10%. Incidence varies among different regions and countries. There is a 30% recurrence rate in subsequent pregnancies.

Pathogenesis

A. The etiology of preeclampsia is unknown, although several theories exist. Generalized vascular endothelial damage is a hallmark of the pathophysiologic responses.

Predisposing Factors

A. Nulliparity
B. Chronic hypertension
C. Age extreme (< 18 years and > 35 years)
D. Race (African American women higher risk)
E. Diabetes mellitus
F. Renal disease
G. Family history of preeclampsia
H. Previous pregnancy with PIH
I. Multiple gestation
J. Hydatidiform mole

Common Complaints

A. Headache unrelieved by analgesics
B. Upper right quadrant pain
C. Severe heartburn unrelieved by antacids
D. Nausea and vomiting
E. Edema
F. Visual disturbances
G. Photophobia

Other Signs and Symptoms

A. **Classic triad of symptoms**
  1. Hypertension.

First trimester signs of PIH need ultrasonographic evaluation for the presence of a gestational trophoblastic disease (molar pregnancy) as well as the other differential diagnoses.

  2. Edema.
  3. Proteinuria: This is not normal and requires evaluation.
B. Brisk deep tendon reflexes (DTRs) or clonus.

Potential Complications

A. Multiple organ involvement.
B. HELLP syndrome: hemolysis, elevated liver enzymes, and low platelets.
C. Intrauterine growth retardation and oligohydramnios are signs of end-organ damage.

Subjective Data

A. Elicit information about headaches, their onset and duration, the progression of headache, and/or other symptoms.
B. What part of the head hurts? Differentiate headache from sinus headache. Note severity and any relief measure tried (acetaminophen, massage, sleep).
C. Is the headache "new"? Does the patient have a previous history of migraines? Is this like a previous migraine?
D. What are other concurrent symptoms: nausea, vomiting, right upper quadrant pain, and visual changes?
E. Question the patient about edema. If edema is present, has it significantly worsened over the past few days? Has she been able to wear rings up to this point? Has she had to wear different shoes due to pedal edema?
F. What are her usual weight and today's weight (on the same scales). Has she gained more than 2 pounds in 1 week?
G. Ask specifics about right upper quadrant pain, sometimes identified as "severe heartburn." Note the duration, severity, and the relief measures tried. Have the patient point to the area of discomfort (midsternum or under right breast).
H. Are there any visual disturbances, such as black dots she can't see through?
I. Review other GI symptoms such as diarrhea, abdominal pain, and gallbladder attack.
J. Review for signs of fever and thyroid storm.
K. Review the patient's history for seizures.

Physical Examination

A. Temperature, blood pressure, pulse and respirations, weight and fetal heart tones.
B. Inspect
  1. Check pedal, hand, and facial edema.
  2. Check fundal height.
C. Palpate
  1. Palpate the abdomen noting any hepatosplenomegaly and RUQ tenderness to the palpation.
  2. Palpate the lower extremities for pitting edema.
D. Percuss
  1. Gently check for liver enlargement.
  2. Perform neurologic exam for hyperreflexia: check DTR and clonus.
E. Auscultate
  1. Auscultate the heart and lungs.
  2. Auscultate the fetal heart tone.

Diagnostic Tests

A. CBC and platelets.
B. ALT and AST.
C. Renal workup
  1. Uric acid, serum creatinine, and urine protein.
  2. Urine culture if proteinuria is present to rule out UTI.
  3. Collect 24-hour urine for total protein and creatinine clearance.
D. Ultrasonography, if indicated, to rule out intrauterine growth retardation and/or oligohydramnios.

Differential Diagnoses

A. Pregnancy-induced hypertension
B. Hyperemesis gravidarum
C. Infection: appendicitis, gastroenteritis, pyelonephritis, glomerulonephritis, hepatitis, and pancreatitis
D. Acute fatty liver of pregnancy
E. Systemic lupus erythematosus
F. Hemolytic uremic syndrome

G. Hepatic encephalopathy
H. Gastrointestinal disorder: peptic ulcer and heartburn
I. Thrombotic or idiopathic thrombocytopenia purpura
J. Gall bladder disease
K. Chronic hypertension
L. Thyroid storm

Plan

A. General interventions
   1. Any patient with an elevated blood pressure should be reassessed in the lateral recumbent position, using proper cuff size, after the patient is allowed to relax for several minutes prior to BP measurement.
   2. If the patient's BP begins to rise above baseline values:
      a. Advise the patient to maintain a modified bed rest schedule (stop working).
      b. Recommend frequent BP evaluation at home.
      c. See the patient weekly or biweekly for further maternal and neonatal assessment; nonstress test (NST) and biophysical profile if appropriate.
   3. If the "classic triad" is present, refer the patient to an obstetrician or perinatologist for further assessment and management. She may need immediate admission to the hospital for inpatient management or delivery.
   4. If the patient has a convulsion, the primary consideration is to protect her. Monitor seizure type and duration. Call for immediate transport to the hospital labor and delivery unit. Place the patient in the lateral recumbent position following the seizure.
   5. Immediately transfer the patient to a hospital for eclampsia after stabilization.
B. Dietary management: Salt restriction does not stop swelling and high blood pressure problems in pregnancy.
C. Pharmaceutical therapy
   1. Diuretics are **not** prescribed during pregnancy for edema.
   2. Angiotensin-converting enzyme (ACE) inhibitors and angiotensin II receptor blockers (ARBs) are not recommended during pregnancy due to the teratogenic effects on the fetus that may occur such as renal dysgenesis and/or fetal death.
   3. Aldomet is commonly used during pregnancy to control chronic or superimposed hypertension during pregnancy.
   4. Inpatient therapy is determined by a physician and may include:
      a. Magnesium sulfate for seizure prophylaxis.
      b. Hydralazine or labetalol are first-line antihypertensive agents if a patient's diastolic BP is greater than 110 mmHg.
      c. Steroids may be given to enhance fetal lung maturity prior to delivery.
      d. In severe PIH, therapy may include cervical ripening agents such as prostaglandins or misoprostol and/or oxytocin induction of labor.
      e. Narcotics may be used for severe headaches.
      f. **Diazepam (Valium) is not recommended for seizures in pregnancy; it causes neonatal thermoregulation problems.**

Follow-up

A. The only "cure" for PIH is delivery. See the patient in 1 week after delivery for BP assessment, or sooner if symptoms persist.

Consultation/Referral

A. If the patient is diagnosed with PIH, refer her to a physician for continued care and delivery.

PRETERM LABOR

Definition

A. Preterm labor is labor that produces documented cervical changes after 20 weeks and prior to 37 completed weeks of gestation.

Incidence

A. Preterm labor occurs in approximately 11% live births in the United States and precedes 50% of the preterm births. It accounts for more than 70% of neonatal mortality.

Pathogenesis

A. Infection and ischemia are common causes of preterm labor. Infection may originate from several sites, including the bladder, kidney(s), cervix, uterus, gastrointestinal tract, and upper respiratory tract. Ischemia may be caused by decreased oxygen delivery to the uterus due to maternal hypoxia, hypovolemia, or vena caval compression. Overdistension of the uterus in the presence of polyhydramnios or multiple gestation may cause preterm labor symptoms. However, in most cases, the cause is unknown.

Predisposing Factors

A. Previous preterm labor or preterm delivery.
B. Preterm rupture of membranes.
C. Uterine anomalies, surgery, and fibroids.
D. Multiple gestations.
E. History of second trimester abortion(s).
F. Incompetent cervix.
G. History of cone biopsy.
H. Recurrent urinary tract and kidney infections.
I. Polyhydramnios.
J. Macrosomatic fetus.
K. Maternal age extremes.
L. Placenta previa.
M. Abruptio placentae.
N. Poor nutritional status and low prepregnancy weight.
O. Maternal dehydration.
P. Maternal race (occurs more frequently in African American population).
Q. Low socioeconomic status.
R. Inadequate prenatal care.
S. Anemia.
T. Substance use/abuse (smoking, drug, alcohol).
U. Vaginal infection.
V. Presence of fetal fibronectin, a protein produced by the trophoblast and other fetal tissues, has been noted in cervical-vaginal secretions between 24–34 weeks' gestation in a subgroup of women that are at increased risk for preterm birth.

Common Complaints

A. Abdominal pain or cramping
B. Low backache
C. Increase or change in vaginal discharge, "gush" of fluid, loss of mucus plug, and bloody show or vaginal spotting
D. Diarrhea
E. "Something not right"

Other Signs and Symptoms

A. Pelvic pressure
B. Contractions or periodlike cramps

Subjective Data

A. Elicit information about the onset, frequency, duration, and course of cramps; presence or absence of backache; how long these symptoms have existed; and whether symptoms began subsequent to a certain event or activity. What, if anything, makes these symptoms better or worse?
B. Question the patient about color, odor, consistency, and amount of vaginal discharge or bleeding: Was there a spot the size of a quarter or a half-dollar? Has she been wearing a perineal pad? How often does she have to change the pad? Is the pad soaked with blood when she changes it?
C. Question the patient about frequency of fetal movements, for fetuses older than 18 weeks' gestation.
D. Question the patient about urinary frequency, presence of urgency or dysuria.
E. Question the patient about recent sexual activity (i.e., has there been recent intercourse?)
F. If the patient complains of diarrhea, ask her if she has a fever, and if anyone else in the family is ill.

Physical Examination

A. Temperature, blood pressure, and fetal heart tones.
B. Inspect: Note general appearance of discomfort.
C. Palpate
   1. Abdomen: Note presence, frequency, intensity of uterine contractions and resting tone. Measure fundal height.
   2. Back: Check for CVA tenderness.
D. Auscultate: Auscultate the heart and lungs (especially if the patient is on tocolysis).
E. Sterile speculum exam: Evaluate rupture of membranes and vaginal discharge or bleeding. **If meconium-stained amniotic fluid is noted, immediately consult a physician and transfer the patient to a hospital. Note if meconium is thin or thick (thick meconium may be associated with breech presentation).**
F. Bimanual exam: If membranes are not ruptured, perform gentle bimanual examination: Note cervical dilation, effacement, station, cervical position, and softness of cervix.
G. Cervical exam during pregnancy: See the Section II Procedure, "Bimanual Examination: Cervical Evaluation During Pregnancy." **Do not perform a digital examination of the cervix if premature rupture of membranes (PROM) is present without active labor.**

Diagnostic Tests

A. WBC, if indicated.
B. Urine dipstick for ketones, leukocyte, esterase, protein, and nitrite.
C. Evaluate vaginal discharge for Ph with phenaphthazine (Nitrazine) tape.
D. Check ferning, if discharge is Nitrazine positive or if PROM is suspected.
E. Wet prep, if indicated.
F. Cervical cultures for STDs.
G. Cervical and rectal culture for group B strep.
H. Fetal fibronectin, where available.
I. Urine culture.
J. Ultrasonography: fetal biometry and dating, cervical length, amniotic fluid volume, biophysical profile, placental location, fetal presentation, ruling out fetal anomalies.
K. Fetal monitoring for contractions.

Differential Diagnoses

A. Preterm labor
B. Preterm, or Braxton Hicks, contractions, with no cervical change
C. Incompetent cervix
D. Preterm rupture of membranes
E. Low back muscle strain
F. Pyelonephritis or UTI
G. Placenta previa
H. Abruptio placentae
I. Gastroenteritis
J. Vaginal infection
K. Maternal dehydration
L. Ketoacidosis

Plan

A. General interventions
   1. Regular uterine contractions with cervical dilation or effacement, with pressure on the lower uterine segment, strongly indicates preterm labor (PTL).
   2. If the cervix is dilated more than 3 cm with contractions upon presentation, the patient is probably having preterm labor. Consult with a physician for hospital admission and tocolysis candidacy.
   3. If the patient is symptomatic with a positive fetal fibronectin test, consult with a physician for maternal transfer to a hospital equipped to care for preterm infants.
B. Second trimester: If the patient shows signs and symptoms of PTL, consider diagnosis of incompetent cervix. Refer the patient to a physician for ultrasonography for cervical length and possible cerclage placement.
C. Outpatient management
   1. Education: see the Section III Patient Teaching Guide for this chapter, "Preterm Labor."
   2. Outpatient bed rest.
   3. Outpatient tocolysis therapy.
   4. Frequent cervical exams, weekly.
   5. Prophylactic treatment against infection.
   6. Administer corticosteroids to enhance fetal lung maturity if less than 34 weeks' gestation. Observe the patient for contractions in the office or have her use a uterine monitoring system at home.

7. Fetal fibronectin testing, where available, using American College of Obstetrics Guidelines.

D. Inpatient management of PTL
1. Observation, possibly with IV hydration.
2. Cervical cerclage.
3. Prophylactic treatment against infection (group B *Streptococci*) until urine and cervical culture results are available.
4. Parenteral tocolysis either to stop PTL or delay delivery long enough to allow transfer to a facility with the ability to care for preterm infants.
5. Administer corticosteroids to enhance fetal lung maturity if less than 34 weeks.
6. Transport the patient to a perinatal center for neonatal care.

E. Patient teaching: See the Section III Patient Teaching Guide for this chapter, "Preterm Labor."

F. Pharmaceutical therapy
1. Tocolytics are generally prescribed from 24–34 weeks' gestation. If the patient is on oral tocolytics, pulse should be less than 120 bpm and lungs should be clear to auscultation; the patient is at risk for pulmonary edema.
2. Suspect pulmonary edema if the patient has pulse greater than 120 bpm, chest pain, shortness of breath, persistent cough, and crackles noted with auscultation.
3. Corticosteroids
   a. Steroids are given to enhance lung maturity in the fetus.
   b. This may be repeated weekly.

Follow-up

A. Depending on the clinical scenario, the patient may need to be seen weekly or biweekly. Fetal fibronectin test may be repeated every 2 weeks. Repeat cultures as indicated, discontinuing antibiotics if cultures are negative. Encourage close phone contact with the patient regarding questions or concerns.

▐ GESTATIONAL DIABETES MELLITUS (GDM)

Definition

A. Gestational diabetes mellitus is abnormal carbohydrate metabolism diagnosed during pregnancy.

Incidence

A. Gestational diabetes (GDM) affects 4% of all pregnancies and occurs 10 times more frequently than overt Type 1 or Type 2 diabetes. It usually resolves after pregnancy.

Pathogenesis

A. Insulin antagonism caused by the placental hormones leads to gestational diabetes. As greater amounts of these hormones are produced with advancing gestation, the diabetogenic effect of pregnancy becomes more pronounced, reaching significant levels in the second trimester. Women with GDM are at risk for later development of Type 1 and, more commonly, Type 2 diabetes. Gestational diabetes may actually be the expression of pregnancy-induced stresses on carbohydrate metabolism in the genetically predisposed patient. Some women have undiagnosed Type 2 diabetes prior to pregnancy.

Predisposing Factors

In Latin American and American Indian populations, almost half of all patients with GDM lack specific risk factors. Factors include the following:

A. Maternal age greater than 30 years
B. Obesity
C. Family history of diabetes
D. Previous birth of a macrosomatic, malformed, or still-born baby
E. Hypertension
F. Glycosuria
G. Previous gestational diabetes

Common Complaints

A. Common complaints of hyperglycemia include excessive thirst and excessive urination. However, gestational diabetes is often asymptomatic.

Other Signs and Symptoms

A. Glycosuria
B. Increased thirst
C. Increased urination
D. Size of fetus greater than average for gestational age
E. Frequent candidal infections
F. Rapid weight gain

Potential Complications

A. Ketoacidosis
1. May develop in GDM.
2. More common in insulin-dependent diabetes.
3. May develop with glucose levels barely exceeding 200 mg/dL.
4. May be present in an undiagnosed diabetic woman receiving β-mimetic agents (such as terbutaline) for tocolysis or steroids to enhance fetal lung maturity. **Fetal mortality rate is 50% in women who come to the hospital in DKA. Ketones cross the placenta.**
5. Therapy hinges on timely, aggressive volume resuscitation and correction of maternal metabolic derangements.

B. Polyhydramnios, or increased risk of premature rupture of membranes and preterm labor, may result from GDM.
C. Increased risk of traumatic birth injury is related to shoulder dystocia and asphyxia associated with fetal macrosomatia.
D. Increased risk for neonatal respiratory problems due to decreased development of lung maturity in the uterus.

Subjective Data

A. Review previous pregnancy history for two or more spontaneous abortions, previous stillbirths, or unexplained neonatal deaths.
B. Review birth weight (macrosomatia) and gestational age of previous children.
C. Review previous pregnancy history for polyhydramnios and/or congenital anomalies.
D. Review the patient's history for a predisposition to infections, especially urinary tract infections and candidal vaginitis.
E. Review previous pregnancy history for gestational diabetes, diet restrictions, and need for insulin therapy.

Physical Examination
A. Blood pressure and weight, blood pressure and pulse.
B. Inspect: Perform speculum exam for wet prep, if indicated.
C. Palpate: Check the patient's fundal height each visit after 20 weeks.
D. Auscultate fetal heart tones after 20-week gestation.

Diagnostic Tests
A. Diabetes screening between 24 and 28 weeks' gestation (earlier if indicated) **or if the patient has a previous history of GDM.**
B. Three-hour glucose tolerance test (GTT) if abnormal diabetes mellitus screen (DMS >129).
C. Day curves (fasting blood sugar [FBS] and pre- and postprandial blood glucose testing).
D. Hgb A1c.
E. Urine dipstick for glucose: Early glycosuria needs further evaluation (i.e., Hgb A1c, urine culture, random glucose "finger stick.").
F. Wet prep, if indicated.
G. Ultrasonography if fetal size is greater than average for gestational date to rule out twins, congenital anomaly such as atresia, and polyhydramnios.

Differential Diagnoses
A. Gestational diabetes
   1. Diabetes mellitus (Type 1)
   2. Diabetes mellitus (Type 2)

Plan
A. General interventions
   1. The American Diabetes Association recommends that all pregnant women be screened.
      a. Diabetes mellitus screen (DMS): 50-gram oral glucose tolerance test
         i. Administer 50-gram oral glucose load (fasting not required).
         ii. Draw blood for glucose assessment 1 hour after glucose load is given.
         iii. Typically performed between 24 and 28 weeks' gestation; performed earlier if the patient has glycosuria or if fetal size is greater than average for gestational date by fundal height measurement, or advanced maternal age.
         iv. Abnormal result is a glucose level 130–140 (use your institutional limits).
         v. Follow up all abnormal results with a 3-hour glucose tolerance test; if DMS is greater than 175 mg/dL, the patient may skip GTT and begin dietary modifications and glucose evaluation for insulin needs.
      b. Three-hour glucose tolerance test (GTT)
         i. The patient must follow a 3-day carbohydrate-loading diet, eating at least 150 g carbohydrates daily prior to the test date. She should have nothing by mouth except water from 10 PM the night before the test until the test is complete. (Four extra slices of bread per day for 3 days may be substituted for the 3-day carbohydrate loading diet.)
         ii. Draw fasting blood glucose first.
         iii. Administer 100-gram glucose load.
         iv. Draw blood for glucose assessment 1 hour, 2 hours, and 3 hours after glucose load is given.
         v. Plasma or serum glucose results:
            (a). Fasting = 95 mg/Dl
            (b). 1 hour = 160 mg/dL
            (c). 2 hours = 155 mg/dL
            (d). 3 hours = 140 mg/dL
         vi. If one or more values of 3-hour GTT are elevated:
            (a). Refer the patient for nutritional counseling. Once the patient is on the American Diabetes Association (ADA) diet, begin testing her weekly for fasting and 2-hour postprandial blood glucose measurements.
   2. Antepartum testing
      a. For women with well-controlled GDM, there is no national consensus with respect to criteria for initiation and timing of testing. Options include weekly biophysical testing beginning at 32–34 weeks. Begin BPP/NST testing at 40 weeks.
      b. For women with insulin-dependent gestational diabetes or whose condition is **not** well controlled, manage as if the patient had pregestational diabetes. Administer twice-weekly nonstress tests beginning by 32 weeks. If a patient's diabetes is poorly controlled, consider fetal assessment earlier and more frequently.
   3. Serial ultrasonography
      a. Evaluate fetal growth, estimate fetal weight, and detect polyhydramnois and malformations.
      b. Repeat at 4- to 6-week intervals to assess growth.
      c. Macrosomia is a leading risk factor for shoulder dystocia at vaginal delivery and cephalopelvic disproportion. Risk of complications rises exponentially when birth weight exceeds 4 kg.
   4. Postpartum contraception
      a. Low-dose oral contraceptives (OCs) may be used in women with GDM who do not have other risk factors.
      b. Rate of subsequent diabetes in OC users is not significantly different from those who do not use OCs.
      c. Consider serial measurement of total cholesterol, low-density lipoprotein, high-density lipoprotein, and triglycerides.
   5. Notify nursery staff of perinatal diabetes history, especially if the patient has a history of insulin-dependent diabetes, so that the neonate can be carefully monitored for hypoglycemia.
B. Patient teaching: Gestational diabetes requires intensive patient and family education to help reduce perinatal complications.
   1. Exercise
      a. If the patient had an active lifestyle prior to pregnancy, encourage her to continue a program of exercise approved for pregnancy such as walking or swimming for 20 min per day.

b. Upper extremity exercise in previously sedentary women with GDM may improve glycemic control.
2. Instruct the patient in self-monitoring blood glucose.
   a. Have her take measurement pre- or postprandially, or both. Fasting blood sugar should be less than 95 mg/dL. Postprandial values should be less than 120 mg/L at 2 hours postprandial.
   b. If the patient is taking multiple doses of insulin, she must take measurements more frequently.
3. See the Section III Patient Teaching Guides for this chapter, "Gestational Diabetes" and "Insulin Therapy During Pregnancy."

C. Dietary management: Place the patient on a diet that is prescribed for preexisting diabetes in pregnancy, such as the American Diabetes Association (ADA) diet, in the following amounts:
1. Current weight less than 80% ideal body weight (IBW): 35–40 kcal/kg/day.
2. Current weight 80%–120% IBW: 30 kcal/kg/day.
3. Current weight 120%–150% IBW: 24 kcal/kg/day.
4. Current weight greater than 150% IBW: 12–15 kcal/kg/day.
5. Dietary consumption should be 50%–60% carbohydrate, 20% protein, 25%–30% fat.

D. Pharmaceutical therapy
1. Insulin therapy is recommended if dietary management does not consistently maintain fasting glucose levels of less than 95 mg/dL. Two-hour postprandial values should be less than 120 mg/dL (see Figure 12.1).
2. While metformin is safe in some trimesters, insulin therapy is most commonly used.
3. In general, insulin therapy in pregnancy is no different from vigorous management of diabetes with insulin in nonpregnant women. Insulin does not cross the placenta.
4. Therapy must respond to the changing insulin requirements during pregnancy.
   a. Women with relatively simple insulin programs may require more complex regimens as the pregnancy progresses.
5. Intensive insulin therapy (as opposed to conventional therapy) is often required in pregnancy.
6. Human insulin (Humulin) is preferred over animal or synthetic insulin.

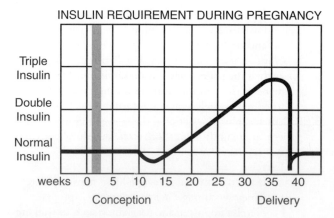

INSULIN REQUIREMENT DURING PREGNANCY

Figure 12.1 Insulin requirement during pregnancy.

7. Instruct the patient to report glucose values by telephone on at least a weekly basis.
8. The blood glucose values should be evaluated at least weekly to adjust to the patient's changing needs.

Follow-up
A. Weekly evaluation of day curves.
B. Fetal testing schedule.
C. For women who develop diabetes during pregnancy, give the patient 75-gram glucose load to evaluate for the development of Type 2 diabetes at the return postpartum visit at 6 weeks after delivery.

Consultation/Referral
A. Consult or comanage the patient with a physician as indicated and if GDM is not controlled by diet and exercise.
B. Refer to a dietician for nutritional consult for carbohydrate counting and teaching the patient dietary and lifestyle changes needed for tight glucose control.

PYELONEPHRITIS IN PREGNANCY

Definition
A. Pyelonephritis is an infection in one or both kidneys, usually involving the entire urinary tract. **Pyelonephritis may evolve into adult respiratory distress syndrome (ARDS) in pregnancy.**

Incidence
A. The incidence of pyelonephritis in pregnancy is 1%–2%. Most cases develop as a consequence of undiagnosed or inadequately treated lower urinary tract infection. Approximately 75%–80% of pyelonephritis cases occur on the right side, with a 10%–15% incidence on the left side. A small percentage of cases are bilateral.

Pathogenesis
A. *E. coli* is the main pathogen in pyelonephritis, though *Klebsiella pneumoniae* and *Proteus* species are also important causes of infection. Occasionally highly virulent gram-negative bacilli, such as *Pseudomonas, Enterobacter,* and *Serratia* are responsible (more commonly noted in immunocompromised patients). Gram-positive cocci do not usually cause upper urinary tract infections such as pyelonephritis. Anaerobes also are unlikely pathogens in pyelonephritis except in cases of chronic obstruction or instrumentation.

Predisposing Factors
A. Pregnancy, due to increased nutrient content of urine and urinary stasis facilitating bacterial growth
B. History of urinary tract infection, cystitis, and pyelonephritis
C. Sickle cell disease

Common Complaints
A. Fever
B. Chills
C. Flank pain or tenderness
D. Urinary frequency or urgency
E. Hematuria and dysuria

Other Signs and Symptoms

A. UTI is associated with urinary frequency, urgency, and dysuria; hematuria; and suprapubic pain.
   1. Chemical reactions to deodorant or douches can affect urination.
   2. Patients with frequent pyelonephritis do **not** complain of frequency and dysuria.
B. Pyelonephritis is associated with fever, palpations, dizziness, backache, and urinary frequency.
   1. Hematuria may be present, especially if the patient has a history of a previous stone.
   2. Dysuria is not always present in upper tract infections.
C. Abdominal pain and uterine contractions, risk of preterm labor and birth.
D. Shortness of breath.

Potential Complications

A. Sepsis and septic shock
B. ARDS: mortality rate 50%–70%
C. Pulmonary embolus, usually presents as sudden onset CVA tenderness

Subjective Data

A. Elicit information on the onset, duration, and progression of symptoms.
B. Elicit problems with voiding. Ask the patient about urinary frequency, urgency, and dysuria.
C. Ask the patient if she has experienced preterm contractions.
D. Ask if the patient is complaining of fever or chills.
E. Ask the patient if her urine has a bad odor.
F. Ask the patient if she has felt more tired than usual.
G. Ask the patient if she has felt more nauseated than usual, or if she has been vomiting.
H. Does she have a backache? Note location (unilateral or bilateral) and what, if anything, makes the backache better or worse.
I. Review the patient's history for sickle cell disease, if appropriate; has she been tested?
J. Review prenatal history for recurrent UTIs, previous pyelonephritis, and any abnormalities of the genitourinary (GU) tract.

Physical Exam

A. Check temperature, pulse, respirations, and blood pressure: fever greater than 100.4°F, tachycardia, tachypnea, hypotension associated with sepsis, septic shock, and ARDS.
B. Inspect: Note general appearance for respiratory distress.
C. Palpate
   1. Back: Check CVA tenderness (right CVA tenderness is more common in pregnancy).
   2. Abdomen
      a. Palpate for uterine tenderness and contractions.
      b. Palpate for suprapubic tenderness.
D. Auscultate
   1. Auscultate the lungs and heart.
   2. Auscultate the fetal heart rate.
E. Bimanual exam: Check for cervical dilation.

Diagnostic Tests

A. CBC with differential or WBC: leukocytosis with left shift on differential seen.
B. Blood culture, if indicated.
C. Respiratory function
   1. ABGs, if indicated.
   2. Pulse oximetry, if indicated.
D. Renal function
   1. Urinalysis
      a. Check urinalysis for WBCs, RBCs, leukocyte esterase, and/or nitrites.
      b. Glucosuria may be normal in pregnancy due to decreased tubular capacity to reabsorb glucose. If it is consistently noted, further testing is needed.
      c. Proteinuria is **not** normal during pregnancy. All cases warrant further investigation.
   2. Urine culture and sensitivity: greater than 100,000 colonies/mL indicate urinary tract infection.
   3. Intravenous pyelogram (IVP), if indicated.
   4. Renal ultrasonography, if indicated.

Differential Diagnoses

A. Pyelonephritis
B. Cystitis
C. Urethritis
D. Urethral stricture
E. Urolithiasis
F. Genital infection
G. Chorioamnionitis
H. Septic abortion
I. Postpartum endometritis
J. Muscular strain
K. Pulmonary embolus
L. Severe upper respiratory tract infection
M. Postprocedural dysuria or urinary frequency (i.e., following bladder catheterization or cystoscopy)
N. Chemical irritants
O. Postpartum septic pelvic thrombophlebitis
P. Renal calculi

Plan

A. General interventions
   1. Rule out other sources of infection.
   2. Assess for preterm labor.
B. Patient education: See the Section III Patient Teaching Guide for this chapter, "Urinary Tract Infection During Pregnancy: Pyelonephritis."
C. Dietary management
   1. Advise the patient to eat a regular diet as tolerated.
   2. Encourage her to drink 8–10 glasses of water a day.
   3. Warn the patient to avoid beverages with caffeine. One hundred percent cranberry juice and cranberry and blueberry capsules are good for urinary tract problems.
D. Pharmaceutical therapy
   1. Broad spectrum antibiotic coverage until cultures and sensitivity results are back.
   2. Drug of choice:
      a. Nitrofurantoin (Macrobid) 100 mg orally every 12 hours for 7–10 days.
      b. Nitrofurantoin macrocrystals (Macrodantin) 100 mg orally every 6 hours for 7–10 days.

3. If dysuria is present: phenazopyridine (Pyridium) 200 mg orally three times daily after meals for 3 days. Warn the patient that phenazopyridine (Pyridium) turns urine orange.
4. Alternative medications:
   a. Ampicillin 500 mg orally four times daily for 10 days.
   b. Cephalexin (Keflex) 500 mg orally four times daily for 10 days.

Follow-up

A. Once antibiotic therapy is initiated, most patients have a decrease in symptoms within 48 hours. By the end of 72 hours, almost 95% of patients are afebrile and asymptomatic.
B. The most likely causes of treatment failure are a resistant microorganism or obstruction; common causes of obstruction in pregnancy are urolithiasis or compression of the ureter by the gravid uterus.
C. Repeat a urine culture at a 2-week follow-up visit.
D. Recurrence rates are very high. After initial antibiotic therapy course is completed, consider a daily prophylactic dose of an antibiotic, such as nitrofurantoin (Macrodantin) 100 mg by mouth at bedtime for recurrent infections.
E. Patients receiving prophylactic antibiotics should have their urine screened for bacteria at each subsequent office visit and be questioned about the recurrence of symptoms.
F. If no prophylactic treatment is undertaken, obtain a urine culture if symptoms recur or if urine dipstick is positive for leukocyte esterase or nitrites.

◨ VAGINAL BLEEDING: FIRST TRIMESTER

Definition

Vaginal bleeding during the first trimester of pregnancy may range from spotting to massive hemorrhage (spontaneous abortion).

Types of abortion:

A. Threatened abortion: vaginal bleeding with absent or minimal pain **and** a closed, long, thick cervix.
B. Inevitable abortion: vaginal bleeding with pain and cervical dilation and/or effacement.
C. Spontaneous abortion: the nonviable products of conception are expelled from the uterus spontaneously.

Incidence

A. Vaginal bleeding occurs in approximately 50% of all pregnancies. Spontaneous abortion, a primary concern in the first trimester, occurs in about 30% of all pregnancies; most occur before the 16th week. Ectopic pregnancy occurs in 1 of every 200 pregnancies; 75% of pregnancies occurring after failure of tubal sterilization are likely to be ectopic.

Pathogenesis

A. Spontaneous abortion: The pathogenesis varies according to cause. In most cases, it is due to embryonic death with resultant decrease in hormone levels and subsequent sloughing of the uterine decidua. Many of the embryonic deaths occur due to chromosomal abnormalities that are incompatible with life.

B. Ectopic pregnancy: Fertilized ovum is prevented or slowed in its progress down the fallopian tube. Pregnancy is implanted outside of the uterus.

Predisposing Factors

A. Spontaneous abortion: in most cases, cause unknown
   1. Advanced maternal age (occurs more often in older women), suggesting that a genetic abnormality in the ovum may contribute
   2. Abnormal uterine environment
   3. Systemic disease
   4. Endocrine or nutritional problems
   5. Immunologic deficiencies
   6. Environmental factors, such as drugs, radiation, and trauma, may play a role.
B. Ectopic pregnancy: caused by previous damage to the fallopian tube; frequently caused by pelvic inflammatory disease, tubal surgery for infertility, or bilateral tubal ligation.

Common Complaints

A. Spontaneous abortion: Vaginal bleeding occurs that may or may not be associated with cramping or uterine contractions. When a pregnancy is greater than 8 weeks' gestation, the presence of uterine bleeding, uterine contractions, and/or pain are indications of a threatened abortion until proven otherwise.
B. Ectopic pregnancy: Vaginal bleeding and pelvic pain occur soon after the first missed period; the patient may be unaware of pregnancy. Sudden, acute, localized abdominal pain is associated with fallopian tube rupture.

Other Signs and Symptoms

A. *Threatened abortion:* Slight bleeding may be present over several weeks; cramping; no passage of tissue; positive pregnancy symptoms present including nausea, vomiting, fatigue, breast tenderness, and urinary frequency.
B. *Inevitable abortion:* Moderate to profuse vaginal bleeding occurs. Tissue may or may not be passed, uterine cramps or abdominal pain, symptoms of pregnancy may be decreased or absent.
C. *Incomplete abortion:* Moderate to profuse vaginal bleeding, sometimes for several weeks; reports of passage of tissue; painful uterine cramping or "contractions" and symptoms of pregnancy often absent.
D. *Complete abortion:* Profuse bleeding, passage of tissue and large clots, abdominal cramping or uterine contractions.
E. *Ectopic pregnancy:* Amenorrhea or irregular vaginal bleeding; abdominal pain is usually present, may be unilateral or generalized and may be associated with vertigo and syncope; shoulder pain, with irritation of phrenic nerve, may be present. Anxiety or palpitations are often noted.

Subjective Data

A. Elicit information about onset, duration, and progression of symptoms.
B. Ask the patient about vaginal bleeding. When did it start? Is it continuous bleeding, "like a period," or is it spotting? How much bleeding has occurred: how many pads have been saturated; what is the size of the blood spots? See Figure 12.2.

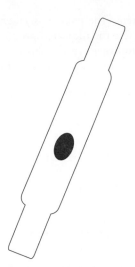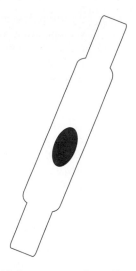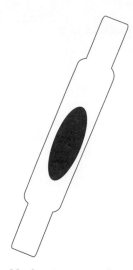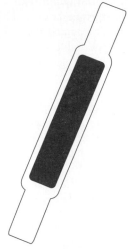

Scant amount: Blood only on tissue when wiped or less than 1-inch stain on peri pad.

Light amount: Less than 4-inch stain on peri pad.

Moderate amount: Less than 6-inch stain on peri pad.

Heavy amount: Saturates peri pad within 1 hour.

Figure 12.2 Estimation of vaginal bleeding.
From *The Lippincott Manual of Nursing Practice,* 9th ed., by S. Nettina, 2010. Philadelphia: Wolters Kluwer Health/Lippincott Williams & Wilkins.

C. What is her current method of birth control? Was the birth control method used consistently? Has she had a tubal ligation or recently used an intrauterine contraceptive device (IUD)?

D. Ask the patient the first day of her last menstrual period to date pregnancy. Did she have a positive pregnancy test? If so, when?

E. Does she have a history of previous ectopic pregnancy or pelvic inflammatory disease?

F. Question the patient regarding the presence or absence of abdominal and/or back pain. If present, is it a continuous discomfort, or intermittent cramping? Was the onset sudden? How severe is the pain?

G. Is she experiencing shoulder pain? This may be referred pain from phrenic nerve irritation due to intraperitoneal bleeding.

Physical Examination

A. Check temperature, pulse, respirations, and blood pressure: Note postural hypotension and tachycardia. Hemodynamic instability may be noted in cases of profuse bleeding; assess vital signs and be alert for hypotension, tachycardia, tachypnea, and/or labored breathing.

B. Inspect
1. Note general overall appearance of discomfort or pain before, during, and after examination.
2. Examine peri pad to determine amount of bleeding, if available.

C. Palpate
1. Perform abdominal examination for rebound tenderness, masses, softness, tenderness, or abdominal wall distension. Sudden, acute, localized abdominal pain with signs of internal hemorrhage suggest rupture of the fallopian tube.
2. Palpate uterine size. Measure fundal height for consistency with pregnancy dates. If fundal height suggests

pregnancy has advanced beyond first trimester, bleeding may be caused by abruption, placenta previa, or rupture of membranes with heavy bloody show.
3. Check iliopsoas and obturator muscle tests.

D. Auscultate: Auscultate the heart, lungs, and bowel sounds to rule out other abdominal problems.

E. Pelvic examination
1. Perform sterile speculum examination: Assess color and amount of bleeding. Tissue and the products of conception may be noted at cervical os or in vaginal vault. Assess for Chadwick's sign. The entire fetus may be noted in the vaginal vault; tissues that remain in the uterus may include portions of fetal membranes or placenta. Look for vaginitis/cervicitis and other signs and symptoms of infection that could be causing the bleeding.
2. Bimanual examination: Check Hegar's sign; elicit this sign cautiously, as false positive result may be related to a rough examination. Evaluate cervical dilation; cervical motion tenderness, often present with ectopic pregnancy; bulging cul-de-sac, which represents a hemoperitoneum. Adnexal mass is present in 50% of ectopic pregnancies.

Diagnostic Tests

A. Pregnancy test: Quantitative serum β human chorionic gonadotropin (HCG); serial tests at least 48 hours apart, making sure to perform test at same lab for accurate results.

B. CBC with differential and platelet

C. Blood type, Rh, antibody screen, and cross match if indicated

D. PT and PTT

E. Doppler ultrasonography for fetal heart tones, for fetuses greater than 11 weeks

F. Ultrasonography: transvaginal and/or abdominal

Differential Diagnoses

A. First trimester vaginal bleeding secondary to
1. Threatened abortion.
2. Inevitable abortion.
3. Incomplete abortion.
4. Complete abortion.
5. Septic abortion.
6. Ectopic pregnancy: There is strong suspicion of ectopic pregnancy or fallopian tube rupture if symptoms present with history of fallopian tube damage (i.e., tubal surgery for infertility, previous ectopic pregnancy), pelvic infection, or IUD use.
7. Hydatidiform mole.
8. Anovulatory bleeding with an antecedent period of amenorrhea.
9. Benign or malignant genital tract lesion.
10. Menstrual bleeding.
11. Genital trauma.
12. Advanced pregnancy with placenta previa or abruptio placentae.
13. Salpingitis.
14. Appendicitis.
15. IUD-related symptoms.
16. Pelvic inflammatory disease.

Plan

A. General interventions: Stabilize maternal condition and then determine the cause of bleeding.
1. Threatened abortion: Expectant management. Bed rest is often prescribed. Symptoms either subside, leading to normal gestation, or worsen, leading to inevitable abortion. If bleeding persists without leading to spontaneous abortion, the patient should be evaluated frequently, usually on a weekly basis, by means of ultrasonography to assess fetal viability. The patient should avoid intercourse and should not use tampons to absorb bleeding.
2. Inevitable abortion: Care may include expectant management or preparation for D and C.
3. Incomplete abortion: Prepare for suction and possible D and C.
4. Complete abortion: If abortion is complete and the products of conception are delivered with complete membranes present and cessation of bleeding has occurred, no surgical intervention is indicated. In these cases, the tissue specimens must be carefully examined for completeness. Send all specimens to the laboratory for further examination. If there is any question regarding complete passing of the placenta, do serial quantitative HCGs until back to nonpregnant levels.
5. Ectopic pregnancy: Consult with a physician regarding possible medical management with methotrexate or refer the patient to a physician for surgical intervention. The physician may perform culdocentesis to assess for hemoperitoneum. If the patient is in shock, resuscitation with intravenous fluids should be started immediately by means of two large-bore angiocatheters. Intravenous fluids such as lactated Ringer's solution or normal saline should be infused at a rapid rate. The patient is taken to the operating room, where the indicated procedure is one that controls hemorrhage in the shortest period of time. Salpingectomy and/or hysterectomy may be included.

B. Patient teaching: See the Section III Patient Teaching Guide for this chapter, "First Trimester Vaginal Bleeding."

C. Pharmaceutical therapy
1. $Rh_O(D)$ immune globulin should be administered to any Rh-negative patient.
2. Acetaminophen (Tylenol) or ibuprofen as needed for discomfort.
3. Ectopic pregnancy: Methotrexate is a folic acid antagonist that has been used to inhibit the growth of trophoblastic cells. This chemotherapy is the treatment of choice for ectopic pregnancy when surgery is contraindicated, or in the management of postoperative persistent trophoblast. Refer the patient to a physician to evaluate her for methotrexate or operative intervention. In most cases, operative intervention is required.

Follow-up

A. Threatened abortion: Follow the patient weekly to assess for interval growth and presence of fetal cardiac motion. Instruct the patient on perineal pad count.

B. Spontaneous abortion: Once the uterine contents have been evacuated, follow up with a 6-week postabortion visit, unless the situation warrants an earlier follow-up visit. Contraception needs to be discussed with the patient. Advise her it is best to wait for two or three menstrual cycles before becoming pregnant again.

C. Ectopic pregnancy: Once the ectopic pregnancy has been removed, the patient should be seen in 2–6 weeks for a postoperative examination, unless the situation warrants an earlier follow-up visit. If methotrexate is used do serial quantitative HCGs until they return to nonpregnant levels.

Consultation/Referral

Consult with a physician if the patient has any frank bleeding, signs of fetal compromise, or maternal shock, or if the cause of bleeding cannot be determined.

VAGINAL BLEEDING: SECOND AND THIRD TRIMESTER

Definition

Bright or dark red vaginal bleeding during the second or third trimester (>12 weeks gestation) may be painless, or it may be associated with uterine contractions or severe abdominal pain. Common causes of bleeding include:

A. Low-lying placenta: the edge of the placenta grows into the area of the lower uterine segment near the cervical os.

B. Placenta previa: implantation of the blastocyst occurs in the lower uterine segment followed by placental growth. Eventually the placenta may partially or completely cover the cervix.

C. Abruptio placentae: partial or premature separation of the placenta.

D. Uterine rupture: complete uterine rupture extends through the entire uterine wall, and the uterine contents are extruded into the abdominal cavity. Incomplete rupture extends through the endometrium and myometrium, but the peritoneum remains intact.

E. Uterine dehiscence: separation of an old surgical scar.

F. Bloody discharge is **not** normal prior to 37 weeks' gestation unless associated with recent sexual intercourse or pelvic exam. Light spotting or bleeding may be caused by recent sexual intercourse, preterm labor, rupture of membranes, or cervicitis.

Incidence

A. Placenta previa: approximately 1:200 pregnancies, more common in parous women.

B. Abruptio placenta: approximately 1:250 pregnancies.

C. Uterine rupture: if uterus is unscarred, incidence is approximately 1:16,849 pregnancies. If uterus has a scar (usually from a previous cesarean section), incidence is approximately 1:100 to 1:200.

Pathogenesis

A. Placenta previa: Placenta previa occurs from defective decidual vascularization, possibly resulting from inflammatory or atrophic changes.

B. Abruptio placenta: Abruptio placenta is initiated by bleeding into the decidua basalis. The decidua then splits, and the placenta is sheared off. Blood may move into and through the myometrium, leading to a board-like uterus.

C. Uterine rupture: Uterine rupture may occur from uterine injury, due to previous surgery or trauma, or anomaly.

Predisposing Factors

A. Placenta previa: late fertilization with delayed implantation, previous uterine scar, advanced maternal age, multiple gestation, large placenta, previous previa, and smoking.

B. Abruptio placenta: pregnancy-induced hypertension, cocaine use, maternal cardiovascular disease, trauma, high parity, sudden decompression of overdistended uterus (i.e., when membranes rupture), smoking, poor nutrition, chorioamnionitis, abdominal trauma, and cephalic version.

C. Uterine rupture: multiparity, previous uterine incision, tetanic contractions, or prolonged labor.

Common Complaints

A. Placenta previa: painless vaginal bleeding, usually in amounts of spotting to frank hemorrhage. Bleeding occasionally is accompanied by cramping or uterine contractions. A "gush" of fluid associated with sudden onset of massive vaginal bleeding may be reported. Painless vaginal bleeding should be treated as a placenta previa until proven otherwise.

B. Abruptio placentae
1. Marginal abruption: vaginal bleeding may be absent or minimal and bright red; there may be some old, dark blood. Abdominal pain is usually mild.

Vaginal bleeding with abdominal pain should be treated as an abruption until proven otherwise.

2. Moderate abruption: vaginal bleeding may be moderate or absent. Abdominal pain is usually significant and associated with contractions.

3. Severe abruption: vaginal bleeding may be moderate, severe, or absent. Abdominal pain is severe. **The patient may have a concealed placental abruption without vaginal bleeding.**

C. Uterine rupture: vaginal bleeding is moderate, severe, or absent. The patient may experience a sudden onset of extreme abdominal pain (commonly at the previous uterine scar site).

Other Signs and Symptoms

A. Nonreassuring fetal heart rate pattern may be seen on the fetal monitor that may include sinusoidal pattern associated with fetal anemia.

B. Placenta previa: uterine resting tone usually relaxed. Fetal status at first exam is usually stable. Recurrence of bleeding is common. First bleeding episode in placenta previa is rarely significant. Second or third bleeding episode is often associated with significant vaginal bleeding.

C. Abruptio placentae: rupture of membranes has bloody show with copious amounts of clear or greenish-brown fluid; the latter is probably meconium-stained fluid, which signifies fetal distress.
1. Marginal abruption: uterine resting tone is usually relaxed. Fetal status on the fetal monitor at first exam is usually stable. Labor progresses rapidly with vaginal bleeding or large amounts of bloody show.

2. Moderate abruption: uterine resting tone is hypertonic. At first exam, the fetus is usually alive. Fetal heart rate may be nonreassuring. Labor progresses rapidly with vaginal bleeding or large amounts of bloody show.

3. Severe abruption: uterine resting tone is hypertonic or "boardlike." At first exam, fetus is frequently dead. If fetus is alive, nonreassuring fetal heart rate pattern is common.

D. Uterine rupture: uterine resting tone may be normal or hypertonic. At first exam, fetus is frequently dead or fetal heart rate pattern is nonreassuring.

Subjective Data

A. Elicit information about onset, duration, and progression of vaginal bleeding. When did it start? Is it continuous bleeding, "like a period," or is it spotting?

B. Ask: How much bleeding has occurred: how many pads have been saturated? What is the size of the blood spots, the size of a quarter or a half-dollar?

C. Elicit information regarding the presence or absence of abdominal pain. If present, review the onset, duration, and progression of pain. Is it a continuous discomfort or intermittent cramping? How severe is the pain? Did it have a sudden onset?

D. Is the patient experiencing shoulder pain? This is likely to be referred pain from phrenic nerve irritation due to intraperitoneal bleeding.

E. Elicit the first day of patient's last menstrual cycle, to date pregnancy.

F. Ask the patient if she feels the baby move, if greater than 18 weeks' gestation.

Physical Examination

A. Check temperature, pulse, respirations and blood pressure; include fetal heart rate.
   1. A pregnant patient does not demonstrate signs and symptoms of hypovolemic shock until she has lost 30% of her circulating volume.
   2. Prepare the patient for emergency transport to a hospital even if she is hemodynamically stable.

B. Inspect: Inspect the patient's general appearance related to discomfort and pain. Observe bleeding characteristics and pooling.

C. Palpate
   1. Check for palpable fetal parts on abdominal wall; note fetal movement.
   2. Palpate the uterus for relaxed or hypertonic uterus. Check for contractions. If present, note frequency, duration, and intensity to palpation.

D. Auscultate
   1. Auscultate the abdomen; check fetal heart tones, or external fetal monitor (EFM) for baseline and periodic fetal heart rate patterns.
   2. Auscultate the maternal heart and lungs.

E. Perform sterile speculum exam to look for the source of bleeding. **Do not perform vaginal bimanual exam until previa is ruled out.**

Diagnostic Tests

A. CBC and platelets.

B. PT, PTT, and fibrinogen.

C. Blood type, Rh status, and type and cross match if indicated.

D. Fetal cell stain, Kleihauer-Betke test. Fetal cell stain can determine the amount of fetal blood in the maternal circulation.

E. Determine if $Rh_O(D)$ immune globulin (RhoGAM) is indicated.

F. Ultrasonography.

G. Nonstress test/electronic fetal monitoring.

Differential Diagnoses

A. Placenta previ

B. Abruptio placentae

C. Uterine rupture

D. Ruptured vasa praevia

E. Rupture of membranes

F. Normal bloody show

G. Rectal hemorrhoidal bleeding

Plan

A. General interventions
   1. Tocolysis may be considered if the patient has no active hemorrhage and reassuring fetal heart rate pattern.
   2. If significant vaginal bleeding is present, the primary goal is to maintain oxygen delivery to the mother and fetus while preparing them for transport. Interventions include maternal positioning to avoid vena caval compression; administering supplemental oxygen; initiating large-bore intravenous line; delivery of fluid bolus of normal saline or lactated Ringer's solution; keeping flow sheet of vital signs, assessments, actions, and responses; maintaining continuous recording of fetal heart rate (FHR) and uterine activity on electronic fetal monitor; and providing emotional support and anticipatory guidance.
   3. If vaginal bleeding is minimal and home management is being considered, discuss risks with the patient and assess her ability to maintain bed rest. Also assess patient's access to telephone and transportation in case of major bleeding episode. Consider the distance from the patient's home to the nearest hospital.

B. Patient teaching: See the Section III Patient Teaching Guide for this chapter, "Vaginal Bleeding, Second and Third Trimester."

C. Pharmaceutical therapy for preterm placenta previa with preterm contractions
   1. Tocolysis options
      a. Terbutaline sulfate (Brethine) 0.25 mg by subcutaneous injection every 15 min times 3 doses if maternal heart rate less than 120.
      b. Terbutaline sulfate (Brethine) 2.5–5.0 mg orally every 4–6 hours, or every 4–6 hours as needed.
      c. Indomethacin 50 mg per rectum followed by 25 mg orally every 6 hours. **Note: Indomethacin should not be given after 32 weeks' gestation, and duration of indomethacin therapy should not exceed 72 hours.**
      d. The patient may be admitted to inpatient antepartum unit for parenteral tocolysis such as magnesium sulfate.
   2. Antenatal steroids may be given if preterm delivery is a possibility within the next week and the EGA is less than 34 weeks.
      a. Betamethasone 12.5 mg may be given by IM injection every 24 hours times two doses.
      b. Dexamethasone 8 mg orally every 12 hours times four doses.
      c. Either regimen may be repeated once a week.
   3. If the patient is Rh-negative, give her $Rh_Q(D)$ immune globulin (RhoGAM) IM by injection after each vaginal bleeding episode.
      a. Full dose $Rh_0(D)$ IM immune globulin, which is adequate.

Follow-up

A. Follow-up depends on patient diagnosis and whether patient hospitalization is needed.

Consultation/Referral

A. Consult a physician for all patients noted to have second and third trimester vaginal bleeding.

B. Consult with a physician if the patient has any frank bleeding, signs of fetal compromise, or maternal shock, or if the cause of bleeding cannot be determined and/or treated by the practitioner.

BREAST ENGORGEMENT

Definition
A. Breast engorgement is swollen, tender breasts caused by overfilling of milk, increased blood flow, and fluids in the breasts.

Incidence
A. Breast engorgement may affect 40% of postpartum mothers.

Pathogenesis
A. **Primary engorgement** is the result of distension and stasis of the vascular and lymphatic circulations occurring 2–4 days following delivery.
B. **Secondary engorgement** is due to distension of the lobules and alveoli with milk as lactation is established. Without stimulation by suckling and removal of milk, secretion of prolactin decreases and milk production decreases and finally ceases.

Predisposing Factors
A. Engorgement often develops if early feedings are not frequent enough, suckling is inadequate, or if breast-feeding is not conducted in a relaxing atmosphere. Engorgement is more likely to develop sooner and more intensely in mothers who have breast-fed a prior child.

Common Complaints
A. Swollen, tender breasts
B. Discomfort when breast-feeding
C. A low-grade fever lasting between 4–16 hours

Other Signs and Symptoms
A. Pain, tenderness, and redness in one area of the breast is associated with mastitis.
B. Physical examination should not be focused just on breast symptoms but should include a general ruling out of other potential problems, such as coexistent urinary tract infection.

Subjective Data
A. Elicit onset, duration, and course of symptoms. Review the frequency of breast-feeding and/or use of breast pump. Is the patient still breast-feeding, or has she stopped due to the discomfort?
B. Exclude other causes of fever, such as UTI, wound infection, and red streaks on one or both breasts, to rule out mastitis.
C. Quantify pain symptoms and relief measures including heat packs, ice packs, breast binder, and analgesics such as Tylenol.

Physical Examination
A. Temperature, blood pressure, and pulse.
B. Inspect: Examine the breasts for erythemic streaks on breasts. Check episiotomy or abdominal incision, if indicated.
C. Palpate:
   1. Examine the breasts for tenderness, hardness, warmth, and lumps.
   2. Palpate axilla for lymphadenopathy.
   3. Check back for CVA tenderness.

Diagnostic Tests
A. Tests generally are not indicated for breast engorgement.
B. Urine culture or wound culture, if applicable.

Differential Diagnoses
A. Breast engorgement
B. Mastitis

Plan
A. General interventions
   1. Encourage the patient to take analgesics prior to breast-feeding (see "Pharmaceutical Therapy" section) and continue breast-feeding.
   2. Encourage ice packs for discomfort and breast-feeding frequently. There should be *no stimulation* to the breasts other than that provided by the baby when nursing, and the patient should take analgesics for discomfort. Reassure her that engorgement is temporary and usually resolves within 24–48 hours.
B. Patient teaching: See the Section III Patient Teaching Guide for this chapter, "Breast Engorgement and Sore Nipples."
   1. Educate the patient regarding milk production.
   2. Advise the patient to breast-feed frequently to reduce chances of engorgement.
   3. Provide reassurance and support for the patient to continue breast-feeding through this temporary period of discomfort. Engorgement may last 2–3 days before milk supply meets demand and continuation of breast-feeding will resolve discomfort and problem.
C. Pharmaceutical therapy: Acetaminophen (Tylenol) two tablets 500–1,000 mg every 4–6 hours, or ibuprofen 400–600 mg orally 30–45 min prior to breast-feeding and as needed.

Follow-up
A. Follow-up may not be required for engorgement.
B. Lactation consultation if indicated.

Individual Considerations
A. Pregnancy loss: It is imperative to discuss breast care and engorgement with women who have a second trimester termination of pregnancy, have a stillbirth, or experience a neonatal loss.

ENDOMETRITIS

Definition
A. Endometritis is an infection of the endometrium (the interior lining of the uterus) that occurs postpartum. Endometritis is the most common cause of puerperal fever in obstetrics.

Incidence
A. The incidence of endometritis has been noted as high as 38.5% after cesarean section; the incidence is 1.2% after vaginal delivery.

Pathogenesis
Onset is usually 3–5 days after delivery, unless it is caused by β-hemolytic streptococcus, in which case the onset is earlier

and more precipitous. Infection is usually polymicrobial in nature. Undiagnosed or unsuccessfully treated infection of the endomyometrium can progress to involve the entire uterus and may spread to accessory pelvic structures. The main pathway for spread of the infection is the broad ligament. Sources of bacteria may be any one or a combination of the following:

A. Endogenous vaginal bacteria, usually pathogenic only when tissue is damaged
   1. β-Hemolytic streptococcus.
   2. *Streptococcus viridans.*
   3. *Neisseria gonorrhoeae.*
   4. *Gardnerella.*
B. Contamination by normal bowel bacteria
   1. *Clostridium perfringens.*
   2. *Escherichia coli.*
   3. *Proteus mirabilis.*
   4. *Aerobacter aerogenes.*
   5. *Enterococcus.*
   6. *Pseudomonas aeruginosa.*
   7. *Klebsiella pneumoniae.*
C. Contamination from environment; staphylococcus is a common organism.

Predisposing Factors

A. Operative delivery: Cesarean section is the major predisposing factor for pelvic infection. The most important determinant of infection for patients undergoing cesarean delivery is the duration of labor.
B. Intrapartum: Prolonged rupture of membranes, numerous vaginal exams in labor, use of internal monitoring devices during labor, use of instruments in delivery, prolonged labor, intrauterine manipulation such as internal rotation or manual removal of placenta can all lead to endometritis.
C. Postpartum: Retained placental fragments or membranes, improper perineal care, and host resistance also predispose a patient to infection.
D. Anemia: This probably represents a marker for poor nutrition.
E. Obesity.

Common Complaints

A. "Feeling ill" with fever or chills
B. Muscle aches
C. Headache
D. Uterine pain and tenderness
E. Foul-smelling lochia

Other Signs and Symptoms

A. Fever (100.4°F–104.0°F).
B. Subinvolution.
C. Uterus may be atonic.
D. Abnormalities of lochia
   1. May be scant and odorless if anaerobic infection.
   2. May be moderately heavy, foul, bloody, or seropurulent if aerobic infection.

Subjective Data

A. Elicit onset, duration, and course of symptoms.
B. Review the color, odor, and amount of lochia.

C. Review the patient's pain or discomfort and the relief measures used.
D. Review other body symptoms to rule out other infections such as UTI, breast engorgement, or mastitis.
E. Review labor and delivery events for complications (see "Predisposing Factors").

Physical Examination

A. Temperature, pulse, and blood pressure: The patient may be tachycardic with heart rate 100–140 bpm.
B. Inspect: Observe color, amount, and odor of lochia. Check abdominal incision, if applicable. Check the perineum for lacerations, breakdown of incision, redness, and drainage.
C. Palpate
   1. Palpate the abdomen; check uterine tenderness.
   2. Palpate the back; check CVA tenderness.
D. Auscultate: Auscultate the heart and lungs.
E. Speculum exam: Inspect the cervix for lacerations, drainage, or redness.
F. Bimanual exam: Check for cervical motion tenderness; palpate adnexa for masses and tenderness; note "heat" of the pelvis.

Diagnostic Tests

A. CBC with differential
B. Blood and urine cultures
C. Cervical cultures, to rule out a sexually transmitted infection (STI), if indicated
D. Wet prep, if indicated

Differential Diagnoses

A. Endometritis
B. Sexually transmitted diseases, such as chlamydia, gonorrhea, or Trichomoniasis
C. Septic pelvic thrombophlebitis
D. Urinary tract infection/pyelonephritis
E. Pneumonitis
F. Extreme breast engorgement "milk fever"
G. Wound infection

Plan

A. General interventions
   1. Instruct on proper hygiene. Teach the patient proper techniques to prevent infection (perineal area, incision site, breast).
   2. Acetaminophen (Tylenol) for fever as needed.
B. Patient teaching: See the Section III Patient Teaching Guide for this chapter, "Endometritis."
C. Pharmaceutical therapy
   1. Antibiotic therapy
      a. Augmentin 500 mg orally four times daily for 10 days.
      b. If the patient is allergic to penicillin and not breast-feeding, doxycycline 100 mg orally every 12 hours for 7 days.
      c. If the patient is allergic to penicillin and breast-feeding, cephalexin (Keflex) 500 mg orally four times daily for 7 days.
      d. Rocephin/ceftriaxone 250 mg IM times 1 with Flagyl 500 mg by mouth twice a day for 7 days

(if breast-feeding pump and dispose of breast milk during treatment)

2. If uterus is boggy and/or bleeding is excessive: methylergonovine maleate (Methergine) 0.2 mg orally every 4 hours for six doses. (Do not give if the patient is hypertensive.)

Follow-up
A. Call the patient in 24–48 hours to evaluate her status.
B. Instruct the patient to call if symptoms do not resolve within 24 hours or if they worsen.

Consultation/Referral
A. Consult with physician if symptoms do not resolve, if they worsen within 24 hours, or if the patient's temperature does not go below 100.0°F after 48 hours on antibiotics. If no significant improvement is seen within 2–3 days, the patient may need to be admitted to the hospital.

HEMORRHAGE, LATE POSTPARTUM

Definition
A. Late postpartum hemorrhage is blood loss of 500 mL or more after the first 24 hours of delivery and within 6 weeks of delivery.

Incidence
A. Incidence is approximately 0.7%.

Pathogenesis
A. Hemorrhage may result from retained placental fragments, subinvolution of the uterus, and/or intrauterine infection.

Predisposing Factors
A. Abnormally adherent placenta
B. Prolonged rupture of membranes leading to infection
C. Overdistended uterus from multiple gestation, and polyhydramnios
D. Hematoma

Common Complaints
A. Heavy red bleeding, or slow reddish-brown oozing
B. Abdominal pain
C. Loss of appetite
D. Fatigue; cannot get enough rest and is unable to complete self-care and child-care activities

Other Signs and Symptoms
A. Lochia rubra is bright-red discharge immediately after delivery (1–3 days) and may contain a few small clots. A continuous trickle of bright-red blood suggests a laceration of the cervix or vagina. Saturation of one perineal pad in less than 15 min (two pads in 30 min, or rapid pooling of blood under the buttocks) is considered excessive bleeding and requires immediate attention.
B. Foul odor: Lochia should not be malodorous. Lochia usually has a "fleshy" odor.
C. Boggy uterus: Check the consistency of the uterus, whether it is firm or boggy. If atony is present, support the lower uterine segment, and massage the uterus or do bimanual compression.
D. Faintness.
E. Tachycardia.
F. Hypotension.

Subjective Data
A. Elicit onset, duration, and course of symptoms.
B. Elicit the amount and color of lochia, including size of blood clot(s).
C. Review symptoms of infection including fever and malodorous lochia.
D. Review labor and delivery events including the date of delivery, use of forceps, or vacuum, weight of baby, manual removal of placenta, complications, and postpartum course.
E. Review pregnancy for predisposing factors such as multiple gestation, polyhydramnios, and so on (as noted above).

Physical Examination
A. Temperature, blood pressure, pulse and respirations.
B. Inspect
   1. Note color and amount of vaginal bleeding. See Figure 12.2.

Lochia may appear heavier when the woman first stands up because the lochia pools in the vagina while she is recumbent. Once the pooled blood is discharged, lochial flow should return to normal.

   2. Inspect episiotomy or abdominal incision.
C. Palpate
   1. Check for consistency of uterus, massaging uterus if boggy.
   2. Express clots, if applicable.
   3. By 2 weeks postpartum, the uterus should have involuted and once again be a "pelvic organ."
   4. Check abdominal tension.
D. Speculum exam: Assess cervical lacerations.
E. Bimanual exam: Rule out retroperitoneal hemorrhage.

Diagnostic Tests
A. Hematocrit or CBC with differential.
B. If bleeding is not under control, type and cross match blood.
C. Coagulation test, if disseminated intravascular coagulation (DIC) is suspected.
D. Blood cultures to rule out infection.

Differential Diagnoses
A. Late postpartum bleeding
B. Normal postpartum bleeding
C. Postpartum infection

Plan
A. General interventions
   1. Perform uterine massage: Support the lower uterine segment during massage to prevent uterine prolapse.
   2. Give IV hydration for hypovolemic shock: hypotension, tachycardia, and faintness.
   3. Hospitalization is usually required for postpartum hemorrhage.

4. Encourage breast-feeding (if applicable) to increase uterine contraction.

5. Advise the patient to rest and increase oral fluids.

B. Pharmaceutical therapy

1. Drug of choice: methylergonovine maleate (Methergine) 0.2 mg orally every 4 hours for six doses. **Do not give if the patient is hypertensive.**

2. For severe hemorrhage

   a. Oxytocin (Pitocin) 10–20 units to 1,000 cc IV fluids.

   b. Methylergonovine maleate (Methergine) 0.2 mg by IM injection, if the patient has no history of hypertension. Advise the patient to take full course of Methergine even if bleeding stops.

   c. **Hemabate: 250 mcg, may repeat every 15–90 min as needed.**

   d. Continue bimanual compression, and notify a physician.

3. If infection is suspected or confirmed, antibiotics are prescribed.

Follow-up

A. Reevaluate the patient 1 week from the date of discharge from the hospital.

B. Repeat hematocrit at postpartum visit.

C. The patient may need iron-replacement therapy, if not already prescribed. If stable at 1-week follow-up visit, have the patient return in 4–6 weeks postpartum for routine postpartum exam.

Consultation/Referral

Immediately consult or refer the patient to a physician for possible hospitalization for dilatation and curettage (D & C).

MASTITIS

Definition

A. Mastitis is an infection of breast tissue with potential for abscess formation.

Incidence

A. Mastitis occurs in 1%–2% of nursing mothers. Ten percent develop abscesses that must be surgically drained. Symptoms seldom appear before the end of the first week postpartum and are most often seen during the first 2 months postpartum.

Pathogenesis

A. During the period of lactation, the breast changes from an essentially nonfunctioning organ to a complex functioning organ of the body. The developing multiductal system becomes a rich environment for the growth of bacteria. The most common offending organism is *Staphylococcus aureus* (95%). The immediate source of the organisms that cause mastitis is almost always the nursing infant's nose and mouth.

Predisposing Factors

Invasion of bacteria in the presence of breast injury including:

A. Bruising from rough manipulation (pumping) or failing to break the neonate's attachment to the areola and nipple before removing from breast

B. Breast engorgement

C. Milk stasis in a duct

D. Cracking or fissures of the nipple

E. Poor hand washing

Common Complaints

A. Breast engorgement, usually bilateral

B. Pain in the breast, usually unilateral

C. Fever

D. Red streak(s)

E. Flulike symptoms: body aches, headache, malaise, and chills

Other Signs and Symptoms

A. Fever: 100.0°F–104.0°F, rapid rise

B. Exquisitely tender breast tissue

C. Hard mass in the breast

D. Tachycardia and tachypnea

E. Axillary lymphadenopathy

Subjective Data

A. Elicit the onset, duration, and course of symptoms.

B. Note the frequency and length of time of the feeding or pumping.

C. Are there any red streaks on the breasts?

D. Are the nipples cracked and bleeding?

E. Quantify pain symptoms, relief measures tried, and results.

F. Review other symptoms to rule out other infections, such as wound infection, episiotomy breakdown, and urinary tract infection.

Physical Examination

A. Temperature and blood pressure, pulse and respirations.

B. Physical exam should not be focused just on breast symptoms but should include a general ruling out of other potential problems, such as coexistent urinary tract infection or endometritis.

C. Inspect

   1. Visually inspect breasts.

   2. Perform breast exam.

   3. Check episiotomy or abdominal incision to rule out infection.

D. Palpate

   1. Perform breast exam. Observe a breast-feeding for adequacy of latch, suck, swallow, jaw glide, and any clicking.

   2. Palpate lymph modes of the neck and axilla.

   3. Palpate the abdomen.

   4. Check CVA tenderness.

E. Auscultate: Auscultate the heart and lungs.

Diagnostic Tests

A. Treatment is usually initiated based on symptoms and exam.

B. CBC: leukocytosis in peripheral smear.

C. WBC, culture and sensitivity of breast milk to identify bacteria for persistent signs of infection or if antibiotic treatment unsuccessful.

D. Urine or wound cultures, if applicable.

Differential Diagnoses

A. Mastitis: fever, chills, and malaise in conjunction with unilateral breast pain
B. Breast engorgement: bilateral presentation of breast discomfort
C. Breast abscess: discharge of purulent exudate from nipple, masses, or reddened areas that develop a bluish hue of the skin over the area of abscess
D. Clogged milk duct
E. Viral syndrome

Plan

A. General interventions: Encourage self-care and support. Advise the family to assist the patient with self-care and infant care during this acute period. The woman may feel extremely ill for the first 24–48 hours of therapy and may find it difficult to continue breast-feeding, self-care, and newborn care activities.
B. Patient education
1. See the Section III Patient Teaching Guides for this chapter, "Mastitis" and "Breast Engorgement and Sore Nipples."
2. Advise the patient to continue to breast-feed or pump to maintain milk supply.
3. Stress the importance of continuation of breast-feeding or pumping despite infection.
C. Dietary management
1. There are no dietary restrictions.
2. Have the patient increase fluid intake with increased temperature (at least 10–12 glasses a day).
3. Encourage her to eliminate caffeine, if possible, or use in moderation.
D. Pharmaceutical therapy
1. Antibiotics:
a. Drug of choice: dicloxaxillin 500 mg by mouth every 6 hours for 10 days.
2. Alternative drug therapy
a. Cephalexin (Keflex) 500 mg by mouth four times daily for 10 days.
b. Amoxicillin and clavulanate (Augmentin) 500 mg by mouth three times daily for 10 days.
3. Advise the patient to complete the full course of antibiotics even if symptoms are improved sooner.
4. Candidal vaginitis may develop secondary to antibiotic therapy. The patient should be aware of the signs and symptoms and treatment plan if it should occur.
5. Acetaminophen (Tylenol) or ibuprofen for pain management.
6. The patient may require pain medication if acetaminophen (Tylenol) or ibuprofen is not effective. Acetaminophen with codeine phosphate (Tylenol No. 3) or propoxyphene napsylate (Darvon-N) 100 mg 1–2 tablets every 3–4 hours as needed for pain may be prescribed.

Follow-up

A. Evaluate the patient in 48 hours if a breast abscess is suspected; assess need for surgical consultation.

Consultation/Referral

A. Consult a physician if a breast abscess is suspected, for persistent signs of infection, or if antibiotic treatment is unsuccessful. Treatment of a breast abscess may include surgical incision and drainage of the abscess.
B. Notify the baby's provider if mastitis is diagnosed.

POSTPARTUM CARE: SIX WEEKS POSTPARTUM EXAM

A. History
1. Chart review
a. Antepartum course, including prenatal laboratory data: Pap smear, cervical cultures, maternal blood type and Rh, rubella and syphilis screen, and CBC
b. Intrapartum course: length of labor, type of delivery, and any maternal complications
c. Neonatal course: gestational age, weight, length, cord gases, admission to normal or intensive care nursery, length of stay in the intensive care nursery, and any neonatal complications
d. Immediate postpartum course: postpartum recovery, any postpartum complications, laboratory data, and length of hospital stay
2. Interval history
a. Number of weeks postpartum
b. General maternal health and well-being including diet or appetite, bowel and bladder function, level of activity, sleep patterns, and pain or discomfort
c. Interval problems: calls to health care provider, visits to emergency room, fever, or illness
d. Adjustment and role adaptation to the baby: motherhood, fatherhood, sibling rivalry, psychosocial assessment of depression, family support, housing or financial issues
e. Resumption of sexual activity: when, problems encountered, comfort measures used, and type of contraception used
f. Family planning: previous method of contraception used, success of method, plans to resume contraception, and options for contraception
g. Status of infant: breast-feeding or bottle feeding, consolability, sleep patterns, voiding and stool patterns
h. Establishment of health care follow-up: pediatrician appointment, immunizations; referral to WIC, public health, and so on, if applicable, or follow-up with nurse practitioner or nurse-midwife
3. Review of relevant systems
a. Breasts: cracked or sore nipples, clogged ducts, engorgement, mastitis; breast care practiced
b. Bladder function: stress incontinence, dysuria, urinary frequency, and flank pain
c. Bowel function: constipation; discomfort, especially if the patient has a history of third- or fourth-degree laceration; relief measures used and results
d. Perineum: problems or discomfort at episiotomy site, problems with wound healing, and signs of infection

e. Lochia: duration, type, odor, presence of clots; or resumption of menses: date, duration, and amount

f. Abdomen: if cesarean delivery, healing of wound, signs of infection; exercises initiated

g. Legs: varicosities, heat, swelling, and calf tenderness

B. Postpartum physical exam
   1. Blood pressure and pulse; temperature, if indicated.
   2. Weight.
   3. Auscultate: Auscultate the heart and lungs.
   4. Breast exam: Examine nipple integrity, masses, inflammation, and engorgement.
   5. Palpate: Palpate the abdomen for tenderness, masses, involution of uterus; examine cesarean section incision for wound integrity and signs of infection.
   6. Examine legs for varicosities and signs of thrombophlebitis.
   7. Examine perineum, healing of episiotomy or lacerations, and abnormalities of Bartholin's gland.
   8. Speculum exam: Note lesions or lacerations of cervix, discharge, signs of infection; obtain Pap smear.
   9. Bimanual exam: Check for abnormalities of cervix, uterus, adnexa; status of involution; presence of cystocele or rectocele; and vaginal muscle tone.
   10. Rectovaginal exam: Check for integrity of episiotomy or laceration if indicated.

C. Laboratory data
   1. Pap smear
   2. Other tests as indicated; CBC if anemia or hemorrhage is documented or suspected

D. Patient teaching: This visit may be the last contact the woman has with the health care delivery system for some time. The practitioner should evaluate any problems and provide appropriate consultations, referrals, interventions, counseling, and teaching.
   1. Explain the necessity of a yearly gynecologic exam.
   2. Encourage regular aerobic, abdominal, and Kegel exercises.
   3. Counsel the patient on choice of contraception.
      a. Abstinence
      b. Natural family planning, calendar method
      c. Spermicides
      d. Barrier methods: condoms, cervical caps, diaphragm
      e. Intrauterine devices
      f. Oral contraceptives
      g. Tubal ligation
      h. Vasectomy
   4. Explain the benefits of a healthy diet, especially if the patient is breast-feeding.
   5. Discuss breast-feeding, if applicable; answer any questions, and address concerns.
   6. Instruct the patient in breast self-exam, and explain the importance of performing this monthly.

E. Follow-up
   1. Administer rubella vaccination if the patient has nonimmune status and administration of vaccine was missed in the hospital stay and she has not had unprotected intercourse since delivery.

2. If a woman's physical exam and laboratory and Pap tests are normal, she does not require a physical for 1 year.

3. Establish a plan for the woman to obtain Pap smear results (follow-up phone call or letter with results).

F. See the Postpartum Examination sheet (Exhibit 12.2) for documentation to use in the patient's chart.

POSTPARTUM DEPRESSION

Definition
A. Postpartum depression is a mood disorder characterized by unexplained tearfulness, sadness, irritability, and disturbances in appetite and sleep patterns, inability to care for self or baby, usually presenting within 2 weeks to 3 months postpartum.

Incidence
A. Reported incidence in the United States is between 10% and 26%.

Pathogenesis
A. It is believed that postpartum depression may be related to psychological, physiologic, and cultural factors. The extreme hormonal changes that occur during the postpartum period may contribute. Postpartum thyroiditis is also a suspected factor. However, no confirmed biologic cause has been found. Some authorities have suggested the mother's feelings of "loss of control" over her own life to be the underlying precipitating factor.

Predisposing Factors
The following may make a mother more likely to experience postpartum depression:

A. Preterm infant
B. Multiple gestation
C. History of postpartum depression or mental illness
D. Social stressors: dissatisfaction in the marriage, financial difficulties, and lack of support in the home
E. Age younger than 20 years
F. Single parent
G. Poor relationship with the father of the baby
H. Evidence of significant emotional problems in the past
I. Having experienced separation from one or both parents during childhood or adolescence
J. Having received poor parental support and attention in childhood or having limited social support in adulthood
K. Low self-esteem

Common Complaints
A. Insomnia
B. Poor appetite
C. Tearfulness
D. Fatigue
E. Anxiety
F. Headaches
G. Difficulty concentrating or confusion

Other Signs and Symptoms
A. Mood swings
B. Despondency, social withdrawal, and feeling of inadequacy

EXHIBIT 12.2 **Postpartum Examination**

Date: _____

History: Age: _____ G_____ PT_____P____ A___L _____

Labs: Blood type & Rh: _____ If negative, was Rhogam workup done and Rhogam given in the hospital if needed?

Rubella: _____ If nonimmune, was she immunized before hospital discharge?_____

Discharge HCT: _____

Medical and antepartum complications: _____

_____

Intrapartum course/complications: _____

_____

Delivery: Date: _____ Type: _____ Sex: _____ Birth weight: _____

Apgars: 1 minute: _____ 5 minutes: _____

Neonatal: Gestational age: _____

Complications: _____

Feeding: Breast/bottle: _____ Current infant status: _____

Surgery: Bilateral tubal ligation (BTL): Yes/No _____

If yes, pathology report reviewed: _____

Postpartum complications: _____

_____

Current status: Medical problems: _____

_____

Sexual intercourse since delivery/problems: _____

_____

Psychosocial/postpartum depression: _____

_____

Medications: _____

_____

Physical exam: B/P: _____ Pulse: _____ Resp: _____ Weight: _____

Breasts: _____

Pelvic: Episiotomy or laceration: _____

Abdomen: _____

Adnexa: _____

Uterus: _____

Vagina: _____

Cervix: _____

Pap smear: Date/results: _____

Plan: Contraception: _____

Referrals: _____

Labs: _____

New prescriptions: _____

Patient Teaching Guides: _____

Other: _____

Signature: _____

C. Guilt
D. Impaired memory
E. Ambivalence about motherhood and baby
F. Inability to care for self and baby
G. Poor grooming of self and/or baby

Subjective Data

A. Elicit onset, duration, and course of symptoms.
B. Review the patient's medical history for predisposing factors (see above).
C. Question the patient regarding her ability to care for her infant, herself, and other family members at home.
D. Review the amount of support in the home. Is she the primary caregiver? Are there any family members or friends that help in the household management, sibling child care, and newborn care?
E. Does the patient get out of bed and dress herself daily?
F. Does the patient have thoughts of harming the infant, herself, or others?

Physical Examination

A. Check temperature, pulse, respirations, and blood pressure.
B. Inspection: Note general overall appearance, including dress, makeup, neatness of hair, tearfulness, and apathy.
C. Observe her interaction with the baby, for example, talking to the baby and tone of voice, eye contact, and so on.

Diagnostic Tests

A. Diagnostic tools are available on the Internet including the Edinburgh Postnatal Depression Scale: http://www.fresno.ucsf.edu/pediatrics/downloads/edinburghscale.pdf
B. If depression is diagnosed, a thyroid profile should be ordered.

Differential Diagnoses

A. Postpartum depression
B. Baby blues: tearfulness, insomnia, fatigue, headaches, poor appetite, and so on; appearing between the birth and 14 postpartum days
C. Postpartum psychosis: extreme emotional lability, agitation, delusions, hallucinations, and sleep disturbances
D. Postpartum panic disorder: extreme anxiety, fear, tightness in the chest, and increased heart rate
E. Postpartum obsessive-compulsive disorder: obsessive thoughts of harming the child, exaggerated fear of being left alone with the infant, anxiety, depression, and/or unnecessarily vigilant protectiveness of the infant
F. Bipolar disorder

Plan

A. General interventions
   1. Assess all patients for postpartum mood disorders at postpartum and all postpartum contacts. See Exhibit 12.3: Kennerley Blues Questionnaire.
   2. Early assessment and treatment is very important. Symptoms that are not treated for several weeks may get progressively worse.
   3. Encourage involvement of the patient's partner and immediate family members in the counseling sessions

so they develop a full understanding of the disease process, learn how to help appropriately, and verbalize their own frustrations and concerns.
   4. If postpartum depression is diagnosed, thyroid levels need to be evaluated.
B. Patient teaching
   1. Advise the patient that she is not to blame for the condition, and that successful treatment is likely.
   2. Discuss participation in a support group.
   3. If prescribed advise the patient that antidepressants may take 4–6 weeks for peak effect. They may produce constipation.
C. Pharmaceutical therapy
   1. Antidepressants may be ordered for women with moderate to severe symptoms of depression when physical and emotional functioning have been compromised. (Refer to the section "Depression" in Chapter 20, "Psychiatric Guidelines."
   2. Citolopram (Lexapro) in a single daily dose, usually taken in the morning. Initial dose 10 mg/day; dosage can be increased at intervals of 1 week to 20 mg.
   3. Sertraline (Zoloft) 50 mg in a single dose at bedtime. Dosage can be increased up to 200 mg/day.
   4. Amitriptyline (Elavil) 75 mg/day in divided doses. Dosage can be increased up to 150 mg/day.

Follow-up

A. If the patient had risk factors for depression noted prior to delivery, a follow-up office visit 3–4 days after hospital discharge is suggested.
B. Frequent telephone contact, or several repeat visits, may be necessary during the course of the depression until the symptoms have improved.
C. Assess the patient for suicidal ideation and child neglect at every contact.

Consultation/Referral

A. Assess the need to refer the patient to a psychiatrist, psychologist, or family counselor.
B. Some patients benefit from group therapy.
C. Consult a psychiatrist about alternative antidepressant therapy if no decrease in signs and symptoms is seen.

Resources

Depression After Delivery patient education sheet from the University of Pittsburgh: http://www.upmc.com/HealthAtoZ/patienteducation/Documents/PostpartumDepression.pdf
Depression After Delivery (DAD) support group: 1-800-944-PPD (4773)
Pacific Postpartum Support Society: http://www.postpartum.org/
Postpartum Support Line: (604) 255-7999

WOUND INFECTION

Definition

A. Infection may occur at the site of cesarean section incision or episiotomy or genital tract laceration. Most wound infections become clinically apparent 5–6 days after delivery.

Incidence

A. Rates of infection after cesarean delivery range from 5–30 times greater than vaginal delivery.

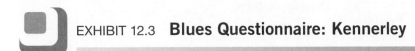

EXHIBIT 12.3 **Blues Questionnaire: Kennerley**

Name: _____ Days Postpartum: _____ Date: _____

Below is a list of words which newly delivered mothers have used to describe how they are feeling. Please indicate HOW YOU HAVE BEEN FEELING TODAY by ticking NO or YES. Then please mark the box which best describes how much there is, if any from your usual self.

	NO	YES	IS THIS	Much less than usual	Less than usual	No difference	More than usual	Much more than usual
Tearful			Is this					
Mentally tense			Is this					
Able to concentrate			Is this					
Low spirited			Is this					
Elated			Is this					
Helpless			Is this					
Finding it difficult to show your feelings			Is this					
Alert			Is this					
Forgetful, muddled			Is this					
Anxious			Is this					
Wishing you were alone			Is this					
Mentally relaxed			Is this					
Brooding on things			Is this					
Feeling sorry for yourself			Is this					
Emotionally numb, without feelings			Is this					
Depressed			Is this					
Over-emotional			Is this					
Happy			Is this					
Confident			Is this					
Changeable in your spirits			Is this					
Tired			Is this					
Irritable			Is this					
Crying without being able to stop			Is this					
Lively			Is this					
Over-sensitive			Is this					
Up and down in your mood			Is this					
Restlessness			Is this					
Calm, tranquil			Is this					

Used with permission. Kennerley, H., & Gath, D. (1989), Maternity Blues. I. detection and measurement by questionnaire. *British Journal of Psychiatry,* 155, 356–362.

Pathogenesis

A. A variety of organisms may be responsible. Examples include group A, B, and D streptococci; gram-negative bacteria such as *E. coli, Staphylococcus aureus, Clostridium, Peptococcus, Peptostreptococcus,* and *Mycoplasma hominis.*

Predisposing Factors

A. Obesity
B. Anemia
C. Malnutrition
D. Smoking
E. Diabetes
F. Substance abuse
G. Susceptible to infection
H. Poor hygiene
I. Lower socioeconomic status

Common Complaints

A. Redness, heat, swelling, and tenderness at site
B. Foul-smelling drainage
C. Elevated temperature

Other Signs and Symptoms

A. Fever and chills
B. Edema
C. Foul-smelling discharge and pus

Subjective Data

A. Elicit onset, duration, and course of symptoms.
B. Review medical history (see "Predisposing Factors"); antepartum history for complications such as diabetes; intrapartum complications for prolonged rupture of membranes, fever in labor, use of internal monitoring devices, length of labor, or frequent cervical examinations.
C. Question the patient regarding hygiene at wound site since delivery, including the frequency of changing perineal pads, use of sitz baths, and showering.
D. Question the patient regarding drainage from wound or episiotomy, noting color, amount, and odor.
E. Review signs and symptoms of breast engorgement and UTI.
F. Review vaginal delivery for third- and fourth-degree episiotomy.

Physical Examination

A. Check temperature, pulse, respirations, and blood pressure.
B. **Examination should not be limited to the incision site. A complete physical is needed to evaluate breasts, lungs, hematomas, and concurrent urinary tract infections.**
C. Inspect: Examine the incision site (episiotomy or abdomen) for drainage, redness or edema, and intactness.
D. Palpate
   1. Perform breast examination.
   2. Palpate suture line (episiotomy or abdomen). Probe incision with cotton-tipped swab to evaluate for hematoma, cellulitis, and/or pus.
   3. Palpate all abdominal quadrants.
   4. Palpate the vagina, to rule out concealed hematoma.
E. Auscultate: Auscultate the heart and lungs.
F. Percuss: Percuss the back to assess CVA tenderness.

Diagnostic Tests

A. CBC with differential
B. Blood culture (optional)
C. Culture of infected area
D. Urinalysis, culture and sensitivity, if indicated

Differential Diagnoses

A. Wound infection.
B. Impending dehiscence. If serosanguinous drainage is noted after the first 24 hours, dehiscence is possible.
C. Episiotomy breakdown.

Plan

A. General interventions
   1. The wound may need to be opened and cleaned.
   2. For an infection at a cesarean section site, wound irrigation and dressing changes several times a day may be necessary.
   3. Home health referral may be needed.
B. Patient teaching: See the Section III Patient Teaching Guide for this chapter, "Wound Infection, Episiotomy, and Cesarean Section."
C. Dietary management
   1. No dietary restrictions are recommended; encourage the patient to eat well-balanced meals. Increase protein in diet for wound healing.
   2. Instruct the patient to increase fluid intake; have her drink at least 10–12 glasses of liquid a day.
D. Pharmaceutical therapy
   1. Augmentin 875 mg twice a day for 7–10 days.
   2. Clindamycin 450 mg every 6 hours for 7–10 days. Safe for breast-feeding.
   3. Cefoxitin 1–2 g by IM injection or IV infusion every 6–8 hours. Safe for breast-feeding.
   4. Acetaminophen (Tylenol) when required for elevated temperature.

Follow-up

A. Reevaluate the patient in 48 hours to assess wound healing.

Consultation/Referral

A. Consult a physician for evaluation and possible surgical closure.

REFERENCES

American Association of Pediatrics and American College of Obstetricians and Gynecologists. (1997). *Guidelines for perinatal care* (4th ed.). Elk Grove Village, IL, and Washington, DC: Authors.

American College of Obstetricians and Gynecologists. (1990). Ectopic pregnancy. *ACOG Technical Bulletin,* Number 150.

American College of Obstetricians and Gynecologists. (1994a). Antenatal corticosteroid therapy for fetal maturation. *ACOG Committee Opinion,* Number 147.

American College of Obstetricians and Gynecologists. (1994b). Diabetes and pregnancy. *ACOG Technical Bulletin,* Number 200.

American College of Obstetricians and Gynecologists. (1995a). Preconceptional care. *ACOG Technical Bulletin,* Number 205.

American College of Obstetricians and Gynecologists. (1995b). Preterm labor. *ACOG Technical Bulletin,* Number 206.

American College of Obstetricians and Gynecologists. (1996). Hypertension in pregnancy. *ACOG Technical Bulletin,* Number 219.

American College of Obstetricians and Gynecologists. (1997). Fetal fibronectin preterm labor risk test. *ACOG Committee Opinion,* Number 187.

American College of Obstetricians and Gynecologists. (1998a). Post-partum hemorrhage. *ACOG Technical Bulletin,* Number 243.

American College of Obstetricians and Gynecologists. (1998b). Vitamin A supplementation during pregnancy. *ACOG Committee Opinion,* Number 196.

American College of Obstetricians and Gynecologists. (2001a). Assessment risk factors for preterm labor. *ACOG Practice Bulletin,* Number 31.

American College of Obstetricians and Gynecologists. (2001b). Gestational diabetes. *ACOG Practice Bulletin,* Number 30.

American College of Obstetricians and Gynecologists. (2003). Management of preterm labor. *ACOG Practice Bulletin,* Number 43.

American College of Obstetricians and Gynecologists. (2004). Nausea and vomiting in pregnancy. *ACOG Practice Bulletin,* Number 52.

American College of Obstetricians and Gynecologists. (2008). Anemia in pregnancy. *ACOG Practice Bulletin,* Number 95.

Anderson, F. W., Hogan, J. G., & Ansbacher, R. (2004). Sudden death: Ectopic pregnancy mortality. *Obstetrics & Gynecology, 103*(6), 1218–1223.

Association of Womens Health, Obstetric & Neonatal Nursing (AWHONN) and Johnson & Johnson Consumer Products. (1996). *Compendium of postpartum care* (pp. 1.17, 1.26–1.29, 1.32–1.33, 4.08–4.09, 5.08). Skillman, NJ: Johnson & Johnson.

Atterbury, J. L., Munn, M. B., Groome, L. J., & Yarnell, J. A. (1997). The antiphospholipid antibody syndrome: An overview. *Journal of Obstetric, Gynecologic, and Neonatal Nursing, 26*(5): 522–530.

Bassetti, M. (1996). Offering a head start to a healthy pregnancy. *Advances for Nurse Practitioners, 4*(7), 22–25.

Beck, C. T. (1995). Screening methods for postpartum depression. *Journal of Obstetric, Gynecologic, and Neonatal Nursing, 24*(4), 308–312.

Beck, C. T. (1998). A checklist to identify women at risk for developing postpartum depression. *Journal of Obstetric, Gynecologic, and Neonatal Nursing, 27*(1), 39–45.

Blackburn, S. T., & Loper, D. E. (1992). *Maternal, fetal, and neonatal physiology: A clinical perspective.* Philadelphia: W. B. Saunders.

Briggs, G. G., Freeman, R. K., & Yagye, S. J. (1994). *Drugs used in pregnancy and lactation* (4th ed.). Baltimore: Williams & Wilkins.

Bung, P., Artal, R., Khodiguian, N., et al. (1991). Exercise in gestational diabetes: An optional therapeutic approach? *Diabetes, 40*(Suppl. 2), 182–185.

Byrne, J., Flagaard-Tillery, K., Johnson, S., Wright, L., & Silver, R. (2009). Group A streptococci puerperal sepsis: Initial characterization of virulence factors in association with clinical parameters. *Journal of Reproductive Immunology, 82*(1), 74–83.

Cash, J. C. (1997). Assessment of the childbearing woman. In J. Weber & J. Kelley (Eds.), *Health assessment in nursing* (pp. 1021–1082). Philadelphia: Lippincott-Raven.

Catalano, P. (2007). Management of obesity in pregnancy. *Obstetrics & Gynecology, 109*(2, Pt. 1), 419–433.

deWeerd, S., Thomas, C., Cikot, R., Steegors-Theunissen, R., deBoo, T., & Steegers, E. (2002). Preconception counseling improves folate status for women planning pregnancy. *Obstetrics & Gynecology, 99*(1), 45–50.

Evans, M., Elixa, L., Landsverger, E., Olbrien, J., & Harrison, H. (2004). Impact of folic acid fortification in the united states: Markedly diminished high maternal serum alpha-fetoprotein values. *Obstetrics & Gynecology, 103*(3), 474–479.

Fuhrmann, K., Reiher, H., Semmler, K., Fischer, F., Fischer, M., & Glockner, E. (1983). Prevention of congenital malformation in infants of insulin-dependent diabetic mothers. *Diabetes Care, 6*(3), 219–223.

Hale, T. W. (2006). *Medications and mother's milk* (12th ed.). Amarillo, TX: Hale Publishing.

Hallak, M., Sharon, A., Diukman, R., et al. (1997). Supplementing iron intravenously in pregnancy: A way to avoid blood transfusions. *Obstetric Gynecology Survey, 52*(11), 666–667.

Hare, J. W. (1994). Diabetes and pregnancy. In C. R. Kahn & G. C. Wier (Eds.), *Joslin's diabetes mellitus* (13th ed., pp. 889–899). Philadelphia: Lea & Febiger.

Henry, T. K. (1997). Pesticide exposure seen in primary care. *Nurse Practitioner Forum, 8*(2), 50–58.

Hill, P. D., & Humenick, S. S. (1994). The occurrence of breast engorgement. *Journal of Human Lactation, 10*(2), 79–86.

Horowitz, I. R., & Gomelia, L. G. (1993). *Obstetrics and gynecology on call* (pp. 289–290). Norwalk, CT: Appleton & Lange.

Kriebs, J. M., & Gregor, C. L. (2005). *Varney's pocket midwife* (2nd ed.). Sudbury, MA: Jones & Bartlett.

Marchesi, D., Bertoni, S., & Maggini, C. (2009). Major and minor depression in pregnancy. *Obstetrics & Gynecology, 113*(6), 1292–1298.

National Institute of Child Health and Human Development Research Planning Workshop. (1997). Electronic fetal heart rate monitoring: Research guidelines for interpretation. *Journal of Obstetrics, Gynecologic, and Neonatal Nursing, 26*(6), 635–640.

Paramsothy, P., Lin, Y., Kernic, M., & Foster-Schubert, K. (2009). Interpregnancy weight gain and caesarean delivery risk in women with a history of gestational diabetes. *Obstetrics and Gynecology, 113*(4), 817–823.

Peaceman, A. M., Andrews, W. W., Thorp, J. M., et al. (1997). Fetal fibronectin as a predictor of preterm birth in patients with symptoms: A multicenter trial. *American Journal of Obstetrics and Gynecology, 177*(1), 13–18.

Perry, L. E. (1996). Preconception care: A health promotion opportunity. *The Nurse Practitioner, 21*(11), 24–41.

Physician ICD–9–CM. (1997). Salt Lake City: Medicode.

Riordan, J. M., & Nichols, F. H. (1990). A descriptive study of lactation mastitis in long-term breast-feeding women. *Journal of Human Lactation, 6*(2), 53–58.

Scoggin, J., & Morgan, G. (1997). *Practice guidelines for obstetrics and gynecology* (pp. 38, 123–125, 174–175, 202–203). Philadelphia: Lippincott-Raven.

Scott, J. R., DiSaia, P. J., Hammond, C. B., et al. (1994). *Danforth's obstetrics and gynecology* (7th ed.). Philadelphia: J. B. Lippincott.

Staff. (2009a). *Anemia in pregnancy.* Retrieved July 10, 2009, from http://www.cdc.org.

Staff. (2009b). *Gestational diabetes.* Retrieved July 9, 2009, from http://www.diabetes.org

Stone, R. (1996). Primary care diagnosis of acute abdominal pain. *The Nurse Practitioner, 21*(12), 19–41.

Timbers, K. A., & Feinberg, R. F. (1997). Recurrent pregnancy loss: A review. *Nurse Practitioner Forum, 8*(2), 77–88.

Tinkle, M. B., & Sterling, B. S. (1997). Neural tube defects: A primary prevention role for nurses. *Journal of Obstetric, Gynecologic, and Neonatal Nursing, 26*(5), 503–512.

Varney, H., Kriebs, J. M., & Gregor, C. L. (2004). *Varney's midwifery* (4th ed.). Sudbury, MA: Jones & Bartlett.

Villers, M., Jamison, M., Castro, L., & James, A. (2008). Morbidity associated with sickle cell disease in pregnancy. *American Journal of Obstetrics and Gynecology, 199*(2), 125:e1–125:e5.

Windsor, R. A., Dalmat, M. E., Orleans, C. T., et al. (1990). *The handbook to plan, implement and evaluate smoking cessation programs for pregnant women.* New York: March of Dimes Birth Defects Foundation.

Wong, A., Blumenfield, Y., El-Sayed, Y., & Druzin, M. (2008). 834: NST surveillance in a large university cohort-rates of nonreassuring tracings by indication. *American Journal of Obstetric and Gynecology, 199*(6, Supp. A), S35.

Gynecologic Guidelines

Rhonda Arthur

AMENORRHEA

Definition

Amenorrhea is absence of menstruation when menstrual periods should occur.

A. Primary amenorrhea
  1. No menstrual period by age 14 in the absence of growth or development of secondary sexual characteristics.
  2. No menstrual period by age 16 regardless of the presence of normal growth and development with the appearance of secondary sexual characteristics.
B. Secondary amenorrhea: No menstrual period for 6 months in a woman who usually has normal periods, or for a length of time equal to three cycle intervals in a woman with less frequent cycles.

Incidence

A. Amenorrhea in a woman who has had menstrual periods is quite common at some time during her reproductive life. Amenorrhea that is a result of agenesis of part of the reproductive system or a chromosomal anomaly is quite rare.

Pathogenesis

A. Physiologic: pregnancy, breast-feeding, and menopause.
B. Disorders of the central nervous system (hypothalamic): Hypothalamic amenorrhea is the most common cause of amenorrhea (28%). There is a deficiency in pulsatile secretion of gonadotropin-releasing hormone (Gn-RH). Examples include a stressful lifestyle (10%); weight loss as in anorexia or bulimia (10%); extreme exercise; medications such as hormones, as in postpill amenorrhea; hypothyroidism (10%); and major medical disease such as Crohn's disease or systemic lupus erythematosus.
C. Disorders of the outflow tract or uterine target organ: Abnormalities in the systems of this compartment are uncommon. Examples include Asherman's syndrome from inadvertent endometrial ablation during D and C (causes 7% of amenorrhea); and agenesis or structural anomalies of the uterus, tubes, or vagina.
D. Disorders of the ovary. Examples include abnormal chromosomes such as Turner's syndrome (0.5%); normal chromosomes (10%) such as in gonadal dysgenesis or agenesis (there may be no or very delayed Tanner stage); premature ovarian failure (premature menopause, before age 40); effect of radiation or chemotherapy; and polycystic ovarian disease.
E. Disorders of the anterior pituitary. Examples include prolactin tumors (7.5%).

Predisposing Factors

A. The disorder can affect any female between the ages of 14 and 55 years.

Common Complaints

A. "I haven't had a period in months." "I have periods only a few times each year."
B. "I have nipple discharge."
C. "I am 16 years old and have never had a menstrual period."

Other Signs and Symptoms

A. Irregular, infrequent menstrual periods
B. Galactorrhea
C. Pregnancy
D. Excessive hair growth

Subjective Data

A. Review complete menstrual history, including age of onset, duration, frequency, regularity, and dysmenorrhea.
B. Review the patient's pregnancy history.
C. Review the patient's contraception history.
D. Note other medications the patient is taking, such as hormones or antidepressants.
E. Ask the patient if she has had a major medical disease or treatment such as chemotherapy for a childhood cancer.
F. Inquire about any breast discharge.
G. Review the patient's weight pattern.
H. Ask the patient to describe her physical self-image. Does she consider herself obese or fat?
I. Review sources of stress in her life.
J. Discuss exercise pattern and history.

Physical Examination

A. Check height, weight, blood pressure, and pulse.
B. Inspect
 1. Note overall appearance. Look at the neck (thyroid). Inspect the breast/genitalia for Tanner staging. See Appendix C: Tanner's Sexual Maturity Stages.
 2. Skin assessment: Check for central hair growth, which is androgen responsive. Areas to inspect for coarse hair include the upper lip, chin, sideburns, neck, chest, lower abdomen, and perineum.
C. Palpate
 1. Palpate the neck for thyroid enlargement.
 2. Palpate the abdomen for enlarged organs or uterine enlargement compatible with pregnancy.
D. Auscultate
 1. Auscultate the heart and lungs.
 2. If pregnancy is suspected, consider auscultating for fetal heart tones.
E. Pelvic examination
 1. Inspect external genitalia. Note pubic hair pattern for Tanner staging. Note any lesions, masses, or discharge.
 2. Speculum examination: Inspect vagina and cervix. Note bluish color, which is Chadwick's sign with pregnancy.
 3. Bimanual examination: Palpate for softening of the cervical isthmus, which is Hegar's sign for pregnancy. Palpate for size of uterus and for adnexal masses.

Diagnostic Tests

A. Urine: pregnancy test.
B. Serum
 1. Serum HCG.
 2. TSH to rule out thyroid disease.
 3. Prolactin: normal less than 20 ng/mL.
 4. FSH: greater than 40 IU/mL indicates ovarian failure.
 5. Consider LH:FSH ratio to rule out polycystic ovaries.
C. Vaginal and/or pelvic ultrasonography.
D. Consider genetic testing/karotype analysis in primary amenorrhea.

Differential Diagnoses

A. Amenorrhea
B. Pregnancy
C. Constitutional delay
D. Hypothyroidism
E. Polycystic ovarian disease
F. Premature ovarian failure, or early menopause
G. Perimenopause
H. Pituitary adenoma
I. Androgen insensitivity syndrome

Plan

A. General interventions
 1. If laboratory values are normal, proceed to progesterone challenge test to rule out hypothalamic amenorrhea.

 2. If the patient is pregnant, counsel regarding pregnancy and begin antepartum care.
 3. If other laboratory information points to an underlying cause for amenorrhea, treat as appropriate.
B. Patient teaching: See the Section III Patient Teaching Guide for this chapter, "Failure to Have a Menstrual Period (Amenorrhea)."
C. Pharmaceutical therapy
 1. Progesterone challenge
 a. Medroxyprogesterone acetate (Provera, Cycrin) 10 mg each day for 5–10 days. Alternatively, progesterone in oil 200 mg by IM injection.
 b. Positive test is any vaginal bleeding. Bleeding usually occurs in 2–7 days after finishing the medicine. A late vaginal bleed may be associated with ovulation.
 c. In the absence of galactorrhea, with a normal prolactin level, normal TSH, and positive progesterone challenge, further evaluation is unnecessary.

All anovulatory patients require therapeutic management. There is a risk of endometrial cancer with unopposed estrogen. There is a short latent period in progression from a normal endometrium to atypia to cancer, even in a young woman.

 A negative withdrawal bleed may be associated with polycystic ovarian syndrome.
 2. Progesterone therapy for hypothalamic amenorrhea
 a. Medroxyprogesterone acetate (Provera, Cycrin) 10 mg for 10 days each month.
 b. Low-dose oral contraceptive pills.
 c. Clomiphene citrate for women desiring pregnancy.
 d. Hormone replacement therapy for perimenopausal women.

Follow-up

A. Reproductive age: The patient should return in 6 months of treatment with progesterone or oral contraceptive pills. Discontinue the hormones and assess for return of normal periods. If this does not occur, reinstitute progesterone or oral contraceptive therapy.
B. Perimenopausal: Maintain hormonal therapy. The patient should return annually.

Consultation/Referral

A. Refer the patient to a physician if there is no withdrawal bleeding from progesterone challenge. The problem is either with the out flow track, which is rare, or with the ovarian production of estrogen or hypothalamic production of gonadotropins. This is usually beyond the scope of the nurse practitioner.
B. Refer the patient to a physician if her prolactin level is elevated (> 20 mg/mL) for further workup to rule out pituitary adenoma.

ATROPHIC VAGINITIS

Definition

A. Atrophic vaginitis is inflammation of the vaginal epithelium due to a lack of estrogen support. Anything that lowers estrogen levels after puberty can result in a loss of vaginal thickness and rugosity and a decrease in the elasticity of the vaginal tissues.

Incidence

A. Atrophic vaginitis is very common. It may occur in three stages of a woman's life: preadolescence, when breast-feeding a baby, and postmenopause.

Pathogenesis

A. Estrogen maintains the vaginal pH in an acidic range. Lack of sufficient estrogen promotes an increase in vaginal pH that supports the development of bacterial infections. Estrogen loss also results in a decrease in vaginal glycogen and a thin-walled epithelium, promoting friability and inflammation.

Predisposing Factors

A. Preadolescence
B. Breast-feeding
C. Postmenopause
D. Ovarian failure

Common Complaints

A. Vaginal dryness, irritation, and/or bleeding
B. Dyspareunia
C. Dysuria

Other Signs and Symptoms

A. Postcoital bleeding
B. Thin vaginal discharge
C. Vaginal itching

Subjective Data

A. Question the patient regarding onset, duration, and course of symptoms.
B. Is this a new problem? If so, review the use of a new soap, laundry detergent, or hygiene products.
C. Describe the color, amount, and odor of vaginal discharge or bleeding.
D. Determine existence of coexisting vasomotor symptoms, such as hot flashes.
E. Is she experiencing dysuria, urinary frequency, vulvar dryness and itching, or dyspareunia? With dyspareunia, question the patient whether discomfort is due to irritation or pain with deep penetration, or both.
F. Determine if the patient is breast-feeding and for what duration.
G. Ask the patient the date of her last menses and if she is having irregular cycles. Determine if the patient had a hysterectomy with oophorectomy or ovarian failure.
H. Review the number of the patient's sexual partners and any new sexual practices.
I. Review the patient's current medications including antidepressants.
J. Explore whether she has stopped hormone replacement therapy.
K. Has the patient tried any self-help measures? Was there any relief?
L. When was the last Pap smear and what were the results?

Physical Examination

A. Check temperature, pulse, and respirations.
B. Inspect: Observe the patient generally for discomfort before, during, and after exam.
C. Palpate: Back: Check for CVA tenderness. Abdomen: Note suprapubic tenderness.

Pelvic Examination

A. Inspect
   1. Examine external genitalia for friability, erythema, lesions, condyloma, and amount and color of discharge.
   2. Sparse and brittle pubic hair, shrinking of the labia minora, and inflammation of the vulva may be noted in menopausal women.
   3. The vulva may appear erythematous, and there may be labial edema.
   4. Excoriation may be present if the woman has complained of pruritus.
B. Palpate: "Milk" urethra for discharge to rule out infection.
C. Speculum examination
   1. Check rugae, friability of vaginal epithelium, color and amount of discharge; evaluate cervix for lesions, friability, erythema.
   2. Typical atrophic symptoms on inspection: thin, friable vaginal epithelium; decreased or absent vaginal rugae; scant vaginal discharge.
D. Bimanual examination
   1. Check for cervical motion tenderness, uterine size and position (if no hysterectomy).
   2. Check adnexa for masses.

Diagnostic Tests

A. Serum follicle stimulating hormone (FSH) level: FSH greater than 40 in IU/mL (check with specific labs) indicates menopause or ovarian failure.
B. Serum estradiol level: estradiol less than 30 pg/mL denotes hypoestrogenemia.
C. Urine culture, if applicable.
D. Vaginal pH; normal pH range is 5.5–7.0.
E. Pap smear with maturation index. (Vaginal wall maturation index evaluation is controversial.)
F. Wet prep
   1. Multiple WBCs indicates inflammation, may show increased bacteria, and may have decreased lactobacillus suggesting atrophic vaginitis.
   2. Test should be negative for *Trichomonas*. Bacterial vaginosis (BV): Whiff test should be negative.
G. Cultures for gonorrhea and chlamydia, if applicable.
H. Ultrasound for uterine lining thickness (less than 4 or 5 mm suggest loss of estrogenic stimulation).
I. Endometrial biopsy, if indicated.

Postmenopausal vaginal bleeding must be thoroughly investigated to rule out the possibility of endometrial hyperplasia or endometrial cancer.

Differential Diagnoses

A. Atrophic vaginitis
B. Trauma
C. Foreign body in the vagina

D. Urinary tract infection
E. Vaginitis from infective cause: fungus, bacteria, or virus
F. Contact irritation: latex (condom); spermicide; lubricant
G. Menopause

Plan

A. General interventions: Treat any underlying infections (gonorrhea, chlamydia, vaginitis, as diagnosed).
B. Patient teaching: See the Section III Patient Teaching Guide for this chapter, "Atrophic Vaginitis."
   1. Preadolescent girls have amelioration of symptoms with increase of endogenous estrogen as puberty approaches.
   2. Women should be reassured that this problem is physical, not emotional.
   3. Discuss the benefits of regular sexual activity to decrease problems of atrophic vaginitis. An important reason for decreased sexual activity is unavailability of partner. Masturbation also facilitates the natural resumption of the production of lubricating secretions by the body. Decline in sexuality is influenced by culture and attitudes as well as physical problems.
   4. Symptomatic relief of dryness during sexual activity may be obtained with the use of water-soluble lubricants and adequate foreplay.
   5. Discuss pregnancy prevention and inform that perimenopausal symptoms do not ensure lack of fertility.
C. Pharmaceutical therapy
   1. Calamine lotion may be applied externally for local symptomatic relief.
   2. Estrogen therapy
      a. Vaginal hormonal therapy

Absolute contraindications to use of estrogen therapy also apply to use of topical estrogen (breast cancer, active liver disease, history of recent thromboembolic event). Vaginal estrogen creams are systemically absorbed. As with use of oral and transdermal estrogen, a progestin must be administered to women who have an intact uterus, secondary to the risk of endometrial hyperplasia or cancer.

      i. Conjugated estrogen (Premarin) cream 0.625 mg/g, use 0.5- to 1.0-g applicator inserted intravaginally at bedtime every night for 1–2 weeks, then every other night for 1–2 weeks, then as needed. **Not for daily use if the patient has an intact uterus.**
      ii. Estradiol (Estrace) 0.1 mg/g, one-half (2 g) to one (4 g) applicator intravaginally at bedtime every night for 1–2 weeks. When vaginal mucosa is restored, maintenance dose is one-quarter applicator (1 g) one to three times weekly in a cyclic regimen. **Not for daily use if the patient has an intact uterus.**

Vaginal estrogen creams are systemically absorbed. As with use of oral and transdermal estrogen, a progestin must be administered to women who have an intact uterus, secondary to the risk of endometrial hyperplasia or cancer.

      iii. Estradiol acetate Transvaginal ring (Femring) 0.5 mg a day to 0.1 mg a day. Insert one ring per vagina and replace every 90 days.
      iv. Estradiol (Estring) 7.5 mcg/24 hours insert one ring per vagina and replace every 90 days.
      v. Estradiol hemihydrate (Vagifem) vaginal tablets 25 mg one tab per vagina each day for 14 days, the tone tablet twice weekly for 10 weeks.
D. Oral estrogen replacement therapy
   1. Conjugated estrogen (Premarin) 0.625 mg orally every day from days 1 through 25 of month. Plus conjugated estrogen (Provera) 10 mg orally on days 13 through 25.
   2. See "Hormone Replacement Therapy" in the "Menopause" section for other regimens.

For long-term estrogen therapy, consider use of oral or patch methods of delivery if the patient shows additional symptoms of hypoestrogenemia (i.e., hot flashes, night sweats).

Follow-up

A. Breast-feeding women should be reevaluated following weaning, especially if symptoms persist (i.e., alternate etiology is suspected).
B. Postmenopausal women should be evaluated for additional etiologies (i.e., endometrial hyperplasia) if vaginal bleeding persists beyond 3–6 months following treatment.
C. The patient should return to clinic 1–2 months after beginning oral or vaginal drug therapy; the patient then needs to be seen in 3–6 months to check side effects, blood pressure, and response to therapy.
D. Perform Pap smears and physical examination per patient health history or risks and symptoms.

Consultation/Referral

A. If bleeding is a symptom in a postmenopausal woman, the practitioner **must** rule out bleeding of uterine origin. If there is **any** doubt, consultation for endometrial biopsy or dilatation and curettage (D and C) must be obtained.

Individual Considerations

A. Breast-feeding women have amelioration of symptoms as weaning progresses unless an alternate etiology exists.
B. Postmenopausal women
   1. Evaluate the patient for other risks of hypoestrogenemia, such as cardiovascular disease and osteoporosis. Continuous systemic estrogen replacement therapy may be indicated.
   2. Vaginitis in the postmenopausal woman is rarely due to any of the organisms responsible for vaginitis in the premenopausal woman (unless she has new sexual partners). Candidiasis, trichomoniasis, and bacterial vaginosis are uncommon after the menstruating years.

BACTERIAL VAGINOSIS (BV, OR *GARDNERELLA*)

Definition

A. Bacterial vaginosis (BV) is an infection of the vagina caused by an alteration in the normal flora of the vagina, with an increase in anaerobes and gram-negative bacilli as well as a decrease in the *Lactobacillus* flora.

Incidence

A. According to the CDC BV is the most common vaginal infection in women of childbearing age and is common in pregnant women. It is not considered exclusively an STD.

Pathogenesis

A. The main etiologic agent in BV is an increase in anaerobes in the vagina. The reason this occurs is unknown. The normal lactobacilli of the vagina decrease and vaginal pH is increased in BV. The organisms present in BV cause the level of vaginal amines to be high. These amines are volatilized when the pH is increased, causing the characteristic "fishy" odor.

B. Bacterial vaginitis is primarily polymicrobial, and the pathogens seen include *Bacteroides* species, *Peptostreptococcus* species, *Eubacterium* species, *Mobiluncus* species, *Gardnerella,* and *Mycoplasma hominis.* The incubation period is unknown.

Predisposing Factors

A. History of sexually transmitted diseases
B. Multiple sexual partners
C. Intrauterine device use
D. Factors that change the normal vaginal flora:
   1. Hormonal changes (menses, pregnancy)
   2. Medications: Oral contraceptive use and antibiotic therapy
   3. Foreign bodies in the vagina (tampons, IUDs), semen, and douching

Common Complaints

A. Vaginal discharge (thin, white, gray, or milky)
B. Fishy vaginal odor
C. Postcoital odor

Other Signs and Symptoms

A. Asymptomatic
B. Increase in odor after menses
C. Itching and burning, occasional

Subjective Data

A. Elicit onset, duration, and course of presenting symptoms.
B. Review any changes in the characteristics and color of vaginal discharge. Does the patient's partner(s) have any symptoms?
C. Review any symptoms of pruritus, perineal excoriation, burning; signs of urinary tract infection.
D. Review medication and medical history.
E. Determine if the patient is pregnant; note date of last menstrual period (LMP).
F. Question the patient for a history of STIs or other vaginal infections.
G. Review previous infection, treatment, compliance with treatment, and results.
H. Note last intercourse date.
I. Elicit information about possible foreign body.
J. Review use of vaginal deodorants or sprays, scented toilet paper, tampons, pads, and douching habits.
K. Review a change in laundry detergent, soaps, and fabric softeners.
L. Review the use of tight restrictive clothing, tight jeans, and nylon panties.
M. Review history for seizures and anticoagulant therapy.

Physical Examination

A. Check temperature, pulse, and respirations.
B. Inspect: Examine external vulva and introitus for discharge, irritation, fissures, lesions, rashes, and condyloma.
C. Palpate
   1. Palpate the abdomen for masses or tenderness. Note enlarged or tender inguinal lymph nodes.
   2. Palpate the external perineal area for vulvar masses.
   3. "Milk" the urethra for discharge.
   4. Check for CVA tenderness.
D. Pelvic examination
   1. Inspect
      a. Note the color, amount, and odor of discharge.
      b. Inspect the cervix.
         i. Bacterial vaginosis is a vaginosis rather than vaginitis. There is usually little or no inflammation of the vaginal epithelium associated with BV.
         ii. Bacterial vaginosis is associated with a pink, healthy cervix; "strawberry cervix" is seen with cervicitis due to *Trichomonas vaginalis.*
         iii. A red, edematous, friable cervix is seen with *Chlamydia trachomatis.*
   2. Speculum examination
      a. Inspect side walls for adhering discharge.
      b. The clinical diagnosis of BV requires the presence of three of the following four signs:
         i. Homogeneous, white, adherent vaginal discharge.
         ii. Vaginal fluid pH greater than 4.5. Take smear for testing from the lateral walls of the vagina, not from the cervix, for accurate pH.
         iii. A fishy, aminelike odor from vaginal fluid before or after mixing it with 10% potassium hydroxide (positive whiff test). Semen releases the vaginal amines; therefore, there is an increase in odor after intercourse.
         iv. Presence of "clue cells" (squamous vaginal epithelial cells covered with bacteria, causing a stippled or granular appearance and ragged, "moth-eaten" borders) or coccobacilli forms both in the fluid and adhering to the epithelial cells.
   3. Bimanual examination: Check for cervical motion tenderness and adnexal masses. **Bacterial vaginosis may be a risk factor for pelvic inflammatory disease.**

Diagnostic Tests

A. Vaginal pH: greater than 4.5 with BV; normal vaginal pH range is 5.5–7.0.
B. Wet prep with 10% potassium hydroxide and normal saline prep; microscopic examination of vaginal secretions should always be done.
C. Herpes culture, if indicated.
D. Urinalysis and culture, if indicated.

Differential Diagnoses
A. Bacterial vaginosis
B. Vulvovaginal candidiasis
C. Trichomoniasis
D. Gonorrhea
E. Chlamydia
F. Presence of foreign body
G. Normal physiologic discharge

Plan
A. General interventions: Inform the patient regarding other modalities for treating BV. These methods include the following:
   1. Vinegar and water douches: 1 tablespoon of white vinegar in 1 pint of water. Douche 1–2 times a week.
   2. *Lactobacillus* and *Acidophilus* culture 4–6 tablets by mouth daily.
   3. Garlic suppositories: one peeled clove of garlic wrapped in a cloth dipped in olive oil inserted vaginally overnight and changed daily.
B. Patient teaching: See the Section III Patient Teaching Guide for this chapter, "Bacterial Vaginosis." Bacterial vaginosis is **not** considered a sexually transmitted infection.
C. Pharmaceutical therapy
   1. Drug of choice
      a. Metronidazole (Flagyl) 500 mg orally twice daily for 7 days or
      b. Metronidazole gel 0.75% one applicator (5g) per vagina at bedtime for 5 days
         i. Metronidazole is less expensive, easier to use, and associated with greater compliance.
         ii. Side effects of metronidazole include sharp, unpleasant metallic taste in the mouth; furry tongue; central nervous system reactions, including seizures; and urinary tract disturbances. Advise the patients to avoid alcohol while taking metronidazole and 24 hours after completing the medication, or they will experience the severe side effects of abdominal distress, nausea, vomiting, and headache.
         iii. Metronidazole may prolong prothrombin time in patients taking oral anticoagulants.
   2. Other medications if the patient is unable to use oral metronidazole
      a. Clindamycin 300 mg by mouth twice daily for 7 days.
      b. Metronidazole gel (MetroGel) 0.75% one applicator vaginally twice daily for 5 days.
      c. Clindamycin 2% cream one applicator vaginally at bedtime for 7 days.

Clindamycin cream is oil-based and may weaken latex condoms for at least 72 hours after terminating therapy.

   3. Special considerations: pregnancy: BV has been associated with adverse pregnancy outcomes; therefore, all symptomatic pregnant women and asymptomatic high risk for preterm delivery women require treatment.

a. Metronidazole 500 mg orally twice a day for 7 days or 250 mg orally three times a day for 7 days or
b. Clindamycin 300 mg orally twice a day for 7 days.

Follow-up
A. Nonpregnant women: no follow-up is recommended unless indicated. Recurrence is common.
B. High risk for preterm delivery pregnant women should be reevaluated 1 month after treatment.
C. Recommendations for treatment of BV in females infected with HIV are the same as for noninfected patients.
D. Consider treatment of the patient's partner(s) in women with recurrent disease.

Consultation/Referral
A. Refer the patient to a physician for recurrence that is unresponsive to therapies.

Individual Considerations
A. Pregnancy: Clindamycin cream may be associated with increased adverse events in newborns and should not be used during the second half of pregnancy.
B. Partners: routine treatment of a patient's partner(s) is not recommended at this time because it does not influence relapse or recurrence rates.

BARTHOLIN CYST OR ABSCESS

Definition
A. The Bartholin's glands are small, round nonpalpable mucous secreting organs. They are located bilaterally in the posterolateral vaginal orifice. Obstruction of the duct causes the gland to swell with mucus and form a Bartholin's cyst. The cause of obstruction is usually unknown but may be due to mechanical trauma, thickened mucous, neoplasm, stenosis of the duct, or infectious organisms not limited to sexually transmitted infections. The cyst may become infected resulting in an abscess. Cysts develop more commonly in younger women and occurrence decreases with aging; therefore, it is important to rule out neoplasm in women over 40 experiencing Bartholoin's cyst.
B. The majority of women with Bartholin's cyst are asymptomatic, but large cysts can case pressure and interfere with walking and sexual intercourse. Abscesses generally develop rapidly over a two- to three-day period and are painful. Some abscesses may spontaneously rupture and often reoccur.

Predisposing Factors
A. History of sexually transmitted diseases
B. Local trauma

Common Complaints
A. Cysts can be asymptomatic and found incidentally on physical exam.
B. Localized pain/irritation.
C. Dysparunia.
D. Difficulty walking or sitting due to edema.

Subjective Data
A. Elicit onset, duration, and course of presenting symptoms.

B. Review any changes in the characteristics and color of vaginal discharge. Does the patient's partner(s) have any symptoms?

C. Review any symptoms of pruritus, perineal excoriation, burning; signs of urinary tract infection.

D. Review the patient's medication and medical history.

E. Determine if the patient is pregnant; note the date of last menstrual period (LMP).

F. Question the patient for a history of STIs or other vaginal infections.

G. Review previous infection, treatment, compliance with treatment, and results.

H. Note last intercourse date.

Physical Examination

A. Examine external vulva and introitus for discharge, irritation, fissures, lesions, and rashes. Bartholin's cyst will appear as a round mass usually near the vaginal orifice causing vulvar asymmetry. Cysts are usually unilateral, tense, nontender, and without erythema. An abscess is usually unilateral, tense, painful, and erythematous.

Diagnostic Tests

A. Culture and sensitivity of purulent abscess fluid

B. Cervical culture for STI (*N. gonorrhea* and *C. trachomotis*)

C. Excisional biopsy in women older than 40

Differential Diagnoses

A. Bartholin's cyst

B. Bartholin's abscess

C. Neoplasm

D. Sexually transmitted infection

E. Sebaceuos cyst

Plan

A. General interventions: Reassurance is indicated for women under 40 with asymptomatic cysts. I& D is often required for symptomatic cysts and abscesses. Because cysts and abscesses often reoccur, surgery to create a permanent opening from the duct to the exterior is often the definitive treatment. Two such surgical methods include placement of a wards catheter or Marsupialization. Referral is indicated for I&D and other surgical intervention if the provider is not experienced with the procedures.

Women over 40 must be referred for surgical exploration and excision biopsy.

B. Warm sitz baths three or four times a day may encourage spontaneous rupture of abscess and provide comfort.

C. Pharmaceutical therapy

1. Abscesses are treated with oral broad spectrum antibiotics such as cephalexin 500 mg four times a day for 7–10 days.

Follow-up

A. Report to care provider if symptoms reoccur.

Consultation/Referral

A. Refer the patient to a physician for recurrence that is unresponsive to therapies. Refer women over 40 with cyst for excisional biopsy.

BREAST PAIN

Definition

A. Benign breast disorders such as mastalgia, masto-dynia, and fibrocystic breast changes are characterized by lumps or pain. The lumps may be physiologic nodularity, a ropy thickening, or distended fluid-filled cysts that are mobile. The pain may be cyclic or noncyclic, and it may be unilateral or bilateral.

Incidence

A. This is a very common problem. Fifty percent or more of menstruating women experience breast pain. Two-thirds of breast pain is cyclic and occurs in women in their 30s; one-third is noncyclic and may occur in women at any age, but it tends to occur in women closer to menopause.

Pathogenesis

A. Dysplastic, benign histologic changes occur in the breast such as hyperplasia of the breast epithelium, adenosis microcysts and macrocysts, duct ectasia, and apocrine metaplasia.

Predisposing Factors

A. Menstruation

B. Ingesting substances containing methyl-xanthines (coffee, tea, chocolate, and cola drinks). Methylxanthines have been noted to contribute to breast pain by clinical observation only.

Common Complaints

A. "My breasts are painful, particularly just before my period."

B. "I have lumps in my breasts, and they hurt."

Other Signs and Symptoms

A. Tender breasts with palpation

B. Ropelike masses, usually bilateral, with mobile, well-circumscribed masses that are cystic or rubbery

Subjective Data

A. Elicit history of pain. Note onset, duration, location, and relation to menstrual period. Ask: Is pain constant or intermittent?

B. What has the patient tried to alleviate the pain? Note what has worked, such as NSAIDs.

C. Note the patient's family history of breast pain, lumps, or cancer.

D. Has there been trauma such as being hit or having rough experience during sex?

E. Do her breasts hurt during or after exercise such as running, aerobics, soccer, or basketball?

F. Does she wear a good, supporting, properly fitted bra generally and for sports?

G. Has she had any breast surgery or biopsy?

H. Note medication history such as oral contraceptives or phenytoin.

Physical Examination

A. Inspect: Examine the breasts, and note masses; dimples; changes in the skin; changes in the way the nipples are pointed while the patient is in the sitting position with arms in neutral position in lap, above the head, or pressing in on hips.

B. Palpate: Palpate the breasts; look for hard, fixed, or cystic masses in the breast, under the nipple, in the tail of the breast, and in the axilla. Use a standardized breast examination technique. Compress the nipple for discharge. Measure masses, and describe them in the patient's record. Use a clock face to describe their location.

Diagnostic Tests

A. Mammogram: may be difficult to interpret in women under 35 years
B. Ultrasonography to differentiate cystic from solid masses
C. MRI useful for detecting tissues with increased blood flow but limited by false positive results
D. Fine-needle aspiration and biopsy
E. Excisional biopsy for solid lumps
F. Pregnancy test

Differential Diagnoses

A. Fibrocystic breast changes with mastalgia
B. Benign breast masses: fibroadenoma and duct ectasia
C. Nipple discharge: duct ectasia, prolactin-secreting pituitary tumors
D. Pain: costal chondritis, chest wall muscle pain, neuralgia, herpes zoster infection, and fibromyalgia
E. Heart: angina pectoris
F. GI: gastroesophageal reflux disease (GERD)
G. Psychologic: anxiety and depression

Plan

A. General interventions: Reassure the patient. Use the term "fibrocystic changes" rather than "fibrocystic disease" to stress the functional nature of the problem. Stress that the pain is real, but not a disease state.
B. Patient teaching: See the Section III Teaching Guide for this chapter, "Fibrocystic Breast Changes and Breast Pain."
   1. Teach the patient breast self-examination. Encourage monthly breast self-exam. Continue clinical breast exams annually.
   2. "Lumpiness" that varies with the menstrual cycle is not abnormal. Breasts may normally be of different sizes. It is a change that is significant.
   3. Consider changing dose or discontinuing HRT for women on HRT with mastalgia.
   4. Symptomatic measures to relieve discomfort
      a. Good supporting bra, properly fitted. Adolescents whose breasts are maturing and perimenopausal women whose body is changing are two groups who often wear improperly fitted bras.
      b. Local heat or ice application (whatever works best).
C. Diet: Elimination of methylxanthines is a good idea, but the relationship of methylxanthines to breast pain is unproven in research studies. Sodium intake restriction has also been advocated, but has not been supported by research.

D. Pharmaceutical therapy
   1. Diuretic: spironolactone (Aldactone) 10 mg twice daily premenstrually.
   2. Oral contraceptive pills: low-dose estrogen (20 jig) pills are recommended.
   3. Topical nonsteroidal anti-inflammatory gel can be used for local mastalgia.
   4. Anti-estrogen treatment.
      a. Danazol (Danocrine) 200 mg daily for 6 months. *Note:* Doses below 400 mg daily may not inhibit ovulation. The patient must use barrier contraceptive or IUD contraceptive measure. Although the side effect profile is significant, long-term symptomatic relief and histologic changes may be achieved.
      b. Tamoxifen citrate 10 mg per day.
   5. Vitamins.
      a. Vitamin E is no longer recommended for treatment of mastalgia.
      b. Research has demonstrated mixed results on the benefits of Vitamin B_6 and Vitamin A.
   6. Herbs.
      a. Flaxseed 25 mg daily may show benefit in the treatment of cyclic mastalgia.
      b. Evening primrose oil: there is insufficient evidence to recommend EPO for the treatment of mastalgia.

Follow-up

A. Young women with fibrocystic changes need to be seen after 1–2 months of pharmacologic therapy to assess for complications and efficacy.
B. Women with atypical hyperplasia on biopsy need close follow-up every 3–6 months by a physician.

Consultation/Referral

A. Consult or refer the patient to a physician when breast masses are identified.
B. Consult with a physician and refer the patient to a surgeon if findings include a suspicious mamographic study, an abnormal needle biopsy, or a solid mass per ultrasonogram.

Individual Considerations

A. Pregnancy: Consider blocked duct or mastitis.
B. Adults: Mammography is indicated annually for women at average risk from age 40–69 and women should be informed of the risks, benefits, and limitations of regular screening. Older women should be individualized considering potential risks, benefits, and limitations of screening. High-risk women may benefit from additional screening including earlier initiation of screening and additional screening modalities such as ultrasound and MRI. When clinical breast examination, mammography, and needle aspiration biopsy are used, breast cancer detection rates are 93%–100%.
C. Geriatric: Breast pain should be worked up as possible cancer.
D. Partners: Pain may inhibit sexual activity involving the breast.

CERVICITIS

Definition
A. Cervicitis is acute or chronic inflammation of the cervix that is visible to the examiner.

Incidence
A. Incidence is unknown due to multiple etiologies.

Pathogenesis
A. Acute cervicitis is primarily due to infection from the following organisms:
  1. Bacteria
    a. *Chlamydia trachomatis*
    b. *Neisseria gonorrhoeae*
    c. *Mycoplasma*
    d. Ureaplasma
  2. Viruses
    a. Herpes simplex virus type 2
    b. Human papillomavirus (HPV)
  3. *Trichomonas vaginalis*
B. Chronic cervicitis is primarily due to the following:
  1. Trauma occurring during childbirth or instrumentation
  2. Infection (see above)
  3. Presence of foreign bodies (IUD)

Predisposing Factors
A. Vaginal delivery
B. Cervical procedures: laser, loop, or other excision procedures
C. IUD
D. Sexually transmitted infections (STIs)

Common Complaints
A. Copious mucopurulent vaginal discharge
B. Postcoital bleeding

Other Signs and Symptoms
A. Asymptomatic; may be found on routine gynecologic exam
B. Thick yellow vaginal discharge
C. Dysuria
D. Dyspareunia
E. Vulvovaginal irritation or pruritus

Subjective Data
A. Determine onset, duration, and course of symptoms. Is there any dyspareunia, pelvic pain, fever, or urinary symptoms?
B. Determine characteristics of the vaginal discharge.
C. Review the patient's history of STIs.
D. Review the patient's sexual history to include number of partners and partner symptoms (if any), use of sex toys, and sexual lifestyle.
E. Note last Pap smear and results. Has the patient ever had an abnormal Pap, and if so, how was it treated?
F. Note date of LMP, use of contraception, and type(s) of contraception.
G. If the patient has recently been pregnant, review her records for cervical cerclage, vaginal delivery with cervical laceration, or other complications.

Physical Examination
A. Check temperature, pulse and respirations.
B. Inspect: Observe generally for discomfort before, during, and after exam.
  1. Observe the external vulva for Bartholin's gland enlargement (Bartholin's gland abscess is due primarily to infection by *Chlamydia*), lesions, irritation, fissures, and condyloma.
  2. Note color, amount, and odor of vaginal discharge.
C. Palpate: Back: Note CVA tenderness. Abdomen: Palpate for enlarged or tender inguinal lymph nodes.
D. Pelvic examination
E. Speculum examination: Inspect cervix for inflammation and ectropion.
  1. **Cervical ectropion is found in 15%–20% of healthy young women (especially in teens and with the use of oral contraceptives). It represents columnar epithelium that is found farther out on the ectocervix, causing the cervix to appear granular and red. Presence of cervical erosion, however, suggests advanced cervical pathology. A "strawberry cervix" (petechiae) is highly suggestive of *Trichomonas vaginalis*.**
  2. Check cervix for friability and bleeding when the cervix is touched with a cotton-tipped swab.
  3. Assess the vagina and cervix for leuko-plakia, lesions, polyps, and discharge. Assess vaginal walls for discharge and rugae.
  4. **Vesicular or ulcerated cervical lesions warrant testing for herpes simplex virus, syphilis, and/or chancroid.**
F. Bimanual examination: Check cervical motion tenderness; adnexal masses; uterine size, consistency, and tenderness.
  1. Milk urethra for discharge.
  2. Palpate Bartholin's glands.

Diagnostic Tests
A. WBC, if indicated
B. Consider testing for syphilis (RPR or VDRI)
C. Wet prep
D. Cervical cultures for GC and chlamydia
E. Pap smear
F. Urine culture and sensitivity, if indicated
G. Herpes culture, if indicated

Differential Diagnoses
A. Cervicitis
B. *Chlamydia*
C. Gonorrhea
D. Bartholin's gland abscess
E. Cervical neoplasm
F. Cervical polyps
G. Herpes simplex virus type 2
H. Urinary tract infection
I. Cervical ulceration, or erosion, from trauma: fingernail, cervical biopsy, postpartum, or sex toys
J. PID

Plan
A. General interventions: Patients whose culture is negative generally respond to a round of doxycycline therapy, which is the drug of choice for nonchlamydial, nongonorrheal cervicitis.

B. Patient teaching
1. Women should be encouraged to obtain routine, annual Pap smear evaluations.
2. Patients should be cautioned to avoid alcohol consumption during and 24 hours after the completion of oral metronidazole due to a disulfiram-like reaction (nausea, vomiting, headache, cramps, and flushing).
3. No sexual intercourse for 1 week.
4. Avoid tampons and douches until antibiotics are completed.
5. Give the patient teaching sheet. See the Section III Patient Teaching Guide for this chapter, "Cervicitis."
C. Pharmaceutical therapy
1. Drug of choice for *Chlamydia:* doxycycline 100 mg twice daily for 7 days. Treat all partners.
2. Drug of choice for gonorrhea: ceftriaxone (Rocephin) 125 mg by IM injection.
3. Drug of choice for herpes simplex virus: acyclovir 200 mg five times daily for current outbreak, or acyclovir 400 mg daily for suppression.
4. Drug of choice for *Trichomonas:* metronidazole 500 mg twice daily for 7 days (treat all partners), or 2 g immediately by IM injection.
5. Drug of choice for urinary tract infection: see the section "Urinary Tract Infection" in Chapter 11, "Genitourinary Guidelines."

Follow-up

A. Recommend "test of cure": reculture 1–2 weeks following pharmacologic therapy.
B. Follow up with Pap smear as mandated by result.

Consultation/Referral

A. Refer the patient to a physician for suspected neoplasm and for cervicitis unresponsive to treatment.
B. If the cervix has a suspicious lesion, the patient should be referred for colposcopy and/or biopsy regardless of cytology results. **On physical examination, the cervix may be edematous and erythematous and may show exposed columnar epithelium. It may be friable. Reddened areas of the cervix may be seen around the cervical os. The irregularity and friability sometimes differentiate them from eversion; other times colposcopy is required to make the distinction.**

Individual Considerations

A. Pregnancy: Cervical inflammation is common in early pregnancy. If an STI is diagnosed, nonteratogenic pharmacologic therapies must be implemented.
B. Partners: A positive STI result warrants treatment of each sexual partner.

CONTRACEPTION

Definition

A. Contraception is the intentional prevention of pregnancy by either or both sexual partners. Contraception can be mechanical, chemical, or surgical and is either reversible or nonreversible. Considerations in counseling regarding contraceptive choices include cost, efficacy, safety, and personal considerations such as personal beliefs systems and ability to use selected method.

Incidence

A. Women frequently visit primary care providers to request contraception and family planning education. Over 11 million women in the United States use oral contraceptive pills. Ninety-eight percent of women aged 15–44 have used at least one contraceptive method. Unfortunately, approximately 50% of all pregnancies in the United States are unintended. Consistent use of a reliable and effective contraceptive method can greatly reduce the unintended pregnancy rate. Easy access and education regarding contraceptive use is a keystone in the prevention of unintended pregnancy.

Subjective Data

A. Review complete menstrual history, including age of onset, duration, frequency, regularity, and dysmenorrhea. Review date of LMP.
B. Review the patient's pregnancy history.
C. Review the patient's contraception and sexual history.
D. Note other medications the patient is taking including over-the-counter medications and supplements.
E. Ask the patient if she has had a major medical disease including hypertension, cardiovascular incident, thromboembolic disease, diabetes, migraine headaches, gallbladder disease, or liver disease.
F. Review substance abuse/use history.
G. Review childhood illness and immunization record.
H. Note allergies.
I. Review pertinent family medical history.

Physical Examination

A. Check height, weight, blood pressure, pulse, and BMI.
B. Inspect.
1. Note overall appearance. Look at neck (thyroid). Inspect breast/genitalia for Tanner staging. See Appendix C: Tanner's Sexual Maturity Stages.
2. Skin assessment: Check for central hair growth, which is androgen responsive. Areas to inspect for coarse hair include the upper lip, chin, sideburns, neck, chest, lower abdomen, and perineum.
C. Palpate.
1. Palpate the neck for thyroid enlargement.
2. Palpate the abdomen for enlarged organs or uterine enlargement compatible with pregnancy.
D. Auscultate.
1. Auscultate the heart and lungs.
2. If pregnancy is suspected, consider auscultating for fetal heart tones.
E. Breast examination.
F. Pelvic examination.
1. Inspect external genitalia. Note pubic hair pattern for Tanner staging. Note any lesions, masses, or discharge.
2. Speculum examination: Inspect vagina and cervix. Note any vaginal discharge. Obtain Pap smear and cervical/vaginal cultures as appropriate.

3. Bimanual examination: Palpate the cervical and check CMT. Palpate for the size of the uterus and for adnexal masses.
4. Consider rectal examination as indicated.

Diagnostic Tests

A. Urine: pregnancy test as indicated/UA as indicated
B. Serum: CBC if indicated by history
C. Pap smear according to ASCP guidelines
D. Vaginal/cervical cultures for STIs as indicated

Plan

A. Patient teaching counseling: Review anatomy and physiology of the menstrual cycle and reproduction with all patients. Review the risks, benefits, costs, and efficacy of contraceptive methods. Review perfect use verses typical use of method selected. Review limitations of STI prevention as related to each method. Review STI prevention with all patients. Together with the patient select the most appropriate method of contraception with regard to cost, efficacy, health status of the patient, ability to use correctly and consistently, and the patient's personal values.

Methods

A. Abstinence: refraining from sexual intercourse
 1. Advantages: Easily accessible and inexpensive. Perfect use offers protections against STIs.
 2. Disadvantages: User dependant.
B. Barrier methods
 1. Male condom
  a. Advantages: Male condoms are easily accessible (over-the-counter with no prescription needed) and relatively inexpensive. Condoms do not require daily intervention and offer some protections against STIs.
  b. Disadvantages: Male condoms are technique dependant for efficacy. Breakage and spillage can occur. Some condoms are made from latex and those with latex allergies need to be aware and carefully check label for latex content. Nonlatex condoms are available. Male condoms are intended for one-time use only.
  c. Efficacy with perfect use of male condoms: approximately 2 in 100 women will become pregnant each year. With typical use of male condoms approximately 15 in 100 women will become pregnant each year.
 2. Female condom
  a. Advantages: Female condoms are easily accessible (over-the-counter with no prescription needed) and relatively inexpensive. Condoms do not require daily intervention and offer some protections against STIs.
  b. Disadvantages: Female condoms are technique dependant for efficacy. Slippage and spillage can occur. The female condom is intended for one-time use only and may be inserted up to 8 hours prior to intercourse.
  c. Efficacy with perfect use of the female condom: approximately 5 in 100 women will become pregnant each year. With typical use of the female condom approximately 21 in 100 women will become pregnant each year.
 3. Diaphragm
  a. Advantages: Diaphragms are nonhormonal and can be used for years with proper care. May be inserted up to 6 hours prior to intercourse.
  b. Disadvantages: Diaphragms must be properly fitted by an experienced health care provider and are user controlled. Placement is crucial to contraceptive benefit and spermicide must be used. Must be removed within 24 hours due to risk of toxic shock syndrome (TSS). The patient must have fit checked after childbirth and weight gain or loss. UTIs may be more frequent in diaphragm users and some women may experience sensitivity or allergy to spermicide. Avoid use during menses.
  c. Efficacy with perfect use of the diaphragm: 6 in 100 women will become pregnant each year. With typical use of the diaphragm 16 in 100 women will become pregnant each year.
 4. Cervical cap
  a. Advantages: cervical caps are nonhormonal and can be used for years with proper care. The cervical cap may be inserted and left in place up to 48 hours.
  b. Disadvantages: cervical caps must be properly fitted by an experienced health care provider and are user controlled. Placement is crucial to contraceptive benefit and spermicide must be used. Must be removed within 48 hours due to risk of toxic shock syndrome (TSS). The Fem cap is made of latex and not appropriate for latex-allergic patients. Some women may experience sensitivity or allergy to spermicide. Avoid use during menses.
  c. Efficacy with use of the cervical cap is similar to the diaphragm.
 5. Vaginal sponge
  a. Advantages: vaginal sponges is a nonhormonal over-the-counter polyurethane sponge that releases the spermicide nonoxynol-9. It can be used for multiple acts of intercourse over 24 hours.
  b. Disadvantages: vaginal sponge is user controlled. Some women may experience sensitivity or allergy to the spermicide. Avoid use during menses.
  c. Efficacy with use perfect use of the vaginal sponge: among parous women 20 in 100 will become pregnant each year and 9 nulliparous women will become pregnant each year. With typical use 32 in 100 parous women and 16 nulliparous women will become pregnant each year.
C. Surgical
 1. Male sterilization.
  a. Advantages: Sterilization is a very effective form of contraception. User does not have to remember to do anything prior to intercourse and it is not user dependant. Sterilization is permanent.
  b. Disadvantages: Sterilization involves a surgical procedure. Insurance may not cover the cost of the procedure.

c. Efficacy with perfect use of male sterilization; 0.1 in 100 women will become pregnant each year. With typical use of male sterilization 0.15 in 100 women will become pregnant each year.

2. Female sterilization is the second most often used contraceptive method in the United States.

   a. Advantages: Sterilization is a very effective form of contraception. User does not have to remember to do anything prior to intercourse and it is not user dependant. Sterilization is permanent.

   b. Disadvantages: Sterilization involves a surgical procedure. If pregnancy does occur there is a higher incidence of ectopic pregnancy. Insurance may not cover the cost of the procedure.

   c. Efficacy with both perfect and typical use of female sterilization: 0.5 in 100 will become pregnant each year.

D. Intrauterine device

1. Hormonal (Mirena)

   a. Advantages: Mirena is a very effective form of contraception. Mirena may be left in place for five years. User does not have to remember to use prior to intercourse. Mirena may reduce menstrual flow.

   b. Disadvantages: Risks of any IUD include uterine perforation; increased spontaneous abortion, ectopic pregnancy, and pelvic pain and infection. Mirena must be inserted by a qualified health care professional. IUD may be spontaneously expelled.

   c. Efficacy with both perfect and typical use of the Mirena: 0.2 in 100 will become pregnant each year.

2. Nonhormonal (ParaGard®)

   a. Advantages: ParaGard is a very effective form of contraception. ParaGard may be left in place for 10 years. User does not have to remember to use prior to intercourse.

   b. Disadvantages: Risks of any IUD include uterine perforation; increased spontaneous abortion, ectopic pregnancy, and pelvic pain and infection. ParaGard must be inserted by a qualified health care professional. IUD may be spontaneously expelled.

   c. Efficacy with use perfect use of the ParaGard: 0.6 in 100 women will become pregnant each year. With typical use of the ParaGard 0.8 in 100 women will become pregnant each year.

Women who are not appropriate candidates for an IUD include those with recent pelvic infections, anatomical uterine abnormalities, and pregnancy. Caution should be exercised when considering an IUD in women who have multiple sexual partners; PID; immunosuppression; undiagnosed, irregular, or heavy menstrual bleeding; abnormal Pap smear; and difficulty obtaining follow-up care. See World Health Organization's IUD Toolkit at http://www.k4health.org/toolkits/iud.

E. Pharmacological

1. Progestin only pills (POP) (also know as mini pill).

   a. Advantages: Progestin only pill is a safe hormonal alternative for women who cannot take estrogen. It is preferred over combined oral contraceptives (COCs) for lactating women as it is not as likely to decrease milk supply. POPs are rapidly reversible and controlled by women.

   b. Disadvantages: Women cannot take POPs if the patient has any contraindications to progestin use. POPs are less effective than COCs and must be taken daily at the same time requiring strict adherence to regime.

   c. Efficacy with use perfect use of POPs: 0.3 in 100 women per year will become pregnant. With typical use 8 in 100 women per year will become pregnant.

2. Injection (Depo-Provera) long-acting progesterone DMPA.

   a. Advantages: Easy to use. The user only has to remember the injection every 3 months. May decrease vaginal bleeding. DMPA is a safe hormonal alternative for women who cannot take estrogen.

   b. Disadvantages: Women cannot use DMPA if they have any contraindications to progesterone use. May cause amenorrhea or irregular vaginal bleeding. May cause increased weight gain. Requires routine (3-month) visits to the provider's office for intramuscular injections. DMPA does not provide protections against STIs. DMPA is associated with reversible decreased bone mineral density.

   c. Efficacy with perfect use of DMPA: 0.3 in 100 women per year will become pregnant. With typical use 3 in 100 women per year will become pregnant.

   d. Depo-Provera should be administered during the first five days of the menstrual cycle, or postpartum prior to resumption of intercourse (preferably after lactation has been established). If this is not possible or if a woman is late for injection, administer pregnancy test and have the patient use condoms for at least one week after injection.

   e. **Absolute Contraindications to Progestogen Therapy**

      i. Active thrombophlebitis or thromboembolic disorders

      ii. Acute liver disease

      iii. Known or suspected cancer of the breast

      iv. Pregnancy

      v. Undiagnosed, abnormal vaginal bleeding

3. Combined estrogen/progesterone contraceptives: Combined estrogen/progesterone contraceptives come in three delivery methods—oral pills, a transdermal patch, and a vaginal ring. Advantages and disadvantages and efficacy are similar regarding hormones but there are some differences in delivery method.

   a. Advantages: Combined contraceptives are easy to use, convenient, rapidly reversible, and controlled by women. The transdermal patch is only changed weekly and the vaginal ring is left in place for 3 weeks. In addition to predictable menses combined contraceptives decrease menstrual flow and length of menses.

   b. Disadvantages: Dependant on user and oral pills must be taken daily. Exposure to hormones may not be suitable for certain women based on health status and risk. See absolute and relative contraindications. See absolute and relative contraindications that are not appropriate for some women. Smoking in conjunction with use of combined contraceptive use increases cardiovascular risk and should be considered. Does not protect against STIs. Other medications such as anticonvulsants and antibiotics may interfere with effectiveness of combined hormonal contraceptives and should be considered in prescribing.

c. Efficacy with perfect use of combined hormonal contraceptive: 0.3 in 100 women per year will become pregnant. With typical use 8 in 100 women per year will become pregnant.

d. Prescribing considerations: Oral contraceptives come in combination extended cycle, combination monophasic, combination biphasic, combination triphasic, and progestin-only formulations. Side effects can be managed in consideration of pill composition. See prescribing reference guides such as the Monthly Prescribing Reference (MRP) at http://www.empr.com. General considerations for pill selection include age, health history/status, and the patient's preference. Because POPs are highly sensitive to consistency in timing reserve prescription of them for women who have contraindications to estrogen. Alternatives for COCs should be considered in women over 35 who smoke due to increased risks of thrombolytic events. In asymptomatic adolescents it is acceptable to prescribe COCs without and initial pelvic exam. For adolescents or anyone who may have difficulty remembering to take a daily pill, consideration should be given to prescription of the vaginal ring, patch, or other methods. See prescriber's reference for complete information on safety side effects and contraindications.

e. **Absolute Contraindications to Estrogen Therapy**
   i. Acute liver disease
   ii. Cerebral vascular or coronary artery disease, MI or stroke
   iii. History of or active thrombophlebitis or thromboembolic disorders
   iv. History of uterine or ovarian cancer
   v. Known or suspected cancer of the breast
   vi. Known or suspected estrogen-dependent neoplasm
   vii. Pregnancy
   viii. Undiagnosed, abnormal vaginal bleeding

f. **Relative Contraindications to Estrogen Therapy**
   i. Active gallbladder disease
   ii. Familial hyperlipidemia

4. Spermicide (foam, film, gel, tablets, and suppositories)
   a. Advantages: spermicide is a nonhormonal over-the-counter preparation and contains nonoxynol-9. It is inexpensive and easily accessible.
   b. Disadvantages: spermicide is user controlled and if not used consistently will lead to contraception failure. Some may experience sensitivity or allergy to spermicide. Spermicide has a high failure rate.
   c. Efficacy with perfect use of spermicide: 18 in 100 women will become pregnant each year. With

typical use of spermicide 29 of 100 women will become pregnant each year.

F. Natural family planning (NFP)
   1. Advantages: NFP is nonhormonal. It is inexpensive and easily accessible.
   2. Disadvantages: NFP is user controlled and depends on regularity of cycle and avoidance of intercourse. Can be complex for user and has a high failure rate. Does not protect against STIs.
   3. Efficacy with use: with typical use of fertility awareness method 25 in 100 women will become pregnant each year.

Additional information, training, and patient teaching may be found at the following Web sites:

Association of Reproductive Health Professionals: http://www.arhp.org/crc/fertility-awareness.html
Institute for Reproductive Health: www.irh.org
Planned Parenthood: www.plannedparenthood.org

G. Withdrawal
   1. Advantages: Withdrawal is nonhormonal. It is inexpensive and easily accessible.
   2. Disadvantages: Withdrawal is user controlled. Withdrawal has a high failure rate and does not protect against STIs.
   3. Efficacy with use: with typical use of withdrawal method 85 in 100 women will become pregnant each year.

Patient Education

A. All patients should be educated on the risks, benefits, and how to correctly use the contraceptive method selected. Warning signs and when to call the care provider information should be provided to all patients. All women of childbearing age should be educated on the availability and proper use of emergency contraceptives. Provide all patients information on the prevention of STIs.

Follow-up

A. The patient should return in 3 months of initiation of oral contraceptives, ring, and patch to assess BP, use, side effects, and satisfaction. Then yearly for health maintenance.
B. Patients on Depo-Provera injections should return every 3 months for follow-up injection and weight evaluation and then yearly for health maintenance.
C. Patients with diaphragm should return for refitting with change in weight or postpartum and for routine health maintenance.

Consultation/Referral

A. If the contraceptive method selected is one the practitioner is not experienced in providing (diaphragm, implant, IUD, surgical sterilization), refer to an experienced appropriate provider.

DYSMENORRHEA

Definition

Dysmenorrhea is painful uterine cramping felt primarily in the lower abdomen but also in the lower back and upper thighs.

A. Primary dysmenorrhea: Not associated with pelvic pathology. Usually associated with ovulatory cycles. Occurs first day or two of the menstrual period. Usually worse the first day. Affects teens and women in their 20s. Often associated with prostaglandin-induced symptoms of diarrhea, nausea, vomiting, and/or headache.

B. Secondary dysmenorrhea: Painful uterine contractions due to a pathologic etiology such as endometriosis or pelvic inflammatory disease (PID). Occurs in women primarily in their 20s, 30s, and 40s.

Incidence

A. Primary dysmenorrhea is very common, affecting virtually 100% of young women to some extent at some time. It is the leading cause of absenteeism from work or school in women under 30. A smaller, but significant group, perhaps 10%, miss days of school or work each month because of the incapacitating pain. The incidence of endometriosis is 8%–30% of women of reproductive age.

Pathogenesis

A. Primary dysmenorrhea is due to myometrial contractions that are caused by prostaglandins in the secretory endometrium. The prostaglandins cause uterine ischemia through platelet aggregation, vasoconstriction, and dysrhythmic contractions.

B. Secondary dysmenorrhea is associated with pathologic conditions such as endometriosis, cervical stenosis, tumors, adhesions, adenomyosis, myomas, polyps, infection (PID), IUD-retained products of conception, or nongynecologic causes. The pain of secondary dysmenorrhea may also be unrelated to menses.

C. In endometriosis, there are islands of endometrium found on peritoneal surfaces of the bladder, broad ligaments, fallopian tubes, ovaries, bowel, and cul-de-sac, as well as distant sites on the abdominal wall, vagina, lung, or other sites.

Predisposing Factors

A. Female
B. Reproductive age
C. Normal menstrual function
D. Cervical stenosis, possibly

Common Complaints

A. "I have painful periods."
B. "My menstrual cramps are terrible, particularly the first day of my cycle."
C. "My cramps are so bad I feel sick to my stomach and have diarrhea."

Other Signs and Symptoms

A. History of menstrual cramps just prior to the onset of the menstrual period and for the first 24–48 hours.
B. Pain beginning earlier; associated with intercourse, defecation, and urination; and lasting throughout the menstrual period is associated with endometriosis or adenomyosis.
C. Acute pain may be associated with infection (PID) or ectopic pregnancy.

Subjective Data

A. Obtain a complete menstrual history: age at menarche; frequency, duration, and regularity of periods; amount of flow, in number of perineal pads or tampons used.
B. Ask the patient about the location of the pain; note radiation and associated symptoms such as nausea, vomiting, or diarrhea.
C. Is pain rhythmic or spasmodic (primary) or steady (secondary)?
D. How old was the patient when the pain began? Primary dysmenorrhea usually begins 2–3 years after menarche.
E. Inquire about the type of contraception used.
F. Obtain obstetric history.
G. Is the pain related to the menstrual period, or does it occur prior to or independent of the menstrual period?
H. Does the patient have dyspareunia?
I. Does she have UTI symptoms?
J. What treatments have been tried, and which were effective?

Physical Examination

A. Height and weight, temperature, blood pressure, and pulse.
B. Inspect.
    1. Examine the general body habitus for female adipose distribution on the buttocks and thighs.
    2. Note breast development (Tanner's stage in Appendix C).
    3. Observe the abdomen for distension.
C. Palpate and percuss: Examine the abdomen for masses or tenderness.
D. Auscultate: Auscultate the heart, lungs, and abdomen for bowel sounds.
E. Pelvic examination.
    1. Inspection: Inspect the external genitalia for pubic hair pattern, lesions, discharge, and odor.
    2. Palpation: Palpate the external genitalia for masses or areas of tenderness.
F. Speculum examination: Inspect the cervix and vagina for discharge, lesions, ectropion, cervical erosion, and IUD string.
G. Bimanual examination.
    1. Palpate the vagina and cul-de-sac areas for tenderness or masses.
    2. Check the cervical position, mobility, and pain with mobility.
    3. Check uterine size, mobility, shape, regularity, masses, position, and tenderness.
    4. Check the adnexa for masses (cystic or solid) and tenderness.
    5. A normal pelvic examination is a significant finding in primary dysmenorrhea and often in endometriosis.

Diagnostic Tests

A. Consider pelvic ultrasonography to rule out pelvic pathology.
B. Laboratory studies: Hgb, HCT, and WBC.
C. Consider vaginal and cervical cultures for *Chlamydia* and gonorrhea, if infection suspected.

Differential Diagnoses

A. Dysmenorrhea: The patient's history and a normal pelvic examination are used to diagnose primary dysmenorrhea.

B. Complication of pregnancy: missed or incomplete abortion or ectopic pregnancy.

C. Endometriosis or adenomyosis.

D. Ruptured ovarian cyst.

E. Infection: endometritis, salpingitis, PID, or pelvic adhesions.

F. Fibroid tumors.

G. Adhesions.

H. UTI.

I. Bowel disease: irritable bowel disease or inflammatory bowel disease.

Plan

A. General interventions: Support patient concerns and identify reality of discomfort. Identify primary source of pain if other diagnoses exist.

B. Patient education: See the Section III Patient Teaching Guides for this chapter, "Painful Menstrual Cramps or Periods (Dysmenorrhea)" and "How to Take Birth Control Pills."

   1. Educate the patient about the physiology of menstruation.

   2. Teach the patient that endometriosis is one of the leading causes of infertility.

   3. Encourage activity and exercise, such as walking or swimming.

   4. Advise warm baths or heating pads to help relieve some pain.

C. Pharmaceutical therapy

   1. Nonsteroidal anti-inflammatory agents (NSAIDs) are the drugs of choice.

      a. They inhibit prostaglandin synthesis in the endometrium, thus decreasing uterine cramping. There is an analgesic effect, also.

      b. The fenamates have been the most effective, followed by the propionic acid derivatives.

      c. The drugs should be started as the menstrual period begins. It is no longer considered standard of care to begin the drugs a few days prior to the onset of the menstrual period.

      d. Prostaglandin inhibitors relieve dysmenorrhea in 80% of women.

   2. Medications of choice for dysmenorrhea

      a. NSAIDs

         i. Arylacetic acid derivatives: naproxen sodium (Aleve) 200 mg every 8–10 hours; naproxen sodium (Anaprox) 275 mg every 6–8 hours, or 550 mg every 12 hours; naproxen as sodium (Naprelan) 1–1.5 g once daily.

         ii. Propionic acid derivatives: ibuprofen (Advil, Motrin, Nuprin) 200–800 mg every 4–6 hours; ketoprofen (Orudis) 12.5–25 mg every 4–6 hours. These are OTC medications.

         iii. Anthranilic acid derivatives: mefenamic acid (Ponstel) 500 mg initial dose, then 250 mg every 6 hours. The treatment maximum is 2–3 days.

         iv. Benzeneacetic acid derivatives: diclofenac potassium (Cataflam) 50 mg three times per day. Initial dose of 100 mg may be given.

      b. Oral contraceptive pills: any combination pill is efficacious.

   3. Medications of choice for endometriosis

      a. NSAIDs

      b. Oral contraceptive pills

      c. With physician consultation or referral, danazol (Danocrine)

      d. With physician consultation or referral, gonadotropin-releasing hormone (Gn-RH) agonists such as nafarelin (Synarel), leuprolide acetate (Lupron, Lupron Depot), and goserelin acetate (Zoladex).

Follow-up

A. Have the patient return in 3 months. Encourage the patient to give the treatment 3 months to determine effectiveness.

Consultation/Referral

A. Consult with a physician if dysmenorrhea does not respond to NSAIDs or oral contraceptives for further workup to determine the source of the pain.

B. Consider consultation with OB/GYN for laparoscopy or hysteroscopy to diagnose endometriosis or adhesions. Laser may be used to destroy endometrial implants or to lyse adhesions.

Individual Considerations

A. Pregnancy: Uterine contractions in pregnancy could be preterm labor.

B. Adolescents: Remember that endometriosis can occur in this age group. It is not an extremely rare finding.

C. Adults: Endometriosis can be a disabling condition interfering with work and sexual relationships. It may continue into the perimenopausal period.

DYSPAREUNIA

Definition

A. Dyspareunia is genital or pelvic discomfort associated with sexual intercourse (entry or deep penetration) and interferes with sexual satisfaction. Dyspareunia may be superficial relating to vulvar and vaginal pain, or it may be deep relating to deep pelvic pain.

Incidence

A. Sixty percent of women have dyspareunia at some time in their life. Up to 30% of women experience chronic dyspareunia.

Pathogenesis

Physical and psychosocial etiologies have been identified.

A. Physical causes

   1. Vulvovaginal anomalies

      a. Thick hymen

      b. Short vagina

      c. Vaginal agenesis

      d. Vaginal septum

   2. Organic dyspareunia

      a. Episiotomy scars

      b. Bartholin's gland cyst

      c. Vulvar dystrophy

      d. Inflammation or infection, STI

e. Vulvovaginal cancer
f. Pelvic disease
   i. PID
   ii. Uterine or ovarian tumors
   iii. Adenomyosis
   iv. Pelvic scarring or adhesions v. endometriosis
3. Musculoskeletal anomalies
   a. Disk disease
   b. Myofascial pain
   c. Coccygodynia
4. Extensive prolapse or organ displacement
5. Urethral syndrome or other urinary tract disorders
6. Vulvodynia
7. Gastrointestinal anomalies
   a. Constipation
   b. Irritable bowel syndrome
   c. Inflammatory bowel disease
   d. Anorexia
8. Hormonal factors
   a. Hypoestrogenemia causing atrophic vaginitis
   b. Breast-feeding
   c. Menopause
B. Psychosocial causes
1. Childhood molestation
2. Fear of pain, infection, or pregnancy
3. Pelvic congestion syndrome
4. Poor partner communication
5. History of sexual assault, including date rape
6. Previous trauma during intercourse
7. Domestic violence

Common Complaints
A. Irritation or burning with intercourse
B. Lack of vaginal lubrication
C. Pain with vulvar or vaginal contact
D. Pain with deep penetration
E. Postcoital bleeding

Other Signs and Symptoms
A. Vulvar pain
B. Vaginal pain or burning
C. Vaginal dryness

Subjective Data
A. Review the onset, duration, and course of presenting symptoms.
B. Review the patient's medical or surgical history for physical causes (see "Pathogenesis").
C. Ask: How often does pain occur: with every intercourse, near periods, in certain sexual positions? What relief measures have been tried; is there improvement with using extra lubrication? How much relief was obtained with each measure?
D. Obtain a complete sexual history including the following:
1. Sexual practices
2. Sexual satisfaction or orgasm
3. Perception of partner satisfaction
4. Age at first coitus
5. History of sexual abuse, molestation, rape
6. Perceptions regarding sexuality
7. Number of sexual partners and preferences

8. Time spent on foreplay
9. History of recent delivery and breast-feeding
10. Age at onset of puberty, date of last menses, and cycle history
11. Current method of birth control and satisfaction with method; previous methods and why they were discontinued
12. Presence of vaginal discharge, odor, dysuria, or other physical symptoms before or after intercourse
13. Medications, including prescription and over-the-counter drugs
14. Can the woman insert a tampon without pain?

Physical Examination
A. Check temperature, pulse, respirations, and blood pressure.
B. Inspection: Observe generally for discomfort before, during, and after examination.

Look for signs of physical or sexual abuse, cuts, bruises, lacerations. For pain greatest upon deep penile penetration, suspect PID, ovarian cyst, endometriosis, pelvic adhesions, relaxation of pelvic support, or uterine fibroids.

C. Auscultate: Auscultate the abdomen for bowel sounds in all quadrants. Auscultation of the abdomen should precede any palpation or percussion due to the changes in intensity and frequency of sounds after manipulation.
D. Palpate.
1. Palpate the abdomen for masses; check for suprapubic tenderness.
2. Examine the back for range of motion.
E. Pelvic examination.
1. Inspect: Perform perineal exam for atrophic vaginitis. Atrophic vaginitis presents as red, shiny, smooth vagina (loss of rugae); vaginal thinning; decreased elasticity of vaginal tissues. Vulvar inflammation may be present. Assess discharge and rugae for hormonal support.
2. Evaluate the patient for vulvovaginitis. Perform vulvar exam for Bartholin's gland enlargement, fissures, condyloma, and herpes. Inspect for anatomic variants: narrowed introitus, congenital malformations (septum), and pelvic relaxation (cystocele and retrocele).
F. Speculum examination: Inspect for cervicitis, friability, and discharge. If the woman can insert a tampon without pain, a mechanical obstruction is unlikely.
G. Bimanual examination: Check cervical motion tenderness; adnexal masses; uterine size, consistency, and position.
H. Rectovaginal examination: Palpate uterosacral ligaments for pain and nodularity and other signs of pelvic inflammatory disease and endometriosis. **In cases of rectal trauma, cultures may be needed to rule out STIs if anal intercourse is practiced.**

Diagnostic Tests
A. CBC
B. Sedimentation rate, if indicated by physical
C. Hormonal assays: FSH, estradiol
D. Wet prep to rule out candidiasis, trichomoniasis, and bacterial vaginosis

E. Cervical cultures for *Chlamydia,* GC
F. Viral cultures of lesions, if any
G. Urine culture, if applicable
H. Stool culture, if applicable
I. Pelvic ultrasonography, if indicated

Differential Diagnoses
A. Dyspareunia
B. See "Pathogenesis"

Plan
A. General interventions.
 1. Detailed physical examination after a thorough history.
 2. Patients should be encouraged to involve their partner(s) in assessment, diagnosis, and treatment of dyspareunia.
 3. A secure, trusting relationship must be established with the care provider before many patients feel comfortable discussing sexuality issues. Continuity with one provider is essential.
 4. Patients with dyspareunia should be evaluated for multiple etiologies. Treat underlying pathologies such as musculoskeletal anomalies, pelvic infection, urinary tract infection, sexually transmitted diseases, hormonal deficiencies, and gastrointestinal etiologies (see specific chapters for treatment plans and drug therapy).
B. Patient teaching: See the Section III Patient Teaching Guide for this chapter, "Pain With Intercourse."
C. Pharmaceutical therapy.
 1. Refer to specific chapter for therapies related to etiology.
 2. Vulvodynia: Consider the use of topical agents applied to the vulva or vestibule, antihistamine therapy, and/or tricyclic antidepressants.
 3. Lidocaine (Xylocaine) 2% gel applied to vulva, vestibule, and fourchette.
 4. Diphenhydramine (Benadryl) 25–50 mg orally at bedtime, or 0.1% triamcinolone acetonide cream twice daily for pruritus.
 5. Amitriptyline 10 mg orally at bedtime.

Follow-up
A. Perform test of cure for all diagnosed infections, if indicated (see specific infection and therapy).
B. Educate the patient on disease and complaints of pain (see the Section III Patient Teaching Guide for this chapter, "Pain With Intercourse").
C. Refer to follow-up plans for specific etiology.

Consultation/Referral
A. Refer the patient to a gynecologist for removal of cysts, endometriomas. Laparoscopy is indicated if endometriosis, adhesions, or an adnexal mass is suspected.
B. Refer the patient to a gynecologist for vulvovaginal anomalies including thickened hymen, shortened vagina, vaginal agenesis; vaginal dilator therapy may be tried.
C. Refer the patient for sexual therapy consultation for continued complaints without an identifiable physical cause.

Individual Considerations
A. Pregnancy or postpartum: Sexual intercourse may continue throughout pregnancy unless there is pain, bleeding, preterm labor, or premature rupture of the membranes. Alternate positions should be suggested by the provider. Sexual intercourse may resume in the postpartum period when the bleeding has decreased or stopped, incision or episiotomy is healed, and the woman is comfortable upon finger insertion and test of vaginal discomfort. Breast-feeding causes hormonal changes that may produce a menopauselike state, and extra lubrication is usually required.
B. Partners: Encourage the patient to have partner(s) participate in sexual health counseling.

EMERGENCY CONTRACEPTION

Definition
A. This is a prospective method of pregnancy prevention when unprotected intercourse occurs.

Incidence
A. Presently, emergency contraception has been used by only 1% of American women. The intent is to increase the use of emergency contraception to reduce the number of unintended pregnancies and thus reduce the number of abortions and deliveries of truly unwanted children. Over 3 million women are not using birth control and are at risk for unintended pregnancy.

Pathophysiology
A. Hormones in oral contraceptive pills temporarily disrupt ovarian hormone production and cause an absent or dysfunctional luteal phase hormone pattern. This results in an out-of-phase endometrium that is unsuitable for implantation. Hormone disruption may likewise interfere with fertilization and cause disordered tubal transport. Hormones or minerals (copper) in an IUD as well as an inflammatory response occur, which make the endometrium unsuitable for implantation and interfere with fertilization and transport.

Predisposing Factors
A. Rape
B. Failure of other means of birth control, including broken condom, dislodged diaphragm or cervical cap, expelled IUD, lost or forgotten pills
C. Unprotected intercourse

Common Complaints
A. "I'm worried that I might get pregnant because the condom broke."
B. "My diaphragm slipped."
C. "I went on vacation and forgot my pills."

Other Signs and Symptoms
A. Unprotected intercourse

Subjective Data
A. Elicit a menstrual history. When was the patient's LMP? Are her periods regular?
B. What form of contraception was used, if any?

C. Has the patient experienced any early signs of pregnancy? If so, discuss.

D. Ask about early symptoms of pregnancy such as frequency of urination, nausea, breast tenderness, and late or missed period.

E. Ask the patient about her feelings or plans if she should get pregnant.

Physical Examination

A. Blood pressure, pulse, and weight.

B. Inspect: abdomen for enlargement compatible with pregnancy.

C. Palpate: abdomen for uterine size; if fundus is palpable, measure for fundal height.

D. Auscultate: heart, lungs, abdomen. If the uterus is enlarged and is measured to be greater than 11 weeks gestation, attempt to hear fetal heart tones with fetal Doppler.

E. Pelvic exam.
1. Inspect the external genitalia for lesions; note female pubic hair pattern.
2. Speculum exam: Observe for bluish color of cervix (Chadwick's sign). Observe vaginal discharge; note color and odor.
3. Bimanual exam: Palpate the cervix for softening associated with early pregnancy. Palpate uterine size.

Diagnostic Tests

A. Pregnancy test: Urine or serum HCG

Differential Diagnoses

A. Unprotected intercourse, potential for pregnancy

B. Pregnancy

C. Dysfunctional uterine bleeding

D. Amenorrhea from anovulation, polycystic ovarian disease, or perimenopause

Plan

A. General interventions
1. Review the patient's past medical history, contraceptive history, date of LMP, estimated date of ovulation, date of unprotected intercourse, and number of hours since the first and most recent unprotected intercourse.
2. Discuss the likely risk of pregnancy.
3. Explore the patient's feeling about continuing pregnancy.
4. Decide whether a physical exam and pregnancy test is needed if there is a possibility of a pregnancy from the previous month.

B. Patient teaching: See the Section III Teaching Guide for this chapter, "Emergency Contraception."
1. Discuss options, risks, failure rates, necessary follow-up, alteration of menstrual period, and warning signs of complications.
2. Discuss interim plan for contraception.
3. Advise the patient to take oral contraceptive pills as prescribed or have IUD inserted within 96 hours of unprotected intercourse.
4. Treatment is most effective if taken within 12–24 hours. **Treatment is not likely to be effective if begun after 72 hours.**

5. Treatment is *not effective* in already established pregnancy.

6. Educate the patient about possibility of menstrual cycle disturbance with the next menstrual period.

7. If menstrual bleeding does not begin within 3 weeks, evaluate for possible pregnancy.

8. Emergency contraception is not associated with an increased incidence of abnormal outcome of pregnancy should pregnancy not be averted. Emergency contraception does not always work.

9. This is **not** to be used as a primary contraceptive method.

10. Have prescription or pack of pills available for an emergency situation.

11. The IUD should be used only for women at low risk for pelvic inflammatory disease and when the woman intends to continue use of the IUD for contraception.

C. Pharmaceutical therapy
1. Emergency contraception medication
   a. Plan B® (levonorgestrel) is available without a prescription for patients age 18 and older. If younger than 18 a prescription is required.
   b. Two doses of a combination of ethinyl estradiol and norgestrel or levonorgestrel, 12 hours apart. Table 13.1 provides the equivalent dosing for Plan B using standard oral contraceptives.
   c. Method must be utilized within 72 hours of unprotected intercourse. Treatment is most effective if taken within 12–24 hours.
   d. Side effects of nausea and vomiting with emergency contraception are common. Take each dose with food. Take antiemetic, dimenhydrinate (Dramamine) 50 mg orally, 30 minutes before dose of medication.
   e. If vomiting occurs within 1–3 hours of taking a dose, take another dose.
   f. Educate the patient about common side effects such as breast tenderness, abdominal pain, headache, and dizziness.

2. Intrauterine device
   a. Copper IUD (Paragard's CUT 380, Ortho Pharmaceuticals) must be inserted within 5–7 days after ovulation in a cycle when unprotected intercourse has occurred. The advantage is that the IUD may be left in place for continuing contraception for 10 years.
   b. Mechanism of action: Two ideas have been proposed.
      i. IUD leads to endometrial changes that prohibit implantation.
      ii. Direct toxic effect of the copper ions on the embryo.

Consultation/Referral

A. Consult with a physician if there is no withdrawal bleed within 4 weeks.

B. Consult with or refer the patient to a physician if necessary to insert IUDs.

TABLE 13.1 Emergency Contraception

Brand	Number of Pills per Dose	Ethynyl Estradiol (µg)/Dose	Levonorgestrel (g) Dose
Ovral	2 white pills	100	0.50
Lo/Ovral	4 white pills	120	0.60
Nordette	4 orange pills	120	0.60
Levlen	4 orange pills	120	0.60
Triphasil	4 yellow pills	120	0.50
Tri-Levlen	4 yellow pills	120	0.50
Alesse	5 pink pills	100	0.50
Plan B	1 white pill	–	0.75

Directions: Take first does within 72 hours after unprotected intercourse, and repeat dose in 12 hours.

C. Here are several ways patients can find emergency contraception:
1. Not 2 Late is operated by the Office of Population Research at Princeton University and the Association of Reproductive Health Professionals: 888-NOT-2-LATE
2. Web sites:
   a. Emergency contraception (you can be included as a provider): http://ec.princeton.edu/
   b. Planned Parenthood: http://www.ppfa.org

Follow-up
A. Have the patient return in 3–4 weeks if she has no menstrual period, or have her return for routine follow-up regardless of whether a menstrual period occurs.

Special Considerations
A. Pregnancy: There is no increased incidence of anomalies if pregnancy does occur.

ENDOMETRIOSIS

Definition
A. Endometriosis is ectopic endometrial tissue that exhibits hormonal responsiveness but is located outside the uterine cavity. Bleeding from this ectopic endometrial tissue causes pelvic inflammation and scarring, resulting in chronic pelvic pain and infertility. Endometrial lesions have been found in the vagina, GI tract (especially the sigmoid colon), thoracic cavity, limbs, and gallbladder.

Incidence
A. The true incidence of endometriosis is unknown. Ranges of 5%–30% have been cited. Positive family history (mother or sister) increases the risk 10-fold. Endometriosis does not have a higher incidence for any particular race or socioeconomic group.

Pathogenesis
A. Retrograde menstruation is the most popular theory for the etiology of endometriosis. Menses are suspected of "flowing backward" through the fallopian tubes, resulting in the "seeding" of endometrial tissue outside the uterus.

Predisposing Factors
A. Positive family history, mother and/or sister
B. History of progressive dysmenorrhea
C. History of prolonged uninterrupted menstrual cycles; first pregnancy at a late age
D. Limited or no prior use of hormonal contraceptives

Common Complaints
A. Pain prior to period
B. Pain with intercourse
C. Pain with bowel movements, may include constipation from the fear or pain of having a bowel movement (dyschezia)
D. Spotting and bleeding

Other Signs and Symptoms
A. Dyspareunia and/or pain that radiates to the thigh
B. Chronic, noncyclic pelvic pain
C. Abnormal vaginal bleeding: premenstrual spotting and dysfunctional uterine bleeding (DUB)
D. Other bowel symptoms: diarrhea and rectal bleeding
E. Urinary symptoms: dysuria, urgency, and hematuria

Subjective Data
A. Review the onset, duration, and course of complaints.
B. Question the patient regarding menstrual history: interval and duration of menstrual cycles and history of dysmenorrhea.
C. Question the patient regarding former use of hormonal contraceptives including levanorgestrel (Norplant System), birth control pills, medroxyprogesterone (Depo-Provera), and progesterone (Progestasert IUD).
D. Question the patient regarding change in bowel patterns or habits or pain with defecation.
E. Question the patient regarding incidence of dyspareunia.
F. Note patient parity and/or history of infertility.

Physical Examination
A. Check temperature, pulse, respirations, and blood pressure.
B. Inspect
1. Note general appearance for discomfort before, during, and after examination.
2. Perform detailed external genitalia exam.
C. Auscultate: Auscultate abdomen for bowel sounds in all quadrants. Auscultation of the abdomen should precede

any palpation or percussion due to the changes in intensity and frequency of sounds after manipulation.

D. Palpate
1. Palpate abdomen for masses.
2. Check for suprapubic tenderness.
3. Back: Check for CVA tenderness.

E. Pelvic examination
1. Speculum examination: Inspect the cervix for cervicitis; friability; discharge color, odor, and amount. Note any cutaneous lesions of the vagina, cervix, perineum that resemble "powder burn or chocolate spots." Laparoscopic findings frequently reveal "powder burn" lesions of endometrial implants along the uterosacral ligament, pelvic peritoneum, ovaries, sigmoid colon, and other pelvic organs.
2. Bimanual examination: Check for cervical motion tenderness, adnexal masses; check uterine size, consistency, position, and mobility.

The most common indicator for endometriosis is a fixed retroverted uterus with nodularity felt along the uterosacral ligaments. Palpation of endometrial implants may result in exquisite pain for the patient.

3. Rectovaginal examination: Palpate uterosacral ligaments for pain and nodularity. Evaluate for masses and polyps of rectum. A rectal examination is done because the uterus is often fixed in a retroverted position due to endometriosis. The endometrial nodules present on the posterior uterine wall, cul-de-sac, and uterosacral ligament may be distinguished better rectally.

Diagnostic Tests

There are no specific diagnostic tests for endometriosis. Definite diagnosis is done by laparoscopy.

A. Serum β HCG, to rule out ectopic pregnancy
B. WBC, to rule out infection
C. Cervical culture for *Chlamydia,* GC, to rule out STI and PID
D. Urine culture, if indicated
E. Transvaginal ultrasonography, to rule out cysts and masses
F. GI series or barium enema, if indicated

Differential Diagnoses

A. Endometriosis
B. Dysmenorrhea
C. Ovarian cysts
D. Pelvic inflammatory disease
E. Premenstrual syndrome
F. Mittelschmerz
G. Trauma
H. Appendicitis
I. Pregnancy: normal, missed abortion, or ectopic
J. GI or GU complaints: diverticular disease, spastic colon, or urinary tract infection

Plan

A. General interventions: After surgical confirmation, the practitioner may comanage endometriosis with a physician.

B. Patient teaching.
1. Treatment goals include prevention of disease progression, alleviation of pain, and establishment or restoration of fertility. Treatment options include the following:
   a. Observation alone
   b. Medical therapy or pharmacologic therapy
   c. Referral or consultation for laparoscopic therapy including laser vaporization and removal of adhesions
2. Continuation or recurrence of pelvic pain may necessitate assisting the woman to manage her chronic pelvic pain and dysmenorrhea with NSAID therapy and/or other nonnarcotic chronic pain therapies, such as visualization and biofeedback.
3. **Hysterectomy and bilateral salpingo-oophorectomy are the only definitive cures for women who do not wish to conserve their reproductive capacity. This should be considered only as a last resort for failed conservative treatment.**

C. Pharmaceutical therapy: Diagnosis must first be confirmed by laparoscopy.
1. Mild endometriosis
   a. Combined oral contraceptive pills are considered first-line therapy. If the patient experiences pain during the week of withdrawal bleeding, she may take active pills continuously, omitting the placebo pills of the "off week."

Combination oral contraceptives are being used to produce a state of pseudopregnancy that should induce regression of the disease.

   b. Medroxyprogesterone acetate 10 mg daily for up to 6 months, or a long-acting progestin (Depo-Provera) 100–200 mg by intramuscular injection each month for 6 months.
2. Moderate to severe complaints
   a. Gonadotropin-releasing hormone (Gn-RH) agonist
      i. Leuprolide acetate (Lupron) 3.75 mg by intramuscular injection every month.
      ii. Nafarelin (Synarel) nasal spray twice daily.

Use of Gn-RH agonist, which acts to suppress ovulation, can result in side effects including hot flashes, mood changes, and other menopausal symptoms. Use is restricted to 6 months to avoid decrease in bone density. Expense of this therapy may preclude its use.

   b. Danazol 200–400 mg twice daily for up to 6 months
      i. **Use of danazol, which acts to produce anovulation and hypogonadotropinism, can result in androgenic side effects including acne, hirsutism, weight gain, and voice changes that may not be reversible.**
      ii. Other side effects, which are reversible, include decreased breast size, atrophic vaginitis, dyspareunia, hot flashes, and emotional liability.

Follow-up

A. Patients must return monthly while receiving Gn-RH agonist or danazol therapies to assess for symptom relief and side effect profile.

Consultation/Referral

A. The workup, evaluation, and medications for endometriosis are expensive. Refer to a gynecologist for initial management. A prudent approach is recommended with conservative treatment option; evaluate the results before trying another.

B. Refer the patient for a surgical consultation for definitive diagnosis. Endometriosis may be suspected based on symptoms and physical examination. It cannot, however, be confirmed unless actually visualized by laparoscopy.

Individual Considerations

A. Pregnancy: Infertility may be a presenting symptom. Treatment may, therefore, be focused on endometriosis abatement and fertility support.

Resources

Endometriosis Association
8585 North 76th Place
Milwaukee, WI 53223
800-992-3636
800-426-2363 (Canada)
http://www.endometriosisassn.org/

Endometriosis Treatment Program
St. Charles Medical Center
2500 North East Neff Road

Bend, OR 97701
800-446-2177, ext. 6904
541-383-6904
9 AM to 5 PM (Pacific time), Monday through Friday

INFERTILITY

Definition

A. Infertility is defined as the inability of a couple to conceive within 12 months of unprotected intercourse. Many clinicians use a 6-month time frame if the woman is older than 35 years of age.

B. A woman who has never been pregnant or a man who has never initiated a pregnancy is said to have "primary infertility."

C. If a previous pregnancy has been achieved and the couple is unable to conceive a subsequent pregnancy, the term "secondary infertility" is applied.

Incidence

A. It is estimated that approximately 2.5 million couples may be classified as infertile. Pelvic inflammatory disease is the leading cause of infertility in the world. Between 5%–20% of infertility is unexplained.

Pathogenesis

Infertility may occur in the male or female. Evaluate both partners:

A. Infrequent intercourse
B. Interpersonal problems
C. Medical. See Table 13.2

TABLE 13.2 Pathogenesis of Infertility

Male Pathogenesis	Female Pathogenesis
A. Faulty sperm production.	A. Advanced maternal age.
1. Azoospermia from:	B. Disorder of ovulation/hypothalamic dysfunction:
a. Cancer therapy.	1. Anovulation.
b. Adult mumps.	2. Amenorrhea.
c. Sertoli-cell-only syndrome.	3. Polycystic ovary triad:
d. Hypogonadism.	a. Acne.
e. Retrograde ejaculation.	b. Obesity.
2. Oligospermia from:	c. Hirsutism.
a. Varicocele.	4. Premature ovarian failure:
b. Small testicular size.	a. Autoimmune.
B. Reproductive tract anomaly:	b. Idiopathic.
1. Blocked vas deferens.	c. Cancer therapy.
2. Varicocele.	5. Luteal phase insufficiency.
3. Congenital obstruction of epididymis.	6. Prolactinoma.
C. Klinefelter's syndrome.	C. Ovarian factors:
D. Physical and chemical agent exposure:	1. Cysts or tumor.
1. Coal tar.	2. Irradiation.
2. Radiation.	

(continued)

TABLE 13.2 *(continued)*

Male Pathogenesis	Female Pathogenesis
E. Endocrine disorders:	D. Tubal disorders/damage/blocked:
1. Diabetes.	1. PID.
2. Low serum testosterone.	2. *Chlamydia trachomatis.*
3. Pituitary tumors.	3. Postpartum infection.
4. Hyperprolactinemia.	4. Pelvic trauma (MVA).
F. Testicular infection.	5. Inflammatory bowel disease.
G. Injury to reproductive organs/tract.	6. Endometriosis.
H. Nerve damage/neurologic disease: spinal cord injury.	7. Adhesions.
I. Impotence/erectile difficulty: performance anxiety.	E. Uterine pathology:
J. Premature ejaculation.	1. Congenital anomalies: duplication.
K. Early withdrawal.	2. Septate.
L. Lifestyle factors:	3. Fibroids.
1. Drugs.	4. IUD.
2. Smoking.	5. Asherman's syndrome.
3. Alcohol.	6. Synechiae.
4. Malnutrition.	F. Cervical factors:
M. Antispermatozoa antibodies.	1. Anatomic abnormalities (hood).
N. Medications:	2. Previous cervical surgery (i.e., conization, which leads to mucus depletion).
1. Antihypertensives.	3. Hostile cervical mucus.
2. Antidepressants.	4. Presence of sperm antibodies in the cervix.
3. Antipsychotics.	5. Infections.
4. Antiulcer agents/antacids.	G. Lifestyle factors:
5. Muscle relaxants.	1. Drugs.
	2. Smoking.
	H. Vaginal factors:
	1. Intact hymen.
	2. Septum.
	3. Absent vagina.
	4. Infection:
	a. *Trichomonas.*
	b. *Candida.*
	c. *Chlamydia.*
	d. *Mycoplasma.*
	e. Bacterial vaginosis.
	f. GC.
	g. Streptococci.
	I. Medications: oral contraceptives.
	J. Medical problems:
	1. Lupus.
	2. Hypothyroidism.
	3. Diabetes.
	4. Antiphospholipid syndrome.

Predisposing Factors

A. Predisposing factors depend on the etiology.

Common Complaints

A. The common complaint is an inability to achieve pregnancy despite frequent acts of intercourse.

Other Signs and Symptoms

A. Dependent on the pathogenesis and history.

Subjective Data

A. Obtain a complete health history including the following:
1. Age of both partners
2. General health of both partners
3. Complete pregnancy history of the female:
   a. Number of pregnancies, term and preterm
   b. Vaginal deliveries or cesarean sections
   c. Recurrent miscarriages, gestational age(s)
   d. Stillbirths
   e. D and C for abortions or miscarriages
   f. Cerclage for incompetent cervix
4. Paternity history of the male
5. Length of infertility, including prior workup, if any
6. Coital history:
   a. Frequency
   b. Timing and adequacy
   c. Use of lubricants; some may be spermicidal
   d. Postcoital habits: douching or voiding
7. Adequacy of intercourse:
   a. Penetration of the vagina
   b. Ejaculation by the male
B. Obtain a complete menstrual history including the following:
1. Age at puberty
2. Regularity of cycles
3. Discomfort during menses
4. Date of last menstrual period
C. Obtain a complete gynecologic history including the following:
1. Contraceptive use
2. Medical and surgical interventions:
   a. D and C
   b. Laparoscopy or endometriosis
3. Anomalies
D. Take a complete nutritional and exercise history; note eating disorders:
1. Anorexia nervosa
2. Bulimia
E. Review male **and** female reproductive tract infections and treatments for past and present partners.
F. Review each individual's habits:
1. Smoking: how much, how often, how long
2. Drugs: how much, how often, how long for each drug
3. Alcohol: how much, how often, how long
4. Use of saunas or hot tubs
5. Exercise, including biking
G. Take a complete medication history, specifically review for the following:
1. Antihypertensives
2. Antidepressants
3. Antipsychotics
4. Antiulcer agents or antacids
5. Muscle relaxants
H. Review for exposure to toxic chemicals, radiation, or known teratogens:
1. Military war exposure
2. Employment exposure
3. Residential exposure:
   a. Microwaves
   b. Pesticides
I. Inquire about DES exposure in utero (for either partner).
J. Review for symptoms of thyroid dysfunction:
1. Weight gain or loss
2. Change of bowel habits
3. Intolerance to heat or cold
4. Appetite changes
K. Review for systemic diseases:
1. Cardiac
2. Collagen vascular diseases
3. Diabetes
L. Make an assessment of the psychosocial context of the infertility including personal, emotional, economic factors; family pressures for children; expectations; timing of pregnancy; consideration of adoption; and stress from failure to conceive.

Signs and Symptoms

A. See "Pathogenesis" and medical history.
B. An initial assessment, including interview, physical examination, and some laboratory tests, is within the scope of function of a primary care provider.
C. Consultation and referral are required for special testing, surgery, and assisted reproductive therapy.

Physical Examination: Male

A. Check temperature, pulse, respirations, and blood pressure. Obtain height, weight, and BMI.
B. Inspect.
1. Note general signs and appearance of underandrogenization: decreased body hair, gynecomastia, and eunuchoid proportions.
2. Test the patient's visual field for possible mass lesion.
3. Examine the penis for hypospadias. Observe urethra for discharge.
C. Percuss: Check deep tendon reflexes (DTRs) for signs of hypothyroidism.
D. Palpate.
1. Neck: Examine thyroid.
2. Genitals: Examine the scrotum for testicular size, absence of vas deferens, and for the presence of varicocele.
E. Rectal examination: Check prostate and seminal vesicles for tenderness and other signs of infection.

Valsalva's maneuver performed while the patient stands helps to reveal small varicocele. Varicocele feels like "a bag of worms" with bluish discoloration visible through the scrotum. Approximately 23%–30% of infertile males have varicocele (usually present on the left side). No treatment is necessary if the semen analysis is normal.

Physical Examination: Female

A. Check temperature, pulse, respirations, and blood pressure.
B. Inspect.
  1. Examine breasts for presence of nipple discharge.
  2. Note general signs and appearance of polycystic ovarian syndrome (PCO).

PCO triad includes acne, obesity, and hirsutism.

C. Auscultate: Abdomen for bowel sounds in all quadrants. Auscultation of the abdomen should precede any palpation or percussion due to the changes in intensity and frequency of sounds after manipulation.
D. Palpate.
  1. Neck: Examine the thyroid.
  2. Check abdomen for tenderness and masses.
  3. Back: Check CVA tenderness.
E. Percuss: Check deep tendon reflexes
F. Pelvic examination
  1. Inspect: Perform detailed external peritoneal exam for signs of infection; lesions; or anomalies of clitoris, labia, Skene's gland, Bartholin's gland, vulva, and perineum.
  2. Speculum examination
    a. Observe length of vagina, position and characteristic of cervix, and any anomalies.
    b. Sound the uterus and cervix for stenosis. Observe the characteristics of cervical mucus: thin and watery or thick and cloudy, odor, or evidence of infection.
  3. Bimanual examination: Check uterine size, consistency, contour, mobility, cervical motion tenderness, and adnexal masses.

A fixed, immobile uterus determined on bimanual exam indicates the presence of pelvic scarring resulting from "old disease" such as endometriosis and pelvic inflammatory disease.

  4. Rectovaginal examination: Palpate uterosacral ligaments for pain and nodularity; evaluate masses and polyps of rectum.

Diagnostic Tests

A. Male factor
  1. Semen analysis
  2. Sperm penetration assay
B. Ovarian factor
  1. Basal body temp (BBT).
  2. Serum progesterone: serum progesterone greater than15 ng/mL indicates ovulation.
  3. Urinary LH for surge.
  4. FSH: a high FSH, greater than 40 m IU/ml, indicates ovarian failure.
  5. TSH.
  6. Serum prolactin.

When nipple discharge is present, check serum prolactin and TSH to rule out hyperprolactinemia and hypothyroidism.

C. Cervical factor
  1. Postcoital test, at LH surge.
  2. Assess for ferning of the cervical mucus.
  3. Assess for spinnbarkeit, during midcycle.

Ferning of cervical mucus, determined by microscopy, indicates preovulatory estrogen. Spinnbarkeit demonstrates estrogenic mucus is thin, clear, and copious in amount and can stretch to introitus from the cervical os.

Just prior to ovulation, the mucus is the thinnest; mucus threads of 6–10 cm from the endocervix are normal.

D. Pelvic or uterine factor
  1. Endometrial biopsy
  2. Hysterosalpingogram (HSG); also done for tubal factor
  3. Ultrasonography
  4. Laparoscopy
E. Other tests
  1. Pap smear with maturation index
  2. Cultures for GC and *Chlamydia*
  3. Pregnancy test, if amenorrhea is present
  4. CBC, sedimentation rate
  5. *Mycoplasma* culture
  6. Wet mount

Differential Diagnoses

A. Infertility
B. Sexual dysfunction
C. Hypothyroidism
D. Hypothalamic dysfunction: amenorrhea
E. Hyperprolactinemia
F. Menopause
G. Ovarian failure
H. Polycystic ovarian syndrome
I. Asherman's syndrome
J. Tubal occlusion
K. Antisperm antibodies
L. Endometriosis
M. Oligo-ovulation
N. Uterine anomalies: fibroids, synechiae, and septa
O. Pelvic adhesions

Plan

A. General interventions
  1. Semen analysis is the first step in an infertility workup. Semen analysis should be performed in a reputable laboratory. If the first evaluation is abnormal, it should be repeated one time. Normal semen analysis includes the following:
    a. Sperm count: greater than 20 million/mL
    b. Volume: 2.6 mL
    c. Motility: greater than 50%
    d. Morphology: greater than 60%
    e. Liquefaction: within 20–30 min of ejaculation
  2. The male physical examination is generally done if semen analysis is abnormal.
  3. **The male should always be evaluated first before a long and expensive female evaluation is begun.**
  4. Female evaluation
    a. Basal body temperature (BBT): Followed for several months to evaluate ovulation. Some patient's

temperatures dip just before the day of ovulation and then rise. Ovulation and the development of the corpus luteum manifest as an increase in BBT by 0.6°F–1°F above the patient's baseline temperature (LH surge). The BBT provides presumptive evidence of normal oocyte production and related hormonal change, as well as guidance for the frequency and timing of intercourse.

   b. Postcoital test (PCT): Evaluates the character, quality, and spinnbarkeit of the cervical mucus. The presence of at least 5–10 motile sperm per high-power field is normal. The PCT should be performed about day 14 or around the time of expected LH surge as determined by the patient's BBT chart. Poor timing of the PCT is a cause of suboptimal mucus. The test should then be repeated.

   c. Endometrial biopsy: Sampling of the uterine lining late in the luteal phase. The test is scheduled 10 days after the BBT increase, or 2–3 days before the onset of the next menses. A normal secretory endometrium and the absence of inflammation indicate that implantation is feasible.

   d. Hysterosalpingogram (HSG; performed in radiology): Evaluates tubal patency and rules out uterine anomalies. The HSG should be scheduled for the interval between cessation of menstrual flow and ovulation to avoid retrograde flow of menstrual tissue into the tubes and the abdominal cavity.

   e. Laparoscopy: Diagnostic if used as the final screening examination for infertility. Performed by a gynecologist, it is usually done in the first 2 weeks of the menstrual cycle to ensure that the patient is not pregnant. Direct visualization of the pelvic organs provides data about degree of adhesion formation, presence of endometriosis or fibroids, and the possibility of surgical repair of damaged tubes.

B. Patient teaching
   1. Infertile couples often require extensive counseling including grief counseling for failure to achieve pregnancy.
   2. See the Section III Patient Teaching Guide for this chapter, "Instructions for Postcoital Testing."
   3. Teach the patient to take basal body temperature measurements.

C. Pharmaceutical therapy
   1. Treatment depends on causative factor(s).
   2. Prescription medications must be supervised by physician and/or specialist due to possible complications such as ovarian hyperstimulation.

Follow-up
A. Follow-up depends on causative factor(s).

Consultation/Referral
A. Consultation and referral is required for special testing, surgery, and assisted reproductive therapy.
B. Immediate referral to a physician is necessary for ovarian hyperstimulation.

MENOPAUSE

Definition
A. Physiologic or natural menopause is the cessation of menses for 12 consecutive months due to the loss of ovarian follicular activity. Natural or physiologic menopause is a retrospective diagnosis recognized 12 months after the final menses. Natural menopause is generally experienced in women between 45 and 55 years of age.
B. Natural menopause before the age of 40 is considered premature.
C. Premature ovarian failure (POF) is the full or intermittent loss of ovarian function before the age of 40. POF is thought to be caused by genetics, autoimmune disorders, or surgical or chemical interventions.
D. Induced menopause is the abrupt cessation of menses related to chemical or surgical interventions.
E. Perimenopause is caused by fluctuations in ovarian function in the years preceding menopause. The average of onset is usually in a woman's 40s but may occur earlier. Due to fluctuations in ovarian function, pregnancy may still occur and unintended pregnancy should be avoided. Perimenopausal symptoms often last several years with the average duration being 5 years.

Incidence
A. Currently 30 million American women are menopausal with another 6 million to become menopausal in the next 10 years.

Pathogenesis
A. Physiologic menopause is due to failure of ovarian follicular development and ovarian hormone depletion. The major endocrine changes include the decreasing negative feedback on the hypothalamic-pituitary system with increasing follicle stimulating hormone (FSH) and luteinizing hormone (LH). When the ovaries cease to produce estrogen they become unable to respond to FSH resulting in the cessation of ovulation and menstruation.

Common Complaints
A. Insomnia
B. Irregular periods
C. Menstrual bleeding that is heavy and prolonged
D. Urogenital atrophy
   1. Vaginal dryness
   2. Dysparunia
   3. Dysuria/frequency
E. Vasomotor hot flashes/night sweats
F. **Intermenstrual or postcoital spotting should be evaluated for pathologic causes.**

Subjective Data
A. Determine onset, duration, and course of presenting symptoms.
B. Obtain complete medical history including medications and assess for risk of osteoporosis, cardiovascular disease, and breast and endometrial cancer.
C. Obtain complete gynecologic history including menarche, interval and duration of menstrual cycles, history of dysmenorrhea, and pregnancy history. Question the

patient regarding sexual history, and contraceptive used (condoms, pills, diaphragm, IUD), frequency of method used.
D. What is the patient's current menstrual pattern? Does she think she is pregnant?
E. Review associated symptoms (hot flashes, insomnia, genitourinary) onset, timing, duration, and impact on daily life.
F. Assess for mood swings and dysphoria.

Physical Examination
A. Check temperature, pulse, respirations, and blood pressure.
B. Inspect: Observe general overall appearance and obtain height, weight, and BMI.
C. Auscultate: heart, lungs, and abdomen. Auscultation of the abdomen should precede any palpation or percussion due to the changes in intensity and frequency of sounds after manipulation.
D. Percuss: Percuss the abdomen for organomegaly.
E. Palpate.
   1. Palpate thyroid gland.
   2. Perform clinical breast exam.
   3. Palpate groin for lymphadenopathy.
   4. Palpate the abdomen for masses.
F. Pelvic examination.
   1. Inspect: Examine vulva for Bartholin's gland enlargement, fissures, condyloma, herpes, pelvic relaxation, and atrophy.
   2. Palpate: "Milk" the urethra for discharge.
   3. Speculum examination: Inspect for cervicitis and friability. Evaluate vaginal discharge and bleeding for color, amount, and odor. Perform cultures and Pap test as indicated.
   4. Bimanual examination.
      a. Check cervical motion tenderness; evaluate the size, contour, mobility, and tenderness of uterus. An enlarged or irregular uterus requires additional evaluation.

Over time it is normal for the postmenopausal uterus to decrease in size.

      b. Palpate the adnexa for tenderness and masses.

Ovaries should not be palpable in postmenopausal women and require further evaluation if masses or ovaries are appreciated.

   5. Rectovaginal examination: with stool for occult blood in women over 50.

Diagnostic Tests
A. FSH greater than 30 IU/L is generally accepted as diagnostic of menopause; however, fluctuations in FSH and 17–2 estradiol (E2) may make use of these markers unreliable.
B. Consider TSH.
C. Consider qualitative β HCG.
D. CBC if excessive vaginal bleeding.
E. Obtain Pap as indicated.
F. Endometrial biopsy as indicated for intermenstrual spotting or vaginal bleeding after menopause.

G. Transvaginal ultrasonography for enlarged or irregular uterus.
H. Additional screening as indicated such as mammogram, hemoccult, cholesterol, and bone mineral density.

Differential Diagnoses
A. Menopause
B. Anemia
C. Cardiac abnormalities
D. Leukemia or other cancer
E. Menstrual irregularity for any cause of secondary amenorrhea
F. Pregnancy
G. Psychosomatic illness
H. Thyroid disorders

Plan
A. General interventions
   1. Provide reassurance and education regarding commonly experienced symptoms.
   2. Provide education regarding healthy lifestyle changes to include regular exercise, weight control, smoking cessation, limiting use of drugs and alcohol, and stress reduction.
   3. Encourage a healthy diet rich in vitamin D and calcium. Supplement diet to achieve calcium 1,200–15,00 mg/day and vitamin D 400–800 IU/day.
   4. Encourage water-soluble vaginal lubricants as needed for vaginal dryness. See section on "Atrophic Vaginitis."
   5. Avoid warm environments, caffeine, alcohol, spicy food, and emotional upset; they may trigger hot flashes.
   6. Encourage sleep hygiene and adequate rest.
   7. Discuss the risks and benefits of hormone replacement therapy (HRT).

Educate the patient to notify care provider if unusual vaginal bleeding, calf pain, chest pain, shortness of breath, hemoptysis, severe headaches, visual disturbances, breast pain, abdominal pain, or jaundice occur on HRT.

   8. Assess and manage women at increased risk for osteoporosis according to current osteoporosis guidelines.
   9. Assess and treat cardiac risk factors including hypertension and lipids as indicated.
   10. Give the patient the relevant teaching guide. See the Section III Patient Teaching Guide for this chapter, "Menopause."
B. Pharmaceutical therapy
   1. Hormone replacement therapy
      a. All women should be counseled regarding the risk, benefits, limitations, and potential increased risks of HRT. Benefits of HRT include the reduction of hot flashes, insomnia, night sweats, vaginal dryness, mood swings and depression. While HRT does reduce the risk of bone loss and fracture, due to potential risks and effective alternative treatments for osteoporosis, HRT is not recommended for the treatment of osteoporosis. (See "Osteoporosis" in Chapter 17, "Musculoskeletal Guidelines.")

Risks of HRT include venous thromboembolism and breast cancer. Long-term unopposed estrogen therapy increases the risk of endometrial cancer. Potential areas of concern with the use of HRT include gallbladder disease and cardiovascular events. The provider should carefully screen and educate the patient prior to initiating HRT.

b. Estrogen and progestogen are recommended for treatment of moderate to severe vasomotor symptoms and moderate to severe vulvar and vaginal atrophy symptoms. For women with an intact uterus progestogen is used with estrogen therapy (ET) to reduce the risk of endometrial hyperplasia and cancer. Postmenopausal women without an intact uterus generally are not prescribed progestogen and are treated with estrogen alone.

c. Oral HRT can be given either sequentially or continuously. The sequential regimen is given daily with progestogen given on days 1 to 12 of the month. It is common to have withdrawal bleed with this regimen. An alternative to this is the continuous regimen in which both estrogen and progestogen are taken daily.

2. Transdermal estrogen
3. Transvaginal estrogen. See Tables 13.3, 13.4, and 13.5.
4. **Absolute contraindications to use of estrogen therapy also apply to use of oral and topical estrogen (breast cancer, active liver disease, and/or history of recent thromboembolic event). Vaginal estrogen creams are systemically absorbed. As with use of oral and transdermal estrogen, a progestin must be administered to women who have an intact uterus, secondary to the risk of endometrial hyperplasia or cancer.**
5. **Absolute Contraindications to Estrogen Therapy**
   a. Acute liver disease
   b. Cerebral vascular or coronary artery disease, MI or stroke
   c. History of or active thrombophlebitis or thromboembolic disorders
   d. History of uterine or ovarian cancer
   e. Known or suspected cancer of the breast
   f. Known or suspected estrogen-dependent neoplasm
   g. Pregnancy
   h. Undiagnosed, abnormal vaginal bleeding

TABLE 13.3 Hormone Replacement Therapy

Name	Active Ingredient	Dosage
Estrogen Sequential or Continuous Combined		
Premarin	Conjugated estrogen	0.625 mg per day
Estratab	Esterified estrogen	0.625 mg per day
Menest	Esterified estrogen	0.625 mg per day
Estrace	Micronized estrodiol	1.0 mg per day
Ortho-est	Estropipate	0.625 mg per day
Progestin Only for Sequential Regimen		
Amen	Medroxyprogesterone	5–10 mg added to estrogen the first 10–14 days of month
Cycrin	Medroxyprogesterone	5–10 mg added to estrogen the first 10–14 days of month
Provera	Medroxyprogesterone	5–10 mg added to estrogen the first 10–14 days of month
Prometrium	Micronized progesterone	100–200 mg added to estrogen the first 10–14 days of month
Progestin Only for Continuous Combined Regimen		
Cycrin	Medroxyprogesterone	2.5 mg a day
Provera	Medroxyprogesterone	2.5 mg a day
Combination Packet for Continuous Combined Regimen		
Prempro	0.625 mg conjugated equine estrogen and 2.5 mg medroxyprogesterone	1 tablet orally each day
Activella	1 mg 17 β-estrdiol and 0.5 mg norethindrone	1 tablet orally each day
FemHrt	5 mcg ethinyl estradiol and 1 mg norethindrone	1 tablet orally each day

See complete prescribing reference or package insert for dosing, titration, contraindications, and side effects.

TABLE 13.4 Transdermal Replacement Therapy

	Name	Active Ingredient	Dosage
Transdermal patch	Climara	Estradiol	0.25 mg/day 0.0375 mg/day 0.05 mg/day 0.06 mg/day 0.075 mg/day Apply one patch weekly (lower abdomen or upper buttocks)
Transdermal patch	Combipatch	Estradiol 0.05 mg and norethidrone acetate 0.14 mg per day Or Estradiol 0.05mg and norethidrone acetate 0.0.25 mg per day	Continuous combined regimen 1 patch twice weekly for 28-day cycle (lower abdomen)
Transdermal patch	Vivelle		1 patch twice weekly to trunk
Gel-Pump	Elestrim	Estradiol	0.06% gel, one pump daily to clean dry skin of upper arm
Gel-Pump	Estrogel	Estradiol	0.75mg/1.25g gel, one pump daily to clean dry skin of upper arm
Spray	Evamist	Estradiol	1.53 mg/spray, one spray daily to inside of arm
	Vivella	Estradiol	0.05/day, 0.1mg/day

See complete prescribing reference or package insert for dosing, titration, contraindications, and side effects.

TABLE 13.5 Transvaginal Replacement Therapy

Delivery	Name	Active Ingredient	Dosage
Cream	Estrace	Micronized 17-β estradiol	0.1 mg/g, one-half (2 g) to one (4 g) applicator intravaginally at bedtime every night for 1–2 weeks. When vaginal mucosa is restored, maintenance dose is one-quarter applicator (1 g) one to three times weekly in a cyclic regimen.
	Premarin	Conjugated equine estrogen	0.625 mg/g, use 0.5- to 1.0-g applicator inserted intravaginally at bedtime every night for 1–2 weeks, then every other night for 1–2 weeks, then as needed
Ring	Estring	Micronized 17 β estradiol	7.5 mg/24 hours insert new ring every 90 days
	Femring	Estradiol acetate	0.05 mg/day–0.1 mg/day insert new ring every 90 days
Vaginal tablet	Vagifem	Estradiol acetate	25 mch once daily for two weeks then twice weekly
IUD	Mirena	Evonorgestrel	20 mcg daily

See complete prescribing reference or package insert for dosing, titration, contraindications, and side effects.

6. **Relative Contraindications to Estrogen Therapy**
   a. Active gallbladder disease
   b. Familial hyperlipidemia
7. Absolute Contraindications to Progestogen Therapy
   a. Active thrombophlebitis or thromboembolic disorders
   b. Acute liver disease
   c. Known or suspected cancer of the breast
   d. Pregnancy
   e. Undiagnosed, abnormal vaginal bleeding
C. Nonhormonal pharmacological therapy for vasomotor symptoms

1. Antidepressants (hot flash relief is almost immediate)
   a. Fluoxetine (Prozac) 20 mg/day
   b. Vanlafaxine (Effexor) 37.5–75 mg/day
   c. Paroxetine (Paxil) 12.5–25 mg/day
2. Anticonvulsant
   a. Gabapentine (Neurontin) 300 mg/day and titrate to three of four a day
3. Antihypertensive
   a. Clonidine 0.05–0.1 mg/twice a day
   For nonhormonal pharmacological therapies review prescribing literature for side effects, titrations, and discontinuation regimens.
D. Nonprescription remedies/herbals

1. Many nonprescription remedies are currently available for the treatment of menopausal symptoms. These remedies include isoflavones (soy and red clover), black cohosh, DonQuai, evening primrose oil (EPO), ginseng, licorice, and vitamin E.
2. The provider should review with the patient the lack of standardization and evidence regarding safety and efficacy of these products. Currently results of research have been insufficient to support or refute the use of these remedies for the treatment of menopausal symptoms.

Follow-up

A. Follow up in 3–6 months to assess response to treatment, and then yearly for physical exam, Pap smear, and lipid panel as indicated.
B. Consider discontinuation of HRT in 5 years based on patient response and risks and benefits.

Consultation/Referral

A. Consult a gynecologist if the patient experiences symptoms resistant to treatment or vaginal bleeding from an unknown source.

PAP SMEAR INTERPRETATION

The Papanicolaou (Pap) smear is a sample of cells taken from the cervix for cytologic evaluation. The Pap smear is a **screening test** designed to increase detection and treatment of precancerous and early cancerous lesions, and to decrease morbidity and mortality from cases of invasive cervical cancer.

In the United States, approximately 14,500 new cases of cervical cancer occur annually. Of these cases, approximately 4,800 deaths occur. Cervical cancer is the seventh most common cancer in women. There has been a 70% reduction in the incidence of cervical cancer due to the use of Pap smear screening.

The following are risk factors for development of cervical cancer:

A. Early age at first intercourse: younger than 18 years.
B. Multiple sexual partners: more than three in a lifetime.
C. High parity.
D. Lower socioeconomic status.
E. Advanced age.
F. Compromised immune system: infection with HIV.
G. Smoking.
H. Male partner with a history of multiple partners or STIs.
I. History of STI, especially HPV.

Sexually transmitted agents, particularly the human papillomavirus (HPV) strains 16, 18, 31, 33, 39, and 42, are strongly associated with the development of cervical cancer. Human papillomavirus DNA is present in 93% of cervical cancer and precursor lesions.

J. DES exposure in utero.

K. Cervical dysplasia; the risk of carcinoma is 100 times greater in women with dysplasia than in those with a normal cervix.

The Pap smear should include sampling from both the ectocervix and the endocervix to be considered "adequate for interpretation." The ectocervix is the cervical portion extending outward from the external cervical os. The endocervix extends upward from the external os to the internal os, where the cervical epithelium meets the uterine endometrium.

Cervical epithelium is composed of squamous and columnar cells. Squamous epithelium, appearing smooth and pink, lines the vagina and continues upward to cover variable amounts of the ectocervix. Columnar epithelium, darker red and more granular in appearance, lines the endometrium and continues downward to the cervix, lining the endocervical canal. The boundary between squamous and columnar epithelium is called the squamocolumnar junction (or transformation zone) and may occur anywhere on the ectocervix or endocervix.

The squamocolumnar junction may regress at various times as a result of hormonal variation, particularly with sexual activity and during pregnancy, through processes known as epidermidalization and squamous metaplasia. Epidermidalization is an upward growth of squamous cells that replace columnar cells. Squamous metaplasia is the differentiation of columnar cells into squamous cells. The area between the original and new squamocolumnar junction is called the transformation zone. When columnar epithelium is visible on the ectocervix, appearing as a granular, red area, it is referred to as eversion, ectropion, or ectopy. This is often seen in pregnancy or with oral contraceptive use.

Cervical cancer is a progressive disease with a number of histologically definable stages. Invasive cancer of the cervix and its precursors are detectable by cytology before becoming symptomatic and before gross clinical signs appear. When symptoms are present, they usually include (in order of frequency) postcoital spotting; intermenstrual bleeding, especially after exertion; and increased menstrual bleeding. Patients with invasive cancer may experience serosanguineous or yellowish vaginal discharge, which may be foul smelling and intermixed with blood.

Advanced disease may cause urinary or rectal symptoms including bleeding. On speculum examination, advanced lesions appear as necrotic ulcers; in invasive disease they may extend upward or protrude into the vagina.

See the Section II Procedure, "Pap Smear and Maturation Index Procedure."

Bethesda System

The 2001 Bethesda system is the most current classification system used to interpret cytologic findings. It includes the following evaluations:

A. Adequacy of the specimen
   1. Satisfactory for evaluation
   2. Presence or absence of endocervical or transformational zone components

3. Quality indicators such as obscuring blood or inflammation
4. Unsatisfactory for evaluation and specific reason

B. General categorization
   1. Negative for intraepithelial lesion or malignancy
   2. Epithelial cell abnormality
   3. Other such as infection

If an infection is indicated as a Pap smear finding, evaluate the patient and treat her accordingly. Pap smears are not diagnostic of vaginal or cervical infection. Institute therapy for infections confirmed through the use of wet prep and/or cultures as guided by cytologic reading. For example, if *Candida* is identified on Pap smear results, evaluate the patient in the office, confirm finding, and treat the patient with appropriate antifungal therapy.

C. Interpretation/result
   1. Squamous cell abnormalities
      a. Atypical squamous cells of undetermined significance (ASCUS): indicates some abnormality but cause is unclear (infection common).
      b. Atypical squamous cells: cannot exclude high-grade squamoous intraepithelial lesion (ASC-H).
      c. Low-grade squamous intraepithelial lesion (LSIL): indicates HPV, mild dysplasia, or cervical intraepithelial neoplasia (CIN) I.
      d. High-grade squamous intraepithelial lesions (HSIL): moderate and severe dysplasia, carcinoma in situ (CIS) or CIN II, and CIN III.
      e. Squamous cell carcinoma.
   2. Glandular cell
      a. Atypical glandular cells (AGC)
      b. Atypical glandular cells favor neoplastic
      c. Adenocarcinoma
   3. Other
      a. Endometrial cells in women over 40

Initial Management of Abnormal Pap Smears

A. ASC-US in women over age 20 is followed by repeat Pap smears (HPV DNA testing preferred) every 6 months for 1 year or colposcopy. If repeat cytology is negative in both screenings, return to annual Pap smear evaluations. If either result is ASC or greater colposcopy is indicated. ASC-US in women age 20 or younger is followed by repeat cytology in 12 months.
B. ASC-H is managed with colposcopy.
C. LSIL in women under 20 is initially managed by repeat cytology in 12 months. For women 20 and over management if LSIL includes colposcopy.
D. HSIL management in women older than 20 includes either immediate loop excision or colposcopy. For women 20 and under colposcopy.
E. AGC management for all subcategories except atypical endometrial cells includes colposcopy.
   1. Atypical endometrial cells management includes endometrial and endocervical sampling.

Pregnant women are considered a special population and at low risk for invasive cervical cancer. Invasive cancer remains the only indication for therapy in pregnant women so it is reasonable to delay colposcopy.

See and download ASCS algorithms for complete management options at http://www.asccp.org

Recommendations

According to the American Cancer Society (ACS) and the U.S. Preventative Task Force (USPTS) guidelines, all women should begin cervical cancer screening three years after beginning vaginal intercourse and no later than age 21 (whichever comes first). The ACS recommends that if the regular Pap test is used patients should be tested yearly, but if liquid-based is used, testing can be done every two years. Beginning at age 30, women who have had 3 normal consecutive Pap tests may decrease Pap test frequency to every 2–3 years.

The American College of Obstetrician/Gynecologists' (ACOG) newest guidelines recommend that cervical screening should begin at 21 years of age to avoid unnecessary treatment in young women who are at low risk for cervical cancer. Cervical screening is recommended every 2 years between 21–29 years of age. Women 30 years and older with no history of abnormal pap smears and 3 consecutive exams may go to every 3-year screenings. (ACOG, December 2009).

Women with special considerations such as DES exposure before birth, previous cervical cancer, and/or immunosuppression should continue annual screening. Women over age 70 with three or more consecutive normal Pap smears may discontinue screening. Refer to Chapter 1, "Health Maintenance Guidelines," for the full recommendations for annual screening.

The Advisory Committee on Immunization practices recommends routine vaccination of females aged 11–12 with three doses of quadrivalent HPV vaccine and states the series can be started as young as 9 years of age. Catch-up vaccination is recommended for females aged 13–26.

Patient education regarding the prevention of cervical cancer by avoiding exposure to HPV should include reduction or elimination of high-risk activities. These high-risk activities include having sexual intercourse at an early age, having multiple sexual partners, having partners with multiple partners, and having sex with uncircumcised males. Use of condoms can reduce the risk of HPV as well as other sexually transmitted infections. Smoking cessation can also reduce the risk of cervical cancer. Identification and treatment of precancerous lesions can reduce the risk of invasive cervical cancer so encourage screening according to ACS guidelines.

Treatment Modalities

Treatment is instituted based on the severity of the lesion and the presence of pathology within the columnar epithelium of the endocervix. Treatment options include the following:

A. Observation and repeat cytology
B. Cryotherapy
C. Loop excision of the transformation zone
D. Laser of the transformation zone
E. Cold-knife conization
F. Observation and repeat cytology

PELVIC INFLAMMATORY DISEASE (PID)

Definition

A. Pelvic inflammatory disease (PID) is an inflammation caused by an infection of the upper genital tract. This inflammation can involve the uterine endometrium (endometritis), fallopian tubes (salpingitis), ovaries (oophoritis), broad ligament or uterine serosa (parametritis), and the pelvic vascular system or pelvic connective tissue.

Incidence

A. Annual incidence is estimated to be approximately 1 million cases in the United States. In women aged 15–24 years, the incidence is projected at 1% annually in the United States.

B. PID is the leading cause of infertility in the world.

Pathogenesis

A. PID is caused by organisms that ascend from the vagina and cervix into the uterus. Menses facilitates gonococcal invasion of the upper genital tract as the luteal phase stimulates gonococcal growth and the cervical mucus barrier is removed. Infection and inflammation spread throughout the endometrium to the fallopian tubes. From there, it extends to the ovaries and peritoneal cavity.

B. The most common organisms cultured from patients with PID are *Chlamydia trachomatis, Neisseria gonorrhoeae, Mycoplasma hominis, Ureaplasma urealyticum, Bacteroides, Peptostreptococcus, E. coli,* and some endogenous aerobes and anaerobes.

C. The incubation period varies with the infective organism.

Predisposing Factors

A. Age: Rates of PID are higher for women at younger ages. It is highest in the under 30-year-old age group (70% incidence under age 25). Teens are particularly susceptible because they have an immature immune system and larger zones of cervical ectopy with thinner cervical mucus.

B. Sexual activity: Women with multiple sexual partners are three times more likely to develop PID, when compared to women with only one partner.

C. Intrauterine devices: IUDs can lead to an iatrogenic development of PID and can promote the spread of vaginal or cervical organisms into the uterus by means of the IUD string.

D. History of PID: Women who have had PID in the past are more likely to have a recurrence.

E. Menstruation: supports the development and spread of PID. Women who are **not** currently menstruating have a decreased risk.

F. History of invasive procedures: These may result in iatrogenic PID. PID is usually seen within 4 weeks of the procedure (D and C, IUD insertion, hysterosalpingogram, and vacuum curettage abortion).

G. There is an increased incidence of PID in African Americans and non-White women and women in lower socioeconomic groups.

H. Cigarette smoking has been implicated in some studies.

I. Frequent vaginal douching has also been implicated in the increase of PID.

Common Complaints

A. Lower abdominal pain
B. Fever or chills
C. Increased vaginal discharge
D. Nausea and vomiting
E. Low back pain

Other Signs and Symptoms

A. Asymptomatic; vague and nonspecific symptoms
B. Minimal to severe pelvic pain
C. Right upper quadrant pain (25%)
D. Abnormal vaginal bleeding

Subjective Data

A. Determine onset, duration, and course of presenting symptoms.

B. Review the character of vaginal discharge (if any); history of recent dysmenorrhea and/or dyspareunia; any intestinal or bladder symptoms.

C. Question the patient regarding sexual history: current number of sexual partners; current or most recent sexual activity; and contraceptive used (condoms, pills, diaphragm, IUD), and frequency of method used.

D. Question the patient as to whether her current sexual partner has experienced any symptoms.

E. What is the patient's current menstrual pattern? Does she think she is pregnant? When did the pain begin in relation to her cycle?

F. Review prior pelvic or abdominal surgeries and procedures (HSG, abortion) and when they were done.

G. Review the history and quality of pain, how long, bilateral or unilateral, what makes it better, and what makes it worse (intercourse, Valsalva's maneuver with BM, movement).

Physical Examination

A. Check temperature, pulse, respirations, and blood pressure.

B. Inspect: Observe general overall appearance for discomfort before, during, and after exam.

C. Auscultate: Auscultate the abdomen for bowel sounds in all quadrants. Auscultation of the abdomen should precede any palpation or percussion due to the changes in intensity and frequency of sounds after manipulation.

D. Percuss: Percuss the abdomen for organomegaly.

E. Palpate.

1. Palpate the groin for lymphadenopathy.
2. Palpate the abdomen for masses.
3. Palpate the levator ani muscle left and right, the urethra, and trigone of the bladder.
4. Perform rebound, involuntary guarding, and jar tests. **The jar test is performed by intentionally hitting or jarring the examination table and watching for a pain response. Pelvic discomfort is exacerbated by the Valsalva's maneuver, intercourse, or movement. Abdominal or pelvic pain with PID is usually bilateral. About 25% of patients complain of right upper quadrant pain; the pain usually occurs within 7–10 days of menses, remains continuously, and is most severe in the lower quadrants.**

F. Pelvic examination.
   1. Inspect: Examine the vulva for Bartholin's gland enlargement, fissures, condyloma, herpes, and pelvic relaxation.
   2. Palpate: "Milk" the urethra for discharge.
   3. Speculum examination: Inspect for cervicitis and friability. Evaluate vaginal discharge and bleeding for color, amount, and odor. Lower abdominal or pelvic pain is the most common symptom of PID and typically is moderate to severe; however, many women may have subtle or mild symptoms that are not readily recognizable as PID, including abnormal bleeding, dyspareunia, or vaginal discharge.
G. Bimanual examination.
   1. Check cervical motion tenderness; evaluate the size, contour, mobility, and tenderness of the uterus.
   2. Palpate the adnexa for tenderness and masses. Classic PID presentation is lower abdominal and adnexal tenderness and cervical motion tenderness (chandelier sign). The pelvic area may feel hot.
H. Rectovaginal examination: Check adnexal thickening and masses.

Diagnostic Tests

A. CBC with differential; WBC greater than 10,500 cell/mm^3
B. Sedimentation rate or C-reactive protein
C. Quantitative β HCG
D. RPR, hepatitis B surface antigen (HBsAg), and HIV
E. Cultures for GC and *Chlamydia*
F. Endometrial biopsy
G. Transvaginal ultrasonography, by referral
H. Laparoscopy, by referral

Always test the patient for quantitative β HCG even if she claims her menses are regular and she is using reliable contraception because of the extreme risk of ectopic pregnancy. Cultures must always be done; lab work (such as HIV) may be done as indicated depending on the patient's history and presentation. Eliciting data in the health history about hysterectomy, previous appendectomy, abortions, and procedures such as hysterosalpingogram (HSG) may provide exclusionary diagnoses.

I. Diagnostic criteria (DC) for clinical diagnosis of PID.
   1. Minimal criteria
      a. Lower abdominal tenderness
      b. Adnexal tenderness
      c. Cervical motion tenderness
   2. Additional routine criteria
      a. Oral temperature greater than 101°F
      b. Abnormal cervical or vaginal discharge
      c. Elevated erythrocyte sedimentation rate (>15 mm/hr)
      d. Elevated C-reactive protein
      e. Laboratory documentation of cervical infection with *Neisseria gonorrhoeae* or *Chlamydia trachomatis*
   3. Elaborate criteria for diagnosing PID
      a. Histopathologic evidence of endometritis on endometrial biopsy

b. Tubo-ovarian abscess on ultrasonogram or radiologic tests
c. Lapasroscopic abnormalities consistent with PID

Differential Diagnoses

A. Gynecologic factors
   1. PID
   2. Ectopic pregnancy
   3. Pelvic endometriosis
   4. Dysmenorrhea
   5. Adenomyosis
   6. Functional ovarian cysts
   7. Endometrial polyps or fibroid
   8. Pelvic relaxation
   9. Anatomic abnormalities
B. Gastrointestinal factors
   1. Acute appendicitis
   2. Irritable bowel syndrome
   3. Ulcerative colitis, Crohn's disease
   4. Diverticulitis
   5. Hernia
C. Genitourinary factors
   1. Cystitis, urethritis interstitial cystitis
   2. Ureteral obstruction
   3. Carcinoma of bladder
D. Musculoskeletal factors
   1. Myofascial pain
   2. Pelvic floor myalgia
   3. Spinal injuries or degenerative disease
E. Neurologic factor: nerve entrapment syndrome

Plan

A. General interventions
   1. A low threshold is needed for diagnosis of PID because of the risk of damage to reproductive health. **Err toward overdiagnosis,** rather than miss treatment of upper tract infection because other common causes of lower abdominal pain, such as irritable bowel syndrome and endometriosis, are not likely to be impaired by empiric antibiotic therapy. The risk of ectopic pregnancy is 6–10 times greater with women with PID compared with uninfected women.
   2. Antibiotic therapy should be instituted promptly, based on clinical diagnosis without awaiting culture results, to minimize the risk of progression of the infection and risk of transmission of the organisms to other sexual partners.
   3. If the patient has an IUD in place, it should be promptly removed.
   4. Ambulatory patients should be monitored closely and reevaluated within 3 days of initiating antibiotic therapy. A decrease in pelvic tenderness should be observed within 3–5 days of initiation of therapy; if not, additional evaluation is warranted.
B. Patient teaching
   1. See the Section III Patient Teaching Guide, "Pelvic Inflammatory Disease (PID)."
   2. Male sexual partners (all partners) of patients with PID must be examined, cultured when possible, and

treated empirically for presumptive gonorrheal and chlamydial infection.

3. Women who do not use any contraception are at the greatest risk. Transmission of STIs can be minimized with effective use of barrier contraceptives. Spermicides prevent infection with chlamydia and gonorrhea. The use of nonoxynol-9 is protective against *N. gonorrhoeae, Treponema-palladium, Trichomonas,* herpes simplex virus, and *Candida.*

4. Oral contraceptive pills are associated with an increase in chlamydia detection in the cervix, but they protect against symptomatic PID.

C. Pharmaceutical therapy. See Table 13.6.

Follow-up

A. Because of the high risk of reinfection, many clinicians recommend reevaluation in 4–6 weeks after completion of therapy. Patients with positive cultures for GC and *Chlamydia* should be recultured in 7–10 days after completing therapy. "Test of cure" is necessary.

B. Hepatitis B immunization should be initiated in previously unvaccinated persons.

Consultation/Referral

Consult a gynecologist if the patient diagnosis is atypical, evidence for a presumptive diagnosis is present, or hospitalization is required. General criteria for hospitalization are the following:

A. Diagnosis is uncertain.
B. Pelvic or tubo-ovarian abscess is suspected.
C. IUD in situ.
D. The patient is pregnant.
E. The patient is an adolescent or believed to be incapable of adhering to outpatient regimen.
F. Outpatient therapy fails; the patient is not better in 48–72 hours.
G. The patient cannot be reevaluated in 48–72 hours.
H. The patient is HIV-positive.
I. There is generalized peritonitis or severe illness.
J. The patient cannot tolerate oral medication therapies.
K. Surgical emergencies cannot be ruled out.

Individual Considerations

A. Pregnancy: Fluoroquinolones are generally contraindicated for pregnant and nursing mothers.
B. Pediatrics: Fluoroquinolones are generally contraindicated for children and adolescents younger than 18 years.
C. Partners: Sexual partners should be evaluated and treated for sexually transmitted infections.

PREMENSTRUAL SYNDROME

Definition

A. Premenstrual syndrome (PMS) is a psychoneuroendocrine disorder with a constellation of symptoms that occur in the luteal phase, beginning particularly from

---

TABLE 13.6   CDC Recommendations for Treating PID

Inpatient Therapy:	Ambulatory Therapy:
Regimen A[a]	**Regimen A**
Cefoteton 2 g IV every 12 hours **or** Cefoxitin 2g **plus** doxycycline 100 mg IV or orally every 12 hours.	Levofloxin 500 mg daily for 14 days **or** Ofloxacin 400 mg orally twice daily for 14 days
	With or Without
This regimen is continued for at least 48 hours after clinical improvement, and followed by doxycycline 100 mg orally twice daily to complete 14-day total course.	Metronidazole 500 mg orally twice daily for 14 days
Regimen B[a]	**Regimen B**
Clindamycin 900 mg IV every 8 hours (15–40 mg/kg/d)	Ceftriaxone 250 g IM once **plus** Doxycycline 100 mg orally twice a day for 14 days **with or without** Metronidazole 500 mg orally twice a day
Plus	**Or**
Gentamicin, loading dose 2.0 mg/kg IV, followed by maintenance 1.5 mg/kg IV every 8 hours. Single daily dosing may be substituted.	Cefoxitin 2 g IM once **plus** Probenecid 2 g in a single concurrent dose **plus** Doxycycline 100 mg orally twice a day for 14 days **with or without** Metronidazole 500 mg orally twice a day
This regimen is continued for at least 48 hours after significant clinical improvement is demonstrated, and it is followed by doxycycline 100 mg orally twice daily to complete a 14-day total course. Alternatively, clindamycin 600 mg orally three times daily may be given to complete a 14-day total course.	

[a]When tubo-ovarian abscess is present, many clinicians use clindamycin because it provides more effective anaerobic coverage than doxycycline.
Note. For women or their partners who cannot tolerate doxycycline or tetracycline, erythromycin 500 mg orally four times daily may be used for 10–14 days.

day 18–21, and interfere with a woman's life. This is followed by a symptom-free period. The American Psychiatric Association (APA) diagnosis is called "luteal phase dysphoric disorder."

Incidence

A. Virtually every menstruating woman experiences some symptoms, sometimes. Twenty percent of menstruating women have symptoms serious enough to interfere with their lives, but only a small percentage have disabling symptoms. Symptoms occur more commonly in women in their 30s and 40s.

Pathogenesis

The basis of PMS is presumably hormonal; there may be a genetic sensitivity to fluctuations of the neurotransmitters. The following are APA diagnostic criteria for luteal phase dysphoric disorder:

A. Symptoms are temporally related to the menstrual cycle, beginning during the last week of the luteal phase and remitting after the onset of menses.
B. The diagnosis requires at least five of the following, and one of the symptoms must be one of the first four:
    1. Affective lability, for example, sudden onset of being sad, tearful, irritable, or angry (mood swings)
    2. Persistent and marked anger or irritability
    3. Marked anxiety or tension
    4. Markedly depressed mood and feelings of hopelessness
    5. Decreased interest in usual activities
    6. Easy fatigability or marked lack of energy
    7. Subjective sense of difficulty in concentrating
    8. Hypersomnia or insomnia
    9. Physical symptoms such as breast tenderness, headaches, edema, abdominal bloating, joint or muscle pain, and weight gain
C. The symptoms interfere with work, usual activities, or relationships.
D. The symptoms are not an exacerbation of another psychiatric disorder.

Predisposing Factors

A. Female of reproductive age

Common Complaints

A. "I've got PMS; I'm so miserable."
B. Feelings of irritability and emotional lability.

Subjective Data

A. Obtain a complete menstrual history:
    1. Menarche; frequency, duration, and regularity of periods.
    2. Ask about premenstrual symptoms that are physical: weight gain, edema, acne, nausea, vomiting, constipation, backache, headache, migraine, syncope, breast tenderness, breast enlargement, hot flashes, paresthesia of hands or feet, aggravation of convulsive disorder, increased appetite, food cravings (sweets, salt, or food in general), and fatigue.
    3. Ask about premenstrual symptoms that are emotional: irritability, emotional lability, anxiety, depression,

crying, palpitations, fatigue, aggression, lethargy, and sleep disturbances.
    4. Ask particularly about the timing of the symptoms. When do the symptoms begin and end in relationship to the menstrual period? Has the patient kept a calendar of symptoms?
B. Ask about symptoms of dysmenorrhea. Some women confuse menstrual cramps and PMS.
C. Note type of contraception the patient uses.
D. Review her obstetric history.
E. Elicit the types of treatment the patient has tried and efficacy of treatment.
F. Ask the patient about the amount and type of exercise she gets. Women with PMS often get little exercise.

Physical Examination

A. Height, weight, and blood pressure.
B. Inspect: Note overall appearance; inspect thyroid.
C. Palpate: Palpate the neck: Note thyroid enlargement or nodules. Palpate the abdomen, noting enlargement, masses, or tenderness.
D. Auscultate: Auscultate the heart, lungs, and abdomen.
E. Pelvic examination.
    1. Inspect the external genitalia for pubic hair pattern, lesions, or discharge.
    2. Speculum examination: Check for discharge and lesions.
    3. Bimanual examination: Check for size, mobility, shape, and tenderness of the uterus and adnexal area.
    4. No physical abnormality or changes are consistent with PMS.

Diagnostic Tests

A. Consider Pap smear and chlamydia and gonorrhea screens.
B. TSH.
C. Research has demonstrated that alterations in hormone levels do not occur.

Differential Diagnoses

A. Premenstrual syndrome.
B. Major depression.
C. Dysmenorrhea.
D. Substance abuse.
E. Perimenopausal symptoms.
F. Sexual dysfunction.
G. Fibromyalgia.
H. There are rarely major medical problems, but hypothyroidism, hyperthyroidism, anemia, and autoimmune disorders (such as systemic lupus erythematosus) must be kept in mind.

Plan

A. General interventions
    1. Have the patient keep a menstrual calendar or diary for at least 3 months to document occurrence of symptoms in the luteal phase.
    2. Symptomatic treatments: Treatment must be individualized.
B. Patient teaching: See the Section III Patient Teaching Guide for this chapter, "Premenstrual Syndrome (PMS)."

1. Diet: Have the patient eat six small meals a day to even out glucose load. Have her avoid caffeine to decrease irritability and facilitate sleep. Encourage her to avoid simple sugars and eat complex carbohydrates to provide a slow, steady source of energy. She should avoid salt to decease edema.
2. Activity: Instruct the patient to increase exercise, preferably aerobic. Have her exercise every day by walking, swimming, and stretching. Encourage her to try stress reduction activities such as imagery or yoga, join a support or counseling group, and avoid or stop smoking. Encourage adequate sleep and rest.
3. Give her the Patient Teaching Guide for this chapter, "Premenstrual Syndrome (PMS)."

C. Pharmaceutical therapy
1. NSAIDs for relief of muscular aches, headaches, and menstrual cramps. Follow directions for the particular NSAIDs, whether OTC or prescription.
2. Minerals
   a. Magnesium 300–500 mg per day.
   b. Calcium 1,000 mg per day.
   c. Chromium 200 µg each day.
   d. Zinc 30 mg each day.
3. Vitamins to decrease anxiety and irritability, food cravings, painful breasts, depression, fatigue, and lethargy.
   a. Vitamin B_6 (pyridoxine) 50–100 mg each day. Some people recommend 400 mg each day.
   b. Multiple vitamin one each day.
   c. Vitamin E 400 mg each day.
4. Herbs: evening primrose oil 500–1,000 mg each day. Because this oil contains vitamin E, do not have the patient take additional vitamin E.
5. See Table 13.7 for other therapies used for PMS.

Follow-up
A. Follow up every 3–4 months to assess or alter therapy.

Consultation/Referral
A. Consult a physician if symptoms are severe or not relieved by first-line measures.
B. Education and encouragement are therapeutic. Acknowledge reality of symptoms.

Individual Considerations
A. Partners: Encourage the patient to have her partner come to a visit. Partner education and support are helpful.

VULVOVAGINAL CANDIDIASIS

Definition
A. Candidiasis (also know as moniliasis) is a common, yeast-like fungal infection of the vulva and vagina. In 90% of the cases, the cause is infection by *Candida albicans*.

Incidence
A. Approximately 75% of all women have at least one episode of candidiasis. It is estimated that 50% of these

---

TABLE 13.7 Medications Used With PMS

Drug	Dose	Purpose
Diuretics		Decreases edema peripherally and, perhaps, centrally.
Spironolactone (Aldactone)	25 mg twice daily as needed	
Hydrochlorothiazide (Hydrodiuril)	25–50 mg once daily as needed	
Antidepressants		Decreases depression and anxiety and improves mood.
Fluoxetine (Prozac)	10–40 mg every day or during the luteal phase (individual dose may vary)	
Paroxetine (Paxil)	10–30 mg every day or during the luteal phase (individual dose may vary)	
Sertraline hydrochloride (Zoloft)	25–30 mg every day or during the luteal phase (individual dose may vary)	
Antianxiety drugs		Decreases anxiety.
Alprazolam (Xanax)	0.25 mg three or four times daily during luteal phase as needed	
Buspirone (BuSpar)	7.5–15 mg twice daily	
Miscellaneous Drugs		
Bromocriptine mesylate (Parlodel)	2.5 mg three times daily during breast luteal phase	Used to decrease tenderness; works slowly.
Oral contraceptive pills (Yaz[a])	Take on a daily basis	Evens the hormonal milieu, blocks ovulation.
Danazol (Danocrine)		Has antiestrogenic effects. *Consult with a physician.*

[a]Has drospirenone and ethinyl estradiol.

women have recurrences. Yeast has been identified with circumcised males, but symptomatic complaints are more common with uncircumcised males.

Pathogenesis

A. Multiple fungal species cause candidiasis, including *Candida albicans* (90%), *C tropicalis, Torulopsis glabrata* (10%), *C parapsilosis,* and *C krusei.*

B. *Candida albicans, C tropicalis,* or *Torulopsis glabrata* are part of the **normal flora** of the mouth, gastrointestinal tract, and vagina. They may become pathogenic with changes in the vaginal pH that encourage the overgrowth of the fungus.

C. The incubation period is 96 hours.

Predisposing Factors

A. Diabetes
B. Systemic antibiotic use
C. Pregnancy
D. Oral contraceptive pill use
E. Obesity
F. Warm climate
G. Immunocompromised
H. HIV
I. Wearing tight, restrictive clothing
J. Corticosteroid use
K. Tub bathing
L. Frequent use of hot tubs or whirlpools

Common Complaints

A. Thick white "cheesy" vaginal discharge
B. Itching, mild to intense vulvar pruritus
C. Vaginal or vulvar irritation, red and swollen
D. Discomfort during and after sexual intercourse

Other Signs and Symptoms

A. Vulvar excoriation
B. Vaginal swelling or inflammation
C. Burning with urination
D. Burning with or during intercourse
E. Increased symptoms near menses

Subjective Data

A. Determine onset, course, and duration of symptoms; note if infection is first occurrence, recurrent, persistent, or chronic.

B. Obtain medication history; include antibiotics, steroids, and birth control pills.

C. Review the patient's past medical history, and review systems for evidence of diabetes, HIV, or any immunocompromise.

D. Review hobbies that include the use of hot tubs, whirlpools, or tight exercise clothing.

E. Review the patient's history of wearing polyester underwear, wearing underwear to bed, or wearing tight jeans.

F. Review previous treatment, self-treatment measures, and compliance to previous treatments.

G. Determine if the patient is pregnant; note first day of last menstrual period (LMP).

H. Review sexual activity and partners. Do the partner(s) have any of the same symptoms, "jock itch," or oral candidiasis?

I. Review the use of vaginal deodorants or spray, scented toilet paper, tampons, pads, and douching.

J. Has there been any change in soaps, laundry detergent, or fabric softeners?

K. Review diet for high sugar content.

Physical Examination

A. Temperature, pulse, and blood pressure.
B. Inspect
   1. Inspect the vulva for inflammation, fissures, lesions, excoriation, rashes, and condyloma.
   2. Examine the hair line and skin folds for inflammation and pediculosis.

Inflammation that spares the skin folds is consistent with contact irritation. Inflammation that is within the skin folds suggests *Candida*.

C. Palpate
   1. Perform external exam for enlarged or tender inguinal lymph nodes, vulvar masses, and lesions.
   2. Back: Check CVA tenderness to rule out bacterial infection.

D. Pelvic examination
   1. Inspect: Observe side walls of vagina. Note amount, smell, and color of the discharge.

Typical discharge with *Candida* is adherent to vaginal side walls and characteristically thick, white, and curdlike (resembles cottage cheese). The discharge has a yeasty to musty smell. Erythema of the side walls may be seen.

   2. Speculum examination: Inspect the cervix for discharge and friability.
   3. Bimanual examination: Check for cervical motion tenderness. Palpate for the size of the uterus and for adnexal masses.

Diagnostic Tests

A. Wet prep with 10% potassium hydroxide and normal saline prep.

Yeast hyphae and/or spores are determined by microscopic examination of vaginal discharge prepared with 10% potassium hydroxide or normal saline. A positive whiff test indicates bacterial vaginosis.

B. Test discharge with nitrazine paper.

The pH with candidiasis remains in the normal range of 3.8 to 4.2.

C. Consider 2-hour glucose testing.
D. Consider testing for GC and *Chlamydia.*
E. Herpes culture, if lesions present.
F. Urinalysis and culture, if indicated.

Differential Diagnoses

A. Vulvovaginal candidiasis
B. Vulvar dystrophy
C. Allergic vulvitis
D. Bacterial vaginosis
E. Urinary tract infection
F. *Chlamydia*

G. Gonorrhea

H. *Trichomonas*

I. Herpes simplex virus type 2

J. Pediculosis pubis

K. Chemical vaginitis

L. Normal physiologic discharge

M. Candidiasis secondary to diabetes

Plan

A. General interventions
1. Although vaginal candidiasis is treated using over-the-counter products, encourage patients with initial presenting symptoms to have an evaluation to rule out other vaginal infections prior to self-treatment.
2. Consider treating partners.

While candidiasis is not considered a sexually transmitted infection, it can be sexually transmitted. The partner should be treated in cases of recurrent infections, even if the partner is asymptomatic.

3. Consider fasting and 2-hour postprandial glucose tests for chronic yeast infections.
4. Consider testing for HIV for chronic yeast infections.
5. Preventive care therapies.
   a. Vinegar and water douche may be effective in mild cases: 1–2 tablespoons vinegar per quart warm water daily for 5 days. Vinegar and water douche may be used each month following completion of the menstrual cycle for **prevention.**
   b. *Acidophilus* capsules 4–6 tablets daily, especially 2–3 days prior to menses.
   c. Vitamin C 500 mg two to four times daily to increase vaginal acidity.
   d. Potassium sorbate 3% douche 1 teaspoon per quart warm water every 1–2 days.
   e. Daily yogurt douches or intravaginal applicator full of yogurt twice a day for 1 week. Have the patient use **plain yogurt** with active cultures.

B. Patient teaching
1. See the Section III Patient Teaching Guide for this chapter, "Vaginal Yeast Infection."
2. Patients should be encouraged to present for evaluation if, after appropriate therapy has been instituted, they continue to have symptoms.
3. Treatment should continue even during menstruation.

C. Pharmaceutical therapy
1. Vaginal antifungal creams: Mild cases may respond to 3 days of therapy; severe cases may require 10–14 days. Some of these preparations are available in vaginal suppository form for a 1- or 3-night regimen with proven efficacy.
   a. Clotrimazole (Gyne-Lotrimin, Lotrimin, Mycelex, Mycelex-G) one applicator full at bedtime for 7 days.
   b. Miconazole (Monistat) one applicator full at bedtime for 7 days.
   c. Butoconazole nitrate (Femstat) one applicator full at bedtime for 7 days.
   d. Terconazole (Terazol) one applicator full at bedtime for 7 days.
   e. Terconazole vaginal antifungal cream is not available over-the-counter. Imidazole drugs (miconazole, clotrimazole, econazole, butoconazole) are not as effective for *non-Candida albicans* infections as are triazole compounds.

2. Oral antifungal agents.
   a. Fluconazole (Diflucan) 150 mg orally once. If treatment is not successful, prescription may be refilled one time; if it is still unsuccessful, consider treating the patient's partner and/or glucose testing for diabetes.
   b. Nystatin one tablet (100,000 units) orally or vaginally for 14 days. Nystatin may be taken twice a day or at bedtime.
   c. Ketoconazole (Nizoral) 200 mg orally in single dose.
      i. Dosage may be increased to 400 mg once daily in patients who don't respond to lower dose.
      ii. Treatment is effective for acute infection, but *very expensive.* It causes hepatic toxicity in 5%–10% of patients; monitor liver function tests. Reserve treatment for long-term suppression of chronic *Candida albicans* infection.

Follow-up

A. The patient who presents with recurrent candidiasis should be evaluated for HIV and/or other immunocompromised etiologies and diabetes.

B. If fasting and 2-hour blood glucose testing is normal, other options for recurrent candidiasis include treatment with clotrimazole one applicator full every other week for 2 months. If the patient remains symptom-free, reduce treatment to once each month, in the week prior to menstrual period.

C. If recurrent candidiasis persists, request laboratory typing of *Candida* for *Torulopsis glabrata* or *C. tropicalis.* If confirmed, treat with prescription of gentian violet-treated tampons. Have the patient use one tampon at bedtime for 12 days.

Consultation/Referral

A. Consult or refer the patient to a physician if there is no response to above treatments and/or in presence of concurrent systemic disease.

Individual Considerations

A. Pregnancy may lead to an increase in vulvovaginal candidiasis because of the increased glycogen content of the vagina and to the stimulatory effects of estrogen and progesterone on candidal growth. Over-the-counter antifungal creams are appropriate for use in this population, if there is no rupture of membranes. Candidiasis may be transmitted from infected mother to newborn at delivery.

B. Partners should be evaluated should the patient present with recurrences. Over-the-counter antifungal creams are appropriate for use in this population.

REFERENCES

Alexander, I. M., & Andrist, L. C. (2006). Menopause. In K. D. Schuiling & F. E. Likis (Eds.), *Women's gynecologic health* (pp. 249–285). Sudbury, MA: Jones and Bartlett.

American Cancer Society. (2008, March 31). *Cervical cancer: Prevention and early detection.* Retrieved July 16, 2009, from http://http://www.cancer.org/docroot/CRI/content/CRI_2_6x_cervical_cancer_prevention_and_early_detection_8.asp?sitearea=PED

American Cancer Society. (2009, March 26). *Detailed guide: Cervical cancer.* Retrieved July 17, 2009, from http://http://foundation.cancer.org/docroot/CRI/content/CRI_2_4_2X_Can_cervical_cancer_be_prevented_8.asp

American College of Obstetricians and Gynecologists. (2006, June). Use of hormonal contraception in women with coexisting medical conditions. *ACOG Practice Bulletin,* Number 73.

American College of Obstetricians and Gynecologists. (2009, December). Cervical cytology screening. *ACOG Practice Bulletin,* Number 109.

American College of Obstetrics and Gynecologists. (2009). *Dysmenorrhea* [Brochure]. Washington, DC: Author.

American Society for Colposcopy and Cervical Pathology. (2007). Consensus guidelines on the management of women with abnormal cervical cancer screening tests. *Journal of Lower Genital Tract Disease, 11*(4), 201–222.

Centers for Disease Control and Prevention. (2006). Sexually transmitted diseases treatment guidelines, 2006. *Morbidity and Mortality Weekly Report, 55*(RR–11), 1–94.

Centers for Disease Control and Prevention. (2007). Quadrivalent human papillomavirus vaccine. *Morbidity and Mortality Weekly Report, 56,* 1–24.

Centers for Disease Control and Prevention. (2008). *Bacterial vaginosis: CDC fact sheet.* Retrieved June 30, 2009, from http://www.cdc.gov/std/bv/STDFact-Bacterial-Vaginosis.htm

Duramed Pharmaceuticals. (2009). *Plan B emergency contraception.* Retrieved July 15, 2009, from http://www.go2planb.com/plan-b-prescribers/emergency-contraceptions.aspx

Efantis, J., & Simon, T. (2008). Menopause. In T. M. Buttaro, J. Trybulski, P. P. Bailey, & J. Sandberg-Cook (Eds.), *Primary care: A collaborative practice* (3rd ed., pp. 877–886). St. Louis: Mosby Elsevier.

Fogel, C. I. (2006). Gynecologic infections. In K. D. Schuiling & F. E. Likis (Eds.), *Women's gynecologic health* (pp. 417–418). Sudbury, MA: Jones and Bartlett.

German, D., & Lee, A. (Eds.). (2008). *Nurse practitioner's prescribing reference.* New York: Haymarket Media.

Gilbert, D. N., Moellering, R. C., Eliopoulos, G. M., Chambers, H. F., & Saag, M. S. (Eds.). (2009). *The Sanford guide to antimicrobial therapy 2009* (39th ed.). Sperryville, VA: Antimicrobial Therapy.

Hatcher, R. A., Trussell, J., Nelson, A. L., Cates, Jr., W., Stewart, F. H., & Kowal, D. (Eds.). (2007). *Contraceptive technology* (19th ed.). New York: Ardent Media.

Master-Hunter, T., & Heiman, D. (2006). Amenorrhea: Evaluation and treatment. *American Family Physician, 73*(8), 1374–1382.

McNeeley, S. (2008). *Bartholin's gland cysts.* The Merk Manuals Online Medical Library. Retrieved July 15, 2009, from http://www.merck.com/mmpe/sec18/ch249/ch249c.html

Mosher, W. D., Martinez, G. M., Chandra, A., Abma, J. C., & Willson, S. J. (2004). Use of contraception and use of family planning services in the United States: 1982–2002. *Advanced Data from Vital and Health Statistics, 350, National Center for Health Statistics.* Retrieved January 15, 2010, from http://www.cdc.gov/nchs/data/ad/ad350.pdf

North American Menopause Society. (2004). Treatment of menopause associated vasomotor symptoms: Position statement of the North American Menopause Society. *Menopause, 11*(1), 11–33.

North American Menopause Society. (2008). Estrogen and progestogen use in postmenopausal women: July 2008 position statement of the North American Menopausal Society. *Menopause, 15*(4), 584–599.

Rosolowich, V., Saettler, E., Szuck, B., Leah, R., Levesque, P., Weisberg, F., et al. (2006). Mastalgia. *Journal of Obstetric and Gynaecology Canada, 28*(1), 49–57.

Saslow, D., Boetes, C., Burke, W., Harms, S., O'Leach, M., Lehman, D., et al. (2007). American Cancer Society guidelines for breast cancer screening with MRI as an adjunct to mammography. *CA: A Cancer Journal for Clinicians, 57*(2), 75–89.

Solomon, D., Davey, D., Kurman, R., Moriarty, A., O'Connor, D., Prey, M., et al. (2002). The 2001 Bethesda System: Terminology for reporting results of cervical cytology. *Journal of the American Medical Association, 287*(16), 2114–2119.

Uphold, C. R., & Graham, M. V. (Eds.). (2003). *Clinical guidelines in family practice* (4th ed.). Gainesville, FL: Barmarrae Books.

U.S. Department of Health and Human Services, U.S. Preventive Task Force. (2003, January). *Cervical cancer screening.* Retrieved July 16, 2009, from http://www.ahrq.gov/clinic/uspstf/uspscerv.htm

Wright, T. C., Massad, S., Dunton, C. J., Spitzer, M., Wilkinson, E. J., & Soloman, D. (2007). 2006 consensus guidelines for the management of women with abnormal cervical cancer screening tests. *American Journal of Obstetrics & Gynecology, 197*(4), 346–355.

Sexually Transmitted Infections Guidelines

Elizabeth Parks

◨ CHLAMYDIA

Definition
A. Chlamydia is a sexually transmitted infection.

Incidence
A. The World Health Organization estimates 50 million cases worldwide with more than 4 million cases annually. Chlamydia is the most common sexually transmitted organism in the United States. It is not a Centers for Disease Control and Prevention (CDC) reportable infection; however, local health department notification is required.

Pathogenesis
A. *Chlamydia trachomatis* is an intracellular bacterium with parasitic properties. It is transmitted by sexual contact or perinatally when a vaginal delivery occurs through an infected birth canal.

Predisposing Factors
A. History of sexually transmitted infections
B. Multiple sexual partners
C. Early age at first coitus
D. Unprotected intercourse

Common Complaints
A. Up to 80% of those infected are asymptomatic.
B. Mucopurulent cervical, vaginal, or urethral discharge.
C. Dysuria.
D. Urinary frequency and urgency.
E. Pelvic pain (dull or severe).

Other Signs and Symptoms
A. Cervical friability
B. Cervical motion tenderness
C. Uterine and/or adnexal tenderness

Subjective Data
A. Elicit history of onset of symptoms, location, frequency, duration, aggravating and alleviating factors, and associated symptomatology.

B. Question the patient about history of other STIs and sexual habits.

Physical Examination
A. Check temperature, pulse, respirations, and blood pressure.
B. Inspect
   1. Males: Observe for anal and/or urethral discharge.
   2. Female pelvic exam: Observe for anal and/or vaginal discharge.
   3. Female speculum exam: Inspect vaginal wall and cervix for discharge and irritation.
C. Palpate
   1. Males
      a. Palpate inguinal lymph nodes.
      b. Milk penis for discharge.
      c. Palpate the groin.
   2. Females
      a. Palpate the inguinal lymph nodes.
      b. Bimanual exam.
         i. Milk urethra.
         ii. Palpate periurethral and Bartholin's glands for exudate.
         iii. Assess for cervical motion tenderness.
         iv. Assess for uterine and adnexal tenderness.

Diagnostic Tests
A. Culture samples from urethra, endocervix, rectum, pharynx, conjunctiva; culture is gold standard for diagnosis.
   1. Insert brush or swab 1–2 cm into endocervix, urethra, or rectum.
   2. Rotate for 30 seconds, withdraw, and place in appropriate culture media for transport.

Differential Diagnoses
A. Chlamydia
B. Gonorrhea
C. Urethritis

Plan

A. General interventions
   1. Culture samples immediately for timely treatment. Consider testing for other STIs such as gonorrhea, trichomoniasis, and so forth.
B. Patient teaching
   1. See the Section III Patient Teaching Guide for this chapter, "Chlamydia."
   2. Inform the patient of the need for partner notification and treatment. Notification is recommended for any partner with whom the patient has had sexual contact within 30 days of the onset of symptoms or 60 days if asymptomatic.
   3. Stress importance of completing treatment regimen.
C. Pharmaceutical therapy
   1. The CDC recommends the following regimens:
      a. Doxycycline 100 mg by mouth twice daily for 7 days.
      b. Azithromycin 1 g by mouth in a single dose.
   2. Alternative regimen:
      a. Ofloxacin 300 mg by mouth twice daily for 7 days.
      b. Erythromycin base 500 mg by mouth four times daily for 7 days.
      c. Erythromycin ethylsuccinate 800 mg by mouth four times daily for 7 days.

Follow-up

A. A test of cure is unnecessary after treatment with doxycycline or azithromycin unless symptoms persist.
B. If an alternative regimen is used for treatment, a test of cure may be considered 3 weeks after completion of the regimen.
C. Test of cure is necessary if the patient is pregnant.
D. It is recommended that the patient be retested in approximately 3 months due to potential for reinfection, which is often directly related to the partner not being treated.

Consultation/Referral

A. Consult or refer the patient to a physician when treatment with the recommended dosage fails if patient noncompliance and reexposure have been ruled out.

Individual Considerations

A. Pregnancy
   1. Doxycycline, ofloxacin, and sulfisoxazole are contraindicated in pregnancy.
   2. The safety and efficacy of azithromycin during pregnancy and lactation has not been established.
   3. The CDC recommends the following regimens for pregnant women:
      a. Erythromycin base 500 mg by mouth four times daily for 7 days.
      b. Erythromycin base 250 mg by mouth four times daily for 14 days.
      c. Erythromycin ethylsuccinate 800 mg by mouth four times daily for 7 days.
      d. Erythromycin ethylsuccinate 400 mg by mouth four times daily for 14 days.
      e. For erythromycin intolerance, Azithromycin 1 g by mouth in a single dose or amoxicillin 500 mg by mouth three times a day for 7 days.

4. A test of cure three weeks after therapy completion is recommended for all pregnant women.
   5. Reexamine the cervix at 34–36 weeks' gestation.
B. Pediatrics
   1. Azithromycin has not been established as safe or effective in persons less than 15 years of age.
   2. Ofloxacin is contraindicated in persons less than 17 years of age.
   3. The CDC recommends the following regimens for children:
      a. Weighing less than 45 kg: erythromycin base or ethylsuccinate 50 mg/kg/day by mouth divided into four doses daily for 14 days.
      b. Weighing more than 45 kg but older than 8: azithromycin 1 g by mouth in a single dose.
      c. Older than 8: azithromycin 1 g by mouth in a single dose or doxycycline 100 mg by mouth twice a day for seven days.
C. Adult: Untreated or long-standing chlamydial infection in women may lead to infertility.

GONORRHEA

Definition

A. Gonorrhea is a sexually transmitted infection.

Incidence

A. The World Health Organization estimates 2.5 million cases worldwide. Gonorrhea is a CDC reportable infection. Male-to-female transmission is estimated at 50%–90%, while female-to-male transmission is estimated at only 20%–25%. Women account for two-thirds of disseminated gonorrhea with joint infection.

Pathogenesis

A. *Neisseria gonorrhoeae,* a gram-negative diplococcus, is the causative organism. The infection begins with adherence of *N. gonorrhoeae* to the mucosal cells in the genitourinary tract or endocervix. The incubation period is typically 2–5 days for urethritis and 5–10 days for cervical infection. Rectal and pharyngeal infections are usually asymptomatic. Transmission during vaginal birth is possible and may result in conjunctivitis and blindness in neonates.

Predisposing Factors

A. History of sexually transmitted infections
B. Multiple sexual partners
C. Early age at first coitus

Common Complaints

A. Dysuria
B. Yellow, white, or mucoid urethral discharge in males
C. Greenish, irritating vaginal discharge in females
D. Menstrual irregularities
E. Pelvic pain
F. Fever

Other Signs and Symptoms

A. Asymptomatic
B. Uterine or adnexal tenderness

C. Mucopurulent discharge from endocervix
D. Polyarthralgias
E. Necrotic skin lesions

Subjective Data

A. Elicit history of onset, duration, and location of symptoms. Note aggravating and alleviating factors and associated symptomatology.
B. Question the patient about history of other STIs and sexual habits.

Physical Examination

A. Temperature
B. Inspect
  1. Inspect the skin for necrotic skin lesions.
  2. Males: Inspect for anal and/or urethral discharge; elicit latter by milking penis.
  3. Females
    a. Inspect anus and introitus for discharge; milk urethra.
    b. Speculum exam: Inspect vaginal walls and cervix for discharge and irritation.
C. Palpate
  1. Examine joints for effusion and swelling.
  2. Males: Palpate inguinal lymph nodes.
  3. Females
    a. Palpate inguinal lymph nodes.
    b. Palpate periurethral and Bartholin's glands for exudate.
    c. Bimanual exam.
      i. Assess for cervical motion, tenderness and friability.
      ii. Assess for uterine and adnexal tenderness.

Diagnostic Tests

A. Culture samples from urethra, endocervix, rectum, pharynx, and conjunctiva.
  1. Thayer-Martin and Genprobe are two of the most commonly used culture media.
  2. Collect exudate with cotton-tipped applicator for Thayer-Martin culture.
  3. Use Dacron-tipped applicator for Genprobe culture.
  4. Obtain endocervix culture samples by rotating swab in endocervix for full 30 seconds.
B. During septic joint stage, gonococci can be recovered from the joint by aspiration for culture.

Differential Diagnoses

A. Gonorrhea
B. Chlamydia
C. Arthritis (rheumatoid or osteoarthritis)

Plan

A. General interventions
  1. Prompt diagnosis is needed to begin treatment.
  2. Report positive test culture to the health department.
B. Patient teaching
  1. See the Section III Patient Teaching Guide for this chapter, "Gonorrhea."
  2. Stress the importance of completing the medication regimen.
  3. Inform the patient of the need for partner notification and treatment. Notification is recommended for any partner with whom the patient has had sexual contact within 30 days of the onset of symptoms or 60 days if asymptomatic.
C. Pharmaceutical therapy
  1. CDC recommendation: ceftriaxone 125 mg by intramuscular injection of a single dose.
  2. Cefixime 400 mg by mouth in a single dose.
  3. Ciprofloxacin 500 mg by mouth in a single dose.
  4. Ofloxacin 400 mg by mouth in a single dose.
  5. Levofloxacin 250 mg by mouth in a single dose
  6. Alternative regimen for possible coinfection with chlamydia: ofloxacin 400 mg in a single dose plus doxycycline 100 mg by mouth twice daily for 7 days.

Follow-up

A. Test of cure is no longer recommended for patients with uncomplicated gonorrhea who are treated with CDC recommended regimen.
B. Individuals infected with gonorrhea are at high risk for reinfection; repeat screening 1–2 months after treatment.

Consultation/Referral

A. Consult with a physician or refer the patient if treatment with the recommended dosage fails and patient noncompliance and reexposure have been ruled out.

Individual Considerations

A. Pregnancy
  1. Treatment with cephalosporins is advised.
  2. Presumed or diagnosed coinfections with chlamydia should be treated with erythromycin.
  3. Quinolones and tetracycline should not be used.
B. Adults
  1. Untreated or long-standing gonorrheal infection in women can lead to infertility.
  2. For patients with allergies to cephalosporins or quinolones: spectinomycin 2 g by intramuscular injection of a single dose.
C. Pediatrics: Sexual abuse should be considered. Suspect chlamydia for conjunctivitis if the infant is 30 days old or younger.
  1. Treatment:
    a. Children less than 45 kg: Erythromycin base 50 mg/kg/day divided in 4 equal doses for 10–14 days. A second course may be needed.
    b. Children greater than 45 kg but younger than 8 years old: Azithromycin 1 g orally single dose.
    c. Children greater than 45 kg but older than 8 years old:
      i. Azithromycin 1 g orally in single dose
      ii. Doxycycline 100 mg twice a day for 7 days

HERPES SIMPLEX VIRUS TYPE 2

Definition

A. Herpes simplex is a recurring viral disease that is transmitted by direct contact with the secretions or mucosa of an infected individual who is shedding the virus. The virus is usually characterized by painful vesicular lesions that form an ulcer, crust over, then dry without scarring.

Incidence

A. The World Health Organization estimates 20 million cases worldwide.

Pathogenesis

A. Herpes simplex virus is the causative organism. Herpes simplex type 1 (HSV-1) produces oral lesions, and type 2 (HSV-2) produces genital lesions. Kissing, sexual contact, vaginal delivery, and autoinoculation are all possible routes of transmission. The virus remains dormant, and outbreaks can be stimulated by several factors, including stress, illness, sunlight exposure, and menstruation.

Predisposing Factors

A. Early age at first coitus
B. Multiple sexual partners
C. History of sexually transmitted infections

Common Complaints

A. Dysuria
B. Pruritus
C. Burning
D. Swelling sensation

Other Signs and Symptoms

A. Primary episode
   1. Painful, vesicular, ulcerated, or crusted oral or genital lesion, singly or in clusters
   2. Flulike syndrome: fever, chills, headache, malaise, and myalgia
B. Recurrent episode: Less painful lesions and little or no systemic symptoms

Subjective Data

A. Elicit history of onset of symptoms; their location, frequency, and duration; aggravating and alleviating factors; and associated symptomatology.
B. Question the patient about history of other STIs and sexual habits.

Physical Examination

A. Check temperature, pulse, respirations, and blood pressure.
B. Inspect: Inspect the head, eyes, ears, nose, throat, and mucous membranes for lesions.
C. Palpate: Palpate the neck for lymphadenopathy.
D. Pelvic exam
   1. Assess external genitalia, perineum, and anus for lesions.
   2. Assess for inguinal lymphadenopathy.

Diagnostic Tests

A. Viral culture.

Clinical diagnosis is often reliable, but confirmation with viral culture should be attempted. Vesicles should be unroofed or crust removed for most reliable sample.

   1. Viral isolation: Obtain vesicular fluid by swabbing lesion with cotton- or Dacron-tipped applicator.
   2. Place applicator in appropriate transport viral medium before drying.
   3. Refrigerate until ready for transport.

B. Serology: HSV-1 and HSV-2 antibodies

Serologic antibodies are present 1–2 weeks after the initial outbreak.

C. Tzanck preparation: Scrape cells from base of lesion with No. 15 blade, then smear them on a microscope slide and stain them with Wright's or Giemsa stain.

Pap smear is not a sensitive test for HSV-2.

Differential Diagnoses

A. Herpes simplex virus
B. Primary syphilis
C. Chancroid
D. Lymphogranuloma venereum (LGV)
E. Folliculitis
F. Candidal fissure
G. Vestibular vulvitis
H. Mucocutaneous manifestations of Crohn's disease

Plan

A General interventions
   1. Culture samples immediately to begin treatment.
B. Patient teaching
   1. See the Section III Patient Teaching Guide for this chapter, "Herpes Simplex Virus."
   2. Advise patients to abstain from sexual activity during prodrome or while lesions are present.
   3. Condom use should be encouraged.
C. Pharmaceutical therapy: The CDC recommends the following treatment regimens:
   1. Primary episode:
      a. Acyclovir 200 mg by mouth five times a day for 7–10 days or until clinical resolution.
      b. Acyclovir 400 mg by mouth three times a day for 7–10 days or until clinical resolution.
      c. Famciclovir 250 mg by mouth three times a day for 7–10 days or until clinical resolution.
      d. Valacyclovir 1 g by mouth twice a day for 7–10 days or until clinical resolution.
   2. Recurrent episode: Begin during prodrome.
      a. Acyclovir 400 mg by mouth three times a day for 5 days.
      b. Acyclovir 800 mg by mouth twice a day for 5 days.
      c. Acyclovir 800 mg by mouth three times a day for 2 days.
      d. Famciclovir 125 mg by mouth two times a day for 5 days.
      e. Famciclovir 1000 mg by mouth two times a day for 1 day.
      f. Valacyclovir 500 mg by mouth two times a day for 3 days.
      g. Valacyclovir 1 g by mouth once daily for 5 days.
   3. Daily suppressive therapy.
      a. Acyclovir 400 mg by mouth twice daily, famciclovir 250 mg by mouth twice a day, or valacyclovir 500 mg by mouth once a day or 1 g by mouth once a day.
      b. Discontinue after 1 year of continuous use to reassess recurrence rate.

Clients receiving daily suppressive therapy of acyclovir 200 mg should use the lowest dose that provides relief from symptoms. Suppressive therapy has been shown to reduce frequency of recurrences by 75% in clients with more than six recurrences per year. It does not eliminate symptomatic or asymptomatic viral shedding or the potential for transmission.

4. Topical acyclovir, famciclovir (Famvir), and valacyclovir (Valtrex) have had mixed results in clinical trials and are not currently recommended by the CDC.

Follow-up
A. Follow-up is not recommended unless it is warranted by clinical presentation.

Consultation/Referral
A. Consult or refer the patient to a physician when there is prolonged ulceration unresponsive to therapy.

Individual Considerations
A. Pregnancy.
1. Acyclovir and Valacyclovir is category B for pregnancy and considered safe to use during pregnancy. These medications can be used for treatment as well as for suppression during pregnancy. The American College of Obstetricians (ACOG) recommends suppressive therapy begin at approximately 36 weeks' gestation to prevent an outbreak of lesions and to increase the chance of having a vaginal delivery. See Table 14.1.
2. Culture lesions if outbreak occurs. Lesion must be crusted for 7 days for vaginal delivery to be an option; otherwise, a cesarean delivery is recommended to avoid transmission of virus to newborn.
3. Pregnant women without genital herpes should be advised to avoid intercourse during the third trimester with partners known or suspected of having genital herpes.
4. Acyclovir allergy: no effective alternatives to acyclovir have been identified.
B. Partners: Symptomatic partners should be evaluated and treated in the same manner as any patient with genital lesions.
C. Geriatric: Genital herpes is rarely seen in the elderly. Recurrent infection of the buttocks region is not uncommon, especially in females.

HUMAN PAPILLOMAVIRUS (HPV)

Definition
A. The human papillomavirus (HPV) is a sexually transmitted infection. Condylomata acuminata, genital warts, and venereal warts are other names for HPV.

Incidence
A. The World Health Organization estimates 30 million cases of HPV infection worldwide.

Pathogenesis
A. The human papillomavirus, a slow-growing DNA virus of the papovavirus family, is the causative organism. Over 70 strains of the virus have been identified, and types 6 and 11 are most associated with genital warts. Types 16, 18, 31, 33, and 35 are high risk and are associated with cervical neoplasia. Warts may appear as early as 1–2 months after exposure, but most infections remain subclinical.

Predisposing Factors
A. Early first coitus
B. Multiple sexual partners
C. History of transmitted infections

Common Complaints
A. Painless genital "bumps" or warts
B. Pruritus
C. Bleeding during or after coitus
D. Malodorous vaginal discharge
E. Dysuria

Other Signs and Symptoms
A. Wartlike growths on genital area that are elevated and rough or flat and smooth
B. Lesions occurring singly or in clusters, from less than 1 mm to cauliflowerlike aggregates
C. Papillomas that are pale pink in color

Subjective Data
A. Elicit history of onset of symptoms, location, frequency, duration, aggravating and alleviating factors, and associated symptomatology.
B. Question the patient about history of other STIs, sexual behaviors, recent change in sexual partner, and partner's history of STIs.

TABLE 14.1 Pharmacological Treatment of Herpes in Pregnancy

Antiviral	Acyclovir Dosage	Valacyclovir Dosage
Initial lesion outbreak	400 mg tid for 7–10 days	1 gm bid for 7–10 days
Recurrent lesions	400 mg tid for 5 days or 800 mg for 5 days	500 mg bid × 3 days
Daily suppression from 36 weeks' gestation until delivery	400 mg tid	500 mg bid

Note. bid = twice a day. tid = three times a day.

Physical Examination

A. Check temperature, pulse, respirations, and blood pressure.
B. Inspect.
   1. Inspect external genitalia, perineum, and anus for lesions.
   2. Females, speculum exam: Inspect vaginal walls and cervix for lesions.
   3. Application of 3% acetic acid whitens lesions.

Diagnostic Tests

A. Visual identification is adequate in most cases.
B. Cytology: Pap smears are useful for screening. Pap results of koilocytosis, dyskeratosis, keratinizing atypia, atypical inflammation, and parakeratosis are all suggestive of HPV.
C. Histology: colposcopy with directed biopsy is diagnostic for subclinical lesions, dysplasia, and malignancy.
D. DNA typing: determination of specific strains is useful in diagnosing subclinical infections (the test is costly and false negatives occur).

Differential Diagnoses

A. Human papillomavirus
B. Condylomata
C. Molluscum contagiosum
D. Carcinoma

Plan

A. General interventions: Make diagnosis promptly to begin treatment.
B. Patient teaching.
   1. See the Section III Patient Teaching Guide for this chapter, "Human Papillomavirus (HPV)."
   2. Explain to the patient that therapy eliminates visible warts but does not eradicate the virus. No therapy has been shown to be effective in eradication of HPV. Ablation of warts may decrease viral load and transmissibility.
   3. Advise the patient to abstain from genital contact while lesions are present.
C. Pharmaceutical therapy.
   1. Therapy is not recommended for subclinical infections (absence of exophytic warts).
   2. Trichloroacetic acid (TCA) 80%–90% solution applied weekly to visible warts by clinician until warts resolve. If unresolved after six applications, consider other therapy. See the Section II Procedure, "Trichloroacetic (TCA)/Podophyllin Therapy."
   3. Podophyllum resin (Podophyllin) 10%–25% in tincture of benzoin compound applied weekly to visible warts by clinician until warts resolve.
      a. Application of petroleum jelly on surrounding skin may be used for protection of unaffected areas.
      b. Advise the patient to wash off resin after 4 hours. If unresolved after six applications, consider other therapy.
   4. Trichloroacetic acid 80%–90% applied to the warts and allowed to dry weekly by clinician until warts resolved.

5. Podofilox 0.5% solution for home treatment, applied to visible warts by the patient twice daily for 3 consecutive days, followed by 4 days without treatment. Cycle is repeated up to four times.
6. Imiquimod 5% (Aldara) cream applied to wart, left on for 6–10 hours, then washed with mild soap. Use daily, three times a week (Mon., Wed., Fri.), until wart resolves or up to 16 weeks.
D. Medical/surgical management: Cryotherapy, electrodesiccation, electrocautery, carbon dioxide laser, and surgical excision are options to be considered for patients with large or extensive lesions or refractory disease.

Follow-up

A. Short-term follow-up is not recommended if the patient is asymptomatic after treatment.
B. **The CDC does not recommend more frequent Pap smears for women with external warts.**
C. Long-term follow-up should include annual Pap smears and pelvic exams. Encourage the patient to self-examine genitalia.

Consultation/Referral

A. Consult or refer the patient to a physician when lesions persist after six consecutive treatments or when cervical or rectal warts are diagnosed.

Individual Considerations

A. Pregnancy: Podophyllum and podofilox are contraindicated during pregnancy.
B. Partners: Treatment recommended if visible lesions are present.
C. Adolescents: Education regarding Gardasil vaccine recommended for girls and boys 9 years to 25 years of age for prevention of acquiring the HPV virus. The vaccination may help to prevent contracting 4 of the viruses (6, 11, 16, 17) that increase the risk of cervical cancer for women.
D. Geriatric.
   1. Verrucous carcinoma and vulvar intraepithelial neoplasia (VIN) can be undistinguishable from condyloma. Older women are more likely to have VIN or carcinoma.
   2. Diagnosis made by biopsy; colposcopy is strongly advised.
   3. Immunocompetence should be investigated in new or recurrent condyloma.

SYPHILIS

Definition

A. Syphilis is a sexually transmitted infection. It is characterized by distinct primary, secondary, and tertiary stages that occur over several years or decades. Latent or inactive periods occur between the stages. Early latent is less than 1 year after infection; late latent is more than 1 year after infection. **Health department notification is required by law in all states.**

Incidence

A. The World Health Organization estimates 4 million cases of syphilis worldwide.

Pathogenesis

A. *Treponema pallidum,* a spirochete bacterium, is the causative organism that infects the mucous membrane.

Predisposing Factors

A. History of sexually transmitted infections
B. Multiple sexual partners
C. Illicit drug use
D. Prostitution

Common Complaints

A. Genital lesion, generalized rash involving palms and soles, mucous patches, and condyloma latum are common.

Other Signs and Symptoms

A. Primary syphilis
   1. Chancre that is painless or minimally painful
   2. Round, indurated lesion with little or no purulent exudate
   3. Regional bilateral lymphadenopathy
B. Secondary syphilis
   1. Generalized maculopapular rash that is nonpruritic and copper colored, on palms or soles; may be erythematous or scaly
   2. Mucous patches; painless, white, mucous membrane lesions
   3. Generalized lymphadenopathy; flulike syndrome including fever, headache, sore throat, and malaise
   4. Patchy alopecia
C. Tertiary syphilis
   1. Gumma: locally destructive granulomatous tumors involving various organs or systems; commonly seen on liver, but can occur on other organs (heart, brain, skin, bone, testis)
   2. Cardiovascular: aortic involvement, aneurysms, and valve insufficiency
   3. Neurologic: tabes dorsalis and general paresis
D. Latent syphilis: Asymptomatic

Latent phase syphilis manifests itself after treatment failure or no history of treatment. Spirochete can lie dormant for years.

E. Congenital syphilis: Symptoms range from asymptomatic to fatal.

Subjective Data

A. Elicit history of onset, location, frequency, duration of symptoms; aggravating and alleviating factors; and associated symptomatology.
B. Question the patient about history of other STIs, illicit drug use, and sexual habits.

Physical Examination

A. Check temperature, pulse, respirations, and blood pressure.
B. Inspect.
   1. Inspect the skin; note lesions and rashes.
   2. Observe the head; note patchy alopecia.
   3. Examine the mouth and throat; note lesions.
   4. Inspect the genital and rectal area; note lesions and rashes.

C. Palpate: Palpate the lymph nodes (neck, supraclavicular, axillary, epitrochlear, and inguinal regions).
D. Auscultate: Auscultate heart and lungs.
E. Neurologic exam.
   1. Assess sensory functioning.
   2. Test cranial nerves, first through twelfth.

Diagnostic Tests

Evaluate for other STIs for patients presenting with syphilis.

A. Serology: Nontreponemal tests
   1. Venereal Disease Research Laboratory (VDRL) test
   2. Rapid plasma reagin (RPR) tests

Results are reactive (positive) or nonreactive (negative). Titers correlate with active disease and should be quantitative. These tests are equally valid but cannot be compared because of titer differences (RPR is slightly higher than VDRL). All reactive results require confirmation with treponemal tests.

B. Serology: Treponemal tests
   1. Fluorescent treponemal antibody absorption (FTA-ABS) test
   2. Microhemagglutination assay for antibody to *T. pallidum* (MHA-TP)

Once FTA-ABS for antibody to *T. pallidum*, VDRL, and RPR are reactive, these tests usually remain reactive for life.

C. Cerebrospinal fluid (CSF) culture to detect neurosyphilis.
D. Microscopy: *Treponema pallidum* cannot be seen with light microscopy; dark-field microscopy exam of the serous exudate from lesions is the definitive test for syphilis. Properly equipped labs with specially trained personnel must be available for this test.

Differential Diagnoses

A. Syphilis
B. Herpes simplex virus

Plan

A. General interventions: Staging of the disease may be difficult but guides management decisions.
B. Patient teaching.
   1. See the Section III Patient Teaching Guide for this chapter, "Syphilis."
   2. Advise the patient to abstain from sexual activity until treatment is completed.
   3. Inform the patients of Jarisch-Herxheimer reaction (fever, headache, myalgia) that may occur within the first 24 hours of treatment. Antipyretics may be prescribed.
   4. Discuss the importance of partner notification.
   5. Stress the importance of complying with follow-up regimen.
C. Pharmaceutical therapy: The CDC recommends the following treatment regimens:
   1. Primary syphilis, secondary syphilis, early latent syphilis:
      a. Adults: benzathine penicillin G 2.4 million units injected intramuscularly in a single dose.
      b. Pediatrics: benzathine penicillin G 50,000 units/kg, up to the adult dose of 2.4 million units, injected intramuscularly in a single dose.

2. Late latent syphilis, latent syphilis of unknown duration, late syphilis (manage with expert consultation):
   a. Adults: benzathine penicillin G 7.2 million units total, administered as three doses (2.4 million units each) injected intramuscularly at 1-week intervals.
   b. Pediatrics: benzathine pencillin G 50,000 units/kg, up to the adult dose of 2.4 million units, injected intramuscularly for three total doses.
3. Neurosyphilis (manage with expert consultation):
   a. Adults: aqueous crystalline penicillin G, 18–24 million units daily, 2–4 million units administered by IV every 4 hours for 10–14 days.
   b. Adults: procaine penicillin 2–4 million units injected intramuscularly daily, plus probenecid 500 mg by mouth four times a day, both for 10–14 days.
   c. Pediatrics: penicillin desensitization, then treatment with recommended regimen.
4. Primary syphilis, secondary syphilis, early latent syphilis, late latent syphilis in (nonpregnant) patient with penicillin allergy: doxycycline 100 mg by mouth twice daily for 2 weeks, or tetracycline 500 mg by mouth four times daily for 2 weeks.
5. Latent syphilis of unknown duration, late syphilis: Treat with above regimen for infections of less than 1 year duration. If greater than 1 year, treat with above regimen for 4 weeks.
6. For pregnant patients with penicillin allergy, penicillin treatment after desensitization is recommended for the following reasons:
   a. Penicillin is effective for preventing transmission and treating the infected fetus.
   b. Doxycycline and tetracycline are contraindicated in pregnancy.
   c. Erythromycin may not cure the infected fetus.

Follow-up

A. Primary and secondary syphilis: Clinical and serologic exams should be conducted at 3 months and 6 months. Absence of fourfold decrease at 3 months is indicative of treatment failure.
B. Latent syphilis: Clinical and serologic exams should be conducted at 6 months and 12 months. Absence of fourfold decrease within 12–24 months is indicative of treatment failure.
C. Late syphilis: Minimal evidence regarding follow-up exists. Follow-up largely depends on nature of lesions.
D. Neurosyphilis: CSF examination should take place every 6 months until cell count is normal.

Consultation/Referral

A. Consult or refer the patient to a physician when the recommended treatment fails and patient noncompliance and reexposure have been ruled out, or when neurosyphilis is diagnosed.

Individual Considerations

A. Pregnancy
   1. Draw blood samples for RPR/VDRL from all prenatal patients.
   2. Administer appropriate regimen for the patient's stage of syphilis.

3. Follow-up: Perform serologic tests monthly until adequacy of treatment has been ensured.
4. The Jarisch-Herxheimer reaction may predispose women to premature labor or fetal distress if treatment occurs in the second half of the pregnancy. Advise these patients to immediately seek medical attention if they experience uterine contractions or changes in fetal movement.
5. Abortions and stillbirths are common.
B. Pediatrics
   1. Congenital syphilis is caused by untreated infection or treatment failure in the mother.
   2. Refer the patient to a physician for infectious disease consultation.
   3. Medication therapy: See "Pharmaceutical Therapy" noted above.
C. Partners: Identify at-risk partners who have had sexual contact with the patient within these time frames:
   1. Primary syphilis: 3 months plus duration of symptoms
   2. Secondary syphilis: 6 months plus duration of symptoms
   3. Early latent syphilis: 1 year
D. Geriatric
   1. Dementia, tremors, and pupillary changes are the result of long-term untreated syphilis.
   2. The CSF should be tested using the FTA-ABS test. The VDRL is usually not adequate.
   3. Syphilis is uncommon in the elderly in developed countries; however, it is very common worldwide.

TRICHOMONIASIS

Definition

A. Trichomoniasis is a sexually transmitted infection. Nonsexual transmission by means of fomites is possible, but rare.

Incidence

A. Trichomoniasis is not a CDC reportable infection. Therefore, exact incidence is unavailable. The World Health Organization estimates 120 million cases worldwide.

Pathogenesis

A. *Trichomonas vaginalis,* a flagellated protozoan, is the causative organism.

Predisposing Factors

A. History of sexually transmitted infections
B. Multiple sexual partners

Common Complaints

A. Copious, yellow-green or watery gray vaginal discharge
B. Vaginal odor
C. Dysuria
D. Dyspareunia
E. Postcoital spotting or bleeding
F. Abdominal discomfort
G. Pruritus

Other Signs and Symptoms

A. Asymptomatic
B. Perineal irritation

Subjective Data

A. Elicit history of onset, location, frequency, duration of symptoms, and aggravating and alleviating factors; note associated symptomatology.
B. Question the patient about history of other STIs or vaginal infections, changes and characteristics of vaginal discharge, and recent change in sexual partner.

Physical Examination

A. Check temperature, pulse, respirations, and blood pressure.
B. Inspect: Inspect introitus for discharge and irritation.
C. Speculum exam.
 1. Inspect the vaginal walls for discharge and irritation.
 2. Inspect the cervix for discharge, erythema, punctate hemorrhages (strawberry-patch cervix), and friability.
D. Bimanual exam.
 1. Assess for cervical motion tenderness.
 2. Palpate for uterine and adnexal tenderness.

Diagnostic Tests

A. Wet prep: presence of motile, flagellated trichomonads. Increased number of white blood cells (>.10 per high-power field) may be present.
B. Culture sample in Diamond's or Kufferberg's medium.
 1. This is the most sensitive and specific diagnostic method.
 2. It is expensive and not widely available.
C. Pap smear: report may include trichomonads, but sensitivity is low.
 1. If trichomonads are noted on Pap smear, the patient should be reexamined and diagnosis confirmed with a wet prep.
D. Vaginal pH is usually greater than 4.5.
E. KOH/wet prep "whiff test" may be positive.

Differential Diagnoses

A. Trichomoniasis
B. Bacterial vaginosis
C. Vulvovaginal candidiasis
D. Chlamydia
E. Gonorrhea
F. Pelvic inflammatory disease
G. Foreign body vaginitis

Plan

A. General interventions: Prompt diagnosis helps to initiate treatment.
B. Patient teaching
 1. See the Section III Patient Teaching Guide for this chapter, "Trichomoniasis."
 2. Advise the patient to abstain from sexual activity until treatment is complete.
 3. Advise the patient to avoid alcohol consumption during and 24 hours after metronidazole treatment due to the possible disulfiramlike (Antabuse) effect.
 4. Inform the patient that urine may darken in color during treatment.
 5. Inform the patient of a possible metallic taste in the mouth during treatment.
C. Pharmaceutical therapy
 1. **Drug of choice: metronidazole or tinidazole 2 g orally in a single dose.**

 2. Alternative regimen: metronidazole 500 mg by mouth twice daily for 7 days. Expected cure rate from either regimen is 95%.
 3. Treatment failure: CDC recommends retreatment with metronidazole 500 mg by mouth twice daily for 7 days.
 4. If repeated failure occurs, treat with metronidazole 2 g by mouth four times daily for 3–5 days.
 5. Metronidazole gel is unlikely to achieve therapeutic levels in the urethra or perivaginal glands. It is a considerably less efficacious treatment than oral preparations and is *not* recommended for use.

Follow-up

A. Immediate follow-up is not recommended if the patient is initially asymptomatic or symptoms are relieved by treatment.

Consultation/Referral

A. Consult or refer the patient to a physician when recommended treatment fails and patient noncompliance and reexposure have been ruled out.

Individual Considerations

A. Pregnancy.
 1. First trimester: metronidazole is contraindicated.
 2. Palliative treatment: clotrimazole 1% vaginal cream one applicator full daily at bedtime for 7 days.
 3. Second and third trimester: metronidazole 2 g by mouth one time.
 4. Lactation: metronidazole 2 g by mouth one time; discontinue breast-feeding during and 24 hours after treatment. Pumping and discarding milk is recommended.
B. Partners: Recommended treatment is metronidazole 2 g orally one time.
C. Geriatric.
 1. Uncommon pathogen in postmenopausal women.
 2. Symptoms are vulvar irritation with discharge.
 3. Diagnose with wet prep.
 4. Treat with metronidazole 1 g in the morning and 1 g in the evening.

REFERENCES

American College of Obestricians and Gynecologists. (2007). Management of herpes in pregnancy. *ACOG Practice Bulletin,* Number 83.

Bennett, E. C. (1994). Vaginitis and sexually transmitted diseases. In E. Q. Youngkin & M. S. Davis (Eds.), *Women's health: A primary care clinical guide* (pp. 203–240). Norwalk, CT: Appleton & Lange.

Centers for Disease Control and Prevention. (1993). Sexually transmitted diseases treatment guidelines. *Morbidity and Mortality Weekly Report, 1993, 42*(No. RR–14): 22–93.

Centers for Disease Control and Prevention. (1998). 1998 Guidelines for treatment of sexually transmitted diseases. *Morbidity and Mortality Weekly Report, January 23,* (47)(No. RR–1).

Centers for Disease Control and Prevention. (2006). Sexually transmitted diseases treatment guidelines 2006. *Morbidity and Mortality Weekly Report, August 4,* (55)(No. RR–11).

Eschenbach, D. A. (1996). Diagnosis and treatment of vaginitis. In M. A. Stenchever (Ed.), *Office gynecology* (pp. 317–342). St. Louis, MO: Mosby Year-Book.

Faro, S. (1995). Inflammatory and sexually transmitted diseases. In D. H. Nichols & P. J. Sweeney (Eds.), *Ambulatory gynecology* (pp. 103–121). Philadelphia: J. B. Lippincott.

Gibbs, R. (2001). Impact of infectious diseases on women's health: 1776–2026. *Obstetrics and Gynecology, 97*(6), 1019–1023.

Gibbs, R. S., & Sweet, R. L. (1995). *Evaluating and treating obstetric and gynecologic infections.* Califon, NJ: Gardiner-Caldwell Synermed.

Hoover, K., & Tao, G. (2008). Missed opportunities for Chlamydia screening of young women in the United States. *Obstetrics and Gynecology, 111*(5), 1097–1102.

Schreiber, C., Meyer, C., Creinin, M., Barnart, K., & Hillier, S. (2006). Effects of long-term use of nonoxynol-9 on vaginalflora. *Obstetrics and Gynecology, 111*(5), 1097–1102.

CHAPTER 15

Infectious Disease Guidelines

Cheryl A. Glass

CAT SCRATCH DISEASE (CSD)

Definition

A. Cat scratch disease (CSD) is a lymphatic infection occurring 3–14 days after a dermal abrasion from a cat scratch. Infection causes unilateral regional adenitis, however, CSD manifestations may also include visceral organ, neurologic, and ocular involvement.

Incidence

A. Incidence is less than 25,000 new cases every year; it is believed to be relatively common. More than 90% of cases have had a history of recent contact with cats, often kittens, which are usually healthy. Multiple cases have been observed in families, presumably resulting from contact with the same animal. There is no documentation of human-to-human transmission. Persons that are immunocompromised are more susceptible to the systemic manifestations. Dissemination to the liver, spleen, eye, or central nervous system occurs in 5%–14% of individuals.

Pathogenesis

A. *Bartonella henselae* is considered to be responsible for most cases of cat scratch disease. *Bartonella henselae* is a fastidious, slow-growing, gram-negative bacterium. Most transmission occurs from feline bites or scratches as well as cat licking to nonintact skin. Other vectors that may be involved in the transmission of *B. henselae* to humans include dogs, monkeys, Ixodes ticks, and fleas from cats or kittens.

B. The incubation period for lesions to appear is 7–12 days after abrasion; lymphadenopathy appears 5–50 days (median = 12 days) after appearance of the primary lesion.

Predisposing Factors

A. Exposure to domestic and outside cats
B. Immunocompromised

Common Complaints

A. **Swollen lymph glands (regional lymph node, groin, axillary, and cervical areas). The predominant sign is regional lymphadenopathy in an otherwise healthy person.**

B. Low-grade fever.
C. Body aches.
D. Fatigue.

Other Signs and Symptoms

A. A skin papule appears 3–10 days after inoculation, often found at the presumed site of inoculation. The papule progresses through the erythematous, vesicular, and popular crusted stages.
B. Headache.
C. Extreme fatigue.
D. Abdominal pain in the presence of hepatosplenomegaly.
E. Arthropathies of the knee, wrist, ankle, and elbows.
F. Visual.
   1. Unilateral eye redness/conjunctivitis is the most common ocular manifestation.
   2. Loss of vision.
   3. Visual disturbances.
   4. Ocular pain (i.e., foreign-body sensation).
   5. Serous discharge.
G. Central nervous.
   1. Changes in level of consciousness.
   2. Persistent high fever.
   3. Seizures within 6 weeks of lymphadenopathy.
H. Cardiac.
   1. Murmur.
   2. Dyspnea.

Subjective Data

A. Review onset and duration of symptoms.
B. Elicit the history of abrasion caused by a kitten/cat or other vectors.
C. Ask the patient about other symptoms such as low-grade fever and body aches.
D. Rule out other illness with review of symptoms (such as pharyngitis and mononucleosis).

Physical Examination

A. Check temperature, pulse, respirations, and blood pressure.
B. Inspect.

1. Examine the skin for scratches, bite marks, erythema, or rash.
2. Conduct an ear, nose, and throat exam.
3. Conduct an eye exam if indicated.
   a. Visual exam: Snellen chart.
   b. Fundoscopic examination may need to be deferred if photophobia is present.
C. Auscultate: Auscultate the heart and lungs.
D. Palpate.
   1. Palpate lymph nodes: preauricular, cervical, axillary, epitrochlear, and inguinal nodes. **Unilateral tender lymph nodes (usually singular) are palpable near scratch site. The area around the affected lymph nodes is typically tender, warm, erythematous, and indurated.**
   2. Palpate the abdomen to rule out organomegaly.
   3. Breast: examine if indicated: mastitis is rare.

Diagnostic Tests

A. Usually none. The cat scratch skin test is no longer recommended. Presenting symptoms may indicate further testing including:
   1. CBC with differential
   2. Sedimentation rate
   3. Bartonella antibody testing
   4. Seminated polymerase chain reaction (PCR) assay
B. Warthin-Starry silver impregnation stain of lymph node, skin, or conjunctival tissue.
C. Biopsy of lymph node (when malignancy is suspected).
D. Abdominal ultrasound or CT in the presence of hepatomegaly, splenomegaly, or hepatosplenomegaly on physical exam.

Differential Diagnoses

A. Cat scratch disease
B. Infectious mononucleosis
C. Kawasaki disease
D. Lyme disease
E. Malignancies that involve lymph nodes such as lymphoma/Hodgkin's disease

Plan

A. General interventions
   1. Management is usually treatment of symptoms. Cat scratch disease is self-limiting with slow resolution in 2–4 months.
   2. Prescribe analgesics for pain.
   3. Rest is advised.
   4. Ice may be applied to the affected nodes.
   5. About 10% of nodes will suppurate, and require aspiration. Incision and drainage is not recommended because of the potential of chronic sinus tract formation. During aspiration, the needle should be moved around in several locations, because microabscesses often exist in multiple septated pockets.
B. Patient teaching
   1. The lymphadenopathy usually regresses within 2–4 months, but may persist for up to 1 year.
   2. Patient education on cats include:
      a. People should avoid playing roughly with cats.
      b. Stray cats should not be handled by children or immunocompromised people.

c. Testing cats is not recommended. Cats do not need to be removed or destroyed.
   d. Always cleanse animal bites or scratches immediately with soap and water to prevent or reduce the transmission of CSD.
3. Disease is not contagious: there is no person-to-person transmission.
4. No vaccination is currently available.
C. Pharmaceutical therapy
   1. Antibiotic therapy is not essential for patients with normal immune systems. Symptoms are usually self-limiting.
   2. Acetaminophen (Tylenol) as needed.
   3. Nonsteroidal anti-inflammatory drugs as needed.
   4. Oral corticosteroids for individuals with atypical symptoms.
   5. Antibiotics may be prescribed if the patient is acutely ill with systemic symptoms, particularly immunocompromised individuals; with hepatosplenomegaly, visual, cardiac, or neurologic symptoms; or with large, painful adenopathy.
      a. Azithromycin dosing for lymphadenitis:
         i. For patients weighing more than 45.5 kg, prescribe 500 mg on day 1, followed by 250 mg for 4 days.
         ii. For patients weighing less than 45.5 kg, prescribe 10 mg/kg on day 1, followed by 5 mg/kg for 4 days.
      b. Clarithromycin may be used as an alternative to Azithromycin for lymphadenitis:
         i. For patients weighing more than 45.5 kg, prescribe 500 mg twice a day for a 7–10 day course.
         ii. For patients weighing less than 45.5 kg, prescribe 15–20 mg/kg divided in 2 doses for a 7–10 day course.
      c. Rifampin may be used as an alternative for lymphadenitis:
         i. In children prescribe 10 mg/kg every 12 hours to a maximum dose of 600 mg/day for a 7–10 day course.
         ii. In adults prescribe 300 mg twice a day for a 7–10 day course.
      d. Timethoprim-sulfamethoxazole may be used an alternative for lymphadenitis:
         i. In children prescribe trimethoprim 8 mg/kg per day, sulfamethozazole 40 mg/kg per day in 2 divided doses for 7–10 days.
         ii. In adults prescribe 1 double strength tablet twice a day.
      e. Hepatosplenic disease and prolonged fever use rifampin (as previously noted) for 10–14 days and add a second agent such as azithromycin or gentamicin:
         i. Azithromycin (as previously noted) for an entire 10–14 day course.
         ii. Gentamicin loading dose 2 mg/kg then 1.5 mg/kg over 8 hours; dose based upon normal renal function and adjusted with monitoring.
      f. Neuroretinitis: the optimal therapy for neuroretinitis is unknown. Consult with the ophthalmologist since the patient will require close monitoring.

g. Neurologic disease: little is known about the optimal therapy for neurologic manifestations of B. henselae infection. Consult with a physician.

h. Endocarditis: the optimal antibiotic therapy and optimal duration of therapy for Bartonella endocarditis is unknown. Consult with a physician.

Follow-up

A. Reevaluate the patient in approximately 6–8 weeks if mild symptoms.

B. Reevaluate in 10 days if placed on antibiotics.

Consultation/Referral

A. Complications are rare; refer the patient to a physician including specialists (neurologist, cardiologist, and ophthalmologist) if infection is systemic or unresponsive to antibiotics.

CYTOMEGALOVIRUS (CMV)

Definition

A. Cytomegalovirus (CMV) is in the herpesvirus family, which includes varicella-zoster (chickenpox) and infectious mononucleosis (Epstein-Barr virus). Differences in CMV genotypes may be associated with differences in virulence. CMV is responsible for a viral infection with a high rate of asymptomatic excretion. Shedding of the virus takes place intermittently. CMV can be isolated in cell culture from urine, pharynx, respiratory secretions, human milk, tears, saliva, semen, cervical secretions, and body fluids such as blood and amniotic fluid. Cytomegalic cells can be found in tissue including the lung, liver, kidney, intestine, adrenal gland, and the central nervous system.

B. Cytomegalovirus persists in latent form after a primary infection, and reactivation can occur years later, particularly under conditions of immunosuppression, transplantation, and pregnancy. CMV is one of the TORCH infections (Toxoplasmosis, Other [i.e., hepatitis and syphilis], Rubella, Cytomegalovirus, and Herpes infections).

Incidence

A. CMV is found worldwide in all age, races, and ethnic groups. Seropositivity increases with age, ranging 40%–100% depending on the geography, cultures, child-rearing practices, and socioeconomic status. Approximately 50% of blood donors have been exposed to CMV, and 10% carry CMV virus in white blood cells. The incidence of horizontal transmission of CMV occurring in settings such as day care ranges from 10% to over 80% from the exposure to saliva and urine. Another increase in CMV is noted in adolescence secondary to sexual activity.

B. The incidence of congenital vertical transmission of CMV ranges from 0.2%–2.5%. Most newborns appear normal and are asymptomatic, however 5%–15% congenitally infected newborns will have symptoms at delivery. Prenatal CMV infections occur from contact with maternal cervicovaginal secretions during delivery or from breast milk ingestion. Preterm infants are at the greatest risk to acquire CMV from breast milk.

Pathogenesis

A. Human CMV, a DNA virus, is a member of the herpesvirus group. This virus is transmitted both horizontally (by direct person-to-person contact with virus-containing secretions) and vertically (from mother to infant before, during, or after birth). Infections have no seasonal correlation.

B. The incubation period for horizontally transmitted CMV infections in households is unknown. Primary CMV infection usually manifests itself 4–7 weeks and may persist as long as 16–20 weeks after initial infection. CMV disease is most likely 30–60 days after transplant.

Predisposing Factors

A. Exposure to young children (especially those in day-care centers).

B. Sexual contact (cervicovaginal secretions and semen).

C. Blood transfusion: **Patients with impaired immune function (e.g., bone marrow and organ transplant recipients, premature babies) are at risk for CMV infection from contaminated transfused blood.**

D. Hospital or occupational exposure: Universal precautions are considered adequate to prevent transmission of CMV within hospitals. Nosocomial transmission from person to person has not been documented. Isolation is not recommended.

E. Pregnancy: Pregnant health care workers are not restricted from caring for CMV-infected patients and should follow universal precautions.

F. Transplacental transmission.

G. Ascending infection from the cervix.

H. Tissue or organ transplantation.

I. Household spread among family members; a young child is most frequently the index case.

J. Breast milk.

Common Complaints

A. Mononucleosis-like syndrome

B. Fever

C. Overwhelming fatigue

D. Pharyngitis

E. Ulcerative lesions in the mouth

Other Signs and Symptoms

A. Mothers: Asymptomatic or mononucleosis-like syndrome

B. Fetuses
1. Intrauterine growth retardation (IUGR)/small for gestational age (SGA)
2. Nonimmune hydrops fetalis
3. Microcephaly noted on ultrasound
4. Intracerebral calcification

C. Infants after congenital exposure
1. Asymptomatic
2. Skin
a. Jaundice at birth
b. Petechiae and purpura of the skin
3. Hepatosplenomegaly
4. Anemia
5. Thrombocytopenia
6. Eyes: chorioretinitis, retinal hemorrhage, optic atrophy

7. Seizure disorders
8. Feeding difficulties
D. Children with congenital exposure
   1. Asymptomatic.
   2. Development: developmental delays, learning disability, and mental retardation.
   3. Ears: progressive hearing loss (usually unilateral). Universal hearing screening programs may identify some of the otherwise asymptomatic infants.
   4. Loss of vision.
E. Adults
   1. Visual changes: floaters or loss of visual fields on one side.
   2. Retinitis.
   3. Arthralgias.
   4. Nausea, abdominal cramping, and vomiting (includes hematemesis).
   5. Prolonged fever.
   6. Mild hepatitis.
   7. Headache.
   8. Gastritis presents with abdominal pain and colitis present as a diarrheal illness. CMV may infect the gastrointestinal tract from the oral cavity through the colon. The typical manifestation of disease is ulcerative lesions. In the mouth, these may be indistinguishable from ulcers caused by HSV or aphthous ulceration.
F. Immunocompromised persons
   1. Bacterial: pneumonia, retinitis, myocarditis, and aseptic meningitis
   2. Anemia
   3. Thrombocytopenia

Subjective Data
A. Review onset of presenting signs, symptoms, and their duration.
B. Review the patient's history for recent upper respiratory infection and mononucleosis-like symptoms.
C. Elicit information concerning contact with any person known to be CMV infected.
D. Review history for other family members with similar symptoms.
E. Ask the patient about any occupational exposure.
F. Review the patient's exposure to children in day-care centers.
G. Review recent blood transfusions and/or organ transplantation.
H. Determine the patient's history for risk factors or presence of HIV.

Physical Examination
A. Check temperature, pulse, respirations, and blood pressure.
B. Inspect.
   1. Inspect skin for jaundice and petechiae.
   2. Evaluate age-appropriate developmental tasks.
   3. Conduct a detailed eye exam. **CMV infection may appear as yellow-white areas with perivascular exudates and hemorrhage a "cottage cheese and ketchup" appearance.**

4. Perform ears, nose, and throat exam.
5. Conduct hearing test.
C. Auscultate: Auscultate the heart and lungs.
D. Palpate.
   1. Palpate the abdomen noting organomegaly.
   2. Pregnancy: palpate fundal height and evaluate for suspected IUGR.
E. Neurologic exam: Assess all cranial nerves.

Diagnostic Tests
A. **Viral culture of specimen from urine, cervix, vagina, nasopharynx, and saliva.**
   1. **Viral culture is the best means of diagnosing acute CMV infections, although it does not distinguish between primary and recurrent disease. Urine contains high titers of the virus because CMV is relatively stable in urine.**
B. CBC with differential: **Differential white blood count reveals increased lymphocytes, many of which are atypical.**
C. Total direct and indirect serum bilirubin.
D. Liver function: ALT and AST.
E. Serology for CMV IgG and IgM: **Only the recovery of the virus from a target organ provides unequivocal evidence that the disease is caused by CMV infection. However, a fourfold or greater rise in IgG-specific antibody titer is usually considered evidence of acute infection.**
F. Amniocentesis for polymerase chain reaction (PCR) to detect CMV DNA is the preferred diagnostic approach for the detection of the infected fetus.
G. Immunocompromised patients, especially transplant recipients, may be monitored for viral surveillance weekly using surrogate markers for viremia-PCR.
H. Chest X-ray if indicated.
I. CT scan if indicated to evaluate abnormalities of the brain in the presence of an abnormal neurologic examination, seizures, and microcephahly.
J. Sensorineural hearing evaluation.

Differential Diagnoses
A. Cytomegalovirus
B. Other TORCH infections (Toxoplasmosis, Syphilis, Hepatitis, Rubella, and Herpes)
C. HIV
D. Viral: autoimmune hepatitis or hepatitis A–E
E. Entroviruses
F. Fever of unknown origin

Plan
A. General interventions
   1. Provide support for the patient and family.
   2. Contact social services if long-term support will be required for these infants/families.
   3. Rest is vital.
B. Patient teaching
   1. Patients with splenomegaly should avoid activity that may increase the risk of injury to the spleen, such as contact sports and heavy lifting.
   2. Mothers infected with CMV should be discouraged from breast-feeding, because CMV virus is secreted in breast milk. CMV-specific IgM antibodies are

present in only 80% of patients with primary CMV infections and in 20% of patients with recurrent infections; therefore, a negative result does not exclude the diagnosis of CMV.

3. Isolation is not required.
4. Use universal precautions, especially good hand washing.
5. Do not share eating or drinking utensils, drinks, or food with toddlers or young children.

C. Pharmaceutical therapy

1. Drug of choice: Ganciclovir (Cytovene) for CMV retinitis is the treatment both for adults and children older than 3 months; treatment is divided into an induction and maintenance phase.

   a. Safety of ganciclovir in pregnancy has not been established.

   b. Patients receiving ganciclovir should have blood counts monitored closely due to dose-dependent bone marrow suppression. Monitor for leukopenia, neutropenia, anemia, or thrombocytopenia. Stop ganciclovir when neutrophil counts are less than 500/mm³. Growth factors may be necessary.

   c. The dose should be decreased in patients with impaired renal function. Monitor creatinine.

   d. Ganciclovir induction: 5 mg/kg per dose intravenously (IV) administered over 1 hour every 12 hours for 14–21 days depending on the clinical and virologic response. Oral ganciclovir should not be used for induction.

   e. Ganciclovir maintenance:

      i. A single daily dose of 5 mg/kg administered intravenously every other day or 5 days a week, skipping the weekend.

      ii. Oral ganciclovir 1 gm orally three times a day may be used for maintenance/prophylaxis in some patients, but poor oral availability makes it less effective than intravenous administration.

   f. Although ganciclovir has appeared to be beneficial in the treatment of some congenitally infected infants, its use is controversial and is considered for high-risk patients with severe congenital CMV.

   g. Newborns: 6 mg/kg per dose administered intravenously over the course of 1 hour. Ganciclovir has been administered in clinical trials for infants at 6 mg/kg IV for 6 weeks.

2. Alternative drug therapy: Foscarnet (Foscavir)

   a. Used in ganciclovir-resistant CMV retinitis and herpes simplex disease.

   b. Use in children is limited and the safe dose is not established.

   c. Safety of Foscarnet in pregnancy has not been established.

   d. Foscarnet is nephrotoxic. Meticulous attention must be paid to renal function. Small changes in creatinine require new calculation for renal clearance. Obtain a 24-hour serum creatinine at baseline and discontinue if serum creatinine is less than 0.4 gL/min/kg.

   e. Patients must be well hydrated.

   f. Foscarnet:

      i. Foscarnet induction: 60mg/kg IV every 8 hours or 90–120 mg/kg IV every 12 hours for 14–21 days for the induction of CMV retinitis.

      ii. Foscarnet maintenance: 90–120 mg/kg IV per day as a single infusion. Infusion rate should not exceed 1 mg/kg/min.

   g. Cytomegalovirus immunoglobulin intravenous (CMV-IGIV): Initial dose is 150 mg/kg and is followed by gradually reduced doses once every 2 weeks for 16 weeks. Currently available antiviral agents do not cure CMV disease in HIV-infected patients.

3. Immune globulin or CMV hyperimmune globulin CytoGam may be utilized for passive immuno-prophylaxis especially in bone marrow and organ transplant recipients to help develop antibodies and protect against CMV infection.

4. CMV vaccines are currently in clinical trials.

Follow-up

A. The patient should be seen for reports of excessive bruising or bleeding, jaundice, or abnormal CNS functioning.

B. Monitor CBC, serum creatinine, and electrolytes (especially calcium and magnesium) every week.

Consultation/Referral

A. Consultation with an infectious disease specialist is indicated for acute infection, especially for immunocompromised patients.

B. Antivirals have many adverse effects and are best managed by a physician who has experience using these drugs.

C. Consultation with a hematologist in severe cases, especially with hemolytic anemia and thrombocytopenia.

D. Consultation with a neurologist for meningitis, encephalitis, polyneuritis, and Guillian-Barré syndrome.

E. Consultation with an ophthalmologist (as indicated).

F. Consultation to a perinatologist is indicated for pregnant patients. Evaluation may include ultrasonography, amniocentesis, and percutaneous umbilical blood sampling (PUBS).

Individual Considerations

A. Pregnancy:

1. Between 55% and 85% of pregnant women are immune to CMV, with a higher prevalence of immunity in lower socioeconomic populations.

2. Susceptible pregnant women have a 2%–2.5% risk of acquiring primary CMV during pregnancy. Those with prior immunity have a 1% chance of reactivation of latent infection.

3. Recovery of CMV from the cervix or urine of women at or before the time of delivery does not warrant a cesarean section.

B. Perinatal transmission of CMV occurs by four routes:

1. In utero transplacental infections
2. Ascending infections from the cervix
3. Exposure to infected secretions from the lower genital tract during delivery
4. Ingestion of infected breast milk

Because CMV is spread by intimate contact with infectious secretions, hand washing after exposure to secretions is particularly important for pregnant health care workers.

C. Pediatrics:
  1. Routine screening for CMV is not recommended for internationally adopted children.
  2. Up to half of all neonates exposed to CMV in the lower genital tract during delivery become infected. Intrapartum or postpartum CMV acquisition does not result in adverse outcomes or sequelae except in very low birth weight infants. Viral excretion from intrapartum or postpartum exposure begins at 3–9 weeks of life; thus, the initial viral cultures are negative.
  3. The child with congenital CMV infection should not be treated differently from other children and should not be excluded from school or child-care institutions since the virus is frequently found in many healthy children.
  4. Sensorineural hearing loss (SNHL) is the most common sequalea following congenital CMV infection. Evaluate for hearing loss at each pediatric visit.
D. Adults:
  1. Occupational exposure: **Risk often appears to be greatest for child-care personnel who care for children younger than 2 years.**
  2. Routine serologic screening for child-care staff is not currently recommended.
  3. Pregnant personnel who may be in contact with CMV-infected patients should be counseled the risk of acquiring CMV infection and about the need to practice good hygiene, particularly hand washing. There is no need for routinely transferring to other work situations.

☐ ENCEPHALITIS

Definition
A. Encephalitis is the inflammation of cerebral tissue caused by viral agents or other toxins.

Incidence
A. Incidence is unknown. Japanese encephalitis occurs in annual epidemics in Asia during the rainy season. The prevalence of Japanese encephalitis (arbovirus) is related to ecologic and climatic conditions that affect the natural transmission cycles during summer months (June–September).
B. Arboviruses (eastern or western equine, St. Louis, and West Nile virus) cause disease when mosquitoes are active, whereas walking in the woods or marshy areas with high tick population might suggest other viral encephalitides such as Colorado tick fever or nonviral etiologies such as Lyme disease or Rocky Mountain spotted fever.
C. Herpes encephalitis has the highest morbidity and mortality of the common viral encephalitides and may occur at any time. The mortality rate for untreated patients is 70%; less than 5% of survivors have normal neurologic function. Herpes simplex type 1 is the most common cause of sporadic encephalitis. The most important viral etiology to rule out is HSV, since this clinical entity is usually fatal if untreated. Survival and recovery from neurologic sequelae are related to the mental status at the time of acyclovir initiation.

Pathogenesis
A. Japanese encephalitis is the most common form of epidemic viral encephalitis. For the past several years, West Nile virus has been the most common cause of proved viral encephalitis in the United States. Encephalitis may occur as a secondary infection from mumps, varicella (chickenpox), rubella, rubeola, rabies, herpes simplex types 1 and 2, Epstein-Barr virus, HIV, and influenza. Postinfectious encephalitis, in contrast to viral encephalitis, typically occurs either as the initial infection is resolving or may appear following subclinical illness that was not appreciated by the patient.
B. The incubation period depends on the pathogen.

Predisposing Factors
A. Military personnel and travelers to Asia
B. Age extremes are highest risk
C. Exposure to vectors such as mosquitoes
D. HIV positive
E. Herpes
F. Rodent-born arenavirus: exposure to the secretions of mice, rats, and hamsters

Common Complaints
A. Severe headache throughout the entire head. **A person with encephalitis has a severe headache throughout the entire head. Over the course of about 48 hours, the person may show a lack of energy and then lapse into a coma.**
B. Stiff neck.
C. Mental changes: altered mental status, altered behavior, and personality changes.
D. Decreased level of consciousness.

Other Signs and Symptoms
A. CNS symptoms:
  1. Nuchal rigidity
  2. Irritability
  3. Hemiparesis: weakness or paralysis on one side of body
  4. Flaccid paralysis
  5. Seizures
  6. Exaggerated deep tendon reflexes
B. Photosensitivity
C. Swollen or protruding eyes
D. Fever
E. Malaise
F. Nausea and/or vomiting

Subjective Data
A. Review the onset, duration, and course of all symptoms.
B. Rule out recent history of chickenpox, rubeola, herpes, or other infections.
C. Ask the patient about recent travel in Asia.
D. Question the patient regarding recent mosquito or animal bites (rule out rabies).
E. Elicit a detailed sexual history.

Physical Examination

A. Check temperature, pulse, respirations, and blood pressure
B. Inspect
  1. Observe general overall appearance.
  2. Conduct an eye exam.
  3. Examine the skin for rash, vesicles, or bites.
    a. Maculopapular rash is seen in approximately half of patients with West Nile virus.
    b. Grouped vesicles in a dermatomal patter suggest varicella-zoster.
  4. Assess dehydration status.
  5. Observe for seizure activity.
  6. Observe for tremors of the eyelids, tongue, lips, and extremities, which may suggest the possibility of St. Louis encephalitis or West Nile encephalitis.
C. Auscultate: Auscultate the lungs and monitor breathing pattern. Auscultate the heart.
D. Palpate
  1. Palpate the lymph nodes: preauricular, posterior auricular, submental and sublingual, anterior cervical chains, and supraclavicular nodes.
  2. Palpate the mastoid bone.
E. Neurologic exam
  1. Assess level of consciousness.
  2. Assess the patient for personality changes.
  3. Assess for meningeal signs:
    a. Signs of meningeal irritation include nuchal rigidity.
    b. Positive Brudzinski's and Kernig's signs:
      i. Brudzinski's sign: Place the patient supine and flex the head upward. Resulting flexion of both hips, knees, and ankles with neck flexion indicates meningeal irritation. (See Figure 15.1.)
      ii. Kernig's sign: Place the patient supine. Keeping one leg straight, flex the other hip and knee to a bent knee to form a 90° angle. Slowly extend the lower leg. This places a stretch on the meninges, resulting in pain and spasm for the hamstring muscle. Resistance to further extension can be felt. (See Figure 15.2.)
  4. Check deep tendon reflexes (exaggerated and/or pathologic reflexes).

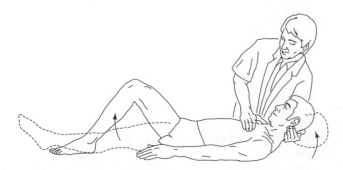

Figure 15.1 Brudzinski's sign.

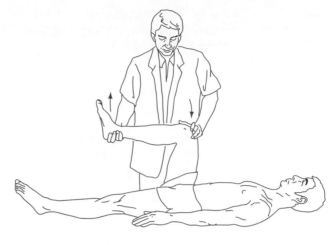

Figure 15.2 Kernig's sign.

Diagnostic Tests

A. CBC with differential.
B. Polymerase chain reaction (PCR) tests for viruses.
C. Serology for arboviruses.
D. Lumbar puncture for the following:
  1. Protein (elevated).
  2. Glucose (usually normal).
  3. White cell count (increased).
  4. Red cell count (usually negative in a nontraumatic tap).
  5. Culture (viral and bacterial): **Detection of virus-specific IgM antibody in cerebrospinal fluid is diagnostic.**
E. EEG.
F. CT scan: useful to rule out space-occupying lesions or brain abscess.
G. MRI: sensitive in detecting demyelination.
H. Brain scan: Imaging studies (CT scan, MRI, brain scan) may be normal early; later, nonspecific abnormalities are seen.
I. Stool or throat cultures may be helpful if enteroviruses are suspected.

Differential Diagnoses

A. Encephalitis
B. West Nile virus
C. St. Louis virus
D. Chickenpox
E. Measles: rubeola or rubella
F. Herpes
G. Rabies
H. Influenza
I. Mumps
J. Meningitis
K. Brain abscess
L. Tuberculosis
M. Syphilis
N. Intracranial hemorrhage
O. Trauma
P. Toxic ingestion
Q. Fungal meningitis
R. Rocky Mountain spotted fever

Plan

A. General interventions: If encephalitis is suspected, hospitalization is recommended for further diagnostic studies and evaluation.

B. Patient teaching.

1. Prevention for vector-borne encephalitis involves mosquito avoidance, use of insect repellents, and vaccination.

2. The Japanese encephalitis (JE) vaccine is an inactivated vaccine derived from infected mouse brain and is recommended for expatriates living in Asia and for certain travelers. It is also recommended for the following:

a. Persons who will be residing in areas where JE virus is endemic or epidemic.

b. Travelers planning prolonged stays (more than 30 days) in endemic areas during the transmission season, especially with activities such as bicycling, camping, or other unprotected outdoor activities in rural areas.

C. Pharmaceutical therapy.

1. Empiric treatment for HSV-1 should always be initiated as soon as possible if the patient has encephalitis without explanation due to the high mortality and morbidity. Acyclovir 10 mg/kg administered intravenously (given over 1 hour) every 8 hours for 14–21 days.

2. Antibiotics for bacterial etiology (refer to diagnosis-specific chapters).

3. Anticonvulsants for seizures.

4. Other pharmaceutical therapies depend on specific causal agent.

Follow-up

A. Follow-up varies and is specific to causal agent.

Consultation/Referral

A. Refer the patient to a physician and/or hospital. Consultations include neurology, infectious disease specialist, and a neurosurgeon for managing elevated intracranial pressure.

Individual Considerations

A. Adult travelers: Advise patient to take mosquito bed nets and aerosol insecticide sprays to reduce the risk of mosquito bites at night.

B. Inactivated Japanese encephalitis vaccine series:

1. Adults: three doses of 1.0 mL each, administered subcutaneously on days 0, 7, and 30. An abbreviated schedule of 0, 7, and 14 days can be used when the longer schedule is precluded by time constraints.

2. Children 1–3 years old: three doses of 0.5 mL each, administered subcutaneously on days 0, 7, and 30. The abbreviated schedule days (0, 7, 14) are the same.

No data are available on vaccine safety and efficacy in infants younger than 12 months.

C. Geriatrics: Elderly patients may be at risk for severe disease.

2009 H1N1 INFLUENZA A

Definition

A. H1N1 influenza A (formerly called swine flu) is an influenza A that causes a highly contagious respiratory disease. H1N1 has been reported worldwide and was designated a phase 6 global pandemic status by the World Health Organization.

B. Persons with flulike symptoms should promptly contact their health care providers. If an antiviral is warranted, it should ideally be started within 48 hours from the onset of symptoms. Viral pneumonia is the primary sign of clinical deterioration.

Incidence

A. In 2009, the World Health Organization declared H1N1 a pandemic. Rate of infection varied by age groups. In the United States the incidence ranged from 1.3 per 100,000 in adults older than 65 years to a high of 26.7 per 100,000 of children aged 5–24.

Pathogenesis

A. H1N1 (swine flu) is a new subtype of influenza A (A/H1N1) virus that is spread by human-to-human transmission. Persons cannot be infected with the H1N1 virus from the consumption of pork. The primary mode of spread is exposure to viral strain respiratory secretions from respiratory droplets (coughing or sneezing) and direct contact of contaminated surfaces. The infectious period is considered to be 1 day prior to the onset of fever and until 24 hours after fever ends.

Predisposing Factors

A. Age

1. Children younger than 5 years, especially those younger than 2 years

2. Adults 25–64 years who have medical conditions that place them at high risk for influenza-related complications

3. Adults age 65 years or older

B. Pregnant women

C. Women up to 2 weeks postpartum

Common Complaints

A. Clinical manifestations of H1N1 influenza depend upon the age and previous experience with the influenza virus. Rapid onset respiratory illness is the most common complaint.

1. Cough

2. Sore throat

3. Dyspnea/wheezing

4. Rhinorrhea

B. Abrupt onset of fever and/or chills (temperature of 100°F [37.8°C] or greater.

C. Headache.

D. Body aches.

E. Altered mental status.

F. Children:

1. Apnea

2. Tachypnea

3. Cyanosis

4. Dehydration

5. Extreme irritability

Other Signs and Symptoms

A. Joint pain

B. Diarrhea (possible)

C. Vomiting (possible)

Subjective Data

A. Review the onset, course, and duration of symptoms, especially fever and respiratory symptoms.
B. Review symptoms of other family members or coworkers who are also ill. Is the onset of acute febrile respiratory illness within 7 days of close contact with a person with a confirmed case of H1N1?
C. If pregnant, establish gestational age.
D. Review for recent travel location, and use of cruise ships/planes.
E. Evaluate living conditions for exposure risks.

Physical Examination

A. Check temperature, pulse, respirations, and blood pressure.
B. Inspect.
   1. Observe general overall appearance.
   2. Assess hydration status.
   3. Conduct an eye, ear, nose, and throat exam.
   4. Children:
      a. Observe for seizure activity.
      b. Note level of activity (playful vs. lethargic).
C. Auscultate: Auscultate the lungs and heart.
D. Palpate: Palpate the neck and lymph nodes: preauricular, posterior auricular, submental and sublingual, anterior cervical chain, and supraclavicular nodes.
E. Neurologic exam
   1. Assess level of consciousness.
   2. Assess for nuchal rigidity.
   3. Assess for meningeal signs:
      a. Signs of meningeal irritation include nuchal rigidity.
      b. Positive Brudzinski's and Kernig's signs (Refer to Figures 15.1 and 15.2.)
         i. Brudzinski's sign: Place the patient supine and flex the head upward. Resulting flexion of both hips, knees, and ankles with neck flexion indicates meningeal irritation.
         ii. Kernig's sign: Place the patient supine. Keeping one leg straight, flex the other hip and knee to a bent knee to form a 90° angle. Slowly extend the lower leg. This places a stretch on the meninges, resulting in pain and spasm for the hamstring muscle. Resistance to further extension can be felt.

Diagnostic Tests

A. Rapid influenza antigen testing. Respiratory swab for H1N1 testing. Swabs should be placed in a refrigerator and the state or local health department will facilitate transport for timely diagnosis. The CDC has defined a confirmed case as an individual with an ILI with laboratory-confirmed H1N1 influenza A detected by real-time reverse transcriptase (rRT)-PCR or culture.
B. CBC with differential.
C. ALT/AST.
D. Bilirubin.
E. Imaging (rule out complications).
   1. Chest X-ray
   2. CT chest imaging

Differential Diagnoses

A. Influenza
   1. H1N1 A (swine flu)
   2. Influenza A
   3. Influenza B
   4. Avian flu (H5N1)
B. Pneumonia
C. Bronchitis
D. Mononucleosis
E. Respiratory syncytial virus (RSV)
F. Early HIV

Plan

A. General interventions
   1. Management is usually treatment of symptoms and is supportive.
      a. Bed rest.
      b. Increased fluids.
      c. Cough suppressants.
      d. Antipyretics and analgesics for fever and myalgias.
      e. Encourage patients to stay home (self-isolate) if they become ill and avoid touching the eyes, nose, and mouth.
   2. Community precautions:
      a. Avoid close contact with those who are sick.
      b. Wash hands often or use alcohol-based hand gels.
      c. The use of face masks may be advisable or required.
      d. Droplet precautions should be used and maintained for 7 days after illness onset or until symptoms have resolved.
B. Pharmaceutical therapy
   1. The 2009 influenza A (H1N1) monovalent vaccine should be administered as prophylaxis.
      a. Target populations for the administration of H1N1 vaccine include:
         i. Pregnant women.
         ii. Children aged 6 months to 18 years.
         iii. Household contacts and caregivers of children younger than 6 months.
         iv. Health care and emergency medical personnel.
         v. Persons aged 25 through 64 years with high-risk medical conditions that would result in complications from the flu.
         vi. Hospitalized patients should be prioritized.
      b. 2009 H1N1 influenza vaccine is available in as an injection (inactivated vaccine) and the 2009 H1N1 nasal spray (made with live, weakened viruses). The dosages vary by age and manufacturer:
         i. Adults: 0.5 mL IM × 1 dose administered in the deltoid *or* for ages 10–49 years: 0.2 mL/dose (0.1 mL per nostril) intranasally × 1 dose
         ii. Pediatrics: Sanofi Pasteur and CSL Limited vaccines *or*
            (a). Ages 6–35 months: 0.25 mL IM in 2 injections administered 4 weeks apart
            (b). Ages 3–9 years: 0.5 mL IM in 2 injections administered 4 weeks apart

(c). Ages 10–17 years: Administer as in adults

iii. Pediatrics: Novaritis vaccine *or*

   (a). Ages 4–9 years: 0.5mL IM in 2 injections administered 4 weeks apart

   (b). Ages 10–17 years: Administer as in adults

iv. Pediatric Intranasal MedImmune vaccine *or*

   (a). Ages 2–9: 0.2 mL/dose (0.1 mL per nostril) in 2 doses administered 4 weeks apart

   (b). Ages older than 9 years: Administer as in adults

c. H1N1 vaccine should be administered IM in the anterolateral aspect of the thigh for infants and in the deltoid muscle of the upper arms in toddlers, children, and adults. Avoid the gluteal muscle.

d. The H1N1 vaccine should not be administered in the same syringe with the seasonal flu vaccine.

e. The seasonal influenza vaccine administered during the flu season is not effective for the H1N1 viral strain.

2. Antiviral therapy.

a. Neuraminidase inhibitors Oseltamivir (Tamiflu) and Zanamivir (Relenza) are used for the treatment of H1N1 influenza A virus.

b. Amantadine and Rimantadine antivirals are not recommended for H1N1 because of resistance to other influenza strains.

c. The WHO recommends that patients with underlying medical conditions and pregnant women should receive treatment with Oseltamivir (oral) or Zanamivir (inhaled) as soon as possible after symptom onset without waiting for laboratory test results.

d. Antiviral therapy recommendations vary by the type of influenza, age groups, renal function, and risk factors. In order to prescribe the most current antiviral therapy, the authors recommend referring to the CDC Web site for the most up-to-date recommendations: http://www.cdc.gov/flu/profes sionals/.

Follow-up

A. Schedule a follow-up visit within 7–10 days if symptoms do not improve.

B. Monitor patient for pulmonary and neurologic complications.

C. H1N1 influenza–associated deaths should be reported to the Centers for Disease Control (CDC) through the state health department.

Consultation/Referral

A. Refer the patient to a physician or neurologist for any complications.

Individual Considerations

A. Pregnancy

1. Pregnancy predisposes the patient to an increased risk for influenzal pneumonia.

2. Flu vaccine may be given to patients in high-risk populations. Because of the risk of influenzal pneumonia, many physicians recommend that pregnant women be vaccinated when an epidemic threatens.

3. Immunization of pregnant women is considered safe at any stage of pregnancy.

4. Both Oseltamivir and Zanamivir are Pregnancy Category C drugs.

B. Pediatrics

1. Influenza A/H1N1 vaccine should be offered/administered prior to flu season (as early as September) to children with asthma, chronic lung problems, or who are immunosuppressed.

2. Infants who are ill with H1N1 influenza A should continue to breast-feed.

3. Aspirin or aspirin-containing products (e.g., bismuth subsalicylate—Pepto Bismol) should not be given to children and young adults with viral illnesses before 21 years of age due to the increased risk of Reye's syndrome.

4. Reye's syndrome has been associated primarily with influenza B, but it is also associated with influenza A infections.

5. Amantadine HCl and Rimantadine HCl are not effective against H1N1 infections and are not FDA-approved for use in children younger than 1 year.

C. Adults: Persons with high-exposure occupations such as teachers, health care workers, police, and firefighters should consider yearly immunization. Vaccine should be offered/administered to persons with chronic metabolic diseases, renal dysfunction, HIV infection, and immunosuppression.

INFLUENZA (FLU)

Definition

A. Influenza is a common, acute, viral infection that is a self-limiting, febrile illness of the respiratory tract. Illness is spread person to person primarily by respiratory secretions that can be spread from infected persons through sneezing, coughing, talking, and by self-inoculation of secretions through direct contact routes. Influenza is one of the top 10 causes of death in the United States when it occurs with pneumonia.

Incidence

A. Epidemics occur yearly, primarily in the winter months in both the northern and southern hemispheres. Travelers should be reminded that the flu season is different by the hemispheres and can occur on cruise ships. Attack rates may be as high as 10%–20% of the population. Mortality is highest in the geriatric population older than 65 years of age, except a shift has been seen during pandemic influenza outbreaks when 50% of deaths occur in individuals younger than 65 years of age. Extraordinarily high attacks have occurred in the institutionalized and semiclosed populations.

Pathogenesis

A. Influenza A and B are viruses that have the ability to undergo periodic antigenic changes of their envelope glycoproteins, the hemagglutinin and neuraminidase. Among influenza A viruses that infect humans, there are three major subtypes of hemagglutinins (H1, H2, and

H3) and two subtypes of neuraminidases (N1 and N2). Influenza A outbreaks typically start abruptly, peak over 2–3 weeks and last approximately 2–3 months. H1N1 (swine flu) is an influenza A virus.

B. The avian flu was the N5N1 and H7N7 viral infections associated with recent exposure to dead or ill poultry. Following exposure, the incubation period for human H5N1 infection is 7 days or less. Clusters of human-to-human transmission of avian flu had a typical incubation period of 3–5 days.

C. Influenza B outbreaks are generally less extensive and less severe. Outbreaks associated with the B virus have been reported in schools, military camps, nursing homes, and cruise ships.

D. *Haemophilus influenzae* is a gram-negative coccobacillus. *H. influenzae* is an invasive bacterial disease that can cause meningitis, otitis media, sinusitis, epiglottitis, septic arthritis, occult febrile bacteremia, cellulitis, pneumonia, and empyema; occasionally, this virulent organism causes neonatal meningitis.

E. The incubation period for *H. influenzae* is from between 18 and 72 hours to 5 days after exposure. The exact period of communicability for *H. influenzae* is unknown, but it may be for as long as the organism is present in the upper respiratory tract.

Predisposing Factors

Primary mode of spread is exposure to viral strain respiratory secretions from respiratory droplets (coughing or sneezing) and direct contact of contaminated surfaces.

A. Adults
1. Aged older than 65 years (dependent on the viral strain)
2. Pregnancy
3. High-exposure jobs: teachers, health care workers, police, and firefighters
4. Recent illnesses or state that has lowered resistance (stress, excessive fatigue, poor nutrition)
5. Immunosuppression from drugs, illness, or chronic illness (transplant recipients, lung disease, heart disease)
6. Crowded living conditions including military camps and institutions such as nursing homes
7. Travel in endemic areas
8. Avian flu: exposure to dead or ill poultry

B. Pediatrics
1. Chronic pulmonary disease including bronchopulmonary dysplasia/chronic lung disease, asthma, cystic fibrosis, or any condition that compromises the respiratory function
2. Congenital heart disease or abnormalities
3. Children younger than 5 years of age

Common Complaints

A. Clinical manifestations of influenza depend upon the age and previous experience with the influenza virus. Children cannot verbalize symptoms such as myalgias and headache. Respiratory symptoms may be less prominent at the onset of illness in children and adults.

B. Rapid onset respiratory illness is the most common complaint.

C. Abrupt onset of fever and/or chills (children tend to run higher fevers).
D. Joint pain.
E. Headache.
F. Conjunctivitis (avian flu).

Other Signs and Symptoms

A. Upper respiratory congestion (watery eyes, clear nasal drainage, headache, sore throat, and hoarseness)
B. Malaise or fatigue
C. Anorexia
D. Swollen lymph nodes
E. Nonproductive cough (persist for weeks)
F. Muscle aches
G. Gastrointestinal symptoms (children tend to have more nausea, vomiting, and poor appetite)
H. Febrile seizures

Subjective Data

A. Review the onset, course, and duration of symptoms, especially myalgia and malaise.
B. Query the patient when his or her last flu vaccination was received.
C. Review symptoms of other family members or coworkers who are also ill.
D. Check immunization status. For children, note whether *H. influenzae* b (Hib) vaccination is up to date.
E. Review for recent travel location and use of cruise ships/planes.
F. Evaluate living conditions for exposure risks.

Physical Examination

A. Check temperature, pulse, respirations, and blood pressure.
B. Inspect.
1. Observe general overall appearance.
2. Assess hydration status.
3. Conduct an eye, ear, nose, and throat exam.
4. Children:
   a. Observe for seizure activity.
   b. Note level of activity (playful vs. lethargic).
C. Auscultate: Auscultate the lungs and heart.
D. Palpate: Palpate the neck and lymph nodes: preauricular, posterior auricular, submental and sublingual, anterior cervical chain, and supraclavicular nodes.
E. Neurologic exam.
1. Assess level of consciousness.
2. Assess for nuchal rigidity.
3. Assess for meningeal signs:
   a. Signs of meningeal irritation include nuchal rigidity.
   b. Positive Brudzinski's and Kernig's signs (Refer to Figures 15.1 and 15.2.)
      i. Brudzinski's sign: Place the patient supine and flex the head upward. Resulting flexion of both hips, knees, and ankles with neck flexion indicates meningeal irritation.
      ii. Kernig's sign: Place the patient supine. Keeping one leg straight, flex the other hip and knee to a bent knee to form a 90° angle. Slowly extend the lower leg. This places a stretch on

the meninges, resulting in pain and spasm for the hamstring muscle. Resistance to further extension can be felt.

Diagnostic Tests

Usually none is required. However, if the patient appears ill, consider the following:

A. White blood count and complete blood count (CBC).
B. Viral RNA cultures: obtain during the first 72 hours of illness because the quality of virus shed subsequently decreases rapidly. There is some evidence that a throat sampling yields an improved specimen. Nasopharyngeal secretions obtained by swab or aspirate should be placed in an appropriate transport medium for culture.
C. Rapid antigen test (usually less sensitive in the detection of influenza A than the PCR; a negative rapid diagnostic test should be confirmed with a viral culture or other means).
D. Monospot test: **Monospot test is negative with the flu and positive with mononucleosis.**
E. Chest radiograph (only if pneumonia suspected).
F. Sputum culture (complications only).
G. Lumbar puncture (complications only).
H. Rapid plasma reagin (RPR) test (for high-risk HIV factors): negative RPR to rule out syphilis.
I. Stool sample if the patient presents with diarrhea.
J. Polymerase chain reaction (PCR) assay (can differentiate between influenza subtypes, it offers high sensitivity and specificity but is not readily available for clinical use).

Differential Diagnoses

A. Influenza
    1. Influenza A
    2. Influenza B
    3. Avian flu (H5N1)
    4. H1N1 (swine flu)
B. Pneumonia
C. Bronchitis
D. Mononucleosis
E. Respiratory syncytial virus (RSV)
F. Early HIV

Plan

A. General interventions
    1. Management is usually treatment of symptoms.
    2. Encourage flu vaccine for patients in susceptible populations prior to flu season. See age-related factors.
    3. *Haemophilus influenzae,* including both type b and non-type b infection, and cases in fully or partially immunized children, should be reported to the Centers for Disease Control and Prevention through the local and state public health department. See Chapter 1, "Health Maintenance Guidelines" for *H. influenzae* b immunization information.
    4. Influenza-associated pediatric deaths should be reported to the Centers for Disease Control (CDC) through the state health department.
    5. Patients should expect to have a persistent cough and malaise after initial acute phase.
B. Patient teaching: See the Section III Patient Teaching Guide for this chapter, "Influenza (Flu)."
C. Pharmaceutical therapy

Influenza can alter the metabolism of certain medications, especially theophylline, possibly resulting in the development of toxicity from high serum concentrations.

    1. Acetaminophen (Tylenol) as needed for fever.
    2. Nonsteroidal anti-inflammatory drugs as needed for body aches.
    3. Antiviral therapy recommendations vary by the type of influenza, age groups, renal function, and risk factors. In order to prescribe the most current antiviral therapy, the authors recommend referring to the CDC Web site for the most up-to-date recommendations, http://www.cdc.gov/flu/professionals/, and referring to the current American Academy Pediatrics' *Red Book: Report of the Committee on Infectious Diseases.*
    4. Zanamivir (Relenza®) is not recommended for persons with underlying airways disease including asthma or chronic obstructive pulmonary disease (COPD). Zanamivir is for uncomplicated acute illness due to influenza A or B in adults and children 7 years and older who have been symptomatic for no more than 2 days.
    5. Oseltamivir (Tamiflu) is for adults and adolescents 13 years or older who have been symptomatic for no more than 2 days. Special dosing is required for children who are younger than 13 and/or weigh less than 80 pounds. Tamiflu is not indicated for the treatment of flu for children less than 1 year of age.
    6. Vaccination.
        a. The CDC's Advisory Committee on Immunization Practice (ACIP) and the American Academy of Pediatrics (AAP) recommend annual influenza vaccination for all children aged 6 months to 18 years.
        b. Flu vaccine should not be administered to persons allergic to eggs.
        c. The vaccine should be administered in the autumn prior to the flu season, at least 6 weeks before the onset of the season.
        d. Immunization is the major means of influenza prevention. There are two types of vaccine available.
            i. Inactivated vaccine (TIV), which is administered intramuscularly.
            ii. Live attenuated, cold-adapted vaccine (LAIV), which is administered intranasally.
        e. The recommended site of vaccination in adults and older children is the deltoid muscle. The anterolateral aspect of the thigh is the preferred site for flu vaccine for small children.
        f. Oseltamivir (Tamiflu®) should not be administered with a live attenuated influenza vaccine within 2 weeks prior to or 48 hours after treatment.

Follow-up

A. Schedule a follow-up visit within 7–10 days if symptoms do not improve.
B. Monitor the patient for pulmonary and neurologic complications.

Consultation/Referral

A. Refer the patient to a physician or neurologist for any complications.

Individual Considerations

A. Pregnancy.
   1. Pregnancy predisposes the patient to an increased risk for influenzal pneumonia.
   2. The flu vaccine may be given to patients in a high-risk population. Because of the risk of influenzal pneumonia, many physicians recommend that pregnant women be vaccinated when an epidemic threatens.
   3. Immunization of pregnant women is considered safe at any stage of pregnancy. Inactivated vaccine (TIV) is safe for breast-feeding mothers and their children.
   4. Amantadine HCl (Symmetrel) is in Pregnancy Category C. It is not recommended for nursing mothers.
   5. Rimantadine HCl (Flumadine) is Pregnancy Category C and should be used with caution in nursing mothers.
B. Pediatrics
   1. Influenza vaccine should be offered/administered prior to flu season (as early as September) to children with asthma, chronic lung problems, or who are immunosuppressed.
   2. The most common pediatric complication of influenza is otitis media. However, in young infants, influenza can produce a sepsislike picture and occasionally can cause croup or pneumonia.
   3. Aspirin or aspirin-containing products (e.g., bismuth subsalicylate—Pepto Bismol) should not be given to children and young adults with viral illnesses before 21 years of age due to the increased risk of Reye's syndrome.
   4. Reye's syndrome has been associated primarily with influenza B, but it is also associated with influenza A infections.
   5. Amantadine HCl and Rimantadine HCl are not effective against influenza B infections and are not FDA-approved for use in children younger than 1 year.
   6. An increased incidence of convulsions has been reported in children with epilepsy who receive Amantadine.
C. Adults: Persons with high-exposure occupations such as teachers, health care workers, police, and firefighters should consider yearly immunization. Vaccine should be offered/administered to persons with chronic metabolic diseases, renal dysfunction, HIV infection, and immunosuppression.
D. Geriatrics.
   1. Influenza vaccine is recommended yearly for patients over the age of 60. The vaccine should be offered to nursing home residents, especially those with a history of cardiopulmonary disease. Factors that contribute to more severe infections include decreased lung compliance and decreased respiration muscle strength.
   2. Pneumococcal pneumonia and influenza are significant causes of mortality and morbidity in the elderly.

KAWASAKI DISEASE

Definition

Kawasaki disease (KD) is an acute febrile illness associated with generalized vasculitis. It is formerly known as mucocutaneous lymph node syndrome. Kawasaki disease is the leading cause of acquired heart disease in U.S. children. Death results from myocardial infarction with coronary occlusion due to thrombosis or progressive stenosis. Approximately 75% of fatalities occur within 6 weeks of the onset of symptoms, but myocardial infarction and sudden death can occur months to years after the acute episode.

Long-term prognosis is unknown. Second episodes rarely occur in previously affected children. Cardiac problems are the primary cause of morbidity and mortality from pericardial effusion, myocarditis, aneurysms, ectasia (coronary artery larger than normal for the child's age), and myocardial infarction.

Although a febrile seizure may occur, there is no evidence that links KD with autism or a long-term seizure disorder.

Diagnostic criteria: Diagnosis of typical syndrome requires fever of at least 5 days' duration, plus four of the following:

A. Mucous membrane changes.
B. Extremity changes.
C. Cervical lymphadenopathy of at least 1 cm in size is the least consistent feature of KD. When present it tends to involve the anterior cervical nodes overlying the sternocleidomastoid muscle.
D. Rash.
E. Bilateral nonexudative conjunctivitis: present in greater than 90% of patients.

Incidence

A. Peak age of occurrence in the United States is between 18 and 24 months. Approximately 80% of patients are younger than 5 years. Children older than 8 years rarely have the disease. Kawasaki disease has been noted worldwide and affects all races. Approximately one child in a hundred has KD a second time.

Pathogenesis

A. Etiology is unknown; it may be caused by viruses, or bacteria such as group A streptococci. A microbial agent is favored because of the disease's acute, self-limited course and community-wide outbreaks. The incubation period is unknown. There is no currently accepted scientific evidence that KD is caused by carpet cleaning or chemical exposure.

Predisposing Factors

A. Asian and Pacific Island ancestry.
B. More common in boys than girls.
C. Epidemics generally occur during the winter and spring seasons.

Common Complaints

A. Long-term fever (1–2 weeks) that doesn't respond to antibiotics. The fever ranges from 101° to above 104° Fahrenheit. Fever may rise and fall for up to 3 weeks.
B. Bilateral bulbar conjunctival injection without exudate.
C. Red, tender hands and soles of feet on day 3–5 following fever.

Classic finding is swollen, indurated, erythematous, and tender palms. Desquamation of the fingers and toes occurs approximately 1–2 weeks after the onset of the fever, and a deep groove may cross the nails (Beau's lines).

D. Cracked, red, dry lip; tongue may appear coated, slightly swollen and looks like a strawberry; and mouth ulcers.
E. Irritability.
F. Decreased food/fluid intake.
G. One or more gastrointestinal symptoms (vomiting, diarrhea, or abdominal pain).
H. One or more respiratory symptoms (rhinorrhea or cough).

Other Signs and Symptoms

A. Tachycardia (disproportionate to fever), gallop rhythms, and EKG changes suggestive of myocarditis.
B. Pericarditis (often subclinical): Coronary aneurysms have been detected as early as 3 days after the onset of symptoms, but in most cases they appear 1–2 weeks later. Carditis can occur at any time during the first 3 weeks of illness and generally resolves by 6–8 weeks.
C. Polymorphous rash that may be maculopapular, scarlatiniform, morbilliform, erythema marginatum, or rarely vesiculopustular; frequently confluent in the perineum, where it undergoes desquamation. **Rash involves the entire body, especially in the perineal region.**
D. Swollen cervical lymph node(s). Patient may have a singular enlarged lymph node, usually a cervical node, up to 1.5 cm.
E. Joint pain.
F. Weakness.
G. Sterile pyuria.

Subjective Data

A. Review onset, course, and duration of symptoms.
B. Elicit the initial site of the rash and the progression to other body areas.
C. Determine if the patient has had any new medication and contact exposures.
D. Rule out other family members with similar symptoms.
E. Review the patient's history for recent strep infection.
F. Take thorough history of symptoms and medication or treatment type and duration.

Physical Examination

A. Check temperature, pulse, respirations, and blood pressure
B. Inspect
   1. Inspect skin, especially hands, feet, and nails.
   2. Conduct a thorough eye examination.
   3. Conduct a thorough ear, nose, throat, and oral exam.
   4. Check hydration status.
C. Auscultate: Auscultate the heart and lungs.
D. Palpate
   1. Palpate the lymph nodes, especially cervical area.
   2. Check the joints for swelling and tenderness.
   3. Males: check for testicular swelling.
   4. Evaluate for splenomegaly.

Diagnostic Tests

No laboratory study proves diagnosis; diagnosis rests on clinical features and exclusion of the other illnesses in the differential diagnosis.

A. CBC with differential: neutropenia.
B. Erythrocyte sedimentation rate (ESR): elevated.
C. C-reactive protein (CRP): elevated.
D. Uric acid.
E. Platelet count: elevated platelet count (1 week after onset).
F. Serum transaminase: elevated.
G. Serum albumin.
H. Specialty tests: quantitative serum immunoglobulins, antinuclear antibody (ANA), rheumatoid factor (RF), VDRL, immune complexes, and complement levels
I. Urinalysis: proteinuria and sterile pyuria.
J. Echocardiogram.
K. EKG.
L. Angiography may be needed.
M. Chest radiograph.

Differential Diagnoses

A. Kawasaki disease
B. Rubeola
C. Cat-scratch fever
D. Drug reaction
E. Rocky Mountain spotted fever
F. Infectious mononucleosis
G. Toxic shock syndrome
H. Other febrile viral exanthemas
I. Syphilis
J. Lyme disease
K. Juvenile rheumatoid arthritis
L. Stevens-Johnson syndrome
M. Staphylococcal scalded skin syndrome

Plan

A. General interventions
   1. The most severe sequelae is the development of coronary artery aneurysm; therefore, prevention and early detection are important.
   2. Initial therapy should be started within 10 days of illness. Management is initially aimed at reducing inflammation.
   3. The use of intravenous immune globulin (IVIG) therapy has drastically reduced the incidence and morbidity and mortality of cardiovascular aneurysm.
B. Patient teaching
   1. Teach parents which signs and symptoms indicate when to contact the office: arthralgias, chest pain, and palpitations.
   2. Disease is not communicable by means of person-to-person contact; therefore, patients do not need to be isolated from other family members.
C. Pharmaceutical therapy
   1. The American Heart Association and the American Academy of Pediatrics recommend: intravenous gamma globulin (2 mg/kg) administered as a single infusion over 8–12 hours within the first 7–10 days of the illness shortens the duration of fever and decreases the frequency of coronary artery aneurysms and other abnormalities.
   2. Up to 20% of patients that receive the IGIV single infusion and aspirin may have a recurrent fever and require retreatment with IGIV 2g/kg within 24–48 hours of persistent fever.
   3. The American Heart Association and the American Academy of Pediatrics recommend initial use of

aspirin (ASA) 30–100 mg/kg/day given orally four times a day until afebrile. The maximum ASA dose should not exceed 4 gm per day. Then ASA 3–5 mg/kg orally per day for 6–8 weeks for its antiplatelet action.

4. Aspirin is continued until laboratory markers for acute inflammation (e.g., platelet count and ESR) return to normal, unless cardiac abnormalities are detected by echo.

5. Aspirin should be rapidly discontinued upon exposure to or sign of varicella or influenza due to the increased risk of Reye's syndrome.

6. Analgesic and antipyretic medications, such as acetaminophen (Tylenol) or ibuprofen, as needed for pain and inflammation.

7. The role of glucocorticoid use remains unclear for treatment of Kawasaki disease. A single pulsed dose of IV methylprednisolone to the single dose of IVIG (2 mg/kg) does not significantly reduce the incidence of cardiac abnormalities.

8. Scheduled routine immunizations of inactivated childhood vaccines may be given at recommended intervals except for live virus vaccines such as varicella-containing vaccines and measles for children that have received IVIG. Varicella and measles vaccination may be given for an outbreak if the child's exposure is high and as long as the vaccination is repeated in at least 11 months after administration of IVIG.

Follow-up

A. The prognosis of patients following Kawasaki depends on the severity of cardiac involvement. Refer the patient to a pediatric cardiologist or physician for follow-up.

Consultation/Referral

A. Consult with a physician if fever persists longer than 5 days and Kawasaki disease is suspected.

B. Refer all affected children to a pediatric cardiologist for coronary artery evaluation.

Individual Considerations

A. Pediatrics
1. Most children are hospitalized for diagnostic evaluation and supportive care. Older children with mild disease may be managed on an outpatient basis.
2. Yearly influenza vaccination is indicated in patients 6 months to 18 years of age who require long-term aspirin therapy, because there is an increased risk for children taking aspirin of development of Reye's syndrome.
3. Children should have limited physical activity during convalescence. Restrictions should be prescribed by the cardiologist.

LYME DISEASE

Definition

A. Lyme disease is a multisystem infection that may be acute or chronic. Lyme disease is the leading vector-borne disease in the United States.

Incidence

A. There is an increased incidence of Lyme disease in southern New England and in the eastern mid-Atlantic states as well as a lower incidence in the upper Midwest. Lyme disease is less common on the West Coast, especially northern California. There is a seasonal increase between the months of April and October; more than 50% of cases occur in June and July. In the United States the incidence is highest among children ages 5–9 years and in adults ages 45–54 years.

Pathogenesis

A. *Borrelia burgdorferi,* a spirochete bacterium, is the infectious agent and is carried by the *Ixodes dammini* deer tick in the east coast and midwestern areas of the United States. Vector transmission is usually from the deer tick to humans. Rodents and pets can also harbor deer ticks.

B. The spirochete enters the bloodstream at the time of tick feeding. The incubation period is 3–32 days, or about 1–3 weeks after bite. Late manifestations occur several months to more than 1 year later.

Predisposing Factors

A. People of all ages are affected.
B. Recreational exposure.
1. Hiking
2. Golfing
3. Hunting
4. Soccer
C. Gardening.
D. Exposure to rodents such as field mice and domestic pets, which may also carry the ticks.

Common Complaints

A. Flulike symptoms
B. Fatigue
C. Headache
D. Joint pain

Other Signs and Symptoms

A. Stage 1: Acute (early localized)
1. Rash: erythema migrans

About 80% of infected persons develop a characteristic expanding erythematous rash, erythema migrans. It usually begins as a red macule at the site of the tick bite and spreads out to form a large annular lesion with red secondary outer rings, an intense red outer border (measuring at least 5 cm), and some clearing at the site of the bite. Appearance is a "bull's-eye" shape. The lesion is generally painless and not pruritic.

2. Body aches
3. Fever or chills
4. Swollen lymph nodes
B. Stage 2: Disseminated infection (early disseminated)
1. Malaise, debilitating fatigue
2. Headache
3. Photophobia
4. Mild neck stiffness
5. Joint or muscle pain
6. Migratory arthralgia

7. Rash: diffuse erythema
8. Itching
9. Transient heart block
   a. In 5%–10% of cases, patients have cardiac involvement: a transient heart block ranging from asymptomatic, first-degree AV block to complete heart block with fainting. Cardiac phase lasts 3–6 weeks.
10. Bell's palsy
    a. A unilateral or bilateral Bell's palsy is the most common cranial nerve deficit.
11. Mild encephalopathy
C. Stage 3: Chronic (late disease)
   1. Prolonged arthritis
      a. Approximately 60% of complaints evolve into frank arthritis. Onset of arthritis is variable but averages 6 months from the time of initial infection. The knee is the most common site and the pattern continues to be oligoarticular.
   2. Chronic neurologic deficits
   3. Distal paresthesia
   4. Radicular pain
   5. Memory loss

Subjective Data

A. Review the onset, course, and duration of symptoms.
B. Ask the patient about any recent outdoor activities such as camping, hiking, gardening, or other activities. Less than half of the people infected remember a tick bite. A history of a tick bite is not necessary for diagnosis.
C. Have other family members had similar symptoms?
D. Review thorough history of medications.
E. Review any history of rash and course of spread.
F. Rule out last symptoms associated with Lyme disease such as arthritis, memory loss, and distal paresthesia.

Physical Examination

A. Check temperature, pulse, respirations, and blood pressure.
B. Inspect.
   1. Observe general overall appearance.
   2. Observe rash pattern and type.
   3. Inspect the skin; observe for targetlike pattern.
C. Palpate.
   1. Palpate the lymph nodes and mastoid bones.
   2. Examine the joints for tenderness, swelling, and range of motion.
D. Auscultate: Auscultate the heart and lungs.
E. Neurologic exam: Evaluate for signs of meningeal irritation by means of Brudzinski's sign and Kernig's signs. (Refer to Figures 15.1 and 15.2.)
   1. Brudzinski's sign: Place the patient supine and flex the head upward. Resulting flexion of both hips, knees, and ankles with neck flexion indicates meningeal irritation.
   2. Kernig's sign: Place the patient supine. Keeping one leg straight, flex the other hip and knee to a bent knee to form a 90° angle. Slowly extend the lower leg. This places a stretch on the meninges, resulting in pain and spasm for the hamstring muscle. Resistance to further extension can be felt.

Diagnostic Tests

A. Complete blood count with differential
B. Sedimentation rate
C. Serum antibody (ELISA) testing for *B. burgdorferi* (not present for several weeks)
D. Western blot if ELISA is positive
E. Lyme titer or culture for spirochete (after 20 days of signs and symptoms)
F. Arthrocentesis for joint effusion
G. Polymerase chain reaction (PCR) testing
H. ALT and AST (may be mildly elevated)
I. Creatine phosphokinase (CPK)

Differential Diagnoses

A. Lyme disease
B. Insect or spider bite
C. Rocky Mountain spotted fever
D. Cellulitis
E. Arthritis
F. Bacterial meningitis
G. Chronic fatigue syndrome
H. Viral syndrome
I. Nummular eczema
J. Tinea corporis (ringworm)

Plan

A. General interventions
   1. **Prophylactic therapy after a tick bite is generally not advised.** It takes 24 hours from the time of tick contact with the skin to transmit the spirochete.
   2. **Start prophylactic treatment with doxycycline for tick bites that are "swollen."**
   3. Wait for the development of symptoms (e.g., erythema migrans) and treat promptly if the patient becomes symptomatic.
B. Patient teaching
   1. See the Section III Patient Teaching Guide for this chapter, "Lyme Disease and Removal of a Tick."
   2. All neurologic signs and symptoms may not completely resolve (such as headache, photophobia, Bell's palsy, and third-stage symptoms).
   3. Patients with active Lyme disease should not donate blood because spirochetemia occurs in early Lyme disease. Patients who have been treated for Lyme disease in the past can be considered for blood donation.
   4. There is not a vaccine for Lyme disease.
   5. Nonspecific symptoms may persist for months after treatment of Lyme disease. There is no evidence that the complaints represent ongoing active infection or need repeated antibiotics.
      a. Headache
      b. Fatigue
      c. Arthralgias
C. Pharmaceutical therapy
   1. Early localized Lyme disease
      a. Doxycycline: 14- to 21-day antibiotic course (warn patient regarding photosensitivity)
         i. Adults: 100 mg, orally, twice daily
         ii. Children older than 8 years of age: 2 mg/kg orally twice daily (maximum 100 mg dose)

b. Amoxicillin: 14- to 21-day antibiotic course
   i. Adults: 500 mg orally three times a day
   ii. Children: 50 mg/kg (maximum of 1.5 g/day) orally divided into three doses
c. Cefuroxime (Ceftin): 14- to 21-day antibiotic course
   i. Adults: 500 mg twice a day
   ii. Children: 30 mg/kg (maximum 1,000 mg/day), divided into two doses

2. Lyme carditis
  a. Ceftriaxone (Rocephin): 75–100 mg/kg (maximum of 2 gm/day), IM or IV infusion for 14–28 days
  b. Penicillin: 300,000 U/kg (maximum of 20 million U/day) given by IV infusion in divided doses every 4 hours for 14–28 days

3. Neurologic manifestations
  a. Facial nerve paralysis: use oral regimen for early disease for 21–28 days.
  b. Lyme meningitis.
    i. Ceftriaxone (Rocephin): 14- to 28-day antibiotic course.
     (a). Adults: 2 gm IM or IV infusion once a day
     (b). Children: 50–75 mg/kg (maximum of 2 gm/day), IM or IV infusion
    ii. Penicillin: 14- to 28-day antibiotic course
     (a). Adults: 18–24 million U per day IV divided into 6 daily doses
     (b). Children: 200,000–400,000 U/kg (maximum 18–24 million U/day) IV divided into 6 daily doses
  c. Possible alternatives for Lyme meningitis: Doxycycline 100 mg by mouth or IV infusion for 14–21 days.

4. Lyme arthritis
  a. Same oral regimen as early localized Lyme disease for a total of 28 days.
  b. Ceftriaxone (Rocephin): 75–100 mg/kg (maximum of 2 gm/day), IM or IV infusion for 14–28 days.
  c. Penicillin: 300,000 U/kg (maximum of 20 million U/day) given by IV infusion in divided doses every 4 hours for 14–28 days.

5. Pregnant women
  a. For localized early Lyme disease, amoxicillin 500 mg three times daily for 21 days.
  b. For disseminated early Lyme disease or any manifestation of late disease, penicillin G 20 million units daily for 14–21 days.
  c. For asymptomatic seropositivity, no treatment is necessary.

6. The Jarisch-Herxheimer reaction, with increased fever, chills, and malaise, can occur transiently when antibiotic therapy is initiated. Nonsteroidal anti-inflammatory agents may be beneficial, and the antimicrobial agent should be continued.

Follow-up

A. Follow-up depends on the stage of disease.
B. Repeat Lyme titer in 1–2 months to determine the need for continuation of antibiotic therapy.

Consultation/Referral

A. Referral to a physician is indicated when the patient with strong clinical evidence of Lyme disease fails to respond to prescribed antibiotics.
B. Consultation with a physician is particularly important for those patients with refractory neurologic deficits or debilitating arthritis.

Individual Considerations

A. Pregnancy
  1. Maternal-fetal transmission of infection with subsequent injury to the fetus has been reported. Antibiotic treatment should be instituted promptly in symptomatic patients.
  2. Tetracyclines are contraindicated in pregnancy. Otherwise, therapy is the same as for nonpregnant persons.
  3. There is no causal relationship between maternal Lyme disease and congenital malformations.
  4. There is no evidence that Lyme disease can be transmitted in breast milk.

MENINGITIS

Definition

A. Meningitis is an acute inflammation of the meninges, or membranes lining the brain and spinal cord. A virus or noninfectious insult, such as blood in the subarachnoid space, causes aseptic meningitis. Three baseline clinical features have been independently associated with an adverse outcome–hypotension, altered mental status, and seizures. Mortality rate varies in part with the organism and if it is a nosocomial or a community-acquired infection.
B. There are currently two meningococcal vaccines for use in children and adults. Temporary protection can be provided in certain cases with chemoprophylaxis.

Incidence

The most common organisms causing bacterial meningitis are presented here.

A. Ages 2 through 18:
  1. *Neisseria (N.) menigitidis* with portal entry in the nasopharynx (60% of cases).
  2. *Streptococcus (S.) pneumoniae* (25%).
  3. *Hemophilus (H.) influenzae* (8%).
  4. Remaining cases are due to *group B streptococcus* and *Listeria (L.) monocytogenes*.
B. Adults up to age 60:
  1. *S. pneumoniae* (adults 60%)
  2. *N. meningitidis* (20%)
  3. *H. influenzae* (10%)
  4. *L. monocytogenes* (6%)
  5. *Group B streptococcus* (4%)
C. Adults 60 years and older:
  1. *S. pneumoniae* (70%)
  2. *L. monocytogenes* (20%)
  3. *N. menigitidis, group B streptococcus, and H influenzae* (3%–4% each)

Acute meningitis due to infectious causes usually does not recur. However, a small number of patients with acute meningitis may develop recurrent attacks between intervals of good health. Chronic meningitis is arbitrarily defined as meningitis lasting for 4 weeks or more.

Pathogenesis

A. An acute inflammation of the meninges can be caused by S. pneumoniae, group B streptococci, H. influenzae, L. monocytogenes, N. menigitidis, gonococci (rare), Mycobacterium tuberculosis, Escherichia (E.) coli, type B, herpes, gram-positive anaerobes, and Bacteroides and as a sequelae of Lyme disease and varicella (chickenpox).

B. The incubation period is variable, depending on the pathogen; usually 1–10 days. Transmission occurs from person to person through droplets from the respiratory tract and requires close contact.

Predisposing Factors

A. Peaks.
   1. Children 2 years of age or younger (peak attack rate: younger than 1 year of age)
   2. Adolescents
   3. Freshman college students living in dormitories
B. Attendance at day care, school, camps, and the military.
C. Sequela of Lyme disease.
D. Odontogenic infection.
E. Sequela of otitis media, *H. influenzae* type B infection, and varicella.
F. Sickle cell disease, asplenia, Hodgkin's disease, and antibody deficiencies.
G. Penetrating wound, spinal tap, surgery, or anatomic abnormality.
H. Maternal predisposing factors: American Academy of Pediatrics lists the following indications for selective intrapartum chemoprophylaxis in group B strep-positive women:
   1. Preterm labor and delivery.
   2. Preterm rupture of membranes.
   3. Rupture of membranes greater than 18 hours before delivery.
   4. Intrapartum fever.
   5. Multiple gestation.
   6. Previous offspring with invasive group B strep disease.

Common Complaints

Classic triad:

A. Nuchal rigidity
B. Fever
C. Altered mental status

Other Signs and Symptoms

A. Neonates or infants:
   1. Decreased level of consciousness (LOC)
   2. High-pitched cry
   3. Irritability, inconsolability
   4. Fever and/or temperature instability
   5. Poor feeding and/or vomiting
   6. Bulging fontanelles
   7. Seizures
   8. Respiratory distress syndrome
B. Children or adults:
   1. Sudden onset of a severe, constant headache affecting the entire head that worsens with movement; CNS symptoms (nuchal rigidity, nausea and/or vomiting, confusion, lethargy, decreased LOC).
   2. Fever or chills.
   3. Backache.
   4. Photophobia.
   5. Difficulty swallowing.
   6. Facial and eye weakness and sagging eyelids.
   7. Seizures.
   8. Rash: the type of rash—macular, maculopapular, petechial, or purpuric—is depended on the virus/organism.
C. Chronic meningitis: usually have subacute onset of symptoms including fever, headache, and vomiting

Subjective Data

A. Review the onset, course, and duration of symptoms including a progressive petechial or ecchymotic rash.
B. Determine current or recent history of ear infections, upper respiratory infection, sinus infection, and chickenpox exposure. Determine recent use of antibiotics.
C. Ask the patient about any recent dental procedures, extractions, and gum procedures.
D. Review the patient's recent history of tick bite and any treatments.
E. Review the patient's recent history of Hib immunization.
F. Evaluate a history of serious drug allergies.
G. Evaluate a history of a recent head trauma.

Physical Examination

A. Check temperature, pulse, respirations, and blood pressure.
B. Inspect.
   1. Observe general overall appearance.
   2. Examine the skin for the presence of a petechial or ecchymotic rash.
   3. Complete an ear, nose, and throat exam.
   4. Examine mouth and teeth for dental diseases and disorders.
   5. Assess the patient for dehydration.
   6. Observe the patient for seizure activity.
   7. Assess level of pain.
C. Auscultate: Auscultate the lungs, monitor breathing pattern, and auscultate heart.
D. Palpate.
   1. Neck: Palpate the lymph nodes.
   2. Head: Palpate the fontanelle in children.
   3. Palpate the mastoid bones.
E. Neurologic exam: Evaluate for signs of meningeal irritation by means of Brudzinski's and Kernig's signs. Positive Brudzinski's and Kernig's signs:
   1. Brudzinski's sign: Place the patient supine and flex the head upward. Resulting flexion of both hips, knees, and ankles with neck flexion indicates meningeal irritation. (Refer to Figures 15.1 and 15.2.)
   2. Kernig's sign: Place the patient supine. Keeping one leg straight, flex the other hip and knee to a bent knee to form a 90° angle. Slowly extend the lower leg. This places a stretch on the meninges, resulting in pain and spasm for the hamstring muscle. Resistance to further extension can be felt.

Diagnostic Tests

A. CBC with differential.

B. Platelet count.

C. Blood cultures × 2.

D. Platelet count.

E. Cerebral spinal fluid tap.

F. Cultures of petechial or purpuric lesion scraping and synovial fluid.

G. MRI or CT scan, with and without contrast (a screening CT is not necessary in the majority of the patients).

Differential Diagnoses

A. Meningitis

B. Neonatal sepsis or pneumonia

C. Lyme disease

D. Herpes

E. Dementia

F. Gonorrhea

G. Otitis media

H. Dental abscess

I. Chickenpox

Plan

A. General interventions

1. Treat aggressively because the progression of disease is often rapid. Antibiotic therapy should be initiated immediately after blood cultures are drawn and the results of the lumbar puncture if the clinical suspicion is high.

2. Dexamethasone should be given shortly before or at the same time as the antibiotics if clinical/laboratory evidence suggest bacterial meningitis.

3. Maintain hydration.

4. In addition to standard precautions, droplet precautions are recommended until 24 hours after initiation of effective antimicrobial therapy.

5. Chemoprophylaxis is warranted for people who have been exposed directly to a patient's oral secretions through close social contact, such as sharing of toothbrushes or eating utensils as well as childcare and preschool contact within 7 days before the onset of the disease in the index case. Throat and nasopharyngeal cultures are of no value in deciding who should receive chemoprophylaxis and are not recommended.

6. Airline travelers with 8 hours of contact, who are seated directly next to an infected person, should receive prophylaxis.

B. Patient teaching

1. If a child suddenly develops a severely stiff neck along with fever and irritability, he or she needs medical help immediately.

2. Advise close contacts of the patient with meningococcal and *H. influenzae* meningitis that prophylactic treatment with rifampin (Rifadin) may be indicated; they should check with their health care providers or the local public health department.

C. Pharmaceutical therapy

1. Dexamethasone therapy should be considered when bacterial meningitis in infants and children (> 1 month old) is diagnosed or strongly suspected on the basis of the CSF tests, *H. influenzae* type B meningitis, and Pneumococcal or meningococcal meningitis.

   a. Dexamethasone should be administered 15–20 min before the first dose of antibiotics.

   b. The recommended Dexamethasone regimen is 0.4 mg/kg every 12 hours for a total of 2 doses by IV infusion for the first 2 days of antibiotic treatment. A regimen of 0.15 mg/kg every 6 hours for 4 days is also appropriate.

2. Antibiotic therapy: Initiate broad-spectrum coverage should be initiated until culture results are available. The doses vary by the organism. All antibiotics should be administered intravenously for at least 7 days. Empiric therapy may require adjustment after the culture results.

   a. Cefotaxime and Ceftriaxone are commonly used as empiric therapy with *S. pneumoniae* and *N. menigitidis* and *H. influenzae*. Vancomycin may be added to Cefotaxime or Ceftriaxone if renal function is normal until culture and susceptibility results are available.

   b. Listeria has traditionally been treated with Ampicillin or penicillin G and gentamicin may be added for its synergistic effect.

   c. Pseudomonas aeruginosa is often resistant to most commonly used antibiotics. Cefazidimine has been the most consistently effective cephalosporin therapy.

3. Chemoprophylaxis in adults includes rifampin, Ceftriaxone, ciprofloxacin, and azithromycin.

4. Vaccinations: There are 2 meningococcal vaccines licensed in the United States with a third being considered for licensure by the Food and Drug Administration.

   a. MPSV4 is administered in a single 0.5 mL dose intramuscularly. For children younger than 18 months of age, 2 doses administered 3 months apart are recommended. MPSV4 can be given concurrently with other vaccines but administered at a different site. In school-aged children and adults, MPSV4 induced protection persists for at least 3–5 years.

   b. MCV4 is used for ages 11 through 55 years and children 2 through 10 years. A single 0.5 mL dose is administered intramuscularly. It can also be given concurrently with other recommended vaccines. Routine childhood immunization with MCV4 is not recommended for children ages 2–10 because the infection rate is low, the immune response is poor, and the duration of immunity is not known. Adolescents 11–18 years and college freshmen living in dormitories should be immunized routinely with a single does of MCV4. MCV4 is given to all military recruits in the United States.

   c. No vaccine is available in the United States for the prevention of serogroup B meningococcal disease.

Follow-up

A. Have the patient return to clinic in 2–3 days if conditions (i.e., otitis media) are not significantly improved with antibiotic therapy.

B. Follow-up is dependent on symptoms. Schedule return visit after completion of antibiotics or 2–3 weeks after initial examination.

C. Sequelae associated with meningococcal disease occur in 11%–19% of patients.
1. Hearing loss
2. Neurologic disability
3. Digit or limb amputations
4. Skin scarring

Consultation/Referral

A. Neonate: Consult with a physician if the patient is younger than 3 months of age. Neonates need hospitalization.

B. Child: Consult with a physician.
1. Exceptions: localized, nonserious infections. Child should be active, playful, drinking, and voiding.
2. The patient needs immediate consultation with a physician if the child is lethargic and inconsolable.

Individual Considerations

A. Pregnancy
1. Maternal: Culture introital or vaginal and anorectal samples for *group B strep,* using a selective medium such as Todd-Hewitt broth. Vaginal colonization *of group B streptococcus* occurs in 5%–40% of pregnant women, of which 40%–70% transmit *group B strep* to their offspring.
2. The most significant problem associated with pregnancy is exposure of the fetus to *group B strep* in the maternal genital tract. In 2002, the CDC, the American Academy of Pediatrics, and the American College of Obstetricians and Gynecologists recommended universal perinatal screening for vaginal and rectal GBS colonization at 35–37 weeks' gestation.
3. Treat patients with positive urine culture only because recolonization occurs frequently. Antibiotics should be administered to women in labor for preterm labor, premature rupture of membranes, positive group B strep cultures (past or present), and preterm premature rupture of membranes in labor.

B. Pediatrics
1. Neonatal sepsis occurs in approximately 1%–2% of cases. In the United States, the risk of developing *H. influenzae* type B invasive disease during the first 5 years of life is about 1:200.
2. Neonatal group B strep infections **usually** present as early onset in the first 2 days of life and as late onset in newborns up to 3 months of age.
3. The premature neonate is at the highest risk for development of symptomatic neonatal disease.
4. Neonates often appear normal at delivery, only to develop a fulminant infection with rapid deterioration. Because of the severity and fulminant course of neonatal group B strep infections, the primary focus is on preventing the vertical transmission of the organism.
5. Infants up to 2 years old may have meningitis without a stiff neck.
6. All infants with meningitis should undergo careful follow-up examinations, including tests for hearing loss and neurologic abnormalities.

MONONUCLEOSIS (EPSTEIN-BARR)

Definition

A. Infectious mononucleosis (IM) is an acute, infectious viral disease caused by Epstein-Barr virus (EBV), with three classic symptoms: fever, pharyngitis, and lymphadenopathy. The spread is via intimate contact between susceptible persons and asymptomatic EBV shedders through the passage of saliva.

Incidence

A. Antibodies to EBV have been demonstrated in all population groups with a worldwide distribution. Approximately 90%–95% of adults are EBV-seropositive. Incidence is unknown; it occurs primarily in adolescents and young adults. The peak incidence of infection is noted in the 15- to 24-year age range. The majority with primary EBV recovers uneventfully.

Pathogenesis

A. Epstein-Barr virus (EBV), a DNA virus, is a herpesvirus and is the primary agent of infectious mononucleosis (IM). EBV persists asymptomatically for life in nearly all adults, and is associated with the development of B cell lymphomas, T cell lymphomas, and Hodgkin lymphoma in certain patients.

B. The incubation period is 4–6 weeks with an average of 11 days; it is communicable during the acute phase, which may be prolonged. Acute symptoms resolve in 1–2 weeks. Pharyngeal excretion may persist for up to 18 months following clinical recovery. And it is estimated that once infected with EBV, the virus may be intermittently shed in the oropharynx for decades.

C. EBV has also been isolated both in the cervix and in male seminal fluid suggesting a possibility of sexual transmission.

Predisposing Factors

A. Age 12–40 years, with peak incidence between 15–24 years of age
B. Exposure through oropharyngeal secretions (kiss, cough, shared food)

Common Complaints

A. Sore throat is the most common symptom.
B. Headache.
C. Fever.
D. Fatigue (may be persistent and severe).

Other Signs and Symptoms

A. Tonsillar pharyngitis: exudate may have a white, gray-green, or necrotic appearance.
B. Generalized aches.
C. Appetite loss.
D. Swollen lymph glands, usually cervical adenopathy, and in the underarm, or groin.
E. Hepatosplenomegaly: mild hepatitis is encountered in approximately 90% of individuals, splenomegaly is noted in approximately 50%. Jaundice is uncommon.
F. Otitis media (infants and children).
G. Abdominal complaints and diarrhea (infants and children).

H. Upper respiratory symptoms (more prominent in young infants).

Subjective Data

A. Review signs, symptoms, and course and duration of symptoms.

B. Assess the patient for recent upper respiratory infection and sore throat.

C. Inquire about any contact with persons known to have mononucleosis.

D. Review the patient's history for other family members with similar symptoms.

E. Carefully review medications. A mononucleosis syndrome with atypical lymphocytosis can be induced by drugs including:

1. Phenytoin
2. Carbamazepine
3. Antibiotics such as isoniazid and minocycline

Physical Examination

A. Check temperature, pulse, respirations, and blood pressure.

B. Inspect.

1. Conduct ear, nose, and throat exam, especially tonsils and palate.
   a. Pharynx shows lymphoid hyperplasia, erythema, and edema.
   b. Tonsillar exudates is present in about 50% of the cases.
   c. Evaluate for petechiae at the junction of the hard and soft palate.
   d. Evaluate for oral hairy leukoplakia (OHL) on the lateral portions of the tongue. OHL appears as white corrugated painless plaques that cannot be scraped from the surface.

C. Auscultate: Auscultate the heart and lungs.

D. Palpate.

1. Palpate the lymph nodes, especially anterior and posterior cervical chains, axilla, and groin. **Firm tender lymph nodes are indicative of mononucleosis; lymphadenopathy is usually symmetric and presents in the posterior cervical chain more than the anterior chain.**

2. Palpate the abdomen, especially the spleen. **Splenomegaly is noted in 50% of cases. Hepatomegaly and tenderness are noted in 10% of cases.**

E. Percuss: Percuss the abdomen, especially the spleen area.

F. Neurologic exam: evaluate for facial nerve palsy or symptoms of meningitis.

Diagnostic Tests

A. CBC with differential and peripheral smear: Complete blood count shows absolute neutropenia (< 500 cells) and atypical lymphocytes.

B. Throat swab for rapid strep; if negative, send for culture.

C. Monospot test.

D. EBV IgM and IgG.

E. Cold agglutinin titer: **Cold agglutinin titer is markedly elevated in the setting of hemolysis (> 1:1000).**

F. Liver function tests: Abnormal liver function tests in a patient with pharyngitis strongly suggest the diagnosis of IM.

G. Abdominal ultrasound if indicated for splenomegaly.

Differential Diagnoses

A. Mononucleosis
B. Strep throat
C. Viral syndrome
D. Hodgkin's disease
E. Hepatitis
F. Cytomegalovirus
G. Secondary syphilis
H. Chronic fatigue syndrome
I. Acute human immunodeficiency virus (HIV)
J. Toxoplasmosis

Plan

A. General interventions

1. Make certain that the patient does not have an upper airway obstruction from enlarged tonsils and lymphoid tissue.
2. Administer analgesics, such as acetaminophen or NSAIDs, for fever, body aches, and malaise.
3. Treat concurrent infections.
4. Isolation is not required with good hand washing and prevention of the spread of pharyngeal secretions.
5. Bed rest is unnecessary.
6. There is no commercially available vaccine to prevent EBV infection.
7. Splenic rupture is rare but potentially life-threatening, occurring in 1–2 cases per thousand. It occurs between the 4th and 21st day of symptomatic illness, but can be the presenting symptom. The typical manifestations are abdominal pain and/or a falling hematocrit.

B. Patient teaching

1. See the Section III Patient Teaching Guide for this chapter, "Mononucleosis."
2. Prolonged communicability may persist for up to 1 year.

C. Pharmaceutical therapy

1. Acyclovir is not recommended for infectious mononucleosis.
2. Antibiotic therapy is reserved for concurrent infections such as streptococcal pharyngitis.
3. Corticosteroids may be considered in the presence of overwhelming infections including IM-related airway obstruction or other complications such as severe hemolytic or aplastic anemia.

Follow-up

A. Examine patient every 1–2 weeks.

B. Initial monospot test may be negative; repeat in 7–10 days.

C. If splenomegaly is present, schedule an appointment to reevaluate the patient prior to the release for contact sports. **Splenomegaly puts patients at risk for rupture secondary to blunt trauma (i.e., sports and motor vehicle accidents).**

Consultation/Referral

A. Consult a physician for marked tonsil enlargement and difficulty swallowing or symptoms lasting longer than 2 weeks. An emergent consultation with an otolaryngologist may be required.

Individual Considerations

A. Pregnancy: Intrauterine infection with EBV is rare.

B. Pediatrics: Primary EBV in young infants and children is common and frequently asymptomatic. Ampicillin and penicillin may cause rashes.

PARVOVIRUS 19 (FIFTH DISEASE)

Definition

A. Parvovirus 19, also known as Fifth disease, is considered one of the TORCH infections (Toxoplasmosis, Other [hepatitis], Rubella, Cytomegalovirus, Herpes).

B. In children, Parvovirus B19 can cause erythema infectiosum (EI), a mild febrile illness with rash. EI is also referred to as "fifth disease" since it represents one of six common childhood exanthems, each named in the order of dates they were first described. In contrast, patients with underlying hemolytic disorders can develop a transient aplastic crisis. Infection during pregnancy can lead to fetal death. It is an acute, communicable, viral infection that is spread by means of respiratory droplet and transplacental transmission. It can be associated with chronic hemolytic anemia and has been associated with fetal death.

Incidence

A. Incidence is unknown; parvovirus occurs worldwide. It is more common in children, and outbreaks are more common in the winter and spring. Because less than 1% of teachers who are pregnant during erythema infectiosum outbreaks are expected to experience an adverse fetal outcome, exclusion of pregnant women from employment in child care or teaching is not recommended.

Pathogenesis

A. Human Parvovirus B19 belongs to the Erythrovirus genus within the Parvoviridae family. Human parvovirus B19 is a DNA virus with preference to erythroid precursor cells. The virus replicates in the erythroid progenitor cell of the bone marrow and blood leading to inhibition of erythropoeises, which can result in symptoms of anemia. The parvovirus associated rash is presumed to be at least partially immune mediated.

B. The incubation period for initial symptoms to develop is 4–10 days after exposure; the rash usually last 5 days but can last as long as 21 days. Parvovirus B19-specific IgM antibodies are detected at day 10–12 and can persist for up to 5 months. Rash and joint symptoms occur 2–3 weeks after acquisition of infection.

Predisposing Factors

A. The only known host for B19 is humans.

B. Exposure to school-aged (through junior high) and daycare populations.

C. Occupational exposure for teachers (16%), day-care workers and homemakers (9% each), and health care workers.

D. Exposure to close contact or crowded conditions.

Common Complaints

A. Clinical presentation is influenced by the infected individual's age and hematologic and immunologic status.

B. Approximately 25% of infected individuals are asymptomatic, 50% have nonspecific flulike symptoms of malaise, muscle pain, and fever.

C. Classic symptoms.
1. Red rash on the face that spreads to the rest of the body. **Erythematous, macular rash on cheeks produces "slap cheek" pattern.**
2. Arthritis: Joint pain most frequently affects the hands, followed by the knees and wrists. Joint symptoms are more common in adults and may be the sole manifestation of infection. Joint pain is more common in women. The arthritis associated with acute B19 infection does not cause joint destruction.
3. Edema.

Other Signs and Symptoms

A. Adults: chronic arthropathy

B. Child
1. Bright red rash on cheeks, may be confused with rubella
2. Maculopapular rash on trunk and extremities, may be pruritic
3. Circumoral pallor
4. Malaise
5. Headache
6. Sore throat and pharyngitis
7. Conjunctivitis
8. Diarrhea

C. Fetus
1. Nonimmune hydrops fetalis
2. Stillbirth
3. Anemia

Subjective Data

A. Review the onset, duration, and course of symptoms.

B. Elicit the initial site of rash and progression to other body areas.

C. Elicit job exposure for schoolteachers and day-care workers.

D. Determine if the patient is pregnant.

E. Determine whether the patient has had any new medication or contact exposures.

F. Rule out other family members with similar symptoms.

G. Ask if the patient has any tattoos or has had a recent tattoo.

Physical Examination

A. Check temperature, pulse, respirations, and blood pressure

B. Inspect
1. Observe rash pattern: "lacy" patterned rash over extremities.
2. Conduct an ear, nose, and throat exam.

C. Palpate
1. Blanch rash area: Rash over extremities blanches with pressure, heat or cold, and sunlight.
2. Palpate spleen: **Splenomegaly is a hallmark sign.**
3. Palpate lymph nodes: Enlarged lymph nodes, especially the posterior cervical nodes, are indicative of infection.

4. Assess joints for tenderness, swelling, and range of motion.

Diagnostic Tests
A. CBC with differential: **Hallmark laboratory finding is the dramatic decrease or absence of measurable reticulocytes.**
B. Parvovirus IgG and IgM antibodies.
C. Polymerase chain reaction (PCR) test.
D. Pregnancy test if necessary.
E. Fetal assessment.
   1. Ultrasonography to evaluate for fetal hydrops. Fetal ascites, pleural and pericardial effusions are evident on ultrasonogram (nonimmune hydrops fetalis).
   2. Percutaneous umbilical sampling (PUBS) to evaluate infection and anemia may be performed.

Differential Diagnoses
A. Parvovirus 19 (Fifth disease)
B. Rubella
C. Aplastic crisis
D. Other viral infection
E. Contact dermatitis
F. Medication allergies
G. Chronic anemia

Plan
A. General interventions
   1. Management is usually supportive treatment of symptoms.
   2. Analgesics for joint pain.
   3. Antipyretic for temperature.
   4. Starch bath for pruritus.
   5. Self-limiting without treatment.
   6. Immunosuppressed patients respond well to intravenous immune globulin (IVIG).
   7. Aplastic crises may require transfusion.
B. Patient teaching
   1. Educate pregnant and immunocompromised patients to avoid exposure.
   2. Routine infection control practices minimize the risk of transmission, including hand washing and droplet precautions. Avoiding sharing food or drinks may partially prevent the spread of B19.
   3. **Disease is most communicable prior to rash; it is not communicable after rash outbreak.**
C. Pharmaceutical therapy
   1. Acetaminophen (Tylenol) for fever.
   2. Nonsteroidal anti-inflammatory drugs for symptomatic relief.
   3. Empiric prescription of a low-dose diuretic (hydrochlorothiazide 12–25 mg/day) for adult joint pain if severe.
   4. Immunoglobulin prophylaxis is not recommended by the CDC at this time. There is no vaccine to prevent parvovirus B19.

Follow-up
A. None is recommended as disease is self-limiting for low-risk population.

Consultation/Referral
A. The incidence of acute B19 in pregnancy is 3.3%–3.8%. Refer pregnant patients to a perinatologist for fetal evaluation for acute exposure in pregnancy.
B. Consult or refer the patient to a physician immediately for exposure of immunocompromised patients, who might require a blood transfusion.

Individual Considerations
A. Pregnancy.
   1. A positive IgG antibody and a negative IgM indicates maternal immunity and the fetus is therefore protected from infection. A positive IgM antibody is consistent with acute parvovirus infection.
   2. Fetal risks are related to the trimester of exposure. Nonimmune hydrops fetalis occurs secondary to hemolysis and inadequate production of erythrocytes. Other risks include spontaneous abortion, intrauterine growth restriction, stillbirth, and neonatal death.
   3. Women who are diagnosed with acute infection beyond 20 weeks' gestation should receive periodic ultrasounds (although serial ultrasounds are commonly performed).
   4. Intrauterine blood transfusion may be performed if severe anemia is confirmed.
   5. Delivery and postnatal management of the hydropic infant should be undertaken in a tertiary care facility. The majority of hydropic infants require respiratory assistance and mechanical ventilation.
B. Pediatrics: Children with abnormal red blood cells (sickle cell disease, hereditary spherocytosis, thalassemia) can develop transient aplastic anemia and may require multiple transfusions.
C. Adults.
   1. Patients may have arthritis and arthralgias lasting months to years after exposure.
   2. Adults may initially be asymptomatic.
   3. Immunocompromised patients may develop severe, chronic anemia.
   4. Working women with young children may benefit from prenatal testing and limiting exposure in pregnancy.

RHEUMATIC FEVER

Definition
A. Acute rheumatic fever (ARF) is an autoimmune inflammatory process that occurs as sequelae of a Group A beta-hemolytic streptococcal (GAS) tonsillopharyngitis. Rheumatic fever is a preventable disease through the detection and adequate treatment of streptococcal pharyngitis.
B. The individual who has had an attack of rheumatic fever is at very high risk of developing recurrences after subsequent GAS pharyngitis and needs continuous antimicrobial prophylaxis to prevent such recurrences (secondary prevention). The most significant complication of ARF is rheumatic heart disease, which occurs after repeated bouts of acute illness.

Incidence

A. Although the incidence of ARF has declined markedly in the United States and Western Europe, the incidence of rheumatic fever is between 0.3%–3.0% following ineffectively treated cases of Group A streptococcal upper respiratory infections (URIs). ARF is most common among children 5–15 years. It is relatively rare in infants and uncommon in preschool-aged children. The incidence of first episodes falls steadily after adolescents and is rare after 35 years of age. The disease does not seem to have a major racial predisposition. About 20% of children diagnosed with rheumatic fever have a positive history of pharyngitis and only 35%–60% recall having any upper respiratory symptoms within the preceding 3 months.

B. Cardiac involvement is the most serious complication. Morbidity due to congestive heart failure (CHF), strokes, and endocarditis is common among individuals with rheumatic heart disease, and about 1.5% of persons with rheumatic carditis die of the disease annually. Mitral stenosis and Sydenham chorea are more common in females who have gone through puberty.

Pathogenesis

A. Rheumatic fever is caused by a preceding infection with Group A streptococcus and *S. pyogenes*. Nonsuppurative inflammatory lesions of the joints, heart, subcutaneous tissue, and central nervous system characterize ARF. The incubation period is between 1–5 weeks and 6 months after a Group A strep pharyngitis.

Predisposing Factors

A. Group A pharyngitis, untreated or inadequately treated
B. Age 5–15 years
C. Crowded living conditions
D. Occupational exposure: teachers, health care providers, and military personnel

Common Complaints

A. Sore throat (generally of sudden onset), pain on swallowing.
B. Joint pain/arthralgias to frank polyarthritis is usually symmetrical and involves large joints such as knees, ankles, elbows, and wrists. Joints feel warm, swollen, and inflamed. **Polyarthritis is the most common manifestation. Both synovitis and periarticular inflammation occur especially in the knees and ankles. There may be erythema of the overlying skin.**
C. Fever varies from 101°F–104°F.

Other Signs and Symptoms

A. Fatigue.
B. Appetite loss.
C. Sydenham Chorea (more common in girls): Chorea, a CNS disorder lasting 1–3 months, is purposeless, involuntary, rapid movements often associated with muscle weakness, involuntary facial grimaces, speech disturbance, and emotional liability. Sydenham chorea usually resolves with permanent damage but occasionally lasts 2–3 years.
D. Subcutaneous nodules are firm, painless nodules that are seen or felt over the extensor surface of certain joints, particularly elbows, knees, and wrists; in the occipital region; or over the spinous processes of the thoracic and lumbar vertebrae. The skin overlying them moves freely and is not inflamed.
E. Erythema marginatum is an evanescent, nonpruritic, pink rash with pale centers and round or wavy margins; lesions vary greatly in size and occur mainly on the trunk and extremities, usually not seen on the face. Erythema is transient, migrates from place to place, and may be brought out by the application of heat.
F. Enlarged lymph nodes.
G. Headache.
H. Carditis: development of new heart murmurs, cardiomegaly, and CHF.
I. Pericarditis, pericardial friction rub, and/or pericardial effusion.
J. Aortic regurgitation, manifested by:
 1. Palpitations
 2. Dyspnea on exertion
 3. Angina at rest

Subjective Data

A. Review a recent history (1–3 months) of sore throat and the onset, duration, severity, and treatment of symptoms.
B. Complete a drug history. Did the patient finish the prescribed antibiotics? Does the patient take aspirin? **Use of aspirin can mask signs of inflammation and tends to prolong the course of the disease.**
C. Assess the patient for signs and symptoms of rheumatic and scarlet fever.
D. Discuss the patient's history of heart problems.

Physical Examination

A. Check temperature, pulse, respirations, and blood pressure.
B. Inspect.
 1. Inspect joints for swelling and warmth.
 2. Observe for signs of chorea.
 3. Conduct a dermal exam, especially the trunk and proximal aspects of the extremities. Individual lesions of erythema marginatum are evanescent, moving over the skin in wavy patterns or with indented margins. The lesions may be macular and can develop and disappear in minutes, appearing to change shape while being examined.
 4. Complete an ear, nose, oral and throat exam. Evaluate tonsillopharyngeal erythema with or without exudates. Observe for beefy red swollen uvula.
C. Auscultate.
 1. Auscultate heart. Note heart murmur, pericardial friction rub, or effusion. Characteristic murmurs of acute carditis include the high-pitched, blowing, hososystolic, apical murmur of mitral regurgitation and a high-pitched, decrescendo, diastolic murmur of aortic regurgitation heard in the aortic area. The features of CHF include tachycardia, a third heart sound, rales, and edema.
 2. Auscultate all lung fields.
D. Palpate.
 1. Palpate the neck lymph nodes.
 2. Palpate the extremities: apical and radial pulses.
E. Neuromuscular exam.

Diagnostic Tests

A. No single specific laboratory test can confirm the diagnosis of acute rheumatic fever (ARF). The throat culture remains the criterion standard for confirmation of Group A streptococcal infection.
   1. If a rapid antigen detection test is negative, obtain a throat culture.
   2. Because of the high specificity, a positive rapid antigen test confirms a streptococcal infection.
B. Erythrocyte sedimentation rate (ESR) is usually elevated at the onset of ARF.
C. C-reactive protein (CRP) is usually elevated at the onset of ARF.
D. EKG or echocardiography. **Note prolonged PR interval.**
E. Chest radiograph can reveal cardiomegaly and CHF.
F. Echocardiology may demonstrate valvular regurgitant lesions.
G. Tests that may rule out differential diagnoses include rheumatoid factor, antinuclear antibody (ANA), Lyme serology, blood cultures, and evaluation for gonorrhea.

Differential Diagnoses

A. Rheumatic fever: Jones Criteria (updated in 1992)
   1. Major criteria
      a. Carditis (based on clinical criteria)
      b. Polyarthritis
      c. Chorea (rare in adults)
      d. Erythema marginatum (uncommon, rare in adults)
      e. Subcutaneous nodules (uncommon, rare in adults)
   2. Minor criteria
      a. Arthralgia
      b. Fever
      c. Elevated ESR or CRP level
      d. Prolonged PR interval
B. Juvenile rheumatoid arthritis
C. Rheumatoid arthritis
D. Gonococcal arthritis
E. Kawasaki disease
F. Systemic lupus erythematous
G. Lyme disease
H. Reiter's syndrome
I. Scarlet fever

Plan

A. General interventions: Bed rest is a traditional part of ARF therapy and is especially important with carditis. Bed rest is needed throughout the acute illness and should continue until the ESR has returned to normal for 2 weeks.
B. Patient teaching.
   1. Reinforce the need to take the complete prescribed course of antibiotics for strep infections.
   2. Adequate treatment for a streptococcal pharyngitis or skin infection is the best prevention against rheumatic fever. Strep infections are contagious, but rheumatic fever is not.
   3. Chorea is usually managed conservatively in a quiet nonstimulatory environment. Valporic acid is the preferred agent if sedation is needed. Although there is no conclusive evidence of their efficacy,

intravenous immunoglobulin, steroids, and plasmapheresis have all been used successfully in refractory chorea.
   4. Diuretics are the mainstay of carditis/heart failure.
C. Pharmaceutical therapy.
   1. Antibiotic treatment in patients who present with acute rheumatic fever is necessary irrespective of the throat culture results to minimize the possible transmission of the rheumatogenic streptococcal strain. The drug of choice is penicillin, but erythromycin or Sulfadiazine may be used in patients who are allergic to penicillin. Use of long-acting intramuscular penicillin G avoids compliance problems of oral regimens.
      a. Benzathine Penicillin G
         i. Adults:
            (a). Primary prophylaxis for treatment of Group A streptococcal pharyngitis: 1.2 million U IM once
            (b). Secondary prophylaxis: 1.2 million U IM every 3–4 weeks
         ii. Pediatrics:
            (a). Primary prophylaxis (< 27 kg): 600,000 U IM once
            (b). Secondary prophylaxis: 600,000 U IM every 3–4 weeks
      b. Penicillin VK
         i. Adults:
            (a). Primary prophylaxis: 500 mg by mouth 2–3 times a day for 10 days
            (b). Secondary prophylaxis: 250 mg by mouth twice a day
         ii. Pediatrics:
            (a). Primary prophylaxis: 250 mg by mouth 2–3 times a day for 10 days
            (b). Secondary prophylaxis: younger than 5 years: 125 mg by mouth twice a day, older than 5 years: 250 mg by mouth twice a day
      c. Erythromycin (EEE, E-Mycin, Ery-Tab)
         i. Adults:
            (a). Primary prophylaxis: 250 mg erythromycin stearate, base or estolate salts (or 400 mg ethylsuccate) every 6 hours by mouth or 500 mg by mouth every 12 hours for 10 days; do not exceed 1 g/day; alternative, 333 mg (as the base) every 8 hours
            (b). Secondary prophylaxis: 250 mg by mouth twice a day
         ii. Pediatrics:
            (a). Primary prophylaxis: 30–50 mg/kg/day (base or ethylsuccinate) by mouth divided every 6–8 hours; not to exceed 1 gm/day for 10 days
            (b). Secondary prophylaxis (base or ethylsuccinate): younger than 5 years: 125 mg by mouth twice a day or older than 5 years: 250 mg by mouth twice a day
      d. Sulfadiazine
         i. Adults: 1 gm by mouth every day for 10 days

ii. Pediatric:
(a). Less than 27 kg: 500 mg by mouth every day for 10 days
(b). Greater than 27 kg: 1 gm by mouth every day for 10 days

2. Codeine is the analgesic of choice for arthritis symptoms.
3. Steroid therapy is reserved for severe carditis.
4. Aspirin (Anacin, Ascriptin, Bayer ASA, Bayer Buffered ASA) is used in patients with moderate-to-severe arthritis and carditis without heart failure. Treatment is administered for at least 8 weeks.
   a. Adults: 90–100 mg/kg/day divided every 6–8 hours for 2 weeks initially, then 60–70 mg/kg/day for 6 weeks; not to exceed 3.6–5.4 g/day
   b. Pediatrics: 60–90 mg/kg/day by mouth divided every 6–8 hours for 8 weeks; adjust according to serum levels

Follow-up

A. The test of cure is a negative throat culture.
B. Pharyngitis patients with a history of rheumatic fever and those who are symptomatic and have a household member with documented Group A streptococcal infection should receive immediate treatment without need for prior testing.
C. Patients need prophylaxis for systemic bacterial endocarditis (SBE) prior to dental and/or surgical procedures.
D. The major complication is cardiac valve disease. Rheumatic fever accounts for the largest number of aortic regurgitation cases. Continuous streptococcus prophylaxis in patients with prior rheumatic fever is the major means of preventing cardiac sequelae.

Consultation/Referral

A. Consult and comanage the patient with a physician.
B. Consult an ear, nose, and throat (ENT) specialist if indicated for patients with intact tonsils and recurrent symptomatic strep infections for consideration of tonsillectomy.
C. Consultation with a cardiologist may be required to manage heart blocks and CHF.
D. Consultation with a neurologist or psychiatrist may be required to confirm the diagnosis of chorea and to assist in its management.

Individual Considerations

A. Pediatrics: Highest risk group; rare in children under 5 years.
B. Adults: Cases are rare for patients over age 40.
C. Pregnancy:
1. Penicillin G is Pregnancy Category B. Fetal risk is not confirmed in humans but has been shown in some studies in animals.
2. Erythromycin is Pregnancy Category B.
3. Sulfadiazine is both a Pregnancy Category B and is not recommended for breast-feeding.
4. Aspirin products are Pregnancy Category D. As fetal risk has been shown in humans, use only if the benefits outweigh the risk to the fetus.

ROCKY MOUNTAIN SPOTTED FEVER

Definition

A. Rocky Mountain spotted fever (RMSF) is a systemic febrile illness with characteristic rash from the bite of an infected tick. It can involve the skin, central nervous system, gastrointestinal tract, and muscles.

Incidence

B. Rocky Mountain spotted fever is the most common rickettsial infection in the United States. The prevalence of RMSF is in the southeastern and southern central states. Although RMSF is more common in rural and suburban locations, it does occur in urban areas. The incidence varies by geographic area. Rocky Mountain spotted fever is more common in the spring and early summer, but has been seen in the cold weather months in the southern United States.

Pathogenesis

A. *Rickettsia rickettsii* is the infectious agent and is transmitted by a tick vector. Rickettsia also infects rodents, squirrels, and chipmunks. Up to one-third of patients with proven RMSF do not recall a recent tick bite or tick contact. Rocky Mountain spotted fever is not transmitted by person-to-person contact.
B. The incubation period is usually about 1 week, but it ranges from 2–14 days after the tick bite. It appears to be related to the size of the rickettsial inoculum.

Predisposing Factors

A. Outdoor activities (hunting, hiking, camping).
B. Tick bite: The tick must attach and feed for 4–6 hours before transmitting the infection.
C. Age is not a predisposing factor, but the disease is more common in children and young adults.
D. Exposure to heavy brush areas.
E. Contact with dogs and other animals with ticks.
F. Transmission has occurred on rare occasion by blood transfusion.

Common Complaints

In early phase, most patients have nonspecific signs and symptoms that may include:

A. Fever.
B. Sudden onset of severe headache.
C. Children may present with prominent abdominal pain that may be mistaken for acute appendicitis, Cholecystitis, or bowel obstruction.
D. Rash usually (90%) occurs between 3–5 days of illness. The typical RMSF rash begins as a pink maculopapular eruption on the ankles and wrists. The rash then spreads both centrally and to the palms of hands and soles of the feet. By the fourth day the rash spreads centripetally and becomes petechial and papular. Hemorrhagic, ulcerated lesions may follow. In a small percentage, the rash is delayed in onset (past 5 days) and/or is atypical (e.g., confined to one body region). **Urticaria and pruritus are not characteristic of RMSF and their presence make the diagnosis unlikely.**
E. Malaise.

F. Myalgias.

G. Nausea with or without vomiting.

Other Signs and Symptoms

A. Deep cough

B. Edema, especially in children

C. Bleeding

D. Conjunctivitis

E. Retinal abnormalities

F. ECG abnormalities

G. Seizures

Subjective Data

A. Review the onset, course, and duration of symptoms.

B. Elicit information about a recent tick bite or removal.

C. Ask the patient about any recent outdoor activities such as camping, hiking, and so on.

D. Rule out similar symptoms in other family members.

E. Review any history of rash and course of spread.

F. Elicit a history of mental or neurologic changes including seizures.

G. Rule out other symptoms associated with Lyme disease such as arthritis, memory loss, and distal paraesthesia.

H. Review the patient's recent history of blood transfusion.

Physical Examination

A. Check temperature, pulse, respirations, and blood pressure

B. Inspect

1. Conduct an ear, nose, and throat exam.

2. Inspect the skin, especially on the wrist, palms, ankles, and the soles of the feet.

3. Note the presence of petechia.

4. Conduct an eye examination.

C. Auscultate

1. Perform complete heart evaluation.

2. Auscultate all lung fields.

D. Palpate

1. Palpate all lymph nodes.

2. Palpate the mastoid bones.

E. Neurologic examination

1. Assess level of consciousness.

2. Evaluate the patient for signs of meningeal irritation, such as nuchal rigidity, positive Brudzinski's and Kernig's signs (see Figures 15.1 and 15.2).

Diagnostic Tests

A. **Antibody titers: A fourfold rise in antibody titer is diagnostic for Rocky Mountain spotted fever. Antibodies typically appear 7–10 days after the onset of the illness.**

B. CBC with differential.

C. Platelet count: As the illness progresses, thrombocytopenia becomes more prevalent and may be severe.

D. Electrolytes.

E. Liver function studies.

F. Bilirubin.

G. Skin biopsy: 3 mm punch biopsy.

H. Lumbar puncture may be indicated.

I. Rickettsial blood cultures are highly sensitive and specific, however, they require specialized laboratories.

Differential Diagnoses

A. Rocky Mountain spotted fever.

B. RMSF is commonly mistaken for an undifferentiated viral illness during the first few days of illness.

C. Viral meningitis.

D. Lyme disease.

E. Mononucleosis.

F. Atypical measles.

G. Viral hepatitis.

F. Parvovirus B19 (Fifth disease).

Plan

A. General interventions

1. Early treatment is necessary; never delay initiation of antimicrobial treatment to confirm clinical suspicion of the disease. This is a life-threatening disease.

2. **Antibiotic therapy (see "Pharmaceutical Therapy"). If penicillin or a cephalosporin is administered empirically in the first few days of the illness, the subsequent rash may be incorrectly diagnosed as a drug reaction.**

3. Hospitalization should be considered for most patients, especially children.

B. Patient teaching

1. See the Section III Patient Teaching Guide for this chapter, "Rocky Mountain Spotted Fever" and the Section II Procedure, "Removal of a Tick."

2. RMSF is not transmissible by person-to-person contact; therefore, isolation is not necessary.

3. Relapse of the illness may occur; the patient should report recurrence of symptoms immediately.

4. Patients who report tick bites should be advised to inform their health care provider if any systemic symptoms, especially fever and headache, occur in the following 14 days.

C. Pharmaceutical therapy

The diagnosis of RMSF can rarely be confirmed or disproved in its early phase; the cornerstone of management is *empiric therapy* based upon clinical judgment and the epidemiologic setting.

1. Drug of choice: doxycycline 100 mg orally or intravenously every 12 hours for 5–7 days for adults or children weighing more than 45 kg. Doxycycline 2.2 mg/kg IV or orally every 12 hours is the dosage for smaller children.

a. Doxycycline 200 mg initial loading dose IV may be given for critically ill patients.

b. Doxycycline is the drug of choice in adults except for pregnant women.

c. Tetracyclines can cause dental staining when administered to children younger than 8 years. Most experts consider the risk of morbidity from rickettsial diseases greater than the minimal risk of dental staining from one short course of doxycycline.

2. Alternative drug therapy: for children 2 weeks old to adult, chloramphenicol (Chloromycetin) 50–100 mg/kg/day in four divided doses for 6–10 days (may discontinue when patient is afebrile for 36 hours).

Chloramphenicol requires frequent serum platelet counts and CBCs.

3. Prophylactic therapy with doxycycline or another tetracycline is not recommended following tick exposure.

Follow-up
A. See the patient 24–48 hours after initial visit and again at the end of antibiotic therapy (unless following lab for chloramphenicol therapy).
B. The patient must be seen for any alteration in mental status, stiff neck, severe headaches, nausea and vomiting, severe weakness, dizziness, or high fever.
C. Hospitalization is indicated in patients who are severely ill or have complications, such as seizures, hypotension, or marked gastrointestinal symptoms.
D. Several rickettsial diseases, including RMSF, are nationally notifiable diseases and should be reported to state and local health departments.

Consultation/Referral
A. Consult a physician for any suspected signs of Rocky Mountain spotted fever because the patient is in danger of vascular collapse and disseminated intravascular collapse.

Individual Considerations
A. Pregnancy: Tetracyclines should not be used in pregnancy.

▣ ROSEOLA (EXANTHEM SUBITUM)

Definition
A. Roseola is a benign viral illness. It is the most common exanthem in infants and young children aged 1–3 years.

Incidence
A. Incidence is unknown; 90% of cases involve children younger than 2 years old. A possible association of HHV-6 and multiple sclerosis has been suggested but is still inconclusive. HHV-6 has been isolated in Kaposi sarcoma (caused by human herpesvirus 8), in which it may contribute to tumor progression. HHV-6 may facilitate oncogenic potential in lymphoma and has been associated with chronic fatigue syndrome.

Pathogenesis
A. Human herpesvirus 6 (HHV-6) is the causative organism. The two variants of HHV-6 are A and B. The genomes of HHV-6A/B have been sequenced. Nearly all primary infections in children appear to be caused by HHV-6B. In the primary infection, replication of the virus occurs in the leukocytes and the salivary glands. It is present in the saliva. The communicable period is most likely during the febrile phase. The incubation period is 5–15 days.
B. Like other herpes viruses, HHV-6 remains latent in most patients who are immunocompetent. Following the acute primary infection, HHV-6 remains latent in lymphocytes and monocytes and has been found in low levels in many tissues. The HHV-6 virus is a major cause of morbidity and mortality in patients who are immunosuppressed, particularly in patients with AIDS and in those who are transplant recipients.

Predisposing Factors
A. Spring and autumn are peak incidence periods.
B. Classic age: 9–12 months (age ranges from 2 weeks to 3 years).
C. Attendance at day-care centers.
D. Transplacental infection occurs in about 1% of cases.

Common Complaints
A. Primary infection with HHV-6 may be asymptomatic, or it may cause the exanthem subitum/roseola syndrome.
B. Child with high fever (up to 105°F) for several (1–3) days: **Abrupt onset of fever followed by rose-pink maculopapular rash with rapid resolution of both is characteristic of roseola. Rash appears after fever is resolved.**
C. Rosie pink rash on chest and body: Rash typically begins on the trunk or chest and spreads to the arms and neck, with mild involvement of face and legs; rash can last several hours to 2 days and fades quickly.
D. Characteristic enanthem (Nagayama spots) consists of erythematous papules on the mucosa of the soft palate and the base of the uvula (usually present on the 4th day).

Other Signs and Symptoms
A. Drowsiness.
B. Seizures (secondary to high fever).
C. Bulging anterior fontanelle (rare).
D. Encephalopathy (rare).
E. Irritability.
F. Gastroenteritis.
G. Patients who are immunocompromised may have malaise and CNS and other organ system involvement.

Subjective Data
A. Ask the parent or caregiver to describe the progression and color of the rash, onset, and duration of all symptoms.
B. Ask about the patient's temperature history and the treatments administered.
C. Review other symptoms such as coryza, cough, sore throat, and watery eyes (rules out roseola).
D. Review family history of others with similar symptoms.
E. Review the patient's history of febrile seizures.
F. Complete a drug history for possible allergic reaction.
G. Inquire regarding recent MMR immunization.

Physical Examination
A. Check temperature, pulse, respirations, and blood pressure.
B. Inspect.
   1. Inspect the skin.
   2. Observe the patient for seizure activity.
   3. Conduct an ear, nose, and throat exam to rule out otitis media.
C. Auscultate: Auscultate the heart and lungs.
D. Palpate.
   1. Palpate the head and fontanelle (if applicable).
   2. Palpate the neck and lymph nodes.
E. Neurologic examination: Check for nuchal rigidity.

Diagnostic Tests

A. None is required unless the diagnosis is unclear.
B. Rule out testing.
   1. CBC with differential
   2. Urinalysis and culture for UTI
   3. Chest radiograph for pneumonia
   4. Blood cultures
   5. Cerebrospinal fluid examination if indicated

Differential Diagnoses

When a child presents with a rash and still has a high fever, consider other diagnoses:

A. Roseola
B. Allergic reaction
C. Cytomegalovirus
D. Rocky Mountain spotted fever
E. Fifth disease (parvovirus)
F. Scarlet fever
G. Meningococcemia
H. Fever of unknown origin
I. Pneumonococcemia

Plan

A. General interventions
   1. Encourage the patient to drink fluids to prevent dehydration (Popsicles, Jell-O, clear fluids).
   2. Watch the patient for lethargy, decreased fluid intake, cough, and irritability.
B. Patient teaching: Treatment is supportive.
C. Pharmaceutical therapy:
   1. At present, no medical antiviral therapy is available for HHV-6 infection.
   2. Acetaminophen (Tylenol) as needed for fever.
   3. Acute or chronic antiseizure medications are not recommended for infants who have had a febrile seizure secondary to roseola.

Follow-up

A. None is required unless other problems occur; resolution is usually rapid.
B. **See the patient immediately for the following:**
   1. Twitching or other signs of seizure
   2. Refusal to drink liquids
   3. Loud and persistent crying, does not stop when consoled
   4. Listlessness and stiff neck

Consultation/Referral

A. Consult and/or refer the patient to a physician if febrile seizures/neurologic signs are present.

Individual Considerations

A. Pediatrics: Children with roseola are often playful without change in appetite, even with high fever.

◨ RUBELLA (GERMAN MEASLES)

Definition

A. Rubella, also known as German measles, is primarily known as a childhood disease. Rubella is considered one of the TORCH infections and is highly contagious. The disease is preventable by immunization. Passive immunity is acquired from birth to 6 months of age from maternal antibodies.

Incidence

A. Rubella is no longer endemic in the United States as a result of an intensive vaccination campaign. The Centers for Disease Control and Prevention (CDC) declared rubella to be eliminated from the United States in 2005. Incidence is unknown. Peak season for rubella is late winter and spring. Insulin dependent diabetes mellitus develops in up to 40% of individuals with congenital rubella infection and progressive encephalopathy has been observed.

Pathogenesis

A. Rubella virus is an enveloped, positive-stranded RNA virus classified as Rubivirus in the Togaviridae family. Humans are the only source of infection. The virus is spread by nasopharyngeal, airborne respiratory droplets, and transplacental routes.
B. The incubation period for postnatally acquired rubella ranges from 14–23 days (usually 16–18 days). It is communicable 1 week before and 4 days after rash and illness. The neonate born with congenital rubella is often highly infectious and should be isolated. Neonates may continue to shed the virus for 1 year or longer.

Predisposing Factors

A. Age 5–9 years
B. Transplacental transmission
C. Never received rubella vaccine
D. Attendance at schools and day-care centers
E. Compromised immune system

Common Complaints

A. Low grade fever.
B. Swollen glands: Posterior auricular, suboccipital, and posterior cervical lymphadenopathy is frequently present 24 hours before rash develops.
C. Rash: Light pink to red macular rash that starts on the face and moves down the body to the trunk. The facial rash clears as the extremity rash erupts. The macular lesions rapidly become papular lesions and fade in 3–4 days. Exanthematous lesions remain discrete and pink, in contrast with the rash of rubeola, which is deep red and becomes confluent (Koplik's spots). Exanthem of rubella is usually preceded by 1–5 days of prodrome symptoms and generally last 3 days, but may persist for as long as 5 days.

Other Signs and Symptoms

A. Headache
B. Sore throat
C. Mild coryza
D. Cough
E. Malaise
F. Conjunctivitis
G. Forchheimer spots in the soft palate
H. Transient polyarthralgia and polyarthritis (older children, adolescents, and women)
I. Itching

Subjective Data

A. Review the onset, duration, and course of symptoms.
B. Rule out similar symptoms in other family members.
C. Review the patient's immunization history (especially recent immunization of MMR).
D. Determine any new medications or contact exposures.
E. Review any history of rash and the course of spread.
F. Determine if the patient is pregnant.

Physical Examination

A. Check temperature, pulse, respirations, and blood pressure.
B. Inspect.
   1. Conduct an ear, nose, and throat exam.
   2. Inspect the mouth for Koplik's spots. Forchheimer spots are reddish spots on the soft palate seen during the prodrome or first day of the rash.
   3. Inspect the skin.
C. Auscultate: Auscultate the lungs and heart.
D. Palpate: Check the lymph nodes, especially the cervical chains.

Diagnostic Tests

A. Blood or urine:
   1. Latex agglutination
   2. Enzyme immunoassay (ELISA)
   3. Passive hemagglutination
   4. Fluorescent immunoassay tests
B. Rubella titer (test initially and repeat 2–4 weeks after exposure)

Serologic rubella titer less than 8 indicates nonimmunity. Rubella titer of greater than 1:32 indicates immunity from a past infection. A fourfold rise in the titer (about 2 weeks after exposure) indicates infection.

C. Pregnancy test if indicated
D. Tissue culture of throat

Differential Diagnoses

A. Rubella (German measles)
B. Rubeola
C. Parvovirus
D. Scarlet fever
E. Allergic reaction, contact dermatitis
F. Roseola

Plan

A. General interventions
   1. Primary prevention is through immunization.
   2. Vaccinating adolescents and adults in college reduces the chance of outbreaks and helps to prevent congenital rubella syndrome.
   3. Generally, the course is mild; however, rest is encouraged.
   4. Treatment is supportive. Have the patient increase oral fluid intake.
   5. Reinforce respiratory and nasal discharge precautions; encourage good hand washing.
   6. Immunize patients preconceptually; advise them to use a method of birth control for 3 months after immunization.
   7. **Rubella cases should be reported to the local health department.**

B. Patient teaching
   1. Patient/children should not to return to work or school for 7 days after the onset of the rash.
   2. Pregnant patients with documented rubella infection should be counseled about the risk of fetal infection and/or compromise.
   3. Children with congenital rubella should be considered contagious until they are at least 1 year of age, unless nasopharyngeal and urine culture are negatively consecutively for rubella virus; infection control precautions should be considered in children up to 3 years of age who are hospitalized for congenital cataract extraction.

C. Pharmaceutical therapy
   1. Acetaminophen (Tylenol) for fever and headache.
   2. Antihistamines: diphenhydramine (Benadryl) for pruritis.
   3. Limited data indicate that intramuscular immune globulin (IG) in a dose of 0.55 ml/kg may decrease clinically apparent shedding and the rate of viremia significantly in exposed susceptible people. The absence of clinical signs in a woman who has received intramuscular IG does not guarantee that infant infection is prevented. The CDC recommends limiting the use of immune globulin to women with known rubella exposure who decline pregnancy termination.
   4. Live-virus rubella vaccine administered within 3 days of exposure has not been demonstrated to prevent illness.
   5. Glucocorticoids, platelet transfusion, and other supportive measures are reserved for patients with complications such as thrombocytopenia or encephalopathy.

Follow-up

A. The disease is self-limiting and has no sequelae (except congenital exposure).
B. Repeat titer 3–4 weeks after exposure.

Consultation/Referral

A. Refer the patient to an obstetrician if the patient is pregnant.

Individual Considerations

A. Pregnancy
   1. Rubella infection has few consequences for an adult, but it presents significant problems for a fetus. Rubella's viral teratogenic effects include cardiovascular malformation, deafness, mental retardation, cataracts, glaucoma, microcephaly, and microphthalmos.
   2. If maternal infection is during the first trimester, 50% of the fetuses infected may abort or have complications. Approximately 30%–50% of fetuses who acquire rubella in the first month of gestation suffer cardiac anomalies. Neural deafness is a common sequela when infection occurs in the second gestational month.
   3. The rubella vaccine is a live, attenuated virus; therefore, it is not safe to give in pregnancy. Immunization may be given postpartum; instruct the patient to avoid

pregnancy for the next 3 months. The rubella vaccine may be given to a woman if she is breast-feeding.

4. Routine prenatal screening for rubella immunity should be undertaken. If a woman is found to be susceptible, the rubella vaccine should be administered during the immediate postpartum period before discharge.

5. Breast-feeding is not a contraindication to postpartum immunization of the mother.

B. Pediatrics

1. The infected neonate must be kept in isolation in the nursery. The neonate may continue to spread the virus for 1 year or longer.

2. Cardiac and eye defects are most frequent when maternal infection occurs before 8 weeks' gestation; hearing loss and growth retardation are observed in maternal infections up to 16 weeks' gestation.

3. Other reported abnormalities include jaundice, hepatosplenomegaly, and thrombocytopenia and dermal erythropoiesis (blueberry muffin lesions).

4. The Advisory Committee on Immunization Practices (ACIP) currently recommends that all children receive two doses of MMR vaccine, separated by at least 28 days, administered on or after the first birthday.

RUBEOLA (RED MEASLES, OR 7-DAY MEASLES)

Definition

A. Rubeola (red measles), also known as hard measles, is a highly communicable viral disease. The disease is preventable by immunization. Passive immunity is acquired from birth to between 4–6 months of age if the mother is immune before pregnancy. Immunity after measles infection is thought to be lifelong.

Incidence

A. Incidence is unknown; widespread measles vaccination has led to its virtual disappearance in the United States.

B. In temperate areas, the peak incidence of infection occurs during late winter and spring.

C. About 5% of all measles cases are due to vaccine failure.

D. There is an increased incidence in two populations: children <5 years of age and college students who have not been immunized.

E. Internationally, approximately 30 million measles cases are reported annually. The U.S. immunization program resulted in a decrease of more than 99% in reported incidence.

F. Rubeola is rarely encountered in pregnancy; however, the reported mortality of congenital measles is 32%.

G. Patients with defects in cell-mediated immunity (AIDS, lymphoma, or other malignancies) are at risk for severe, progressive measles infection.

H. A generalized immunosuppression that follows measles frequently predisposes patients to complications such as otitis media and bronchopneumonia. Laryngotracheobronchitis (croup), and diarrhea occur more commonly in young children. Two rare neurologic syndromes are

associated with measles: acute disseminated encephalomyelitis (ADEM) may occur soon after the initial clinical manifestations of measles has resolved; and subacute sclerosing panencephalitis (SSPE) presents 7 to 10 years after initial infection.

Pathogenesis

A. Paramyxovirus (an RNA virus) is the causative agent and is spread by respiratory droplet, direct skin contact, or transplacental passage. The incubation period lasts 10–14 days from exposure to onset. It is communicable a few days before fever to 4 days after rash appears. The measles virus replicates locally, spreads to regional lymphatic tissues, and is then thought to disseminate to other reticuloendothelial sites via the bloodstream.

Predisposing Factors

A. Age less than 5 years and not immunized.

B. Schools: College age and not immunized with two doses. In 1989, the United States adopted a two-dose strategy; revaccination with measles, mumps, and rubella (MMR) vaccine is recommended for all students and their siblings.

C. Late winter and early spring time.

D. Transplacental passage; presents clinically in the first 10 days of life.

E. Crowded living conditions.

F. Measles has been attributed to poor nutritional status and Vitamin A deficiency.

Common Complaints

A. Suspected case: febrile illness accompanied by a rash.

B. Clinical case: **The patient is usually very ill with a fever and the three Cs: cough, coryza, and conjunctivitis. The patient generally recovers rapidly after the first 3–4 days.**

1. Fever greater than 101°F and often exceeding 104°F.

2. Respiratory symptoms: coryza and cough. The cough may persist for 1–2 weeks after the measles infection.

3. Conjunctivitis.

C. Rash: **Macular rash develops on the face and neck; then lesions become maculopapular and spread to the trunk and extremities in 24–48 hours. The rash may appear red brown or purple red at the hairline. The rash lasts 4–7 days.**

D. Koplik's spots on buccal mucosa: Koplik's spots are pathognomonic for measles. Bluish-gray specks or "grains of sand" on a red base.

E. Probable case: meets clinical case definition but is not linked epidemiologically to a confirmed case and lacks serologic or virologic proof of disease.

F. Confirmed case meets the laboratory criteria for measles or meets the clinical case definition and is epidemiologically linked to a confirmed case.

Other Signs and Symptoms

A. Loss of appetite

B. Bronchitis

C. Photophobia

D. General lymphoid involvement

Subjective Data

A. Review the onset and duration of symptoms such as cough, conjunctivitis, coryza, and Koplik's spots.

B. Rule out similar symptoms in other family members.
C. Review the patient's immunization history.
D. Determine any new medications or contact exposures.
E. Review any history of rash and the course of spread.
F. Elicit the presence of chest pain, ear pain, and confusion (signs of complications).
G. Determine if the patient is pregnant.
H. Review the patient's history of tick bite (recent camping, hiking, and so forth).

Physical Examination

A. Check temperature, pulse, respirations, and blood pressure.
B. Inspect.
  1. Conduct a dermal exam.
  2. Conduct an ear, nose, and throat exam.
  3. Examine the mouth for Koplik's spots; they appear on buccal mucosa within 12 hours. Koplik's spots are tiny (1–3 mm) bluish-white spots on an erythematous base that cluster adjacent to the molars on the buccal mucosa. Koplik's spots often begin to slough when the exanthem appears.
  4. The characteristic rash is maculopapular and blanches; it begins on the face and spreads centrifugally to involve the neck, upper trunk, lower trunk, and extremities. The lesions may become confluent, especially in the face where the rash develops first. The palms and soles of the feet are rarely involved.
C. Auscultate: Auscultate the lungs and heart.
D. Palpate: Palpate the neck and lymph nodes: generalized lymphadenopathy and splenomegaly are uncommon.
E. Neurologic exam:
  1. Check for nuchal rigidity.
  2. Complete a mental status exam.

Diagnostic Tests

A. Serologic procedures are not routinely done; however, leukopenia and T-cell cytopenia often occurs and thrombocytopenia may also been seen.
B. Antibody titer at the onset of the rash; repeat antibody titer every 3–4 weeks.
  1. Rubeola IgG and IgM antibody levels. The World Health Organization (WHO) has recommended the diagnosis of measles be confirmed with laboratory testing.
  2. Serum IgM alone is the standard test to confirm the diagnosis of measles. At least a fourfold increase in antimeasles antibody titer is indicative of infection.
C. Chest X-ray if indicated: may show interstitial pneumonitis.

Differential Diagnoses

A. Rubeola (red, or 7-day, measles).
B. During the prodomal period measles may resemble a common cold, except a fever is present.
C. Rubella (German measles).
D. Roseola (exanthem subitum).
E. Rocky Mountain spotted fever.
F. Scarlet fever.
G. Mononucleosis.
H. Drug reaction.

I. Kawasaki disease.
J. Parvovirus B19.
K. Toxic shock syndrome.

Plan

A. General interventions
  1. Primary prevention is through immunization.
    a. **Rubeola cases should be reported to the local health department since one case is considered an outbreak.**
    b. In order for vaccination to be considered adequate for school outbreaks, two doses of measles vaccine must have been administered after the age of 12 months and separated by at least 28 days.
    c. Those who are properly vaccinated may reenter school immediately after vaccination.
  2. Encourage the patient to rest.
  3. The patient must be isolated 4 days from the onset of the rash, up to 21 days.
  4. Encourage respiratory and nasal discharge precautions.
  5. There is no specific treatment for rubeola; however, otitis media and pneumonia both due to bacterial superinfection should be treated with appropriate antibiotics.
  6. Monitor the patient for signs of complications.
B. Patient teaching
  1. Tell the patient to avoid bright lights with photophobia; may need sunglasses.
  2. Reinforce the need to comply with immunization schedule.
C. Pharmaceutical therapy
  1. Vitamin A is recommended by the World Health Organization and UNICEF to all children with measles in areas where vitamin A deficiency is prevalent or where the mortality from measles exceeds 1 percent.
    a. For children 6 months to 12 months, 100,000 IU (50,000 IU/mL) in a single dose. This high dose may be associated with vomiting and headache for a few hours.
    b. For children 1 year and older, 200,000 IU (50,000 IU/mL) in a single dose. The higher dose may be associated with vomiting and headache for a few hours.
    c. For children with ophthalmologic evidence of vitamin A deficiency, the vitamin A dosage should be repeated on day 2 and day 28.
  2. Treatment for exposed persons:
    a. Give live measles vaccine if exposure was within 72 hours. Dose is 0.5 mL by subcutaneous injection in the outer aspect of the upper arm.
    b. Give immunoglobulin 0.25 mL/kg/dose (0.5 mL/kg for patients with HIV); by intramuscular injection (maximum dose is 15 mL) to induce passive immunity and to prevent or modify symptoms within 6 days of exposure. If immune globulin dose exceeds 10 mL, divide dose into several muscle sites to reduce local pain.
      i. **Do not give immunoglobulin with the live measles vaccine.**

c. Immunoglobulin is especially indicated for susceptible persons in the household, pregnant women, immunocompromised persons, and children under 1 year of age.

d. Measles is susceptible to ribavirin in vitro; however, further studies are clearly need to determine whether or not this treatment should be recommended.

3. Live measles virus vaccine should be given (except in pregnant women) approximately 3 months after immunoglobulin administration as long as they are at least 15 months of age at that time and there is no contraindication to vaccination.

4. Children and adolescents with symptomatic HIV infection who are exposed to measles should receive immunoglobulin (IG) 0.5 mL/kg regardless of vaccination status.

5. Exposure to measles is not a contraindication to vaccination. Available data suggest that live measles virus vaccine, if given within 72 hours of measles exposure, provides protection in some cases. If the exposure does not result in infection, the vaccine should induce protection against subsequent measles infection.

Follow-up

A. See the patient daily for mental status exam and examination of chest to rule out complications such as encephalitis and pneumonia.

B. Follow-up is needed 3–4 days after onset of exanthem.

C. Investigate immune status of family and other immediate contacts; prescribe vaccine if necessary.

Consultation/Referral

A. Refer the patient to a physician if fever lasts over 4 days; it is indicative of complications. Hospitalization may be indicated for treatment of measles complications (e.g., bacterial superinfection, pneumonia, dehydration, or croup).

Individual Considerations

A. General

1. A history of anaphylaxis after ingestion of gelatin is associated with an increased risk of anaphylaxis from the MMR or measles vaccine. This history should warrant a skin test for gelatin allergy.

2. Individuals with anaphylaxis, excluding contact dermatitis, from neomycin should not receive these vaccines because they contain a small amount of this antibiotic.

3. A history of anaphylaxis after egg ingestion is **not** a contraindication to measles immunization.

B. Pregnancy

1. Susceptible pregnant women who are exposed to rubeola should receive the immunoglobulin (see "Pharmaceutical Therapy" section) in an attempt to modify or prevent the infection.

2. Although no increase in risk of birth defects has been observed in mothers who were given live measles or MMR vaccine during pregnancy, there is a theoretical risk of such events. Measles vaccine is a live attenuated vaccine and is contraindicated in pregnancy.

3. Measles in the mother during delivery does not necessarily lead to measles in the neonate. Congenital measles (defined by the appearance of the measles rash within 10 days of birth) and postnatally acquired measles (rash appears 14–30 days of birth) have been associated with a spectrum of illness ranging from mild to severe disease.

4. Measles vaccine may be administered postpartum to nonimmune mothers.

C. Pediatrics

1. Immunoglobulin 0.25 mL/kg should be given to infants delivered from mothers with measles in the last of week of pregnancy or the first postpartum week.

2. Children without evidence of measles immunity are recommended not to be admitted to school until the first dose of MMR has been administered.

3. A childhood maintenance visit between ages 11–12 years is recommended to update vaccinations.

4. Concern has been raised periodically about the possible link between receipt of MMR and autism. A number of studies have now been performed that fail to demonstrate any such association.

5. Pediatric immunization.

a. Children older than 6 months: 1.5 mL in the outer aspect of the upper arm. Trivalent measles-mumps-rubella (MMR) vaccine should be used unless contraindicationed in adults and children older than 12 months of age.

SCARLET FEVER (SCARLATINA)

Definition

A. Scarlet fever is an acute infectious disease with vascular response to bacterial exotoxin usually associated with Group A beta-hemolytic streptococcal pharyngitis. Scarlatina may be present with pharyngitis. Development of the scarlet fever rash requires prior exposure to S. pyogenes. Scarlet fever was previously known as Scarlatina in older literature references.

Incidence

A. Scarlet fever is uncommon in children under the age of 2 years. Highest incidence is in children 4–8 years of age. By the time children are 10 years old, 80% have developed lifelong protective antibodies against streptococcal pryogenic exotoxins.

Pathogenesis

A. Group A hemolytic streptococcus and some strains of staphylococcus are spread by respiratory droplet means and occasionally by direct physical contact from infected wounds, skin, or burns.

B. The incubation period is 1–4 days. It is communicable during the incubation period and clinical illness (around 10 days) and no longer infectious after 24 hours of antibiotic therapy.

C. Exotoxin-mediated streptococcal infections range from localized skin disorders (e.g., bullous impetigo) to the systemic rash of scarlet fever to the uncommon but highly lethal streptococcal toxic shock syndrome.

Predisposing Factors
A. Strep throat pharyngitis; family history of recurrent strep infections
B. Direct physical contact with sputum or infected skin
C. Crowded situations (e.g., schools, institutional settings) or unsanitary living conditions

Common Complaints
A. Abrupt onset of fever
B. Headache
C. Sore throat
D. Bright red rash
E. Nausea and vomiting

Other Signs and Symptoms
A. **Day 1:** High fever (as high as 103°F–104° F), red sore throat, swollen tonsils (may have exudate), enlarged lymph nodes in neck, cough, and vomiting. Fever peaks by the second day and gradually returns to normal in 5–7 days. Fever abates within 12–24 hours after initiation of antibiotic therapy.
B. **Day 2:** The characteristic rash appears 12–48 hours after onset of fever. Bright red rash on the face, except around the mouth. **Bright red rash blanches on pressure, has rough sandpaper texture, and appears first on flexor surfaces then rapidly becomes more generalized. The rash lasts 4–10 days followed by desquamation of the hands and feet that disappears by the end of 3 weeks. Rash is typically present on the face, which usually has a flushed appearance with circumoral pallor. The rash is most marked in the skin folds. The rash often exhibits a linear petechial character in the antecubital fossae and axillary folds, known as Pastia's lines.**
C. **Day 3:**
   1. Strawberry tongue; rash on the body increases, spreads to neck, chest, back, then the entire body.
   2. Strawberry tongue appears as a thick white coat with hypertrophied red papillae 24–48 hours after infection.
D. **Days 4–5:** The white coating disappears from the tongue.
E. **Day 6:** Rash fades, and skin begins to peel; continues for 10–14 days; the palms of the hands and the soles of the feet are usually spared.

Subjective Data
A. Ask the patient about the onset and progression of the rash, its color and duration, and all other symptoms.
B. Review other symptoms related to complications, such as ear pain, chest pain, and edema.
C. Review family history and possible contact with infected wounds or others with similar symptoms of pharyngitis.
D. Determine any new medications or contact exposures.
E. Determine if the patient is allergic to penicillin.
F. Review patient's recent history of impetigo.

Physical Examination
A. Check temperature, pulse, respirations, and blood pressure.
B. Inspect.
   1. Conduct an ear, nose, throat exam.
   2. Inspect the mouth
      a. Exudative tonsillitis preceding scarlet fever is often accompanied by erythematous oral mucous membranes, along with petechiae and punctuate red macules on the hard and soft palate and uvula (i.e., Forchheimer spots).
      b. Day 1 or 2, a white coating covers the dorsum of the tongue with reddened papillae projecting through: white strawberry tongue.
      c. Distinctive facial finding: circumoral pallor.
   3. Inspect the skin; note the texture of the rash. The rash is most marked in the skin folds of the inguinal, axillary, antecubital, and abdominal areas and about pressure points.
C. Auscultate: Auscultate the heart and lungs.
D. Palpate.
   1. Palpate the abdomen for organomegaly.
   2. Palpate lymph nodes in the neck.

Diagnostic Tests
A. Throat culture remains the criterion standard for confirmation of Group A streptococcal upper respiratory infection. Vigorously swab the posterior pharynx, tonsils, and any exudates with a cotton or Dacron swab under strong illumination; avoid the lips, tongue, and buccal mucosa.
B. Rapid antigen detection testing (RADT) strep throat swab.
C. White blood count (WBC) in scarlet fever may increase to 12,000–16,000 per mm³, with a differential up to 955 polymorphonuclear lymphocytes.

Differential Diagnoses
A. Scarlet fever: staphylococcal scarlet fever can be differentiated from streptococcal scarlet fever in the following ways:
   1. There is no circumoral pallor or strawberry tongue with staphylococcal scarlet fever.
   2. The erythematous skin is often painful or tender with staphylococcal infection.
   3. Desquamation of the superficial epidermis occurs as with the streptococcal illness; if the superficial skin separates and sloughs after only a few days, the patient should be classified as having scalded skin syndrome. Desquamation, one of the most distinctive features of scarlet fever, begins 7–10 days after the resolution of the rash and may continue up to 6 weeks.
B. Kawasaki disease: Kawasaki disease needs to be carefully differentiated from scarlet fever; Kawasaki disease has additional signs of conjunctivitis, cracking lips, and diarrhea.
C. Rubeola.
D. Rubella.
E. Toxic shock syndrome.
F. Drug reaction.

Plan
A. General interventions.
   1. Have the patient rest with no work or school. Infection is contagious for 24 hours after antibiotic therapy is begun.

2. Prepare the patient for skin desquamation.
3. Throat cultures on other household members may be necessary.
4. Acetaminophen (Tylenol) for temperature and pain relief.

B. Patient teaching: Reinforce the need to comply with full antibiotic treatment.

C. Pharmaceutical therapy.
1. Tetracyclines and sulfonamides should not be used.
2. Drug of choice for streptococcal infections is penicillin by mouth or intramuscular injection. Erythromycin may be substituted for patients with penicillin allergies.
    a. Adults:
        i. Penicillin V (Pen-Vee K): 250 mg orally three or four times daily for 10 days.
        ii. Penicillin G benzathine (Bicillin L-A): 1.2 million units by IM injection in one dose.
        iii. Erythromycin (EES, E-mycin or Ery-Tab): 250 mg every 6 hours orally before meals, or 500 mg orally every 12 hours before meals for 10 days.
    b. Children:
        i. Children younger than 12 years: Penicillin V (Pen-Vee K) 25–50 mg/kg/day orally divided in three or four doses for 10 days; do not exceed 3 g/day.
        ii. Children older than 12 years: administer Penicillin V as adults.
        iii. Children less than 27 kg: Pencillin G benzathine 600,000 units IM as one dose.
        iv. Children greater than 27 kg: administer Pencillin G benzathine as in adults.
        v. Amoxicillin is often used in place of oral penicillin in children, since the taste of the oral suspension is more palatable. Administration of 50 mg/kg (maximum 1,000 mg) in a single dose orally for 10 days is effective as oral penicillin V or amoxicillin given in multiple times per day for 10 days. **However, strict adherence on once-daily dosing must be ensured.**
        vi. Erythromycin (E-mycin or Ery-Tab): 30–50 mg/kg four times a day for 10 days.

Follow-up

A. No follow-up is needed for patients with uncomplicated illnesses.

Consultation/Referral

A. Refer the patient to a physician, (i.e., ENT or infectious disease specialist) for complications, such as unresolved otitis media, sinusitis, bacteremia, rheumatic fever, and glomerulonephritis.

TOXOPLASMOSIS

Definition

A. Toxoplasmosis is caused by an intracellular protozoan parasite, Toxoplasma gondii. Cats are the primary host in which T. gondii can complete its reproductive cycle. Humans are the intermediate host. Toxoplasmosis is acquired through contact with infected cat feces, by eating raw or undercooked meat, and by eating soil-contaminated fruit or vegetables. In less developed countries, contaminated unfiltered water is an important source of infection, as well as by receiving a transfusion or organ transplantation from an infected donor (rare).

B. Emphasis should not be placed on prior exposure to cats, since patients can acquire toxoplasma without direct contact with felines. Toxoplasmosis is one of the TORCH infections. Toxoplasmosis causes CNS disease in patients with AIDS and has perinatal consequences. Latent infection can persist for the life of the host.

Incidence

A. Toxoplasmosis has a worldwide distribution. There is no association with cat ownership. The incidence of seropositivity in adults ranges from 9% (U.S.) to 85% (Europe). Adults most commonly acquire toxoplasmosis by environmental exposure, that is, ingestion of infectious oocysts usually from soil contamination with feline feces.

B. Once a person is infected, the parasite lies dormant in neural and muscle tissue and will never be eliminated. Approximately 50% of all pregnant women in the United States have been previously infected and are immune, whereas those who keep cats as pets have a higher seropositivity rate. The rate of primary infection during pregnancy ranges from 1–8 per 1,000. The greatest risk to the fetus is vertical transmission in the first trimester.

Pathogenesis

A. *Toxoplasma gondii* is the causative agent and an intracellular protozoan parasite. *T. gondii* is worldwide in distribution; cats, birds, and domesticated animals serve as reservoirs. *T. gondii* is recognized as a major cause of opportunistic infection in AIDS.

B. Routine screening for toxoplasmosis in pregnancy is not currently recommended. Maternal toxoplasmosis infection is acquired orally. Fetal infection results from transmission of parasites via placenta (vertical transmission).

Predisposing Factors

A. Eating raw or undercooked meats, especially mutton, lamb, and pork.

B. Exposure to contaminated soil or garden, kitty litter, and cats.

C. AIDS.

D. *T. gondii* has been documented as being acquired from blood or blood product transfusion and organ (i.e., heart) or bone marrow transplant from a seropositive donor with latent infection.

Common Complaints

A. 80%–90% of acute T. gondii infectious hosts are asymptomatic.

B. Bilateral, symmetrical, nontender cervical adenopathy.

C. 30% of symptomatic patients have generalized lymphadenopathy.

Other Signs and Symptoms

A. Usually subclinical infection
1. Fever
2. Arthralgia, malaise, and myalgia

3. Headache
4. Sore throat/pharyngitis
5. Skin rash: diffuse nonpruritic maculopapular rash
6. Hepatosplenomegaly
7. Chorioretinitis: Ocular pain and loss of visual acuity (most frequent, permanent manifestation of toxoplasmic infection)

B. Pregnancy.
1. Intrauterine growth restriction (IUGR) or low birth weight
2. Hydrocephaly
3. Microcephaly
4. Anemia

C. CNS toxoplasmosis
1. **Headache, dull and constant, is an almost universal symptom of cerebral lesions in AIDS patients.**
2. Fever.
3. Lethargy.
4. Altered mental state.
5. Seizures.
6. Weakness.
7. Hemiparesis.
8. Cranial nerve disturbances.
9. Sensory abnormalities.
10. Movement disorders.
11. Neuropsychiatric manifestations: Toxoplasmosis is a significant factor in the causation of mental retardation and blindness.

Subjective Data

A. Review onset, course, and duration of symptoms.
B. Determine if the patient is pregnant.
C. Review presence of indoor cat and contact with kitty litter.
D. Rule out other illness with review of symptoms such as pharyngitis (mononucleosis).
E. Elicit initial site of rash and progression to other body areas.
F. Determine any new medications and contact exposures.
G. Rule out other family members with similar symptoms.
H. Review HIV status.

Physical Examination

A. Check temperature, pulse, respirations, and blood pressure.
B. Inspect
1. Conduct ear, nose, and throat exam and careful funduscopic exam.

Funduscopic exam may reveal yellow-white areas of retinitis with fluffy borders. Diagnosis of ocular toxoplasmosis is based on observation of characteristic retinal lesions in conjunction with toxoplasma specific serum IgG or IgM antibodies.

2. Complete a dermal exam.
C. Auscultate: Auscultate lungs and heart.
D. Palpate.
1. Palpate all lymph nodes, especially cervical nodes. Lymph nodes are usually smaller than 3 cm in size and nonfluctuant.
2. Palpate the abdomen.
3. Palpate the joints.
E. Neurologic exam: Conduct a mental status evaluation.

Diagnostic Tests

A. Enzyme-linked immunosorbent assay (ELISA) is the most commonly employed due to overall performance and cost for Toxoplasmosis IgG and IgM antibody titer. Maternal infections usually are confirmed by a fourfold rise in the serum IgG.
B. Serial titers: no single level of IgG antibody can be used to determine the duration of the infection.
C. CBC with differential.
D. HIV (rule out).
E. Pregnancy test if indicated.
F. Culture: Tissue smears, tissue section, and body fluids for presence of *T. gondii* may be considered in neonates. It takes 3–6 weeks to confirm the diagnosis.
G. CT scan or MRI (usually superior to CT scan).

Differential Diagnoses

A. Toxoplasmosis
B. Epstein-Barr virus
C. CMV (CMV retinitis)
D. Cat scratch disease
E. Tuberculosis
F. Syphilis
G. Sarcoidosis
H. Hodgkin's disease
I. Lymphoma
J. Viral syndrome
K. HIV
L. Mononucleosis
M. *Pneumocystis carinii* pneumonia (PCP)
N. Varicella-zoster
O. Fungal infection of eye

Plan

A. Patient teaching: See the Section III Patient Teaching Guide for this chapter, "Prevention of Toxoplasmosis."
B. Pharmaceutical therapy.
1. Treatment is rarely necessary since most clinical illness resolved spontaneously; the exception is during pregnancy.
2. Treatment is usually given for 2–4 weeks.
a. Nonpregnant adults: one of two regimens is typically prescribed:
i. Pyrimethamine: 100 mg loading dose then 25–50 mg by mouth daily; *plus* Sulfadiazine 2–4 gm/day by mouth in divided doses; *plus* Leucovorin calcium (folinic acid) 10–25 mg by mouth daily.
ii. Pyrimethamine: 100 mg loading dose then 25–50 mg by mouth daily; *plus* Clindamycin 300 mg by mouth four times a day; *plus* Leucovorin calcium (folinic acid) 10–25 mg by mouth daily.
b. Pregnancy: Despite the lack of evidence of treatment efficacy, prenatal treatment is usually offered to pregnant women who are diagnosed with toxoplasmosis.
i. Spiramycin alone: 1 gm orally every 8 hours without food. The drug is available in the United States for use in pregnancy from

Rhone-Poulenc (Montreal, Quebec) if an Investigation New Drug (IND) number is obtained from the Food and Drug Administration (FDA) under the "compassionate use" pathway.

   ii. Three-week course of Pyrimethamine 50 mg once a day orally or 25 mg twice a day; *and* Sulfadiazine 3 gm/day orally divided in two or three doses; *alternating* with a 3-week course of Spiramycin 1 gm orally three times a day until delivery.

   iii. Pyrimethamine 25 mg once per day by mouth *and* sulfadiazine 4 g/day orally divided into 2–4 doses until term.

   iv. Leucovorin calcium (folinic acid) 10–25 mg/day orally is added during Pyrimethamine and Sulfadiazine administration to prevent bone marrow suppression.

c. Children:

   i. Trimethoprim-sufamethoxazole 150–750 mg/m^2/day in two divided doses daily.

   ii. For children 1 month of age or older: Dapsone 2 mg/kg (maximum of 25 mg, orally every day; *plus* Pyrimethamine 1 mg/kg, orally every day; *plus* Leucovorin 5 mg orally every 3 days).

d. Persons with compromised immune system:

   i. Trimethoprim 10 mg/kg/daily *plus* Sulfamethoxazole 50 mg/kg/daily by mouth. May be considered as a nonpyrimethamine alternative for AIDS patients if unable to tolerate usual adult therapy noted above.

   ii. **Administering dapsone with pyrimethamine appears to provide effective chemoprophylaxis in HIV patients seropositive for T. gondii who have CD4 cell counts lower than 200. However, rash, fever, and hemolytic anemia are common adverse effects, often necessitating cessation of therapy.**

   iii. For AIDS patients, after primary therapy, lifelong prophylaxis for recurrence of toxoplasmosis is required for as long as they are immunosuppressed.

Follow-up

A. Follow up in 1 week to evaluate for secondary complications.

B. Pyrimethamine is a folic acid antagonist that can cause dose-related bone marrow suppression with resultant anemia, leukopenia, and thrombocytopenia. Sulfadiazine is another folic acid antagonist, works synergistically with Pyrimethamine, and can cause bone marrow suppression and reversible acute renal failure. Patients should return for laboratory monitoring (CBC and platelet counts) weekly.

Consultation/Referral

A. Consultation is needed for all patients; comanage with a physician.

B. Refer the patient to an obstetrician if she is pregnant.

C. Ophthalmologist-medication recommendation depends on the size of the eye lesion, the location, and the characteristics of the lesion (active acute versus chronic not progressing).

Individual Considerations

A. Pregnancy

1. Routine prenatal screening is not standard of care secondary to costs. Many women have antibodies prior to pregnancy that protect the fetus.

2. Transplacental infection increases the incidence of first trimester spontaneous abortion, intrauterine growth retardation, preterm birth, neonatal anomalies, and stillbirth.

3. Pyrimethamine is a folic acid antagonist and should not be given in the first trimester.

4. Sulfadiazine should not be given in the third trimester secondary to the increased incidence of jaundice in the neonate.

B. Pediatrics

1. 70%–90% of affected infants with congenital infection may be asymptomatic at birth or may present with low birth weight, enlarged liver and spleen, jaundice, and anemia.

   a. Signs of congenital toxoplasmosis at birth can include maculopapular rash, generalized lymphadenopathy, hepatomegaly, splenomegaly, jaundice, and thrombocytopenia.

   b. Cerebral calcifications may be demonstrated by radiography, ultrasound, or CT of the head.

   c. Characteristic retinal lesions (chorioretinitis) develop in up to 85% of young adults after untreated congenital infection. Acute ocular involvement manifests as blurred vision.

   d. Ocular disease can become reactivated years after the initial infection in health and immunocompromised people.

2. Complications including visual impairment from chorioretinitis or learning disabilities or mental retardation damage may develop several years later.

3. Treatment consists of drug therapy for the first year of life (see "Pharmaceutical Therapy"), which appears to limit further central nervous system injury but does not reverse the prenatal damage already sustained by the neonate.

4. Corticosteroids also may be administered to infants with chorioretinitis.

C. AIDS patients

1. Patients with AIDS who have antibodies to *T. gondii* and a CD4 count of 100 cells/mm^3 should be considered at high risk for development of clinical disease. Reactivation of latent infection in the CNS is a common HIV- and AIDS-related complication.

2. Patients with a CD4 count less than 100 cells/mm^3 should receive prophylaxis against toxoplasmosis.

3. The use of serology in HIV-infected patients is mainly to identify those at risk for developing toxoplasmosis. Therefore, all HIV-positive patients should be tested for the presence of IgG antibodies.

VARICELLA (CHICKENPOX)

Definition

A. Varicella, commonly called chickenpox, is a viral disease with a vesicular rash that occurs in crops. It manifests as a generalized, pruritic, vesicular rash. Varicella-zoster virus (VZV) infection causes two clinically distinct forms of disease: varicella (chickenpox) and herpes zoster (shingles). Primary VZV results in the diffuse vesicular rash of chickenpox.

B. Varicella is considered one of the TORCH infections. Varicella infection can be fatal for an infant if the mother develops varicella from 5 days before to 2 days after delivery. A newborn is protected for several months from chickenpox if the mother had the disease prior to or during pregnancy. The immunity diminishes in 4–12 months.

Incidence

A. Infants are generally protected in the first few months through passive immunity. The peak incidence shifting from children younger than 10 years of age to children between 10 and 14 years of age demonstrates the highest incidence following the implementation of universal immunization in 1995. Varicella tends to be more severe in adolescents and adults. Hemorrhagic varicella is much more common among immunocompromised patients. Immunity is generally considered lifelong.

B. The rate of herpes zoster after varicella vaccination was 2.6/100,000 by 1998 CDC unpublished data. The incidence of herpes zoster after natural varicella infection among healthy children less than 20 years old is 68/100,000; for all ages the incidence is 215/100,000.

C. Seasonal incidence of VZV peaks in the months of March through May.

Pathogenesis

A. Varicella-zoster virus (VZV) is a herpes virus. Humans are the only source of infection for this highly contagious virus infecting over 90% of susceptible household contacts. Person-to-person transmission occurs primarily by direct contact with a patient with varicella or zoster, and it occasionally occurs by airborne droplet spread, from respiratory secretions spread onto the conjunctival or nasal/oral mucosal, and from direct contact with vesicular zoster lesions. In utero infections also occur from transplacental passage of the virus during maternal varicella infection.

B. The incubation period is 10–21 days. It is communicable 1 day to 1 week before macular eruption and until lesions crust over (about 1 week).

Predisposing Factors

A. Exposure to someone with the varicella virus:
   1. Direct contact with skin lesions or by respiratory tract secretions.
   2. Direct contact with patients with shingles can induce chickenpox in susceptible health care workers.

B. Compromised immune system.

C. Nosocomial transmission is well documented in pediatric units, but transmission is extremely rare in newborn nurseries.

D. Late winter and early spring.

Common Complaints

A. Low-grade fever.

B. Mild malaise.

C. Skin lesions or rash: Characteristic rash is pruritic, vesicular exanthem occurring in crops that begin on the head and neck and progress to involve the trunk and extremities. Blisters collapse within 24 hours to 1 week and crust over to form scabs. Skin eruptions appear almost anywhere on the body including the scalp; penis; and inside the mouth, nose, throat, and vagina.

D. Itching.

E. Myalgia 1–4 days before onset of rash.

Other Signs and Symptoms

A. Children may have a mild prodrome to bacterial infections.

B. Adults may develop varicella pneumonitis. (The risk of pneumonitis is higher in smokers than nonsmokers.)

C. Cough.

D. Headache.

E. Respiratory symptoms: cough and chest discomfort. Respiratory symptoms usually develop shortly after cutaneous eruption. Respiratory failure in pregnancy can be rapid.

F. Abdominal pain lasting 1–2 days.

Subjective Data

A. Review the onset, duration, and course of symptoms.

B. Elicit exposure information when noting characteristic rash, when it started, spread of the rash or lesions, and characteristic changes.

C. Review any pulmonary or nervous system problems that occur as complications.

D. Determine if the person has HIV, is immunocompromised, or is pregnant.

E. Determine caregiver's immunity status to varicella.

Physical Examination

A. Check temperature, pulse, respirations, and blood pressure.

B. Inspect.
   1. Conduct a dermal exam, especially hairline.
   2. Inspect the buccal mucosa.
   3. Conduct an ear, nose, and throat exam, and a detailed eye exam.
   4. Shingles: note location of lesions; usually involves only one to three dermatomes.

C. Auscultate: Auscultate the heart and lungs.

D. Palpate: Palpate the neck and lymph nodes.

Diagnostic Tests

A. Diagnosis is usually determined by the appearance of the skin eruptions, and laboratory tests are not necessary.

B. ELISA.

C. Tissue culture of vesicular fluid or tissue biopsy (requires up to a week for result).

D. Varicella IgG and IgM: VZV-specific IgM is present within 5 days of onset of the rash and lasts 4–5 weeks. A significant increase in varicella IgG antibody by standard serologic assay can confirm a diagnosis retrospectively. These antibody tests are not as reliable in immunocompromised people.

E. Pregnancy test if indicated; if positive, order the following:
   1. Anti-VZV IgG to establish immunity
   2. Tzanck smear of suspicious lesions
   3. Culture lesion for herpes simplex
F. PCR of vesicular swabs or scrapings, scabs for crusted lesions, or tissue biopsy.

Differential Diagnoses

A. Varicella, or chickenpox
B. Herpes simplex
C. Scabies
D. Impetigo
E. Coxsackievirus
F. Insect or spider bite
G. Drug reaction
H. Secondary syphilis

Plan

A. General interventions
   1. Avoid contact with persons infected with chickenpox. Patients with varicella should avoid contact with others. Health care workers should be immune to varicella. Determine immunity status with varicella IgG antibody titer if status unknown.
   2. Strict isolation should be enforced. Varicella is contagious 1 week before outbreak and until the lesions crust over (about 1 week). Isolation is a precaution until the vesicles dry.
   3. Oatmeal baths (Aveeno) for comfort. Spray starch may also be sprayed on lesions to assist with severe itching.
B. Patient teaching
   1. See the Section III Patient Teaching Guide for this chapter, "Chickenpox (Varicella)."
   2. Lesions that can be covered pose little risk to a susceptible person because transmission usually occurs from direct contact with the fluid from the lesion. Clothing or a dressing should cover lesions until they have crusted.
   3. Scarring can occur from secondary infection of lesions; encourage good hand washing and no scratching.
C. Pharmaceutical therapy
   1. Acetaminophen (Tylenol) as needed for fever. No aspirin products should be administered due to the potential for Reye's syndrome.
   2. Acyclovir therapy is **not** recommended routinely for treatment of uncomplicated varicella in otherwise healthy children.
   3. Acyclovir is recommended, if it can be initiated within the first 24 hours after the onset of rash, in the following groups:
      a. Otherwise healthy, nonpregnant individuals 13 years of age or older
      b. Children older than 12 months with a chronic cutaneous or pulmonary disorder, and those receiving long-term salicylate therapy
      c. Children receiving short, intermittent, or aerosolized course of corticosteroids (if possible, discontinue corticosteroids)

4. If therapy can be initiated within the first 24 hours of rash onset, prescribe oral acyclovir 20 mg/kg/dose in four divided doses for 5 days (maximum dose is 800 mg per dose four times daily); the usual dose for adults is 800 mg four times a day. **Patients on oral acyclovir should be well hydrated during therapy.**
5. Acyclovir by IV infusion is recommended for treatment of immunocompromised patients and patients with serious complications such as varicella pneumonia or encephalitis. Acyclovir IV dosage is 10 mg/kg every 8 hours for 7 days.
6. Varicella-zoster immune globulin is no longer available. The only manufacturer of this product has ceased production.
7. Systemic antipruritic: Diphenhydramine HCl (Benadryl).
   a. Adults: 25–50 mg every 4–6 hours (maximum adult dosage 300 mg/day).
   b. Children:
      i. Not recommended for neonates.
      ii. Children younger than 6 years of age: dosage must be individualized.
      iii. Children 6–12 years of age: 12.5–25 mg every 4–6 hours (maximum children dosage 150 mg/day).
8. Varicella vaccine may be given simultaneously with MMR vaccine, but separate syringes and injection sites must be used. If not given simultaneously, the interval between administration of varicella vaccine and MMR should be at least 1 month.
9. Antihistamines are helpful in the symptomatic treatment of pruritus.

Follow-up

A. No follow-up is necessary in uncomplicated cases.
B. Have the patient return to the office for any secondary skin infections, conjunctival involvement, CNS problems such as encephalitis and meningitis, or pneumonia.

Consultation/Referral

A. Refer the patient to a physician if pregnant; varicella pneumonia in pregnancy is a medical emergency.

Individual Considerations

A. Pregnancy
   1. Varicella vaccine should not be administered to pregnant women. A pregnant mother or household member is not a contraindication for immunization for a child in the household.
   2. When postpubertal females are immunized, pregnancy should be avoided for at least 1 month after immunization.
   3. Varicella-zoster immune globulin (VZIG): Maternal therapy's aim is to reduce maternal morbidity; whether it protects the fetus is unknown.
   4. Reporting by telephone of inadvertent immunization when the varicella-zoster-containing vaccine is given during pregnancy is encouraged: 1-800-986-8999 or via the Internet at www.merckpregnancyregistries.com/varivax.html.

5. Maternal complications of active varicella infection may include preterm labor, encephalitis, and varicella pneumonia. Mortality rate in gravid females is 10%. The profound maternal hypoxia that occurs in varicella pneumonia is associated with increased risk of spontaneous abortion and stillbirth.

6. Fetal complication of active varicella infection may include intrauterine growth retardation, limb reduction defects, and eye defects.

7. Acyclovir is a Category B drug based on Food and Drug Administration (FDA) Drug Classification in pregnancy. Intravenous Acyclovir is recommended for the pregnant patient with serious complications of varicella. VariZIG or IGIV can be used during pregnancy for susceptible women who are exposed to VZV.

B. Pediatrics

1. Varicella can develop between 1 and 16 days of life in infants born to mothers with active live varicella at delivery.

2. Neonates usually have no prodrome or mild signs and symptoms with slight malaise and low-grade fever. Neonatal varicella is a serious illness associated with up to 25% mortality rate. Complications include conjunctival involvement, secondary bacterial infection, viral pneumonia, encephalitis, aseptic meningitis, myelitis, Guillian-Barré syndrome, and Reye's syndrome.

3. Children entering day care facilities and schools should have received varicella vaccine or have evidence of immunity.

4. Children with varicella should not receive salicylates or salicylate-containing products due to the risk for Reye's syndrome.

5. Children with varicella who have been excluded from childcare may return when all lesions have dried and crusted.

C. Adults

1. Adult patients usually have a prodrome and more severe illness than children. Adults have 25% increased risk of mortality.

2. Shingles (reactivated chickenpox) appears as grouped vesicular lesions distributed in one to three sensory dermatomes, sometimes accompanied by pain localized to the area. Systemic symptoms are few.

3. A recommendation for varicella vaccination includes persons at high risk for exposure, which include adolescents and adults who live in households with children.

D. Immunocompromised: Intravenous antiviral therapy is recommended for immunocompromised patients, including patients being treated with chronic corticosteroids. Therapy initiated early in the course of illness, especially within 24 hours of rash onset, maximized efficacy. Oral Acyclovir should not be used to treat immunocompromised children with varicella because of poor bioavailabilty.

REFERENCES

Albrecht, M. A. (2009a, January 1). Epidemiology of varicella-zoster virus infection: Chickenpox. *UpToDate Online 16.3*. Retrieved June, 11 2009, from http://www.uptodate.com/online/content/topic.do?topicKey=viral_in/2110&selectedTitle=5-150&source=search_result

Albrecht, M. A. (2009b, January 1). Treatment of varicella-zoster virus infection: Chickenpox. *UpToDate Online 16.3*. Retrieved June, 11 2009, from http://www.uptodate.com/online/content/topic.do?topicKey=viral_in/6256&selectedTitle=10-150&source=search_result

American Academy of Pediatrics. (2009a). Cat-scratch disease (Bartonella henselae). In L. K. Pickering (Ed.), *Red Book: 2009 Report of the Committee on Infectious Diseases* (26th ed., pp. 249–250). Elk Grove Village, IL: Author. Retrieved June 27, 2009, from http://aapredbook.aappublications.org.proxy.library.vanderbilt.edu/cgi/content/full/2009/1/3.25

American Academy of Pediatrics. (2009b). Cytomegalovirus. In L. K. Pickering (Ed.), *Red Book: 2009 Report of the Committee on Infectious Diseases* (26th ed., p. 180). Elk Grove Village, IL: Author. Retrieved June 27, 2009, from http://aapredbook.aappublications.org.proxy.library.vanderbilt.edu/cgi/content/full/2009/1/2.10.2

American Academy of Pediatrics. (2009c). Cytomegalovirus infection. In L. K. Pickering (Ed.), *Red Book: 2009 Report of the Committee on Infectious Diseases* (26th ed., pp. 275–280). Elk Grove Village, IL: Author. Retrieved June 27, 2009, from http://aapredbook.aappublications.org.proxy.library.vanderbilt.edu/cgi/content/full/2009/1/3.35

American Academy of Pediatrics. (2009d). Group A streptococcal infections. In L. K. Pickering (Ed.), *Red Book: 2009 Report of the Committee on Infectious Diseases* (26th ed., pp. 173–174). Elk Grove Village, IL: Author. Retrieved July 19, 2009, from http://aapredbook.aappublications.org.proxy.library.vanderbilt.edu/cgi/content/full/2009/1/3.125

American Academy of Pediatrics. (2009e). Influenza. In L. K. Pickering (Ed.), *Red Book: 2009 Report of the Committee on Infectious Diseases* (26th ed., pp. 400–412). Elk Grove Village, IL: Author. Retrieved June 27, 2009, from http://aapredbook.aappublications.org.proxy.library.vanderbilt.edu/cgi/content/full/2009/1/3.64

American Academy of Pediatrics. (2009f). Kawasaki disease. In L. K. Pickering (Ed.), *Red Book: 2009 Report of the Committee on Infectious Diseases* (26th ed., pp. 413–418). Elk Grove Village, IL: Author. Retrieved June 27, 2009, from http://aapredbook.aappublications.org.proxy.library.vanderbilt.edu/cgi/content/full/2009/1/3.66

American Academy of Pediatrics. (2009g). Lyme disease (Lyme Borreliosis, Borrelia burgdorferi infection). In L. K. Pickering (Ed.), *Red Book: 2009 Report of the Committee on Infectious Diseases* (26th ed., pp. 430–435). Elk Grove Village, IL: Author. Retrieved June 27, 2009, from http://aapredbook.aappublications.org.proxy.library.vanderbilt.edu/cgi/content/full/2009/1/3.73

American Academy of Pediatrics. (2009h). Meningococcal infections. In L. K. Pickering (Ed.), *Red Book: 2009 Report of the Committee on Infectious Diseases* (26th ed., pp. 455–463). Elk Grove Village, IL: Author. Retrieved June 27, 2009, from http://aapredbook.aappublications.org.proxy.library.vanderbilt.edu/cgi/content/full/2009/1/3.78

American Academy of Pediatrics. (2009i). Parvovirus B19 (Erythema infectiosum, fifth disease). In L. K. Pickering (Ed.), *Red Book: 2009 Report of the Committee on Infectious Diseases* (26th ed., pp. 491–493). Elk Grove Village, IL: Author. Retrieved June 27, 2009, from http://aapredbook.aappublications.org.proxy.library.vanderbilt.edu/cgi/content/full/2009/1/3.92

American Academy of Pediatrics. (2009j). Prevention of tickborne infections. In L. K. Pickering (Ed.), *Red Book: 2009 Report of the Committee on Infectious Diseases* (26th ed., pp. 191–193). Elk Grove Village, IL: Author. Retrieved June 27, 2009, http://aapredbook.aappublications.org.proxy.library.vanderbilt.edu/cgi/content/full/2009/1/3.73

American Academy of Pediatrics. (2009k). Rocky Mountain spotted fever. In L. K. Pickering (Ed.), *Red Book: 2009 Report of the Committee on Infectious Diseases* (26th ed., pp. 573–575). Elk Grove Village, IL: Author. Retrieved June 27, 2009, from http://aapredbook.aappublications.org.proxy.library.vanderbilt.edu/cgi/content/full/2009/1/3.114

American Academy of Pediatrics. (2009l). Rubella. In L. K. Pickering (Ed.), *Red Book: 2009 Report of the Committee on Infectious Diseases*

(26th ed., pp. 579–584). Elk Grove Village, IL: Author. Retrieved June 27, 2009, from http://aapredbook.aappublications.org.proxy.library.vanderbilt.edu/cgi/content/full/2009/1/3.116

American Academy of Pediatrics. (2009m). *Toxoplasmosis Gondii* infections. In L. K. Pickering (Ed.), *Red Book: 2009 Report of the Committee on Infectious Diseases* (26th ed., pp. 593–596). Elk Grove Village, IL: Author. Retrieved July 5, 2009, from http://aapredbook.aappublications.org.proxy.library.vanderbilt.edu/cgi/content/full/2009/1/3.138

American Academy of Pediatrics. (2009n). Varicella-zoster infections. In L. K. Pickering (Ed.), *Red Book: 2009 Report of the Committee on Infectious Diseases* (26th ed., pp. 714–727). Elk Grove Village, IL: Author. Retrieved June 27, 2009, from http://aapredbook.aappublications.org.proxy.library.vanderbilt.edu/cgi/content/full/2009/1/3.150

American Heart Association. (n.d.). *Kawasaki disease: Signs, symptoms, and diagnosis.* Retrieved June 14, 2009, from http://www.americanheart.org/presenter.jhtml?identifier=984.

Aronson, M. D., & Auwaerter, P. G. (2009, January 1). Infectious mononucleosis in adults and adolescents. *UpToDate Online 16.3.* Retrieved July 27, 2009, from http://www.uptodate.com/online/content/topic.do?topicKey=viral_in/27361&selectedTitle=17-150&source=search_result

Baker, A. L., Minich, L. M., Atz, A. M., Klein, G., Korsin, R., Lambert, R., et al. (2008, April 10–12). *Associated symptoms at presentation in Kawasaki disease (KD).* Paper presented at the Ninth International Kawasaki Disease Symposium, Taipei, Taiwan. Abstract retrieved June 14, 2009, from http://www.americanheart.org/downloadable/heart/1208894314097Kawasaki%20Abstracts.pdf

Balentine, J., & Lombardi, D. P. (2009).Scarlet fever. *emedicine.* Retrieved July 19, 2009, from http://emedicine.medscape.com/article/785981-print

Barinaga, J. L., & Skolnik, P. R. (2009, January 1). Clinical presentation and diagnosis of measles. *UpToDate Online 16.3.* Retrieved June 11, 2009, from http://www.uptodate.com/online/content/topic.do?topicKey=global/4540&selectedTitle=1-150&source=search_result

Bekhor, D., Barinaga, J. L., & Skolnik, P. R. Prevention and treatment of measles. *UpToDate Online 16.3.* Retrieved June 11, 2009, from http://www.uptodate.com/online/content/topic.do?topicKey=global/2539&selectedTitle=3-150&source=search_result

Bronze, M. S. (2010, January 5). H1N1 influenza (swine flu). *emedicine.* Retrieved January 17, 2010, from http://emedicine.medscape.com/article/1673658-print

Centers for Disease Control and Prevention. (1999, May 28). Prevention of varicella updated recommendation of the Advisory Committee on Immunization Practices (ACIP). *MMWR Weekly, 48*(RR06), pp. 1–5. Retrieved July 5, 2009, from http://www.cdc.gov/mmwr/preview/mmwrhtml/rr4806a1.htm

Centers for Disease Control and Prevention. (2008, August 19). *Removing ticks.* Retrieved July 1, 2009, from http://www.cdc.gov/ticks/tick_removeal.html

Centers for Disease Control and Prevention. (2010, January 15). *2009 H1N1 flu.* Retrieved January 17, 2010, from http://www.cdc.gov/h1n1flu/

Centers for Disease Control and Prevention. (n.d.). *Influenza antiviral medications: Summary for clinicians.* Retrieved June 3, 2009, from http://www.cdc.gov/flu/professionals/

Centers for Disease Control and Prevention. (n.d.). *Seasonal influenza information for health professionals.* Retrieved June 1, 2009, from http://www.cdc.gov/flu/professionals/

Centers for Disease Control and Prevention. (n.d.). *Toxoplasmosis.* Retrieved July 14, 2009, from http://www.cdc.gov/toxoplasmosis/index.html

Chen, S.S.P., & Fennelly, G. F. (2009, June 10). Measles. *emedicine.* Retrieved July 19, 2009, from http://emedicine.medscape.com/article/966220-print

Demmler, G. J. (2009, January 1). *Cytomegalovirus infection and disease in newborns, infants, children, and adolescents.* Retrieved April 12, 2010, from http://www.uptodate.com/online/content/topic.do?topicKey=pedi_id/12521&selectedTitle=1-150&source=search_result

Dolin, R. (2009, January 13). Epidemiology of influenza. *UpToDate Online 16.3.* Retrieved June 1, 2009, from http://www.uptodate.com/online/content/topic.do?topicKey=pulm_inf/17274&selectedTitle=3-150&source=search_result

Ernst, D., & Lee, A. (Eds.). (Summer 2009). *NPPR: Nurse practitioners' prescribing reference.* New York: A Haymarket Media Publication.

Fekete, T., & Quagliarello, V. (2009, January 1). Treatment and prevention of bacterial meningitis in adults. *UpToDate Online 16.3.* Retrieved June 28, 2009, from http://www.uptodate.com/online/content/topic.do?topicKey=cns_infe/5161&view=print

Florin, T. A., Zaoutis, T. E., & Zaoutis, L. B. (2008). Beyond cat scratch disease: Widening spectrum of Bartonella henselae infection. *Pediatrics, 121,* e1413–e1425.

Friel, T. J. (2009, January 1). Diagnosis of Cytomegalovirus. *UpToDate Online 16.3.* Retrieved May 25, 2009, from http://www.uptodate.com/online/content/topic.do?topicKey=viral_in/16156

Gerber, M. A., Baltimore, R. S., Eaton, C. B., Gewitz, M., Rowley, A. H., Shulman, S. T., et al. (2009). Prevention of rheumatic fever and diagnosis and treatment of acute streptococcal pharyngitis: A scientific statement from the American Heart Association Rheumatic Fever, Endocarditis, and Kawasaki Disease Committee of the Council on Cardiovascular Disease in the Young, the Interdisciplinary Council on Functional Genomics and Translational Biology, and the Interdisciplinary Council on Quality of Care and Outcomes Research: Endorsed by the American Academy of Pediatrics. *Circulation, 119,* 1541–1551.

Gilbert, R., & Williams, K. (2009, January 1). Toxoplasmosis and pregnancy. *UpToDate Online 16.3.* Retrieved June 11, 2009, from http://www.uptodate.com/online/content/topic.do?topicKey=pregcomp/16134&selectedTitle=4-150&source=search_result

Hall, C. B. (2009, January 28). Influenza vaccination in children. *UpToDate Online 16.3.* Retrieved June 1, 2009, from http://www.uptodate.com/online/content/topic.do?topicKey=pedi_id/10944&selectedTitle=7-150&source=search_result

Hall, C. B. (2009, February 5). Clinical features and diagnosis of influenza in children. *UpToDate Online 16.3.* Retrieved June 1, 2009, from http://www.uptodate.com/online/content/topic.do?topicKey=pedi_id/14498&selectedTitle=2-150&source=search_result

Hay, C. M. (2009, January 1). Rubella. *UpToDate Online 16.3.* Retrieved June 11, 2009, from http://www.uptodate.com/online/content/topic.do?topicKey=viral_in/19982&selectedTitle=2-150&source=search_result

Heller, H. M. (2009, January 1). Toxoplasmosis in immunocompetent hosts. *UpToDate Online 16.3.* Retrieved June 11, 2009, from http://www.uptodate.com/online/content/topic.do?topicKey=parasite/18915&selectedTitle=3-150&source=search_result

Hibberd, P. L. (2009, January 15). Influenza vaccination in adults. *UpToDate Online 16.3.* Retrieved June 1, 2009, from http://www.uptodate.com/online/content/topic.do?topicKey=pulm_inf/17544&selectedTitle=6-150&source=search_result

Jani, A. A., & Kallen, A. J. (2009). Japanese Encephalitis. *emedicine.* Retreivied June 1, 2009, from http://emedicine.medscape.com/article/233802-print

Johnson, R. P., & Gluckman, S. J. (2009, February 11). Viral encephalitis in adults. *UpToDate Online 16.3.* Retrieved June 1, 2009, from http://www.uptodate.com/online/content/topic.do?topicKey=cns_infe/2236&view=print

Jordan, J. A. (2008, April 15). Clinical manifestations and pathogenesis of human parvovirus B19 infection. *UpToDate Online 16.3.* Retrieved June 11, 2009, from http://www.uptodate.com/online/content/topic.do?topicKey=viral_in/10455&selectedTitle=1-131&source=search_result

Jordan, J. E. (2008, September 24). Treatment and prevention of parvovirus B19 infection. *UpToDate Online 16.3.* Retrieved June 11, 2009, from http://www.uptodate.com/online/content/topic.do?topicKey=viral_in/4441&selectedTitle=2-131&source=search_result

Kawasaki Disease Foundation: http://www.kdfoundation.org/

Lawes, R. (2009). Cat scratch disease. *Nursing, 39,* 72.

Ledbetter, E. (2009). Quick care tips: Assessment and treatment of influenza. *Advance for Nurse Practitioners, 17,* 40.

Lexi-Comp. (n.d.). *Cytomegalovirus immune globulin (Intravenous-human): Patient drug information.* Lexi-Comp, Inc. 1978–2006.

Retrieved May 25, 2009, from http://www.uptodate.com/online/content/topic.do?topicKey=pat_drug/335306&selectedTitle=22~150&source=search_result

Mango, S. L., & Spatar, L. (2009). Cat scratch disease in primary care. *The Journal of Nurse Practitioners, 5,* 353–358.

MMWR Recommendations and Reports. (1989, February 17). *Current trend risks associated with human parvovirus B19 infection.* Centers for Disease Control and Prevention. Retrieved June 21, 2009, from http://www.cdc.gov/mmwr/preview/mmwrhtml/00001348.htm

MMWR Recommendations and Reports. (1993, January 8). *Inactivated Japanese encephalitis virus vaccine recommendations of the Advisory Committee on Immunization Practices. (ACIP).* Centers for Disease Control and Prevention. Retrieved June 20, 2009, from http://www.cdc.gov/mmwr/preview/mmwrhtml/00020599.htm

MMWR Weekly. (2005, July 22). *Disparities in universal prenatal screening for group B streptococcus—North Carolina, 2002–2003.* Centers for Disease Control and Prevention. Retrieved August 19, 2009, from http://www.cdc.gov/mmwr/preview/mmwrhtml/mm5428a3.htm

Nervi, S. J., Kapila, R., Ressner, R. A., Horvath, L. L., & Drayton, J. R. (n.d.). Catscratch disease. *emedicine.* Retrieved May 19, 2009, from http://emedicine.medscape.com/article/214100-overview

Newburger, J. W., Takahashi, M., Gerber, M. A., Gewitz, M. H., Tani, L. Y., Burns, J. C., et al. (2004). Diagnosis, treatment, and long-term management of Kawasaki disease: A statement for health professionals from the Committee on Rheumatic Fever, Endocarditis and Kawasaki Disease, Council on Cardiovascular Disease in the Young, American Heart Association. *Circulation, 110,* 2747–2771.

Pichichero, M. E. (2009a, January 1). Complications of streptococcal tonsillopharyngitis. *UpToDate Online 16.3.* Retrieved June 11, 2009, from http://www.uptodate.com/online/content/topic.do?topicKey=upp_resp/4610&selectedTitle=1~18&source=search_result

Pichichero, M. E. (2009b, January 1). Treatment and prevention of streptococcal tonsillopharyngitis. *UpToDate Online 16.3.* Retrieved July 19, 2009, from http://www.uptodate.com/online/content/topic.do?topicKey=upp_resp/5468&view=print

Rance, K. S. (2009). Influenza's widening scope: Dangers prompt broader vaccination. *Advances for Nurse Practitioners, 17,* 39–42, 57.

Riley, L. E. (2009a, January 1). Rubella in pregnancy. *UpToDate Online 16.3.* Retrieved June 11, 2009, from http://www.uptodate.com/online/content/topic.do?topicKey=viral_in/23790&selectedTitle=1~150&source=search_result

Riley, L. E. (2009b, January 1). Varicella-zoster virus infection in pregnancy. *UpToDate Online 16.3.* Retrieved June, 11 2009, from http://www.uptodate.com/online/content/topic.do?topicKey=viral_in/4765&selectedTitle=2~150&source=search_result

Riley, L. E., & Fernandes, C. J. (2008, December 16). Parvovirus B19 infection during pregnancy. *UpToDate Online 16.3.* Retrieved June 11, 2009, from http://www.uptodate.com/online/content/topic.do?topicKey=viral_in/12853&selectedTitle=3~131&source=search_result

Sexton, D. J. (2009a, January 1). Approach to the patient with chronic meningitis. *UpToDate Online 16.3.* Retrieved June 11, 2009, from http://www.uptodate.com/online/content/topic.do?topicKey=cns_infe/10731&selectedTitle=1~150&source=search_result

Sexton, D. J. (2009b, January 1). Clinical manifestations of Lyme disease in adults. *UpToDate Online 16.3.* Retrieved June 11, 2009, from http://www.uptodate.com/online/content/topic.do?topicKey=tickflea/7919&selectedTitle=1~150&source=search_result

Sexton, D. J. (2009c, January 1). Clinical manifestations and diagnosis of Rocky Mountain spotted fever. *UpToDate Online 16.3.* Retrieved June 11, 2009, from http://www.uptodate.com/online/content/topic.do?topicKey=tickflea/4723&selectedTitle=3~36&source=search_result

Sexton, D. J. (2009d, January 1). Treatment of Lyme disease. *UpToDate Online 16.3.* Retrieved June 11, 2009, from http://www.uptodate.com/online/content/topic.do?topicKey=tickflea/11121&selectedTitle=5~150&source=search_result

Sexton, D. J. (2009e, January 1). Treatment of Rocky Mountain spotted fever. *UpToDate Online 16.3.* Retrieved June 11, 2009, from http://www.uptodate.com/online/content/topic.do?topicKey=tickflea/6884&selectedTitle=1~36&source=search_result

Shapiro, E. D. (2009, January 1). Lyme disease: Clinical manifestations in children. *UpToDate Online 16.3.* Retrieved June 11, 2009, from http://www.uptodate.com/online/content/topic.do?topicKey=pedi_id/38385&selectedTitle=3~150&source=search_result

Spach, D. H. (2009, January). Endocarditis caused by Bartonella. *UpToDate Online 16.3.* Retrieved May 26, 2009, from http://www.uptodate.com/online/content/topic.do?topicKey=endocard/6776&selectedTitle=1~150&source=search_result

Spach, D. H., & Kaplan, S. L. (2009, January 1). Treatment of cat scratch disease. *UpToDate Online 16.3.* Retrieved May 19, 2009, from http://www.uptodate.com/online/content/topic.do?topicKey=oth_bact/4699&selectedTitle=1~41&source=search_result

Stephenson, I. (2008, October 12). Clinical manifestations and diagnosis of avian influenza. *UpToDate Online 16.3.* Retrieved June 1, 2009, from http://www.uptodate.com/online/content/topic.do?topicKey=pulm_inf/15905&selectedTitle=10~150&source=search_result

Sullivan, J. L. (2009, January 1). Clinical manifestations and treatment of Epstein-Barr virus infection. *UpToDate Online 16.3.* Retrieved June 11, 2009, from http://www.uptodate.com/online/content/topic.do?topicKey=viral_in/13539&selectedTitle=3~150&source=search_result

Sundel, R. (2008, June 3). Clinical manifestations and diagnosis of Kawasaki disease. *UpToDate Online 16.* Retrieved June 14, 2009, from http://www.uptodate.com/online/content/topic.do?topicKey=pedirheu/5411&selectedTitle=2~150&source=search_result#

Sundel, R. (2009, January 30). Initial treatment and prognosis of Kawasaki disease. *UpToDate Online 16.* Retrieved June 14, 2009, from http://www.uptodate.com/online/content/topic.do?topicKey=pedirheu/7206&selectedTitle=1~150&source=search_result

Thorner, A. R. (2009a, May 29). Treatment and prevention of swine H1N1 influenza. *UpToDate Online 16.3.* Retrieved June 1, 2009, from http://www.uptodate.com/online/content/topic.do?topicKey=pulm_inf/19054&selectedTitle=1~150&source=search_result

Thorner, A. R. (2009b, December 23). Treatment of pandemic H1N1 influenza ("swine influenza"). *UpToDate.* Retrieved January 17, 2010, from http://www.uptodate.com/online/content/topic.do?topicKey=pulm_inf/19054&view=print

Thorner, A. R. (2010, January 8). Epidemiology, clinical manifestations, and diagnosis of pandemic H1N1 influenza ("swine influenza"). *UpToDate.* Retrieved January 17, 2010, from http://www.uptodate.com/online/content/topic.do?topicKey=pulm_inf/18836&view=print

Tremblay, C. (2009, January 1). Cytomegalovirus infection in pregnancy. *UpToDate Online 16.3.* Retrieved May 25, 2009, from http://www.uptodate.com/online/content/topic.do?topicKey=viral_in/23892&selectedTitle=4~150&source=search_result

Wallace, M. R., & Lutwick, L. I. (2009, April 13). Rheumatic fever. *emedicine.* Retrieved July 26, 2009, from http://emedicine.medscape.com/article/1007946-print

White, R. W., & Gorman, C. R. (2009*). Roseola infantum.* Retrieved July 19, 2009, from http://emedicine.medscape.com/article/1133023-print

Willis, T. S. (2009, April 28). Cytomegalovirus. *emedicine, infectious diseases.* Retrieved May 25, 2009, from http://emedicine.medscape.com/article/215702-print

Systemic Disorders Guidelines

Julie Adkins

CHRONIC FATIGUE

Definition

A. Fatigue is one of the most common symptoms confronting the practitioner in an office practice. A patient with chronic fatigue is characterized as having fatigue with multiple associated symptoms for longer than 6 months in which these symptoms have a profound impact on daily activities.

Incidence

A. Fatigue accounts for 1%–3% of visits to generalists as an isolated symptom or diagnosis. Psychiatric disorders are involved in less than 50% of cases. Chronic fatigue has a reported frequency in excess of 20%. Fatigue is seen predominately in young adults and in more females than males.

Pathogenesis

A. Fatigue is a sensitive but nonspecific indicator of underlying medical and/or psychological pathology. It is reportedly more often due to unknown cause or to psychiatric illness than to physical illness, injury, medications, drugs, or alcohol.

Predisposing Factors

A. Hyperthyroidism
B. Hypothyroidism
C. Cardiac disease: congestive heart failure
D. Neurally mediated hypotension
E. Infections: endocarditis, hepatitis
F. Respiratory disorders: COPD and sleep apnea
G. Anemia
H. Arthritides and related disorders
I. Cancer
J. Alcoholism
K. Side effects from drugs such as sedatives and β-blockers
L. Psychologic conditions such as insomnia, depression, anxiety, and somatization disorder
M. Female gender
N. Epstein-Barr virus

Common Complaints

A. Lack of energy
B. Listlessness
C. Fatigue that interferes with participation in family, work, or even leisure activities

Other Signs and Symptoms

A. Weakness
B. Overexertion
C. Poor physical conditioning
D. Inadequate quality or quantity of sleep
E. Undernutrition and poor appetite
F. Stress
G. Obesity
H. Emotional problems: depression, anxiety, and somatization disorder

Subjective Data

A. Review history for onset, duration, and course description of the fatigue.
B. Ask the patient about significant losses, low self-esteem, and occurrence of crying spells and suicidal thoughts. **High prevalence of depression and suicide is present in this patient population.**
C. Ask the patient about a history of any abuse of hypnotic drugs, alcohol, or tranquilizers.
D. Review medications, both over-the-counter and prescription drugs.
E. Review the patient's medical history for cardiac, thyroid, and other medical conditions.
F. Review sleep and insomnia history.
G. Review history for family illness, new baby or postpartum.
H. Establish last menses to rule out pregnancy.
I. Review exercise patterns.
J. Review diet with 24-hour recall.
K. Elicit history of fever, night sweats, weight loss, and enlarged lymph node(s).
L. Inquire about recent major life changes, such as moving or a change in job.
M. Establish usual weight, and review recent weight gain or loss, over what period.

N. Review any recent infections, flu, or mononucleosis.

O. Review high-risk sexual practices and intravenous drug use to rule out HIV exposure.

P. Review recent history for transfusion of blood products to rule out hepatitis or HIV exposure.

Q. Obtain history of the patient's daily living and working habits.

Physical Examination

A. Check temperature, pulse, respirations, blood pressure and weight; check for postural hypotension.

B. Inspection.
1. Observe general overall appearance. Skin: Conduct dermal exam for changes in pigmentation, purpura, dryness, rashes, jaundice, pallor, splinter hemorrhages, or petechiae.
2. Eyes: Conduct a funduscopic exam to rule out Roth's spots and tuberculoma.
3. Check sclerae for icterus.
4. Throat: Inspect pharynx for petechiae at the junction of hard and soft palate, to rule out mononucleosis.
5. Extremities: Inspect the joints for inflammation.

C. Palpate.
1. Palpate the neck, to rule out goiter.
2. Palpate all lymph nodes (neck, axilla, and groin) for size, degree of tenderness, and distribution.
3. Complete clinical breast exam for masses.
4. Palpate the abdomen for organomegaly, masses, and ascites.
5. Palpate the joints for tenderness.
6. Assess the genitalia for masses and tenderness, to rule out infection.

D. Percuss: Percuss the abdomen for organomegaly, masses, ascites, and hepatic tenderness.

E. Auscultate: Auscultate the heart and lungs.

F. Neurologic exam: Complete mental status assessment.

G. Rectal exam: Assess for masses, prostatic pathology, and occult blood.

Diagnostic Tests

A. CBC with differential and peripheral smear.

B. Erythrocyte sedimentation rate (ESR).

C. Calcium, albumin, BUN, and creatinine.

D. Glucose.

E. Transaminase (aminotransferase): viral hepatitis is associated with elevation in transaminase.

F. HIV serum test.

G. Thyrotropin (TSH) to rule out hyperthyroidism or hypothyroidism.

H. Heterophile test to rule out acute mononucleosis.

I. Monospot.

J. Epstein-Barr virus.

Differential Diagnoses

A. Chronic fatigue syndrome.

B. Hypercalcemia.

C. Mild renal failure.

D. Early diabetes mellitus.

E. Hypothyroid or hyperthyroidism.

F. Cardiac disease.

G. Anemia.

H. Anicteric hepatitis.

I. Connective tissue disease.

J. Immune hyperactivity.

K. Disturbed sleep.

L. Occult neoplasm.

M. Infection: history of fever, sweats, weight loss, and diffuse adenopathy. These symptoms also suggest HIV, especially with high-risk behaviors (see "Human Immunodeficiency Virus [HIV]" section).

N. CDC criteria for chronic fatigue syndrome diagnosis:
1. **Major criteria (must meet both):**
   a. New onset fatigue greater than 6 months with 50% decrease in activity
   b. Exclusion of other medical or psychological conditions that produce similar presentations
2. **Minor criteria, symptoms (must have at least 4 or more symptoms plus 2 physical findings):**
   a. Mild fever
   b. Sore throat
   c. Painful cervical or axillary adenopathy
   d. General muscle weakness
   e. Myalgia
   f. Headache
   g. Prolonged fatigue after exercise
   h. Migratory arthralgia
   i. Sleep disturbance
   j. Neurologic or psychological complaint (one or more)
   k. Photophobia
   l. Scotoma
   m. Forcefulness
   n. Irritability
   o. Confusion
   p. Difficulty with concentration
   q. Depression
   r. Rapid onset of main symptom
3. **Minor criteria, physical signs (must have 2, or 8 of above 11 *symptoms*):**
   a. **Low-grade fever**
   b. Pharyngitis, nonexudative
   c. Palpable or tender anterior or posterior cervical or axillary adenopathy documented by a physician

O. Mononucleosis.

Plan

A. General interventions
1. Find out the patient's view of his or her illness before proceeding with patient education.
2. Manage underlying disease (refer to specific chapters).
3. Treat the patient with nutritional or vitamin supplementation, as indicated.
4. There are no therapies that provide prompt relief from symptoms.
5. Strong patient-provider alliance is essential.
6. Evaluate the patient for the possibility that he or she is confusing focal neuromuscular disease with generalized lassitude.

B. Patient teaching
1. Discuss and review the evidence for the diagnosis, and offer a careful explanation of symptoms. Many

patients think they have a medical problem producing fatigue symptoms.

2. Review the diagnostic criteria for depression (see Chapter 20, "Psychiatric Guidelines"), and describe the neurochemical mechanisms by which depression leads to fatigue. Refer the patient for individual counseling or group therapy.
3. Review the idiopathic nature of chronic fatigue syndrome and its nonprogressive nature. Inform the patient it has a gradually improving clinical course and the chance of full recovery. Symptoms are self-limited, usually clearing within 12–18 months.
4. Encourage the patient to begin a gentle exercise program and to engage in life's activities.
5. Provide nutritional education.

C. Pharmaceutical therapy
1. For postural hypotension:
   a. Increase dietary sodium.
   b. Antihypotensive agent: fludrocortisone 0.1 mg daily.
2. Low-dose antidepressant therapy for disordered sleep:
   a. Amitriptyline HC1 25 mg every bedtime.
   b. Imipramine HCl 25–50 mg at bedtime. May increase dosage up to 300 mg daily.
   c. Doxepin HCl 10–20 mg every bedtime.
   d. Short-term hypnotic: zolpidem (Ambien) 5–10 mg at bedtime.
3. NSAIDs for symptomatic relief of myalgia, arthralgia, or headache.
4. Correct anemia with iron supplements, if applicable.

Follow-up

A. **Follow up in 2 weeks to reevaluate status and then monthly depending on signs and symptoms.**
B. Follow closely if the patient is depressed.

Consultation/Referral

A. Consult a physician if no improvement is seen with therapies. Emphasize the legitimacy of the patient's symptoms and summarize the workup, its rationale, and findings.
B. Refer the patient to a mental health professional as indicated by depression and/or suicidality.

Individual Considerations

A. Adults: Fatigue is most often explained by common factors such as overexertion, poor physical conditioning, inadequate quantity or quality of sleep, obesity, undernutrition, stress, and emotional problems.

Resource

Chronic Fatigue Immune Dysfunction Syndrome (CFIDS) Association
PO Box 220398
Charlotte, NC 28222-0398
800-442-3437
24 hours a day, 7 days a week

FEVERS OF UNKNOWN ORIGIN (FUO)

Definition

A. The criteria for fevers of unknown origin (FUO) are an illness of at least 3-week duration, fever over 101.0°F (38.3°C) (Ferri, 2004, p. 338) on several occasions, and remaining undiagnosed after 1 week of study in the hospital. Because of cost factors, the criterion requiring 1 week of hospitalization is often bypassed.

Incidence

A. In adults, infections account for 20%–40% of the cases. Cancer accounts for 7%–20% of the cases of FUO. In children, infections are the most common cause of FUO, accounting for 30%–50% of the cases; cancer is a rare cause of FUO in children. Autoimmune disorders occur with equal frequency in adults and children. Infection, cancer, and autoimmune disorders combined account for 20%–25% of FUO in patients who have been febrile for 6 months or longer. Various miscellaneous diseases account for another 25%. Approximately 50% of FUO remain undiagnosed but have a benign course with symptoms eventually resolving.

Pathogenesis

There are five categories of causes of FUO:

A. Infection: Most common systemic infections are tuberculosis and endocarditis.
B. Neoplasms: Most common are lymphoma and leukemia.
C. Autoimmune disorders: Most common are Still's disease, systemic lupus erythematosus, and polyarteritis nodosa.
D. Miscellaneous causes: These include hyperthyroidism, thyroiditis, sarcoidosis, Whipple's disease, familial Mediterranean fever, recurrent pulmonary emboli, alcoholic hepatitis, drug fever, factitious fever, and others.
E. Undiagnosed FUO.

Predisposing Factors

A. Upper respiratory infection
B. Urinary tract infection
C. Viral illnesses
D. Drug allergy, especially to antibiotics
E. Connective tissue disease

Common Complaints

A. The patient feels "sick all over," with malaise and fatigue.
B. Chills all over the body with high fever.

Other Signs and Symptoms

A. Tachycardia
B. Sensation of warmth or flushing
C. Piloerection
D. Myalgias
E. Mild inability to concentrate, confusion, delirium, or even stupor
F. Labial herpes simplex outbreak, or fever blisters
G. Children: seizures

Subjective Data

A. Review the onset, course, and duration of symptoms.
B. Review family, occupational, and social history.
C. Review sexual practices, including monogamy and oral, rectal, and vaginal sexual habits, and recreational habits and any new changes.
D. Elicit information regarding use of intravenous drugs.
E. Review if the patient has had this before. How was it treated?

F. Review travel during the last month.

G. Review any new hobbies, changes at home or work, or other new events.

H. Review the patient's history for contact with any friends or family members that have been sick and do not seem to be getting any better.

I. Review the patient's history for eating any uncooked meat and dietary changes during the past month.

J. Review the child's history specifically for febrile seizures.

K. Review for risk factors for thrombophlebitis (see Chapter 9, "Cardiovascular Guidelines").

Physical Examination

A. Check temperature, pulse, respirations, blood pressure, weight, and height

B. Inspect
  1. Conduct funduscopic exam to rule out retinopathy, Roth's spots, and choroidal tubercles.
  2. Examine the ears, nose, and throat. Inspect the mouth.
  3. Observe the skin and mucous membranes.

C. Palpate
  1. Palpate the neck, axilla, and groin for lymphadenopathy.
  2. Elderly: Palpate the scalp for tender arteries of cranial arteritis.
  3. Children: Palpate the fontanelles.
  4. Palpate the thyroid gland.
  5. Palpate the abdomen for organomegaly, masses, tenderness, guarding, rebound, suprapubic tenderness, and CVA tenderness.
  6. Palpate the musculoskeletal system for bone or joint swelling, tenderness, increased warmth; check lower extremities for evidence of phlebitis, asymmetrical swelling, calf tenderness, and palpable cord.

D. Percuss
  1. Percuss the sinuses for tenderness, and transilluminate for evidence of sinusitis.
  2. Percuss the chest for consolidation.
  3. Percuss the abdomen.

E. Auscultate
  1. Auscultate the heart for murmurs and rubs.
  2. Auscultate the lungs for rales, consolidation, and effusion.

F. Neurologic exam
  1. Assess for signs of meningeal irritation (Brudzinski's and Kernig's signs), and presence of focal deficits.
  2. Conduct mental status exam.

G. Genitorectal exam, if applicable
  1. Female: Conduct pelvic exam for cervical discharge, adnexal masses, lesions, and PID symptoms.
  2. Male: Conduct prostate and testicular exam for tenderness and masses; check penis for discharge, rash, and lesions.
  3. Both: Conduct rectal exam for discharge, tenderness, and masses; check stool for occult blood specimen.
  4. Skin: rashes or wounds.

Diagnostic Tests

A. CBC with differential.

B. Sedimentation rate.

C. Urinalysis and urine culture.

D. Blood glucose.

E. Liver function test.

F. Blood cultures.

G. Consider serology for suspected infections or pathology (refer to Chapter 15, "Infectious Disease Guidelines"). Suspected infections include Epstein-Barr virus, Q fever, Lyme disease or other tick-borne diseases, hepatitis, syphilis, and cytomegalovirus.

H. Suspected collagen disease: antinuclear antibodies (ANA) and rheumatoid factor.

I. Suspected tuberculosis: tuberculin skin test, sputum and urine cultures.

J. Immunologic studies: ELISA, Western blot test, and antistreptolysin O (ASLO) titer.

K. Suspected mononucleosis: heterophile antibody test.

L. Suspected *Salmonella:* Widal's test.

M. Suspected thyroiditis: thyroid profile.

N. Suspected malaria or relapsing fever: direct examination of blood smears.

O. Imaging: depends on suspected infection.
  1. Chest, sinus radiographic films.
  2. GI studies: proctosigmoidoscopy, evaluate gallbladder function.
  3. CT scan of abdomen and pelvis, abdominal ultrasonography.
  4. MRI is better than CT scan for detecting lesions of the nervous system.

P. Suspected embolism: ventilation-perfusion (V/Q) scan.

Q. Suspected endocarditis or atrial myxoma: echocardiography.

R. Radionuclide studies: gallium scan and radium-labeled immunoglobulin useful in detecting infection and neoplasm.

S. Laparotomy in the deteriorating patient if the diagnosis is elusive despite extensive evaluation. Any abnormal finding should be aggressively evaluated: headache necessitates a lumbar puncture to rule out meningitis; biopsy any skin from an area of rash to look for cutaneous manifestations of collagen vascular disease or infection; enlarged lymph nodes should be aspirated or biopsied and examined for cytologic features to rule out neoplasm and send for culture.

Differential Diagnoses

A. Fevers of unknown origin

B. Systemic and localized infections

C. Neoplasms

D. Autoimmune disorders

E. Thrombophlebitis

F. Miscellaneous causes (see "Definition")

Plan

A. General interventions: Observe the patient taking own temperature to document the presence of a fever to make sure the temperature is not self-induced.

B. Patient teaching.
  1. Instruct the patient to keep a record of temperatures, preferably rectal, taken each evening, when elevations are most likely to occur.
  2. Reassure the patient that there is nothing abnormal about temperatures in the range of 97.0°F–99.3°F.

3. Instruct the patient on use of physical cooling aids, such as exposure of skin to cool ambient temperature, bedside fan, and sponging with cool water or alcohol.
4. Explain to the patient that immersion in an ice water bath may be indicated for hyperthermic emergencies.

C. Pharmaceutical therapy.
1. Start therapeutic trials if a diagnosis is strongly suspected.
    a. Antituberculous drugs for tuberculosis.
    b. Tetracycline for brucellosis.
    c. If the patient shows no clinical response in 2 weeks, stop therapy and reevaluate.
2. Symptomatic antipyretic therapy: salicylates or acetaminophen every 4 hours.

Follow-up

A. Follow up in 24–48 hours.
B. Indications for admission to the hospital: fever remains elevated beyond 101°F for weeks, and ambulatory diagnostic efforts have been unsuccessful.

Consultation/Referral

A. Consult with a physician for diagnosis and comanagement if indicated.
B. Refer the patient to a specialist if unable to differentiate definitive diagnosis.

Individual Considerations

A. Pregnancy
1. Refer the patient for perinatal consultation.
2. High fevers early in the first trimester have been associated with an increase in neural tube defects.
3. Maternal fevers may cause fetal tachycardia.
B. Pediatrics
1. Toxic-appearing infants and children should be hospitalized and given parenteral antibiotic therapy following prompt diagnostic testing that includes WBC; urinalysis; and cultures of blood, urine, and cerebrospinal fluid. Consult a physician.
2. Infants under 28 days regardless of appearance are generally hospitalized and given parenteral antibiotic therapy following prompt diagnostic testing with WBC, urinalysis, and cultures.
3. Aspirin products should not be given to children due to the risk of Reye's syndrome.
4. Consider inflammatory bowel disease in older children and adolescents.
C. Geriatrics
1. Common causes of FUO include TB, Hodgkin's lymphoma, and temporal arteritis.
2. Elderly patients commonly present with nonspecific symptoms.

HUMAN IMMUNODEFICIENCY VIRUS (HIV)
by Beverly R. Byram

Definition

A. Acquired immunodeficiency syndrome (AIDS) is a chronic, life-threatening condition caused by the human immunodeficiency virus (HIV). HIV is a retrovirus that targets helper T (CD4) cells and contains a viral enzyme called reverse transcriptase that allows the virus to convert its RNA to DNA then integrate and take over the cell's own genetic material. Once taken over the new cell begins to produce new HIV retrovirus. This process kills the CD4 cells that are the body's main defense against illness. This interferes with the body's ability to fight off infection—bacteria, viruses, and fungi—that cause disease. AIDS is the term used to define a severely compromised immune system.

Incidence

A. According to the Centers for Disease Control and Prevention (CDC) by the end of 2003 there were approximately 1 million persons living with HIV in the United States. Approximately 25% of those were unaware of their HIV status. An estimated 47% of those living with HIV are African American, 34% White, and 17% Hispanic. Asians/Pacific Islanders and American Indians/Alaskan Natives each represent 1%.
B. The largest population living with HIV comprises men having sex with men (MSM), followed by persons infected by high-risk heterosexual contact, those infected by intravenous drug users (IVDU), and those exposed through both MSM and IVDU.
C. Worldwide of those infected with HIV, 46% are women and 50% of all new infections worldwide are in women. Of these, 83% are infected heterosexually. In the United States, of the number of women infected, more than 80% are either African American or Hispanic. HIV/AIDS remains the leading cause of death in African American women ages 25–34 in the United States, whereas AIDS is the 10th leading cause of death in White women in the same age group.
D. Due to the rapidity of changing technology and knowledge, refer to the Web sites for the newest statistics.

Pathogenesis

A. HIV belongs to a subgroup of retroviruses called lentiviruses or "slow" viruses. The course of infection of the virus is characterized by a long interval between infection and the onset of serious symptoms. CD4 cells are the primary target of the HIV.
B. Primary HIV infection is followed by a burst of viremia during which the virus is easily detected in peripheral blood per HIV PCR viral load. During the "window period," the first 2–6 weeks following infection, persons may test negative for the HIV antibody with the ELISA and Western Blot tests. During this time the person can be highly infectious to sexual partners. In this time of early infection with high viral load the CD4 cells can decrease by 20–40%. Within 2–4 weeks after exposure to the virus up to 70% of infected patients experience a flu-like illness related to acute infection. The immune system fights back to reduce the HIV levels with killer T cells (CD8) that attack and kill the infected cells. The patient's CD4 cell count may rebound by 80–90%. A patient can remain symptom-free for a long time, often years. During this time there is low-level replication of HIV but ongoing deterioration of the immune system. Enough of

the immune system remains intact to prevent most infections. The patient is infectious during this time.

C. The final phase of HIV occurs when a sufficient number of CD4 cells are destroyed and when production of new CD4 cells cannot match destruction. Patients exhibit fatigue, fever, and weight loss. This failure of the immune system leads to AIDS.

D. An HIV-infected person can live an average of 8–10 years before developing clinical symptoms. HIV disease is not uniformly expressed in all people. A small portion of patients develop AIDS and die within months of infection. Approximately 5% of infected patients, known as "long-term nonprogressors," have no signs of disease after 12 or more years.

E. Most AIDS defining conditions are marked by a CD4 count of less than 200 cells or the appearance of one or more of the opportunistic infections (OI). Bacteria, viruses, or fungi that would not cause illness in a healthy immune system cause opportunistic infections. These infections are often severe and sometimes fatal.

Predisposing Factors

A. Gay or bisexual men or prostitutes
B. Needle sharing by IV drug users (IVDU)
C. Perinatal infection: mother to child transmission
D. Open wound and mucous membrane exposure to body fluids of infected person
E. Recipients of transfusion of contaminated blood or blood products (rare since 1985)

Common Complaints

A. Fatigue: often severe
B. Fever: longer than 1 month
C. Night sweats: drenching
D. Loss of appetite
E. Weight loss
F. Rash

Other Signs and Symptoms

A. Lymphadenopathy: enlarged lymph nodes often involving at least two noncontiguous sites
B. Anemia
C. Neutropenia
D. Thrombocytopenia
E. Cough
F. Dyspnea
G. Asymptomatic whitish patches on sides of tongue: hairy leukoplakia
H. Thrush: oral candidiasis
I. Odynaphagia: esophageal candidiasis, CMV esophagitis
J. Chronic vaginal candidiasis
K. Skin changes: rashes, dry skin, and seborrheic dermatitis
L. Purplish, nonblanching nodules found on the skin, mucous membranes, and viscera: Kaposii's sarcoma
M. Muscle wasting
N. Chronic diarrhea: longer than 1 month
O. Hepatosplenomegaly
P. Cardiomyopathy
Q. Chronic bacterial infections including community-acquired pneumonias
R. Tuberculosis
S. Sexually transmitted infections (STIs)
T. Peripheral neuropathy
U. Dementia
V. Children: failure to thrive

Subjective Data

A. Review symptoms: onset, course, and duration.
B. Ask about previous HIV testing: dates and reasons for testing.
C. Past medical history review: hospitalizations, comorbidities, immunizations, normal weight, pain, chronic lymph node disorders, and any changes of skin overlying lymph nodes.
D. Past surgical history review.
E. Sexual history: number of partners in the past year, number of lifetime partners, any previous partner known HIV positive, STIs, and any previous partners known to have been incarcerated.
   1. Women: history of abnormal paps, contraception, and condom use with partner.
   2. Men: MSM, heterosexual, bisexual, receptive anal intercourse, and condom use.
F. Past mental health history: past and current mental health diagnosis and treatment.
G. Substance use: tobacco, alcohol, and drugs.
H. History of IVDU: needle sharing and when last used drugs.
I. Transfusion or blood product history prior to 1985.
J. Lived or traveled outside of the United States: when and for how long.
K. Assess the presence of persistent fever with no localizing symptoms.
L. Assess the patient's support system: who knows diagnosis?

Physical Examination

A. Height, weight, blood pressure, pulse, respiratory rate, and temperature
B. General observation: general appearance, including fat distribution, signs of wasting
C. Inspect
   1. Skin: evaluate for rashes, seborrhea, folliculitis, moles, Kaposii's scarcoma, warts, herpes, dry skin, skin cancer, fungal infections, molluscum contagiosum, jaundice, and needle marks.
   2. Head and neck; eyes, ears, nose, and throat (HEENT)
      a. Assess visual acuity.
      b. Retina exam for CMV.
      c. Evaluate sclera foricterus.
      d. Oral exam for thrush, hairy leukoplakia, mucosal Kaposii's sarcoma, gingivitis, aphthous ulcers, and dental health.
D. Auscultate
   1. Pulmonary auscultation for air movement and abnormal breath sounds
   2. Cardiac evaluation for normal and abnormal heart sounds
E. Palpate
   1. Palpate the thyroid.
   2. Lymphatic evaluation of regional versus generalized swelling: specific location, size and texture of nodes.

3. Palpate the abdomen to evaluate the presence of hepatosplenomegaly, masses, tenderness, pain, or rebound tenderness.
4. Breast examination (female).

F. Rectal/vaginal examination
   1. Both genders: inspect for the presence of ulcers and warts in the vagina, perineum, and rectum.
   2. Females: perform bimanual examination, pap smear, obtain specimens for STI testing, and perform a digital rectal exam.
   3. Males: testicular exam, digital rectal exam, consider an anal pap if indicated (currently not in guidelines).

G. Neurologic examination
   1. Assess mental status.
   2. Assess cranial nerves including gait, strength, deep tendon reflexes, evaluation of proprioception, vibration, pinprick, temperature, and sensation in distal extremities.

H. Psychiatric examination: screen for depression

Diagnostic Tests

A. Repeat HIV ELISA and Western Blot
B. CBC, with differential, including platelets
C. Complete chemistry profile
D. Fasting lipid profile
E. VDRL and RPR
F. Serologies for toxoplasmosis and cytomegalovirus (CMV IgG)
G. CD4/CD8 cells and CD4/CD8 ratio
H. HIV RNA viral load
I. HIV resistance genotype
J. HLA-B 5701 (risk for Abacavir hypersensitivity reaction syndrome)
K. Hepatitis serologies: HAV serology (antibody); HBV serology (HBsAb, HBeAb, HBsAb); and HCV serology (antibody)
L. Cultures for STIs—anal, vaginal (culture pharynx if history indicates oral sex)
M. Urinalysis
N. Pap smear
O. Tuberculin skin tests: chest X-ray if history of positive PPD

Differential Diagnoses

A. HIV
B. Other diseases that lead to immune suppression or are related to symptoms
C. Cancer
D. Chronic infections
E. TORCH infections
F. Syphilis
G. Tuberculosis
H. Endocarditis
I. Infectious enterocolitis
J. Bowel disorders: antibiotic-associated colitis, inflammatory bowel disease, or malabsorptive symptoms
K. Endocrine diseases
L. Neuropathy
M. Alcoholism
N. Liver disease
O. Renal disease
P. Thyroid disease
Q. Vitamin deficiency
R. Chronic meningitis

Plan

A. General interventions.
   1. Refer and comanage the patient with HIV/AIDS clinician.
   2. Identify and treat substance abuse.
   3. Explain to the patient that at each visit you will review history, conduct a physical exam, and run laboratory studies to assess health status.
   4. Discuss health habits: smoking, nutrition, and exercise.
   5. Discuss treatment plan.
      a. Highly active antiretroviral therapy (HAART)
      b. Therapy for opportunistic infections and malignancies
      c. Prophylaxis for opportunistic infections: PCP and MAC
      d. Managing side effects of medications and comorbidities
      e. Immunizations

B. Patient teaching:
   1. Discuss living with HIV disease.
   2. Discuss transmission prevention strategies: safer sex practices and condom use.
   3. Provide contact information for AIDS social service organizations (ASO).
   4. Discuss the patient's concerns including notification of sexual partner(s) and needle-sharing partner(s).
   5. See the Section III Patient Teaching Guide for this chapter, "Reference Resources for Patients With HIV/AIDS.

C. Discuss birth control and family planning issues.
D. Pharmaceutical therapy.
   1. Treatment with Highly Active Anti-retroviral Therapy (HAART). Always consult with an infectious disease HIV/AIDS specialist for treatment options.
      a. HAART: At this time there are 24 individual medications from 5 classes of drugs as well as 5 pills that are combinations of 2 or 3 of these medications. Recommendations are a minimum of 3 drugs from a minimum of 2 classes (Public Health Service Task Force Guidelines for the Use of Antiretroviral Agents in HIV-1 Infected Adults and Adolescents). Classes:
         i. Nucleoside/Nucleotide Reverse Transcriptase Inhibitors (NRTIs)
         ii. Non-Nucleoside Reverse Transcriptase Inhibitors (NNRTIs)
         iii. Protease Inhibitors (PIs)
         iv. Integrase Inhibitors (INIs)
         v. Fusion Inhibitors (FIs)
         vi. CCR5 Inhibitors (CIs)
         vii. Combination Antiretrovirals (NRTIs + NNRTIs)
   2. Prophylaxis and treatment for opportunistic infections (OIs). May discontinue prophylaxis if sustained immune reconstitution on HAART.

a. Pneumocystis Pneumonia (PCP). Prophylaxis if CD4 count less than 200 or has oral candidiasis.
   i. First line: Bactrim DS (TMP-SMZ) 1 tab 3 times weekly or 1 tab daily (if Toxoplasmosis positive)
   ii. Alternatives: Dapsone, Atovaquone, and Aerosolized Pentamidine
b. Mycobacterium Avium Complex (MAC) Prophylaxis if CD4 count less than 75.
   i. First line: Zithromax 1,200 mg weekly
   ii. Alternative: Clarithromycin
3. Managing side effects of HAART and complications of HIV therapy: Multiple complications of long-term HIV infection and treatment with HAART.
   a. Lipodystrophy syndrome, bone marrow suppression, cardiovascular disease, CNS side effects, GI intolerance, hepatic failure, hepatoxicity, hyperlipidemia, insulin resistance, diabetes, lactic acidosis/hepatic steotosis, nephrotoxicity, osteonecrosis, osteopenia, peripheral neuropathy, nephrolithiasis, urolithiasis, crystalluria, hypogonadism, and psychiatric complications
4. Immunizations.
   a. Hepatitis A and B series
   b. Tetanus
   c. Pneumococcal vaccine
   d. Yearly influenza vaccines
   e. Gardasil series for women (currently no guidelines for men)

Follow-up

A. Schedule return visit 4 weeks after initial visit to discuss staging HIV/AIDS and living with HIV/AIDS.
B. PPD yearly unless history of positive PPD then yearly chest X-ray.
C. Pap smear.
   1. Initially, if normal repeat in 6 months, then yearly if remains normal.
   2. If abnormal follow Guidelines by the American Society of Colposcopy and Cervical Pathology (ASCCP).
D. Some clinicians advocate for anal pap smears for men but there are no set guidelines at present.

Consultation/Referral

A. Refer the patient to a specialist in HIV for management of continued care and pharmacologic therapy.
B. Refer the patient to a nutritionist for baseline evaluation and diet counseling.
C. Refer pregnant women to a perinatologist.
D. Ophthalmology exam yearly for CMV screening and vision changes.
E. Dental referral.
F. Hepatology referral if chronic, active hepatitis B and/or C.

Individual Considerations

A. Preconception counseling
   1. Preconception counseling: The goal is to avoid transmission of HIV to partner and baby. Use ovulation kits (basal body charts) to determine the most fertile time for pregnancy.

a. Discordant couples
   i. HIV positive female and HIV negative male
   ii. Self-insemination (methods: syringe, turkey baster, cervical cap)
b. HIV positive male and HIV negative female
   i. Sperm washing/IVF: very expensive; often cost-prohibitive.
   ii. HIV positive male partner on HAART and HIV viral load as close to undetectable as possible.
   iii. Unprotected sex during ovulation times only and no other.
c. HIV positive male and HIV positive female: avoid superinfection
   i. Both partners on HAART and vial loads as close to undetectable as possible.
   ii. Unprotected sex during ovulation times only and no other.
B. Pregnancy recommendations for use of antiretroviral drugs in pregnant HIV-infected women for maternal health and interventions to reduce perinatal HIV transmission in the United States:
   1. Antepartum
      a. HAART starting at 10–12 weeks gestation or maintaining treatment if already on pregnancy-approved HAART.
      b. Goal of therapy is undetectable HIV viral load.
      c. Sustiva should not be used in pregnancy.
      d. Vaginal delivery can be offered if HIV viral load is less than 1,000.
   2. Intrapartum
      a. Continue oral HAART.
      b. Zidovudine IV 2 mg/kg in the first hour then 1 mg/kg throughout delivery.
      c. C-section if HIV viral load greater than 1,000.
   3. Postpartum
      a. HAART for mother is continued depending on immunologic status.
      b. Infant receives Zidovudine 2 mg/kg every 6 hours for the first 6 weeks of life.
      c. Breast-feeding is contraindicated.
C. Pediatrics
   1. Perinatal transmission in the United States has been reduced to less than 2% due to HAART.
   2. Infants born to HIV-infected mothers test positive for HIV antibody ELISA test. Transplacentally acquired antibody may persist in the child for up to 18 months.
   3. Clinical and laboratory evaluation of the child must continue until the infant has cleared the mother's antibodies. HIV viral loads are drawn at birth, 3 weeks, 6 weeks, 3 months, 6 months, and 12–15 months.
   4. Children who are HIV positive from vertical transmission should be followed by pediatric infectious disease clinicians.
   5. All routine immunizations are recommended for HIV-infected children except for severely immunocompromised HIV-infected children who should not receive live virus vaccines.

D. Adults: occupational postexposure prophylaxis (PEP)
1. Depending upon exposure type and severity postexposure ART should be started as quickly as possible and be taken for 4 weeks postexposure.
2. Expert consultation should be obtained as quickly as possible. (National HIV/AIDS Clinician's Consultation Center PEPline: 1-888-448-8765.)
3. Follow with occupational health for regular clinical assessment and labs.
4. Perform HIV testing: baseline, 6 weeks, 3 months, 6 months, and 1 year.
5. HIV testing with HIV RNA viral load if an illness compatible with seroconversion illness occurs (fever, lymphadenopathy, pharyngitis, rash).
6. Advise transmission precautions during first 3–6 months postexposure (use condoms, refrain from donating blood, discontinue breast-feeding).

IDIOPATHIC (AUTOIMMUNE) THROMBOCYTOPENIC PURPURA (ITP)

Definition
A. Idiopathic thrombocytopenic purpura (ITP) is an autoimmune disorder in which an IgG autoantibody is formed that binds to platelets. The platelet count is less than 150,000 mm³.

Incidence
A. Acute ITP occurs commonly in childhood, frequently precipitated by a viral infection. Peak age of incidence is between 20 and 50 years. There is a 2:1 female to male predominance. The adult form is usually a chronic disease (> 6 months) and seldom follows a viral infection.

Pathogenesis
A. ITP is due to production of antiplatelet antibodies that leads to peripheral destruction and sequestration of platelets. It is not clear which antigen on the platelet surface is involved. Platelets are not destroyed by direct lysis even if the antiplatelet antibody binds complement. Destruction takes place in the spleen, where splenic macrophages with Fc receptors bind to antibody-coated platelets.

Predisposing Factors
A. Infections
B. Chronic alcoholism
C. Sepsis
D. AIDS
E. Immune disorders, such as systemic lupus erythematosus (SLE)
F. Drug use
G. Chronic lymphocytic leukemia (CLL)
H. Pregnancy

Common Complaints
A. Purple spots and bruises on skin
B. Nosebleeds
C. Mouth and gums bleeding

Other Signs and Symptoms
A. Purpura, petechiae, and hemorrhagic bullae in the mouth.
B. Tendency to bleed easily.
C. Menorrhagia.
D. No systemic illness; the patient feels well and is not febrile.

Subjective Data
A. Determine when the patient or caregiver first noticed symptoms; note if the symptoms have changed or progressed.
B. Rule out pregnancy as cause of nosebleeds.
C. Ask if the patient is feeling well except for the bleeding or bruising.
D. Determine if the patient has a fever.
E. Obtain medication history for over-the-counter and prescribed medications.
F. Determine the patient's history of immune disorders, recent infections, alcoholism, and pregnancy.
G. Establish usual weight and any recent weight loss.

Physical Examination
A. Check temperature, pulse, respirations, blood pressure, and weight.
B. Inspect.
1. Observe general appearance.
2. Conduct dermal exam for purpura and petechiae.
3. Conduct eye exam; check sclera for hemorrhages.
4. Examine the mouth for dental carries and poor hygiene, mouth petechiae, and hemorrhagic bullae.
C. Palpate.
1. Palpate the abdomen, liver, and spleen.

Normally, the spleen should not be palpable.

2. Palpate the cervical, axillary, and groin lymph nodes for adenopathy.
D. Percuss: Percuss the abdomen, liver, and spleen.
E. Auscultate.
1. Auscultate the heart and lungs.
2. Auscultate the abdomen for bowel sounds and bruits.

Diagnostic Tests
A. Platelet count

The major concern during the initial phase is risk of cerebral hemorrhage when platelet count is less than 5,000 platelets/μL.

B. IgG

Increased levels of IgG appear on the platelet count in the presence of thrombocytopenia.

C. CBC with differential and peripheral smear

Peripheral smear shows normal WBCs and RBCs, platelets low in count with large size.

D. Bleeding time
E. Coagulation tests: PT, PTT, and fibrinogen

Coagulation studies are normal.

F. Referral for bone marrow aspiration

Bone marrow may appear normal or have increased megakarocytes with thrombocytopenia.

Differential Diagnoses

Thrombocytopenia may be produced two ways: by abnormal bone marrow function or by peripheral destruction of platelets.

A. Abnormal bone marrow function
1. Aplastic anemia.
2. Hematologic malignancies.
3. Myelodysplasia; this can only be ruled out by examining the bone marrow.
4. Megaloblastic anemia.
5. Chronic alcoholism.
B. Nonbone marrow disorders
1. Immune disorders
a. Idiopathic thrombocytopenic purpura
b. Drug induced from medications being taken
c. Secondary to CLL and SLE
d. Posttransfusion purpura
2. Hypersplenism resulting from liver disease (Ferri, 2004, p. 473)
3. Disseminated intravascular coagulation
4. Thrombotic thrombocytopenic purpura
5. Sepsis
6. Hemangiomas
7. Viral infection, AIDS
8. Pregnancy
9. Hypothyroidism

Plan

A. General interventions: Comanage the patient with a physician for medication therapy.
B. Patient teaching.
1. Instruct the patient to avoid trauma; tell him or her **no contact sports.**
2. Instruct the patient to avoid salicylates; they impair platelet function.
3. Prednisone therapy benefits.
a. Prednisone increases platelet count by increasing platelet production.
b. Long-term therapy may decrease antibody production.
c. Bleeding often diminishes 1 day after beginning prednisone.
d. Platelet count usually begins to rise within a week; responses are almost always seen within 3 weeks.
e. About 80% of patients respond, and the platelet count usually returns to normal.
C. Medical or surgical management.
1. Splenectomy is the most definitive treatment. Most adults ultimately undergo splenectomy.
2. Splenectomy is indicated if patients do not respond to prednisone initially or require unacceptably high doses to maintain an adequate platelet count.
D. Pharmaceutical therapy.
1. Initial treatment.
a. Prednisone 1–2 mg/kg/day.
b. High-dose therapy should be continued until the platelet count is normal, and the dose should then be gradually tapered.
2. In most patients, thrombocytopenia recurs if prednisone is completely withdrawn.

3. High-dose therapy should not be continued indefinitely in an attempt to avoid surgery.
4. Alternative drug therapy.
a. High-dose intravenous immunoglobulin 400 mg/kg/day for 3–5 days is highly effective in rapidly raising the platelet count.
b. This treatment is expensive, costing approximately $5,000.
c. The beneficial effect lasts only 1–2 weeks.
d. This therapy should be reserved for emergency situations such as preparing a severely thrombocytopenic patient for surgery.
5. Danazol 600 mg/day.
a. Danazol is used for patients who fail to respond to prednisone and splenectomy.
6. Platelet transfusions are an option that is rarely used.

Exogenous platelets survive no better than the patient's own platelets. In many cases, platelets survive less than a few hours. This therapy is reserved for cases of life-threatening bleeding in which enhanced hemostasis for even an hour may be of benefit.

Follow-up

A. The patient must be monitored very closely by a physician. Perform daily to weekly platelet counts; frequency depends on the severity and course.
B. Prognosis for acute ITP: 80% respond and fully recover within 2 months; 15%–20% progress to chronic ITP.
C. Prognosis for chronic ITP: 10%–20% recover fully; remainder continue to have low platelet counts and may see a remission or relapses over time.
D. The principal cause of death from ITP is intracranial hemorrhage (Ferri, 2004, p. 473).

Consultation/Referral

A. After diagnosis, refer the patient to a hematologist.

Individual Considerations

A. Pregnancy
1. Rule out HEELP syndrome, infection, and DIC as causes of thrombocytopenia.
2. There is an increased incidence of spontaneous abortions and hemorrhage at the time of delivery from genital tract injury.
3. Antepartum management: Conduct fetal blood sampling and testing when the mother has a known history of ITP.
4. Intrapartum management.
a. Avoid fetal hypoxia, which can decrease the fetal platelet count.
b. Avoid prolonged labor.
c. Conduct continuous fetal monitoring.
d. Epidural anesthesia may be used if the platelet count is at least 100,000 cells/mm^3.
5. Postpartum management: Breast-feeding is not recommended because of the possible transmission of antiplatelet antibodies through breast milk.
B. Pediatrics
1. ITP is frequently precipitated by a viral infection.
2. It usually has an acute course that is self-limited.
C. Geriatrics: ITP is uncommon in this population; there is usually another cause for low platelets in geriatrics.

IRON DEFICIENCY ANEMIA (MICROCYTIC, HYPOCHROMIC)

Definition

A. Microcytic anemia is characterized by small, pale red blood cells (RBCs), and depletion of iron (Fe) stores. The hematocrit (HCT) is less than 41% in males with a hemoglobin (Hgb) less than 13.5 g/dL. In females, the HCT is less than 37% with a Hgb less than 12 g/dL. Usually mild, it can become moderate or severe.

Incidence

A. Iron deficiency is the most common cause of anemia worldwide; it is particularly prevalent in women of child-bearing age. It is estimated to occur in 20% of adult women, 50% of pregnant women, and 3% of adult males in the United States.

Pathogenesis

A. Anemia is acquired; it develops slowly and in stages. Iron loss exceeds intake so that stored iron is progressively depleted. As stored iron is depleted, a compensatory increase in absorption of dietary iron and in the concentration of transferrin occurs. Iron stores can no longer meet the needs of the erythroid marrow; the plasma transferrin level increases and the serum iron concentration declines, resulting in a decrease in iron available for red blood cell formation.

Predisposing Factors

A. Female with heavy menses
B. Chronic blood loss, gastrointestinal blood loss
C. Family history or personal history of anemia
D. Poor diet
E. Closely spaced pregnancies
F. Lactation
G. Pica
H. Chronic hemoglobinuria due to an abnormally functioning cardiac valve
I. Chronic aspirin use
J. Repeated blood donation
K. Decreased iron absorption due to gastric surgery

Common Complaints

A. Fatigued all of the time
B. Heart feels like it is racing, beating hard
C. Out of breath on exertion
D. Loss of appetite, nausea and vomiting
E. Headaches throughout day
F. Weak and dizzy

Other Signs and Symptoms

Clinical presentation depends on severity, patient's age, and the ability of the cardiovascular and pulmonary systems to compensate for decreasing oxygen carrying capacity of the blood.

A. Initial: Exercise-induced dyspnea and mild fatigue symptoms may be minimal until the patient has significant anemia.
B. As HCT falls: Dyspnea and fatigue increase.
  1. Malaise
  2. Drowsiness
  3. Sore tongue and mouth
  4. Skin pallor
  5. Pale mucous membranes and conjunctiva
  6. Pale fingernail beds
  7. Tachycardia
  8. Palpitations
  9. Tinnitus
C. Severe anemia.
  1. Atrophic glossitis, cheilitis (lesions at the corner of the mouth)
  2. Koilonychia (thin concave fingernails with raised edges)

Subjective Data

A. Inquire about onset, course, and duration of symptoms.
B. Ask the patient about past history of GI bleeding.
C. Take careful history of gastrointestinal complaints that might suggest gastritis, peptic ulcer disease, or other conditions that might produce GI bleeding.
D. Ask if there has been a change in stool color or bleeding from hemorrhoids.
E. In menstruating women, ask about blood loss during menses.
F. Ask about dietary intake of iron-rich foods and pica.
G. Obtain medication history, especially use of aspirin and other NSAIDs.
H. Rule out history of anemia, blood-clotting problems, sickle cell disease, glucose-6-phosphate dehydrogenase (G6PD) deficiency, or other hereditary hemolytic disease.
I. Review occupation, hobbies, and so on with exposure to lead or lead paint.
J. Has the patient experienced palpitations, chest pain, dizziness, or shortness of breath?

Physical Examination

A. Check temperature, pulse, respirations, blood pressure, and weight. Check for postural hypotension. Children: plot weight, height, and head growth parameters on growth chart. See Table 16.1.
B. Inspect.
  1. Inspect general appearance; the patient may be pale, lethargic, or without overt signs if anemia is mild.
  2. Conduct eye exam; check conjunctivae for paleness.
  3. Examine oral mucosa, corners of the mouth (for cheilitis); note appearance of the tongue (atrophy of the papillae; smooth, shiny, beefy red appearance), angular stomatitis, or pale gums.
  4. Examine the skin for dryness and perfusion.
  5. Examine nails for brittleness, flattening, ridges, and concave or spoon shape.
C. Palpate: Palpate the abdomen for tenderness and enlargement of the liver and spleen.
D. Percuss: Percuss the abdomen.
E. Auscultate: Auscultate the heart for systolic flow murmurs.
F. Rectal exam: Assess for masses, and obtain stool for occult blood.

Diagnostic Tests

A. Initial
  1. CBC with differential and peripheral smear
  2. Serum ferritin level, serum iron, total iron-binding capacity (TIBC), Retic count

TABLE 16.1 Normal Hemoglobin and Hematocrit Values for Children

Age	Hgb	HCT
1–2 years old	> 11.0%	> 33.0%
2–5 years old	> 11.2%	> 34.0%
5–8 years old	> 11.4%	> 34.5%
8–12 years old	> 11.6%	> 35.5%
12–18 years old	> 12.0%	> 36.0%

3. Serum iron concentration: absent iron stores equals ferritin value less than 30 ng/mL
4. Urinalysis
5. Stool for occult blood
B. Follow-up
   1. Total iron-binding capacity: serum total iron-binding capacity (TIBC) rises, serum ferritin.
   2. HCT 3–4 weeks after treatment. Treatment should continue for at least 4–6 months after the HCT returns to normal.
   3. GI series, if indicated.
   4. Endoscope, if indicated.
   5. Ultrasonography, if indicated.

Differential Diagnoses

A. Iron deficiency anemia
B. Inadequate intake of iron
C. Any condition that causes acute or chronic blood loss
D. Hemolytic diseases such as sickle cell and G6PD deficiency
E. Anemia of chronic disease, thalassemia, and sideroblastic anemias
F. Lead poisoning
G. Neoplasm

Plan

A. General interventions: Identify source of anemia. Discuss dietary sources of iron-rich foods. Infants should be ingesting formula enriched with iron and iron-enriched cereals.
B. Patient teaching.
   1. See the Section III Patient Teaching Guide for this chapter, "Iron Deficiency Anemia."
   2. Stress the importance of dietary intake of foods high in iron, which is absorbed better than most vitamins. Orange juice increases absorption of iron. Tea and milk reduce iron absorption.
   3. Provide iron supplements.
   4. Encourage the patient to stop smoking.
C. Pharmaceutical therapy.
   1. Oral iron replacement
      a. Adult
         i. Begin 6-month trial of ferrous sulfate tablets 300–325 mg three times daily before meals or with orange juice 1 hour before meals. Food decreases iron delivery by 50% (Springhouse Guide, 1997, pp. 151–153).
         ii. Iron supplement (Slow Fe) one time-release capsule daily.
      b. Children
         i. Liquid iron 3 mg/kg/day in a single dose.
         ii. Chewable vitamin with an iron supplement one tablet every day for mild cases.
   2. Alternative drug therapy: Parenteral iron is indicated if the patient cannot tolerate or absorb oral iron or if iron loss exceeds oral replacement.
      a. Iron dextran injection (Imferon)
      b. Iron sorbitex injection (Jectofer)
         i. Parenteral iron therapy is expensive.
         ii. It is associated with significant side effects: anaphylaxis, phlebitis, regional adenopathy, serum sickness-type reaction, and staining of intramuscular injection sites.
         iii. Dose is based on the patient's weight.
         iv. Do not administer parenteral iron along with oral iron.

Follow-up

A. Follow-up of adults is variable, depending on source of blood loss. Manage signs of anemia.
B. It is advisable to see the patient after 3–4 weeks, both to monitor the hematologic response and to answer questions about the medication, which may result in improved compliance.
C. If the patient's hemoglobin level has increased by 1.0 g/dL in 3–4 weeks, continue iron supplementation for additional 3–6 months.
D. Determine effectiveness of iron replacement therapy during the first 2 weeks of therapy by checking the reticulocyte count.

Consultation/Referral

A. Refer the patient to a physician for the following:
   1. Hemoglobin is not increased by 1.0 g/dL after 1 month of treatment.
   2. The therapeutic trial should not be continued beyond 1 month because the hemoglobin concentration has not increased and patient compliance with recommended regimen is not a factor.
   3. There is a steady downward trend in HCT despite treatment.
   4. There is a significant drop in HCT over previous readings (rule out lab error first).
   5. Lab findings show Hgb less than 9.0 g/dL or HCT less than 27%. Suspect underlying inflammatory, infectious, or malignant disease.
B. Refer the patient for nutrition consultation, if indicated.

Individual Considerations

A. Pregnancy
   1. Check HCT at initial prenatal visit, 28 weeks, and 4 weeks after initiating therapy.
   2. Lab findings of Hgb greater than 13 g/dL and HCT greater than 40% may indicate hypovolemia. Be alert for signs of dehydration and preeclampsia.
   3. Counsel the patient on proper diet and refer her to a dietitian.
   4. Recommend one to two iron tablets a day in addition to prenatal vitamin containing iron.

5. If unable to tolerate vitamins, recommend children's Chewable Flintstones vitamins with iron, 2 orally, daily.

B. Pediatrics
1. Place medication in back of mouth to reduce staining of teeth.
2. All infants must be on iron-fortified formula or breast milk.
3. Inform caregiver not to give cow's milk to infants less than 12 months old.
4. Educate parents about iron-rich foods that are age-appropriate: cereals, bran, dried fruit, red meat, and beans.
5. Obtain height and weight of infants and children, plot on growth chart, and compare with previous parameters.

C. Adults
1. Bleeding is the usual cause of anemia in adults. In adult men and postmenopausal women, bleeding is usually from the GI tract.
2. In premenopausal women, menstrual loss may be the underlying cause of anemia.
3. Smokers may have higher Hgb levels; therefore, anemia may be masked if standard Hgb levels are used.

LYMPHADENOPATHY

Definition

Lymphadenopathy is enlargement of a lymph node, manifested in benign, self-limiting diseases and in those that are incurable and fatal. Only small lymph nodes in the neck, axilla, and groin are palpable in normal individuals. Palpable nodes in other regions, or any node exceeding 0.5 cm (Ferri, 2004, p. 1299) in size, are potentially abnormal.

There are different categories of lymphadenopathy:

A. Localized adenopathy.
B. Hilar adenopathy.
C. Generalized lymphadenopathy.
D. Other lymphatic abnormalities that present in other ways, such as lymphangitis, lymphadenitis, and lymphedema.

Incidence

A. Lymphadenopathy is a very common presenting symptom. Age is an important diagnostic factor: in patients under the age of 30, the cause proves to be benign in 80% of cases; in patients over age 50, the rate of benign disease falls to 40%.

Pathogenesis

A. Inflammation and infiltration are responsible for pathologic enlargement. Localized lymphadenopathy may represent the spread of disease from an area of drainage. The left supraclavicular node is referred to as the "sentinel" node, which is in contact with the thoracic duct and drains much of the abdominal cavity. The right supraclavicular node drains the mediastinum, lungs, and esophagus. Generalized lymphadenopathy often results from infection, malignancy, hypersensitivity, and metabolic disease.

Predisposing Factors

A. Factors posing high risk for HIV infection
1. Homosexuality and bisexuality
2. Intravenous drug abuse
3. Hemophilia, conditions requiring multiple transfusions
4. Prostitution
5. Haitian ancestry

B. Occupational exposure
C. History of pharyngitis, upper body infections (head and neck), or intraoral infection
D. Exposure to animals: cats, sheep, cattle, rodents, deer ticks
E. Travel to the southwest United States
F. Exposure to bird droppings
G. Lacerations sustained from gardening
H. Exposure to tuberculosis
I. History of sexual exposure resulting in sexually transmitted infections
J. History of tobacco abuse
K. Cancer
L. Anticonvulsant drugs that cause skin rash, fever, hepatosplenomegaly, and eosinophilia; for example, phenytoin (Dilantin)
M. Other medications
1. Hydralazine
2. Para-aminosalicylic acid
3. Allopurinol

Common Complaints

A. Sore throat
B. Fever
C. Fatigue and malaise
D. Loss of appetite
E. Loss of weight
F. Swollen, painless lumps in neck

Other Signs and Symptoms

A. May feel "good" except for finding enlarged lymph node.
B. Node location(s): For inguinal enlargement, rule out conditions that may resemble inguinal or femoral lymphadenopathy: hernias; ectopic testicular, endometrial, or splenic tissue; lipomas; varices; and aneurysms. If inguinal area is painful and tender, it is most frequently caused by sexually transmitted infections.
C. Skin rash.
D. Bruising or petechiae.
E. Pruritus.
F. Erythema of skin or scalp.
G. Skin eruption.
H. Night sweats.
I. Enlarged and tender abdomen, abdominal pain.
J. Joint pain.

Subjective Data

A. A comprehensive and detailed history is necessary for diagnosis (see "Predisposing Factors"). Review the onset, course, and duration of symptoms.
B. What does the patient note with respect to location, tenderness or painfulness, softness or hardness, and mobility

of lymph nodes? Has the patient noticed more than one enlarged lymph node?

C. Review the patient's history of intravenous drug use. Review risk factors for HIV.

D. Review history for hobbies, specifically gardening and camping, and occupation (see "Toxoplasmosis" and "Lyme Disease" in Chapter 15, "Infectious Disease Guidelines").

E. Review medications: prescription, over-the-counter, and herbal remedies.

F. Determine whether the patient has a fever or a known valvular heart disease.

G. Review any other associated symptoms or signs.

H. Review any recent exposure to family and friends with infections. Has the patient had recent immunizations?

I. Review recent dental problems or abscessed teeth.

J. Note whether the patient is a smoker. If so, how much, for how long, and when did the patient quit smoking?

K. Review the patient's history for recent cat scratches (see "Cat Scratch Disease (CSD)" in Chapter 15, "Infectious Disease Guidelines").

L. Review the patient's history for recent travel.

M. Review the patient's history for new sexual partners, to rule out STIs.

N. Review usual weight and any recent weight loss, noting how much over what period of time.

O. Elicit information about similar symptoms in the past, when they occurred, how they were treated (antibiotics, biopsy), and the success of the treatment.

P. Elicit information about alcohol intake, noting how much, how long, and if the patient has quit, how long ago.

Physical Examination

A. Check temperature, pulse, respirations, blood pressure, and weight.

B. Inspect.
1. Conduct a funduscopic exam.
2. Examine the eyes, ears, nose, and throat.
3. Conduct a dermal exam, and check mucous membranes for a primary inoculation site; this may be clue to a diagnosis of cat scratch disease.

C. Palpate.
1. Palpate the abdomen.
2. Conduct a clinical breast exam. Palpate mass to determine if it is a lymph node, if applicable.
3. Palpate all nodal areas for localized and generalized lymphadenopathy.
   a. Hard, fixed nodes suggest metastasis, and a biopsy should be taken promptly. Size alone is not itself diagnostic; any node larger than 3 cm suggests neoplastic disease.
4. Palpate the scalp in the elderly for the tender arteries of cranial arteritis.
5. Palpate the neck for thyroid gland tenderness.

D. Percuss: Percuss sinuses for tenderness, and transilluminate for evidence of sinusitis.

E. Auscultate: Auscultate the heart and lungs.

F. Musculoskeletal system exam
1. Assess for bone or joint swelling, tenderness, and increased warmth.
2. Examine lower extremities for evidence of phlebitis: asymmetric swelling, calf tenderness, and palpable cord.

G. Genitorectal exam.
1. Conduct careful external evaluation for herpetic lesions, masses, discharge, erythema, chancroid, scabies, and pediculosis.
2. "Milk" urethra for discharge.
3. Note any folliculitis if the patient regularly shaves genital area.
4. Female pelvic exam: Look for cervical discharge, cervical motion tenderness, adnexal tenderness, and mass or "heat" in the pelvis.
5. Males: Examine the prostate and testicles for tenderness and masses, the penis for discharge and rash.
6. Examine rectum for discharge, tenderness, masses, and fistulas.

Diagnostic Tests

A. CBC with differential.

B. Peripheral blood smear: the most useful laboratory test; may be helpful in the diagnosis of chronic leukemia, infectious mononucleosis, and other viral illnesses.

C. Blood chemistries.

D. Liver function tests, especially alkaline phosphatase.

E. Angiotensin converting enzyme (ACE).

F. Antinuclear antibody (ANA) and rheumatoid factor.

G. RPR and MHA-TP, to rule out syphilis.

H. Heterophile test, to rule out mononucleosis.

I. ELISA and Western blot, to rule out HIV.

J. Uric acid: elevations may reflect lymphoma or other hematologic malignancies.

K. Blood cultures.

L. Urethral or cervical cultures and smears.

M. Throat culture.

N. Chest X-ray.

O. Mammogram with ultrasonography of suspicious breast area, if indicated.

P. After consultation.
1. Abdominal ultrasonography or CT scan, if indicated.
2. Biopsy or fine-needle aspiration: Fine-needle aspiration is used to obtain a cytologic diagnosis of a suspected cancer. False-negative results may occasionally occur.
3. Lymph node biopsy: Lymph node biopsy is the definitive test to confirm or rule out a suspected neoplastic process.
4. Mediastinoscopy.

Q. Tuberculin skin testing (PPD) and the angiotensin converting enzyme (ACE) determination can facilitate assessment.
1. If the patient tests *negative for ACE and PPD* and is Caucasian, then bronchoscopy and mediastinoscopy may be necessary to rule out lymphoma. If the patient tests *positive for ACE but negative for PPD,* then the probability is very high that sarcoidosis is the cause.
2. If the patient tests *negative for ACE but positive for PPD,* then primary TB is likely.

Differential Diagnoses

A. There are four general categories for lymphadenopathy:
1. Infections
   a. Mononucleosis.

b. AIDS or AIDS-related complex (ARC): Generalized adenopathy in an asymptomatic HIV-infected patient indicates a high risk of progression to AIDS. The lymphadenopathy represents follicular hyperplasia in response to HIV infection.
   c. Toxoplasmosis.
   d. Secondary syphilis.
2. Hypersensitivity reactions
   a. Serum sickness
   b. Phenytoin and other drugs
   c. Vasculitis: lupus and rheumatoid arthritis
3. Metabolic diseases
   a. Hyperthyroidism
   b. Lipidoses
4. Neoplasia
   a. Leukemia
   b. Hodgkin's disease, advanced stages
   c. Non-Hodgkin's lymphoma

B. Causes can be isolated by site of the enlarged nodes. See Table 16.2.

Plan

A. General interventions.
   1. Pay careful attention to nodal history and characteristics on physical examination.
   2. Make a careful assessment to establish the palpable mass is a lymph node. Chronicity alone is not always serious.

TABLE 16.2 Causes of Lymphadenopathy by Site of Enlarged Nodes

Anterior Auricular	**Epitrochlear**
Viral conjunctivitis	Syphilis (bilateral)
Trachoma	Hand infection (unilateral)
Posterior Auricular	**Inguinal**
Rubella	Syphilis
Scalp infection	Genital herpes
	Lymphogranuloma venereum
Submandibular or	Chancroid
Cervical (Unilateral)	Lower extremity or local
Buccal cavity infection	infection
Pharyngitis (can be bilateral)	
Nasopharyngeal tumor	**Any Region**
Thyroid malignancy	Cat-scratch fever
	Hodgkin's disease
Cervical (Bilateral)	Leukemia
Mononucleosis Sarcoidosis	Metastatic cancer
Toxoplasmosis Pharyngitis	Sarcoidosis
	Granulomatous infections
Supraclavicular (Right)	
Pulmonary malignancy	**Hilar Adenopathy**
Mediastinal malignancy	Sarcoidosis (unilateral or
Esophageal malignancy	bilateral)
	Fungal infection
Supraclavicular (Left)	(histoplasmosis,
Intra-abdominal malignancy	coccidioidomycosis)
Renal malignancy	Lymphoma (unilateral or
Testicular or ovarian	bilateral)
malignancy	Bronchogenic carcinoma
	(unilateral or bilateral)
Axillary	Tuberculosis (unilateral or
Breast malignancy	bilateral)
Breast infection	
Upper extremity infection	

B. Patient teaching: as indicated by the particular disease process causing the lymphadenopathy. See the relevant guidelines.
C. Pharmaceutical therapy: dependent on the diagnosis.

Follow-up

A. Follow the patient closely to evaluate resolution of lymphadenopathy and disease process.
B. Follow-up depends on the diagnosis.

Consultation/Referral

A. Consultation with a physician may be useful if a period of observation is needed.
B. Refer the patient to a specialist after initial workup, if indicated.
C. Refer the patient to an oncologist or oncologic surgeon if the patient is suspected of having a malignancy, to consider the need for biopsy or best approach to obtaining a tissue diagnosis.

Individual Considerations

A. Pediatrics.
   1. Palpable nodes in the anterior cervical triangle of the neck are common in children and usually suggest infection as a cause.
   2. Kawasaki disease is seen among children and young adults; it is also known as mucocutaneous lymph node syndrome (see Chapter 15, "Infectious Disease Guidelines"). Hodgkin's lymphoma is one of the most common cancers of young adults.
B. Geriatrics: Regional lymphadenopathy occurs often when carcinomas metastasize to lymph nodes in the elderly.

PERNICIOUS ANEMIA (MEGALOBLASTIC ANEMIA)

Definition

A. Pernicious anemia is a megaloblastic, macrocytic, normochromic anemia caused by a deficiency of intrinsic factor in the gastric juices produced by the stomach, which results in malabsorption of Vitamin B_{12} necessary for DNA synthesis and maturation of RBCs. There is the production of abnormally large and oval red cells with a mean corpuscular volume in excess of 100 fL (femtoliters). The anemia can be severe, with hematocrits as low as 10%–15%.

Incidence

A. Pernicious anemia is common in people of northern European descent. Both sexes are equally affected. It is most prevalent in Scandinavian and English-speaking populations. It usually occurs in the fifth and sixth decades of life; it is rarely seen in persons under age 35 years, but it can occur in individuals in their 20s. There is an increased incidence in those with other immunologic disease.

Pathogenesis

A. Pernicious anemia is possibly due to an autoimmune reaction involving the gastric parietal cell that results in nonproduction of intrinsic factor and atrophy of gastric mucosa. Vitamin B$_{12}$ deficiency can result from inadequate intake, impaired absorption, increased requirements as in pregnancy, or faulty utilization. Poor intake is rare, occurring most often in strict vegetarians.

Predisposing Factors
A. People of northern European descent
B. Ages 50–60 years
C. Immunologic disease
D. Loss of parietal cells following gastrectomy
E. Overgrowth of intestinal organisms
F. Crohn's disease
G. Ileal resection or abnormalities
H. Fish tapeworm
I. Congenital enzyme deficiencies
J. Diet: strict vegetarian diets
K. Medications such as aminosalicylate sodium
L. Alcoholism
M. Hashimoto's thyroiditis

Common Complaints

Classic presentation involves sore tongue and numbness and tingling in the extremities, hands, or feet.

A. Weakness and dizziness
B. Tongue is sore, red, and shiny
C. Numbness, burning, tingling sensation of arms or legs
D. Feel heart "jumping out of skin"
E. Edema of lower extremities
F. Anorexia
G. Diarrhea

Other Signs and Symptoms
A. Dyspnea on exertion
B. Pallor
C. Fatigue
D. Tachycardia
E. Exercise intolerance
F. Angina
G. Glossitis
H. Mucositis
I. Peripheral paresthesia
J. Palpitations
K. Abdominal tenderness, organomegaly
L. Advanced stages: dementia and spinal cord degeneration

Subjective Data
A. Inquire about onset, duration, and course of presenting symptoms.
B. Ask the patient to describe usual bowel habits. Has there been any blood in stools?
C. If GI complaints are present, inquire about presence of red, burning tongue; abdominal complaints; presence of diarrhea or constipation.
D. If neurologic complaints are present, inquire about presence of pins-and-needles paresthesia and weakness, unsteadiness due to proprioceptive difficulties, lethargy, and fatigue.
E. Inquire about dietary intake, using 24-hour recall.
F. Ask about alcohol consumption: How much? How long?

G. Obtain medication history: OTC and prescription drugs.
H. Obtain past medical history, specifically if the patient has history of gastrectomy, resection of ileum, or other GI disorders.
I. Review usual weight and recent loss.

Physical Examination
A. Check temperature, pulse, respirations, blood pressure, weight, and height for children; plot on graph.
B. Inspect.
   1. Observe general, overall appearance; observe walking.
   2. Conduct oral exam for characteristic red, shiny tongue.
   3. Conduct dermal and eye exams for color: affected patients are slightly icteric.
   4. Evaluate the look of the person related to age: affected patients show premature aging or graying.
C. Palpate.
   1. Palpate the abdomen for masses.
   2. Evaluate pedal edema.
D. Percuss: Percuss the abdomen for tenderness and organomegaly.
E. Auscultate.
   1. Auscultate heart sounds and lungs.
   2. Auscultate the abdomen for bowel sounds.
F. Neurologic exam: Assess deep tendon reflexes (DTRs) and mental status.
   1. Look for paresthesia involving hands and feet, gait disturbances, memory loss (mild forgetfulness to dementia or altered thought processes). Poor finger-nose coordination may be seen; positive Romberg's and Babinski's signs may be present.

Diagnostic Tests
A. CBC with differential and peripheral smear: **Macro-ovalocytes and hypersegmented neutrophils may be present on peripheral blood smear. (They are absent in the setting of concurrent iron deficiency.)**
B. Serum Vitamin B$_{12}$ level: less than 100 pg/mL.
C. Serum folic acid levels, serum iron, serum ferritin, and TIBC.
D. Serum intrinsic factor antibody.
E. LDH.
F. Urinalysis.
G. Stool for occult blood.
H. Oral Schilling test with and without intrinsic factor.
I. GI radiographic studies.
J. Gastric analysis: Achlorhydria is found on stimulation testing.
K. Bone marrow aspiration.

Differential Diagnoses
Differential diagnosis of anemia by red cell morphology can be undertaken (MCV = mean corpuscular volume, MCHC = mean corpuscular hemoglobin concentration). Common causes of each type of anemia are as follows:

A. Normochromic, normocytic: normal MCV = 80–100, MCHC = 32%–36%
   1. Aplastic anemia
   2. Chronic disease

3. Early iron deficiency
4. Hemolysis
5. Hemorrhage
B. Microcytic: MCV = 50–82, MCHC = 24–32
   1. Chronic disease
   2. Iron deficiency
   3. Thalassemia
C. Macrocytic: MCV > 100, MCHC > 36
   1. Antimetabolites
   2. Folic acid deficiencies
   3. Vitamin B_{12} deficiencies
   4. Chronic alcoholism

Plan

A. General interventions
   1. Most common method of determining Vitamin B_{12} deficiency is by serum Vitamin B_{12} assay.
   2. Most common method of demonstrating folate deficiency is by measurement of serum folic acid levels.
   3. Red cell indices and peripheral smear should be done to determine classification of anemia to facilitate workup.
   4. Red cell distribution width (RDW) determination can assist in detecting red cell heterogeneity previously available only by exam of the peripheral smear. The RDW determination overcomes the problems of detecting coexisting microcytic and macrocytic anemias.
B. Patient teaching
   1. See the Section III Patient Teaching Guide for this chapter, "Pernicious Anemia."
   2. Neurologic symptoms usually improve with treatment; however, some neurologic deficits may not be reversible.
C. Pharmaceutical therapy
   1. Vitamin B_{12} (cyanocobalamin or hydroxocobalamin) 100 mg intramuscularly or subcutaneous administration daily for 1 week.
      a. Decrease frequency and administer a total of 2,000 mg during the first 6 weeks of therapy (weekly for 1 month).
      b. **Maintenance treatment requires lifelong administration of 100 mg IM injection monthly depending on B12 levels. Some people may require lifelong administration at different intervals such as every 2 weeks.**
      c. Nascobal (intranasal cyanocobalamin) one spray in one nostril one time per week (Ferri, 2004, p. 65).
   2. Recommended daily allowance for Vitamin B_{12}:
      a. Neonates and infants up to 6 months: 0.3 μg/day.
      b. Children older than 6 months to 1 year: 0.5 μg/day.
      c. Children 1–3 years: 0.7 μg/day.
      d. Children 4–6 years: 1.0 μg/day.
      e. Children 7–10 years: 1.4 μg/day.
      f. Adults and children older than 11 years: 2.0 μg/day.
      g. Pregnant women: 2.2 μg/day.
      h. Breast-feeding women: 2.6 μg/day.

3. Concomitant iron supplementation during first month of therapy. Rapid blood cell regeneration increases iron requirements and can lead to iron deficiency.

Follow-up

A. The patient must be seen in 2 weeks to determine response to treatment: increased reticulocyte count and increased hematocrit; diminution in neurologic signs and symptoms.
B. Evaluate the patient monthly when giving Vitamin B_{12} injections.
C. **Endoscopy every 5 years is used to rule out gastric carcinoma (Disease Management, 2002).**
D. Check the patient every 6 months for hematocrit, and check his or her stool for occult blood.
E. Hematocrit value rises 4%–5% per week in uncomplicated cases.

Consultation/Referral

A. Refer the patient to a dietitian.
B. Rapid reticulocytosis should be seen following treatment; it peaks in 7–10 days.
C. Consult a physician if no change is seen.

Individual Considerations

A. Pregnancy.
   1. Lactovegetarians and ovolactovegetarians do well in pregnancy.
   2. Vegetarian women who eat neither eggs nor milk products should take Vitamin B_{12} supplements during pregnancy and lactation.
B. Pediatrics: Congenital disorder usually is seen prior to 3 years of age.
C. Adults: Disorder rarely is seen in patients under age 35 years.
D. Geriatrics.
   1. Disorder most commonly is seen in the geriatric population.
   2. Follow up elderly patients with assessment of cardiovascular symptoms 48 hours after initiating therapy.
   3. Rapid blood cell regeneration increases iron requirements and can lead to iron deficiency.

SYSTEMIC LUPUS ERYTHEMATOSUS (SLE)

Definition

Systemic lupus erythematosus (SLE) is a chronic, inflammatory autoimmune disorder. It may affect multiple organ systems. The body's immune system forms antibodies that attack healthy tissues and organs. The clinical course is marked by spontaneous remission and relapses. Severity varies from a mild episodic disorder to a rapidly fulminating fatal disease. The three types of lupus are as follows:

A. Discoid lupus erythematosus (DLE) affects the skin, causing a rash, lesions, or both.
B. Systemic lupus erythematosus (SLE) attacks body organs and systems, such as joints, kidneys, brain, heart, and

lungs. SLE is usually more severe than DLE and can be life-threatening.

C. Drug-induced lupus symptoms usually disappear when medication is discontinued.

Incidence

A. The incidence of SLE in relation to sex, ancestry, and familial history has been repeatedly documented. About 85% of patients with SLE are women; it affects mainly young women after menarche and before menopause. The majority of patients who develop SLE during childhood or after age 50 are also women. SLE occurs in 1:1000 White women and 1:250 Black women. The disorder is concordant in 25%–75% of identical twins. The risk of developing the disease if a mother has SLE for a daughter is 1:40, for a son is 1:250. Positive antinuclear antibody is seen in asymptomatic family members, and the prevalence of other rheumatic diseases is increased among close relatives of patients. There is a high frequency of specific genes in SLE. Ten percent of DLE patients go on to develop SLE.

Pathogenesis

A. Clinical manifestations of SLE are secondary to the trapping of antigen-antibody complexes in capillaries of visceral structures, or to autoantibody-mediated destruction of host cells such as thrombocytopenia.

Predisposing Factors

A. Female gender
B. African, Asian, Hispanic ancestry
C. Childbearing age
D. Positive family history of SLE
E. Drug use
   1. Procainamide
   2. Hydralazine
   3. Isoniazid

Common Complaints

A. Joint pain: Joint symptoms occur in 90% of patients.
B. Fever.
C. Loss of appetite.
D. Fatigue.
E. Weight loss.
F. Hair loss.
G. Rash and skin lesions over areas exposed to sunlight.

Other Signs and Symptoms

A. Discoid lupus erythematosus:
   1. Rash: erythematous, round, scaling papules 5–10 mm in diameter, appearing as "butterfly" shape across bridge of nose
   2. Rash, commonly on the trunk, extremities, scalp, external ear, and neck
   3. Photosensitivity
B. Systemic lupus erythematosus
   1. Malar rash
   2. Discoid rash
   3. Weight loss
   4. Fatigue
   5. Photosensitivity
   6. Oral ulcers
   7. Acute or subacute abdominal pain
   8. Alopecia
   9. Arthritis, generally bilateral, symmetric especially in hands and wrists
   10. Tendon involvement
   11. Serositis
   12. Frequent UTIs, chronic renal problems as indicated by proteinuria and cellular casts
   13. Fever and malaise
   14. Lymphadenopathy
   15. Other complications
      a. Hashimoto's thyroiditis
      b. Hemolytic anemia
      c. Thrombocytopenia purpura
      d. Arterial and venous thrombosis
      e. Recurrent pleurisy
      f. Pleural effusion, pneumonitis
      g. Pulmonary embolism
      h. Pericarditis, endocarditis, myocarditis
      i. Hypertension
      j. Splenomegaly
C. CNS problems
   1. Chronic headaches (migraine)
   2. Seizures or epilepsy
   3. Personality changes, chronic brain syndrome
D. Decreased Hgb, WBC, and platelets

Subjective Data

A. Determine systemic features and onset, course, and duration of symptoms (see "Signs and Symptoms").
B. Obtain medication history (see "Predisposing Factors").
C. Determine family history of rheumatoid diseases.
D. Review the patient's recent history for possible allergen exposure.

Physical Examination

A. Check temperature, pulse, respirations, and blood pressure
B. Inspect
   1. Observe general overall appearance and generalized movement of extremities.
   2. Conduct dermal exam for color, petechiae, rashes and lesions, and hair loss.
   3. Conduct funduscopic exam; note photosensitivity.

Funduscopic exam: Cotton-wool exudates are the most common eye lesion.

   4. Examine mouth for lesions.
   5. Observe for pericardial lifts and heaves.
C. Palpate
   1. Palpate the back for tactile fremitus; palpate the heart for lifts, heaves, and thrills.
   2. Palpate the neck for thyroid enlargement.
   3. Palpate the neck, axilla, and groin for lymphadenopathy.
   4. Palpate the abdomen for organomegaly, masses, and tenderness; check suprapubic tenderness and CVA tenderness.

D. Percuss
1. Percuss the chest, anterior and posterior lung fields for consolidation.
2. Percuss the abdomen for splenomegaly.
E. Auscultate
1. Auscultate the heart.
2. Auscultate the abdomen.
F. Musculoskeletal exam
1. Examine for bone or joint swelling, tenderness, and increased warmth.
2. Check lower extremities for evidence of phlebitis, asymmetrical swelling, calf tenderness, and palpable cord.
G. Neurologic exam: Complete neurologic exam with mental status exam

Diagnostic Examination
A. CBC with differential.
B. Platelets.
C. Antinuclear antibody (ANA): positive ANA, erythrocyte sedimentation rate (ESR).
D. Complement levels (decreased C3 and C4).
E. Rheumatoid factor.
F. Lupus erythematosus (LE) cell prep: positive.
G. Anti-DNA antibodies.
H. Rapid plasma reagin (RPR) for syphilis.
I. Thyroid profile.
J. Urinalysis and urine culture.
K. Collect 24-hour urine for protein and creatinine clearance.
L. Skin biopsy.
M. Follow-up Coombs' test: positive.
N. MHA-TP to confirm reactive syphilis for positive RPR: False-positive serologic test for syphilis needs follow-up.
O. Chest X-ray film may show changes.
P. X-ray films for nondestructive arthritis.

Differential Diagnoses
A. Lupus.
B. DLE.
C. SLE.
D. Drug-induced lupus.
E. Rheumatoid arthritis: Lupus can resemble rheumatoid arthritis (RA), especially early in the course of SLE. Unlike RA, the arthritis is nonerosive: there is no joint destruction.
F. Vasculitis.
G. Scleroderma.
H. Chronic active hepatitis.
I. Acute drug reactions.
J. Polyarteritis.
K. Infection.
L. Influenza.
M. Rosacea.
N. Neoplasm.

Plan
A. General interventions: After diagnosis, refer the patient to and comanage with a physician.
B. Patient teaching: See the Section III Patient Teaching Guide for this chapter, "Lupus."

C. Pharmaceutical therapy
1. NSAIDs for arthritis symptoms.
2. Prednisone 40–60 mg initially for the control of thrombocytopenic purpura, hemolytic anemia, myocarditis, pericarditis, convulsions, and nephritis.
3. Always give the lowest dose that controls the condition.
4. Corticosteroids can usually be tapered to low doses, 10–15 mg/day, during disease inactivity.
5. Antimalarial drug, hydroxychloroquine sulfate every day, may help treat lupus rashes and joint symptoms that do not respond to NSAIDs. Do not exceed 400 mg/day. **Consult with a specialist.**
6. Alternative drug therapy: Immunosuppressive agents such as cyclophosphamide, chlorambucil, azathioprine are used in cases resistant to corticosteroids. The exact role of immunosuppressive agents is controversial.

Follow-up
A. Very close follow-up by a physician specialist is needed when immunosuppressants are employed.
B. Monitor the patient for infections, especially with opportunistic organisms.

Infections are the leading cause of death secondary to the depression of WBCs, followed by active SLE, chiefly due to renal or CNS disease.

Consultation/Referral
A. After diagnosis, refer the patient to a medical specialist, a rheumatologist.
B. Refer the patient to a perinatologist for pregnancy management.

Individual Considerations
A. Pregnancy
1. Infertility: 25% of patients have a problem getting pregnant.
2. Patients with SLE experience frequent miscarriages and stillbirths.
3. Patients are considered "high-risk" patients who need consultation and management with a perinatologist.
4. Thirty-three percent of patients have an antibody (anti-cardiolipin) that is associated with early failure of the placenta.
5. Ten percent have a related antibody (lupus anticoagulant) that allows early pregnancy, but compromises fetal growth as the placenta fails.
6. Twenty-five percent of the remaining pregnancies deliver prematurely.
7. Family planning,
a. Barrier methods or IUD are best and safest.
b. Birth control pills may exacerbate lupus. However, they are safer than an unwanted pregnancy.
8. Exacerbations of lupus are sometimes caused by pregnancy.
B. Pediatrics
1. Prematurity is the greatest danger of lupus' effects on the baby.

2. There are no known congenital abnormalities related to lupus.
3. Three percent of all lupus patients have a baby with neonatal lupus. This is a syndrome, not SLE, and it is transient.
C. Geriatrics: Males are affected more than females.

VITAMIN D DEFICIENCY *by Jill C. Cash*

Definition
A. Vitamin D deficiency is defined as having a serum 25 (OH)D level lower than 15 ng/mL. Vitamin D insufficiency is defined as having a serum 25 (OH)D level lower than 30 ng/mL. Vitamin D deficiency is also known as hypovitaminosis D.

Incidence
A. Vitamin D deficiency is seen in all ages. It is highest in the elderly, institutionalized, and/or hospitalized. It is found to be more common in women than in men (83% vs. 48%), the difference most likely being less skin exposure to the sun and higher incidence in the winter months, again due to less sun exposure in the winter months.

Pathogenesis
A. Vitamin D is obtained from direct sunlight exposure from the sun to direct skin and by ingesting Vitamin D-rich foods. The liver is responsible for breaking it down, it hydroxylates the Vitamin D to storage form, 25-hydroxyvitamin D (25[OH]D), which then breaks down into the next step in the kidney into the bioactive form, 1,25-dihydroxyvitamin D (1,25[OH]2D). The 1,25(OH)2D is regulated by the parathyroid hormone and causes calcium absorption to occur in the intestine, which in return affects bone metabolism and muscle function. When any part of this cascade is interrupted, the cascade does not occur flow and Vitamin D deficiency occurs.

Predisposing Factors
A. Race (darker skin population).
B. Age: elderly population highest risk.
C. Long-term institutionalized individuals (nursing home).
D. Obese individuals.
E. Decreased sun exposure (individuals who spend very little time outdoors in the sun).
F. People with certain medical conditions with serious nervous or digestive disorders (chronic kidney disease and malabsorption problems).
G. Medications: drugs such as dilantin, phenobarbital, rifampin induce hepatic p450 enzymes and accelerate catabolism of Vitamin D.

Common Complaints
A. Complaints vary from being no complaints to severe.
B. Chronic muscle aches/pain/fatigue/weakness.
C. Joint pain and bone pain.
D. Waddling gait, leg bowing, kyphosis, scoliosis, and protrusion of acetabuli.

Other Signs and Symptoms
A. Fracture of bone.
B. Frequent falls and muscle weakness.
C. The most severe form of Vitamin D deficiency can cause nutritional rickets.

Subjective Data
A. With patients presenting with complaints, assess onset, duration, and course of complaints.
B. Assess daily nutritional habits. Does the patient get enough calcium and Vitamin D in current diet?
C. Does the patient live in the home or an institution? Is the patient allowed to spend time outdoors in sunlight? What time of the season/year is it, allowing 20–30 min in the sun without sunscreen reasonable?
D. Is the patient currently taking any vitamin supplements? If so, review vitamin and ingredients in that particular vitamin.
E. Review the patient history and determine if the patient has chronic condition, malabsorption condition, chronic kidney condition, or medications interfering with absorption. If no current diagnosis of gastrointestinal problem, inquire regarding food intolerances, stool patterns, constipation, and diarrhea history.
F. Does the patient currently take a Vitamin D and/or calcium supplement?
G. Has the patient had a recent Vitamin D level drawn?
H. Inquire regarding the patient's fatigue level.
I. Assess for muscle weakness, frequent falls, especially if a pattern is noticed that this occurs more commonly in the winter months.
J. Has the patient been diagnosed with osteoporosis? If so, the patient needs to be screened for Vitamin D deficiency.

Physical Examination
A. Check pulse and blood pressure.
B. Inspect.
   1. Observe the patient walk in the room and assess for stability.
   2. Observe the skin color and overall appearance and type of skin texture.
   3. Note any deformities in the spine.
      a. Kyphosis
      b. Bowing of the legs
      c. Waddling of gait
C. Palpate.
   1. Joints or areas of complained tenderness that the patient presented with.
   2. Palpate the abdomen if suspected intestinal absorption problems and workup needed.
D. Auscultate the heart and lungs.

Diagnostic Tests
A. Serum 25 (OH)D Normal (30–80 ng/mL)
B. Parathyroid hormone Normal (14–72 pg/mL)
C. Calcium level Normal (8.5–10.2 mg/dL)

Differential Diagnoses
A. Vitamin D deficiency
B. Osteoporosis
C. Rickets
D. Cystic fibrosis

E. Malabsorption syndrome

F. Chronic kidney disease

Plan

A. Inadequate sun exposure: recommend 20–30 min of sunlight during summer months without use of sunscreen.

B. Vitamin D₂: 50,000 IU weekly for 8 weeks and recheck Vitamin D level. If still less than 30 ng/mL at that point, repeat dose for another 8 weeks and recheck again when second course is finished.

C. When Vitamin D levels are > 30 ng/mL, prescribe Vitamin D 2000 IU daily.

D. For malabsorption problems, refer to gastrointestinal specialist for work-up.

E. Diet must be increased with foods high in Vitamin D. A few foods high in Vitamin D include: fish oil, cod liver, salmon, milk fortified with Vitamin D, and cereals fortified with Vitamin D.

F. Calcium should also be taken with Vitamin D on a daily basis for the prevention of osteoporosis.

Follow-up

A. Follow-up should be performed according to recommendations based on laboratory results. Initial laboratory results should be repeated in 8 weeks with initial treatment. Once Vitamin D levels are stable, repeat labwork routinely to confirm that levels remain within normal range. If levels continue to fall, refer to a specialist.

Consultation/Referral

A. Consult with a physician or refer to a gastrointestinal specialist for patients who consistently have low Vitamin D levels.

Individual Considerations

A. Pregnancy: No contraindications for treatment during pregnancy. The same prescribing dose is safe for pregnancy and breast-feeding patients.

B. Pediatrics:

1. Up to 1 year of age, Vitamin D₂ or D₃, 1,000–2,000 IU per day with calcium supplementation recommended.

2. American Academy of Pediatrics recommends infants fed exclusively by breast milk should have Vitamin D supplementation.

3. Ages 1–18 years: 50,000 IU Vitamin D₂ every week for 8 weeks.

C. Geriatrics: Commonly seen in this population. All patients diagnosed with osteoporosis should be assessed for Vitamin D deficiency.

REFERENCES

AIDSmeds. (2008, October 22). *Currently approved drugs for HIV: A comparative chart.* Retrieved February 13, 2010, from http://www.aidsmeds.com/articles/DrugChart_10632.shtml

AIDSmeds. (2010, March 4). *Treatment for HIV & AIDS.* Retrieved February 13, 2010, from http://www.aidsmeds.com/list.shtml

American Academy of HIV Medicine. (2007). *Fundamentals of HIV medicine for the HIV specialist.* Washington, DC: Author. Retrieved March 31, 2010, from www.AAHIVM.org

American Society for Colposcopy and Cervical Pathology. (2006a). *Consensus guidelines 2006: Consensus guidelines for the management of women with abnormal cervical cancer screening tests.* Retrieved December 12, 2009, from http://www.asccp.org/pdf/consensus/algorithms_cyto_07.pdf

American Society for Colposcopy and Cervical Pathology. (2006b). *Consensus guidelines 2006: Consensus guidelines for the management of women with cervical intraepithial neoplasia or adenocarcinoma in situ.* Retrieved December 12, 2009, from http://www.asccp.org/pdf/consensus/algorithms_hist_07.pdf

Barker, L., Buron, J., & Zeive, P. (Eds.). (1995). *Principles of ambulatory medicine.* Baltimore: Williams & Wilkins.

Casey, C. F., Slawson, D. C., & Neal, L. R. (2010). Vitamin D supplementation in infants, children and adolescents. *American Family Physician, 81*(6), 745–781.

Centers for Disease Control and Prevention. (2003, July 18). *MMWR recommendations and reports: Incorporating HIV prevention into the medical care of persons living with HIV.* Retrieved November 14, 2009, from http://aidsinfo.nih.gov/contentfiles/HIVpreventioninmedcare_TB.pdf

Centers for Disease Control and Prevention. (2005, September 30). *MMWR recommendations and reports: Management of occupational exposures to HIV and recommendations for postexposure prophylaxis.* Retrieved January 9, 2010, from http://aidsinfo.nih.gov/contentfiles/healthcareoccupexpoGL.pdf

Centers for Disease Control and Prevention. (2006, October 19). *Questions and answers: Men on the down low.* Retrieved March 6, 2010, from http://www.cdc.gov/hiv/topics/aa/resources/qa/print/downlow.htm

Centers for Disease Control and Prevention. (2007, June 28). *HIV/AIDS and African Americans.* Retrieved November 14, 2009, from http://www.cdc.gov/hiv/topics/aa/print/index.htm

Centers for Disease Control and Prevention. (2008, August 3). *HIV and AIDS in the United States: A picture of today's epidemic.* Retrieved November 14, 2009, from http://www.cdc.gov/hiv/topics/surveillance/print/united_states.htm

Centers for Disease Control and Prevention. (2008, August 26). *HIV infection reporting.* Retrieved November 14, 2009, from http://www.cdc.gov/hiv/topics/surveillance/print/reporting.htm

Centers for Disease Control and Prevention. (2008, September 11). *HIV incidence.* Retrieved November 14, 2009, from http://www.cdc.gov/hiv/topics/surveillance/print/incidence.htm

Centers for Disease Control and Prevention. (2008, December 5). *MMWR recommendations and reports: Revised surveillance case definitions for HIV infection among adults, adolescents, and children aged < 18 months and for HIV infection and AIDS among children aged 18 months to < 13 years—United States, 2008. Morbidity and Mortality Weekly Report, 57*(RR–10), 1–8. Retrieved November 14, 2009, from http://www.cdc.gov/mmwr/preview/mmwrhtml/rr5710a1.htm?s_cid=rr5710a1_e

Centers for Disease Control and Prevention. (2009, February 2009). *HIV/AIDS basic statistics.* Retrieved November 14, 2009, from http://www.cdc.gov/hiv/topics/surveillance/print/basic.htm

Centers for Disease Control and Prevention. (2009, April 10). *MMWR recommendations and reports: Guidelines for prevention and treatment of opportunistic infections in HIV-infected adults and adolescents. Morbidity and Mortality Weekly Report.* Retrieved December 12, 2009, from http://aidsinfo.nih.gov/contentfiles/adult_OI_041009.pdf

Centers for Disease Control and Prevention. (2009, September 25). *HIV/AIDS and men who have sex with men (MSM).* Retrieved November 14, 2009, from http://www.cdc.gov/hiv/topics/msm/print/index.htm

Centers for Disease Control and Prevention. (2009, October 27). *NHBS: HIV risk and testing behaviors among young MSM.* Retrieved November 14, 2009, from http://www.cdc.gov/hiv/topics/msm/print/ymsm.htm

DHHS Panel on Antiretroviral Guidelines for Adults and Adolescents. (2009, December 1). *Guidelines for the use of antiretroviral agents in HIV-1-infected adults and adolescents* (pp. 1–168). Retrieved December 12, 2009, from http://aidsinfo.nih.gov/contentfiles/AdultandAdolescentGL.pdf

Disease Management for Nurse Practitioners. (2002). Springhouse, PA: Springhouse Corporation.

Dowd, T. R., & Stewart, F. M. (1994). Primary care approach to lymphadenopathy. *Nurse Practitioner, 19,* 36–43.

Fauci, A., Braunwald, E., Isselbacher, K., & Wilson, J., et. al., (Eds.). (1998). *Harrison's principles of internal medicine.* New York: McGraw-Hill.

Ferri, F. (2004). *Ferri's clinical advisor.* Philadelphia: Mosby.

Furniss, K. (1997). Battered women: How nurses can help. *Lifelines, August,* 12–14.

Horn, T., & Urbina, A. (2008, October 22). *The POZ and AIDSmeds drug chart.* Retrieved March 6, 2010, from http://www.aidsmeds.com/lessons/DrugChartHighRes.pdf

International AIDS Society. (n.d.). *Optimizing HIV treatment.* Retrieved March 6, 2010, from http://www.iasociety.org/Defautl.aspx?pageID=389

Jones, A., & Hansen, K. (2009). Recognizing the musculoskeletal manifestations of vitamin D deficiency. *The Journal of Musculoskeletal Medicine, 26,* 289–296.

National HIV/AIDS Clinician's Consultation Center. Retrieved from www.ncc.ucsf.edu

National Osteoporosis Foundation. Retrieved March 10, 2010, from http://www.nof.org/prevention/vitaminD.htm

Perinatal HIV Guidelines Working Group. (2009, April 29). *Public Health Service Task Force recommendations for use of antiretroviral drugs in pregnant HIV-infected women for maternal health and interventions to reduce perinatal HIV transmission in the United States,* pp. 1–90. Retrieved March 6, 2010, from http://aidsinfo.nih.gov/ContentFiles/PerinatialGL.pdf

The AIDS Infonet. *Reliable, up-to-date treatment information.* Retrieved December 12, 2009, from www.aidsinfonet.org

The Body. (n.d.). *Approved HIV medications by class.* Retrieved March 6, 2010, from http://www.thebody.com/index/treat/classes.html

The Body. (n.d.). *First steps to HIV/AIDS treatment.* Retrieved March 6, 2010, from http://www.thebody.com/index/treat/first.html

The Body. (n.d.). *HIV/AIDS medication basics.* Retrieved March 6, 2010, from http://www.thebody.com/content/art40488.html

The Body. (n.d.). *HIV drug-drug interactions.* Retrieved March 6, 2010, from http://www.thebody.com/index/treat/interactions.html

The Body. (n.d.). *Side effects of HIV/AIDS and HIV medications.* Retrieved March 6, 2010, from http://www.thebody.com/index/treat/side_effects.html#general

Tierney, L., McPhee, J., & Papadakis, M (Eds.). (2007). *Current medical diagnosis and treatment* (46th ed.). New York: McGraw-Hill.

U.S. Food and Drug Administration. (n.d.). *Antiretroviral drugs used in the treatment of HIV infection.* Retrieved March 6, 2010, from http://www.fda.gov/ForConsumers/byAudience/ForThe patient Advocates/HIVandAIDSActivities/ucm118915.htm

Working Group on Antiretroviral Therapy and Medical Management of HIV-Infected Children. (2009, February 23). *Guidelines for the use of antiretroviral agents in pediatric HIV infection,* pp. 1–139. Retrieved March 6, 2010, from http://aidsinfo.nih.gov/ContentFiles/PediatricGuidelines.pdf

World Health Organization. (2009a, November). *Rapid advice: Antiretroviral therapy for HIV infection in adults and adolescents.* Retrieved March 6, 2010, from http://www.who.int/hiv/pub/arv/rapid_advice_art.pdf

World Health Organization. (2009b, November). *Rapid advice: Use of antiretroviral drugs for treating pregnant women and preventing HIV infection in infants.* Retrieved March 6, 2010, from http://www.searo.who.int/LinkFiles/HIV-AIDS_Rapid_Advice_MTCT%28web%29.pdf

CHAPTER 17

Musculoskeletal Guidelines

Julie Adkins

FIBROMYALGIA

Definition

Fibromyalgia syndrome is a clinical condition characterized by generalized aching and stiffness, associated with the finding of numerous tender points in characteristic locations. The most current guidelines for diagnosis are the **1990 Criteria for the Classification of Fibromyalgia (Wolfe et al., 1990):**

A. **Widespread pain for longer than 3 months.** (It requires bilateral pain, above and below the waist, axial skeletal pain. Low back pain is regarded as being below the waist.)

B. **Pain on digital palpation (using at least 4 kg of force on palpation) in at least 11 of 18 of the following points:**
   1. Occiput: bilateral, at the suboccipital muscle insertions.
   2. Low cervical: bilateral, at the anterior aspects of the intertransverse spaces at C5–C7.
   3. Trapezius: bilateral, at the midpoint of the upper border.
   4. Supraspinatus: bilateral, at origins, above the scapula spine near the medial border.
   5. Second rib: bilateral, at the second costochondral junction, just lateral to the junction on upper surfaces.
   6. Lateral epicondyle: bilateral, 2 cm distal to the epicondyle.
   7. Gluteal: bilateral, in upper outer quadrants of buttocks in anterior fold of muscle.
   8. Greater trochanter: bilateral, posterior to the trochanteric prominence.
   9. Knee: bilateral, at the medial fat pad proximal to the joint line.

Areas palpated are considered positive if the patient verbalized area as being "painful" when palpated.

Incidence

A. Fibromyalgia affects females more than males at a ratio of 10:1 and patients with an average age of 47 years. Five percent of the population are affected with fibromyalgia. It has a usual onset between 20 and 50 years; however, it has also been diagnosed in the young as well as the elderly. Often patients have symptoms for longer than 5 years before finally being diagnosed. The prevalence of fibromyalgia in rheumatology practice is 20%.

Pathogenesis

A. The cause is unclear. Studies of sleep physiology, neurohormonal function, muscular function, and psychologic factors support a central mechanism for the disorder linked to depression. Other research suggests a pathophysiologic and psychological disorder.

Predisposing Factors

A. Life stress
B. Depression
C. Female gender
D. Age: mid-30s and older

Common Complaints

A. Common complaints are multifocal pain present longer than 3 months, moderate to extreme fatigue, morning stiffness, nonrestorative sleep, pain worsening with stress, exposure to cold, inactivity or overactivity, sensitivity to touch, light and sound, cognitive difficulties, and changes in barometric pressure.

Other Signs and Symptoms

A. Numbness
B. Swelling
C. Reactive hyperemia of skin
D. Raynaud's phenomenon
E. Irritable bowel syndrome and bladder
F. Headaches
G. Restless leg syndrome
H. Anxiety/depression

Subjective Data

A. Determine onset, duration, and course of complaints.
B. Does fatigue interfere with the patient's daily activity?
C. Note sleep quality. Does the patient feel rested after sleeping?
D. Do exacerbations of discomfort occur with stress, activity, and cold?

E. Has the patient experienced stress and/or depression in the past?

F. Does she have a family history of rheumatoid disease?

G. Has she ever been diagnosed with chronic fatigue syndrome, Lyme disease, or thyroid disease?

Physical Examination

A. Check temperature, pulse, and blood pressure.

B. Inspect
1. Observe overall appearance.
2. Observe the nails, skin, mucous membranes, eyes, joints, and spine. If clubbing is noted and tender points are minimal, consider hypertrophic osteoarthropathy.

C. Palpate: Palpate the muscles as outlined in above criteria for classification of fibromyalgia. Note the following when palpating for tender points:
1. Pressure should be insufficient to produce pain in normal patients or at uninvolved sites in affected patients.
2. Pain on digital palpation must be present in at least 11 of 18 tender point sites.
3. "Positive pain reaction" is related to the patient stating that palpation causes pain. Tender is not to be considered as pain.
4. Painful points must be differentiated from trigger points of myofascial syndrome, which produce referred pain on compression.
5. Control areas not expected to be tender in fibromyalgia, such as middle of the forehead and fingertips, should be examined to exclude psychologic pain or malingering.

D. Auscultate the heart and lungs.

Diagnostic Tests

A. Antinuclear antibody (ANA)

B. Sedimentation rate

C. TSH

D. Creatinine phosphokinase

E. Lyme titer if history of rash, arthritis, or deer tick exposure is present

Differential Diagnoses

A. Fibromyalgia

B. Rheumatoid arthritis

C. Osteoarthritis

D. Polymyalgia rheumatica

E. Ankylosing spondylitis

F. Myositis

G. Lupus erythematous

H. Hypothyroidism

I. Chronic fatigue syndrome

Plan

A. General interventions: Routine follow-up is recommended. Multiple therapies may be beneficial for controlling symptoms. Stress importance of daily exercises and therapy to control pain. Support groups are beneficial for patients and families.

B. Patient teaching: See the Section III Patient Teaching Guide for this chapter, "Fibromyalgia." Teach the patient that fibromyalgia is a recognizable syndrome that does not progress or cripple and does not warrant further testing. The patient can be assured it is not "all in her head."
1. Exercise: Encourage the patient to exercise daily, including stretching programs along with walking, low-impact cardiovascular conditioning such as cycling, and low-impact aerobics. Initially, pain may increase with the first 2 weeks of exercise, then it improves with a routine exercise program.
2. Pain control: Pain may improve with exercise, hot baths, heating pads, warm weather, and stress reduction.

C. Pharmaceutical therapy
1. Amitriptyline 10–50 mg at bedtime for sleep.
2. Cyclobenzaprine 10–40 mg daily.
3. NSAIDs 200–600 mg every 4–6 hours. Maximum dose is 1.2 g a day.
4. Analgesics such as acetaminophen (Tylenol) as needed.
5. Selective serotonin reuptake inhibitors (SSRIs) if depression is present.
6. Lyrica 75 mg twice a day to 150 mg twice a day. Maximum dose of 450 mg a day.
7. Cymbalta 30–60 mg once a day
8. Savella titrated dose 12.5 mg on day 1, 12.5 mg twice a day for 2 days, days 4–7 25 mg twice a day, then 50 mg twice a day (recommended dose). Maximum dose 100 mg twice a day. Withdraw gradually. Precautions with renal impairment.

Follow-up

A. Schedule regular visits in initial 2–4 weeks to evaluate how therapy is helping. Educate the patient each visit, and stress positive reinforcement and supervision of treatment regimen. Visits may then be scheduled every 3 months to monitor progress.

Consultation/Referral

A. Consult with a physician if the patient has abnormal laboratory results.

B. Consult or refer the patient to a physician if depression is suspected and current medication therapy is unsuccessful.

GOUT

Definition

A. Gout is an inflammatory disease of the joints, caused by high concentrations of uric acid in the joints and bones.

Incidence

A. Gout is most common in men from ages 30–60.

Pathogenesis

A. Primary: High levels of uric acid result from either increased production or decreased excretion rates of uric acid.

B. Secondary: Hyperuricemia results from primary disease processes such as hypertension, renal failure, kidney disorders, enzyme deficiencies, and skin disorders.

C. Medications can also cause hyperuricemia.

Predisposing Factors

A. Obesity
B. Renal disease
C. Hypertension
D. Skin disorders
E. Blood disorders
F. Medications (diuretics, acetylsalicylic acid, alcohol, nicotinic acid, ethambutol, pyrazinamide)
G. Men older than 30 years old
H. Lead poison

Common Complaints

A. Redness, swelling, warmth, and/or pain in the joint (usually one joint only)

Other Signs and Symptoms

A. Tophi seen from several years of untreated gout.
B. Fever may be present in acute stages.

Subjective Data

A. Note when initial symptoms began.
B. Review the patient history of gout.
C. Determine what makes the symptoms worse or better.
D. List medications/therapies used and the result of the different therapies used.

Physical Examination

A. Check temperature, pulse, respirations, and blood pressure.
B. Inspect
   1. Inspect the joints.
   2. Note the presence of tophi on other joints.
C. Palpate: Palpate the joints for tenderness or pain.

Diagnostic Tests

A. CBC: white blood cell count elevated
B. Erythrocyte sedimentation rate (ESR): elevated in gout
C. Serum uric acid level: uric acid greater than 7.0 mg/dL
D. 24-hour urine uric acid excretion: greater than 900 mg/24 hours
E. Rheumatoid factor titer
F. Joint fluid aspiration for urate crystals

Differential Diagnoses

A. Gout
B. Infectious arthritis
C. Rheumatoid arthritis
D. Hyperparathyroidism
E. Pseudogout
F. Bursitis
G. Cellulitis

Plan

A. General interventions
   1. Rest the joint area; no heavy lifting or weight-bearing activity.
   2. **Aspirin products should not be used.**
B. Patient teaching
   1. Increase fluid intake to at least 8 glasses of water daily.
   2. See the Section III Patient Teaching Guide for this chapter, "Gout."

C. Pharmaceutical therapy
   1. Analgesia
      a. Indocin 50 mg every 8 hours for 8 doses, then 25 mg every 8 hours until pain-free.
      b. Naproxen, 750 mg initially, followed by 250 mg every 8 hours.
      c. Colchicine 0.5 mg every 1–2 hours until symptoms improved (not to exceed 5 mg/24 hours). Colchicine must be taken within 24 hours of acute attack to be effective. Colchicine warnings: be aware of contraindications. Caution regarding drug interactions. Probenecid effects with other drugs include penicillin and methotrexate.
   2. For hypersecretion of uric acid, long-term therapy is needed to decrease uric acid production: yloprim is the drug of choice. The goal is to keep the uric acid level less than 6.5 mg/dL.
   3. For reduced excretion rates of uric acid, consider Benemid 250 mg by mouth twice a day for 1 week, then increase to 500 mg by mouth twice a day. Increased consumption of fluids must be encouraged.
   4. Chronic gout: If patients have three or more attacks per year, consider long-term therapy; low dose of NSAIDs or allopurinol for 2–12 months.

Follow-up

A. The patient should be contacted within 24 hours for evaluation.
B. Follow-up visit in 1 month to reevaluate status.
C. Chronic gout: obtain yearly uric acid levels; before initiating long-term therapy, obtain baseline blood urea nitrogen (BUN), serum lipid profile, and CBC.

Consultation/Referral

A. Consult a physician for aspiration of joint fluid.

Individual Considerations

A. Pregnancy: Colchicine not recommended.
B. Pediatrics
   1. Colchicine not recommended.
   2. If gout is seen in this population, consider underlying primary cause (i.e., inborn error of metabolism).
C. Geriatrics
   1. Reformation in joint areas may be seen in patients who have a history of gout from the uric acid deposits.

NECK AND UPPER BACK DISORDERS

Definition

A. Nonspecific disorders: self-limited, usually benign disorders with unclear etiology, such as regional upper back and neck pain and shoulder pain adjacent to the neck
B. Degenerative disorders: consequences of aging or repetitive use, or a combination thereof, such as degenerative disk disease and osteoarthritis
C. Potentially serious neck or upper back disorders: fractures, dislocation, infection, tumor, progressive neurologic deficit, or cord compression

Incidence

A. Exact numbers are unknown.

Pathogenesis

A. Cervical strain is irritation and spasm of the upper back and cervical muscles. The upper portion of the trapezius and the levator scapulae muscles, rhomboid major and minor muscles, and the long cervical muscles are most often affected.

Predisposing Factors

A. Whiplashlike injuries
B. Cervical strain
C. Cervical arthritis

Common Complaints

A. Aching neck
B. Tightness and tenderness in neck area
C. Stiffness and tightness in shoulders
D. Stiff neck and a headache upon awakening

Other Signs and Symptoms

A. Limited range of motion
B. Back pain: guarding with cervical motion
C. Numbness in upper extremities
D. Muscle weakness

Subjective Data

A. What are presenting symptoms? Note pain, numbness, weakness, or stiffness.
B. Was there any type of injury, either recently or in the past?
C. Is the pain located primarily in the neck, upper back, or shoulder? Is there any radiation noted?
D. How do these symptoms limit the patient's activity?
E. How long can the patient sit, stand, walk, or do overhead work?
F. Is the patient able to lift? If so, how much weight is bearable? Compare to normal weight.
G. How long has the patient had these symptoms?
H. How have the symptoms evolved, from the beginning of discomfort until now?
I. If the patient has a previous history of similar or the same pain, what therapy was used in the past and what were the results?
J. Does the patient have any medical problems?

Physical Examination

Infection may include severe cervical spasms (nuchal rigidity), elevated temperature, chills, hypotension, and tachycardia.

A. Check temperature, blood pressure, and pulse.
B. Inspect: Observe stance and gait. Note the patient's coordination and use of extremities.
C. Palpate
1. Palpate trigger points in upper back, paracervical and rhomboid muscles.
2. Palpate for any bony tenderness in neck, shoulders, and upper back.
3. Perform range of motion tests.
4. Assess the patient for reduced ipsilateral and contralateral bending of the neck.
5. Check for fracture, or inability to move neck due to pain, and severe cervical midline vertebral pain.

Note tenderness, the patient holding head for stability; look for possible neurologic deficits.
D. Assess DTRs bilaterally.
1. Biceps reflex tests fifth and sixth cervical nerve root.
2. Brachioradialis reflex tests fifth and sixth cervical nerve root.
3. Triceps reflex tests seventh and eighth cervical nerve root.
E. Test muscle strength in shoulders.
F. Abduction, elbow flexion, or supination tests fourth and fifth cervical disks.
G. Check for weakness of radial wrist extension, indicating fifth and sixth cervical disk problems. Check for weakness of elbow extension and ulnar wrist flexion, indicating seventh cervical nerve impairment. Check weak finger abduction and adduction, indicating seventh and eighth cervical nerve impairment. Measure circumference at forearm and upper arm for muscle atrophy. Dominant arm is 1/4 inch greater than nondominant arm.
H. Sensory: Test light touch, pinprick, pressure sensations in forearm and hand. Possible cervical spinal cord compromise is indicated by paresthesia of upper extremities, weakness of upper or lower extremities, and difficulty walking.
I. Percuss back, spine, and neck areas. Tumor is indicated by tenderness to vertebral percussion, cachexia.
J. Auscultate heart and lungs.

Diagnostic Tests

A. Radiography of cervical spine

Differential Diagnoses

A. Regional neck pain
B. Cervical strain
C. Cervical arthritis
D. Cervical nerve root compression with radiculopathy
E. Rotator cuff tendinitis
F. Rotator cuff tendon tear
G. Postlaminectomy syndrome
H. Spinal stenosis

Plan

A. General interventions
1. Correct posture and lifestyle modifications (exercise, strengthening, etc.) are imperative for the patient to remain free of pain. Patient education and therapy depend on individual diagnosis.
B. Patient teaching
1. Teach the patient to use local applications of cold packs during the first 3 days of acute complaints and hot pack applications thereafter.
2. Encourage the following changes in lifestyle:
   a. Sitting straight with shoulders held high.
   b. Sleeping with the head and neck aligned with the body and a small pillow under the neck.
   c. Driving with arms slightly shrugged, using arm rests.
   d. Avoiding carrying objects with a strap over shoulders.
3. Suggest adjustments in tasks at work and at home.

4. Encourage daily stretching exercises, including shoulder roll, scapular pinch, and neck stretches.
5. Have the patient perform range of motion exercises daily.
6. Tell the patient to avoid extremes of range of motion, prolonged periods in one position, and any other aggravating activity.
7. Explain relaxation techniques and stress reduction.
8. Give the patient the Section III Teaching Guide for this chapter, "RICE Therapy and Exercise Therapy," if applicable.

C. Pharmaceutical therapy
   1. Nonprescription medications: acetaminophen or NSAIDs.
   2. Prescription medications: NSAIDs and/or muscle relaxants for nighttime use.

Follow-up

A. Evaluate the patient after 2 weeks of conservative treatment. If pain continues after 2–3 weeks despite adequate therapy, order radiography and physical therapy, including ultrasonography, massage, and gentle cervical traction beginning at 5 pounds for 5–10 min once a day. Soft cervical collar may be worn while doing physical work.

Consultation/Referral

A. Consult or refer the patient to a physician if there is still no improvement after adequate time for healing and no relief noted with physical therapy and medications.

OSTEOARTHRITIS

Definition

A. Osteoarthritis (OA), formerly degenerative joint disease, is a chronic noninflammatory disease that affects the movable joints. Osteoarthritis is characterized by destruction of the cartilage with resultant decrease in the joint spaces and bony overgrowth. Osteoarthritis is considered to be primary when there are no underlying conditions, and secondary to conditions such as trauma, septic arthritis, inflammatory arthritis, metabolic disorders, or congenital or acquired joint abnormalities.

Incidence

A. It is estimated that up to 12% of the general population between the ages of 25 and 74 have osteoarthritis. The incidence clearly increases with age as up to 85% of the general population over the age of 65 has radiographic changes suggestive of OA. Ninety percent of all people have radiographic features of osteoarthritis on weight-bearing joints by age 40 (Tierney, McPhe, & Papadakis, 2007).

Pathogenesis

A. Damage to the articular cartilage and subchondral bone may be due to local trauma and results in chondrocyte injury. Chondrocytes release proteolytic enzymes that assist in repair of the cartilage. In OA, the remodeling process of chondrocytes and the release of enzymes is impaired and results in a loss of strength and greater trauma and destruction of the subchondral bone. The end result is joint destruction and bony overgrowth (Noble, 1996).

Predisposing Factors

A. Increasing age: among patients over the age of 55.
B. Gender: women are more commonly affected and exhibit greater disease severity.
C. Genetic predisposition; distal interpha-langeal (DIP) joint involvement.
D. Trauma such as previous fractures, ligamentous injuries; occupationally related repetitive stress.
E. Altered joint anatomy or instability.
F. Obesity: mechanical injury in the knee may increase OA.
G. Secondary inflammation such as infections, inflammatory arthropathies, and metabolic disorders.

Common Complaints

A. Unilateral joint pain frequently involving the finger joints
B. Morning stiffness lasting less than 1 hour

Other Signs and Symptoms

A. Unilateral joint pain involving the distal (DIP) and proximal interphalangeal (PIP) joints, first carpometacarpal joint, hips, knees, cervical and lumbar spine, and first metatarsophalangeal joint
B. Mild osteoarthritis, or early disease, pain that increases with joint use and decreases with rest
C. Severe osteoarthritis, or late disease, pain that is present with rest

Subjective Data

A. Elicit the patient's age at onset of pain.
B. Has the pain gradually gotten worse over the months or years?
C. How long does the pain last in the morning? Does the pain get worse with joint use and better with rest?
D. What joints are involved?
E. Is the joint pain described as "aching"?
F. What does the patient take to relieve the pain?
G. Is there any joint deformity, redness, swelling, or warmth?
H. Is there any decrease in range of motion of the joint?
I. Is there any family history of osteoarthritis?

Physical Examination

A. Check temperature, pulse, and blood pressure.
B. Inspect the joints for enlargement, edema, and erythema.
C. Palpate
   1. Palpate the joints, noting temperature, edema, and tenderness. Joints are cool; bony enlargement may be present in the PIP (Bouchard's nodes) or DIP joints (Heberden's nodes) and other weight-bearing joints.
   2. Palpate extremities. Perform assisted and active range-of-motion (ROM) exercises. With exam, limited ROM of the joint and/or pain on palpation may be present, along with crepitus.

Diagnostic Tests

A. Erythrocyte sedimentation rate (ESR): OA does not cause an increase of the ESR (Tierney, McPhe, & Papadakis, 2007).
B. Chemistry profile.
C. CBC.
D. Rheumatoid factor (RF).

E. Routine radiography: confirms disease severity and presence of joint narrowing.

F. CT scan or MRI: considered with nerve impingement syndrome (spine) or spinal stenosis.

Differential Diagnoses

A. Inflammatory osteoarthritis
B. Rheumatoid arthritis
C. Gout or pseudogout
D. Septic arthritis
E. Bursitis or tendonitis
F. Systemic lupus erythematous
G. Fracture or trauma

Plan

A. General interventions
   1. Confirm diagnosis.
   2. Provide the patient support and education to improve patient well-being and reduce discomfort.
   3. Physical therapy and/or occupational therapy should be initiated, if indicated.

B. Patient teaching
   1. See the Section III Patient Teaching Guide for this chapter, "Osteoarthritis."
   2. Reinforce the importance of joint protection; avoid repetitive stress or trauma.
   3. Encourage daily exercises and strengthening.
   4. Encourage weight loss if the patient is obese.

C. Pharmaceutical therapy
   1. First-line agents: The goal of treatment is to preserve joint mobility. First-line agents should be used in a stepwise approach.
      a. Acetaminophen up to 1 g four times daily. In early disease, this may be given on an as-needed basis.
      b. NSAIDs if acetaminophen has failed to control the pain. Use with caution. Consider renal function and risk factors for peptic ulcer disease (PUD).
         i. For high-risk patients, an H_2 receptor blocker may decrease gastritis and be helpful in preventing duodenal ulcers. Consider Arthrotec 50: one tablet three times a day.
         ii. **Misoprostol may be considered in patients who are at high risk for gastric ulcers. It should not be used by pregnant women. It is considered high risk for fetal death and possible congenital abnormalities.**
      c. Topical capsaicin or methyl salicylate creams applied to the affected area. Capsaicin creams may cause local burning at the site of application for the first several days.
   2. Second-line agents: Second-line agents, such as intra-articular corticosteroid injections, may prevent some joint erosion and decrease pain. The same joint should not be injected more than 3–4 times a year in 3-month intervals. If the joint is injected at this frequency for more than 1 year, alternative options, such as surgery, should be considered.

Follow-up

A. Follow-up is based on disease severity and therapeutic treatment. If the patient is treated with first-line agents, follow up on pain control, nonpharmoco-logic interventions, and possible side effects of medications within 2–4 weeks.

Consultation/Referral

A. Give the patient a surgical referral, if indicated.

Individual Considerations

A. Pregnancy: NSAIDs should not be used in pregnancy unless clearly indicated. Misoprostol should be used with great caution in women of childbearing age due to its potential for fetal abnormalities and abortive properties.

B. Adults and Geriatrics: Patients on chronic NSAIDs should be monitored closely for toxicity such as renal insufficiency, gastritis, and PUD. This is especially true for the elderly and those with preexisting GI disease, diabetes, congestive heart failure, and cirrhosis.

OSTEOPOROSIS

Definition

A. Osteoporosis is a condition of reduced bone mass resulting in bone fragility and fracture. The World Health Organization has defined it as "spinal or hip bone mineral density (BMD) of 2.5 standard deviations or more below the mean for healthy, young women (T-score of –2.5 or below) as measured by dual energy x-ray absorptiometry" (Sweet, Sweet, Jeremiah, & Galazka, 2009, p. 193).

B. Osteopenia is defined as a spinal or hip BMD between 1 and 2.5 standard deviations below the mean (Sweet et al., 2009).

Incidence

A. Fifty to sixty percent of 50-year-old women sustain osteoporosis-related fractures during their remaining life. Spinal fractures occur in 25% of White women by age 65, causing pain, deformity, and disability. Most common fractures include 25% at distal radius (Colles' fracture), 50% in vertebrae, and 25% in the hip.

B. One-third of all women and 17% of men suffer a hip fracture before age 90, and 20% of those who sustain a fracture die within 3 months of the event.

Pathogenesis

A. Osteoporosis is due to bone reabsorption being greater than bone formation.

Predisposing Factors

A. Hypogonadal states, particularly menopause
B. Small body frame
C. Smoking
D. Low calcium intake
E. Lack of weight-bearing exercise
F. Family history
G. Excessive alcohol intake
H. Asian or Caucasian
I. Secondary causes include:
   1. Hyperparathyroidism
   2. Hyperthyroidism
   3. Cushing's syndrome
   4. Multiple myeloma
   5. Thyroid replacement therapy

6. Corticosteroid therapy
7. Renal disease

Common Complaints
A. Loss of height
B. Kyphosis, or dowager's hump
C. Back pain as a result of a fracture

Other Signs and Symptoms
A. Cervical lordosis
B. Fracture with little or no trauma
C. Crush fracture of vertebra
D. Pain

Subjective Data
A. Explore history of the following:
  1. Loss of height
  2. Low initial bone mass
  3. Early menopause, oophorectomy, postmenopause, or amenorrhea
  4. European or Asian family origin
  5. Family history of spinal fractures and osteoporosis
  6. Sedentary lifestyle with little weight-bearing activity
  7. Endocrine disorders
  8. Medications taken, specifically corticosteroids, barbiturates, heparin, and thyroid hormone
  9. Low calcium and vitamin D intake
  10. Increased alcohol, caffeine, and protein intake
  11. Renal disease/dialysis
B. Determine onset, duration, location, and characteristic of pain.
C. Has the patient had any recent falls?

Physical Examination
A. Check pulse, blood pressure, height, and weight.
B. Inspect
  1. Compare present height to previous height.
  2. Observe presence of dorsal kyphosis.
  3. Observe physical abnormalities that interfere with mobility.
C. Palpate the joints and over bone for pain.

Diagnostic Test
A. TSH.
B. Serum calcium.
C. Glucose.
D. Estrogen, to rule out endocrine disease.
E. CBC, ESR, and serum protein electrophoresis, to rule out multiple myeloma and leukemia.
F. Serum 25-hydroxy vitamin D level and alkaline phosphatase to assess for Vitamin D deficiency and to rule out a common form of osteomalacia.
G. Bone mineral density (BMD) can measure bone density of the spine or hip. Medicare will reimburse for BMD every 2 years.
H. The WHO Fracture Risk Assessment Took, or FRAX, was developed to determine the absolute fracture risk of breaking a bone in the next 10 years. This tool may be used with the BMD results to determine who needs to be treated with medication for prevention of fracture when treatment is unclear.
I. Radiography, if vertebral fracture is suspected.

Differential Diagnoses
A. Osteoporosis
B. Osteoarthritis
C. Secondary causes
  1. Thyroid disease
  2. Glucocorticoid therapy
  3. Malabsorption syndromes
  4. Renal or collagen disease
  5. Vitamin D deficiency
  6. Metastatic cancer
  7. Multiple myeloma

Plan
A. General interventions: Lifestyle changes should be introduced to the patient.
B. Patient teaching
  1. Educate the patient regarding calcium intake in diet.
    a. Dietary intake of calcium should be 1,000 mg per day to age 40. Women need 1,500 mg of calcium after menopause if they are not on hormone replacement therapy. Sources high in calcium include salmon or sardines with bones, low-fat yogurt and skim milk, green vegetables, and cheese.
    b. Tell the patient to avoid increased protein intake to minimize increased urinary output of calcium.
    c. Encourage the patient to eliminate alcohol and caffeine from diet.
  2. Encourage the patient to eliminate cigarette smoking.
  3. Prescribe regular moderate exercise, such as 30 min of walking at least three times per week, at minimum. Walking 50–60 min three times per week provides optimal benefits.
  4. Tell the patient to avoid medications that may cause drowsiness and may precipitate falls.
  5. Use extra light at night in the bathroom to help prevent falls.
  6. Remove all scatter rugs and clutter: make the home safer including installing hand rails on steps.
C. Pharmaceutical therapy
  1. Calcium supplements:

Calcium supplements may be contraindicated in patients who have a history of renal stones.

    a. Calcium carbonate (Os-Cal) 500 mg orally 1–3 times per day, or Turns 1 tablet orally 2–3 times a day.
    b. Supplementation of 400–600 mg orally per day plus dietary intake provides adequate daily calcium intake.
  2. Hormone replacement therapy (HRT):
    Estrogen therapy and progesterone therapy are available as tablet or transdermal patches and come in a wide variety of doses.
    a. Postmenopausal women with uterus should take conjugated estrogen (Premarin) 0.625 mg orally daily, or medroxyprogesterone (Provera) 10 mg orally daily. Premarin in doses less than 0.625 mg may not be protective against osteoporosis.

b. Postmenopausal women without uterus should take conjugated estrogen (Premarin) 0.625 mg orally daily.

c. Begin at least at cessation of menses and continue for at least 7–10 years.

d. Women with progressive disease should be given HRT plus calcium supplementation up to 2,000 mg per day.

e. Evaluate women closely based on history and risk factor for needed benefit of HRT for treatment of osteoporosis. The Women's Health Initiative study indicated significant increased risk of cardiovascular events and breast cancer for women taking estrogen and progestin therapy combined (*ACOG Practice Bulletin*, 2004).

3. Selective estrogen receptor modulator (SERM):

a. Raloxifene (Evista) 60 mg orally daily. For postmenopausal women. Prevents osteoporosis, cardioprotective, and appears to decrease estrogen-recepted breast cancer by 65% over 8 years (National Osteoporosis Foundation, n.d.). May note side effect of increased vasomotor symptoms and increased risk of venous thromboembolism.

4. Calcitonin:

a. Intranasal calcitonin (Miacalcin) 200 IU 1 puff in alternating nostrils daily.

b. Calcitonin injections (Calcimar) 100 IU by subcutaneous injection three times per week at bedtime.

c. Fortical (Calcitonin-salmon) 200 U/spray: nasal spray 1 spray in nostril daily, alternate nostrils.

5. Bisphosphonates:

a. Acts by reducing bone resorption and bone loss by preventing osteoclast activity.

b. May be given daily, weekly, or monthly.

i. Alendronate sodium (Fosamax) 70 mg weekly.

ii. Risedronate (Actonel) 150 mg monthly; Boniva (Ibandronate) 150 mg monthly.

iii. Zoledronic (Reclast) 5 mg/100 mL IV infusion once yearly. IV infusion given once a year over 15-min infusion. The creatinine and calcium must be checked prior to infusion.

c. Give the patient instructions to take medication with 6–8 oz water one-half hour before breakfast or any medication for the day. Have her stand or sit upright after taking medication. Tell her not to eat food for 30 min after taking the medication. Precautions should be used for patients who have upper gastrointestinal side effects.

6. Parathyroid hormone:

a. Recombinant human PTH rebuilds bone density and increases strength of bone. Approved for severe osteoporosis for postmenopausal women and men with the diagnosis of osteoporosis who have failed antiresportive therapy and not able to tolerate bisphosphanates.

b. Forteo (Teriparatide) 250 mcg/mL injection: 20 mcg subcutaneous daily. Taken for a maximum of 2 years. Check calcium and renal function before prescribing.

Follow-up

A. If the patient is on calcium supplements, check urinary calcium excretion two times per year. If it is below 250 mg per day, nephrocalcinosis and the risk of renal stones is decreased.

B. Bone density test recommended every 2 years to evaluate effectiveness of medical plan.

Consultation/Referral

A. If fracture is suspected, consult with a physician.

Individual Considerations

A. Geriatrics: Osteoporosis is seen primarily in this population.

◧ PLANTAR FASCIITIS

Definition

A. Plantar fasciitis is an inflammatory condition in the plantar fascia (foot) that causes pain in the arch of the foot and radiates to the heel.

Incidence

A. The incidence is unknown, but plantar fasciitis is the most common cause of heel pain in the United States.

Pathogenesis

A. Repetitive small tears in the plantar fascia causing collagen breakdown at the medial tubercle of the calcaneus.

Predisposing Factors

A. Athletes: overuse injury from running

B. Tight or weak muscles/tendons (Achilles tendon, heel cord, gastrecnemius, soleus muscle)

C. Poor arch support/improper footwear (poor support in shoes)

D. Anatomic abnormalities (low arch support, flat foot, high arch, tibial torsion, overpronated foot, leg length discrepancy, forefoot varus, thinning of fat pad)

Common Complaints

A. Severe foot pain in the bottom of the foot, especially first thing in the morning

B. Burning pain when walking

C. Stiffness in foot/heel

D. May be worse in the morning, improve during day, and then get painful at the end of day

Other Signs and Symptoms

A. Both heels may be affected.

B. Pain located medial tubercle of calcaneus, medial of longitudinal arch.

C. Heel spurs may or may not be present.

D. Pain worsens with standing for long periods of time.

Subjective Data

A. Ask the patient when pain began, when it occurs, and how long it lasts.

B. Does pain occur with walking, running, and standing?

C. Is pain constant, stabbing pain? Rate pain on pain scale of 1–10.

D. Locate pain site, does pain radiate into toes or leg?

Physical Examination

A. Check pulse and blood pressure.

B. Inspect
1. Examine feet bilaterally.
2. Note swelling, discoloration, or rash.

C. Palpate
1. Palpate both feet, noting tenderness at point tenderness. Point tenderness will be noted over insertion on medial heel (calcaneus medial tubercle).
2. Perform passive dorsiflexion of toes and ankle. Have the patient stand on tips of toes to see if this elicits pain.

D. Auscultate the heart and lungs

Diagnostic Tests

A. X-ray may be performed, but is often normal and not needed. Perform if tumor, spur, or fracture is suspected.

B. MRI if thickening of proximal plantar fascia noted or rupture of proximal fascia suspected.

Differential Diagnoses

A. Plantar fasciitis

B. Heel pain

C. Heel spur

Plan

A. Conservative treatment includes no long periods of standing for the next 6–8 weeks.

B. Arch support: Encourage the patient to get a pair of good supportive shoes with good arch supports. Arch supports are imperative for relief and shoes may need additional arch support in addition to new shoes.

C. Shoe inserts are suggested. Suggest getting proper shoe fitting for running if the patient is an athlete.

D. The patient should avoid walking on hard surfaces and never go barefoot. Avoid wearing sandals and flip-flops.

E. NSAIDS such as ibuprofen (Motrin) 800 mg three times daily or naproxen (Naprosyn) 500 mg by mouth twice a day for comfort.

F. Ice therapy may help with pain control and swelling.

G. For severe cases, a corticosteroid lidocaine injection 1–1.5 mL injected directly into the most tender area on sole of foot may be helpful.

H. Exercises:
1. Roll foot arch with a tennis ball for 20–30 min each evening to help stretch plantar fascia.
2. Perform calf stretches against a wall, leaning forward against the wall, extending one leg behind you, one leg in front of you, stretch the leg, and reverse.

Follow-up

A. Recommend follow-up in 4 weeks following treatment. Pain should slowly improve with aggressive treatment management. The patient must be compliant with instructions given for improvement. May take 6–12 months for complete resolution.

B. If pain worsens, consider diagnostic workup (X-ray or MRI).

Consultation/Referral

A. Refer to a podiatrist if conservative treatment therapy failed after 6 weeks.

Individual Considerations

A. None

⬚ SCIATICA

Definition

A. Sciatica is a sharp or burning pain, usually associated with numbness that radiates down the posterior or lateral leg that can result in neurosensory and/or motor deficits. Sciatica indicates abnormal function of the lumbosacral nerve roots or one of the nerves in the lumbosacral plexus.

Incidence

A. The prevalence of sciatica in the general population is 40%, though only 1% have any neurosensory or motor deficits. The most common cause of sciatica is herniated disks, 95% of which occur at the L4–L5 or L5–S1 level.

Pathogenesis

A. Pressure on the nerve from a herniated disk, from bony osteophytes, a compression fracture, or any other extrinsic pressure (e.g., pelvic mass or epidural process, "wallet sciatica") causes progressive sensory, sensorimotor, or sensorimotor visceral loss.

Predisposing Factors

A. Inflexibility

B. Obesity

C. Trauma

D. Bony osteophytes

Common Complaints

A. Pain around the buttock area

B. Pain often associated with numbness traveling down the lateral or posterior leg

C. Numbness

D. Paresthesia

Other Signs and Symptoms

A. Difficulty walking with affected leg

B. Positive straight leg raises

C. Decreased sensation

Subjective Data

A. Elicit onset of symptoms, duration, and what makes pain better or worse.

B. Inquire about previous episodes of pain or trauma.

C. Have the patient point to the area of pain, numbness, or tingling.

D. Are symptoms unilateral or bilateral?

E. Question the patient about loss of bowel or bladder control or other deficits and/or changes.

F. Does the patient notice leg weakness or difficulty walking?

Physical Examination

A. Check pulse and blood pressure.

B. Inspect gait and movement of back and extremities.

C. Palpate spinous processes.

D. Examine flexion and extension of spine. Assess sensation, DTRs, muscle strength, and motor weakness of lower extremities.

E. Examine neurologic function of back and lower extremity.
   1. Straight leg raising sign is positive.
   2. Dorsiflexion of ankle is positive.
   3. Check for loss of sensation in radicular pattern. Light touch pinprick and two point discrimination are not present.
   4. Look for decrease or loss of deep tendon reflexes.
   5. Check muscle strength of lower extremities.
   6. Check motor weakness.
   7. Check for cauda equina syndrome, indicated by urinary retention, radicular symptoms, and saddle anesthesia.

Cauda equina syndrome is a surgical emergency, characterized by bowel and bladder dysfunction; saddle anesthesia at the anus, perineum, or genitals; and widespread or progressive loss of strength in the legs or gait disturbances.

F. Percuss for tenderness over the spinous processes.

Diagnostic Tests
A. Radiography, when red flags for fracture, cancer, or infection are present.
B. CT scan or MRI, when cauda equina, tumor, infection, or fracture is suspected; MRI is test of choice for patients with prior back surgery.

Differential Diagnoses
A. Sciatica of unknown etiology
B. Lumbosacral strain
C. Herniated disk
D. Bony osteophytes, spinal stenosis
E. Compression fracture
F. Neoplasm of spine
G. Pelvic mass
H. Epidural process causing progressive sensory, sensorimotor, or sensorimotor visceral loss
I. Meralgia paresthetica

Plan
A. General interventions: Care for these patients should evolve over a three-step process.
   1. Step 1 (2–4 days)
      a. Bed rest for severe radiculopathy only.
      b. Limit walking and standing to 30–40 min each day.
      c. Recommend application of heat or cold packs to site as needed.
   2. Step 2 (7–14 days)
      a. Reevaluate neurologic and back exam; tell the patient "Let pain be your guide" when resuming normal daily activities.
      b. Have him or her perform gentle stretching exercises.
      c. Encourage walking on flat surfaces.
      d. Educate him or her regarding proper care of the back, with regard to exercises, posture, and so forth.
      e. Provide handouts on back exercises/stretches for the patient. See Section III Patient Teaching Guide, "Back Stretches."
      f. Physical therapy may be implemented at this time if no significant improvement is noted.
   3. Step 3 (2–3 weeks)
      a. Reevaluate the patient, noting degree of improvement with exam.

   b. Continue muscle toning and reconditioning exercises.
   c. If improvement noted, gradually increase physical activities.
   d. Reinforce healthy care of the back.
   e. Continue physical therapy until the patient can perform exercises without assistance or until released by the physical therapist.
B. Pharmaceutical therapy
   1. NSAIDs as needed: naproxen (Naprosyn) 500 mg initially, followed by 250 mg every 6–8 hours.
   2. Acetaminophen may also be used as needed, especially if the patient is not able to tolerate ibuprofen.
   3. For more severe pain not relieved by NSAIDs, consider acetaminophen (Tylenol) with codeine for short duration. Narcotics should not be used for more than 2 weeks.
   4. Muscle relaxants: Muscle relaxants should not be used for more than 2 weeks.
      a. Cyclobenzaprine (Flexeril) 10 mg 1–3 times daily.
      b. Muscle relaxants place patients at risk for drowsiness. Warn the patient not to mix medications with alcohol because it may potentiate the medication.

Follow-up
A. Initial follow-up is needed in 1–2 weeks. See recommendation of stepwise approach.

Consultation/Referral
A. If cauda equina syndrome is suspected, prompt referral to a physician is necessary.
B. If pain is severe enough that narcotics are needed, consult with a physician.
C. If bilateral sciatica is associated with vertebral collapse, osteoporosis, neoplasia, and/or vascular disease, consult with a physician.

Individual Considerations
A. Pregnancy: Sciatica pain is common due to physiologic changes of the pelvis as pregnancy progresses to term. Avoid use of NSAIDs. Physical therapy may be used as indicated.
B. Adults: For adults over 50 years presenting with no prior history of backache, consider differential diagnosis of neoplasm. Most common metastasis is secondary to primary site of breast or prostate, or to multiple myeloma. Pain is most prominent in recumbent position and rarely radiates into buttock or leg.
C. Geriatrics: Bilateral sciatica is associated with vertebral collapse, osteoporosis, neoplasia, and/or vascular disease. Refer the patient to a physician immediately. Use caution when prescribing medication to the elderly due to the risk for drowsiness and potential falls.

◘ SPRAINS: ANKLE AND KNEE

Definition
Sprains are ligament stretching or partially tearing from forceful stress on the joint. Sprains are categorized as the following:
A. Grade 1: Microscopic tears without ligament tearing or joint instability

B. Grade 2: Partial tearing of involved ligaments and laxity of joint with moderate function loss

C. Grade 3: Ligament tearing with severe function loss and joint instability

Incidence

A. **Ankle** sprains are among the most common injuries seen in primary care.

B. **Knee** injuries are among the 10 most common causes of occupational injury and worker compensation claims.

Pathogenesis

A. Sudden stress to a supporting ligament causes ligament stretching or tearing. Sprains are usually the result of jumping, falling, or rotating a joint.

B. Ankle sprains are most often inversion sprains with symptoms on the lateral side of the joint.

C. Eversion injuries affect the medial side.

D. Knee sprains most often involve the patellofemoral joint.

Predisposing Factors

A. Previous injury to ankle or knee

B. Athletic activities

C. Patellofemoral instability

Common Complaints

A. "I twisted my ankle or knee."

B. "I stepped off of a step and came down on the side of my foot."

C. Swelling, pain, weakness of ankle or knee from a previous injury.

Other Signs and Symptoms

A. First degree: Minimal pain; mild to moderate pain with stress, little swelling; minimal tenderness with palpation; little functional loss; unimpaired weight bearing or walking; internal microdamage with full continuity

B. Second degree: Moderate pain with range of motion; swelling; marked tenderness on palpation; moderate loss of function; difficulty with weight bearing or walking; mechanical dissociation with partial loss of continuity

C. Third degree: Severe pain, especially with passive inversion; severe swelling, marked tenderness; marked decrease in range of motion; intolerant of weight bearing or walking; joint instability; discoloration of skin; complete rupture of a ligament

Subjective Data

A. Inquire about history of trauma.

B. Have the patient describe the injury: time, place, activity, predisposing factors, and time symptoms developed.

C. Determine if the symptoms are acute or chronic.

D. Inquire about the type and location of the pain.

E. Have the patient describe the pain, and what conditions aggravate or relieve pain.

F. Ask if there are symptoms of popping, clicking, locking, recurrent swelling, or giving way of joint.

G. Ask if there is pain or other symptoms elsewhere, such as low back, hip, or leg.

H. Explore history of any previous ankle or knee injury.

I. Determine if the current injury was evaluated and treated previously.

J. Have the patient describe ability to bear weight on extremity and to tolerate range of motion.

K. Review the patient's medical history for arthritis, gout, cancer, autoimmune disorders, or metabolic disease.

Physical Examination

A. Check temperature, pulse, respirations, and blood pressure.

B. Inspect
  1. Observe ambulation. Note overall appearance and facial grimaces during exam.
  2. Inspect injured area for swelling, discoloration, and deformity. Compare injured side to uninjured side.

C. Palpate
  1. Palpate the injured site for tenderness.
  2. Palpate the joints above and below the injured site.
  3. Perform range of motion (active and passive), resisted ROM to evaluate strength.
  4. Check for catching or locking of the knee on extension.
  5. Assess neurovascular status of the knee or ankle and distal extremity.
  6. **Ankle:** Palpate for tender sulcus in anterolateral aspect on inversion of the ankle. Assess for pain aggravated by forced ankle inversion. Perform isometric test of plantar flexion and eversion. Perform anterior drawer test, talar tilt test.
  7. **Knee:** Palpate for tenderness on the medial and lateral joint line. Perform McMurray's test to detect a torn meniscus (see Section II, "Evaluation of Sprains"). Symptoms of sprained knees:
     a. Meniscus tear: locking of knee with flexion and giving way of knee.
     b. Collateral ligament tear or strain: pain at lateral or medial sides.
     c. Anterior cruciate tear: popping sound at injury site and immediate swelling.
     d. Posterior cruciate tear or strain: pain in interior knee.
     e. Patellofemoral syndrome: popping or snapping, pain under patella with motion, and pain on stairs or hills.
     f. Tendinitis: pain over patellar tendon.
     g. Prepatellar bursitis: swelling over patella with inability to kneel due to swelling.
     h. Nonspecific effusion: effusion worse with exercise.
  8. See the Section II Procedure, "Evaluation of Sprains."

Diagnostic Tests

A. Radiography of extremity, if fracture is suspected.

B. MRI, if mechanical symptoms and effusion persist.

C. Bone scans or MRI are usually reserved for those who have failed to respond after 6–12 weeks of therapy.

Differential Diagnoses

A. Ankle sprain
  1. Fracture
  2. Acute dislocation
  3. Infection
  4. Ligament strain

   5. Tendinitis or tenosynovitis
   6. Nonspecific foot or ankle pain
B. Knee sprain
   1. Fracture
   2. Dislocation
   3. Septic arthritis
   4. Infected prepatellar bursitis
   5. Inflammation
   6. Tumor
   7. Meniscus tear
   8. Collateral ligament tear
   9. Anterior cruciate tear
   10. Posterior cruciate tear
   11. Collateral ligament strain
   12. Cruciate ligament strain
   13. Patellofemoral syndrome, or chondromalacia
   14. Effusion, nonspecific
   15. Patellar tendinitis
   16. Prepatellar bursitis
   17. Nonspecific knee pain

Plan

A. General interventions: Reinforce the degree of injury and the need to take care of extremity to prevent further damage.
B. Patient teaching
   1. See the Section III Patient Teaching Guide for this chapter, "RICE Therapy and Exercise Therapy."
   2. Give the patient the Section III Patient Teaching Guide for this chapter, "Ankle Exercises" or "Knee Exercises."
C. Pharmaceutical therapy
   1. Drug of choice
      a. Nonsteroidal anti-inflammatory drugs to reduce pain and inflammation.
      b. Consider one of the following: aspirin, ibuprofen, indomethacin, or piroxicam.
      c. If there is increased risk for bleeding, acetaminophen with codeine may be used for pain.
   2. Injectable medication
      a. Methylprednisolone acetate (Depo-Medrol) may be used if symptoms continue to be present 6–8 weeks after injury.
      b. Repeat injection in 4–6 weeks if symptoms have not been reduced by 50%.

Follow-up

A. Schedule initial follow-up in 2 weeks to evaluate current therapy or sooner if problems arise.

Consultation/Referral

A. Refer the patient to a physician if fracture is suspected.
B. Refer the patient to a physician or orthopedic surgeon if therapy is unproductive and symptoms have not begun to regress within 6 weeks.

Individual Considerations

A. Pediatrics: In prepubertal or peripubertal patients, knee ligaments usually do not tear. Instead, the growth plate may open up on one side. This age group needs stress radiography to check for fracture of the growth plate.

REFERENCES

American College of Obstetricians and Gynecologists. (2004). ACOG practice bulletin. Clinical management guidelines for obstetrician-gynecologists. Number 50, January 2003. *Obstetrics and Gynecology, 103,* 203–216.

Bellantoni, M. (1996). Osteoporosis prevention and treatment. *American Family Physician, 1,* 986–991.

Bigos, S., Bowyer, O., Braen, G., Brown, K., Deyo, R., Haldeman, S., et al. (1994). *Acute low back problems in adults: Clinical Practice Guideline Number 14,* AHCPR Publication No. 95–0642. Rockville, MD: Agency for Health Care Policy and Research, Public Health Service, U.S. Department of Health and Human Services.

Birrer, R. B., Bordelon, R. L., & Sammarco, G. J. (1992, February 29). Ankle: Don't miss a sprain. *Patient Care, 26,* 6–28.

Chow, R., Qaseem, A., Snow, V., Casey, D., Cross, Jr., T., Shekelle, P., et al. (2007). Clinical guidelines: Diagnosis and treatment of low back pain. *A Joint Clinical Practice Guideline from the American College of Physicians and the American Pain Society, 147*(7), 478–491.

Daily, P., Bishop, G., Russell, I., & Fletcher, E. M. (1990). Psychological stress and the fibrosistic/fibromyalgia syndrome. *Journal of Rheumatology, 17,* 1380.

Daniels, J. (1997). Treatment of occupationally acquired low back pain. *American Family Physician, 2,* 587–596.

Deyo, R. A., Loeser, J. D., & Bigos, S. J. (1990). Herniated lumbar intervertebral disc. *Annals of Internal Medicine, 112,* 598–603.

Emkey, G., & Reginato, A. (2009, October). All about gout and pseudogout: Meeting a growing challenge. *The Journal of Musculoskeletal Medicine,* S17–S23.

Ernst, D., & Lee, A. (Eds.). (2009). *NPPR: Nurse practitioners' prescribing reference.* New York: A Haymarket Media Publication.

Jones, A. (1997). Primary care management of acute low back pain. *The Nurse Practitioner, 22*(7), 50–68.

Kalaci, A., Cakici, H., Hapa, O., Yanat, A. N., & Sevinc, T. T. (2009). Treatment of plantar fasciitis using four different local injection modalities: A randomized prospective clinical trial. *Journal of the American Podiatric Medical Association, 99*(2), 108–113.

Kinkade, S. (2007). Evaluation and treatment of acute low back pain. *American Family Physician, 75*(8), 1181–1188.

Lewiecki, E. M., & Watts, N. B. (2009). New guidelines for the prevention and treatment of osteoporosis. *Southern Medical Journal, 102*(2), 175–179.

McGee, C. (1997). Secondary amenorrhea leading to osteoporosis. *The Nurse Practitioner, 22*(5), 22, 38, 41–45, 48.

Mufson, M., & Regestein, Q. (1993). The spectrum of fibromyalgia disorders. *Arthritis and Rheumatism, 35*(5), 647–649.

Muma, R., Lyons, B., Newman, T., & Carnes, B. (1996). *Patient education: A practical approach.* Stamford, CT: Appleton & Lange.

National Fibromyalgia Association. (n.d.). Fibromyalgia fact sheet. Retrieved July 28, 2009, from http://www.fmaware.org

National Osteoporosis Foundation. (n.d.). Prevention: Vitamin D. Retrieved March 10, 2010, from http://www.nof.org/prevention/vitaminD.htm

National Osteoporosis Foundation. (n.d.). *Medications to prevent & treat osteoporosis.* Retrieved April 3, 2010, from http://www.nof.org/patientinfo/medications.htm#Raloxifene

National Osteoporosis Foundation. (1998). *Physician's guide to prevention and treatment of osteoporosis.* Retrieved March 3, 2010, from http://www.nof.org/professionals/clinicals-Guide

Neufeld, S. K., & Cerrato, R. (2008). Plantar fasciitis: Evaluation and treatment. *The Journal of the American Academy of Orthopaedic Surgeons, 16*(6), 338–346.

Noble, J. (1996). *Textbook of primary care medicine* (2nd ed.). St. Louis: Mosby.

PDR Health. (2009). Retrieved July 28, 2009, from www.pdrhealth.com

Pham, A. N., Colon-Emeric, C. S., & Weber, T. J. (2009). Osteoporosis in older women. *Clinical Geriatrics, 17*(10), 20–28.

Ross, C. (1997). A comparison of osteoarthritis and rheumatoid arthritis: Diagnosis and treatment. *The Nurse Practitioner, 22*(9), 20–39.

Sweet, M. G., Sweet, J. M., Jeremiah, M. P., & Galazka, S. S. (2009). Diagnosis and treatment of osteoporosis. *American Family Physician, 79*(3), 193–200.

Tierney, L., McPhe, S., & Papadakis, M. (2007). *Current medical diagnosis and treatment* (46th ed.). New York: McGraw-Hill.

Turk, D., & Wilson, H. (2009). Managing fibromyalgia: An update on diagnosis and treatment. *The Journal of Musculoskeletal Medicine,* S1–S7.

U.S. Department of Health and Human Services. (2004). *Bone health and osteoporosis: A report of the Surgeon General.* Retrieved March 1, 2010, from http://www.surgeongeneralgov/library/bonehealth/content.html

Wolfe, F., Smythe, H., Yunus, M., Bennett, R. M., Bombardier, C., Goldenberg, D. L., et al. (1990). The American College of Rheumatology 1990 criteria for the classification of fibromyalgia: Report of the Multicenter Criteria Committee. *Arthritis and Rheumatism, 33,* 160–173.

Neurological Guidelines

Jill C. Cash

⌐ ALZHEIMER'S DISEASE

Definition
A. Alzheimer's disease is a permanent, progressive decline in several dimensions of cognitive functioning, including memory disturbance, that severely interferes with the person's everyday living but has no decrease in level of consciousness. Insidious onset, gradually progressive decline in intellectual functioning, and absence of other specific causes of dementia are also present.

Incidence
A. There are over 4 million cases of Alzheimer's disease per 350 million people. Among the elderly, approximately 40% of those over 85 years of age are affected. Of all types of dementias, Alzheimer's dementia includes 70% of those affected, with the other 30% affected by atypical dementia.

Pathogenesis
A. The disease is a degenerative process involving cell loss from the basal forebrain, cerebral cortex, and other areas.

Predisposing Factors
A. Advanced age greater than 50 years
B. Severe head trauma
C. Abnormal genetic makeup, Down syndrome
D. Positive family history of Alzheimer's disease

Common Complaints
A. Significant memory loss

Other Signs and Symptoms
A. Loss of language and social skills in later stages
B. Loss of all intellectual capacities
C. Change in personality
D. Aphasia
E. Apraxia
F. Agnosia
G. Sleep and mood disorders
H. Fecal and urinary incontinence
I. Delusions
J. Weight loss
K. Seizures

Subjective Data

Family members are a good resource for obtaining an accurate history.

A. Determine onset, course, and duration of symptoms.
B. Note loss of immediate, recent, or remote memory, such as trouble remembering appointments, difficulty recalling recent events, and inability to find personal belongings.
C. Determine the patient's ability to make reasonable judgments, such as answering the phone when it rings, and so forth.
D. Is the patient able to carry on daily functions of living, including cooking meals and cleaning house?
E. Discuss the patient's sleep-wake cycle.
F. Assess the patient for decreased appetite, lack of pleasure in usual activities, melancholy mood, or other symptoms associated with depression.
G. Note language difficulties and problems expressing self.
H. Note any recent physical illness.
I. Review the patient's medication history.
J. Discuss alcohol intake and abuse factors.
K. Review past medical history of head trauma, hypertension, cerebrovascular accident (CVA), cancer, metabolic problems, neurologic disease, infections, gastric surgery (vitamin B_{12} deficiency), and emotional or psychiatric problems.

Physical Examination
A. Check temperature, pulse, respirations, blood pressure, and weight.
B. Inspect: Inspect overall appearance for hygiene and nutritional status.
C. Auscultate: Auscultate the heart and lungs.
D. Neurologic exam: Perform a complete neurologic exam.
E. Perform mental status exam with screening tool. Clock drawing test may also be administered and used with the screening tool.

Rule out other specific causes of dementia, including cerebrovascular disease. Diagnosis requires the presence of characteristic clinical features involving two or more areas of cognitive function, such as language impairment, apraxia or agnosia, as well as progressive worsening of memory.

Diagnostic Tests

A. Hachinski ischemic score (see Table 18.1): Results of 4 or less indicate Alzheimer's disease, and scores of 7 or greater indicate multi-infarct dementia.
B. CBC.
C. Chemistry profile.
D. Thyroid function studies.
E. Folate and B_{12} levels.
F. VDRL for syphilis.
G. Chest radiography.
H. CT scan of brain.

Differential Diagnoses

A. Alzheimer's disease
B. Drug interactions
C. Delirium
D. Depression
E. Cerebrovascular disease

Plan

A. General interventions
 1. Provide supportive measures.
 2. Treatment may include treating coexisting diseases, thyroid disease, and vitamin B_{12} deficiency.

TABLE 18.1 The Modified Hachinski Ischemic Score

Feature	Points*
Abrupt onset of symptoms	2
Stepwise deterioration (e.g., decline-stability-decline)	1
Fluctuating course	2
Nocturnal confusion	1
Personality relatively preserved	1
Depression	1
Somatic complaints (e.g., body aches, chest pain)	1
Emotional lability	1
History or presence of hypertension	1
History of stroke	2
Evidence of coexisting atheroscleroisis (e.g., peripheral arterial disease [PAD], MI)	1
Focal neurologic symptoms (e.g., hemiparesis, homonymous hemianopia, aphasia)	2
Focal neurologic signs (e.g., unilateral weakness, sensory loss, asymmetric reflexes, Babinski's sign)	2

*Total score is determined:
< 4 suggests primary dementia (e.g., Alzheimer's disease)
4–7 = indeterminate
> 7 suggests vascular dementia

3. Cognitive stimulation has been shown to slow down the degenerative process. Therefore, encourage musical therapy, occupational therapy, and mind-stimulating activities.
 4. Ensure that the patient has a safe environment; measures may need to be taken for environmental safety, such as locks on doors, alarms on doors, and so on.
 5. Daily exercise should be encouraged.
B. Patient teaching
 1. Support groups are encouraged for the patient and spouse. Therapy sessions for each may be beneficial.
 2. Patient support group:
 Alzheimer's Association
 National Office, 225 N. Michigan Ave., Fl. 17
 Chicago, IL 60601, 312-335-8700
 Fax: 866-699-1246
 Alzheimer's Disease Education and Referral Center
 800-438-4380 or 800-272-3900 or (www. Alz.org)
 3. Families needing legal and financial advice should seek this out early and not wait for a crisis. 24/7 helpline: 1-800-272-3900: Alzheimer's Disease Family Relief Program 800-437-2423
C. Pharmaceutical therapy
 1. Cholinesterase inhibitors
 a. Rivastigmine (Exelon) 1.5–6 mg twice a day or patch starting at 4.6 mg/24 hours and then titrate up to 9.5 mg/24 hours.
 b. Donepezil (Aricept) then 10 mg/day may be given after 1 month.
 c. Galantamine (Razadyne) 4 mg twice a day with meals for 4 weeks, then may titrate to max of 12 mg twice a day. For missed doses, will need to retitrate doses.
 2. NMDA receptor antagonist
 a. Memantine (Namenda) 5–20 mg/daily.
 3. Assess the patient for secondary behaviors of dementia. Psychosis, delusions, hallucinations, anxiety, depression, and insomnia may occur and should be treated accordingly. Cognitive and behavioral interventions should be initiated in assisting the patient in controlling these behaviors. The benefits and risks must be weighted and for some patients pharmacological treatment may be necessary for those patients exhibiting extreme, aggressive behaviors with irritability and/or insomnia. Treatment with antipsychotics is very controversial due to the side effects and extreme complications that may occur with these medications.
 4. Treatment of depression. Nortriptyline (Pamelor) 30–50 mg daily, sertraline (Zoloft), paroxetine (Paxil), or escitalopram (Lexapro). Monitor SSRI for weight loss, decrease in seizure threshold, tremors; not used with MAO-I. Monitor coumadin and lithium levels closely.

Follow-up

A. Follow-up is variable, depending on patient status and needs of the patient and family. Follow-up is recommended every 3 months to follow progression of disease. If medications are being introduced, monitor the patient more frequently.

Consultation/Referral

A. Consider visiting nurse, social worker, occupational and physical therapy.

B. Consult a physician for medication treatment for secondary behavioral symptoms.

Individual Considerations
A. Adults: Estrogen replacement therapy and antioxidant therapy (Vitamin E) are being studied for their effectiveness in prevention and delay of Alzheimer's disease.
B. Geriatrics
   1. Alzheimer's disease is primarily seen in this population.
   2. Long-term prognosis: Average patient lives 7–10 years after early symptoms, but life span while demented can be 20 years or more.

BELL'S PALSY

Definition
A. Bell's palsy, also known as idiopathic peripheral facial palsy, is characterized by an acute onset of unilateral facial paralysis. It accounts for approximately 75% of all cases of facial paralysis.

Incidence
A. Bell's palsy has an incidence of 25:100,000. Approximately 5% of those affected experience recurrence. Both sexes are affected, as well as all ages, but most patients are in their middle years, older than 30 years.

Pathogenesis
A. The pathogenesis of Bell's palsy is unknown, but some possible etiologies include genetic, metabolic, autoimmune, and vascular causes. An increasing body of evidence reveals that Bell's palsy may be a virally induced neuritis. A triggering event or stressor induces activation of a latent virus, most likely herpes zoster or herpes simplex virus, present within the geniculate ganglion of the facial nerve. Viral activation results in reexpression of dormant viral particles and neural inflammation leading to entrapment, ischemia, and degeneration of the facial nerve.

Predisposing Factors
A. Diabetes
B. Pregnancy
C. Recent infection
D. Positive family history
E. Hypertension
F. Hypothyroidism

Common Complaints
A. Acute onset of unilateral facial weakness with inability to close one eye
B. Sagging of one eyebrow
C. Loss of nasolabial fold
D. Mouth drawn to affected side

Other Signs and Symptoms
A. Ipsilateral retroauricular pain with or preceding paralysis
B. Hyperacusis or hypersensitivity to sound
C. Dysgeusia, or perversion of taste, in the anterior two-thirds of the tongue
D. Facial paresthesia
E. Drooling

Subjective Data
A. Elicit onset, duration, and course of symptoms.
B. Have the patient describe all neurologic symptoms present.
C. Note associated symptoms such as disruption of taste and disturbances in visual function or hearing.
D. Note predisposing factors such as trauma, infection, or pregnancy.
E. Review the patient's family history for presence of Bell's palsy.
F. Review the patient's medical history; especially note cerebrovascular or cardiac risk factors. A focused history should include contraindications to use of steroids.

Physical Examination
A. Check temperature, pulse, respirations and blood pressure.
B. Inspect
   1. Note facial appearance.
   2. Observe symmetry of eyes. Check corneal reflex (decreased). Assess ears, nose, and throat; assess the skin for lesions. Assess in and behind ears for zosteriform lesions.
   3. Complete ear exam to rule out infection. **Assess paralysis of all the muscles supplied by one facial nerve. Paralysis may be of varying degrees and need not be complete.**
C. Auscultate: Auscultate the heart and lungs.
D. Neurologic exam: Perform a complete neurologic exam; test all cranial nerves.

Subjective decreased sensation may be present in the trigeminal distribution.

Diagnostic Tests
A. Lyme titer: positive in patients with secondary facial weakness from Lyme disease.
B. Skull radiography, CT scan, or MRI: negative in Bell's palsy, but may show evidence of fracture line, bony erosion by either infection or neoplasm, stroke, or tumor.
C. Electromyographic (EMG) studies: occasionally performed to predict prognosis and progression. EMG is reserved for severe cases of paralysis lasting longer than 1 week.
D. Lumbar puncture: indicated only when other conditions are suspected. CSF should be sent for cytology.

Differential Diagnoses
A. Bell's palsy
B. Cerebellopontine angle mass lesion
C. Stroke
D. Craniocerebral trauma
E. Lyme disease
F. Ramsay Hunt syndrome, herpes zoster oticus
G. Acoustic neuroma
H. Middle ear disease such as purulent otitis media or neoplasms
I. Guillain-Barré syndrome
J. Sarcoidosis
K. Carcinomatous meningitis

Plan
A. General interventions
   1. Provide eye protection by means of the following:
      a. Methylcellulose drops as needed and ocular lubricant (Lacri-Lube) at bedtime.

b. Tape eye closed, especially at night.
c. Wear dark glasses when outdoors to minimize exposure.
2. Physical therapy may be beneficial.
3. Ensure the patient gets reassurance and emotional support.

Recovery may take 3–6 months or longer and is complete in approximately 80% of the cases.

B. Patient teaching: See the Section III Patient Teaching Guide for this chapter, "Bell's Palsy."
C. Medical and surgical management.
   1. Consider operative decompression by an otologic surgeon; this is controversial.
   2. Operative anastomosis of the twelfth cranial nerve to the seventh cranial nerve; this may cause difficulty with eating and has a limited role in facial restoration.
D. Pharmaceutical therapy.
   1. Prednisone: adults take 80 mg every day with breakfast for first 3 days, then decrease dosage to 40 mg for 3 days, then to 20 mg daily for 3 days, then stop.

Recent studies suggest that a brief course of prednisone conveys modest benefits with minimal risks.

   2. Use of oral acyclovir in conjunction with prednisone, at a dosage of 400 mg five times per day for 10 days, is controversial. Consider acyclovir for patients without renal insufficiency and with no other contraindications to therapy.
   3. Analgesics, such as acetaminophen, for ear pain.

Follow-up
A. For patients with severe symptoms, follow up in 3–4 days, then again in 2 weeks.
B. If symptoms worsen or do not resolve within 4 weeks, have the patient return to the clinic.

Consultation/Referral
A. Consult a neurologist for the following:
   1. Failure to resolve significantly after 4–6 weeks. Only 5%–8% report distressing residual signs and symptoms, including contracture of facial muscles at rest and synergistic mass innervation due to defective nerve regeneration, manifested as either crocodile tears secondary to abnormal secretory fibers intended for the salivary glands or ipsilateral eyelid shutting.
   2. Other cranial nerve involvement or other abnormalities on neurologic exam.
   3. Recurrence of facial palsy: about 5%–7% of patients experience recurrence of symptoms. Known causes of recurrent palsy include sarcoidosis, diabetes, leukemia, and infectious mononucleosis.
   4. Bilateral facial palsies.
B. Consult an ophthalmologist for persistent ocular pain or development of a corneal abrasion or ulceration.

Individual Considerations
A. Pregnancy: The incidence of Bell's palsy is increased in pregnancy, with the highest incidence in the third trimester or immediately postpartum. May treat with prednisone during pregnancy.

CARPAL TUNNEL SYNDROME

Definition
A. Carpal tunnel syndrome (CTS) is a nerve entrapment condition of the median nerve of the wrist.

Incidence
A. Carpal tunnel syndrome occurs in approximately 1% of the general population. It is primarily seen in 30- to 60-year-old adults.

Pathogenesis
A. CTS occurs from compression of the median nerve in the carpal canal. Compression occurs due to swelling of the flexor tenosynovium, and the pressure blocks the nerve fibers, which produces numbness and discomfort in the hands. Repetitive flexion and extension of the wrists create increased pressure in the carpal canal.
B. Potential causes of CTS include blunt trauma or structural changes; tumors; systemic diseases, such as rheumatoid disorders, diabetes mellitus, thyroid disorders, endocrine diseases, and so forth; mechanical overuse syndrome; infectious diseases, such as TB and leprosy. Consider multifactorial causes of CTS.

Predisposing Factors
A. Women
B. Hobbies or jobs that require repetitive wrist or hand movement and the use of vibratory tools
C. Pregnancy

Common Complaints
A. Pain
B. Tingling
C. Numbness sensation in the wrists, hands, and fingers that radiates up into the forearm

Other Signs and Symptoms
A. Paresthesia in wrists, hands, and fingers.
B. Localized pain of radial three digits of the hand.
C. Weakness with grasp.
D. Decreased dexterity.
E. Night pain in wrists.
F. Referred pain to elbow and/or shoulder.
G. Long-term pressure in the carpus can produce ischemic changes and may lead to axonal death, muscular atrophy, and pain. Long-term nerve compression may produce irreversible changes.

Subjective Data
A. Determine onset, duration, and course of presenting symptoms.
B. Note the progression of symptoms since the initial occurrence.
C. Assess whether the symptoms increase with hand or wrist activity and decrease with the joint at rest.
D. Identify what factors precipitate symptoms, what makes symptoms worse, and what alleviates symptoms.
E. Inquire whether the patient awakens at night with numbness and tingling sensations.
F. Have the patient describe the pain, and note if radiation is present. Are symptoms bilateral?

G. Note the patient's occupation, hobby, and/or daily routines that require hand or wrist use.

H. Identify what treatment and/or relief measures have been used, and note results.

Physical Examination

A. Check temperature, pulse, respirations, and blood pressure.

B. Inspect: Inspect the hands for deformities. Note wasting or atrophy.

C. Palpate: Perform sensory motor evaluation of the hand and arm:
   1. Perform Tinel's test: Tap over transverse carpal ligament; result is positive if tingling in fingers is noted.
   2. Perform Phalen's test: Have patient place elbows on flat surface and hold forearms in vertical position, then flex wrists; result is positive if pain, numbness, or tingling is noted within the next 60 seconds.

Diagnostic Tests

A. EMG, or electromyography.

B. Nerve conduction velocity studies.

C. If an underlying systemic illness or condition exists, consider the following:
   1. Erythrocyte sedimentation rate (ESR).
   2. Blood glucose.
   3. Thyroid profile.
   4. Inflammatory disease studies.

Differential Diagnoses

A. Carpal tunnel syndrome

B. Peripheral neuropathy

C. Cervical spondylosis and cervical disk herniation

D. Brachial plexus lesion

E. Trauma

F. Thenar atrophy and neuropathy

G. Osteoarthritis

H. Neurologic disorders: polyneuritis, multiple sclerosis, tumors, and so on

Plan

A. General interventions
   1. Help the patient identify causative agents, eliminate activity if possible, decrease repetitive use, or use alternative methods to accomplish the same task.
   2. Have him or her rest arms and wrists as much as possible.
   3. Encourage him or her to perform daily stretching exercises.
   4. Instruct him or her to splint wrists, especially at bedtime while sleeping.

B. Patient teaching
   1. Instruct the patient how to splint his or her wrists.
   2. Demonstrate stretching exercises.
   3. Stress the importance of rest and elimination of the causative activity.

C. Pharmaceutical therapy
   1. NSAIDs as needed. Ibuprofen (Motrin) 600–800 mg by mouth three times daily or naproxen (Naprosyn) 500 mg by mouth twice a day.
   2. Vitamin B_6 100 mg/day.
   3. Consider corticosteroid injections in carpal canal (40 mg/mL with 1% lidocaine 1 mL)

Follow-up

A. Depending on treatment, consider follow-up in 1 month to evaluate status.

Consultation/Referral

A. Refer the patient to a physician for severe cases requiring evaluation for surgery.

B. Refer the patient to a surgeon for severe symptoms that could require carpal tunnel release.

B. Consider occupational therapy consult.

Individual Considerations

A. Pregnancy: CTS is the most frequent complaint during pregnancy. About 15% of the cases will progress and continue several months postpartum.

DEMENTIA

Definition

A. Dementia is a syndrome of acquired persistent cognitive impairment that affects the content, but not the level, of consciousness.

Incidence

A. Dementia is present in 5%–20% of persons older than 60 years, and in up to 40% of those 75 years and older. It accounts for more than 50% of nursing home admissions and is the condition most feared by aging adults.

Pathogenesis

A. The most common cause of dementia is Alzheimer's disease (70%), with the other cases due to mixed causes (30%), such as multi-infarct or vascular dementia. There are a number of other diseases that alter cerebral metabolism resulting in dementia, such as Huntington's and Parkinson's diseases. A variety of diseases that can produce or mimic dementia may be arrested or reversed. These are classified as pseudodementia, such as hypothyroidism or depression.

Predisposing Factors

A. Genetic predisposition

B. Metabolic disorders

C. Nutritional deficiencies

D. Alcoholism

E. Vascular disorders

Common Complaints

DSM–IV criteria for diagnosis of dementia:

A. The development of multiple cognitive deficits manifested by both of the following:
   1. Memory impairment
   2. One (or more) of the following cognitive disturbances:
      a. Aphasia, or language disturbances
      b. Apraxia, or impaired ability to carry out motor activities despite intact motor function
      c. Agnosia, or failure to recognize or identify objects despite intact sensory function
      d. Disturbance in executive functioning, planning, organizing, sequencing, and abstracting

B. Considerable impairment in social or occupation functioning

Other Signs and Symptoms
A. Insidious onset
B. Diminished ability to concentrate and recall recent events
C. Impairment of judgment and difficulty with conversation
D. Agitation and depression
E. Inability to perform activities of daily living
F. Paranoia, hallucinations, and delusions

Impairment of remote memory carries a graver prognosis than the loss of recent memory alone.

Subjective Data
A. Elicit onset and duration of symptoms; commonly, this information comes from family members.
B. Question the family members and/or caregivers regarding personality changes in the patient, or any changes in personal hygiene.
C. Review the patient's history for sexually transmitted infections.
D. Is there a loss of interest in things the patient used to find important?

Physical Examination
A. Check temperature, pulse, respirations, and blood pressure.
B. Inspect
   1. Observe general appearance; note grooming, interest in conversation, and apathy.
   2. Note the presence of slurred speech and slowed body movements.
   3. Inspect the nail beds and mucous membranes for anemia.
C. Palpate: Assess the thyroid.
D. Neurologic exam: Perform a complete neurologic exam, including cranial nerves, gait, motor function, and cerebellar function.

Diagnostic Tests
A. Pfeiffer's short, portable, mental status questionnaire or mental exam of choice.
B. Rule out possible reversible causes of dementia; not all are required, so use discretion:
   1. Thyroid function tests, to rule out either hypothyroidism or hyperthyroidism
   2. CBC
   3. Vitamin B_{12} level: anemia or B_{12} deficiency
   4. Serum chemistry profile: hyponatremia
   5. Toxicology screen or serum drug screen: toxicity or intoxication
   6. VDRL, FTA-ABS, or MHA-TP (CSF) to confirm syphilis
   7. HIV-1 antibody titer: AIDS dementia complex
   8. Liver function tests: liver disease
   9. CT scan or MRI: vascular dementia, tumor, chronic subdural hematoma, normal pressure hydrocephalus, and AIDS dementia complex
   10. EKG: Creutzfeldt-Jakob disease

The history is the key to the diagnosis of dementia. The physical exam may be normal. Dementia is *not* a normal part of aging; normal aging intelligence scores decrease by only about 10% by age 80. A thorough search for a potentially reversible cause is required.

Differential Diagnoses
A. Completely reversible dementia, rarely.
B. Depression and adverse reactions to medications are the most common reversible causes of dementia. Use the DEMENTIA pneumonic suggested by Ouslander, Osterweil, & Morley (1997):
   D: Drugs or depression
   E: Emotional upset
   M: Metabolic, for example, vitamin B_{12} deficiency or hypothyroidism
   E: Ear or eye impairment or sensory impairment
   N: Normal pressure hydrocephalus
   T: Tumors or masses, for example, subdural hematoma
   I: Infection or sepsis
   A: Anemia

Plan
A. General interventions
   1. The goal is to treat identifiable abnormalities.
   2. Supportive care for the family and patient should be arranged.
   3. No general measures are available to improve cognitive function; medications are of limited use.
   4. A safe environment, respite for the caregiver, and information on support groups for the caregiver and family are very helpful.
   5. See "Alzheimer's Disease" section for treatment and care for families needing legal and/or financial assistance.
B. Patient teaching
   1. See the Section III Patient Teaching Guide for this chapter, "Dementia."
   2. Recommended handbooks for the family include:
      a. *The 36 Hour Day: A Family Guide to Caring for Persons With Alzheimer's Disease, Related Dementing Illness, and Memory Loss in Later Life,* by Nancy Mace and Peter Rabins (Johns Hopkins University Press, 2006).
      b. "Guidelines for Dignity" and "Family Guide." Both can be ordered through the Alzheimer's Disease and Related Disorders Association or its local chapters. The national headquarters can be contacted at the following address:
      Alzheimer's Disease and Related Disorders Association
      919 North Michigan Avenue
      Suite 1000
      Chicago, IL
      60611-1676
      800-272-3900
C. Pharmaceutical therapy
   1. No general measures are available to improve cognitive function in patients with advanced dementia.
   2. See treatment strategies under Alzheimer's dementia.

3. Research is underway on hormone replacement therapy and cognitive function, but as yet no approved or recommended therapy exists. See the section on "Alzheimer's Disease" for medication treatment for appropriate needs.

Follow-up
A. Routine follow-up is based on identified cause and treatment plan for the dementia, reversible pseudodementia, or dementia of the Alzheimer's type.

Consultation/Referral
A. Refer the patient to a physician that specializes in the care of dementia.
B. Consult a physician when dementia is a symptom of a reversible disease.
C. Consider social work consult for family assessment.

Individual Considerations
A. Pediatrics: A patient who presents at a young age with dementia requires a thorough workup to evaluate the cause of the symptoms.

B. Adults: Irreversible dementia or Alzheimer's disease begins in the fourth to fifth decade of life and is characterized by loss of recent memory, inability to learn new information, language problems, mood swings, and personality changes.

GUILLAIN-BARRÉ SYNDROME
by Cheryl A. Glass

Definition
Guillain-Barré syndrome (GBS) is an acute immune-mediated polyneuropathy of the peripheral nervous system. GBS often follows an infection. It usually presents with ascending, progressive, multifocal, symmetric muscle weakness, and paraesthesia. GBS was considered monophasic and remits spontaneously but may also reoccur in 2%–5% of patients. Twenty to thirty percent of patients will have persistent disability measured by tools such as the overall disability sum score (ODSS). See Table 18.2.

TABLE 18.2 Overall Disability Sum Score (ODSS)

Area of Body	Activities	Functional Ability for Each Activity	Disability Scale Grade
Arm disability	A. Dressing upper part of body (excludes buttons/zippers) B. Washing and brushing hair C. Turning a key in a lock D. Using a knife and fork (use of spoon applies if never used a fork/knife) E. Doing/undoing buttons and zippers	Not affected; Affected but does not prevent activity; Prevents activity	0 = Normal function for all activities 1 = Minor signs/symptoms (S/S) in 1 or both arms but does not affect the activity 2 = Moderate S/S in 1 or both arms affecting but not preventing any activity 3 = Severe S/S in 1 or both arms preventing at least 1 but not all activities 4 = Severe S/S in both arms preventing all functions, purposeful movements still possible 5 = Severe S/S in both arms preventing all purposeful movements

Leg disability	A. Do you have any problems walking?
	B. Do you walk with a walking aid?
	C. How do you get around for 25 feet (10 meters):
	  1. Without aid
	  2. With one stick or crutch or holding someone's arm
	  3. With two sticks or crutches or one stick and a crutch and holding to someone's arm
	  4. With a wheelchair
	D. If you use a wheelchair, can you stand and walk a few steps with help?
	E. If you are restricted to bed most of the time, are you able to make some purposeful movements?
		No; Yes; Does not apply	0 = Walking is not affected
			1 = Walking is affected but does not look abnormal
			2 = Walks independently but gait looks abnormal
			3 = Usually uses unilateral support (stick, crutch, one arm) to walk 25 feet (10 meters)
			4 = Usually uses bilateral support (stick, crutch, two arms) to walk 25 feet (10 meters)
			5 = Usually uses a wheelchair to travel 25 feet (10 meters)
			6 = Restricted to wheelchair, unable to stand and walk a few steps with help but able to make some purposeful leg movements
			7 = Restricted to wheelchair or bed most of the day, preventing all purposeful movements of the legs (e.g., unable to reposition legs in bed)

Adapted from "Clinimetric Evaluation of a New Overall Disability Scale in Immune Mediated Polyneuropathies," by I. Merkies, P. Schmitz, F. G. A. van der Meche, J. Samihn, & P. A. van Doorn, 2002. *Journal of Neurological Neurosurgery Psychiatry, 72,* 597.

There are several variants of GBS:

A. Miller Fisher syndrome (MFS) often follows an infection, especially *Campylobacter jejuni* (*C. jejuni*) gastroenteritis.
B. Acute Inflammatory Demyelinating Polyradiculoneuropathy (AIDP): approximately two-thirds occur after an infection including *C. jejuni*, CMV, *Mycoplasma pneumonia*, or influenza virus.
C. Acute motor axonal neuropathy (AMAN)
D. Acute sensorimotor axonal neuropathy (AMSAN)

Incidence

A. The incidence of GBS is 0.6–2.4 per 100,000 adults.
B. The lifetime individual incidence is 1:1000.
C. GBS occurs in all age groups.
D. The incidence of GBS in children is 0.38–0.91 cases per 100,000.
E. 80%–90% become nonambulatory during the illness.
F. Relapses are not uncommon in adults that have been treated with IVIG and plasma exchange.

Pathogenesis

A. GBS is believed to be an immune mediated response linked to an antecedent infection wherein a patchy demyelination of the motor component of multiple peripheral nerves occurs. This causes a failure of neuromuscular transmission and leads to abrupt, distal weakness and symmetrical onset of paresthesias. The sensory disturbance is quickly followed by a rapid progressive limb weakness and sometimes paralysis. Most patients are able to identify a specific date of onset of sensory and motor symptoms.

Predisposing Factors

A. Up to two-thirds of patients with GBS have experienced a viral upper respiratory infection or gastroenteritis 10–14 days before onset.
  1. *C. jejuni* gastroenteritis
  2. Cytomegalovirus (CMV)
  3. Epstein-Barr virus (EBV)
  4. *Mycoplasma pneumonia*
  5. HIV
  6. *Haemophilus influenza*
  7. Entroviruses
  8. Hepatitis A and B
  9. Herpes simplex
  10. *Chamydophila* (formerly *Chlamydia*) pneumonia
B. Trauma.
C. Surgery.
D. Parturition.
E. Immunization.
F. There is no genetic factor for GBS.

Common Complaints

A. The classic clinical features:
  1. Progressive, fairly symmetric muscle weakness
    a. Difficulty walking
    b. Nearly complete paralysis including:
      i. All extremities, generally starts in the proximal legs
      ii. Facial muscles/oropharyngeal weakness
      iii. Respiratory muscles
      iv. Bulbar (ocular) muscles

  2. Accompanying absent or depressed deep tendon reflexes
B. Acute weakness in hands, dropping things, trouble picking up small objects or buttoning buttons
C. Acute onset of persistent tingling or pins and needles sensation in feet, possibly in hands
D. Prominent severe lower back pain

Other Signs and Symptoms

A. Sinus tachycardia or other arrhythmias
B. Bilateral generally symmetric muscle weakness not improved by rest
C. Urinary retention
D. Ileus-gastric motility disorders
E. Severe residual fatigue that may persist for years
F. Loss of sweating

Subjective Data

A. Ask the patient about any dyspnea. If there is shortness of breath (SOB), assess the need to go immediately by ambulance to a hospital.
B. Elicit information regarding the onset and duration of symptoms.
C. Question the patient regarding change or progression of symptoms.
D. Ascertain if the patient has had recent URI, flu, gastroenteritis, other infections, recent trauma, or surgery: determine if there was an associated fever.
E. Look for paresthesias preceding weakness by approximately 24–48 hours.
F. Look for recent exposure to environmental hazards: lead, pesticides, volatile solvents, or ticks.

Physical Examination

A. Check temperature, pulse, respirations, and blood pressure (persistent hypotension, hypertension alternating with hypotension, or orthostatic hypotension).
B. Inspect: Observe overall appearance; look for gait disturbance and respiratory distress.
C. Auscultate
  1. Note heart rate and rhythm: tachycardia is common; bradycardia and other arrhythmias may be noted.
  2. Auscultate the lung fields.
  3. Abdomen assessment for bowel sounds/dysfunction.
D. Palpate
  1. Palpate the extremities.
  2. Note muscle tone, normal muscle bulk.
  3. Assess DTRs, muscle strength, areflexia (lack of reflexes) or hyporeflexia (diminished).
  4. Look for symmetric weakness. Incidence of weakness in the ankle and knee is greater than biceps and triceps.
  5. Palpate the abdomen: assess urinary retention.
E. Neurologic exam
  1. Perform complete neurologic exam: generally no sensory deficits to touch or pinprick are noted. Decreased proprioception or vibration may be seen. In approximately 50% of clients, GBS may progress rapidly, sometimes within hours, to severe respiratory muscle weakness and respiratory failure.

Diagnostic Tests

Prompt treatment mandates the clinician make the diagnosis of GBS solely on history and examination. Testing done in the inpatient setting include:

A. Lumbar puncture
B. Needle electromyelogram (EMG)
C. Nerve conduction studies
D. Antibody testing

Differential Diagnoses

A. Guillain-Barré syndrome
B. Myasthenia gravis (MG)
C. Poliomyelitis
D. Acute intermittent porphyria
E. West Nile encephalomyelitis
F. Tick paralysis: Lyme neuroborreliosis
G. Diphtheria
H. HIV
I. Cervical myelopathy
J. Sarcoidosis
K. Poisoning
   1. Heavy metal poisoning (arsenic, lead, thallium)
   2. Hexacarbon abuse (glue sniffing neuropathy)
   3. Organophosphate poisoning
   4. Botulism

Plan

A. General interventions: Early diagnosis is crucial to appropriate management. A possible diagnosis of GBS requires *immediate* hospitalization at a facility with ICU capabilities and consultation with a neurologist who has experience managing GBS.
B. Hospital medical management
   1. Plasmapheresis.
   2. Intravenous immunoglobulin (IVIG) administration.
   3. Steroids have not been shown to be helpful and may be detrimental.
   4. Because of the associated autonomic instability, hypertension should be treated with short-acting intravenous agents.
   5. The presence of at least 4 of the 6 predictors indicate the need for support/mechanical ventilation:
      a. Onset of symptoms less than 7 days
      b. Inability to cough
      c. Inability to stand
      d. Inability to lift the elbows
      e. Inability to lift the head
      f. An increase in liver enzymes
   6. Heparin and support/pressure stockings are used for nonambulatory patients due to the risk of deep vein thrombosis (DVT) and pulmonary embolus (PE).
C. Pharmaceutical therapy
   1. Pain therapy
      a. Gabapentin (Neurontin) 15 mg/kg/day.
      b. Carbamazepine (Tegretol) 300 mg/day.
      c. Narcotics may be necessary.
      d. Tricyclic antidepressants.
   2. Immunizations

   a. Immunizations are not recommended during the acute phase and up to approximately 1 year after the onset of GBS.
   b. Influenza, tetanus, and typhoid immunizations have been most commonly associated with relapse of GBS symptoms.

Follow-up

A. Patients generally follow up with a neurologist once they have been discharged from the hospital or rehabilitation facility.
B. Full recovery can take up to 2 years with severe cases, and a small percentage of patients experience recurrence.
C. Physical rehabilitation with a multidisciplinary team focused on proper limb positioning, posture, orthotics, exercise, and nutrition.

Consultation/Referral

A. Consult with a physician if Guillain-Barré syndrome is suspected.

Individual Considerations

A. Ninety percent of people with GBS make a complete recovery. GBS severe enough to require mechanical ventilation is associated with both incomplete recovery and up to 20% mortality.

HEADACHE *by Cheryl A. Glass*

Definition

A. Headache is a discomfort of the head that is produced from inflammation and/or tightness of the arteries, nerves, and/or muscles of the cranium. Primary headaches are a major cause for missed school and work, presenteeism, and disability in children and adults.
B. There are multiple types of headaches-including tension-type headaches, trigeminal autonomic cephalalgias including cluster headaches-and chronic daily headaches (see Table 18.3). Migraines are discussed in a separate section. Posttraumatic headaches occur within 7 days after head trauma. Tension headaches are the most frequent type, occurring as part of postconcussive syndrome.

Incidence

Headaches are very common and their incidence depends on age, gender, and type of headache.

A. Tension-type headaches (TTH) are the most common primary headache affecting 31%–74% of the population.
B. Headaches occur in 90% of school-aged children.
C. Cluster headaches have been reported in children as young as age 3. The prevalence is in less than 1% of the population, with men affected more than women.
D. Chronic daily headaches are more common in girls than in boys.
E. Medication overuse headaches are reported in 20%–36% of adolescents with daily headaches.

TABLE 18.3 International Headache Society Classification of Headaches (ICHD–II)

Tension-Type Headache (TTH)[a]	Cluster Headache	Mediation Overuse Headache (MOH)[b]
Episodic headache lasting minutes to days. Pain is mild to moderate, typically bilateral, pressing or tightening quality. Pain does not worsen with activity.	Episodic or chronic attacks separated by pain-free periods lasting a month or longer. Pain almost always recurs on the same side during a cluster period. May be provoked by alcohol, histamine, or nitroglycerine.	Variable headache that often has a peculiar pattern with characteristics shifting, even within the same day, from migrainelike to tension-type headaches.

Diagnostic Criteria (Tension-Type Headache):

A. At least 10 episodes, < 1 day per month on average and fulfills B–D criteria:
B. Headache lasts 30 min to 7 days
C. At least 2 of the following characteristics:
   1. Bilateral location
   2. Pressure/tightening, nonpulsating quality
   3. Mild to moderate intensity
   4. No increase with routine physical activity such as walking or climbing stairs.
D. Both of the following:
   1. No nausea or vomiting
   2. No more than one photophobia or phonophobia
E. Not attributed to another disorder

Diagnostic Criteria (Cluster Headache):

A. At least 5 attacks that fulfills B–D criteria:
B. Severe or very severe unilateral orbital, supraorbital, and/or temporal pain lasting 15–180 min if untreated.
C. Accompanied by at least 1 of the following:
   1. Ipsilateral conjunctival injection and/or lacrimation
   2. Ipsilateral nasal congestion and/or rhinorrhea
   3. Ipsilateral eyelid edema
   4. Ipsilateral forehead and facial sweating
   5. Ipsilateral miosis and/or ptosis
   6. Restlessness or agitation (usually unable to lie down and characteristically pace the floor)
D. Attacks have a frequency from 1 every other day to 8 per day.
E. Not attributed to another disorder.

Diagnostic Criteria (Mediation Overuse Headache):

A. Present on ≥ 15 days/month that fulfills C–D criteria:
B. Regular overuse for ≥ 3 months of 1 or more drugs that can be taken for acute/or symptomatic treatment of headaches.
C. Developed or markedly worsened during medication overuse.
D. Headache resolves or reverts to its previous pattern within 2 months after discontinuing the overused medication.

Example of medications include Ergotamine, triptans, analgesics, opioids, and combination analgesics.

[a] Previously called common, muscle contraction, stress, ordinary, or psychogenic headache.
[b] Previously called rebound, drug-induced, or medication misuse headache.
Adapted from the International Headache Society Classification of Headaches (ICHD–II).

Pathogenesis

A. Because there are different types of headaches, the origin of each type differs. Many people have a combination of the different types of headaches. Headache causes range from systemic illness, such as infections; medical disorders, such as tumors or hemorrhage; medications; drug use; and/or stress. Tension headaches are headaches that occur due to contracted muscles of the scalp and neck. Cluster headaches have an uncertain etiology; however, they appear to be caused by extracerebral vasodilation.

Predisposing Factors

A. Tension, stress
B. Cervical, or back, disorders
C. Medications (e.g., nitroglycerine)
D. Bruxism
E. Sleep disorders (e.g., snoring, insomnia)
F. Foods/caffeine/alcohol
G. Hormonal changes
H. Family history of headaches
I. Sexual activity
J. Cough
K. Exertion/exercise
L. Viral/infectious etiologies

Common Complaints

A. Depending on type of headache, other symptoms may coexist, such as lacrimation, nasal congestion, restlessness, and visual changes.

Other Signs and Symptoms

A. Crying
B. Behavioral problems

Subjective Data

A. Use the following acronym for subjective information, PQRST:
   P: Provocation, or worsening of factors stimulating headaches
   Q: Quality of pain, severity of pain
   R: Region of headache
   S: Strength of pain, evaluate pain on scale of 1–10
   T: Time, including onset, frequency, and duration of headaches
B. Assess whether the patient frequently has migraine headaches. Is this the first or worst headache ever experienced by the patient?
C. If recurrent headaches exist, note frequency and patterns of similar headaches.

D. Note whether the patient has ever identified potential triggers of recurring headaches such as dietary, stressors, and odors (i.e., perfumes, cigarette smoke).

E. Identify the location of pain, along with radiation if present.

F. Describe the type of pain: throbbing, constant, or burning.

G. Assess the presence of associated symptoms: nausea or vomiting, photophobia, or noise sensitivity.

H. Determine whether the patient experiences any neurologic symptoms and/or prodromal symptoms prior to a headache.

I. Review the methods used in the past to abort and/or prevent headaches and the results.

J. Inquire about past diagnostic evaluations for headaches.

K. Note a family history of headaches.

L. List current medications, including over-the-counter medications and herbals.

M. Review the patient's medical history for head trauma, infection, allergies, presence of a VP shunt, or other neurologic diagnoses.

Physical Examination

Physical exam may be normal unless patient presents with a headache.

A. Check blood pressure, pulse, and respirations (temperature if meningeal signs are present).

B. Inspect
   1. Observe overall appearance for the presence of discomfort, photosensitivity (use of sunglasses indoors), and level of consciousness.
   2. Examine the eyes; perform funduscopic exam.
   3. Inspect the ears, nose, and throat.

C. Auscultate
   1. Listen for bruit at neck, eyes, and head for clinical signs of arteriovenous (AV) malformation.

D. Palpate
   1. Palpate the head, eyes, ears, TMJ, sinus cavities, temporal and neck arteries.
   2. Palpate cervical vertebrae, cervical muscles, and shoulder regions. Identify potential trigger areas: occipital nerves leave halfway between the middle of the neck at the back of the neck and lateral to this area. When palpating this trigger area, pain may be reproduced with palpation.
   3. Examine the spine and neck muscles.
   4. Assess cervical range of motion (ROM).

E. Perform neurologic exam.
   1. Extraocular movements (EOM)
   2. Pupil response
   3. Getting up from a seated position without any support
   4. Walking on tiptoes and heels
   5. Tandem gait
   6. Romberg test
   7. Symmetry on motor, sensory, deep tendon reflexes (DTRs), and coordination tests

Diagnostic Tests

Tests are selected based on history and physical exam.

A. Sinus films to rule out sinusitis or a lesion.

B. Consider sleep studies for obstructive sleep apnea.

C. CT scan or MRI: needed if headache is severe, no results are achieved with drug therapy, and/or aura is present.

D. People, especially children, with any positive neurologic signs of an intracranial process should have neuroimaging.

E. Lab tests are rarely need for headaches, unless an infectious process is suspected.

Differential Diagnoses

A. Headache
   1. Tension
   2. Cluster
   3. Medication overuse
   4. Migraine
   5. Combination headache

B. Sinusitis

C. Meningitis: meningism, acute headache with fever, lethargy, nausea or vomiting, irritability, photophobia, and systemic infection

D. Space-occupying lesion: subacute and progressive pain, new onset for adults older than 40 years

E. Temporal arteritis: new onset progressive headache for adults older than 50 years, with presenting symptoms of temporal artery swelling, pain, pulselessness, visual changes, mental sluggishness, systemic symptoms (fever, anorexia, malaise), and ESR greater than 50 mm/hour

F. Carotid dissection: sudden headache with neck pain, radiating to the face, ear, or eye; onset related to neck movement or trauma, Horner's syndrome, tinnitus, ipsilateral tongue weakness, cervical bruit or tenderness, diplopia, and syncope

G. Temporomandibular joint syndrome: jaw claudication, clicking, and locking sensation

Plan

A. General interventions
   1. Encourage the patient to restrict associated triggers, such as food, alcohol, and odors.
   2. Encourage the patient to exercise daily.
   3. Have the patient begin a stress management routine, including yoga, meditation, and massage.
   4. Tell the patient to take medications as prescribed.
   5. Cluster headaches can be exacerbated by alcohol.
   6. Use ice/heat for muscular tension.

B. Patient teaching
   1. Encourage the patient to keep a diary of headaches and associated factors to try to pinpoint headache triggers.
   2. Teach patients who have menstrual headaches to avoid precipitating factors, such as alcohol, tyramine or phenylethylamine foods, missed meals, and sleeping late.
   3. For muscular headaches that are nonmenstrual, biofeedback, breathing exercises, and visualization are helpful. Prevention must be stressed. Encourage lifestyle changes and daily exercise.
   4. When patients overuse various analgesics for headaches, paroxysmal migraines can convert into chronic daily headaches. Caution patients regarding this effect.
   5. Medication overuse headaches (MOH) occur with the highest incidence with opioids, butalbital-containing

combinations, and ASA/acetaminophen/caffeine combinations as well as triptans. Withdrawal of the overused medication is the treatment of choice for MOH.

C. Pharmaceutical therapy: Therapy should be started at the lowest dosage and titrated up as tolerated, avoiding overuse.

1. Nonsteroidal anti-inflammatory medications:
   a. Acetylsalicylic acid (ASA) 650–1,000 mg orally. Maximal dose 4 g/day.
   b. Ibuprofen (Advil) 400–800 mg every 8 hours. Maximum dose 2.4 g/day.

2. Combination medications:
   a. Acetaminophen, butalbital, and caffeine (Fioricet) with or without codeine 1–2 tablets every 4 hours as needed. Maximum dose is 6 tablets per day.
   b. ASA, butalbital, and caffeine (Fiorinal) 1 or 2 tablets every 4 hours as needed. Caution the patient regarding dependency patterns.
   c. Isometheptene mucate, dichloralphenazone, and acetaminophen (Midrin) 2 capsules at onset. Then 1 capsule every hour if needed up to 5 capsules in a 12-hour period.
   d. Acetaminophen, ASA, and caffeine (Excedrin) 2 tablets every 6 hours. Maximal dose of 4 g of aspirin or acetaminophen.

3. Cluster or vascular headaches:
   a. Verapamil is the agent of choice for prevention therapy with cluster headaches.
   b. Propranolol (Inderal) or carbamazepine 80 mg daily in divided doses. Maximum range 160–240 mg daily.
   c. Oxygen 100% therapy has been effective for cluster headaches.

4. Menstrual headaches:
   a. Estrogen supplements or continuous cycling is used to decrease headaches. Have the patient start taking estrogen 2 days before expected migraine and use for 7 days.
   b. Naproxen 275–550 mg every 2–6 hours (maximum dose 1.5 mg/day) starting 7 days as needed before menses.
   c. Ibuprofen 600 mg three times daily.
   d. Fluoxetine (Prozac) 10–20 mg daily is also used for patients with premenstrual syndrome with luteal phase defect.

5. Antidepressants may also be utilized for preventive treatment.

Follow-up

A. See the patient in 2 weeks to evaluate how therapies have worked.

B. Evaluate the patient's "headache log" to assist him or her in identifying headache triggers, if present.

Consultation/Referral

A. Consult a physician if headaches are caused by acute problems other than migraine and/or tension headaches.

B. Severe episodes need to be evaluated by a physician for opioid agonists and antagonists, narcotics, and neuroleptics.

C. If medications do not help with headaches, refer the patient to a neurologist.

Individual Considerations

A. Pediatrics
   1. Antihistamines are useful as a preventive agent, as are biofeedback and relaxation techniques.
   2. Avoid using aspirin-containing products due to the potential of Reye's syndrome. Differentiating the causative factor is essential for this population.

B. Adults: Patients who are premenopausal may see improvement when their estrogen levels are constant, instead of being cyclic.

C. Geriatrics
   1. Headaches decrease with age. Serious causes of headaches increase with age.
   2. Consider imaging studies in the elderly with unusual presentations of headaches.
   3. Consider chronic subdural hematomas with patients who have frequent falls; perform CT scan or MRI for evaluation.
   4. Elderly patients may not exhibit any symptoms other than a headache.
   5. When medicating the elderly, start dosages low and increase as tolerated.
   6. Consider all contraindications when prescribing medications; many elderly patients have cardiovascular disease, which is contraindicated with ergot derivatives.

▣ MIGRAINE HEADACHE *by Cheryl A. Glass*

Definition

A. Migraine headaches are a common medical complaint responsible for a significant disability and loss of quality of life. The economic impact involves loss of workdays, school, social interaction, and loss of productivity while at work (presenteeism). There are three types of migraines described by the International Headache Society (IHS) by type and diagnostic criteria (see Table 18.4).

Incidence

Headaches are one of the most common medical complaints. The exact incidence of migraines is unknown since patients self-treat, are underdiagnosed, and are commonly misdiagnosed. Twelve to sixteen percent is the overall estimated incidence of migraines in North American and Europe; however, several subset of migraineurs are noted in the literature:

A. 1%–3% incidence in preschoolers.

B. 4%–11% incidence in school-aged children.
   1. Boys outnumber girls before age 7.
   2. Boys are equally likely to have migraines between ages 7 and 11.

C. 8%–23% incidence in adolescents.

D. 2% of the population has chronic migraines.

Pathogenesis

A. Migraines have broad sensory processing dysfunction, with a prominent perception of pain in the dense somatosensory innervation of intracranial vessels. Current pathophysiologic concepts of migraine and migraine aura include a possible dysfunction of neuromodulatory structures in the brainstem and cortical spreading depression (CSD). Different receptors, including calcitonin

TABLE 18.4   International Headache Society Classification of Migraines (ICHD–II)

Migraine Without Aura	Migraine With Aura (There Are 6 Subtypes)	Chronic Migraine*
Recurrent headache attack lasting 4–72 hours meeting the diagnostic criteria	Recurrent disorder manifesting reversible focal neurological symptoms that usually develop gradually over 5–20 min and last for less than 60 min. Typical aura consists of visual and/or sensory and/or speech symptoms	Chronic migraine that meets the criteria for migraine without aura that occurs with a frequency of at least 15 headache days per month for longer than 3 months' duration.

Diagnostic Criteria:

Migraine Without Aura:

A. At least 5 attacks that fulfill criteria B–D
B. Headache attacks last 4–72 hours (untreated or unsuccessfully treated)
C. Has at least 2 of the following:
   1. Unilateral location
   2. Pulsating quality
   3. Moderate or severe intensity
   4. Aggravated by or causing avoidance of routine physical activity
D. During headache at least 1 of the following:
   1. Nausea and/or vomiting
   2. Photophobia and phonophobia
E. Not attributed to another disorder

Diagnostic Criteria:

Migraine With Aura:

A. At least 2 attacks that fulfill criteria B–D
B. Aura consist of at least 1 of the following but no motor weakness:
   1. Fully reversible visual symptoms including positive features (e.g., flickering lights, spots, or lines) and/or negative features (i.e., loss of vision)
   2. Fully reversible sensory symptoms including positive features (i.e., pins and needles) and/or negative features (i.e., numbness)
   3. Fully reversible dysphasic speech disturbance
C. At least 2 of the following:
   1. Homonymous visual symptoms (i.e., additional loss or blurring of central vision) and/or unilateral sensory symptoms
   2. At least 1 aura symptom develops gradually over $\geq$ 5 min and/or different aura symptoms occur in succession over $\geq$ 5 min
   3. Each symptom last $\geq$ 5 min and $\leq$ 60 min
D. Headache fulfilling criteria B–C: Migraine without aura begins during the aura or follows the aura within 60 min
E. Not attributed to another disorder

Diagnostic Criteria:

Chronic Migraine:

A. Headache, in the absence of medication overuse headache (MOH), on $\geq$ 15 days per month for at least 3 months.
B. Occurring in a patient who has had at least 5 attacks fulfilling criteria for migraine without aura.
C. On $\geq$ 8 days per month for at least 3 months headache fulfills C1 and/or C2 criteria noted below.
C1. Has at least 2 of the following:
   (a) Unilateral location
   (b) Pulsating quality
   (c) Moderate or severe pain intensity
   (d) Aggravation by or causing avoidance of routine physical activity
   and at least 1 of the following:
   (a) Nausea and/or vomiting
   (b) Photophobia and phonophobia
C2. Treated and relieved by triptan(s) or ergot before the expected development of C1 symptoms
D. No medication overuse and not attributed to another causative disorder

*A proposed alternative criteria is defined as a chronic headache for at least 4 migraine days and at least 15 total headache days, with at least 50% of headache days meeting criteria for migraine.
Adapted from the International Headache Society ICHD–II.

gene-related peptide (CGRP), TRPVI, and glutamate receptors, are currently being targeted for migraine therapeutics.

Predisposing Factors

A. Family history of migraines.
B. Chronic use of over-the-counter analgesics (rebound).
C. Post-head trauma.
D. Food, odor, light, sound, sleep, weather changes, hormonal changes, and stress triggers.
E. Menstruation.
F. Obesity.
G. Daily habitual snoring is a modest risk factor.

Common Complaints

A. Unilateral headache (bilateral in children)
B. Frontotemporal area (occipital in children)
C. Photophobia, or sensitivity to light (young children may cover their eyes)
D. Phonophobia, or sensitivity to sound (young children may cover their ears)
E. Osmophobia, or hypersensitivity/aversion to smells/odors
F. Nausea with/without vomiting

G. Prodrome phase: fatigue, reduced concentration, agitation, craving, fatigue, irritability, depression, frequent yawning, or hyperexcitability hours to days before the onset of aura and headache.

Other Signs and Symptoms

A. Muscle tension and neck pain
B. Cutaneous allodynia (pain from stimulus to normal skin or scalp)
C. Sinus congestion
D. Prodrome phase can last 25 hours accompanied by fatigue and a "hangover" headache

Subjective Data

A. Use the following the acronym used for subjective information, PQRST:
   P: Provocation, or worsening of factors stimulating headaches
   Q: Quality of pain, severity of pain
   R: Region of headache
   S: Strength of pain, evaluate pain on a scale of 1–10
   T: Time, including onset, frequency, and duration of headaches

B. Assess whether the patient frequently has migraines headaches. Is this the first or worst headache ever experienced by the patient?

C. If recurrent headaches exist, note frequency and patterns of similar headaches.

D. Note whether the patient has ever identified potential triggers of recurring headaches such as dietary, stressors, and odors (i.e., perfumes and cigarette smoke)

E. Identify the location of the pain, along with radiation if present.

F. Describe the type of pain: throbbing, constant, or burning.

G. Assess the presence of associated symptoms: nausea or vomiting, photophobia, and noise sensitivity.

H. Determine whether the patient experiences any neurologic symptoms and/or prodromal symptoms prior to headache.

I. Review the methods used in the past to abort and/or prevent headaches and the results.

J. Inquire about past diagnostic evaluations for headaches.

K. Note a family history of headaches.

L. List current medications, including over-the-counter medications and herbals.

M. Review the patient's medical history for head trauma, infection, allergies, presence of a VP shunt, or other neurologic diagnoses.

Physical Examination

Physical exam may be normal unless the patient presents with a headache.

A. Check blood pressure, pulse, and respirations (temperature if meningeal signs are present).

B. Inspect
 1. Observe overall appearance for the presence of discomfort, photosensitivity (use of sunglasses indoors), and level of consciousness.
 2. Examine the eyes; perform funduscopic exam.
 3. Inspect the ears, nose, and throat.

C. Auscultate
 1. Listen for bruit at neck, eyes, and head for clinical signs of arteriovenous (AV) malformation.

D. Palpate
 1. Palpate the head, eyes, ears, TMJ, sinus cavities, temporal and neck arteries.
 2. Palpate cervical vertebrae, cervical muscles, and shoulder regions. Identify potential trigger areas: occipital nerves leave halfway between the middle of the neck at the back of the neck and lateral to this area. When palpating this trigger area, pain may be reproduced with palpation.
 3. Examine the spine and neck muscles.
 4. Assess the cervical range of motion (ROM).

E. Perform neurologic exam
 1. Extraocular movements (EOM)
 2. Pupil response
 3. Getting up from a seated position without any support
 4. Walking on tiptoes and heels
 5. Tandem gait
 6. Romberg test
 7. Symmetry on motor, sensory, deep tendon reflexes (DTRs), and coordination tests

Diagnostic Tests

A. Neuroimaging is based on the history and physical examination:
 1. In adults and children stable headaches, a normal examination, and the absence of seizures does not require neuroimaging.
 2. Neuroimaging should be considered for children with headaches with abnormal neurologic examination and/or seizures.
 3. Neuroimaging should be considered for children with severe headaches, change in headaches, or associated neurologic dysfunction.
 4. An emergent noncontrast CT should be obtained when the patient complains of "the worst headache ever" or when focal neurologic findings, nuchal rigidity, or altered mental status exist.
 5. The presence of personality changes, depression, and a migraine may indicate a temporal lobe tumor.
 6. The presence of orbital bruit requires neuroimaging.
 7. Neuroimaging is recommended for adults with onset of headache after age 40.
 8. Onset of headache with exertion, cough, or sexual activity should be considered for neuroimaging.

B. A lumbar puncture may be indicated in children, and altered mental status or focal findings.

C. Sinus films to rule out sinusitis or a lesion.

D. Drug screen may be indicated.

Differential Diagnoses

A. Migraine
 1. Migraine with aura
 2. Migraine without aura

B. Other types of headaches
 1. Medication overuse headache (MOH)
 2. Common headache
 3. Cluster headache
 4. Combination headache
 5. Chronic daily headache

C. Sinusitis

D. Space-occupying lesion: subacute and progressive pain, new onset for adults older than 40 years

E. Temporal arteritis: new onset progressive headache for adults older than 50 years

F. Carotid dissection: sudden headache with neck pain radiating to the face, ear, or eye

G. Temporomandibular joint (TMJ) syndrome

Plan

A. General interventions: There are four main approaches to migraine therapy:
 1. Nonpharmacologic interventions:
  a. Adjust habits to maintain a routine pattern of sleeping. This is especially important to maintain on weekends and vacations.
  b. Do not skip breakfast. Eat regular meals with 1 or 2 snacks
  c. Avoid food triggers identified by the patient's migraine diary.
  d. Encourage drinking no more than 2 caffeinated beverages/day.

e. Hydration is important.

f. Encourage at least 30 min of exercise 3–7 days a week.

g. Cold compresses

2. Behavioral interventions:

a. Use relaxation techniques such as yoga, deep breathing, meditation, and guided imagery.

b. Biofeedback is an adjunct to relaxation training.

c. Cognitive behavioral therapy.

d. Psychiatric therapy.

3. Complementary and alternative interventions:

a. Acupuncture.

b. Nutraceuticals, including magnesium, coenzyme Q10, and butternut root extract.

c. Vitamins: Riboflavin (B$_2$).

d. Herbal (nonregulated by the FDA), including feverfew and butternut root extract.

e. Physical therapy.

f. Hypnosis.

g. TENS, chiropractic manipulation, botulinum toxin type-A (BoNT-A), and occlusal adjustment are also noted in the literature.

4. Pharmacologic interventions: Patients should be counseled to take medications as prescribed. When patients overuse various analgesics for headaches, paroxysmal migraines can convert into chronic daily headaches.

B. Patient teaching: Encourage the patient to keep a headache diary; an example of a migraine diary is available at http://www.webmd.com/migraines-headaches/guide/headache-diary.

1. Examples of food triggers are aspartame, red wine, alcohol, chocolate, aged cheese, oranges, tomatoes, avocado, nuts, onions, tyramine, phenylethylamine, monosodium glutamate (MSG), and nitrates and nitrites found in hot dogs, luncheon meat, and sausage.

2. Examples of odor triggers include tobacco smoke, perfumes, and strong odors.

3. Examples of visual triggers include strobe lights, bright lights/sunlight, fluorescent lights, and glare.

4. Other triggers are medications, barometric weather changes, too much/too little sleep, and high altitude.

C. Pharmaceutical therapy (see Table 18.5)

1. Many drugs commonly utilized for migraines are not FDA approved for migraine therapy, including amitriptyline, nortriptyline, and selective serotonin reuptake inhibitors (SSRIs).

2. Antiepileptic medications, including valproic acid (Depakote) and topiramate (Topamax), are FDA approved for migraine prophylaxis. Topiramate should not be prescribed or discontinued for a history of kidney stones.

3. Beta-blockers are approved for migraine prophylaxis; however, they must be used with caution for patients with comorbidities such as asthma, depression, diabetes, and thyroid disease.

4. There are currently seven triptans and one triptan/NSAID combination. Triptans are widely used for menstrual migraines. Triptans should be used cautiously in patients with cardiovascular comorbidities and some are not approved for children. Triptans should not be given within 24 hours of an ergot.

5. Dihydroergotamine mesylate (Migranal) is not to be used for patients during pregnancy or with heart disease, or ischemic or vasospastic circulatory disease. Use ergot derivatives selectively. These medications are not to be used on a long-term basis or more than three times per week. There is an associated risk of strokes when using these medications due to the vasoconstrictive mechanisms of the medications.

6. Ergots and triptans should not be given within 14 days of an MAO inhibitor.

7. Antiemetics are prescribed as needed for nausea/vomiting associated with migraines.

Follow-up

A. See the patient in 2 weeks to evaluate how therapies have worked.

B. Evaluate the patient's headache diary to assist him or her in identifying headache triggers or patterns, such as prior to menstruation.

C. Monitor liver enzymes and CBC periodically with antiseizure medication prophylaxis.

Consultation/Referral

A. Consult a physician if headaches are caused by acute problems other than migraine and/or tension headaches.

B. If medications do not help with headaches, refer the patient to a neurologist.

C. Send the patient to the emergency department for any neurologic, life-threatening signs.

Individual Considerations

A Pregnancy: many medications are contraindicated in pregnancy.

B. Pediatrics

1. Avoid using aspirin-containing products due to the potential of Reye's syndrome.

2. Differentiating the causative factor is essential for this population.

3. Adolescents may see improvement when their estrogen levels are constant instead of cyclic.

C. Geriatrics

1. Headaches decrease after age 50. Headache onset after age 50 is associated with epilepsy, essential tremor, ischemic stroke, mood disorders, asthma, and patent foramen ovale.

2. Consider imaging studies for elderly patients that present with unusual headaches.

3. Consider chronic subdural hematomas with patients who have frequent falls; perform CT scan or MRI for evaluation. Elderly patients may not exhibit any symptoms other than a headache.

4. Consider all contraindications when prescribing medications; many elderly patients have cardiovascular disease, which is contraindicated with ergot derivatives.

TABLE 18.5 Oral Medications for Migraines

Medication	Class	Instructions for Oral[a] Adult Dosing	Acute vs. Prophylaxis
Sumatriptan (Imitrex)	Triptan	Initially 25–100 mg. May repeat in 2-hour intervals. (Maximum dose 200 mg/24 hours) Also available subcutaneous and intranasal	Acute treatment
Rizatriptan (Maxalt)	Triptan	Initially 5–10 mg. May repeat in 2-hour intervals. (Maximum dose 30 mg/24 hours) Available in oral or disintegrating tablets	Acute treatment
Zolmitriptan (Zomig)	Triptan	Initially 2.5–5 mg. May repeat in 2 hours. (Maximum dose 10 mg/24 hours) Available in oral or disintegrating tablets	Acute treatment
Naratriptan (Amerge)	Triptan	Initially 1–2.5 mg. May repeat in 4 hours. (Maximum dose 5 mg/24 hours)	Acute treatment
Alomtriptan (Axert)	Triptan	Initially 6.25–12.5 mg. May repeat in 2 hours. (Maximum dose 25 mg/24 hours)	Acute treatment
Eletriptan (Replax)	Triptan	Initially 40 mg. May repeat in 2 hours. (Maximum dose 80 mg/24 hours)	Acute treatment
Frovatriptan (Frova)	Triptan	Initially 2.5 mg. May repeat in 2 hours. (Maximum dose 7.5 mg/24 hours)	Acute treatment
Sumatriptan with Naproxen sodium (Treximet)	Triptan + NSAID	1 tablet = sumatriptan 85 mg + 500 mg naproxen sodium. Initially 1 tablet. May repeat in 2 hours. (Maximum dose 2 tabs/24 hours)	Acute treatment
Dihydroergotamine mesylate (Migranal)	Ergot derivative	[a]Only available in intranasal spray Initially 1 spray in each nostril. May repeat in 15 min. (Maximum 6 sprays/24 hours with a maximum of 8 sprays/week)	Acute treatment
Cafergot	Ergot derivative	Initially 2 tablets at onset. May repeat 1 tablet every half hour. (Maximum dose 6 tablets/24 hours with a maximum of 10 tablets/week) Also available in suppositories	Acute treatment migraines and cluster headaches
Propranolol (Inderal)	Beta-blocker	Initially 80 mg/day. May titrate up to 240 mg/day	Migraine prophylaxis
Topiramate (Topamax)	Antiseizure	Requires titration: Week 1: 25 mg every bedtime Week 2: 25 mg/AM and 25 mg/at bedtime Week 3: 25 mg/AM and 50 mg/at bedtime Week 4: 50 mg/AM and 50 mg/at bedtime (Maximum 100 mg/24 hours)	Migraine prophylaxis
Valproic acid (Depakote)	Antiseizure	500 mg/daily for 1 week, then increase up to 1 g/day	
Amitriptyline	Antidepressant	Initially 75 mg/day in divided doses or 50–100 mg/at bedtime (Maximum 150 mg/24 hours)	Migraine prophylaxis
Nortriptyline (Pamelor)	Antidepressant	Initially 25 mg, 3–4 times a day. (Maximum dose 150 mg/day)	Migraine prophylaxis
Fluoxetine (Prozac)	SSRI	Initially 20 mg/AM. Increase if needed after several weeks. Doses > 20 mg/day should be given in divided doses in the AM and at noon. (Maximum 80 mg/24 hours)	Migraine prophylaxis

MILD TRAUMATIC BRAIN INJURY (MTBI)
by Kimberly D. Waltrip

Definition

Head injury is defined as any physical damage (i.e., a blow, a jolt, a bump) or functional impairment of the cranial contents, including the scalp, skull, meninges, blood vessels, or brain. Mild traumatic brain injury (MTBI) results in a disruption of brain function. *Concussion* is a commonly used term to describe MTBI; 90% of patients with concussive injuries do not experience decreased level of consciousness (LOC). Serious complications of minor head injury include asymptomatic extradural hematomas, fatal thrombosis of the basilar artery, and hemorrhage from existing conditions such as fibrous dysplasia or essential thrombocytopenia.

The American Academy of Neurology offers guidelines for grading the severity of concussions as follows:

A. Grade I: Confusion, symptoms last less than 15 min, no loss of consciousness
B. Grade II: Symptoms last longer than 15 min, no loss of consciousness
C. Grade III: Loss of consciousness (IIIa, unresponsive period lasts seconds; IIIb, unresponsive period lasts minutes)

Incidence

A. An estimated 1.4 million head injuries occur in the United States each year. Of these, approximately 75%–90% are classified as mild traumatic brain injuries.

Predisposing Factors

A. Motor vehicle accidents
B. Assaults
C. Sports and recreation-related trauma
D. Male gender
E. Ages of increased incidence
   1. 0–4 years
   2. 5–24 years
   3. 75 years and older
F. Military occupation (i.e., war zones: exposure to blasts)
G. Falls

Pathogenesis

A. Head-injured patients can potentially sustain two different types of injuries: *primary* (impact) injury and *secondary* injury. A primary injury is a direct result from the injury and occurs at the time of initial insult. This type of injury is purely mechanical and may be focal (contusion or laceration, bone fragmentation), or diffuse, as in concussion or diffuse axonal injury (DAI). These injuries do not require surgical intervention.
B. Secondary injury is caused by a flow-metabolism mismatch. It is a complication of primary brain damage. This includes ischemic and hypoxic damage; cerebral edema; intracranial hemorrhage (ICH), and the impact of prolonged increased intracranial pressure (ICP), hydrocephalus, and infection. Secondary injury has a delayed onset, occurring in a matter of seconds, minutes, hours, or days.

Common Complaints

A. Headaches that are often constant, generalized, or frontal; may last for days or weeks
B. Brief amnestic epoch surrounding impact
C. Faintness
D. Nausea/vomiting
E. Changes in vision, often slight blurring
F. Drowsiness
G. Loss of consciousness

Other Signs and Symptoms

Other presenting symptoms and complaints are identified in four categories as follows: physical, emotional, cognitive, and sleep-cycle disturbances.

A. Physical
   1. Reported or observed injury to the head
   2. Dizziness
   3. Fatigue
   4. Decrease/change in balance
   5. Photophobia
   6. Sensitivity to noise
   7. Numbness/tingling
   8. Seizures, delayed onset status post injury
B. Emotional
   1. Irritability
   2. Nervousness
   3. Depression
C. Cognitive
   1. Difficulty concentrating
   2. Memory impairment
      a. Short-term memory loss
      b. Repetition
   3. Confusion
   4. Slow responses/difficulty processing
D. Sleep-cycle disturbance
   1. Feeling "drowsy"
   2. Difficulty falling asleep
   3. Sleeping more or less than usual

Subjective Data

A. Obtain a description of injury from the patient or witness of the traumatic event, if possible. Identify the cause of the head injury, how it occurred (direct or indirect injury), and what type of force was exerted.
B. Confirm the patient's level of consciousness at the time of injury and after injury. Inquire about amnesia (retrograde and anterograde), which might predict increased severity of the injury. Ask about the occurrence, whether it was observed by others, and duration.
C. Review initial and current symptoms (see common complaints, signs and symptoms). Include description, location, severity, and onset of symptoms. It is important to note what has happened since the actual injury. It is not uncommon for patients to report symptoms that re-emerge or worsen with exertion.
D. Obtain the patient's medical history, especially of previous head injuries. Learning disabilities (e.g., ADHD), developmental disorders, depression, anxiety, sleep disorders, and mood disorders should also be noted since these can affect recovery.
E. Review current medications; certain medications, such as warfarin (Coumadin), can be a predisposing factor that can lead to complications.
F. Document any drug and alcohol history.
G. Ask significant others if they have noticed any additional signs or symptoms, behavioral changes, or evidence of seizure activity.

Physical Examination

A. Check temperature, pulse, respirations, and blood pressure.
B. Inspect
   1. Observe overall appearance. Note level of consciousness.
   2. Inspect the skin and head for obvious injury. Periorbital ecchymosis ("raccoon's eyes"), postauricular/mastoid

ecchymosis (Battle's sign), or evidence of a cerebrospinal fluid leak (otorrhea, rhinorrhea) suggests a basilar skull fracture.

3. Examine the eyes for the presence of papilledema (indicates increased ICP), proptosis, and periorbital edema.

4. Examine the ears (hemotympanum or possible laceration to the external canal), nose, and throat.

5. Examine for facial fractures.

6. Examine for any trauma to the spine.

C. Auscultate

1. Auscultate over the globes of the eyes if warranted (bruit may indicate traumatic carotid-cavernous fistula).

2. Auscultate carotid arteries bilaterally if warranted (bruit may indicate carotid dissection).

3. Auscultate the heart and lungs if cardiovascular etiology is suspected.

4. Auscultate the abdomen, if other injuries have occurred from incidental injury such as a contact sport or motor vehicle accident.

D. Palpate

1. Palpate for instability of the facial bones, including the zygomatic arch: can have a palpable step-off with orbital rim fractures.

2. If appropriate, palpate the abdomen to rule out any other incidental injury.

E. Neurologic examination

1. Assess mental status and memory. Determine whether the patient is awake, alert, cooperative, and oriented (to person, place, time, and situation). Temporary impairment of memory is one of the most common deficits after a head injury.

2. Assess cranial nerve function
   a. Opthalmoscopic/visual exam (cranial nerve II)
   b. Pupillary response (cranial nerve III)
   c. Extraocular movements (cranial nerves III, IV, VI)
   d. Facial sensation and muscles of mastication (cranial nerve V)
   e. Facial expression and taste (cranial nerve VII)

3. Perform a motor examination on all four extremities.

4. Perform a sensory exam on all four extremities.

Diagnostic Tests

A. A plain film of the skull is usually not obtained for a minor traumatic injury. If the patient has suspected skull fracture or clinical indications for imaging, a CT scan is preferred. This type of imaging will usually reveal any linear or basilar skull fractures.

B. CT scan is indicated for patients with the following:

1. Decreasing consciousness during or after the injury
2. Focal neurologic symptoms
3. Potential, penetrating, or depressed skull fractures
4. Increasing or persistent severe headache with nausea or vomiting
5. Seizures postinjury
6. Alcohol or prescription intoxication
7. Amnesia status post injury
8. Unreliable or questionable accuracy regarding the history of the injury

C. Consider AP and lateral spine films for suspected soft tissue injury, or vertebral fracture, especially if the patient has experienced an amnestic episode or cannot recall the accident.

D. Drug screen

E. Blood alcohol level

Differential Diagnoses

A. Concussion (mild traumatic brain injury)
B. Contusion
C. Intracranial hemorrhage (ICH)
D. Shearing injury
E. Skull fracture
F. Subdural hematoma (SDH)
G. Epidural hematoma (EDH)
H. Vascular occlusion or dissection
I. Diffuse axonal injury (DAI)

Plan

A. General interventions

1. Admit to the hospital for decreased LOC, seizure activity, focal deficits, penetrating or depressed skull fracture, vomiting, serious facial injuries, and positive head CT findings.

2. Hospitalization may be required if the patient has an injured middle meningeal artery or if venous sinus or fractures posteriorly in the skull are suspected. Posterior fossa hematomas may present suddenly (will see a wide pulse pressure).

3. Consider possible secondary injuries, including cerebral edema, cerebral infarction, cerebral hemorrhage, hydrocephalus, and infection.

4. The patient should not be impaired from alcohol or other drugs when leaving the clinic, which can impact and potentially mask neurologic function or changes.

5. Hospital admission should be considered for patients without home observation/supervision.

6. Discuss suspected abuse in private with the patient.

B. Patient teaching

1. See the Section III Patient Teaching Guide for this chapter, "Mild Head Injury."

2. Provide instruction regarding safety and accident prevention, including:
   a. Use of safety helmets.
   b. Use of safety belts.
   c. Never driving under the influence.
   d. Use of age-appropriate car seats and booster seats for children.
   e. Removal of scatter rugs and other objects that would increase fall risks.
   f. Use nonslip mats in the shower/bathtub.
   g. Install grab bars for the shower/bathtub.
   h. Use safety gates at the bottom and top of stairs in homes with small children.
   i. Always keep stairs, floors, and hallways clean and clear from clutter.
   j. Install handrails for steps.
   k. Wear the correct protective gear related to athletic games and work.

C. Pharmaceutical therapy
1. Analgesics: acetaminophen 650 mg every 4 hours as needed for headache.
2. Tricyclic antidepressants may be used for posttraumatic migraines.

Follow-up
A. Patients with injuries mild enough to be discharged may be observed. Patients with normal examinations in the outpatient setting generally do not require routine follow-up.

Consultation/Referral
A. Refer all patients to the ED for the following:
1. Focal neurologic deficit(s)
2. Decreasing level of consciousness
3. Persistent headaches, nausea, and vomiting
4. Seizures or other evidence of skull fractures
5. Neuropsychological dysfunction
B. Refer to a neurologist to evaluate postconcussive syndrome for continued complaints (i.e., irritability, fatigue, headaches, difficulty concentrating, dizziness, and memory problems). Further evaluation such as MRI and EEG testing may needed.
C. Refer to a psychologist trained in neuropsychological testing (indicated for patients with a mild head injury). The assessment tool evaluates brain function in the areas of attention/concentration, initiation/planning, motor/sensory skills, visual perception, learning and memory, language, speed of processing information/reaction time, and complex problem solving.

Resources
Brain Injury Association of America: http://www.biausa.org; http://www.biausa.org/elements/BIAM/2009/2009_sports_concussions_fact_sheet.pdf
Brain Injury Resource Center: http://www.headinjury.com/
Brain Injury Resource Foundation, 1841 Montreal Road, Suite 220, Tucker, GA 30084, 678-937-1557, www.birf.info
TBI Resource Center: http://www.braininjuryresources.org/

MULTIPLE SCLEROSIS
by Kimberly D. Waltrip

Definition
Multiple sclerosis (MS) is an autoimmune degenerative disease that targets the white matter of the brain and spinal cord. The process of inflammatory demyelination varies in progression, with recurrent relapse and remission of symptoms over time. The most common symptoms include visual disturbances, spastic paraparesis, and bladder dysfunction. The course of MS is typically intermittent with periodic exacerbations in various areas of the central nervous system. MS can also present more acutely in severity, progression, and variety of symptoms. Early diagnosis is difficult. Complete recovery after the first attack is common; however, subsequent exacerbations lead to lesser return of function over time.

The loss of myelin leads to neurologic deficits in vision, speech, gait, writing, memory, and swallowing or cough reflex. Patients typically present in the ED when they experience relapse, and 80% of these patients have exacerbations of previous, rather than new, deficits.

Relapsing-remitting multiple sclerosis (RRMS) affects 70%–85% of patients. There are four categories of MS:
A. Relapsing-Remitting (RR)
B. Primary Progressive (PP)
C. Secondary Progressive (SP), which many patients with RR will progress to over time.
D. Progressive-Relapsing (PR), a pattern combining relapsing-remitting and relapsing progressive. PR is intermediate in clinical severity.

Incidence
A. In 2009, the Multiple Sclerosis Foundation estimated that 350,000–500,000 people in the United States have a diagnosis of MS, with a total of 2.5 million cases worldwide. U.S. physicians are not required to report new cases of MS. The signs and symptoms of MS can go unrecognized for some time and therefore may affect the accuracy of the statistics.

Pathogenesis
The cause of MS is unknown. Autoimmune attacks on the myelin sheaths of nerves initiate an inflammatory response, followed by eventual plaque formation and scarring, the hallmark characteristic of the disease. There is a loss of saltatory conduction. Axonal death occurs during this acute inflammatory response, explaining any permanent disability. The associated inflammation and edema around a MS lesion, along with myelin and axonal loss, contribute to the associated neurologic deficit. A limited amount of remyelination and the eventual resolution of inflammation will allow some degree of recovery with remission. Over time, multiple plaques will continue to develop in diffuse areas of the CNS. With each attack, there is a lesser degree of recovery, with subsequent decrease in function.

Predisposing Factors
A. Family history of MS.
B. Female gender (two times more likely than men to develop MS).
C. Age 20–50 (onset can vary from age 10–59, regarding onset).
D. Caucasian race (Northern European ancestry).
E. Environment (living in temperate zones, e.g., Canada, northern United States, Europe: this is associated with prevalence, no direct link has been established at this time; it is suspected that this distance from the equator causes a vitamin D deficiency secondary to a lack of direct sunlight, contributing to the development of MS).
F. Previous viral infection (e.g., Epstein-Barr virus, varicella zoster) *may* increase susceptibility.
G. Smoking.

Common Complaints
A. Sensory loss (e.g., paresthesias) is often reported early in the course of the disease.

B. Visual disturbances (diplopia on lateral gaze occurs in 33% of patients, blurred vision, loss of vision, eye pain).

C. Urinary incontinence, frequency, hesitancy, or urgency.

D. Fatigue (70% of cases).

E. Weakness in one or more extremities.

F. Gait disturbance.

Other Signs and Symptoms

A. Babinski sign.

B. Spasticity.

C. Depression (nearly 50% of cases).

D. Hyperreflexia.

E. Loss of proprioception.

F. Impotence (males).

G. Impaired cognition: subjective difficulties with attention span, concentration, short-term memory, planning, and judgment; dementia is reported in 3% of patients (late-stage MS).

H. Dysarthria.

I. Reduced libido (both sexes).

J. Constipation.

K. Pain.

L. Trigeminal neuralgia (rare).

M. Dysphagia.

Subjective Data

A. Establish location and onset of symptoms. Is this the first time the patient has experienced the symptom in question? Was the onset acute or insidious?

B. Ask the patient to describe the quality and severity of the symptom, and how it has evolved over time, including the duration. Is there a relapse/remitting pattern? Is there progression of the symptom?

C. Ask the patient if there are any factors that aggravate or alleviate the symptom. Does hot weather (also including hot tubs, saunas, overexertion) aggravate the condition? Does rest help? Did the symptom resolve on its own?

D. Establish if there have been any known viral or bacterial infections prior to symptoms.

E. Evaluate visual complaints, including the presence of scotoma, decreased color perception, diplopia, decreased acuity, or painful extraocular eye movements. Is visual deterioration induced by exercise, a hot meal, or a hot bath (Uhthoff phenomenon)?

Physical Examination

A. Check temperature, blood pressure, pulse, and respirations.

B. Inspect

1. Conduct a complete eye exam (Snellen eye chart, test cranial nerves II, III, IV, and VI).

   a. 50% of patients present with retrobulbar involvement, yet fundoscopy results are normal.

   b. Anterior involvement causes papillitis; look for presence of macular star.

   c. Assess pupillary response bilaterally; look for pendular nystagmus or sinusoidal involuntary oscillations of one or both eyes, and/or loss of smooth eye pursuit.

2. Conduct a neurologic and musculoskeletal exam.

   a. Sensory: test for perception of sharp vs. dull stimulus, heat vs. cold stimulus, local pain stimulus, proprioception, utilize the tuning fork to evaluate sense of vibration.

   b. Motor strength (test all extremities): observe for increased tone (spasticity), clonus, and tremors.

   c. Heel-to-toe tandem gait testing (evaluate for ataxia, cerebellar involvement); Romberg test.

   d. Finger-to-nose testing, heel-to-shin testing (r/o dystaxia).

   e. Check deep tendon reflexes (DTRs); may present with Babinski sign, hyperreflexia.

   f. Assess mental status (orientation to person, place, time, and situation); also test short-term memory and ability to plan (impaired planning is another cognitive issue with MS patients).

   g. Assess for pain: location, onset, duration, timing/setting, aggravating factors, alleviating factors, and associated data.

   h. Assess for depression especially with progression of symptoms.

Diagnostic Tests

A. There is no specific confirmatory test for MS.

B. MRI is the test of choice to support the clinical diagnosis of MS. MRI of the head will reveal associated plaques, if present, but cannot determine whether these lesions are specific to MS (other diseases may have similar radiographic findings).

C. Cerebral spinal fluid (CSF) analysis: characteristics of MS are the presence of oligoclonal bands, increased IgG (> 12%), and increased WBCs (> 5%).

D. Evoked response test (ERT) or evoked potential (EP): there are several different tests that evaluate brain function and nerve conduction/velocity; can detect subtle changes in brainstem function (BAER), visual interpretation and perception (VEP or VER), and sensation (SSEP).

E. CBC with differential.

F. Serum glucose to rule out hypoglycemia and chronic hyperglycemia as causes of neurologic findings.

Differential Diagnoses

A. Multiple sclerosis

B. CNS lymphoma

C. CNS infection

D. Acute disseminated encephalomyelitis (ADEM)

E. Tumor: brainstem, cerebellar, or spinal cord

F. Amyotropic lateral sclerosis (ALS)

G. Systemic lupus erythematosus (SLE)

H. Syringomyelia

I. Progressive multifocal leukoencephalopathy

J. Sarcoidosis

K. Sjogren's syndrome

L. Acute transverse myelitis

M. Myasthenia gravis (MG)

N. Guillain-Barré (GB)

O. Cerebrovascular accident (CVA)

P. Diabetes

Q. Cord compression (stenosis, ruptured disc)

R. Behcet disease

Plan

A. Patient teaching
1. Educate on heat sensitivity and how it can aggravate symptoms: avoid hot tubs, saunas, prolonged exposure in hot/humid weather; choose appropriate clothing for the season.
2. For visual disturbances, resting the eyes at various times during the day can be helpful; for double-vision, an eye patch can be used temporarily.
3. Stress the importance of exercise and its effect on MS-related fatigue and spasticity; overactivity/overwork is another issue to address at this time. Rest periods will be needed during exacerbations.
4. Teach Kegel's exercises and timed-voiding to improve bladder function; avoid alcohol and caffeinated beverages.
5. Increase water intake, dietary fiber intake, and physical activity to increase bowel motility.
6. Educate on signs and symptoms of infection, especially UTIs, and how it can trigger exacerbation. Around 60% experience heat sensitivity, which causes a "pseudoexacerbation," that is, MS symptoms may become worse, but do not necessarily cause further axon/myelin issues.
7. Teach self-intermittent catheterization for urinary retention.
8. Discuss the purpose and availability of local MS support groups.
9. Discuss counseling for adaptive coping techniques, improving family dynamics/relationships with significant others, adjustment to physical disability, and addressing anticipatory grief issues.
10. Educate on all medications, side effects, and any associated follow-up laboratory testing that is needed.
11. Suggest strategies regarding short-term memory and planning ability: the patient can write things down, make lists, draw pictures, and take more time when devising plans.

B. Pharmaceutical therapy: prescribed according to the type of MS and may include a combination of the following:
1. Disease-modifying drugs suppress the immune system in order to slow the progression of MS (lessen the frequency and severity of exacerbations, reduce MS plaques). Interferon (beta-1a and -1b), mitoxantrone, and glatiramer acetate are in this category.
2. Natalizumab (Tysabri) may be considered for relapsing, remitting MS (RRMS). It is prescribed by, or in consultation with, a neurologist who specializes in MS treatment. The Food and Drug Administration (FDA) generally recommends natalizumab for patients who have had an inadequate response to, or are unable to tolerate, other MS therapies. In 2006, the FDA approved sale under strict treatment guidelines involving infusions centers.
3. Short-term steroid use (methylprednisolone) can shorten a period of exacerbation. Long-term use is not recommended. Intravenous steroids may be prescribed initially, then transition to oral steroids (prednisone, Decadron) and taper off over time.
4. Baclofen, Zanaflex, Valium (watch for sedation, dependence), Dantrium (would use only when other drugs are ineffective, as it can cause liver damage), and clonidine are drugs used for associated spasticity.
5. Botulinum toxin injections may be used for treatment of spasticity.
6. Intrathecal pump placement may be used for administration of baclofen or clonidine for spasticity.
7. Stool softeners (Colace, Peri-Colace), bulk-forming agents (Metamucil), or laxatives (Milk of Magnesia, MiraLAX) can be taken for complaints of constipation.
8. Flomax or Hytrin can be used to improve urine outflow.
9. Ditropan, Tofranil, and Detrol are drugs commonly used to treat bladder spasms.
10. SSRIs (Zoloft, Prozac) or SSNRIs (Cymbalta, Effexor) for treatment of depression. Patients with protracted, painful, progressive medical conditions are at risk for suicide.
11. Provigil or Symmetrel can be used to treat fatigue symptoms.
12. Stem-cell transplantation is noted in the literature as a consideration for future treatment of RRMS.

Follow-up

A. A neurologist who specializes in MS management should coordinate and prescribe therapies for MS patients. NP comanagement with primary care physician for follow-up depends on the presentation, diagnosis, and therapies.

Consultation/Referral

A. Neurology consultation/referral for the management of MS.
B. Ophthalmology for visual disturbances, optic neuritis.
C. Urology for GU disturbances (impotence in males, urinary hesitancy, frequency, incontinence, and urgency, UTIs).
D. Occupational therapy can address any issues with performing activities of daily living, including fine motor skills (coordination, strength), and prescribe any necessary adaptive equipment.
E. Speech therapy can address any issues with language, cognition, or swallowing.
F. Physical therapy can address gait disturbances, motor weakness, spasticity, range of motion (ROM), and prescribe assistive devices for impaired physical mobility.
G. Psychiatry consultation for pharmacologic management of depression, dementia if indicated; psychology or licensed professional counselor referral for counseling.
H. Social work referral to assist with insurance issues, locating community resources, applying for disability, arranging home health care, placement in a skilled nursing facility, and providing counseling for the individual and the family.

Individual Considerations

A. Pregnancy:
1. Symptoms of MS may stabilize or remit during pregnancy, but 20%–40% of patients have a relapse within 3 months after delivery.

2. No evidence suggests that pregnancy affects the long-term course of MS. There is no acceleration in the rate of disability or disease progression postpartum.

3. Neither epidural anesthesia nor breast-feeding has an adverse effect on the rate of relapse or progression of disability.

4. There are no accepted guidelines for recommending for or against pregnancy in women with MS. Each patient's MS history and current neurologic deficits should be considered independently.

5. Pregnancy may affect the choice of therapy since some drugs used to treat MS are known teratogens. Glucocorticoids may cause neonatal adrenal suppression and maternal glucose intolerance.

B. Pediatrics:
1. MS is a rare diagnosis in children younger than 16 years.
2. Children with MS generally have a similar clinical presentation to adults.

C. Geriatrics: The occurrence of MS is rare in those older than 60 years.

Resources

Multiple Sclerosis Association of America: http://www.msassociation.org
Multiple Sclerosis Foundation: http://www.msfocus.org
National Multiple Sclerosis Society: http://www.nationalmssociety.org

MYASTHENIA GRAVIS *by Jill C. Cash*

Definition
A. Myasthenia gravis (MG) is a chronic autoimmune disorder that affects the neuromuscular junction and is characterized by fatigability and weakness of voluntary muscles.

Incidence
A. The prevalence is 0.5–11.5 cases per 1 million people. There are two peaks in MG incidence that are age- and gender-related: one is women in their 20s and 30s, and the other is men in their 60s and 70s.

Pathophysiology
A. MG is believed to be an antibody-mediated autoimmune attack that destroys variable numbers of acetylcholine receptors (AChR) at the postsynaptic junction. The decrease in AChRs results in weakness with repeated activities and recovery after rest. MG is often associated with thymic hyperplasia or tumors; the thymus plays an unclear role in the autoimmune process of MG.

Predisposing Factors
A. No predisposing factors have been identified.

Common Complaints
A. Classic triad: ptosis, diplopia, and dysphagia
1. Fluctuating symptoms such as droopy eyelid(s).
2. Blurry or double vision.
3. Sense of choking.
B. Difficulty chewing.
C. Slurring of speech.

D. Easy fatigability.
E. Symptoms are more pronounced with fatigue or in the evening.

Other Signs and Symptoms
A. Selected voluntary muscles that fatigue with activity.
B. Motor function that improves with rest but then decreases with use.
C. Sign of impending MG crisis:
1. Sudden onset of inspiratory distress.
2. Difficulty swallowing.
3. Visual difficulty.
4. Tachycardia.
5. Rapid onset of weakness.

Subjective Data
A. Establish onset of symptoms and possible progression.
B. Ask the patient what makes the symptoms better or worse: does rest help?
C. Ask if the patient feels better in the morning or in the afternoon or evening.
D. Look for difficulties with chewing or swallowing.
E. Investigate medications the patient is currently taking or has recently taken, such as antibiotics.

Physical Examination

The presentation and course of MG are both highly variable, and MG can therefore be very difficult to diagnose.

A. Check temperature, pulse, respirations, and blood pressure.
B. Inspect
1. Observe overall appearance.
2. Perform complete eye exam. Subtleties of eye movement dysfunction are often key in differentiating MG from other disorders.
C. Palpate: Assess DTRs; note normal to increased reflexes.
D. Neurologic exam
1. Perform complete neurologic exam.
2. Test the following:
a. Muscle strength: weakness is increased with repetition or sustained activity; arm raise cannot be sustained.
b. Eyes: upward or lateral gaze cannot be maintained for longer than 30 seconds.
c. Eyes: ptosis occurs with repetitive lid closure.
d. Voice: voice quality or speech changes when counting out loud to 100.

Normal coordination, normal sensory perception, and normal pupillary response are noted in MG.

Diagnostic Tests
A. Antibody titer for acetylcholine receptor: positive in 90% of patients with MG
B. Cholinesterase-inhibiting drug test: improvement in strength following injection of edrophonium (Tensilon)
C. Repetitive muscle stimulation test: decremental response
D. Single-fiber electromyography (EMG): jitter

Initial diagnostic tests may be equivocal with some negative test results, but this does not absolutely rule out myasthenia.

Differential Diagnoses

A. Myasthenia gravis: the most common disorder of neuromuscular transmission. **It is important to maintain a high index of suspicion and include MG in the differential diagnosis of any patient presenting with variable muscle weakness even without eye signs.**

B. Incomplete extraocular nerve palsy.

C. Polymyositis.

D. Brain stem transient ischemic attack (TIA).

E. Amyotrophic lateral sclerosis (ALS).

F. Brain stem vascular accident: "dizziness" is a symptom rarely seen with MG but often associated with brain stem ischemia.

G. Guillain-Barré syndrome.

H. Brain stem tumor.

I. Hyperthyroidism or hypothyroidism.

J. **Cholinergic crisis: While it is useful to distinguish myasthenic crisis (weakness from MG exacerbation) from cholinergic crisis (weakness from too much medication), both can rapidly lead to respiratory failure. Transportation to an emergency room for evaluation should not be delayed by attempts to differentiate the two.**

K. Eaton-Lambert myasthenic syndrome: often associated with bronchogenic carcinoma but may precede detection of the carcinoma by as many as 2 years.

Plan

A. General interventions
1. MG is primarily managed by a neurologist given the difficulty in diagnosing it, the variable course of the disease, and the highly individualized medication regimen required.
2. The course of MG fluctuates most during the first 3–5 years after diagnosis.

B. Patient teaching
1. See the Section III Patient Teaching Guide for this chapter, "Myasthenia Gravis."
2. Patients should have a MedicAlert tag and always carry a list of their medications and dosing schedules in case of an emergency.

C. Medical and surgical management
1. Thymectomy is an early consideration; an MRI of the chest is obtained once the diagnosis is made to assess for thymic enlargement.

Thymectomy lessens the severity of MG but rarely results in complete elimination of the need for medication.

2. Plasmapheresis, or plasma exchange to remove antibodies, is used emergently for the management of myasthenic crisis. Opinion is mixed regarding its use in the long-term management of myasthenia.

D. Pharmaceutical therapy
1. **Many medications can cause worsening of myasthenic symptoms, so changes and additions of any medication require consultation with the patient's neurologist. Cholinesterase-inhibiting medications:**
   a. Pyridostigmine (Mestinon) 60 mg and 180 mg SR titrate as needed, with usual dose up to 600mg/day.
   b. Neostigmine methylsulfate (Prostigmin) 0.25–0.5 and 1.0 mg/mL concentrations titrated with starting dose 0.5 mg SC or IM every 3–4 hours.
2. Steroids may be used when inpatient and then tapered on an outpatient basis, tapering every 3 days.
3. Effectiveness of medication regimen is gauged by changes in ptosis, diplopia, dysphagia, chewing ability, and muscle fatigue.
4. Care should be used with use of medications that may worsen symptoms of weakness.

Follow-up

A. Patients with MG require lifelong management by a neurologist, given the variable course both of the disease and the patient's response to treatment.

B. The patient is initially followed every 1–2 months, then every 3–4 months.

Consultation/Referral

A. If myasthenia gravis is suspected, consult with a physician and consider neurologic referral.

Individual Considerations

A. Pregnancy
1. MG is considered high risk for both the woman and the fetus.
   a. Pregnancy requires management by the patient's neurologist and a perinatologist.
2. MG frequently manifests for the first time during pregnancy. Refer to a perinatologist.

B. Pediatrics
1. MG is associated with prematurity, and the infant may have transient neonatal myasthenia. The patient will need a neonatology consult.
2. Myasthenia is less severe and commonly remits spontaneously in children, so thymectomy is not recommended.

C. Adults: Oral contraceptives may worsen myasthenic symptoms.

NEUROLOGIC EMERGENCY: FEBRILE SEIZURES *by Cheryl A. Glass*

Definition

Febrile seizures are of short duration, usually less than 5 min, and are generalized tonic-clonic convulsions; 4%–16% have focal features. The seizures are associated with fever in the absence of central nervous system infection, acute electrolyte imbalance, or any other defined cause for a seizure. The majority of children with febrile seizures do not develop epilepsy.

There are two types of febrile seizures, simple and complex.

A. Simple seizures are brief (< 15 min), generalized (without a focal component), and occur once during a 24-hour period.

B. Complex febrile seizures have at least one of the following features: duration lasting longer than 15 min, multiple seizures in 24 hours, and focal features.

Incidence

A. Three to eight percent of the populations of children up to the age of 7 develop seizures with a febrile illness. Twenty to thirty percent of children have recurrent febrile seizures during subsequent illnesses. Twenty-four percent of children have a family history of febrile seizures and 4% have a family history of epilepsy.

B. The risk of febrile seizures has been noted to increase after administration of the diphtheria, tetanus, toxoid, and whole-cell pertussis (DTP) and the measles, mumps, and rubella (MMR) vaccines.

Pathogenesis

A. Fever is characterized by a cytokine-mediated rise in core temperature as well as immunologic, neurologic, endocrinologic, and physiologic changes. A febrile seizure is an abnormal electrical discharge of neurons in the cerebral cortex causing tonic-clonic muscular contractions, induced by fever in children.

B. Febrile seizures have been identified from a combination of genetic and environmental factors. It is related to an autosomal dominant inheritance, and a few other genes and chromosomal loci have been identified. Iron insufficiency may play a role in the pathogenesis of febrile seizures.

Predisposing Factors

A. Fever
   1. Temperature of a least 100.4°F (38°C)
   2. More likely to occur with the maximal rate of temperature rise
   3. May occur early or late in the course of the febrile illness
   4. May occur before fever is apparent
B. Family history of febrile seizures
C. Family history of seizures
D. Age
   1. Occurs between 6 months and 6 years
   2. Median age of onset is 18 months
   3. 50% of children have febrile seizures between 12 and 30 months
E. Attendance in day care
F. Other neurologic abnormalities
G. Viral infections
H. Bacterial infections

Common Complaints

A. Fever
B. Generalized tonic-clonic seizure lasting less than 5 min

Other Signs and Symptoms

A. An altered state of consciousness after the seizure
B. Vomiting
C. Decreased feeding

Subjective Data

A. Ascertain whether the child had a fever at the time of the seizure.
B. Ask the caregiver to describe how the child appeared prior to the seizure: lethargic, normal, or irritable.
C. Review what happened during the seizure: jerky movements of one extremity, blinking, and general convulsions with loss of consciousness.
D. After the seizure, determine whether the child was very sleepy, confused, or normal.
E. Review what other symptoms, such as vomiting or diarrhea, the child has and what treatment(s) have been given prior to presentation.
F. Note if this has ever happened before. If so, was it the same?
G. Assess the patient's medical history and developmental course.
H. Elicit information about any family history of any type of seizures.
I. Is anyone else in the family/day care ill?

Physical Examination

A. Check temperature, pulse, respirations, blood pressure, and capillary refill.
B. Inspect
   1. Observe overall appearance: observe for seizure activity and level of consciousness: unable to arouse or if able to arouse, is the patient having trouble staying awake?
   2. Presence of difficulty breathing, grunting, and retractions.
   3. Presence and quality of crying: weak, high-pitched, or continuous crying.
   4. Inspect the head for the presence of bulging fontanelle (if applies).
   5. Evaluate the eyes for the presence of petechiae; are they sunken?
   6. Ears: evaluate the tympanic membrane.
   7. Nasal examination for signs of sinusitis and nasal flaring.
   8. Oral exam for dry mucous membranes, erythema, and enlarged tonsils.
   9. Dermal exam: evaluate for the presence of cyanosis, pallor, check skin tone and turgor, evaluate for the presence of a rash.
   10. Nails: check for prolonged capillary refill. A capillary refill of 3 seconds or greater is an intermediate risk for serious illness such as meningococcal disease.
   11. Check for nuchal rigidity/stiffness.
C. Auscultate
   1. Auscultate the heart.
   2. Auscultate all lung fields for crackles and decreased breath sounds.
   3. Auscultate all quadrants of the abdomen.
D. Palpate
   1. Fontanels (if applies).
   2. Evaluate lymphadenopathy.
   3. Palpate the abdomen for masses, tenderness, and rebound.
E. Neurologic exam: Perform complete neurologic exam, assessing all cranial nerves. Be alert for signs and symptoms of CNS infection: stiff neck, lethargy, and confusion are highly indicative of CNS infection. The neurologic exam should be normal. Any abnormal neurologic findings are inconsistent with febrile seizures.

Diagnostic Tests

A. Pulse oximetry.
B. CBC.

C. Blood chemistries are not indicated with febrile seizures unless electrolyte imbalance or other specific indications exist. Seizures that continue more than 5 min should have electrolytes and glucose evaluated.

D. Urinalysis.

E. EEG is not indicated for febrile seizures; however, if neurologic signs are present or seizures are recurrent, an EEG and neurologic workup should be done.

F. Lumbar puncture indicated if there are positive neurologic signs, especially in children 12–18 months and infants younger than 12 months who present after their first febrile seizure.

G. Consider chest X-ray for respiratory problems.

H. Consider stool cultures if indicated for diarrhea.

I. CT and MRI imaging is not required for children with simple febrile seizures.

Differential Diagnoses

A. Febrile seizure

B. Shaking chills from fever

C. Metabolic imbalances: hypoglycemia, hyponatremia, and hypomagnesemia

D. Syncope

E. CNS infection: encephalitis, meningitis, and abscess

F. Epilepsy

G. Brain tumor

Plan

A. General interventions
   1. Tepid sponge baths have not be shown to be effective in the prevention of febrile seizures and are not recommended for the treatment of fever.
   2. Children with fevers should not be undressed or overwrapped.
   3. Support the patient with positioning to prevent aspiration; maintain airway, and administer oxygen. Do *not* try to pry the jaws open to place an object between the teeth.

B. Patient teaching
   1. Give the Section III Patient Teaching Guide for this chapter, "Febrile Seizures."
   2. Neurologic sequelae, intellectual impairment, and behavioral disorders are rare following febrile seizures.

C. Pharmaceutical therapy
   1. Antipyretic agents do not prevent febrile seizures and are not utilized for prophylaxis. Ibuprofen (Motrin) or acetaminophen (Tylenol), using age/weight appropriate doses every 4 hours, may be given for temperature elevation of 104°F (37.9°C).
   2. Antibiotics are not indicated for a fever without an apparent source.
   3. The American Academy of Pediatrics Committee on Quality Improvement and Management, Subcommittee on Febrile Seizures concluded that on the basis of the risks and benefits of effective therapies, neither continuous nor intermittent anticonvulsant therapy is recommended for children with 1 or more simple febrile seizures.

Follow-up

A. See the patient for repeat seizures and as needed.

Consultation/Referral

A. Consult a neurologist for uncontrolled or repeated seizures. When no fever is present, it may be the onset of epilepsy and should be referred.

B. When meningitis cannot be eliminated by history and physical examination, the child should be admitted to the hospital.

C. If seizures are continuous, this is a medical emergency. The patient should be sent to the hospital immediately by ambulance, and a neurologist should be consulted.

Individual Considerations

A. Geriatrics:
   1. Twenty to thirty percent of older adults have blunted or absent fever response to infection.
   2. Alteration in cognitive function, especially delirium, may be present before (or in the absence of) of fever in older adults with an infection.
   3. The use of antipyretics for adults with a fever is the presence of severe coronary artery disease. Shivering is strenuous on the heart and circulatory system.
   4. Adverse consequences of fever are rare in older adults. There is little evidence that a fever increases an older adults risk for long-term neurological symptoms.

PARKINSON'S DISEASE

Definition

A. Parkinson's disease is an idiopathic, progressive, chronic neurologic syndrome characterized by a combination of akinesia or bradykinesia, or reduction of spontaneous activity and movement; rigidity, or increase in spontaneous muscle tone and involuntary movements; tremor; and postural instability.

Incidence

A. One percent of the population over age 50 has Parkinson's disease. The mean age of onset is 55–60 years. Only 5% is seen between the ages of 21–40. There is no gender difference in prevalence. Parkinson's disease (PD) is seen most frequently in people of European ancestry.

Pathophysiology

A. For reasons that are unclear, degenerative changes occur in the basal ganglia and deplete the dopaminergic neurons in the substantia nigra, resulting in dopamine reduction in the striatum. This interrupts neuronal circuits and produces akinesia and rigidity. The pathophysiology of tremor is less clear, but thalamic involvement is implicated.

Predisposing Factors

A. Antecedent encephalitis

B. Arteriosclerosis

C. Trauma

D. Toxins

E. Drugs, particularly phenothiazines

F. Familial neurodegenerative diseases in which parkinsonism is a prominent feature

Common Complaints

Cardinal symptoms:

A. Tremor at rest
B. Cogwheel resistance with tremor
C. Dyskinesias: bradykinesia, or slow voluntary movement, especially with daily activities such as cutting food, dressing self, and so forth
D. Postural instability: stooped posture
E. Difficulty walking, with tendency to fall

Other Signs and Symptoms

A. Micrographia (handwriting that decreases in size when writing out name).
B. Voice changes: fading, softness, hoarseness, and mumbling.
C. Saliva escaping mouth, especially at night.
D. Dysphagia.
E. Difficulty turning in bed.
F. Lability of mood.
G. Oily, greasy skin.
H. Excessive perspiration.
I. Constipation.
J. Urinary hesitancy or frequency.
K. Memory loss: a significant percentage of PD patients develop dementia; it can also be a medication side effect most often seen with anticholinergics or tricyclic antidepressants.

Subjective Data

A. Elicit information regarding onset of symptoms. Note changes in progression of symptoms.
B. Talk with the patient and family to establish if there have been behavioral changes, problems with activities such as eating or getting out of chairs, or personality changes.
C. Determine if other family members have had similar symptoms.
D. Ascertain the patient's medical history, including current medications, both prescription and OTC.
E. Particularly in patients younger than 55 years, investigate substance abuse and exposure to herbicides or pesticides.

Physical Examination

A. Check temperature, pulse, respirations, blood pressure, and weight: note orthostatic hypotension.
B. Inspect
   1. Observe overall appearance.
   2. Note asymmetric tremor at rest.
   3. Note subtle facial masking, decreased frequency and amplitude of eye blinks.
   4. Note posture and gait disturbances: festination, or shuffling, increasingly tiny steps; usually walking with arms down to side; difficulty turning; freezing, or inability to continue to move.
C. Palpate: Palpate extremities, noting increased tone in resting muscles.
D. Neurologic exam
   1. Perform complete neurologic exam. Assess all cranial nerves. Assess DTRs.
   2. Assess rapid alternating movements. Note difficulty with rapid alternating movements such as tapping fingers or turning palm alternately up and down.

3. Check cogwheel phenomenon, which is stepwise rigidity of movement with passive range of motion rather than anticipated smooth movement through range of motion. Best tested in wrists.
4. Perform mental status exam.
5. Assess the progression of the disease state with the scale of choice. Scales commonly used include:
   a. Unified Parkinson's Disease Rating Scale available at http://www.mdvu.org/library/ratingscales/pd/
   b. MDS–UPDRS (Movement Disorder Society Scale) available at http://www.movementdisorders.org/UserFiles/New%20UPDRS%207%203%2008%20final.pdf
   c. Hoehn and Yahr Scale available at http://neurosurgery.mgh.harvard.edu/Functional/pdstages.htm
   d. Scales for Outcomes in Parkinson's Disease—Psychiatric Complications (nonmotor evaluation) and Nonmotor Symptom Screening Questionnaire available at http://www.neurology.org/cgi/content/abstract/61/9/1222

Diagnostic Tests

A. There is no definitive diagnostic test for PD.
B. Urinalysis to rule out UTI with any urinary symptoms.
C. Speech therapy evaluation of dysarthria and dysphagia to assess aspiration risk.
D. Brain CT scan or MRI to exclude mass lesion, multiple infarcts, or normal pressure hydrocephalus.
E. MRI of cervical spine if there is increased gait disturbance after a fall.

Differential Diagnoses

A. Parkinson's disease
B. Essential tremor
C. Multi-infarct dementia
D. Alzheimer's disease
E. Brain tumor
F. Progressive supranuclear palsy
G. Normal pressure hydrocephalus
H. Shy-Drager syndrome
I. Hypothyroidism
J. Hereditary disease such as Huntington's chorea or Wilson's disease
K. Medication side effect, particularly dopamine-receptor blockers such as antipsychotics or antiemetics
L. Chorea: not generally seen in PD; its development in a patient with PD is generally a medication side effect and should be discussed with the patient's neurologist.

Plan

A. General interventions
   1. Encourage regular exercise to maintain or improve flexibility.
   2. The patient should follow a diet that is high in fiber and calcium, with adequate fluid intake, to limit complications due to constipation and osteoporosis. In some patients, protein intake may need to be timed to limit interactions with levodopa.
   3. PD can be neither cured nor arrested; treatment is aimed at minimizing symptoms with minimal drug side effects.

4. Recommend group support and patient and family education.
5. Home safety evaluations are recommended because the symptoms of PD place patients at high risk for falls and accidental injury.
B. Patient teaching: See the Section III Patient Teaching Guide for this chapter, "Managing Your Parkinson's Disease."
C. Medical and surgical management
   1. Surgery, such as pallidotomy or thalamotomy, is an option for severe PD in which tremor is poorly controlled with medications.
   2. Fetal dopaminergic neural transplants remain investigational.
D. Pharmaceutical therapy
   1. Polypharmacy is the hallmark rather than the exception with PD. Always comanage with a neurologist.
   2. Lower doses of several medications, rather than high doses of a single agent, aid in maximizing function while minimizing side effects.
   3. Drug dosages are always tapered, not stopped abruptly.
   4. First-line drug:
      a. Levodopa, combined with a decarboxylase inhibitor, is the mainstay of treatment. Sinemet is the levodopa and carbidopa combination drug most often used.
         i. The dose and dosing frequency are very individualized.
         ii. Patients are often on a combination of sustained release and short-acting preparations.
         iii. See literature for individual dosing. Titrate dose up every 3 days for adjustments.
         iv. Long-term use is often associated with adverse effects requiring careful medication dosage.
   5. Second-line therapy: Dopamine agonists: generally given in conjunction with levodopa, these allow use of lower doses of levodopa that can delay or reduce levodopa-associated problems.
   6. Ergot derivatives include:
      a. Bromocriptine and pergolide are the two dopamine agonists most often used.
         i. Bromocriptine mesylate (Parlodel) is initiated at 1.25 mg daily or twice a day and slowly increased to 10–25 mg daily.
         ii. Pergolide mesylate (Permax) is initiated at 0.05 mg daily and increased slowly to 2–3 mg in divided doses three times a day.
      b. Non-ergot drugs are preferred due to fewer side effects:
         i. Pramipexole (Mirapex) 0.125 mg three times daily up to 4.5 mg/day maximum useful for tremors or Ropinirole (ReQuip) 0.25 mg three times daily, max 24 hours period.
   7. Neuroprotective agents: selegiline (Eldepryl), monoamine oxidase (MAO-B) inhibitor 5 mg at breakfast and at lunch, may have neuroprotective effects and slow progression of symptoms.
      a. Often an initial treatment, a drug is usually continued throughout the disease course. Maximum dose is 10 mg/day.
      b. Amantadine (Symmetrel) is used as short-term monotherapy in patients younger than 60 years with mild to moderate PD in which akinesia and rigidity are more prominent than tremor.
         i. Its effects tend to wane, and it should be tapered once other antiparkinsonian drugs are started.
         ii. The usual dose is 100–300 mg twice daily. Adjust the dose gradually.
   8. Anticholinergics: these are useful for treating resting tremor but not akinesia or impaired postural reflexes.
      a. The centrally acting drug trihexyphenidyl HCL (Artane) is the most common anticholinergic used.
         i. Drug is usually started at 0.5–1.0 mg twice daily with food and slowly increased to 2–3 mg three times daily.
         ii. Dosage should always be tapered, never stopped abruptly.
         iii. Use is not recommended in patients older than 60 years or with dementia.
      b. Benztropin mesylate (Cogentin) 0.5–1 mg at bedtime may also be used in PD. Maximum is 6 mg/day. Increase every 6–7 days.
   9. Sleep disorders are common in PD and respond well to tricyclic antidepressants (TCAs), benzodiazepines, diphenhydramine, or low-dose chloral hydrate.
   10. Excessive daytime sleepiness should first be evaluated as a symptom of depression before it is attributed to medications or effects of PD.

As PD progresses, patients often develop clear "on" and "off" times of medication effectiveness and functional ability, so medication schedules are very carefully customized to maximize "on" times.

Follow-up

A. Parkinson's disease requires lifelong management by a neurologist.
B. Frequency of appointments depends on severity of disease and response to medication. Depression and neuropsychiatric side effects of medications are often seen in patients with PD, so any office visit should involve screening for these. Inquire particularly about memory loss, vivid dreams or nightmares, hallucinations, symptoms of depression or anxiety, and occurrence of panic attacks. Discuss findings with the patient's neurologist, as medication adjustments could be required.

Consultation/Referral

A. Managing PD requires referral to a neurologist to initiate and adjust medications.
B. If a PD patient requires the addition of medication for other conditions, consult the patient's neurologist to evaluate for possible serious adverse effects.
C. Involvement with a support group can be helpful for the patient and family. Information about Parkinson's disease and local support groups can be obtained from:
   1. The American Parkinson's Disease Association, Inc.
      60 Bay Street, Suite 401
      Staten Island, NY 10301
      800-223-2732

2. National Parkinson Foundation
1501 NW 9th Ave., Bob Hope Road
Miami, FL 33136-1494
800-433-7022

Individual Considerations

A. Pediatrics: When Parkinson's is seen in this age group, it is usually due to secondary factors.
B. Geriatrics: Most commonly seen in this population.

SEIZURES *by Cheryl A. Glass*

Definition

Accurate classification of seizures is dependent on observations of witnessed seizures, full medical history including comorbidities, and clinical findings. Epilepsy is not diagnosed until the patient has more that one seizure secondary to an underlying condition in the brain. Status epilepticus is a continuous state of seizure and is usually defined as 30 min of uninterrupted seizure activity.

A. Infantile spasms begin at 3 months to 2 years of age. They are characterized by clusters of quick, sudden movements, including the head falling forward, arm flexion, and knees drawn up to the chest.
B. Partial (focal) seizures generally only involve one portion of the brain. They are the most common type of seizures and may be accompanied by visual or auditory hallucinations.
   1. Simple partial seizures (SPS) are not associated with altered consciousness.
   2. Common SPS includes jerking of a limb and may be preceded by an aura, including epigastric discomfort, fear, or unpleasant smells.
   3. Complex partial seizure (CPS) is notable for impaired consciousness. Confusion, fatigue, and headaches may follow a CPS.
   4. A simple partial seizure may last a few seconds and develop into a CPS with symptoms that include staring, repetitive motor behaviors, clouded consciousness, and automatisms (swallowing, chewing, or lip smacking).
C. Generalized seizures are notable for electroencephalographic (EEG) changes since both hemispheres of the brain are involved. Almost all generalized seizures involve loss/impaired consciousness. There are four subtypes of generalized seizures:
   1. Tonic-clonic, also known as grand mal seizures, generally last 1–2 min and are notable for falls, cries, rigidity (tonicity), jerking (clonicity), and possible cyanosis.
   2. Absent seizures, also called petit mal seizures, last 2–15 seconds and are notable for beginning and ending abruptly. Symptoms noted include staring, eye flutters, and automatisms. First aid is not required.
   3. Myoclonic seizures are characterized by rapid, brief contraction of muscles (sudden jerks or clumsiness) usually on both sides of the body, arm, or sudden jerk of a foot during sleep. First aid is generally not required.
   4. Atonic seizures, also called drop seizures, are characterized by abrupt loss of muscle tone, loss of posture, or sudden collapse. These seizures tend to be resistant to medication. Protective headgear may be needed. Generally first aid is not required unless an injury occurs.
D. Lennox-Gastaut syndrome (LGS) is a rare form of epilepsy consisting of multiple seizure types. Types include cognitive impairment and drop seizures. LGS patients may require antiseizure medications, steroids or immune globulin, vagus nerve stimulation, surgical resection, and ketogenic diet.
E. Eclampsia occurs anytime in pregnancy from the second trimester to the puerperium. It is notable for the occurrence of one or more generalized convulsions and/or coma in women with preeclampsia (in the absence of other neurologic conditions).
   1. Eclampsia is self-limited and delivery is the treatment.
   2. The tonic-clonic seizure generally lasts 60–75 seconds.
   3. Fetal bradycardia last 3–5 min, but does not necessitate an emergent cesarean section delivery. Compensatory fetal tachycardia and transient fetal heart rate decelerations occur. Delivery should be considered for the lack of improvement in 10–15 min after maternal/fetal resuscitative interventions.
   4. Seizures due to eclampsia generally resolve within a few hours to days postpartum. HELLP syndrome (Hemolysis, Elevated Liver Enzymes, Low Platelets) develop in approximately 10%–20% of women with preeclampsia/eclampsia.

Incidence

A. 2.5 million Americans are affected by epilepsy.
B. Seniors: 300,000 (most rapid population with epilepsy).
C. Eclampsia
   1. Mild preeclampsia 0.5%.
   2. Severe preeclampsia from 2%–3%.
   3. 48 hours postpartum up to 33%.

Pathogenesis

A. Epilepsy is a functional disorder of the brain when neurons signal abnormally. The exact cause of epilepsy and eclampsia is unknown.

Predisposing Factors

A. Tumors
B. Alcohol/drug
C. Cerebral infarction/stroke
D. Hypoglycemia
E. Alzheimer's disease
F. Posttrauma (head injury)
G. Surgery
H. Pregnancy (eclampsia)
I. Febrile illness
J. Photosensitivity
K. Risk factors for recurrent seizures
   1. Identifiable brain disease
   2. Mental retardation
   3. Abnormal neurologic examination/EEG

4. Seizures onset after age 10
5. Multiple types of seizures
6. Family history/genetics
7. Poor response to AEDs/combination therapy at time of withdrawal
8. Chronic alcoholism
L. Eclampsia risk factors
   1. Nulliparous
   2. Pregnancy-induced hypertension
   3. Teens to lower 20s and again older than 35 years
   4. Other conditions to be ruled out include:
      a. Stroke
      b. Hypertensive disease
      c. Space-occupying lesion
      d. Metabolic disorders (hypoglycemia, uremia, water intoxication)
      e. Meningitis or encephalitis
      f. Drug use (Methamphetamine, cocaine)
      g. Idiopathic epilepsy
      h. Thrombotic thrombocytopenia purpura (TTT)

Common Complaints

A. Aura: epigastric discomfort, fear, or unpleasant smells
B. Automatisms (swallowing, chewing, fumbling, picking clothes, or lip smacking)
C. Stiffing then jerking of limbs
D. Staring with/without repetitive motor behaviors
E. Eclampsia
   1. Headache: severe or persistent frontal or occipital
   2. Blurred vision
   3. Photophobia
   4. Right upper quadrant pain/epigastric pain
   5. Altered mental status
   6. Nausea and vomiting
   7. Hyperreflexia

Other Signs and Symptoms

A. Lack of memory of seizure
B. Impaired consciousness.
C. Postictal
   1. Confusion
   2. Amnesia
   3. Fatigue
   4. Headaches
   5. Loss of urine or bowel control

Subjective Data

A. Obtain a history from the patient or a person that witnesses the seizure.
   1. Have the witness describe the duration, part of the body affected, and qualities of the seizure.
B. Evaluate if the patient has ever had seizures, and ask was this an isolated event.
C. Did the patient have a fever or an active/recent infection?
D. Do a thorough review of the patient's medical history, including head injury, pregnancy, diabetes, and cancer.
E. Ask if there is a family history of seizures.

Physical Examination

A. Blood pressure, pulse, respirations, and temperature

B. Inspect: level of consciousness, orientation, general overall exam for secondary injuries from fall or striking objects.
C. Auscultate: lungs for possible aspiration
D. Palpation (if applicable for any injuries)
E. Neurological examination: full examination.

Diagnostic Tests

A. Diagnosis is confirmed by the patient's history, witness accounts, neurological examination, blood work, and clinical testing, such as EEG.
B. Electroencephalograph (EEG).
C. Neuroimaging CT or MRI.
D. Blood glucose.
E. Drug/alcohol screen.

Differential Diagnoses

A. Seizures
B. Brain tumor
C. CNS infection
D. Drug/alcohol use
E. Stroke
F. Hypoglycemia
G. Trauma

Plan

A. Emergency transport may be required. Seizures longer than 5–10 min require emergent care.
B. Obtain a consultation with a neurologist for a thorough evaluation.
C. States vary on the driving requirements/restrictions for patients with epilepsy. Individual state driving requirements are noted on the Epilepsy Foundation Web site: http://www.epilepsyfoundation.org/living/wellness/transportation/drivinglaws.cfm.
   1. A person with epilepsy has the risk of a motor-vehicle accident (MVA) while driving. It is considered similar or slightly higher than in patients with other medical conditions (diabetes, cardiovascular disease) and compares with the risk of MVA with persons with sleep apnea, alcoholism, dementia, and cellular phone use.
   2. Regulatory agents, as a measure of driving risk, require having a seizure-free interval of 3–12 months (state dependent). In studies the seizure-free interval was the strongest predictor of MVA.
   3. Clinicians must warn patients about possible driving risks after reduction of medications or missing AED doses and must consider the patients' neurologic deficits other than seizures (e.g., cognition and visual field deficits) when making recommendations about driving. The risk factors for an MVA for persons with epilepsy are:
      a. Medication noncompliance
      b. Recent history of alcohol or drug abuse
      c. Uncorrectable brain functional or metabolic disorder
      d. Structural brain disease
      e. Frequent seizure recurrence after seizure-free intervals
      f. Prior crashes caused by seizures

Patient Teaching

A. Keeping a seizure diary is extremely helpful in identifying seizure trends, drug compliance, monitoring side effects, and evaluating the need for changing the course of therapy. The frequency or time of day that seizures occur is used in the adjustment of AED dosage and timing of administration.

B. Seizure triggers:
1. Most common cause is missed AED and/or sudden discontinuation of meds.
2. Sleep deprivation.
3. Alcohol/drug intake.
4. Stress.
5. Hormone fluctuations.
6. Pregnancy.
7. Photosensitivity/strobe or flashing light/intense lights.
8. TV and video games (flicker frequency).
9. Contrasting visual patterns (grids, checkerboard, stripes).

C. Review the importance of medication adherence.
1. Give oral and written dosing instructions.
2. Refill the prescription prior to running out.
3. Take the medication on a schedule (set a watch alarm, use a pill container, mark off the calendar). Taking an extra pill when a seizure aura occurs will not stop the seizure, since it is not absorbed fast enough.
4. New prescription interaction profiles should be evaluated before starting new drugs.
5. Patients should not use supplements, herbal, or over-the-counter medications without checking with their health care provider.

D. Excessive alcohol use (> 3 drinks/day) increases the likelihood of seizures. Patients should have not more than 1–2 drinks/day.

E. First aid for grand mal seizure includes:
1. Stay calm.
2. Time the seizure. Call 911 if the seizure lasts longer than 5–10 min.
3. Clear the area to prevent harm with surrounding objects.
4. Turn the person to the side and do not put anything in his or her mouth.
5. Do not hold the person down.
6. Place a soft object under the head to prevent head injury.
7. CPR is not necessary unless the person stops breathing after the seizure.
8. Stay with the person and reassure him or her.
9. Help get the person home; call family or friends.
10. Immediate transport to the ER is necessary for known conditions such as:
   a. Diabetes/hypoglycemia
   b. Heat exhaustion
   c. Pregnancy
   d. Infection/high fever
   e. Poisoning
   f. Head injury

F. First aid for petit mal seizures:
1. Stay calm.
2. Guide the patient away from any dangers.
3. Block access to hazards.
4. Do not restrain the person.
5. Stay with the person until full awareness returns.

Pharmaceutical Therapy

A. There is controversy concerning whether to start antiepileptic drug (AED) therapy for the first seizure. AEDs are generally started after a second seizure.

B. The prescription of AEDs should be individually weighed with a risk-versus-benefit decision that includes such factors as age; gender; family planning/desire for pregnancy; current driver; type/recurrence of seizure; abnormal EEG; concurrent medications used for other comorbid conditions; history of depression, anxiety, suicidal ideation, and hepatic and renal disease; cost; patient preference and lifestyle issues; and side effect profile of mediation(s). See Table 18.6.

C. A neurologist consultation should be obtained for full evaluation and prescription of AED with a neurologist or primary health care providers managing subsequent follow-up.

D. A single agent AED is started and titrated slowly to the lowest dose that is the most effective in seizure control with the least number of side effects.
1. Ideally the patient should be maintained on one AED; however, combination therapy may be required or the first agent discontinued.
2. When a second AED is required, the second additional medication is started by titration, a therapeutic level is achieved, and the first AED is subsequently tapered off. During this period of time there is an increase in side effects.
3. Switching to a generic formulation has been noted to increase seizure activity.
4. Rectal diazepam gel (Diastat) may be prescribed to use at home for patients with a history of prolonged seizures.

E. Stevens-Johnson syndrome (SJS) and toxic epidermal necrolysis (TEN) can occur up to 4 months after the institution of AEDs, including carbamazepine (Tegretol), oxcarbazepine (Trileptal), phenytoin (Dilantin), and lamotrigine (Lamictal).

F. Women should be routinely prescribed folate supplements of 0.4–0.8 mg/day. The folic acid recommendation is 4 mg/day for 1–3 months prior to conception when the patient is on valproate or carbamazepine (Tegretol).

Follow-up

A. Follow-up by primary health care providers is dependent on the frequency of seizures, toxicity profile of AED, and other comorbid conditions.

B. Subsequent visits include the evaluation:
1. Drug compliance.
2. Seizure log/diary.
3. Drug concentrations, blood counts, and hepatic and renal function.
4. Premenstrual serum levels when there is an increase in seizure activity the week before menstruation.
5. Yearly drug levels are required for patients on a stable dose with no seizures.

C. There is an increased risk of suicide associated with several AEDs. Evaluation of the patient 1 week after

TABLE 18.6 Antiepileptic Medications

Drug	Seizure Type	First-Line Treatment
Rufinamide (Banzel)	Lennox-Gastaut syndrome (LGS)	Adjunctive treatment
Divalproex sodium (Depakote)	Absence seizures Complex partial seizure	First-line treatment
Phenytoin (Dilantin)	Tonic-clonic seizures Psychomotor and neurosurgical induced seizures	First-line treatment
Felbamate (Felbatol)	Partial seizures Lennox-Gastaut syndrome	Not first line in partial seizures and used as an adjunctive for LGS
Tiagabine (Gabitril)	Partial seizures	Adjunctive treatment
Levetiracetam (Keppra)	Partial onset seizures Myoclonic seizures Generalized tonic-clonic seizures	Adjunctive treatment for all types of seizures
Clonazepam (Klonopin)	Absence seizures Lennox-Gastaut syndrome Myoclonic seizures	First-line treatment
Lamotrigine (Lamictal)	Partial seizures Lennox-Gastaut syndrome	First-line treatment for LGS
Pregabalin (Lyrica)	Partial onset seizure	Adjunctive treatment
Primidone (Mysoline)	Focal and psychomotor seizures Tonic-clonic seizures	Not first-line treatment
Gabapentin (Neurontin)	Partial seizures	Adjunctive treatment
Carbamazepine (Tegretol)	Partial or mixed seizures Generalized tonic-clonic seizures	First-line treatment
Topiramate (Topamax)	Partial onset seizures Generalized tonic-clonic seizures Lennox-Gastaut syndrome	First-line treatment and adjunctive for LGS
Oxcarbazepine (Trileptal)	Partial seizures	Monotherapy or adjunct treatment
Valproate	Lennox-Gastaut syndrome	First-line treatment in LGS
Magnesium Sulfate (MgSO4)	Eclamptic tonic-clonic seizure	First-line treatment

institution of therapy is prudent. Instructions should be given to notify the office concerning depression.

D. Bone loss is noted with long-term therapy with AEDs; therefore, a DEXA scan is warranted.

E. Patients taking AEDs need regular dental/oral care.

F. Each state has the legal prerogative to grant driving privileges. Clinicians cannot grant or suspend driving privileges.
1. Six states require clinicians to report their patients with seizures (CA, DE, NV, NJ, OR, and PA).
2. Some states require a letter sent to the Motor Vehicle Administration stating, "My patient has seizures and has been advised not to drive."
3. All states require drivers with epilepsy or seizures to report their condition.
4. Commercial driving restrictions are stricter. Restrictions for commercial vehicles involved in intrastate commerce vary among individual states.

G. Chronic hypertension develops in up to 78% of women with preeclampsia/eclampsia.

Consultation/Referral
A. A neurology consultation is necessary for the evaluation and medication initiation and the use of a ketogenic diet.

B. A neurosurgical consultation is necessary to evaluate a vagus nerve stimulator.

Individual Considerations
A. Women
1. Preconception counseling and a planned pregnancy is imperative.
   a. Discuss the teratogenicity of AEDs.
   b. Increase folic acid to 4 mg/day to help prevent neural tube defects.
   c. Stress the need for regular prenatal care.
2. Oral contraceptives are less effective on AEDs. The failure rate is 0.7–3.1 per 100 women. Women taking enzyme-inducing AEDs should use a back-up method or alternative birth control. Enzyme-inducting AEDs include:
   a. Dilantin (phenytoin)
   b. Phenobarbital
   c. Tegretol (carbamazepine)
   d. Zarontin (ethosuximide)
   e. Felbatol (felbamate)
   f. Topamax (topiramate)
   g. Trileptal (oxcarbazepine)

3. Estrogen and progesterone act on the temporal lobe where partial seizures often begin. Seizure patterns may change during menopause.
B. Pediatrics: A ketogenic diet may be prescribed under a physician's care.
C. Geriatrics
   1. Seizures are likely to begin from 60–80 years of age.
   2. Management may be more difficult dependent upon comorbidities and the use of other medications.
   3. Older patients have an increase of falls and loss of independence.

TRANSIENT ISCHEMIC ATTACK (TIA) *by Cheryl A. Glass*

Definition
A. Transient ischemic attacks (TIAs) are brief focal brain deficits, spinal-cord, or retinal ischemia (without acute infarction) caused by vascular occlusion. Symptoms generally last less than an hour; however, they may have permanent sequelae. TIAs are a risk factor for recurrent risk of stroke. Approximately 15% of diagnosed strokes are preceded by TIAs.

Incidence
A. The prevalence of TIAs in the United States is between 200,000 and 500,000 per year. The early risk of stroke is approximately 4%–5% at 2 days and as high as 11% at day 7 after a TIA. The risk from death from coronary artery disease and stroke is as high as 6%–10%, depending on other risk factors.

Pathogenesis
A. The pathogeneis is a neurologic event secondary to a temporary reduction of blood flow to the brain from a partially occluded vessel or related to an acute thromboembolic event.

Predisposing Factors
A. Hypertension
B. Atherosclerosis
C. African American
D. Age older than 40 years
E. Hypotensive episodes
F. Oral contraceptives
G. Atrial fibrillation
H. Smoking
I. Familial hyperlipidemia
J. Diabetes mellitus
K. Valvular heart disease
L. Infective endocarditis
M. Migraine with aura

Common Complaints
A. Acute onset of focal neurologic deficit

Other Signs and Symptoms
A. Dysarthria
B. Dysphagia
C. Near syncope
D. Hemiparesis
E. Temporary monocular blindness
F. Behavior changes
G. Vertigo
H. Dizziness
I. Ataxia
J. Diplopia

Subjective Data
A. Ask detailed questions about symptoms before, during, and after the spell.
   1. Review the exact timing of onset of symptoms.
   2. How intense were the symptoms?
   3. What was the duration and the presence of any fluctuation of symptoms?
   4. Has there been a pattern that is becoming more frequent or escalating in symptoms?
B. Interview the patient, family members, witnesses, and emergency personnel for their description to behavior, speech, gait, memory, and movement.
C. Focus on precipitating factors and state of consciousness after the acute event.
D. Question the patient about risk factors such as hypertension, smoking, cardiac disease, and heredity.
E. Review all medications, including anticoagulants, over-the-counter, and herbals.
F. Review the medical history.
   1. Recent surgeries specifically carotid or cardiac surgeries
   2. Seizures
   3. Central nervous system infection
   4. Illicit drug use
   5. Presence of any metabolic disorders
   6. Recent trauma (blunt or torsion injury to the neck)
   7. Atrial fibrillation

Physical Examination
A. Check temperature, pulse, respirations, and blood pressure, including orthostatic blood pressure and pulse and pulse oximetry.
B. General observation: Observe overall appearance, level of consciousness, ability to interact, language, difficulty swallowing, tremors, spasticity, as well as memory skills.
C. Inspect
   1. Dermal exam
      a. Overall hydration status.
      b. Look for postcarotid endarterectomy scars, presence of a pacemaker, implantable cardioverter defibrillator, or other cardiac surgical scars.
   2. Check pupil size and reactivity to light.
   3. Perform a fundoscopic exam to evaluate optic disc margins, retinal plaques, and pigmentation.
D. Auscultate
   1. Heart for rate, rhythm, murmurs, or rubs.
   2. Lungs: note respiratory rate and pattern.
   3. Carotid arteries for the presence of bruit.
E. Palpate
   1. Palpate extremities for pulses and peripheral edema.
F. Neurologic exam
   1. Cranial nerve testing
      a. Wrinkle forehead/raise eyebrows.

  b. Smile and show teeth.

  c. Stick out the tongue/lateral tongue movement.

  d. Ocular movements.

  e. Visual field.

 2. Motor strength

  a. Shrug shoulders.

  b. Test muscle strength: grasp hands and squeeze.

  c. Check reflexes of biceps, triceps, patellar, brachioradial, and Achilles.

 3. Sensory testing: pinprick

 4. Gait and posture (cerebellar system evaluation)

  a. Ocular movements

  b. Gait

  c. Finger-to-nose

  d. Heel-to-knee

Diagnostic Tests

A. Pulse oximetry.

B. Laboratory tests:

 1. Glucose

 2. Electrolytes and creatinine

 3. Serum chemistry

 4. CBC

 5. Lipid profile

 6. Cardiac enzymes

 7. Erythrocyte sedimentation rate (ESR)

 8. PT/PTT

 9. Coagulation and hypercoagulablity testing

C. Consider drug testing.

D. MRI or CT scan within 24 hours of symptom onset.

E. Carotid Doppler ultrasonography identifies patients with urgent surgical needs.

F. Cardiac imaging to evaluate cardioembolic sources.

G. EKG to evaluate dysrhythmias (i.e., atrial fibrillation).

H. Lumbar puncture to rule out infection, demyelinating disease, and subarachnoid hemorrhage.

I. EEG as indicated for seizure activity.

Differential Diagnoses

A. Transient ischemic attack

B. Ischemia stroke

C. Subarachnoid hemorrhage/subdural hematoma

D. Migraine

E. Hypoglycemia

F. Epilepsy

G. Malignant hypertension

H. Brain tumor

I. Bell's palsy

J. Multiple sclerosis

Plan

A. General interventions

 1. Carefully assess the patient to timely diagnose TIA.

 2. Perform a full workup to determine the underlying disease process.

 3. Prevent stroke by modification of risk factors.

B. Patient teaching: See the Section III Patient Teaching Guide for this chapter, "Transient Ischemic Attacks (TIAs)."

C. Medical and surgical management

 1. Treat TIAs with antiplatelet drugs as soon as intracranial bleeding is ruled out.

 2. Consider carotid endarterectomy.

 3. Lipid control.

 4. Glucose control.

 5. Smoking cessation.

 6. Eliminate or reduce alcohol consumption.

 7. Start exercise plan/lose weight.

D. Pharmaceutical therapy

 1. Antiplatelet therapy

  a. Aspirin 50–325 mg/day.

  b. Dipyridamole (Persantine) 200 mg/day. May be given as an adjunct with warfarin therapy.

  c. Aspirin + Dipyridamole extended release (Aggrenox) 25/200 mg twice a day.

  d. Clopidogrel (Plavix) 75 mg/day. Aspirin is not routinely recommended with Clopidogrel due to the risk of hemorrhage.

  e. Ticlopidine (Ticlid) 250 mg twice a day.

  f. Warfarin (Coumadin) 5–15 mg titrate for a goal INR of 2.0–3.0.

 2. Antihypertensive therapy as indicated.

Follow-up

A. Rapid transfer is essential for a patient with positive symptoms for risk stratification.

B. Specific follow-up depends on etiology, severity, frequency, and duration of TIAs.

C. Follow-up laboratory testing as indicated (i.e., CBC, INR).

D. Monitor the patient for occult bleeding if started on antiplatelet, antithrombic medications.

Consultation/Referral

A. TIA should be viewed as a medical emergency because these patients have salvageable neurologic function; consult with a physician.

B. Cardiology and neurology consultations should be obtained when cardioembolic TIAs are treated with anticoagulation therapy.

C. Ophthalmologic consultation is indicated to assess the nature of transient visual symptoms.

D. Vascular surgeon consultation is necessary for patients with significant stenosis or occlusion.

Individual Considerations

A. Adults: TIAs that occur in the younger adult population should be evaluated for embolism.

B. Geriatrics: TIAs are most commonly seen in this population.

VERTIGO

Definition

A. Vertigo is the illusion of self or environmental movement, typically rotating. Vertigo is often classified as either central or peripheral in origin.

Incidence

B. It is estimated that approximately 0.5% of the population consult their primary health care provider each year regarding vertigo. Both sexes, as well as all age groups, are affected.

Pathogenesis

A. Distinguishing between peripheral and central vertigo is critical because the evaluation, treatment, and progress vary significantly. Central vertigo suggests brain stem dysfunction affecting the vestibular nuclei or their connections. This may be secondary to a structural lesion such as neoplasm or ischemia.

B. Vertigo due to vascular insufficiency is rarely isolated, and other symptoms of brain stem involvement are usually seen, such as diplopia, dysphagia, motor weakness, or disruption in sensation. Neoplasms are usually slow growing, and the vestibular dysfunction is often insidious. Other considerations for causes of central vertigo include multiple sclerosis (MS), seizures, and migraines.

C. Vertigo of peripheral origin is more common and may be caused by dysfunction of the inner ear or vestibular nerve. Benign paroxysmal positional vertigo (BPPV) is the most commonly diagnosed of peripheral vestibular disorders. The cause of BPPV is unknown. The most common explanation is free otoconia within the semicircular canals are dislodged by trauma, infection, or degeneration. The debris relocates when the head is repositioned and provokes vertigo. Causes of labyrinthine dysfunction include infection, trauma, ischemia, or toxins such as drugs or alcohol.

D. Other possible causes of vertigo are psychogenic, cardiovascular, and metabolic.

Predisposing Factors

A. Head or body movement
B. Fear or anxiety
C. Stress
D. Recent infection, usually upper respiratory in cases of vestibular neuronitis
E. Family history, especially in cases of vertiginous migraine

Common Complaints

A. Dizziness with or without change in body positioning
B. Nausea
C. Tinnitus
D. Aural fullness
E. Hearing loss

Other Signs and Symptoms

A. Central origin, including vascular insufficiencies, strokes, neoplasms, migraine, MS, seizures
   1. Double vision
   2. Dysarthria
   3. Dysphagia
   4. Paresthesias
   5. Changes in motor or sensory exam
   6. Mild to moderate vertigo
   7. Multiple episodes of vertigo lasting seconds to minutes in duration with vascular insufficiency and seizures
   8. Constant complaints of vertigo with neoplasms or strokes
   9. Multiple episodes of vertigo lasting hours with migraines
   10. Single episodes of vertigo with MS
   11. Dix-Hallpike test: Habituation common with delayed nystagmus

B. Peripheral origin, including BPPV, Meniere's disease, labyrinthitis, vestibular dysfunction, vestibular neuritis, and acoustic neuroma
   1. No associated signs of brain stem dysfunction.
   2. Vertigo, usually described as severe.
   3. Multiple episodes of vertigo lasting hours with Meniere's disease.
   4. Single or multiple episodes of vertigo with labyrinthitis.
   5. Vestibular dysfunction, described as constant vertigo.
   6. Severe nausea or vomiting.
   7. Hearing loss or tinnitus, aural fullness may be present, as well as a roaring sound.
   8. Triad of vertigo, tinnitus, and hearing loss is suggestive of Meniere's disease.
   9. Dix-Hallpike test: no habituation: nystagmus occurs immediately.

Subjective Data

A. Elicit onset, frequency, duration, and course of presenting symptoms.
B. Elicit from the patient a verbal description of the sensation(s) experienced.
C. Note triggering and alleviating factors.
D. Query the patient regarding associated symptoms such as hearing loss, tinnitus, nausea, difficulty with gait, aural fullness, or other neurologic manifestations such as nystagmus.
E. Review the patient's past medical history, including recent infections; trauma; medications; risk factors for cardiovascular disease such as smoking, diabetes, and hyperlipidemia.
F. Review medication use: aminoglycoside, antibiotics, diuretics, antihypertensives, and antidepressants.

Physical Examination

A. Check temperature, pulse, respirations, and blood pressure; note orthostatic hypotension.
B. Inspect
   1. Observe overall appearance.

Generalized muscle weakness may be observed.

   2. Note gait: difficulty with tandem gait.
   3. Inspect the eyes, ears, nose, and mouth. Assess for nystagmus; a few beats of nystagmus on extreme lateral gaze may be normal.
C. Palpate
   1. Palpate extremities; note pulses and edema.
   2. Perform Rinne test and Weber's tests.
D. Neurologic exam
   1. Perform complete neurologic exam.
   2. Assess cranial nerves.

Brain stem involvement is frequently seen with detailed neurologic exam. Signs of cerebellar dysfunction include difficulty with finger-to-nose testing, rapid alternating supination or pronation of hands, and gait disturbance.

    3. Perform Romberg's test: The patient stands with feet together and closes his or her eyes. Positive result is when the patient sways. This may be seen with vestibular disease and acoustic neuroma.

E. Auscultate
    1. Auscultate the heart, lungs, neck, and carotid arteries.

Physical examination may reveal cardiovascular abnormalities, such as a carotid bruit.

    2. Auscultate the abdomen.

Diagnostic Tests

A. Thyroid function studies.
B. VDRL: to rule out secondary or early tertiary syphilis, which can have symptoms similar to Meniere's disease.
C. CT scan.
D. MRI with and without contrast to assess for mass, especially if a central origin is suspected.
E. Caloric test: definitive procedure for identifying vestibular pathology.
F. Electronystagmography: most useful in chronic peripheral disorders to determine the degree and progression of vestibular deficit.
G. Audiogram: test for possible hearing loss.
H. Rotating chair test: interprets the slow component velocity of the nystagmus response with bilateral canals stimulated.
I. Bárány's maneuver test: with patient sitting, turn his or her head to the right and quickly lower him or her to supine position with head over the edge 30° below the horizontal level. Repeat on the other side.
    1. Central nystagmus is not suppressed by fixation and rarely has torsional components. Latency to evoked nystagmus with provocative maneuvers (Bárány's maneuvers) is shorter with longer duration.
    2. Peripheral nystagmus is suppressed by fixation and commonly has torsional components. Latency to evoked nystagmus with provocative maneuvers is longer with shorter duration.

Differential Diagnoses

A. Vertigo
B. Vascular insufficiencies
C. Stroke
D. Neoplasms
E. Migraine
F. MS
G. Seizures
H. BPPV
I. Meniere's disease
J. Labyrinthitis
K. Vestibular dysfunction
L. Vestibular neuritis
M. Acoustic neuroma
N. Syncope
O. Multiple sensory defects
P. Parkinson's disease

Plan

A. General interventions: Treatment of vertigo depends upon the underlying pathology and duration of the symptoms.
    1. Acute vertigo: Maintain the patient on bed rest, with the reassurance that most patients with acute vertigo recover spontaneously over a period of several weeks to months.
    2. Chronic vertigo: Refer the patient for physical therapy with emphasis on vestibular rehabilitation.
        a. Cawthorne Cooksey physical exercise regimen encourages eye, head, and body movements to facilitate recalibration of the vestibulo-ocular and vestibulospinal reflexes.
        b. Encourage ambulation when tolerated to induce central compensatory mechanism.
    3. Meniere's disease: The patient needs bed rest in the acute phase and nutritional therapy with restrictions of sodium, caffeine, alcohol, and tobacco.
    4. Benign paroxysmal positional vertigo (BPPV)
        a. The patient needs bed rest for acute symptoms.
        b. Canalith repositioning procedures (CRP) provide immediate resolution of vertigo in 85%–95% of patients. Epley procedure: The canalith repositioning procedure is safe, simple, inexpensive, quick, and easy to perform. It is likely to be unsuccessful in patients with bilateral positional nystagmus, and it is not recommended for patients with acute vertigo, many of whom may have vestibular neuronitis. See the Section II Procedure, "Epley Procedure for Vertigo."
        c. Instead, meclizine is used for 1–2 weeks, and then the patient is reassessed. Stop meclizine on the day the patient returns; it may suppress the positional nystagmus.
        d. For patients with severe positional vertigo during the Dix-Hallpike maneuver, premedicate with a prochlorperazine (Compazine) 25 mg suppository 1 hour prior to performance of the CRP.
        e. If the Dix-Hallpike is positive on the left, use a left-sided CRP. Conversely, if it is positive on the right, use a right-sided CRP. If the patient has bilateral disease, refer him or her to an otolaryngologist or treat the more symptomatic side first.
        f. Epley recommends wearing a cervical collar for 2 nights after the maneuver, plus some other special instructions, to try to prevent the otoconia returning to the posterior semicircular canal.
B. Patient teaching: Encourage compliance with bed rest and exercises.
C. Pharmaceutical therapy
    1. Acute vertigo:
    Antiemetic: prochlorperazine (Compazine) 5–10 mg by mouth or IM injection, or 25 mg per rectum; dose may be repeated in 6–8 hours as needed.
        a. Dimenhydrinate (Dramamine) 25–100 mg by mouth, IM or IV every 4–8 hours.
        b. Promethazine (Phenergan) 12.5–25 mg orally, IM, or rectally every 4–12 hours.
        c. Vestibular sedative

i. Cinnarizine 15 mg orally, may be repeated every 8 hours as needed.

ii. Meclizine (Antivert) 12.5–50 mg every 4–8 hours as needed.

iii. Diazepam (Valium) 2–10 mg every 6–8 hours as needed.

2. Chronic vertigo
   a. Cinnarizine 15 mg orally, may be repeated every 8 hours as needed.
   b. Clonazepam (Klonopin) 0.5–1.0 mg every 8 hours as needed. Dosage may be increased 0.5–1.0 mg every 3 days until desired response, not to exceed 20 mg/day.
   c. Carbamazepine (Tegretol) 100 mg twice daily; dosage may be increased 100 mg every 12 hours, not to exceed 1.2 g/day.

3. Meniere's disease
   a. Consider diuretics such as hydrochlorothiazide and triamterene (Diazide) together will help with vertigo but may not reduce hearing loss.
   b. Tricyclic antidepressants may be used in resistant cases.

4. Benign paroxysmal positional vertigo: Symptomatic relief can be achieved with medications described under acute vertigo.

Follow-up

A. Follow up as needed according to origin of the diagnosis and the patient's needs.

Consultation/Referral

A. Refer to a physician if the patient does not experience improvement in 2–4 weeks. If symptoms worsen, consider referring to an ENT specialist.

REFERENCES

All about multiple sclerosis. (n.d.). Retrieved August 25, 2009, from http://www.mult-sclerosis.org/

American Academy of Pediatrics Steering Committee on Quality Improvement and Management, Subcommittee on Febrile Seizures. (2008, June). Febrile seizures: Clinical Practice Guideline for the long-term management of the child with simple febrile seizures. *Pediatrics, 121*(6), 1281–1286.

American Psychiatric Association. (1994). *Diagnostic and statistical manual of mental disorders* (4th ed.). Washington, DC: Author.

Bajwa, Z. H., & Sabahat, A. (2009, October 15). Headache syndromes other than migraine. *UpToDate.* Retrieved January 21, 2010, from http://www.uptodate.com/online/content/topic.do?topicKey=headache/5253&view=print

Bajwa, Z. H., & Wootton, R. J. (2009, July 10). Evaluation of headache in adults. *UpToDate.* Retrieved January 21, 2010, from http://www.uptodate.com/online/content/topic.do?topicKey=headache/5074&view=print

Bauer, C. A., & Coker, N. J. (1996). Update on facial nerve disorders. *Otolaryngologic Clinics of North America, 29,* 445–454.

Bear, M. F., Connors, B. W., & Paradiso, M. A. (Eds.). (2007). *Neuroscience: Exploring the brain.* (3rd ed.). Philadelphia: Lippincott, William & Wilkins.

Berlit, P. (1996). *Memorix neurology.* London: Chapman & Hall Medical.

Besdine, R., Rubenstein, L., & Snyder, L. (Eds.). (1996). *Medical care of the nursing home resident: What a physician needs to know.* Philadelphia: American College of Physicians.

Blass, J. P. (1996). Age-associated memory impairment and Alzheimer's disease. *Journal of the American Geriatric Society, 44,* 209–211.

Bonthius, D. J., & Lee, A. G. (2009, September 27). Approach to the child with headache. *UpToDate.* Retrieved January 21,

2010, from http://www.uptodate.com/online/content/topic.do?topicKey=gen_pedi/13001&view=print

Burke, M. E. (1993). Myasthenia gravis and pregnancy. *Journal of Perinatal and Neonatal Nursing, 7,* 11–21.

Burns, T. M. (2008). Guillain-Barré syndrome. *Seminary in Neurology, 28,* 152–167.

Calhoun, A. H., Ford, S., Millen, C., Finkle, A. G., Truong, Y., & Nie, Y. (in press). The prevalence of neck pain in migraine. *Headache.*

Centers for Disease Control and Prevention. (2006, July). *Facts about traumatic brain injury.* Retrieved December 22, 2009, from http://www.biausa.org/elements/aboutbi/factsheets/factsaboutbi_2008.pdf

Centers for Disease Control and Prevention. (2008, April 1). *Traumatic brain injury.* Retrieved December 22, 2009, from http://www.cdc.gov/traumaticbraininjury/tbi_concussion.html

Centers for Disease Control and Prevention. (2009, March 20). *First aid for seizures.* Retrieved February 27, 2010, from http://www.cdc.gov/epilepsy/basics/first_aid.htm

Centers for Disease Control and Prevention. (2010, February 2). *Epilepsy.* Retrieved February 27, 2010, from http://www.cdc.gov/epilepsy/

Centers for Disease Control and Prevention. (n.d.). *Facts about concussion and brain injury.* Retrieved December 22, 2009, from http://www.cdc.gov/NCIPC/tbi/tbibook.pdf

Cognitive dysfunction. (n.d.). Retrieved August 25, 2009, from http://www.mult-sclerosis.org/cognitivedysfunction.html

Coutin, I., & Glass, S. (1996). Recognizing uncommon headache syndrome. *American Family Physician, 54,* 2247–2252.

Cruse, R. P. (2009, January 8). Overview of Guillain-Barré syndrome in children. *UpToDate.* Retrieved February 21, 2010, from http://www.uptodate.com/online/content/topic.do?topicKey=ped_neur/9790&view=print

Cucchiara, B. L., & Messé, S. R. (2009, June 18). Antiplatelet therapy for secondary prevention of stroke. *UpToDate.* Retrieved January 21, 2010, from http://www.uptodate.com/online/content/topic.do?topicKey=cva_dise/12856&view=print

Cummings, J. L. (2008). The black book of Alzheimer's disease, part 2. *Primary Psychiatry, 15,* 69–90.

DeGowin, R. (1994). *Diagnostic examination* (6th ed.). New York: McGraw-Hill.

Dematteis, J. A. (1996). Guillain-Barré syndrome: A team approach to diagnosis and treatment. *American Family Physician, 54,* 197–300.

Diamond, S. (2005). Prevention and symptomatic relief of migraine: Which drugs to choose? *Clinical Advisor, April*(Suppl.), 9–14.

Dodick, D. (1997). Headache as a symptom of ominous disease. *Postgraduate Medicine, 101,* 46–66.

Donofrio, P. D., Berger, A., & Brannagan, T. H., et.al. (2009). Consensus statement: The use of intravenous immunoglobulin in the treatment of neuromuscular conditions report of the AANEM Ad Hoc Committee. *Muscle & Nerve, 40,* 890–900.

Donohoe, K. M. (1994). Nursing care of the patient with myasthenia gravis. *Neurologic Clinics of North America, 12,* 369–385.

Edmeads, J. (1997). Headaches in older people. *Postgraduate Medicine, 101,* 91–100.

Epilepsy Foundation. (n.d.). *Diagnosing epilepsy.* Retrieved February 27, 2010, from http://www.epilepsyfoundation.org/about/diagnosis/

Epilepsy Foundation. (n.d.). *Driver information by state.* Retrieved February 27, 2010, from http://www.epilepsyfoundation.org/living/wellness/transportation/drivinglaws.cfm

Epilepsy Foundation. (n.d.). *Epilepsy and seniors.* Retrieved February 27, 2010, from http://www.epilepsyfoundation.org/living/seniors/latercauses.cfm

Epilepsy Foundation. (n.d.). *Epilepsy treatment for seniors.* Retrieved February 27, 2010, from http://www.epilepsyfoundation.org/living/seniors/latertreatment.cfm

Epilepsy Foundation. (n.d.). *First aid for seizures.* Retrieved February 27, 2010, from http://www.epilepsyfoundation.org/about/firstaid/

Epilepsy Foundation. (n.d.). *Photosensitivity and epilepsy.* Retrieved February 27, 2010, from http://www.epilepsyfoundation.org/about/photosensitivity/gerba.cfm

Epilepsy Foundation. (n.d.). *Prolonged or serial seizures (status epilepticus).* Retrieved February 27, 2010, from http://www.epilepsyfoundation.org/about/types/types/statusepilepticus.cfm

Epilepsy Foundation. (n.d.). *Seizure triggers and precipitants.* Retrieved February 27, 2010, from http://www.epilepsyfoundation.org/about/types/triggers/livingtrigger.cfm\

Epilepsy Foundation. (n.d.). *Senior's health issues.* Retrieved February 27, 2010, from http://www.epilepsyfoundation.org/living/seniors/

Epilepsy Foundation. (n.d.). *The treatment decision.* Retrieved February 27, 2010, from http://www.epilepsyfoundation.org/about/diagnosis/decision.cfm

Epilepsy Foundation. (n.d.). *Treatment.* Retrieved February 27, 2010, from http://www.epilepsyfoundation.org/about/treatment/

Epilepsy Foundation (n.d.). *Types of seizures.* Retrieved February 27, 2010, from http://www.epilepsyfoundation.org/about/types/types/index.cfm

Epilepsy Foundation. (n.d.). *Women's health issues.* Retrieved February 27, 2010, from http://www.epilepsyfoundation.org/living/women/index.cfm

Ernst, D., & Lee, A. (Eds.). (2009–2010, Winter). *NPPR: Nurse practitioners' prescribing reference.* New York: A Haymarket Media Publication.

Farrell, M. A. (in press). Medical management of Lennox-Gastaut syndrome. *CNS Drugs.*

Fettes, I. (1997). Menstrual migraine. *Postgraduate Medicine, 101,* 67–80.

Fishman, M. A. (2009, September 28). Febrile seizures. *UpToDate.* Retrieved January 21, 2010, from http://www.uptodate.com/online/content/topic.do?topicKey=ped_neur/22060&view=print

Goldstein, J. N. (2009, November 17). Transient ischemia attack. *emedicine.* Retrieved January 21, 2010, from http://emedicine.medscape.com/article/794281-print

Greenberg, M. (1994). *Handbook of neurosurgery* (3rd ed.). Lakeland, FL: Greenberg Graphics.

Greenberg, M. S. (1997). *Handbook of neurosurgery* (Vol. 1). Lakcland, FL: Greenberg Graphics.

Gunner, K. B., Smith, H. D., Cromwell, P. F., & Yetman, R. J. (2007). Practice guideline for diagnosis and management of migraine headaches in children and adolescents: Part one. *Journal of Pediatric Health Care, 21,* 327–332.

Gunner, K. B., Smith, H. D., & Ferguson, L. E. (2008). Practice guidelines for diagnosis and management of migraine headaches in children and adolescents: Part two. *Journal of Pediatric Health Care, 22,* 52–59.

Haefner, H., & Fitzsimmons, M. (1997). Carpel tunnel syndrome. *The Female Patient, 22,* 21–31.

Hall, G. R., Gallagher, M., & Dougherty, J. (2009). Integrating roles for successful dementia management. *The Nurse Practitioner, 34,* 35–41.

Hayes, Inc. (2009, February 2). *Hayes news service: Stem cell transplantation and relapsing-remitting multiple sclerosis.* Retrieved August 28, 2009, from https://www.hayesinc.com/subscribers/displaySubscriberArticle.do?articleId=9219&searchStore=%24search_type%3Dall%24icd%3D%24keywords%3Dmultiple%2Csclerosis%24status%3Dall%24page%3D1%24from_date%3D%24to_date%3D%24report_type_options%3D%24technology_type_options%3D%24organ_system_options%3D%24specialty_options%3D%24order%3DsearchRelevance

Hayes, Inc. (2009, April 13). *Health Technology Brief: Natalizumab (Tysabri®, Biogen Idec and Elan Pharmaceuticals) for relapsing remitting multiple sclerosis.* Retrieved August 28, 2009, from https://www.hayesinc.com/subscribers/displaySubscriberArticle.do?articleId=9617&searchStore=%24search_type%3Dall%24icd%3D%24keywords%3Dmultiple%2Csclerosis%24status%3Dall%24page%3D1%24from_date%3D%24to_date%3D%24report_type_options%3D%24technology_type_options%3D%24organ_system_options%3D%24specialty_options%3D%24order%3DsearchRelevance

Hershey, A. D. (2010). Current approaches to the diagnosis and management of paediatric migraine. *Lancet Neurology, 9,* 190–204.

Hickey, J. V. (1997). *The clinical practice of neurological and neurosurgical nursing* (4th ed., pp. 613–625). Philadelphia: Lippincott.

Hoole, A. J., Pickard, C. G., Jr., Ouimette, R. M., Lohr, J. A., & Greenberg, R. A. (1995). *Patient care guidelines for nurse practitioners* (4th ed., pp. 70–73). Philadelphia: Lippincott.

Hopkins, L. C. (1994). Clinical features of myasthenia gravis. *Neurologic Clinics of North America, 12,* 243–26l.

Hughes, R.A.C., Wijdicks, E.F.M., & Benson, E., et. al. (2005). Supportive care for patients with Guillain-Barré syndrome. *Archives of Neurology, 62,* 1194–1198.

Hund, E. F., Borel, C. O., Cornblath, D. R., Hanley, D. F., & McKhann, G. M. (1993). Intensive management of severe Guillain-Barré syndrome. *Critical Care Medicine, 22,* 433–446.

International Headache Society ICHD–II. (n.d.). *Chronic migraine.* Retrieved February 18, 2010, from http://www.ihs-classification.org/en/

International Headache Society ICHD–II. (n.d.). *Cluster headache.* Retrieved February 20, 2010, from http://www.ihs-classification.org/en/

International Headache Society ICHD–II. (n.d.). *Medication overuse headache.* Retrieved February 20, 2010, from http://www.ihs-classification.org/en/

International Headache Society ICHD–II. (n.d.). *Migraine.* Retrieved February 17, 2010, from http://www.ihs-classification.org/en/

International Headache Society ICHD–II. (n.d.). *Tension-type headache.* Retrieved February 20, 2010, from http://www.ihs-classification.org/en/

Isselbacher, K. J., Braunwald, E., Wilson, J. D., Martin, J. B., Fauci, A. S., & Kasper, D. L. (1994). *Harrison's principles of internal medicine* (13th ed., p. 2227). New York: McGraw-Hill.

Johnson, R. T., & Griffin, J. W. (1997). *Current therapy in neurologic disease* (5th ed.). New York: Mosby.

Jones, H. R. (1996). Childhood Guillain-Barré syndrome: Clinical presentation, diagnosis, and therapy. *Journal of Child Neurology, 11,* 4–12.

Kistler, J. P., Furie, K. L., & Ay, H. (2009, October 13). Initial evaluation and management of transient ischemic attack and minor stroke. *UpToDate.* Retrieved January 21, 2010, from http://www.uptodate.com/online/content/topic.do?topicKey=cva_dise/6023&view=print

Knox, G. W., & McPherson, A. (1997). Meniere's disease: Differential diagnosis and treatment. *American Family Physician, 55,* 1185–1190.

Koller, W. C., Silver, D., & Lieberman, A. (1994). An algorithm for the management of Parkinson's disease. *Neurology, 44,* S1–S52.

Krumholz, A., & Hopp, J. (2009, June 10). Driving restrictions for patients with seizures and epilepsy. *UpToDate.* Retrieved January 21, 2010, from http://www.uptodate.com/online/content/topic.do?topicKey=epil_eeg/7166&view=print

Kuitwaard, K., van Koningsveld, R., & Ruts, L., et al. (2009). Recurrent Guillain-Barré syndrome. *Journal of Neurology Neurosurgery Psychiatry, 80,* 56–59.

Kutcher, J., Lee, M. J., & Hickenbottom, S. (2009, May 1). Neurologic disorders complicating pregnancy. *Online 16.3.* Retrieved August 28, 2009, from http://www.uptodate.com/online/content/topic.do?topicKey=medneuro/8805&view=print

Lazoff, M. (2009, July 16). Multiple sclerosis. *emedicine.* Retrieved August 28, 2009, from http://emedicine.medscape.com/article/793013-print

Levin, B. E., Tomer, R., & Rey, G. J. (1992). Cognitive impairments in Parkinson's disease. *Neurologic Clinics, 10,* 471–485.

Lieberman, A. (1992). An integrated approach to patient management in Parkinson's disease. *Neurologic Clinics, 10,* 553–565.

Lonergan, E. (Ed.). (1996). *Geriatrics.* Stamford, CT: Appleton & Lange.

Loteze, T. E. (2009, May 1). Pathogenesis, clinical features, and diagnosis of pediatric multiple sclerosis. Retrieved August 28, 2009, from http://www.uptodate.com/online/content/topic.do?topicKey=ped_neur/8027&view=print

Luxon, L. M. (1996). Vertigo: New approaches to diagnosis and management. *British Journal of Hospital Medicine, 55,* 519–541.

Mandel, S., Sataloff, R. T., & Schapiro, S. R. (1993). *Minor head trauma: Assessment, management, and rehabilitation.* New York: Springer-Verlag.

McMahon-Parkes, K., & Cornock, N. A. (1997). Guillain-Barré syndrome: Biological basis, treatment, and care. *Intensive and Critical Care Nursing, 13,* 42–48.

Merkies, I. S. J., Schmitz, P. I. M., van der Meché, F. G. A., Samihn, J., & van Doorn, P. A. (2002). Clinimetric evaluation of a new overall disability scale in immune mediated polyneuropathies. *Journal of Neurology Neurosurgery Psychiatry, 72,* 596–601.

Meyer, H. (2009, December). Pharmacological management for the adult migraine sufferer. *Journal of Neuroscience Nursing, 41,* 348–352.

Morrell, M. J. (1993). Differential diagnosis of seizures. *Neurologic Clinics, 11,* 737–754.

Mukerji, S., Aloka, F., & Farooq, M. U., et. al. (2009). Cardiovascular complication of the Guillain-Barré syndrome. *American Journal of Cardiology, 104,* 1452–1455.

National Institute of Health and Clinical Excellence, National Collaborating Centre for Women's and Children's Health. (2007, May). *Feverish illness in children: Assessment and initial management in children younger than 5 years.* Clinical Guideline No. 47. Retrieved February 13, 2010, from http://www.nice.org.uk/nicemedia/pdf/CG47Guidance.pdf

National Institute of Neurological Disorders and Stroke. (n.d.). *NINDS multiple sclerosis information page.* Retrieved August 28, 2009, from http://www.ninds.nih.gov/disorders/multiple_sclerosis/multiple_sclerosis.htm

National Institutes of Health. (n.d.). *NIH stroke scale.* Retrieved February 20, 2010, from http://www.ninds.nih.gov/doctors/NIH_Stroke_Scale.pdf

Norwitz, E. R. (2009, June 30). Eclampsia. *UpToDate.* Retrieved January 21, 2010, from http://www.uptodate.com/online/content/topic.do?topicKey=cc_obst/3033&view=print

Nutt, J., & Wooten, G. F. (2005). Diagnosis abdominal initial management of Parkinson's disease. *New England Journal of Medicine, 353,* 1021–1027.

Olek, M. J. (2009, February 27). Diagnosis of multiple sclerosis in adults. *UpToDate Online 16.3.* Retrieved August 28, 2009, from http://www.uptodate.com/online/content/topic.do?topicKey=demyelin/4438&view=print

Ouslander, J., Osterweil, D., & Morley, J. (1997). *Medical care in the nursing home* (2nd ed.). New York: McGraw-Hill.

Outzen, M. (2009). Management of fever in older adults. *Journal of Gerontological Nursing, 35,* 17–25.

Parry, G. (1993). *Guillain-Barré syndrome.* New York: Thieme Medical Publishers.

Patten, J. P. (1996). *Neurological differential diagnosis* (2nd ed.). New York: Springer.

Pestauro, K. A. (2009). Modern management of the migraine headache. *American Journal of Lifestyle Medicine, 3,* 147–159.

Poewe, W. (1993). Clinical features, diagnosis, and imaging of parkinsonian syndromes. *Current Opinion in Neurology and Neurosurgery, 6,* 333–338.

Pulec, J. L. (1995). Surgical treatment of vertigo. *Acta Otolaryngol, 519,* 21–25.

Rains, J. C. (2008). Chronic headache and potentially modifiable risk factors: Screening and behavioral management of sleep disorders. *Headache, 48,* 32–39.

Reichel, W. (Ed.). (1995). *Care of the elderly* (4th ed.). Baltimore: Williams & Wilkins.

Reilly, P., & Bullock, R. (1997). *Head injury.* London: Chapman & Hall.

Rosenfield, D. (1995). Headaches: How to distinguish neck induced from vascular pain, and what to do. *Consultant, 35,* 1495–1500.

Ruckenstein, M. J. (1995). A practical approach to dizziness. *Postgraduate Medicine, 97,* 70–81.

Ryan, C. (1996). Evaluation of patients with chronic headaches. *American Family Physician, 54,* 1051–1057.

Sadleir, L. G., & Scheffer, I. E. (2007). Febrile seizures. *British Medical Journal, 334,* 307–311.

Sanders, D. B., & Scoppetta, C. (1994). The treatment of patients with myasthenia gravis. *Neurologic Clinics of North America, 12,* 343–367.

Schachter, S. C. (2009, September 24). Overview of the management of epilepsy in adults. *UpToDate.* Retrieved January 21, 2009, from http://www.uptodate.com/online/content/topic.do?topicKey=epil_eeg/4878&view=print

Scott, B. L., & Stacy, M. A. (2009, June). The management of Parkinson's disease in the primary care setting. *Clinician Reviews* (Self Study Supplement), 1–12.

Siderowf, A., & Stern, M. (2003). Update on Parkinson's disease. *Annals of Internal Medicine, 138,* 651–658.

Smith, T. R., & Stoneman, J. (2006 April). What do you recommend to a patient taking analgesics for headache on a daily basis? *Clinician Reviews* (Suppl. Migraine Management FAQs), 6–10.

Soreff, S. (2009, April 9). Suicide. *emedicine.* Retrieved August 31, 2009, from http://emedicine.medscape.com/article/288598-print

Sprenger, T., & Goadsby, P. J. (2009). Migraine pathogenesis and state of pharmacological treatment options [Electronic version]. *BMC Medicine, 7.* Retrieved February 13, 2010, from http://www.biomedcentral.com/content/pdf/1741-7015-7-71.pdf

Stacy, M., & Jancovic, J. (1992). Differential diagnosis of Parkinson's disease and the parkinsonism plus syndromes. *Neurologic Clinics, 10,* 341–359.

Stewart, D. P., Kaylor, J., & Koutanis, E. (1996). Cognitive deficits in presumed minor head-injured patients. *Academic Emergency Medicine, 3,* 21–26.

Strengell, T., Uhari, M., Tarkka, R., Uusimaa, J., Alen, R., Lautala, P., et al. (2009). Antipyretic agents for preventing recurrences of febrile seizures. *Archives of Pediatric Adolescent Medicine, 163*(9), 799–804.

Swoboda, K. J., & Drislane, F. W. (1994). Seizure disorders: Syndromes, diagnosis, and management. *Comprehensive Therapy, 20,* 67–73.

Tabaton, M. (1994). Research advance in the biology of Alzheimer's disease. *Clinical Geriatric Medicine, 10,* 249.

Tanner, C. M. (1992). Epidemiology of Parkinson's disease. *Neurologic Clinics, 10,* 317–329.

Taylor, F. R. (2008, February 11). Tension-type headache in adults: Acute treatment. *UpToDate.* Retrieved January 21, 2010, from http://www.uptodate.com/online/content/topic.do?topicKey=headache/8484&view=print

The Merck Manuals for Healthcare Professionals. (2007). *Dementia.* Retrieved April 3, 2010, from http://www.merck.com/mmpe/sec16/ch213/ch213c.html#tb_213-003

Treiman, D. M. (1993). Current treatment strategies in selected situations in epilepsy. *Epilepsia, 34,* S17–S22.

U.S. Department of Health and Human Services, Centers for Disease Control and Prevention. (2008a, December 23). *Acute Concussion Evaluation (ACE).* Retrieved December 22, 2009, from http://cdc.gov/NCIPC/tbi/ACE-a.pdf

U.S. Department of Health and Human Services, Centers for Disease Control and Prevention. (2008b, December 23). *Heads up: Brain injury in your practice, a tool kit for physicians.* Retrieved December 22, 2009, from http://cdc.gov/NCIPC/tbi/physicians_tool_kit.htm

U.S. Department of Health and Human Services, Centers for Disease Control and Prevention. (2008c, December 23). *Heads up: Facts for physicians about mild traumatic brain injury.* Retrieved December 22, 2009, from http://cdc.gov/NCIPC/tbi/Facts_for_Physicians_booklet.pdf

U.S. Department of Health and Human Services, Centers for Disease Control and Prevention. (n.d.). *Heads up: Preventing concussion.* Retrieved January 23, 2010, from http://cdc.gov/NCIPC/tbi/Heads_Up_factsheet_english.pdf

Visser, L. H., van der Meche, F.G.A., Meulstee, J., Roth-Barth, P. P., Jacobs, B. C., Schmitz, P.I.M., et al. (1996). Cytomegalovirus infection and Guillain-Barré syndrome: The clinical, electrophysiologic, and prognostic factors. *Neurology, 47,* 668–673.

Vriesendorp, F. J. (2009a, June 9). Treatment and prognosis of Guillain-Barré syndrome in adults. *UpToDate.* Retrieved February 21, 2010, from http://www.uptodate.com/online/content/topic.do?topicKey=muscle/8595&view=print

Vriesendorp, F. J. (2009b, July 22). Clinical features and diagnosis of Guillain-Barré syndrome in adults. *UpToDate.* Retrieved February 21, 2010, from http://www.uptodate.com/online/content/topic.do?topicKey=muscle/14568&view=print

WebMD. (2010). *Migraines & headaches guide.* Retrieved February 15, 2010, from http://www.webmd.com/migraines-headaches/guide/headache-diary

Widner, H., & Rehncrona, S. (1993). Transplantation and surgical treatment of parkinsonian syndromes. *Current Opinion in Neurology and Neurosurgery, 6,* 344–349.

Wright, W. (2005a). Practitioners on the frontline: Assessing patients for migraine. *Clinical Advisor, April*(Suppl.), 3–8.

Wright, W. (2005b). Serotonin agonists target the pathogenesis of migraine. *Clinical Advisor, April*(Suppl.), 15–20.

Endocrine Guidelines

Lynn Followell

⬛ ADDISON'S DISEASE

Definition
A. Primary adrenal insufficiency resulting in glucocorticoid and mineralocorticoid insufficiency.

Incidence
A. Approximately 1–4/100,000 persons; men and women equally affected.

Pathogenesis
A. Autoimmune dysfunction of the adrenals accounts for up to 80% of cases; 10%–20% of cases are attributed to tuberculosis. At least 90% of the adrenal gland is destroyed, resulting in chronic cortisol deficiency, reduced aldosterone, and decreased adrenal androgens. As a result, volume and sodium depletions occur with potassium excess.

Predisposing Factors
A. Other autoimmune disorders
   1. Insulin-dependent diabetes mellitus
   2. Pernicious anemia
   3. Thyroid disorders
B. Disseminated tuberculosis
C. Gonadal failure
D. Hypoparathyroidism
E. Vitiligo
F. Alopecia areata
G. Chronic active hepatitis
H. Metastatic disease (especially lung and breast cancer)
I. Acquired immunodeficiency syndrome (AIDS)
J. Certain medications (e.g., ketoconazole, anticoagulant)
K. Fungal disease
L. Bleeding diathesis (e.g., disseminated intravascular coagulation [DIC])
M. Sepsis
N. Metabolic stress
O. Trauma

Common Complaints
A. Weakness
B. Fatigue
C. Anorexia
D. Nausea
E. Diarrhea
F. Abdominal pain
G. Weight loss
H. Hyperpigmentation

Other Signs and Symptoms
A. Proximal muscle weakness
B. Failure to gain weight (children)
C. Muscle and joint pain
D. Reduced axillary/pubic hair in women
E. Amenorrhea
F. Hypotension
G. Anemia with
   1. Lymphocytosis
   2. Eosinophilia
   3. Neutropenia
   4. Hyponatremia
   5. Hyperkalemia
   6. Hypoglycemia
   7. Hypercalcemia
H. Positive antiadrenal antibodies
I. Low plasma cortisol or failure to rise after corticotropin (ACTH) administration
J. EKG changes: decreased voltage, prolonged PR and QT intervals, and general slowed rhythm

Acute adrenal crisis, medical emergency: sudden low back, abdominal, or leg pain; severe vomiting or diarrhea; hypotension; and loss of consciousness.

Subjective Data
A. Determine extent of fatigue.
B. Elicit degree and location of weakness.
C. Question the patient regarding appetite, nausea, or diarrhea.
D. Evaluate food intake.
E. Determine the amount of weight loss or weight gain (children).
F. Discuss hypopigmentation or hyperpigmentation and whether it occurs on unexposed areas as well as exposed areas of the skin.

G. Note presence of abdominal, muscle, and joint pain.

H. Assess for lightheadedness and/or fainting and when it occurs.

I. Inquire about the patient's history of cancer or fungal infections.

J. Note last date of tuberculosis evaluation (purified protein derivative [PPD]) and results.

K. Determine human immunodeficiency virus (HIV) status or risk.

L. For women, discuss pubic and axillary hair distribution and note menstrual patterns.

M. Inquire about libido.

N. Inquire regarding cold intolerance.

Physical Examination

A. Check temperature, pulse, respirations, and blood pressure; pulse and blood pressure seated and standing, weight.

B. Inspect
1. Observe overall appearance.
2. Note hair distribution and skin pigmentation.

C. Auscultate
1. Auscultate the heart, lungs, and abdomen.

D. Palpate
1. Palpate the abdomen.

E. Musculoskeletal: perform complete musculoskeletal examination.

Diagnostic Tests

A. Serum chemistry and electrolytes.

B. Complete blood count (CBC).

C. PPD.

D. Rapid ACTH test: Rapid ACTH stimulation test excludes or establishes adrenal insufficiency but does not differentiate between primary and secondary adrenal insufficiency; with abnormal results (plasma cortisol < 18–20 µg/dL), proceed to plasma ACTH levels.

E. Plasma ACTH level.

Plasma ACTH level differentiates between primary (adrenal) and secondary (pituitary) or tertiary (hypothalamus) etiologies (high plasma ACTH with primary whereas normal or low with secondary insufficiency). The clinician can use corticotropin-releasing hormone (CRH) to distinguish between pituitary and hypothalamic etiologies.

F. Antiadrenal antibodies: A negative adrenal antibody test is observed in 30%–50% of persons with idiopathic Addison's disease and does not rule out adrenal insufficiency of autoimmune etiology.

G. Computed tomography (CT) scan of adrenals.

Differential Diagnoses

A. Secondary adrenal insufficiency (usually after exogenous glucocorticoid therapy)

B. Hypothalamic/pituitary lesions

C. Diabetic coma

D. Salt-losing nephritis

E. Acute infections

F. Occult cancer

G. Anorexia nervosa

H. Hemochromatosis

I. Acute poisoning

J. Myasthenia gravis

K. Pigmentation due to racial/ethnic variations

L. Premature primary ovarian failure

M. Testicular failure

N. Pernicious anemia

O. Cancer

P. Iatrogenic Cushing's syndrome

Plan

A. General interventions
1. If primary adrenal insufficiency is established, and the cause is not apparent, order adrenal CT scan to look for metastatic disease, sarcoidosis, and tuberculosis.

B. Patient teaching
1. See the Section III Patient Teaching Guide for this chapter, "Addison's Disease."
2. Teach the patient regarding adrenal crisis and encourage treatment before symptoms begin.
3. Encourage the patient to avoid contacts that predispose him or her to infections.

C. Pharmaceutical therapy
1. Hydrocortisone (drug of choice) or prednisone in three doses (every 8 hours), or two-thirds in the morning and the remainder in the afternoon or early evening; 12–15 mg cortisol/m^2 body surface area; most adults need a total of 20–30 mg/day.
2. Increase hydrocortisone dose or add prednisone if ill; if accompanied by diarrhea, excessive sweating, or fever, the patient should double routine dose.
3. Simultaneously decrease fludrocortisone about 50% to avoid salt retention and elevated blood pressure.
   a. Total daily stress dose is about 100–400 mg hydrocortisone.
4. If serum aldosterone is undetectable, mineralocorticoid replacement is likely necessary in addition to glucocorticoid.
5. Abrupt discontinuation of exogenous glucocorticoid administration after course as short as 3 weeks may induce temporary secondary adrenal insufficiency, leading to decreased cortisol but normal or near-normal aldosterone production. This may occur up to 12 months after discontinuation of glucocorticoid therapy.
6. Pediatrics
   a. Hydrocortisone 10–20 mg/m^2/d in three to four divided doses; with adrenal enzyme defects: 25% in morning and afternoon and 50% at night.
   b. Fludrocortisone acetate typically 0.05–0.2 mg/day every day or two divided doses for children.

Follow-up

A. Plasma renin activity: when less than 10 ng/mL, this is a probable indication of adequate fludrocortisone dose.

B. Serum and urinary cortisol and serum ACTH to monitor hydrocortisone dose. Urinary free cortisol greater than 70 µg/24 hours indicates excessive hydrocortisone dose, whereas values less than 20 µg/24 hours indicate inadequate hydrocortisone dose.

C. Monitor blood pressure and serum electrolytes to determine fludrocortisone dose.

D. Do annual adrenal function studies.

Consultation/Referral

A. If Addison's disease is suspected, consult with a physician.
B. Consider Addison's disease in any patient with hypotension and hyperkalemia.

Individual Considerations

A. Pregnancy
1. Due to changes in plasma cortisol, diagnosis is based on lack of rise in plasma cortisol concentration after ACTH administration.
2. If nausea and vomiting are problems, intramuscular glucocorticoid may be necessary.
3. Delivery requires increased glucocorticoid dose similar to surgery.
B. Pediatrics
1. Leading causes of Addison's disease are hereditary enzymatic defects resulting in congenital adrenal hyperplasia, as well as idiopathic causes.
C. Geriatrics
1. Urinary excretion rate of cortisol decreases by about 25%; serum level and response to ACTH stimulation are unchanged.

CUSHING'S SYNDROME

Definition

A. Cushing's syndrome is a cluster of symptoms, signs, and biochemical abnormalities arising from glucocorticoid overproduction. Iatrogenically induced Cushing's syndrome is the type most frequently observed clinically.

Incidence

A. For endogenous cases, 2–4 new cases per 1,000,000 annually; it is five times more frequent in women.

Pathogenesis

The cause is exogenous (chronic glucocorticoid or ACTH administration) or endogenous (increased ACTH secretion). The endogenous type is due to either excessive pituitary or ectopic ACTH secretion (ACTH dependent) resulting in signs of androgen excess or autonomous cortisol overproduction (ACTH independent [of ACTH regulation]) resulting in depressed ACTH production and absent signs of androgen excess. The etiology of spontaneous Cushing's (adults) comprises:

A. 70%–80% pituitary ACTH hypersecretion (90% pituitary adenoma, 10% pituitary hyperplasia).
B. 10%–15% autonomous adrenal tumor (adenoma or carcinoma).
C. 5%–15% ectopic ACTH secretion (nonpituitary neoplasm, usually lung).
D. less than 1% bilateral nodular hyperplasia without ACTH.
E. Among children younger than 12 years, the cause is usually iatrogenic. Cortisol excess precipitates generalized protein catabolism, reduced intestinal calcium reabsorption, elevated hepatic glucogenesis and glycogenosis, impaired collagen production leading to atrophy of connective and fatty tissues, impaired immune and inflammatory responses, and accelerated atherosclerosis.

Predisposing Factors

A. Exogenous glucocorticoid administration
B. Excess alcohol intake
C. Pituitary adenoma
D. Thoracic tumors
E. Adrenal neoplasms
F. Tumors of the pancreas
G. Thyroid and thymus disease
H. Pheochromocytoma

Common Complaints

A. Excessive coarse hair on face, chest, and back
B. Rapid weight gain
C. Easy bruising
D. Muscle weakness
E. Oligo- or amenorrhea
F. Impotence

Other Signs and Symptoms

A. Cervicodorsal and supraclavicular fat pad
B. Hirsutism in women
C. Acne and/or folliculitis
D. Increased intraocular pressure
E. Purple striae
F. Increased blood pressure
G. Polydipsia/polyuria, increased serum glucose and glycosuria
H. Osteopenia/osteoporosis
I. Mood lability/changes
J. Growth deceleration (children)
K. Delayed skeletal maturation (children)
L. Spontaneous hypokalemia
M. Erythrocytosis

Subjective Data

A. Ask if the patient has taken exogenous glucocorticoids.
B. Determine whether the onset of complaints was acute or subacute.
C. Assess for bruising and determine if bruising was precipitated by trauma.
D. Assess for muscle weakness and, if present, whether it is proximal weakness.
E. Review the patient's menstrual history, including characteristics of menstrual periods.
F. Identify the patient's family history of similar problems.
G. Question the patient regarding any vision impairment.
H. Rule out the presence of abdominal pain.
I. Review the patient's history of neoplasms and location.
J. Identify the current pattern of sexual function.
K. Question the patient regarding mood swings or recent treatment for psychiatric disorder.
L. Identify the pattern of weight gain and effectiveness of weight loss interventions, if implemented.
M. Assess for the presence of leg or arm pain.
N. Review the patient's history of fractures, especially if postmenopausal.
O. Determine the amount of alcohol consumed.

Physical Examination

A. Temperature, pulse, height, and weight.
B. Inspect

1. Inspect the skin, noting hair distribution, lesions, bruising, and striae.
2. Observe the face and note shape.
3. Observe the neck.

Note that "moon-shaped" face and fat pads in posterior neck ("buffalo hump") are characteristics of patients with Cushing's syndrome.

4. Complete funduscopic examination. Be alert for cataracts, glaucoma, and/or signs of benign intracranial hypertension.
C. Auscultate
   1. Auscultate the heart and lungs.
D. Musculoskeletal
   1. Complete musculoskeletal examination. Be alert for septic necrosis of femoral and/or humeral head.

Diagnostic Tests

A. Serum electrolytes.
B. CBC and glucose.
C. Overnight dexamethasone test.

The overnight dexamethasone suppression test has a false-positive rate of 20%–30%; false positives can occur with obesity, stress, depression, alcoholism, pregnancy, or medications that increase the hepatic metabolism of cortisol and dexamethasone (e.g., antiseizure drugs, estrogen, and rifampin). The false-negative rate is less than 3%. Use the low-dose dexamethasone test as an alternative.

D. Plasma ACTH.

The hallmark sign is the presence of measurable plasma ACTH in persons with clinical and biochemical hypercortisolism.

1. If elevated cortisol levels are confirmed, cause is determined by plasma ACTH level response to high-dose dexamethasone.
   a. No cortisol suppression with undetectable to low ACTH levels suggests adrenal Cushing's syndrome.
   b. Suppression to less than or equal to 50% of baseline cortisol with normal to elevated ACTH suggests pituitary Cushing's syndrome.
E. 24-hour free urine cortisol.

The 24-hour urinary free cortisol is the most sensitive and specific test and is the best choice for screening.

F. High-dose dexamethasone test.
G. Bone density studies.
H. Magnetic resonance imaging (MRI) (if pituitary source suspected).
I. CT scan of abdomen/chest (if adrenal source suspected). Due to small size, CT and MRI are only able to identify 30%–50% of pituitary adenomas.
J. CRH test.

Differential Diagnoses

A. Iatrogenically induced Cushing's syndrome
B. Depression
C. Severe obesity
D. Chronic stress
E. Familial cortisol resistance
F. Medication induced (e.g., phenytoin, phenobarbital, primidone)
G. Pituitary adenoma
H. Adrenal and other neoplasms
I. Alcoholism
J. Nephrolithiasis
K. Psychosis

Plan

A. General interventions
   1. Taper glucocorticoid dose as appropriate for underlying disease.
   2. Begin alcohol detoxification if applicable.
   3. Consider hormone replacement therapy for postmenopausal women.
B. Patient teaching
   1. See the Section III Patient Teaching Guide for this chapter, "Cushing's Syndrome."
C. Medical/surgical management
   1. If noniatrogenic etiology, surgery is the treatment of choice followed by irradiation and/or chemotherapy.
D. Pharmaceutical therapy
   1. Calcium 1,000 mg/day and vitamin D 400 IU/day.
   2. Mitotane (Lysodren) 2–6 g daily or aminoglutethamid for control of adrenocortical carcinoma progression.
   3. Metyrapone inhibits adrenal steroid biosynthesis.
   4. Trilostane, ketoconazole (most useful for blocking adrenal steroidogenesis), and suramin inhibit adrenal steroid biosynthesis.
      a. For ketoconazole begin with 200 mg and increase every 4–7 days.
   5. Hydrocortisone may be given in physiologic doses to avoid adrenal insufficiency.

Most persons on daily steroid program for over 2–4 weeks have some degree of hypothalamic-pituitary-adrenal axis suppression.

   6. Mifeprisone (RU 486) is given for ectopic ACTH production or adrenal carcinoma.
   7. Cyproheptadine and bromocriptine may induce biochemical and clinical remission in a small number of persons.

Follow-up

A. At the provider's discretion, 1–2 weeks after tests are complete, follow up to discuss results and possible therapy.

Consultation/Referral

A. If Cushing's syndrome is suspected, consult with a physician regarding treatment and therapy.

Individual Considerations

A. Pregnancy
   1. Urinary free cortisol increases in the third trimester but women still have normal 17-hydroxycorticosteroids and normal diurnal variability of serum cortisol.

B. Pediatrics
   1. It is possible to differentiate between exogenous obesity and Cushing's syndrome by the child's growth rate; exogenous obesity is characterized by normal or slightly increased growth rate.

Resources

Addison and Cushing International Federation (ACIF)
PO Box 52137
2505 CC The Hague, The Netherlands
http://www.pslgroup.com/dg/6253e.htm

DIABETES MELLITUS

Definition
Diabetes is a group of diseases characterized by high levels of blood glucose with a defect in insulin secretion or action caused by a chronic disorder of carbohydrate, fat, and protein metabolism. There are three main types of diabetes: type 1, type 2, and gestational.

A. Type 1 diabetes, formerly referred to as insulin-dependent diabetes mellitus (IDDM), type I, or juvenile-onset diabetes, is an endocrine condition in which there is complete destruction of pancreatic beta cells or a complete absence of insulin.
B. Type 2 diabetes, formerly referred to as non-insulin-dependent diabetes mellitus (NIDDM), type II, or adult-onset diabetes, describes a condition in which individuals have an impairment in insulin production and/or insulin resistance.
C. Gestational diabetes is diagnosed during pregnancy. It usually disappears when the pregnancy is completed. It will increase the woman's risk of developing type 2 diabetes later in life.

Incidence
A. It is estimated that more than 15.7 million Americans have diabetes, 5.9% of the population. Diagnosed cases account for 10.3 million with an estimated 5.4 million who have not been diagnosed. Type 1 diabetes accounts for less than 10% of diagnosed cases. There are 798,000 new cases reported a year.

Pathogenesis
A. Type 1 diabetes is an inherited defect causing an alteration in immunologic integrity, placing the beta cell at risk for inflammatory damage. The mechanism of damage is autoimmune. Environmental factors that may influence the etiology of diabetes include mumps, coxsackie virus, cytomegalovirus, and hepatitis. Other factors that may influence the disease include diets high in dairy products, emotional and physical stress, and/or environmental toxins.
B. Type 2 diabetes involves impaired insulin secretion, insulin resistance, and/or an abnormally elevated glucose production by the liver. Genetics and obesity are important factors that influence its development.
C. The severity of carbohydrate intolerance in gestational diabetes is unknown. Women identified at risk have screening done during the 24th and 28th weeks of gestation.

Predisposing Factors
A. First-degree relative with type 1 or type 2 diabetes
B. Obese individuals being greater than 120% of ideal body weight
C. Body mass index (BMI) greater than or equal to 27 kg/m²
D. History of recurrent skin, genital, or urinary infections
E. Native American, Hispanic, Asian, and African American heritage
F. Hypertension with systolic pressure greater than 140 and diastolic pressure greater than 90 mmHg
G. High-density lipoprotein level of 35 mg/dL or less and/or triglyceride level of greater than or equal to 250 mg/dL
H. History of giving birth to babies larger than 9 lb or gestational diabetes
I. History of impaired glucose tolerance or fasting glucose
J. Medications: steroids, hormones, diuretics, some hypertensive medications, decongestants, diet pills, nonsteroidal anti-inflammatory drugs (NSAIDs), nicotine, caffeine, sugar-containing syrups, and fish oil

Common Complaints
A. Classic triad of symptoms
   1. Polyuria
   2. Polydipsia
   3. Polyphagia
B. Weight loss
C. Lack of energy
D. Recurrent infections (urinary tract, vaginal, skin breakdown that is slow to heal)
E. Asymptomatic

Other Signs and Symptoms
A. Weakness
B. Fatigue
C. Nausea and vomiting
D. Abdominal pain
E. Anorexia
F. Sexual dysfunction, including impotence or dyspareunia
G. Itching
H. Visual disturbances
I. Signs and symptoms related to nephropathy, neuropathy, and/or retinopathy

Subjective Data
A. Obtain a detailed history regarding onset, duration, and course of presenting symptoms.
B. Question the patient regarding all characteristic signs and symptoms of diabetes.
C. Determine the patient's nutritional status, 24-hour recall, weight history, and eating patterns.
D. Review the family history of diabetes or other endocrine disorders.
E. Note predisposing factors to diabetes.
F. Review the patient's social history, including smoking, alcohol, and exercise.

Physical Examination
A. Check temperature, pulse, respirations, blood pressure, and weight.
B. Inspect
   1. Observe overall appearance.

2. Perform oral examination. Diabetic patients are prone to thrush, gingivitis, plaque, and infections. A dental examination should be done every 6 months.
3. Complete funduscopic examination. Proliferative diabetic retinopathy is the leading cause of new blindness in adults in the United States. It occurs 60% of the time in those with type 1 and 30% of the time in those with type 2 diabetes. Patients with diabetes are 25 times more at risk for blindness and have a four to six times the increased risk for cataracts and twice an increased risk for glaucoma.
4. Inspect the skin, including feet, hands, fingers, and insulin injection sites.

C. Auscultate
1. Auscultate the heart. The incidence of cardiovascular disease is two to four times higher in adults with diabetes. The risk of stroke is two to four times higher because 60%–65% of the patients have hypertension.
2. Auscultate the lungs.

D. Percuss
1. Percuss the chest, abdomen, and deep tendon reflexes.

E. Palpate
1. Palpate the neck (thyroid).
2. Palpate the abdomen.
3. Palpate the extremities and check pulses.

Diagnostic Tests

A. Fasting plasma glucose: greater than or equal to 126 mg/dL. All patients should have a baseline fasting blood sugar performed at 45 years of age, then repeated every 3 years. The baseline should be performed earlier if any predisposing factors exist.
B. Random plasma glucose: greater than or equal to 200 mg/dL with symptoms of diabetes.
C. Oral glucose tolerance test: After 75 g glucose load, a 2-hour plasma glucose greater than or equal to 200 mg/dL; impaired glucose tolerance is a fasting plasma glucose of greater than or equal to 126 mg/dL.
D. HgbA1c.

According to the Diabetes Control and Complications Trial, an gbA1c of 7.2% or below decreases the risk of retinopathy, neuropathy, and nephropathy by 50%–70%.

Differential Diagnoses

A. Diabetes mellitus
B. Benign pancreatic insufficiency
C. Pheochromocytoma
D. Cushing's syndrome
E. History of corticosteroid use
F. Stress hyperglycemia
G. Acromegaly
H. Hemochromatosis
I. Somogyi phenomenon: early morning hyperglycemia due to very early morning (2:00–3:00 AM) hypoglycemia

Plan

A. General interventions
1. Establish, review, and evaluate individual goals with the patient on a routine basis.

2. Center goals around normal metabolic control and the prevention and delay of complications while maintaining a flexible, normal, high-quality life.
3. After a new diagnosis is made and treatment begun, be alert for an initial remission or honeymoon phase with decreased insulin needs and better control that may last 3–6 months.
4. Include the following in the treatment plan:
   a. Exercise plan
      i. Develop a consistent, individualized exercise plan with the patient to improve insulin sensitivity, blood sugars, weight reduction, and reduction of cardiovascular complications.
      ii. Evaluation by a health care provider, including a complete physical examination and EKG, must precede any exercise program.
      iii. The goal of exercise should be three to four times a week for 20–45 min.
      iv. Exercise should not be done if the fasting blood sugar is greater than 250 mg/dL and ketones are present in the urine or if the glucose level is greater than 300 mg/dL at any time regardless of the presence of ketones.
      v. Because exercise can lower blood sugar concentration, special precautions such as medication adjustment and meal planning should be done before and after exercise if the patient is taking insulin or a glucose-lowering medication.
   b. Self-monitoring blood glucose (SMBG): The process of monitoring the patient's blood gives valuable information to the patient on a daily basis and assists the provider in identifying trends.
      i. Several different meters are available with a variety of options. A certified diabetes educator can show examples of different types before the patient purchases one.
      ii. Frequency of testing depends on the type of medication the patient is taking and the patient's compliance and motivation.
      iii. Additional testing should be done at times of changes in medication, meal plans, and/or exercise; and during illness or stress.
   c. Psychosocial support: It is important from the beginning of treatment to give the patient a sense of control.
      i. Consistent involvement of family members will influence compliance. Assess and discuss psychosocial issues at each visit.

B. Patient teaching
1. See the Section III Patient Teaching Guide for this chapter, "Diabetes."
2. Topics in the educational plan include the pathophysiology of diabetes, procedures for self-monitoring blood glucose and medication therapies, recognition and treatment of hypoglycemia, and instructions for special situations such as illness and traveling.
3. Include preventive care, instructions for family members, and the importance of wearing a Medic-Alert tag.

C. Dietary management
1. Nutritional plan: The patient should meet with a dietitian who has experience with diabetes nutritional therapy.
2. Nutritional recommendations include protein 10%–20% (less if nephropathy), carbohydrates 55%–60%, and fat 20%–25%.
3. Involve the family to improve compliance with the individualized meal plan.

D. Pharmaceutical therapy
1. Type 1 diabetes depends on exogenous insulin for treatment.
2. Treatment for type 2 diabetes is usually begun with an exercise program and nutrition plan. If glycemic goals are not reached in 2 or 3 months, monotherapy of medications is considered.
   a. Monotherapy
      i. Sulfonylurea: first-generation (Orinase, Diabinese) and second-generation (Micronase, Glucotrol, Amaryl), Biguanide: metformin (Glucophage), Thiazolidinedione: troglitazone (Rezulin), α-Glucosidase inhibitor: acarbose (Precose).
      ii. Insulin: the onset and peaks are dependent on the type of insulin.
      iii. Avandia 4 mg every day (monotherapy or combination).
      iv. If monotherapy is not successful in 2 or 3 months then combination therapy is used.
   b. Combination therapy
      i. Sulfonylurea + biguanide
      ii. Sulfonylurea + insulin
      iii. Sulfonylurea + α-glucosidase inhibitor; sulfonylurea + biguanide + insulin; thiazolidinedione + insulin
      iv. Biguanide + α-glucosidase inhibitor; biguanide + insulin
      v. α-Glucosidase inhibitor + insulin
      vi. Incretin Mimetics + Biguanide

Although patients with type 2 diabetes do not depend on exogenous insulin, many will require supplemental insulin during times of stress, illness, or pregnancy or routinely along with oral medication. See Tables 19.1 and 19.2.

c. Additional medications that may need to be considered
   i. Angiotensin-converting enzyme (ACE) inhibitors are the antihypertensive drug of choice.
   ii. Calcium channel blockers may reduce microalbuminuria and proteinuria.
   iii. Aspirin has been found to decrease cardiovascular risk in patients.
d. Some medications adversely affect diabetes:
   i. Nicotinic acids affect glycemic control by increasing insulin resistance.
   ii. β-Blockers increase the risk of hypoglycemia episodes in patients taking oral hypoglycemia.
   iii. Thiazide diuretics act the same as β-blockers.

Follow-up

A. Determine follow-up appointments by the type of diabetes, age, patient compliance, any treatment changes, and presence of any complications related to diabetes or other health problems.
B. A glycosylated hemoglobin determination every 3–4 months can assist the provider in measuring control even if the patient is not seen in the office. There are several computer software packages that print the glucometer readings for assessing compliance; this can be done by the provider or the patient.
C. The American Diabetes Association blood glucose goals are:
1. Preprandial glucose 80–120 mg/dL
2. 1–2 hours after meals a glucose level of less than 180 mg/dL
3. A bedtime glucose level of 100–140 mg/dL
4. HgbA1c less than 7%
5. Blood pressure should be less than 130/85 mmHg
6. Cholesterol less than 200 mg/dL, triglycerides less than 200 mg/dL, high-density lipoproteins greater than 35 mg/dL, and low-density lipoproteins less than 130 mg/dL and less than 100 mg/dL if heart disease is present
D. Annual tests or examinations should include a dilated funduscopic examination by an ophthalmologist, an annual EKG, Carville foot examination, flu vaccination, thyroid studies, serum creatinine, lipid panel, urinalysis,

TABLE 19.1 Action Times of Insulin

Insulin	Onset	Peaks	Duration
Lispro	10 min	1.5 h	3 h
Regular	20 min	3–4 h	8 h
NPH	1.5 h	4–12 h	22 h
Lente	2.5 h	7–15 h	24 h
Ultralente	4 h	10–24 h	36 h
70 NPH/30 Reg	0–1 h	Dual	12–20 h
50 NPH/50 Reg	0–1 h	Dual	12–20 h

TABLE 19.2 Diabetes Medication/Class (Alphabetical Order)

Drug	Brand Name	CM Drug Class
ActosPlus Met	Pioglitazone + Metformin	Thiazolidinedione plus Biguanide
Amaryl	Glimepiride	Sulfonylurea
Apidra	Insulin glulisine	Rapid-acting insulin
Avandamet	Rosiglitazone + Metformin	Thiazolidinedione plus Biguanide
Avandaryl	Rosiglitazone + Glimepiride	Thiazolidinedione plus Sulfonylurea
Avandia	Rosiglitazone	Thiazolidineodione
Byetta	Exenatide	Incretin mimetic
Diabeta	Glyburide	Sulfonylurea (2nd generation)
Duetact	Pioglitazone + Glimepride	Thiazolidinedione plus Sulfonylurea
Glucagon	—N/A—	Antihypoglycemic
Glucophage XR	Metformin ext. release	Biguanide
Glucotrol XL	Glipizide ext. release	Sulfonylurea (2nd generation)
Glucovance	Glyburide + Metformin	Sulfonylurea plus Biguanide
Glynase PresTab	Glyburide micronized	Sulfonylurea (2nd generation)
Gylset	Miglitol	Alpha-glucosidase inhibitor
Humalog	Insulin lispro	Rapid-acting insulin
Humulin 70/30	NPH/Regular insulin	Short-and intermediate-acting insulin
Humulin 50/50	NPH/Regular insulin	Short-and intermediate-acting insulin
Humulin R	Regular insulin	Rapid-acting insulin
Humulin N	NPH insulin	Intermediate-acting insulin
Janumet	Sitagliptin + Metformin	Dipeptidyl peptidase-4 inhibitor plus Biguanide
Januvia	Sitagliptin	Dipeptidyl peptidase-4 inhibitor
Lantus	Insulin glargine	Long-acting insulin
Levemir	Insulin detemir	Long-acting insulin
Metaglip	Metformin + Glipizide	Biguanide plus Sulfonylurea
Micronase	Glyburide	Sulfonylurea (2nd generation)
Novolin 70/30	Insulin isophane + Regular insulin	Short- and intermediate-acting insulin
Novolog	Insulin Aspart	Rapid-acting Insulin
Novolog Mix 70/30	Insulin Aspart Protamine/Insulin Aspart	Short- and intermediate-acting insulin
Humalog Mix 75/25	Insulin Lispro Protamine/Insulin Lispro	Short- and intermediate-acting insulin
Humalog Mix 50/50	Insulin Lispro Protamine/Insulin Lispro	Short- and intermediate-acting insulin
Novolin N	Insulin Isophane Suspension NPH	Intermediate-acting insulin
Onglyza	Saxaglipn	Dipeptidyl peptidase-4 inhibitor
Prandimed	Repaglinde + Metformin	Meglitinide analogue plus Biguanide
Prandin	Repaglinde	Meglitinide analogue
Precose	Acarbose	Alpha-glucosidase inhibitor
Starlix	Nateglinide	Insulin secretagogue
Symlin	Pramlintide	Amylin analogue/amylinomimetic

and urine for microalbuminuria. Additional tests may be needed if complications develop.

Consultation/Referral
A. Refer to the physician if the patient experiences:
1. Diabetic ketoacidosis.
2. Severe or frequent hypoglycemia that is unresponsive to conventional pharmaceutical therapy.
3. Hyperosmolar hyperglycemic nonketotic syndrome.
4. Pregnancy.
5. Symptoms from an acute complication related to retinopathy.
6. Nephropathy develops 35%–45% of the time in type 1 and 20% of the time in type 2 diabetes; it is the leading disease requiring kidney dialysis.
7. Neuropathy: 60%–70% of patients experience impaired sensation or pain in feet/hands, carpal tunnel syndrome; over half of all amputations of lower extremities are related to diabetes.

Individual Considerations
A. Pregnancy/preconceptual
1. Women considering pregnancy should be switched to insulin before conception and during pregnancy.
   a. Fetal anomalies increase proportionally to uncontrolled diabetes.
   b. HgbA1c goal prior to conception is less than 7%.
2. Hypertensive medications may need to be changed if considering pregnancy because ACE inhibitors, β-blockers, and diuretics are contraindicated.
3. Increased monitoring of blood glucose is necessary during pregnancy.
B. Pediatrics: Children with diabetes should see an endocrinologist or diabetologist.

GALACTORRHEA

Definition
A. The production of a milky discharge excreted from the nipple, occurring beyond the 6-month period of pregnancy and/or breast-feeding cessation.

Incidence
A. It is estimated that 1%–50% of reproductive women will experience galactorrhea at some time in their life.

Pathogenesis
A. The pathogenesis depends on the etiology. Physiologic galactorrhea is caused by pregnancy. The anterior pituitary gland secretes prolactin, which stimulates milk production. Milk production is normal for 6 months after pregnancy and/or after breast-feeding has ceased.

Predisposing Factors
A. Reproductive women (15–50 years old)
B. Medications: oral contraceptions, phenothiazines, haloperidole (Haldol), metoclopramide (Reglan), Isoniazid, Reserpine, methyldopa (Aldonet), and imipramine (Tofranil)

Common Complaints
A. Milky discharge from the nipple

Subjective Data
A. Note the onset, duration, and course of presenting symptoms.
B. Ask whether the patient has been pregnant and/or breast-fed within the past 6 months. If so, how long did she nurse?
C. Review her menstrual history and pattern.
D. Ask her to describe the discharge, noting color, consistency, and/or presence of blood.
E. Determine the mechanism of production of discharge: spontaneous or with manual expression.
F. Assess for any palpable mass in the breast.
G. Review current medications, including use of oral contraceptives.
H. Note any previous experience with galactorrhea. If so, discuss testing performed and treatment, if any.
I. Identify any family history of breast cancer or other tumors.

Physical Examination
A. Check temperature, pulse, respirations, and blood pressure.
B. Inspect
1. Inspect the breast.
2. Assess the discharge.
3. Inspect the skin; note dimpling, retraction, and irregularities.
4. Eyes: Complete funduscopic examination.
5. Perform visual field testing.
C. Palpate
1. Palpate the breasts for masses and fibrocystic changes.
2. Squeeze the nipple to induce discharge.
3. Palpate the axillary lymph nodes.
4. Palpate the neck, thyroid, and lymph nodes.

Diagnostic Tests
A. Prolactin level: normal level is 1–20 ng/mL.
B. Thyroid-stimulating hormone (TSH).

Many cases of galactorrhea are considered idiopathic. Usually endocrine studies will be normal.

C. β human chorionic gonadotropin (β HCG).
D. Hemocult of breast discharge.
E. Breast discharge for pathology.
F. CT/MRI of sella turcica if pituitary mass is suspected.
G. Mammogram if tumor is suspected.

Differential Diagnoses
A. Galactorrhea
B. Fibrocystic disease
C. Mastitis
D. Breast tumor
E. Medication induction
F. Breast cancer: bloody nipple discharge, painless, firm fixed mass
G. Pituitary adenoma: can produce permanent visual field loss and headaches
H. Hypothalamic disorders
I. Chiari-Frommel: galactorrhea occurring after 6 months postpartum

Plan

A. General interventions
1. Treat underlying cause of nipple discharge.
2. If induced by medications, stop medications.
3. If benign cause, no treatment is necessary with medication. Monitor symptoms. If symptoms progress, reevaluate.
B. Patient teaching
1. Teach self-examination of the breast.
C. Pharmaceutical therapy
1. If treatment needed: Parlodel 2.5 mg by mouth daily with food. May increase to three times daily if needed.
2. Do not use bromocriptine (Parlodel) in patients with a history of hypertension, preeclampsia, or sensitivity to ergot alkaloids.

Follow-up

A. Monitor prolactin level every 6–12 months.
B. Yearly vision evaluation.
C. MRI at 1 year, then every 2–5 years if symptoms persist.

Consultation/Referral

A. Consult a physician if breast tumor is suspected with bloody discharge or palpable mass noted.

Individual Considerations

A. Pregnancy
1. Galactorrhea during pregnancy is a normal physiologic response.
2. If galactorrhea persists after pregnancy/lactation has ceased for 6 months, a full workup evaluation is required.
B. Adults: Men: Galactorrhea is rare in men; however, it can occur with prolactinoma.

GYNECOMASTIA

Definition

A. Gynecomastia is an enlargement of the breast tissue in males.

Incidence

A. Approximately 40%–60% of adolescent boys will experience breast enlargement. It is also seen in older men (65 years) with excessive weight gain.

Pathogenesis

A. Male breast duct proliferation occurs due to a hormonal imbalance of estrogen. Pathologic conditions such as pituitary tumors, systemic disorders, kidney disease, thyroid disorders, and liver disease can cause symptoms to occur. Medications can also induce symptoms. These medications include antidepressants, cimetidine, hormones, and sedatives.

Predisposing Factors

A. Newborns
B. Puberty
C. Age (men older than 65 years) with excessive weight gain
D. Family history
E. Klinefelter's syndrome
F. Malnutrition with severe weight loss
G. Peutz-Jeghers syndrome

Common Complaints

A. Enlargement of breast tissue with or without discomfort

Other Signs and Symptoms

A. Asymptomatic
B. Type I: nodule present under areola tissue area
C. Type II: nodule palpable under and beyond areola area
D. Type III: breast enlargement without contour separation of tissue

Subjective Data

A. Identify when breast development first appeared.
B. Determine whether enlargement is unilateral or bilateral.
C. Review the progression of enlargement.
D. Note any pain, discharge, or masses that are palpable.
E. List current medications, drugs, alcohol, and substance abuse.
F. Review the patient's medical history.
G. Note the patient's family history of gynecomastia.
H. Explore nutritional intake.
I. Discuss the patient's level of physical activity (sports, hobbies, etc).

Differential Diagnoses

A. Gynecomastia
B. Obesity: fatty breast enlargement without glandular involvement
C. Breast cancer: fixed, firm nodule in tissue with dimpling and/or breast discharge
D. Neurofibroma
E. Lipoma

Plan

A. General interventions
1. Identify any pathologic condition. If none is identified, reassure the patient that normal resolution will occur over time.
B. Patient teaching
1. Reinforce weight reduction if weight gain is a factor in the condition.
C. Pharmaceutical therapy
1. Antiestrogens (tamoxifen)
2. Danazol: pubertal boys
3. Diethylstilbestrol (DES): elderly men

Follow-up

A. Follow-up is dependent on etiology and/or patient needs.
B. Follow up pubertal boys every 4–6 months for evaluation of development or regression.

Consultation/Referral

Consult a physician or refer to an endocrinologist if the male patient:

A. Is noted to have breast enlargement for longer than 2 years.
B. Is a pubertal boy without genital development.

Individual Considerations

A. Newborns: commonly seen in newborns due to the maternal estrogen. This breast enlargement spontaneously regresses over time.

HIRSUTISM

Definitions

A. An excessive production of an androgenic hormone that causes the development of male features in females, particularly hair distribution.

Incidence

A. Approximately 8%–10% of women develop hirsutism after puberty.

Pathogenesis

A. The pathogenesis depends on the etiology: excessive amounts of androgenic hormones from the ovary, adrenal gland, and/or a hormonal imbalance. The two major adrenal gland conditions responsible for hirsutism or virilism are congenital adrenal hyperplasia and Cushing's syndrome.

Predisposing Factors

A. Females who have a family history of endocrine disorders
B. Usually occurs in the second to third decade of life
C. Southern European ancestry
D. Anovulation

Common Complaints

A. An excessive amount of hair production on the upper lip, chin, and/or chest

Other Signs and Symptoms

A. Irregular periods
B. Infertility
C. Acne
D. Virilization (temporal hair recessation, large muscle mass, deep voice)

Subjective Data

A. Note the age of onset, duration, and distribution pattern of the excessive hair growth.
B. Review any previous experiences with similar symptoms. What were the diagnosis, treatment, and results?
C. Note the patient's menstrual history. Note amenorrhea and galactorrhea. Has the patient ever had a history of infertility?

Physical Examination

A. Check temperature, pulse, respirations, and blood pressure.
B. Inspect
   1. Look for excessive hair growth on face, breasts, abdomen, back, and shoulders.
   2. Assess for signs of virilization.
C. Palpate: Perform a pelvic examination to assess for enlarged ovaries or masses.

Diagnostic Tests

A. Total testosterone (200 ng/dL, need further workup)
B. Free serum testosterone
C. TSH, follicle-stimulating hormone (FSH), luteinizing hormone (LH), and prolactin levels
D. Dehydroepiandosterone (DHEA) sulfate
E. 24-hour urine: 17-ketosteroid assay
F. Pelvic ultrasound
G. CT of ovaries/adrenal gland if abnormally elevated blood tests

Differential Diagnoses

A. Hirsutism: can be secondary to primary diagnosis (idiopathic, hypothyroidism, infertility, obesity, ovarian disease, hyperprolactinemia).
B. Hypothyroidism: elevated TSH.
C. Ovarian tumor: testosterone level greater than 200 ng/dL.
D. Adrenal tumor: DHEA greater than 800 µg/dL.
E. Excessive steroid use: the patient medicates self with excessive steroids.
F. Cushing's disease: centripetal obesity and muscle wasting.

Plan

A. General interventions
   1. Medications are not recommended for mild cases. Hair removal by other mechanisms is recommended as the patient desires (plucking, waxing, bleaching, etc).
   2. Moderate to severe cases require treatment with medications. Drug therapy may stop excessive hair growth. Current hair growth will not spontaneously resolve. Hair removal may also be desired until the drug shows an effect.
   3. If acne is severe, institute appropriate therapy (see "Acne Vulgaris" in Chapter 3, "Dermatology Guidelines").
B. Patient teaching
   1. If obese, reinforce weight loss management. Consider nutritional consult.
   2. Educate the patient that it may take 3–6 months on medication to see results.
C. Pharmaceutical therapy
   1. Use oral contraceptives daily; any brand is effective.
   2. Use high-estrogen pills to increase steroid-binding globulins.
   3. Use high-progesterone pills to influence the clearance of testosterone.

Ovarian and/or adrenal tumor must be ruled out before medication therapy is instituted.

Follow-up

A. Follow-up depends on the treatment. If medication is used, follow up in 3 months to evaluate effectiveness.

Consultation/Referral

A. Consult a physician if abnormally elevated laboratory results exist or if Cushing's disease is suspected.
B. Refer to a physician if there is no improvement after 3 months of medication treatment.
C. Refer patients who have virilization and elevated testosterone levels to an endocrinologist.

Individual Considerations

A. Pregnancy
   1. If conception occurs, discontinue medications, which may be teratogenic to the fetus.

2. If anovulation is diagnosed, fertility measures are needed if pregnancy is desired.
B. Geriatric
   1. Hirsutism may be seen in women after menopause.
   2. Hirsutism that occurs in the middle to late years in life should be closely monitored for adrenal hyperplasia and adrenal and/or ovarian tumors.

HYPERTHYROIDISM *by Cheryl A. Glass*

Definition
A. Hyperthyroidism is a condition in which thyroid hormone exerts greater than normal responses. Hyperthyroidism may be subclinical and may not be easily recognized or exhibit overt symptoms. The most common hyperthyroid conditions are Graves' disease and toxic multinodular goiter. The American Thyroid Association recommends that adults be creased for thyroid dysfunction (TSH) beginning at age 35 and every 5 years thereafter. However, Medicare does not cover a screening TSH in an asymptomatic patient.

Incidence
A. Overall incidence of hyperthyroidism is 1.3%.
B. Female gender
   1. 5:1 ratio higher in women than men.
   2. Older women 4%–5% incidence.
   3. Graves' disease is more common in younger women.
   4. Toxic nodular goiter is more common in older women.
C. Children
   1. Graves' disease in children 0.02% (1:5000)
   2. Most often occurs in 11- to 15-year-olds
D. Elderly: toxic multinodular goiter (Plummer disease) occurs in 15%–20% of patients with thyrotoxicosis.
E. Symptomatology incidence
   1. Ophthalmopathy is more common in smokers.
   2. Atrial fibrillation 10%–25% incidence and is more common in the elderly.

Pathogenesis
Hyperthyroidism is one form of thyrotoxicosis in which an excess of hormone is excreted by the thyroid gland. The diseases that can cause hyperthyroidism include Graves' disease, toxic multinodular goiter, thyroid cancer, and increased secretion of TSH. Thyrotoxicosis not related to hyperthyroidism may be subacute thyroiditis, ectopic thyroid tissue, and ingestion of excessive thyroid hormone. Postpartum thyroiditis can precipitate a short-term mild hyperthyroidism, which has an onset at 2–6 months postpartum. Severe thyrotoxicosis of any cause is called thyrotoxic crisis or storm.

In Graves' disease, the normal feedback mechanisms that regulate hormone secretion are taken over by some abnormal thyroid-stimulating mechanism. Thyroid autoantibodies of the immunoglobulin G (IgG) class are present in more than 95% of patients with Graves' disease. The hyper functioning of the thyroid gland causes suppression of TSH and thyrotropin-releasing hormone (TRH). There are profound increases in iodine uptake and thyroid gland metabolism, which are believed to be the causes of the gland enlargement. The resulting increase in the level of circulating thyroid hormone is responsible for the thyrotoxic symptoms.

In the condition called toxic multinodular goiter, the thyroid gland enlarges in response to some bodily need such as puberty, pregnancy, iodine deficiency, and immunologic, viral, and genetic disorders. As TSH levels rise, the gland enlarges; when the condition demanding increased thyroid hormone resolves, TSH levels usually return to normal and the gland slowly returns to its original size.

Predisposing Factors
A. Graves' disease
   1. Women in the second through fifth decades of life
   2. Familial autoimmune thyroid disease
   3. Concomitant disorders believed to be autoimmune
   4. Increased in Trisomy 21
   5. Higher incidence in smokers
B. Toxic multinodular goiter
   1. Older people
   2. Recent exposure to iodine-containing medications (amiodarone and radiocontrast dye)
   3. Long-standing simple goiter
   4. Conditions such as puberty, pregnancy, iodine deficiency, immunologic, viral, or genetic disorders

Common Complaints
A. Grave's disease
   1. Prominence/protrusion of the eye (exophthalmos)
   2. Prominent "stare"
   3. Visual changes
      a. Diplopia
      b. Photophobia
      c. Eye irritation: gritty feeling or pain
B. Weight loss with no change in diet or an increase in appetite
C. Anorexia (may be prominent in the elderly)
D. Weakness and fatigue
E. Tachycardia
F. Decreased tolerance to heat
G. Thinning scalp hair
H. Fingernails separation from the nail bed
I. Smooth, thin skin
J. Heart palpitations (atrial fibrillation)
K. Bowel symptoms
   1. Increase in frequency and loose bowel movements (not diarrhea)
   2. Constipation (more frequent in the elderly)
L. Swelling of feet and ankles

Other Signs and Symptoms
A. Goiter: **Approximately 50% of patients will not have an enlargement of the thyroid gland. Elderly patients are less likely to have a goiter.**
B. Periorbital edema.
C. Flushing, warm skin.
D. Fine hand tremors.
E. Dyspnea.
F. Exertional fatigue/exercise intolerance.
G. Insomnia.

H. Irritability.

I. Nervousness.

J. Mood swings.

K. Inability to concentrate.

L. Depression and apathy (elderly).

M. Hyperactivity (children).

N. Decreased menses.

O. Impotence and decreased libido in men.

P. Gynecomastia.

Q. Galactorrhea (TSH-mediated hyperthyroidism).

R. Atrial dysrhythmias (atrial fibrillation), left ventricular dilation.

S. Urinary frequency and nocturia (enuresis is common in children).

T. A combination of these noted symptoms should lead to the assessment of hyperthyroidism.

Subjective Data

A. Identify when symptoms began, duration, and any change or progression.

B. Identify whether the patient has noticed enlargement of the thyroid gland, difficulty swallowing, or change in voice.

C. Assess for change in weight over the last 3 months, last 6 months, and last year. Ask the patient whether his or her appetite has changed.

D. Explore the patient's family history of thyroid problems.

E. Obtain the patient's medical history of associated diseases (especially those of autoimmune pathogenesis: pernicious anemia, type 1 diabetes mellitus, myasthenia gravis, rheumatoid arthritis, ulcerative colitis).

F. Review the patient's medication history, including amiodarone, interferon alfa, levothyroxine (overdose), expectorants, and health food supplements containing seaweed.

G. Ask the patient to identify any changes in bowel habits, loose (nondiarrhea) stools, frequency of bowel movements, or constipation.

H. Ask about moods, changes in concentration, feelings of restlessness, nervousness, anxiety, and change in sleep habits.

I. Assess for any cardiac symptoms, such as palpitations, chest pain, shortness of breath, and decreased tolerance for activities previously done.

J. Ask whether the patient has noticed any swelling or puffiness anywhere.

K. Determine whether the patient has experienced changes in vision and/or eye irritation.

L. Assess for hand tremors, increase in the moistness and coolness of the skin, flushing, and blushing.

M. Ask the patient to identify any menstrual changes or whether the patient has had a recent pregnancy, or is in the postpartum period.

N. Review for a recent history of a viral infection.

O. Review recent trauma to the neck (significant trauma can cause thyrotoxicosis).

Physical Examination

A. Check temperature, pulse (tachycardia), respirations (dyspnea), blood pressure (systolic hypertension), and weight. Children: Plot height/weight on growth curve. (Accelerated growth is noted.)

B. Inspect

1. Observe overall appearance: Does the patient have any difficulty with breathing, including dyspnea, or difficulty swallowing from tracheal obstruction secondary to a large goiter?

2. Note eyelid retraction, lid lag, and exophthalmos. The clinician may see periorbital edema and an elevated upper eyelid, which leads to decreased blinking and a staring quality in Graves' disease.

3. Note tremors, which are best demonstrated from outstretched hands.

4. Inspect the skin for temperature and texture.

5. Inspect the fingernails for:
   a. Onycholysis, also known as Plummer's nails (loosening of the nails from the nailbeds).
   b. Softening of the nails.

6. Inspect scalp hair.

7. Assess Tanner Stage: puberty may be delayed.

C. Auscultate

1. Auscultate the thyroid for bruits.

2. Auscultate the heart, pulse rate. Patients with subclinical hyperthyroidism frequently present with atrial fibrillation.

3. Auscultate the carotid arteries for bruits.

4. Auscultate bowel sounds.

D. Palpate

1. Palpate the neck and thyroid for nodules, thrills, and enlargement. Depending on the etiology of the hyperthyroidism, the thyroid may range from normal to massive (Graves' disease or toxic multinodular goiter). Palpation of the thyroid can induce the gland to release increased hormone; be alert for signs and symptoms of thyroid storm.

2. If the thyroid is tender and painful to palpation, granulomatous thyroiditis may be the etiology of hyperthyroidism.

3. Palpate the heart for thrills.

4. Palpate extremities for edema. Pretibal myxedema is noted in Graves' disease.

E. Neurologic examination

1. Assess deep tendon reflexes.

2. Tests for lid lag
   a. Have the patient follow your finger as it moves up and down.
   b. Have the patient look down and observe if sclera can be seen above the iris.

3. Have the patient stick out the tongue to observe for presence of tremors.

Diagnostic Tests

A. TSH, free thyroxine (T_4), triiodothyronine (T_3). See Table 19.3.

B. Radioactive iodine (^{131}I) uptake (RAIU) if needed. If the patient has ophthalmopathy, clinical symptoms of hyperthyroidism, and a diffusely enlarged thyroid gland, the RAIU test is not necessary to confirm Graves' disease.

C. Consider additional laboratory testing:

TABLE 19.3 Test Results in Hyperthyroidism

Disorder	TSH	Free T$_4$	T$_3$	RAIU & Thyroid Scan
Overt hyperthyroidism	L	H	H	H
Graves' disease	L	H	H	H
Multinodular goiter	L	H	–	H
T$_3$ thyrotoxicosis (may be caused by antithyroid drug therapy)	L	N or H	H	N or H

Note. H = High, L = Low, N = Normal

1. CBC (may have normochromic, normocytic anemia).
2. Serum ferritin (may be high).

D. If T$_4$ and T$_3$ are high, but TSH is normal or high a pituitary MRI should be ordered to look for a pituitary mass.

E. An echocardiogram should be considered if an irregular heart rate and signs of heart failure are noted on examination.

Differential Diagnoses

A. Hyperthyroidism
   1. Graves' disease
   2. T$_3$-toxicosis
   3. T$_4$-toxicosis
   4. Thyroid adenoma
   5. Drug-induced hyperthyroidism, that is, iodine-rich amiodarone
   6. Subclinical hyperthyroidism
   7. TSH-induced hyperthyroidism (TSH-secreting pituitary adenoma)
   8. Hyperthyroidism during pregnancy
   9. Hashitoxicosis (combination of Hashimoto and thyroidtoxicosis), rare autoimmune thyroid disease
B. Cardiovascular disease such as coronary artery disease and heart failure
C. Gastrointestinal disorders such as irritable bowel syndrome, ulcerative colitis, and Crohn's disease
D. Cancer: testicular germ cell tumors
E. Neurologic disorder
F. Hydatidiform mole (molar pregnancy)
G. Psychological disorder

Plan

A. General interventions
   1. Carefully assess for complications of hyperthyroidism: cardiac, ophthalmologic, gastrointestinal, musculoskeletal, and psychological and address each area identified.
   2. Patients with tachycardia, palpitations, tremors, anxiety, and eyelid lag can be treated with a β-adrenergic antagonist for some relief from those symptoms until they become euthyroid.
B. Patient teaching
   1. Patients taking propylthiouracil (PTU) or methimazole (MMI) should be instructed to immediately report any side effects, including rash, hives, fever, jaundice, abdominal pain, and clay-colored stools.
   2. Less than 1% of patients develop agranulocytosis, but all patients should be instructed to call the provider immediately if a fever, sore throat, or joint aches develops due to their susceptibility to serious infection.
   3. Patients receiving radioactive iodine (RAI) should be informed that they most likely will need to take lifelong hormone replacement after the RAI treatment is completed.
   4. Teach safety measures to guard against the possibility of fractures due to bone density loss secondary to hyperthyroidism.
   5. Inform patients that an episode of serious depression may follow successful treatment of hyperthyroidism.
   6. No special diet is required; however, patients should be told to avoid herbal supplements and sushi that contains seaweed.
C. Medical/surgical management
   1. Radioactive Iodine (RAI) is a common choice of therapy for adults. It is administered in capsule form or in water.
      a. One dose is usually sufficient; however, a second dose may be given if necessary.
      b. Permanent hypothyroidism requiring lifelong hormone replacement is the only notable complication.
   2. Surgical removal is seldom used except in limited patient conditions.
      a. Pregnancy if women are noncompliant or cannot tolerate thionamides because of allergies or agranulocytosis.
      b. Severe hyperthyroidism in children.
      c. Patients who refuse radioactive iodine therapy.
      d. Refractory amiodarone-induced hyperthyroidism.
      e. Patients with unstable cardiac conditions that require quick normalization of thyroid function.
D. Pharmaceutical therapy
   1. Antithyroid drugs; the choice of drugs depends on clinician experience, the severity of the disease, and patient preference. Provide titration of antithyroid drug dose every 4 weeks until thyroid function normalizes and to ensure the patient does not become hypothyroid. Graves' disease may go into remission after treatment for 12–18 months and drug therapy can be discontinued.

a. Propylthiouracil (PTU)
   i. Initial dose 100–150 mg by mouth three times daily. Dosage decrease is almost always required at 4–8 weeks of start.
   ii. Thyroid storm: 150–200 mg orally every 4–6 hours
   iii. Not a first-line agent in pediatrics
b. Methimazole (MMI) (Tapazole)
   i. Adults: 20–40 mg/day or in divided twice-a-day dose. Maintenance doses are 2.5–15 mg/day
   ii. Pediatrics: 0.2 mg/kg/day
2. Radioactive iodine therapy is one of the most common treatments in adults. It is administered orally as a single dose. Radioactive iodine is contraindicated in pregnancy and lactation.
3. Beta-Blockers such as propranolol (Inderal) are also used for hyperthyroidism.
4. Atrial fibrillation treatment is directed to restoring a euthyroid state. Other therapies include:
   a. Beta blockers (unless contraindicated, including COPD and asthma).
   b. Calcium channel blockers if unable to utilize beta blocker.
   c. Oral anticoagulation (INR 2–3) to prevent systemic embolism.
   d. Antiarrhythmic drugs and cardioversion may be unsuccessful until euthyroid.

Follow-up

A. Depending on the experience of the clinician, a specialist best performs therapy, including radioactive iodine and antithyroid medication.
B. Patients receiving PTU or MMI should be seen in the office every 3–4 weeks for evaluation and have blood drawn for serum TSH and free T_4 measurements until euthyroid state is achieved and maintained.
C. Patients are usually maintained on these drugs for 1–2 years, with office visits every 3 months. The drug is then gradually withdrawn and 25%–90% of patients experience permanent remission.
D. Patients with RAI therapy should be seen in the office to monitor thyroid levels. It is anticipated that most of them will require lifelong hormone replacement medication following treatment.
E. Dexa scans to evaluate osteopenia/osteoporosis.
F. Consider testing for impaired glucose intolerance in untreated patients.

Consultation/Referral

A. Ophthalmology consultation for patients with ophthalmologic involvement.
B. If surgery is the choice of treatment, refer the patient to an endocrinologist and a surgeon.
C. An experienced obstetrician or perinatologist should follow pregnant women.

Individual Considerations

A. Pregnancy
   1. Pregnant patients with mild hyperthyroidism may be followed with treatment.

2. If an antithyroid drug is necessary, PTU is the drug of choice in the first trimester. Methimazole (MMI) has been associated with congenital anomalies such as tracheoesophageal fistula and choanal atresia. After the first trimester mothers may be switched to MMI.
3. Monitor thyroid function every 4 weeks during pregnancy.
4. RAI therapy is contraindicated during pregnancy and breast-feeding.
5. Thyrotoxicosis may improve during pregnancy; however, symptoms may relapse during the postpartum period.
6. Hyperthyroidism in the third trimester may increase the risk of low birth weight.
7. Prolonged high-dose iodine therapy can cause fetal goiter.
8. Ultrasounds should be preformed to evaluate fetal hyperthyroidism such as goiter, poor growth, cardiac failure, and hydrops.
B. Pediatrics
   1. Low thyroid function at birth is present in approximately half of the neonates whose mother received PTU or MMI during pregnancy.
   2. Graves' disease can occur in prepubescent girls. Symptoms can be vague and include hyperactivity or slowness and fatigue.
   3. Carefully assess for goiter in children who present with a variety of symptoms otherwise unexplained.
   4. PTU should not be used in pediatrics unless there is allergy to, or intolerance of, methimazole and other options are not available.
C. Adults: sympathetic activation (anxiety, hyperactivity, etc.) is seen in adult years more commonly than in the elderly population.
D. Geriatrics
   1. Older patents exhibit only three clinical signs (tachycardia, fatigue, and weight loss), whereas younger patient may exhibit as many as 12 symptoms.
   2. Rare signs in this population include atrial fibrillation, hyperactive reflexes, increased sweating, heat intolerance, tremors, nervousness, polydipsia, and increased appetite. Goiter is much less common.
   3. Elderly women with hyperthyroidism are at increased risk for accelerated bone loss.

HYPOTHYROIDISM *by Cheryl A. Glass*

Definition

A. Hypothyroidism is a condition in which the body does not produce enough thyroid hormone. In general hypothyroidism is considered permanent, requiring lifelong therapy to restore a euthyroid state. The most common physical finding is a goiter. The most common worldwide cause of hypothyroidism is iodine deficiency, while the most common cause in the United States is Hashimoto thyroiditis, an autoimmune thyroid disease.

Incidence

A. 0.1%–2% of overt hypothyroidism.
B. Occurs in women more than men (5–8 times higher).
C. 5%–15% in women over age 65.
D. 6% of adolescents have acquired hypothyroidism.
E. 10% of patients with type 1 diabetes will develop chronic thyroiditis.
F. Up to 10% develop lymphocytic thyroiditis in the post-partum period (up to 10 months postpartum).
G. 1:4000 newborns have congenital hypothyroidism (cretinism).

Pathogenesis

Hypothyroidism is caused by an insufficient production of thyroid hormones by the thyroid gland, either by a primary or a secondary cause.

A. Primary causes include decreased hormone production caused by autoimmune thyroiditis, endemic iodine deficiency, congenital defects, or decreased thyroid activity after treatment for hyperthyroidism.
B. Secondary causes are much less common but may include insufficient stimulation from the pituitary or hypothalamus and peripheral resistance to thyroid hormones.

The most common cause of primary hypothyroidism is chronic autoimmune thyroiditis called Hashimoto's thyroiditis. In this disease, circulating thyroid antibodies and the infiltration of lyphocytes destroy thyroid tissue. Autoimmune thyroiditis may also be a result of an inherited immune defect.

Acute thyroidism is a rare cause of hypothyroidism in which the cause is an acute bacterial infection. Subacute thyroiditis, a nonbacterial inflammation of the thyroid, is often preceded by a viral infection. Both of these conditions cause inflammation of the thyroid gland by lymphocytic and leukocytic infiltration into the thyroid tissue, resulting in hypothyroidism.

Predisposing Factors

A. Iodine deficiency.
B. Women over the age of 40 are at the highest risk.
C. Presence of other autoimmune disorders (diagnosed and previously undiagnosed).
D. Recent acute bacterial or viral infection.
E. Treatment with RAI for thyroid gland problems.
F. Surgical removal of thyroid gland.
G. Exposure to external radiation.
H. Evidence of pituitary or hypothalamic disease.
I. Postpartum.
J. Type 1 (autoimmune) diabetes mellitus.
K. Chromosomal disorders
   1. Down syndrome.
   2. Turner's syndrome.
   3. Klinefelter's syndrome.
L. Celiac disease.
M. Drug-induced
   1. Amiodarone.
   2. Interferon alpha.
   3. Thalidomide.
   4. Lithium.
   5. Stavudine.
   6. Dopamine.

Common Complaints

A. Weight gain/obesity
B. Fatigue/sluggishness
C. Cold intolerance
D. Constipation
E. Dry and flaky skin
F. Coarseness or loss of hair, inability of hair to hold a curl, hair loss at eyebrows, and reduced growth of hair
G. Reduced growth of nails
H. Hoarseness
I. Memory or mental impairment, difficulty concentrating, and slowed speech or thinking
J. Periorbital edema and facial puffiness
K. Irregular or heavy menses and infertility
L. Muscle aching and stiffness
M. Children
   1. Short stature
   2. Delayed skeletal maturation
   3. Overweight
   4. Delayed puberty
   5. Some adolescent have sexual precocity
      a. Girls: breast development
      b. Boys: macro-orchidism

Other Signs and Symptoms

A. Asymptomatic if subclinical hypothyroidism and have no overt symptoms.
B. Delayed reflexes.
C. Elevated blood pressure.
D. Hyperlipidemia.
E. Jaundice.
F. Painful subacute thyroiditis
   1. Sudden neck pain with sore throat, radiates to jaw and ears, and pain shifts to sides of the neck.
   2. Late stage: myxedema, thick scaly skin, muscle weakness/joint pain, enlarged tongue, hearing loss, bradycardia, cardiac hypertrophy, pleural effusion, and ascites.
G. Pituitary or hypothalamic failure
   1. Loss of axillary and pubic hair.
   2. Cessation of menses.
   3. Postural hypotension.
H. Exercise intolerance.
I. Carpal tunnel syndrome is a common occurrence.
J. Depression.
K. Ataxia.
L. Decreased concentration/memory impairment.

Subjective Data

A. Note history of recent illness and/or pregnancy.
B. Evaluate the patient's medical/surgical history for any treatment of hyperthyroid, including radioactive treatment or thyroidectomy.
C. Review dietary and weight history, how much weight has been gained and over what period of time.
D. Review any changes in health status or symptoms associated with other body systems (thyroid symptoms usually involve multiple body systems).
E. Review any history of obstructive sleep apnea.
F. Assess for pain or swelling of the neck or difficulty swallowing.

G. Inquire as to the patient's history of super-voltage X-ray therapy to the neck for nonthyroid cancer or for polio.

H. Identify family history:
1. Does the patient have a first-degree relative with thyroid disease?
2. Is there a family history of any endocrine problems, including thyroid, type 1 diabetes mellitus, and/or rheumatoid arthritis?

I. Review the patient's medication history for current medication, over-the-counter (OTC) medications, vitamins, or herbal supplements.

J. Review the patient's menstrual history or history of infertility.

Physical Examination

A. Check temperature, pulse (bradycardia), respirations, blood pressure (decreased systolic BP and increased diastolic BP), and weight. Plot height/weight on growth curve for children.

B. General observation
1. Gait problems such as ataxia or rigidity and spasticity of the trunk and proximal extremities
2. Quality of the patient's voice (hoarseness)
3. Signs of depression, decreased concentration, or memory impairment

C. Inspection
1. Inspect the skin (dry/flaky) or presence of jaundice.
2. Inspect the hair (coarse, thin, brittle) and decrease in pubic/axillary hair pattern.
3. Oral examination for evaluation of macroglossia (enlarged tongue).
4. Inspect the face/eye for periorbital puffiness/edema.
5. Inspect the neck for the presence of a goiter and surgical scar.
6. Child: Assess Tanner Stage of puberty.

D. Auscultate
1. Auscultate the thyroid and carotids.
2. Auscultate the heart.
3. Auscultate the lungs.
4. Auscultate the abdomen for bowel sounds in each quadrant (hypoactive).

E. Palpate
1. Palpate the neck, thyroid gland, and lymph nodes.
2. Palpate the abdomen for presence of abdominal distention, ascites, and hepatomegaly.
3. Palpate/evaluate extremities for edema.

F. Musculoskeletal examination: Perform a detailed musculoskeletal examination.

G. Neurologic examination
1. Check visual fields (restricted with hypothyroidism).
2. Test hearing
   a. Whisper words and have the patient repeat.
   b. Ticking watch.
   c. Using a tuning fork:
      i. Weber test: place vibrating fork on top midline of head (sound hearing equally in both ears).
      ii. Rinne test: place vibrating tuning fork on mastoid, begin counting, and ask the patient to tell you when he or she no longer hears; then quickly reposition 1/2 to 1 inch from the ear and ask the patient when he or she no longer hears (hearing should be twice as long as bone conduction).
3. Check for loss or reduction of deep tendon reflexes (DTRs).
4. Evaluate proximal muscle weakness/strength.
5. Test for abnormal tandem gait: have the patient walk across the room in a heel-toe, heel-toe fashion.
6. Check for sensory loss.
   a. Evaluate the first 3 fingers and one-half of the fourth finger on testing loss of sensation from carpal tunnel syndrome.
   b. Evaluate sensory loss of the feet/legs (generally symmetrical in a "stocking-glove" distribution).

Diagnostic Tests

A. TSH.
B. When a high TSH is noted, repeat the test and add a Free T_4.
C. T_3 resin uptake.
D. Thyroid antibodies. See Table 19.4.
E. TSH assay (if TSH assay is elevated, it indicates hypothyroidism).
F. Thyroid scan.
G. CBC (anemia).
H. Lipid profile.
I. Ultrasound of the neck and thyroid to detect nodules (not a first-line test).

Differential Diagnoses

A. Hypothyroidism
1. Hashimoto's thyroiditis.
2. Subclinical hypothyroidism.

TABLE 19.4 Test Results in Hypothyroidism

Disorder	TSH	Free T_4	T_3	RAIU & Thyroid Scan	Peroxidase Antibodies
Hypothyroid	H	L	Sometimes L	N or L	n/a
Hashimoto's disease	H or variable	N or L	Not helpful	Variable	Positive
Subacute hypothyroidism	L	H	H or variable	L or absent	Usually thyroiditis
Silent lymphocytic thyroiditis (usually postpartum)	L when toxic H when hypothyroid	H when toxic L when hypothyroid	n/a	L when toxic	Positive

Note. H = High, L = Low, N = Normal, RAIU = Radioactive iodine uptake.

3. Hypothyroidism secondary to treatment/intervention for hyperthyroidism.
4. De Quervain thyroiditis.
5. If TSH and Free T_4 both low, consider hypothyroidism secondary to pituitary or hypothalamic failure.

B. Obesity: Patients with elevated total cholesterol levels or triglyceride levels are often misdiagnosed by assuming that these symptoms are caused by obesity and high fat diets.
C. Depression.
D. Ischemic heart disease.
E. Nephrotic syndrome.
F. Cirrhosis.
G. Side effects/adverse effects of medications.
H. Constipation.
I. Sleep apnea/sleep disorder.
J. Fibromyalgia.
K. Infectious mononucleosis.

Plan

A. General interventions
1. The American Thyroid Association clinical practice guideline for detection of both subclinical and symptomatic hypothyroidism recommends that all adults age 35 and older be screened for hypothyroidism every 5 years to identify thyroid disease in the early stages. However, Medicare does not cover a screening TSH in an asymptomatic patient.
2. Patients with underactive thyroids require lifelong treatment with levothyroxine.
3. In patients with subacute thyroiditis, relatively large doses of nonsteroidal anti-inflammatory drugs (NSAIDs) or prednisone may be prescribed.
4. For patients with enlarged thyroid glands, surgery may be recommended if the gland begins obstructing the airway.
5. The treatment of patients with malignant thyroid nodules depends on the type of cancer.
B. Patient teaching
1. Teach the patient about the nature and course of the disease, as well as the signs and symptoms. Frequently patients are relieved that their perceived symptoms are real and that there is treatment. This may also improve patient compliance.
2. Teach the patient to report any side effects of the drug:
   a. Tachycardia
   b. Palpitations
   c. Chest pain
3. Emphasize the need for lifelong treatment with levothyroxine and the dangers of noncompliance.
4. Thyroid replacement should be taken on an empty stomach.
5. The beneficial effects of thyroid replacement occur in about 3 days to 1 week; the patient may not feel the clinical effects for several months.
6. When switching brands or using a generic, the serum TSH should be checked in 6 weeks.
C. Pharmacological therapy

1. Patients requiring therapy with levothyroxine should be treated with the same brand/generic consistently since potency varies between brand and generics.
   a. Levothyroxine (Synthroid, Levoxyl, Levothroid, Unithroid)
      i. Adults 1.6 µ/kg/day by mouth.
      ii. Elderly with comorbid CAD or severe COPD should be started at 25–50 µ/day.
      iii. Maintenance dose 50–200 µ by mouth every morning.
      iv. Pediatric dosing is age and weight dependent.
   b. Desiccated thyroid (Armour Thyroid)
      i. Adult initial dosing 30 mg/day by mouth and increased by 15–30 mg/day every 4 weeks.
      ii. Maintenance dose 60–180 mg/day.
      iii. Pediatric dosing is age and weight dependent.
2. The medication should be titrated to the lowest dosage needed to maintain euthyroidism and a nonelevated serum TSH and a normal or slightly elevated T_4.
3. Elderly patients and those with cardiovascular disease should be started on very low doses (25 µg/day) of levothyroxine; doses are increased very gradually, over 8–12 weeks, as tolerated. Close monitoring for the development of cardiac complications such as angina, arrhythmias, and myocardial infarction needs to be undertaken.
4. Thyroid hormones should be taken on an empty stomach in the mornings to avoid insomnia.
5. Other drugs can reduce the effectiveness/affect absorption of thyroid hormone:
   a. Cholesterol-reducing drugs.
   b. Cholestyramine interferes with absorption in the gut.
   c. Calcium carbonate.
   d. Aluminum hydroxide.
   e. Sucralfate (Carafate).
   f. If taking one of these drugs and levothyroxine, they should be taken 4–6 hours apart.
6. Dietary fiber can interfere with levothyroxine absorption. Coffee reduces the absorption of levothyroxine.
7. Pharmacologic treatment of the patient with subclinical hypothyroidism is controversial. If a goiter is present, treatment may be considered.

Follow-up

A. Patients who are not treated with medication should be seen every 6–12 months for reevaluation.
B. When medication is instituted, monitor laboratory values and patient well-being in the office every 4–6 weeks.
C. After the dosage is stabilized, the patient with an elevated serum TSH level should be seen every 6–12 months.
1. Undetectable TSH levels are indicative of overmedication.
2. High TSH levels are indicative of insufficient medication or patient noncompliance.
D. After the TSH is normalized, regular annual follow-up visits are required.
E. DEXA scan as indicated.

Consultation/Referral

A. Consult with an endocrinologist is recommended for:
   1. Children/teens younger than 18 years.
   2. Patients unresponsive to therapy.
   3. Pregnant patients.
   4. Presence of goiter, nodule, or other structural changes in the thyroid.
   5. Compression symptoms of dysphagia.
   6. Any patient with myxedema, significant cardiac disease, or involvement or hypothyroidism secondary to pituitary or hypothalamic failure should be managed in consultation with a physician or should be referred to an endocrinologist for continued care.
   7. If fine-needle aspiration biopsy is required.

Individual Considerations

A. Pregnancy
   1. Pregnancy: monitor TSH levels monthly during the first trimester.
   2. Small increases in medication dosage may be required.
   3. Some women develop postpartum thyroiditis and hypothyroidism after taking hyperthyroid medication during pregnancy or immediately thereafter.
   4. Postpartum: monitor TSH level at 6 weeks' postpartum examination.
   5. A common cause of congenital hypothyroidism is maternal and infant iodine deficiency.
   6. Monitor the TSH to avoid overtreatment in postpartum women because excess thyroid hormone levels increase the risk of osteoporosis.

B. Geriatrics
   1. Some elderly patients who are actually hyperthyroid exhibit symptoms of hypothyroidism.

METABOLIC SYNDROME/INSULIN RESISTANCE SYNDROME

Definition

Metabolic syndrome is an association of several complex disorders: Obesity, insulin resistant type 2 diabetes, hypertension, and hyperlipidemia. This coexistence of conditions leads to atherosclerotic cardiovascular disease. Metabolic syndrome is considered a proinflammatory and prothrombotic state. Elevated triglycerides and low HDL cholesterol are strong predictors of vascular events. Triglycerides and the waist circumference are considered the strongest predictors for the development of metabolic syndrome.

The inclusion of type 2 diabetes in the definition of metabolic syndrome is debated. Currently there is no consensus definition for metabolic syndrome in children. The Adult Treatment Panel (ATP) III defines metabolic syndrome in adults as the coexistence of any three of five conditions. See Table 19.5.

Complications associated with metabolic syndrome include fatty liver disease, cirrhosis, chronic kidney disease, polycystic ovarian syndrome (PCOS), obstructive sleep apnea (OSA), and gout.

Metabolic syndrome is noted in the literature under other names, including insulin resistance syndrome and obesity dyslipidemia syndrome. Previously the term "Syndrome X" was used; however, Syndrome X is noted to have normal coronary arteries and the occurrence of angina.

Incidence

A. Age-dependent increase in incidence; however, with the increase in childhood obesity metabolic syndrome is being diagnosed in children. The incidence in children is 4.2%–8.4% (dependent on ethnicity).

TABLE 19.5 ATP III Criteria for Metabolic Syndrome

Metabolic Syndrome Traits	Definition

Central/abdominal obesity	Adult waist circumference:
	  Men > 40 inches (102 cm)
	  Women > 35 inches (88 cm)
	Obesity in children 6 years to < 10 years: waist circumference ≥ 90th percentile
	Obesity ages 10 to < 16 years: ≥ 90th percentile ≥ 16 years use adult criteria

Serum triglycerides	Adults: ≥ 150 mg/dL *or* drug treatment for elevated triglycerides Children: > 100 mg/dL
Serum HDL cholesterol	Adults: < 40 mg/dL in men; < 50 mg/dL in women; *or* drug treatment for low HDL-C Children: ≤ 35 mg/dL
Blood pressure	Adults: ≥ 130/85 *or* drug treatment for hypertension Children: ≥ 90th percentile for age, sex, and height
Fasting plasma glucose (FPG)	Adults: ≥ 100 mg/dL *or* drug treatment for elevated blood glucose Children: ≥ 110 mg/dL

From "Third Report of the Expert Panel on Detection, Evaluation, and Treatment of High Blood Cholesterol in Adults (ATP III Final Report)," by the National Institutes of Health, 2002. Bethesda, MD: National Institutes of Health.

B. Ethnic background
   1. Native Americans are at the greatest risk (19% prevalence).
   2. Mexican Americans have the highest prevalence (12.9%).
   3. Non-Hispanic Whites (10.9% prevalence).
   4. Non-Hispanic Blacks (2.9% prevalence).

Pathogenesis

A. The exact etiology is unknown; however, abdominal obesity has been associated with insulin resistance. Vascular endothelial dysfunction occurs secondary to insulin resistance, hyperglycemia, hyperinsulinemia, and adipokines. Along with high blood pressure and abnormal lipids, vascular inflammation places the individual at high risk for a cardiovascular insult.

Predisposing Factors

A. Genetic predisposition
B. Weight gain, especially central/abdominal obesity
C. Females, especially postmenopausal
D. Smoking
E. High carbohydrate diet, especially soft drink consumption
F. Lack of exercise
   1. Sedentary lifestyle
   2. Television watching in children and adults

Common Complaints

A. Complaints are all related to the individual coexisting comorbid symptoms.

Other Signs and Symptoms

A. All are related to the individual coexisting comorbid symptoms.

Subjective Data

A. Review the patient's medical history related to comorbid conditions, including obesity, hypertension, and any abnormal laboratory testing (lipids, and triglycerides and glucose tolerance tests).
B. Review the patient's family history.
C. Review all prescription medications, over-the-counter drugs, and herbals.
D. Review the patient's current level of exercise.
E. Review the patient's usual diet (24-hour recall) noting high fat and high glucose consumption.
F. Review the patient's reproductive history.

Physical Examination

A. Height, weight, waist circumference, blood pressure, pulse, and respirations.
B. Calculate the body mass index and waist-to-hip measurement. Several Internet sites have BMI, body fat, and waist-to-hip ratio calculators.
C. General observations for Acanthosis nigricans and skin tags (insulin resistance).
D. A full physical examination is guided by the patient's medical history and presenting signs and symptoms.

Diagnostic Tests

A. Fasting glucose.
B. Fasting lipid panel.
C. Triglycerides.
D. Consider thyroid function.
E. Consider C-reactive protein (CRP) (optional).

Differential Diagnoses

A. Metabolic syndrome
   1. Obesity
   2. Hypertension
   3. Hyperlipidemia
   4. High fasting plasma glucose

Plan

A. Aggressive lifestyle modification focusing on increased physical activity and weight reduction is a cornerstone for treatment.
   1. Dietary recommendations include a low-fat, low-cholesterol and/or DASH diets. Decrease simple sugar and saturated and trans fats and cholesterol (see Appendix B).
   2. Exercise recommendations include a minimum of 30 min a day of walking at a brisk pace or other activity at a moderate intensity. Starting by using a pedometer, walking at breaks, or household work.
   3. Weight loss of 5%–10% or more. Gradual weight loss of 1–2 kg per month. Even small amounts of loss are associated with health benefits.
   4. Blood pressure control strategies include a low-sodium diet (DASH), smoking cessation, and alcohol in moderation.
   5. Counsel on smoking cessation.
   6. Abdominoplasties do not lower the risk for CAD or insulin sensitivity.
B. Pharmaceutical therapy
   1. Currently the treatment for metabolic syndrome is the treatment of each individual component/diagnoses for the individual.
   2. Insulin resistant patients usually are not treated by insulin.
   3. Nicotinic acid is the most common drug used for elevated triglycerides and fibrates, and nicotinic acid is used for low HDL-C.
      a. Niacin (Niaspan) 1.5–6 g/day by mouth at bedtime or in divided three times daily dosing. May need to add aspirin therapy for flushing. Aspirin should be taken at least a half-hour before dosing.
      b. Pediatric dose has not been established.
   4. A low-dose aspirin may be prescribed related to the patient's risk of cardiovascular disease's prothrombotic state. Clopidogrel (Plavix) may be used if unable to take aspirin.
   5. Oral hypoglycemic agents used to treat type 2 diabetes are not currently recommended for the **prevention** of metabolic syndrome. However, they are used for insulin resistance to improve glucose tolerance.
      a. Metformin (Glucophage) may be considered for increased fasting glucose (IFG and IGT)
         i. Adult: 500 mg by mouth twice a day, may increase to 850 mg by mouth three times daily if necessary. Titrate slowly due to side effects. Metformin must be stopped prior to any procedure with radiographic dye.

ii. Not recommended in pediatric population.
b. Thiazolidinediones such as rosiglitazone (Avandia) 8 mg/day orally.

Follow-up

A. Follow-up involves assessing patients for metabolic syndrome at 3-year intervals for anyone with one or more risk traits. Follow-up testing includes:
1. BMI calculation
2. Waist-to-hip calculation
3. Fasting lipid profile
4. Fasting glucose
5. Blood pressure

Consultation/Referral

A. Refer to an obstetrician-gynecologist for consultation and management for infertility/pregnancy.
B. Refer to a specialist for any comorbid condition as needed.

Individual Considerations

A. Individual considerations for pregnancy, pediatrics, and geriatrics are specific to their comorbid condition.

OBESITY *by Cheryl A. Glass*

Definition

A. Obesity is a multifactorial disease with physical, psychological, and social consequences. The body mass index (BMI) is a standard measuring tool. The BMI is calculated by using the formula: weight in kilograms divided by height in meters squared (weight [kg]/height [m]^2). In adults, obesity is defined by a BMI greater than 30 kg/m^2.
B. The BMI for children is calculated the same way as for adults but is interpreted using age- and gender-specific percentages (BMI-for-age) clinical charts (see Tables 19.6 and 19.7). The CDC defines childhood obesity by percentiles. Children charts are available on the Centers for Disease Control's (CDC) Web site at http://www.cdc.gov/growthcharts/.

Incidence

A. More than one-third of the adults in the United States are obese, and 16% of U.S. children are obese. Obesity rates cross all groups in society, irrespective of age, sex, race, ethnicity, socioeconomic status, educational level, or geographic group.

Pathogenesis

Numerous factors contribute in the development of obesity, including:

A. Imbalance between energy intake and energy output
B. Genetics (40%–70% presumed explanation)
C. Environmental factors
D. Drug-induced obesity
1. Tricyclic antidepressants
2. Oral contraceptive
3. Antipsychotics
4. Sulfonylureas
5. Anticonvulsants (sodium valproate, carbamazepine)
6. Glucocorticoids

Predisposing Factors

A. Consuming too many calories/high-fat diet
B. Poor dietary choices
C. Readily available food sources, especially fast foods
D. Lack of exercise/sedentary lifestyle
E. Decreased/elimination of physical education requirements in public schools
F. Television (TV), computer, and hand-held game use more than 3 hours/day
G. Increased leisure time
H. Lack of funding and planning for community parks and recreation areas
I. Ethnic background: African American, Hispanic
J. Family history of obesity
K. Pregnancy

Common Complaints

A. Difficulties with ADLs or functional impairment
B. Lack of interest/inability to tolerate exercise
C. Shortness of breath and/or asthma exacerbations
D. Difficulty with personal hygiene
E. Urinary incontinence
F. Desire to loose weight

Other Signs and Symptoms

A. Obstructive sleep apnea (OSA)
B. Increased asthma symptoms
C. Infertility/polycystic ovarian syndrome

TABLE 19.6 Childhood Obesity by Percentiles

Childhood Obesity Category	BMI Definitions by Percentiles
Underweight	Less than the 5th percentile
Healthy Weight	5th to less than 85th percentile
Overweight	85th to less than 95th percentile
Obese	Equal to or greater than 95th percentile

TABLE 19.7 Adult Obesity by BMI

Classification of Adult Obesity by BMI	BMI (kg/m^2)
Underweight	< 18.5
Normal	18.5–24.9
Overweight (Pre-obese)	25.0–29.9
Obesity	30.0–34.9
Severely Obese	> 40.0
Morbid Obese	40.0–49.9
Super Obese	> 50.0
Super-Super Obese (SSO)	≥ 60.0

D. Symptoms associated with cholelithiasis

E. Hypertension

F. Early sexual maturity in girls

Subjective Data

A. Review onset of weight gain and duration of obesity. Identify when the patient first noticed the weight gain.

B. Ask the patient about other symptoms secondary to obesity.

C. Review full medical history.

D. Review medications, including over-the-counter herbals and diet products.

E. Review the patient's previous history of weight loss attempts.

F. Assess ADL and function limitations and the presence of exercise intolerance.

G. Elicit history of sleep disorders (i.e., snoring and obstruction, sleep apnea).

H. Review 24-hour dietary recall. Review the patient's normal average meals per day, including snacks.

I. Review consumption of high caloric drinks and alcohol intake.

J. Assess for history of binge eating, purging, lack of satiety, food-seeking behaviors, and other abnormal feeding habits.

K. Assess for depression.

L. Assess for readiness and commitment for weight loss.

M. Ask the patient to describe his or her activity level, exercise routine, and daily activity (work activity).

Physical Examination

A. Pulse, respirations, and blood pressure.

B. Measure height and weight to calculate BMI.

C. Measure waist and hip circumferences to calculate the waist-to-hip circumference ratio. The waist-to-hip ratio is the strongest anthropometric measure that is associated with myocardial infarction risk, and is a better predictor than BMI.

D. Inspect
   1. Observe the overall appearance and note body fat distribution.
   2. Examine the skin.
   3. Mouth and teeth: assess dental enamel for signs of purging.

E. Palpate the neck and thyroid.

F. Auscultate: Auscultate the heart, lungs, and abdomen.

G. Palpate the extremities: note edema.

Diagnostic Tests

A. Thyroid function.

B. Lipid panel.

C. Triglycerides.

D. Pregnancy test.

E. Fasting blood sugar/3 hour glucose tolerance test (GTT).

F. Sleep study (if indicated).

G. Consider genetic testing.

Differential Diagnoses

A. Obesity

B. Pseudo cerebri

C. Binge eating

D. Genetic syndrome (e.g., Prader-Willi syndrome)

E. Cushing's syndrome

F. Diabetes mellitus

G. Insulin resistance syndrome

Plan

Manage obesity as a chronic relapsing disease, including the comanagement of other diseases secondary to obesity (i.e., diabetes, hypertension).

A. General interventions
   1. Reinforce the positive impact that weight loss measures (diet, exercise) can have and the overall health benefits of weight loss.
   2. Identify and monitor any cardiovascular complications.
   3. Behavior modification
      a. Dietary plan
         i. Low calorie
         ii. Increase in fruits and vegetables
         iii. Eliminate alcohol and sugar-containing beverages
         iv. Reduction of high glycemic foods such as candy
         v. Reduction in high caloric foods and drinks
         vi. Reduction of fat intake
         vii. Reduction of portion sizes
         viii. Increase water intake
      b. Exercise plan
         i. Children and adolescents should do 60 min or more of physical activity every day. Exercise should include moderate- or vigorous-intensity aerobic physical activity 3 days/week and muscle and bone strengthening physical activity at least 3 days/week.
         ii. Adults should strive to do the equivalent of at least 150 min a week of moderate intensity or 75 min of vigorous-intensity aerobic physical activity. Aerobic activity should be performed in episodes of at least 10 min, and preferably spread throughout the week.
      c. Obtain counseling on stimulus control, goal setting, self-monitoring, and contracts that reward behaviors.

B. Patient teaching on obesity treatment modalities
   1. Keep a food diary to identify food triggers.
   2. Counsel about pharmaceutical therapy drug side effects and the lack of long-term safety data, and the temporary nature of the weight loss achieved with medications. Typical weight loss is modest, less than 5 kg at 1 year.

C. Pharmaceutical therapy
   1. After an adequate trial (minimum of 6 months) of diet and exercise therapy, consider pharmaceutical therapy.
   2. There are no data to determine whether one drug is more efficacious than another, and there is no evidence for increased weight loss with combination therapy.
   3. The choice of a pharmaceutical agent depends on the side effect profile of the drug and tolerance of the side effects.
   4. The Food and Drug Administration (FDA) has not approved any weight-loss drug for use beyond

2 years in adults. Appetite suppressants include phentermine, benzphetamine, and phendimetrazine that are FDA approved for short-term (12-week) use. Sibutramine (Meridia®, Reductil®) is FDA approved for 1-year use. Orlistat (Xenical®) is FDA approved for 2-year use.

5. Appetite suppressants
   a. Phentermine (Adipex-P) 37.5 mg orally once daily before or 1–2 hours after breakfast, or 18.75 mg 1–2 times per day for initial BMI greater than 30 kg/m², or BMI greater than 27 kg/m² in the presence of risk factors.
      i. Avoid late evening dosing.
      ii. Not recommended for children younger than 16 years.
      iii. Not recommended in the presence of hypertension, hyperthyroidism, cardiovascular disease, and drug or alcohol abuse.
      iv. Do not prescribe during or within 14 days of monoamine oxidase inhibitors (MAOIs).
   b. Benzphetamine (Didrex) 25–50 mg orally initially in the mid-morning or mid-afternoon. Increase if needed to 25–50 mg 1–3 times a day.
      i. Not recommended in children or adolescents.
      ii. Not recommended in the presence of hypertension, hyperthyroidism, cardiovascular disease, and drug or alcohol abuse.
      iii. Do not prescribe during or within 14 days of monoamine oxidase inhibitors (MAOIs).
      iv. Pregnancy Category X: known to cause fetal abnormalities or toxicity in animal and human studies.
   c. Phendimetrazine (Bontril PDM) 35 mg orally 2 or 3 times daily 1 hour before meals. May reduce to 17.5 mg/dose. Maximum dose 210 mg/day in 3 evenly divided doses. Also available in slow-release 105 mg in the morning 30–60 min before breakfast.
      i. Not recommended in children or adolescents.
      ii. Not recommended in the presence of hypertension, hyperthyroidism, cardiovascular disease, and drug or alcohol abuse.
      iii. Do not prescribe during or within 14 days of monoamine oxidase inhibitors (MAOIs).
   d. Sibutramine (Meridia) 10 mg orally once a day. After 4 weeks may titrate to 15 mg once a day.
      i. Not recommended in children or adolescents younger than 16 years old.
      ii. FDA approved for use up to 2 years.
      iii. Not recommended for nursing mothers.
      iv. Blood pressure and pulse should be monitored regularly during therapy. Consider discontinuing sibutramine with sustained blood pressure and pulse increases.
      v. Not recommended with severe renal or hepatic dysfunction or with a history of narrow-angle glaucoma.
6. Lipase inhibitor
   a. Orlistat (Xenical) for use with a low-fat diet. Recommend 30% of calories spread over 3 main meals.
      i. Take one 120 mg capsule orally during or up to 1 hour after main meals up to three times per day.
      ii. If a meal is missed or had no fat, skip dosage.
      iii. May decrease absorption of fat-soluble vitamins and beta-carotene.
      iv. Orlistat carries an FDA warning regarding safety and efficacy for use in patients younger than 12 years and in pregnancy and lactation since it interferes with the absorption of fat-soluble vitamins.
      v. Supplement diet with a multivitamin.
      vi. FDA approved for up to 2 years' use in adults.
      vii. Gastrointestinal side effects include fatty/oily stools, oily spotting, flatus with discharge, fecal urgency, and fecal incontinence.
      viii. Contraindicated in chronic malabsorption syndrome and cholestiasis.
      ix. May affect doses for antidiabetic medications.
      x. Monitor warfarin and cyclosoporine levels.
   b. Alli®, a lipase inhibitor, is the only FDA-available over-the-counter (OTC) weight loss product.

Follow-up

A. Reevaluate the patient in approximately 1 month if started on pharmaceutical therapy.
B. Maintain the recommended schedule for comorbid conditions.
C. If a candidate for bariatric surgery, follow recommended pretreatment/preauthorization guidelines required by the payer and bariatric center.

Consultation/Referral

A. Refer for a nutrition/registered dietitian consultation.
B. Consider a referral to a bariatric center/surgical consultation and evaluation of bariatric surgery.
C. Consider a psychology consultation (may be required prior to bariatric surgery).
D. If the family is eligible refer to the Women, Infant and Children (WIC) program.

Individual Considerations

A. Pregnancy
   1. Benzphetamine (Didrex) is a Category X drug.
   2. Council patients regarding appropriate weight gain with pregnancy.
B. Pediatrics
   1. The cornerstone for the management for obesity in children is modification of dietary and exercise habits.
   2. The first step for overweight children older than 2 years is maintenance of baseline weight if there is no secondary complication of obesity (i.e., diabetes and hypertension).
   3. Weight loss goal should be approximately 1 pound per month to a BMI below the 85th percentile.
   4. Decrease sedentary behaviors (i.e., watching TV, surfing the Internet, and playing video games).
   5. Incorporate exercise into family time.
   6. Long-term safety and effectiveness of low-carbohydrate, high-protein diets such as the Atkins diet have not been adequately studied in children.

7. Use of pharmacotherapies in children and adolescents requires further research, unless noted above under drug therapies.
C. Geriatrics
   1. All adults should avoid inactivity. Some exercise is better than none.

POLYCYSTIC OVARIAN SYNDROME (PCOS)

Definition

Polycystic ovary syndrome (PCOS) is characterized by ovulatory dysfunction and hyperandrogenism. PCOS was previously called Stein-Leventhal syndrome. PCOS is a risk factor for metabolic syndrome, infertility, glucose intolerance, and type 2 diabetes mellitus. PCOS itself is not considered a disease; instead it is a syndrome of coexisting conditions (see Table 19.8).

The Androgen Excess Society diagnostic criteria for PCOS is:

A. Hyperandrogenism
B. Ovarian dysfunction
C. Exclusion of other androgen excess or related disorders

Although obesity is one of the hallmarks of PCOS, lean women may also have insulin resistance/PCOS. The diagnosis of PCOS is based on medical history, physical examination, and laboratory tests. Aggressive lifestyle modification is the mainstay of all adolescents and women with PCOS.

Incidence

A. The incidence of PCOS is 6.5% up to 10% in the literature. It is the one of the most common endocrinopathies in women, with 5–7 million women in the United States experiencing the effects of PCOS.

Pathogenesis

A. The exact etiology is unknown; however, PCOS is noted to have insulin resistance and abnormal pituitary function, as well as abnormal steroidogenesis.

Predisposing Factors

A. Obesity
B. Genetic predisposition
C. Metabolic syndrome

TABLE 19.8 PCOS Associated Symptoms

Cutaneous signs	Hirsutism Severe acne Alopecia
Menstrual irregularity	Oligomenorrhea Amenorrhea Dysfunctional uterine bleeding
Obesity	> 35 inches (88 cm) waist circumference for women and adolescents ≥ 16 years ≥ 90 percentile for ages 10 to < 16 years
Polycystic ovaries	Noted on ultrasound

Common Complaints

A. Hirsutism
B. Menstrual problems
C. Obesity
D. Infertility

Other Signs and Symptoms

A. Acne
B. Alopecia (male pattern)
C. Hyperhidrosis
D. Acanthosis nigricans
E. Seborrhea

Subjective Data

A. Review the patient's menstruation history:
   1. Premature puberty (before age 8)
   2. Primary amenorrhea: lack of menses by age 15
   3. Oligomenorrhea: missing 4 periods/year
   4. DUB: bleeding at irregular intervals, heavy cycles, periods longer than 7 days
B. Review the patient's history of weight gain, increased waist circumference, and obesity.
C. Review the patient's history of any skin/hair changes.
D. Review the family history for the presence of diabetes, metabolic syndrome, and infertility.

Physical Examination

A. Check height, weight, waist circumference, blood pressure, pulse, and respirations.
B. Calculate the body mass index and waist-to-hip measurement. Several Internet sites have BMI, body fat, and waist-to-hip ratio calculators.
C. Inspect
   1. Skin:
      a. Evaluate hirsutism (upper lip, chin, nape of the neck, periareolar, abdomen-linea alba).
   2. Observe fat distribution.
D. Perform pelvic examination to evaluate enlarged ovaries and pelvic masses.

Diagnostic Tests

A. Fasting glucose
B. Oral glucose tolerance test (OGTT) if fasting glucose is elevated between 100 mg/dL and 125 mg/dL
C. Thyroid function tests (TSH, Free T_4)
D. Random serum cortisol to rule out Cushing's syndrome
E. Serum LH and prolactin to rule out hypothalamic and pituitary diseases
F. Ultrasound to rule out ovarian pathology (as indicated: not required for definitive diagnosis)
G. Insulinlike growth factor (IGF-I)
H. Dehydroepiandrosterone sulfate (DHEAS) to rule out adrenal hyperandrogenism
I. Free and total testosterone
J. Lipid profiles
K. Endometrial biopsy if indicated for women without menses for 1 year
L. Pregnancy test prior to start of pharmaceutical therapy and history of anovulation

Differential Diagnoses

A. PCOS

B. Adrenal disorders
1. Congenital adrenal hyperplasia (CAH)
2. Cushing's syndrome
3. Cortisol resistance
C. Hyperprolactinemia
D. Acromegaly
E. Insulin resistance (types 1 and 2 diabetes)
F. Thyroid dysfunction
G. Virilizing tumors
H. Drug-induced
1. Anabolic steroids
2. Valproic acid

Plan

A. Aggressive lifestyle modification focusing on increased physical activity and weight reduction is a cornerstone for treatment.
1. Exercise recommendations include a minimum of 30 min a day of walking at a brisk pace or other activity at a moderate intensity. Starting by using a pedometer, walking at breaks, or household work.
2. Weight loss of 5%–10% or more. Gradual weight loss of 1–2 kg per month. Even small amounts of loss are associated with health benefits.
3. Weight loss may cause a resumption of ovulation and the ability to get pregnant.
4. High fiber, low fat, and reduction of refined sugar diet.
B. Hair removal can be achieved with shaving, waxing, or use of depilatories. Electrolysis and laser treatment are more expensive therapies for hirsutism.
C. Pharmaceutical therapy
1. Oral contraceptives (OCPs) are the most commonly used treatment for endometrial prevention and hirsutism.
   a. Due to sodium and water retention, weight reduction while on OCPs is more difficult.
   b. Oral contraceptives that contain 30–35 μ of ethinyl estradiol and progestins such as norethindrone (Ortho Micronor®), norgestimate (Ortho-Tri-Cyclen®), desogestrel (Desogen® and Ortho-Cept®), or dirospirenone (Yasmin®) are prescribed for PCOS.
2. Metformin (Glucophage) is used to manage oligomenorrhea, weight loss, lowering insulin levels, and ovulation induction for women with PCOS.
   a. Start metformin 500 mg at the evening meal. The dosage can be increased by 500 mg per week in divided doses up to the maximum of 2,000 mg/day.
   b. Titrate slowly due to the gastrointestinal side effects.
   c. Check a metabolic panel before and every 3–6 months to evaluate for lactic acidosis.
   d. Metformin is contraindicated in patients with renal impairment; assess renal function prior to instituting metformin and monitor regularly.
   e. Metformin must be stopped prior to any procedure with radiographic dye.
3. Thiazolidinediones such as rosiglitazone (Avandia) 4 mg twice a day for 2 months may be used for insulin sensitivity. Liver panels should be performed prior to beginning any thiazolidinedione due to hepatoxicity.
4. Medroxyprogesterone acetate (Provera) is used for a withdrawal bleed 5–10 mg daily for 10 days every 1–2 months or micronized progesterone (Prometrium®) 100–200 mg by mouth at bedtime for 7–10 days/month are used to protect the endometrium.
5. Spironolactone (Aldactone) 100–200 mg twice a day is utilized after a 4- to 6-month oral contraceptive trial as antiandrogen therapy.
   a. Spironolactone is also a good alternative when OCPs are contraindicated. However, spironolactone can be used in combination with OCPs.
   b. Alternative methods of birth control should be used when spironolactone is used alone secondary to abnormal development of the male fetus external genitalia.
   c. Monitor potassium during spironolactone therapy.
6. Eflornithine (Vaniqa) topical may be prescribed to prevent facial hair regrowth.
7. Clomiphen citrate (Clomid) is used for ovulation induction. Weight loss should be attempted prior to starting ovulation induction treatment.

Follow-up

A. Glucose tolerance needs to be evaluated regularly for type 2 diabetes in women with PCOS. See Table 19.9.

Consultation/Referral

A. Refer to an obstetrician/gynecologist or a reproductive endocrinologist for consultation and management for:
1. Infertility/pregnancy
2. Menstrual bleeding that is not controlled despite OCPs.
B. An endocrinologist may be an appropriate consultation.
C. Consider a nutritional consultation.

⬛ RAYNAUD PHENOMENON

Definition

Raynaud phenomenon (RP) is an idiopathic disease in which an exaggerated vascular response occurs in extreme measures (heat, cold, and stress) and is manifested by bilateral blanching and discomfort in the fingers, followed by cyanosis, then erythema after warming the digits.

Having cold hands and feet are very common complaints. Raynaud phenomenon involves both cutaneous color change and cool skin temperature. Although the hands are the most common area of attacks, it also can occur in the toes, ears, nose, face, knees, and nipples. A Raynaud attack typically begins in a single finger and spreads symmetrically; however, the thumb is often spared.

RP may be either primary or secondary. Spontaneous remission may occur with primary RP.

A. Criteria for diagnosis of primary RP include:
1. Symmetric episodic attacks
2. No evidence of peripheral vascular disease
3. No tissue gangrene, digital pitting, or tissue injury
4. Negative nailfold capillary examination
5. Negative antinuclear antibody test
6. Normal erythrocyte sedimentation rate (ESR)

TABLE 19.9	Androgen Excess Society Screening and Treatment Requirements for Impaired Glucose Tolerance (IGT)

All patients with PCOS, regardless of BMI, should be screened for IGT using a 2-hour oral glucose tolerance test (OGTT).

Patients with a normal glucose test should be rescreened at least once every 2 years or earlier if additional risk factors are identified.

Patients with IGT should be screened annually for the development of type 2 diabetes mellitus.

Adolescents with PCOS should be screened for IGT using a 2-hour OGTT every 2 years. If IGT develops, the treatment with metformin should be considered.

The mainstay of treatment with PCOS and IGT is intensive lifestyle modifications (diet, exercise, and weight loss).

Insulin-sensitizing agents should be considered for patients with PCOS and IGT.

Adapted from the 2007 Androgen Excess Society Position Statement (Kelsey et al., 2007).

B. Indications of secondary RP
 1. Age on onset older than 40 years
 2. Painful severe attacks with signs of ulceration/ischemia
 3. Ischemic signs/symptoms proximal to the fingers or toes
 4. Asymmetric attacks
 5. Abnormal laboratory, suggesting vascular or autoimmune disorders

Incidence
A. 3%–20% in women
B. 3%–14% in men
C. 3% in African Americans
D. Wide global differences from the United States

Pathogenesis
A. Primary Raynaud: Speculated theories include digital microvascular vasospasm due to increased response of α_2-adrenergic receptors and a high sympathetic vascular tone.
B. Secondary Raynaud: Symptoms occur as a secondary manifestation from other diseases such as connective tissue disorders, systemic sclerosis, atherosclerotic diseases, and neurovascular disorders such as carpal tunnel syndrome. Symptoms may be unilateral and may only affect one for two fingers. Secondary Raynaud usually has poorer morbidity than primary disease.

Predisposing Factors
A. Primary Raynaud
 1. Female
 2. Onset of symptoms after menarche (15–30 years)
 3. Smoking
 4. Emotional stress
B. Secondary Raynaud
 1. Onset after age 40
 2. Male gender
C. Family history: multiple family members
D. Frostbite
E. Vascular trauma (distal ulnar artery)
F. Vibration-induced/occupation exposure (jackhammers, pneumatic drills)
G. Medication-associated RP (see Table 19.10).

Common Complaints
A. Paleness of the fingertips after exposure to cold temperatures, followed by redness and discomfort after warming fingers.
B. "White attack": sharp, demarcated color of skin pallor
C. "Blue attack": cyanotic skin
D. White or blue attack usually lasts 15–20 min
E. Age of onset between 15 and 30 years of age

Other Signs and Symptoms
A. Paresthesias and numbness
B. Clumsiness of the aching hand/finger
C. Loss of pulp in pads of fingers (severe cases)

Subjective Data
A. Determine the age of onset, time, duration, and course of presenting symptoms.
B. Question the patient regarding location and symptoms, noting blanching, followed by erythema and pain after hands are warm.
C. Note frequency of attacks.
D. Review the presence of any other skin alterations that have occurred. Do they also note skin mottling of the arms and legs? Livedo reticularis is a lilac or violet mottling or reticular pattern during a cold response.
E. Ask the patient to identify any events that precipitate occurrences, and what makes symptoms worse or better.
 1. Air-conditioning
 2. Grocery cold/freezer food sections
 3. Cold weather
 4. Cold water
 5. Emotional stress
 6. Sudden startling

TABLE 19.10	Drugs That Induce Raynaud Phenomenon

Amphetamines	Clonidine	Interferon-alpha
Beta blockers	Cocaine	Nicotine
Bleomycin	Cyclosporine	Vinblastine
Cisplatin	Ergot	Vinyl chloride

F. Identify any other symptoms that occur at the same time, such as migraine headaches.

G. Review the patient's health history for underlying disorders such as hypothyroidism and connective tissue disease.

H. Review current or past occupation (especially those that include the use of vibratory tools).

I. Review current medications, stimulants, herbals, and over-the-counter medications.

Physical Examination

A. Check temperature, pulse, respirations, and blood pressure.

B. Inspect
1. Dermal examination: note malar/petechial rash, telangiectasias, digital pallor, or erythema. Examine for any ulceration or signs of ischemia.
2. Inspect joints for swelling or redness and overall ischemic changes.
3. Examine several fingernails using a microscope or ophthalmoscope; examine capillaries at nailfold.
   a. Normal: fine red capillaries, lined in the same direction.
   b. Abnormal: capillaries dilated, tortuous, irregularly spaced. Avoid using the index finger for evaluation.

C. Auscultate the heart and lung fields.

D. Palpate joints for tenderness and peripheral pulses bilaterally.

E. Neurologic examination: sensory function
1. Sensory discrimination (hot/cold, sharp/dull).
2. Location of sensation (proximal/distal to previous stimuli).
3. Vibratory sensation with tuning fork (distal to proximal joints).
4. Graphanesthesia (draw a number or letter in palm of the hand with a blunt object such as a pencil, applicator stick, or pen and have the patient identify the letter/number).

Diagnostic Tests

A. There is no gold standard diagnostic test.

B. History alone is accepted as diagnostic since no office test application consistently triggers an attack. A history of at least two color changes, pallor, and cyanosis after cold exposure is adequate for the diagnosis of RP.

C. The cold water challenge test is no longer recommended.

D. Tools to assess vascular response (usually not readily available)
1. Nailfold capillaroscopy
2. Videomicroscopy
3. Thermography
4. Angiography
5. Laser Doppler
6. Direct measures of the skin temperature and local blood flow

E. Laboratory tests
1. Antinuclear antibody
2. ESR
3. Thyroid profile if hypothyroidism is suspected
4. Other tests, depending on suspected etiology
   a. CBC
   b. Chemistry profile with renal and liver function
   c. Urinalysis
   d. Rheumatoid factor
   e. Complement (C3 and C4)
   f. ANA

Differential Diagnoses

A. Raynaud phenomenon (primary vs. secondary)
B. Scleroderma
C. Systemic lupus erythematosus
D. Occupational trauma
E. Medication induced
F. Peripheral vascular disease
G. Neurovascular processes (diabetes, atherosclerosis, thrombosis obliterans)

Plan

A. General interventions
1. If ulcerations are present monitor for secondary infections. Consider topical/systemic antibiotics if secondary infection. Debridement may be necessary.
2. Biofeedback and relaxation techniques are frequently used for treatment.

B. Patient teaching
1. Stress the importance of not smoking.
2. Keep the body warm.
   a. If in extreme temperatures, wear extra clothing (thermal underwear) to maintain temperature.
   b. Wear mittens instead of gloves to protect hands and keep them warm.
   c. Wear a hat to conserve heat.
3. If possible, stop all medications that could be inducing symptoms. Other drugs that should be avoided include:
   a. Decongestants
   b. Herbs that contain ephedra
4. If vibrator injury is present, stop the repetitive activity that induces symptoms. Consider alternative methods of work. If unable to totally stop the activity, decrease time spent using the vibratory equipment.

C. Surgical therapy
1. Temporary sympathectomy involving a local chemical block with lidocaine or bupivacaine (without epinephrine) relieves the pain.
2. Botulinum toxin A has been used for chemical sympathectomy.
3. Cervical sympathectomy (primary RP).
4. Localized digital sympathectomy.
5. Vascular reconstruction.

D. Pharmaceutical therapy
1. Therapy may be required only during the winter months.
2. Long-acting calcium channel blockers are used.
   a. Nifedipine 30–180 mg/day
   b. Amlodipine 5–20 mg/day
3. Low-dose aspirin antiplatelet therapy 75–81 mg/day may be considered in secondary RP with a history of ischemic ulcers or other thrombotic events.

Follow-up

A. Follow up in 1 month or as needed by patient symptoms.

Consultation/Referral

A. Consult a physician if signs of ischemia present and/or if refractory symptoms are present.
B. Refer to a rheumatologist if there is a moderate/high suspicion of secondary RP.
C. Refer for surgical therapies.

Individual Considerations

A. Pediatrics: Raynaud is commonly seen in children with systemic lupus erythematous and scleroderma.
B. Adults: onset of Raynaud after age 40 is commonly associated with an underlying disease.

RHEUMATOID ARTHRITIS

Definition

Rheumatoid arthritis (RA) is a chronic systemic disease that involves articular inflammation of the joints. The disease is generally insidious and symmetrical involvement of joints is a characteristic feature. Typically the interphalangeal joints of the fingers and thumbs are noted; however, other joints involved include the elbows, shoulders, ankles, knees, and toes.

Rheumatoid arthritis is not limited to the joints; extra-articular features of RA include anemia, pleuropericarditis, neuropathy, myopathy, splenomegaly, Sjögren's syndrome, scleritis, vasculitis, and renal disease. Most patients with extra-articular symptoms also have the classic RA joint symptoms. Patients with RA are at increased risk for carpal tunnel syndrome, development of carpal tunnel syndrome, stroke, an osteoporotic fracture, and renal disease (secondary to drug toxicity).

The American College of Rheumatology criteria for RA require that five of the seven symptoms must be present, with the first four symptoms being continuous for at least 6 weeks:

A. Morning stiffness longer than 1 hour for more than 6 weeks
B. Arthritis of at least three joint groups with soft tissue swelling or fluid longer than 6 weeks
C. Swelling of at least one of the following joints: proximal interphalangeal, metacarpophalangeal, or wrists longer than 6 weeks
D. Symmetrical joint swelling longer than 6 weeks
E. Subcutaneous nodules
F. Positive rheumatoid factor test
G. Radiographic changes consistent with RA
There are four stages of RA:

A. Stage 1: No symptoms or signs, normal activity. Antigen is present.
B. Stage 2: Morning stiffness, warmth at joint, normal activities of daily living, minimal limitation in joint use. Increase T cells, B cells, antibody production, and synovial cells.
C. Stage 3: Morning stiffness, warmth at joint, and extra-articular manifestations. Marked limitation in activities of daily living. Increase T cells, B cells, antibody production, and synovial cells.
D. Stage 4: Same as stage 3 plus proliferating synovial membrane involved causing injury to the bone, tendons, and cartilage. Incapacitated or confined to wheelchair.

Incidence

A. RA occurs in approximately 1%–2% of the population.

Pathogenesis

A. The cause is unknown. Articular inflammation results in joint damage. Antibody formation in the joint area results in inflammation in the joint area.

Predisposing Factors

A. Family history
B. Female gender
C. Ages 20–50 years
D. Recent systemic illness or trauma

Common Complaints

A. Joint pain
B. Stiffness
C. Swelling and warmth of the joints, especially fingers, hands, wrists, elbows, shoulders, ankles, and/or knees.

Other Signs and Symptoms

A. Fatigue
B. Malaise
C. Subcutaneous nodules
D. Joint deformities
   1. Proximal interphalangeal joints: boutonniere deformities
   2. Fingers: swan neck contractures
   3. Wrists: loss of extension
   4. Hips: loss of internal rotation, followed by flexion contractures
   5. Knees: suprapateller pouch distention
   6. Elbows: decreased extension, olecranon bursitis
   7. Shoulders: limited movement
   8. Cervical spine: subluxation rare
   9. Temporomandibular joint: pain with biting
E. Depression
F. Low-grade fever
G. Weight loss
H. Myalgia
I. Anemia
J. Carpal tunnel syndrome

Subjective Data

A. Review when joint pains began and identify the joints involved.
B. Elicit the patient's description of pain and a description of how the pain interferes with activities of daily living (walking, climbing stairs, using the toilet, getting up from a chair, opening a jar).
C. Review the family history of RA.
D. Has the patient ever had any type of injury to the specific joint area? Rule out recent injuries.
E. Identify what make the pain worse and alleviating factors.
F. Review list of medications, including herbal and over-the-counter. What therapies have specifically been used and what were the results?
G. Review the patient's history for recent infections.
H. Does the patient use any assistive devices, including cane, crutches, walker, wheelchair/power mobility device, kitchen devices/grips, and so forth?

Physical Examination

A. Check temperature, pulse, respirations, blood pressure, and weight.
B. General observation
   1. The patient getting up and down in the chair.
   2. The patient walking (may have a tendency to bear weight on heels and hyperextend toes secondary to tenderness to the metatarsophalangeal joints).
   3. Observe the patient handling objects in his or her hands.
   4. Observe for signs of depression.
C. Inspect
   1. Inspect all joints, noting deformities, erythema, and temperature. (Heat and redness are not prominent features of RA.)
   2. Evaluate for pitting edema in the hand (may have a "boxing glove" appearance).
   3. Inspect for subcutaneous rheumatoid nodules (elbow is most common site).
   4. Evaluate skin for ulcerative lesions (secondary from venous stasis and neutrophilic infiltration), skin atrophy and ecchymosed from glucocorticoids, and petechiae (side effect from medications causing thrombocytopenia).
   5. Eye examination
      a. Episcleritis: acute redness and pain without discharge
      b. Scleritis: deep ocular pain with dark red discoloration
D. Auscultate
   1. Auscultate the heart.
   2. Auscultate the lungs (at risk for infectious complications from immunosuppression and pulmonary toxicity from methotrexate and gold salts).
E. Percuss
   1. Patellar tap to evaluate synovial thickening/effusion of the knee.
F. Palpate
   1. Palpate the lymph nodes.
   2. Oral exam to palpate the salivary glands (may have lymphocytic infiltration).
   3. Palpate all joints to evaluate for tenderness with pressure, pain with movement of the joint, and "bogginess" of the joint (synovial thickening).
   4. Palpate the popliteal fossa for evidence of a popliteal (Baker's) cyst.
   5. Abdominal examination for splenomegaly.
G. Musculoskeletal examination
   1. Assess grip (a reduced grip is a useful parameter in evaluating disease activity and progression).
   2. Assess the strength of the extremities.
   3. Assess the range of motion (active and passive) and flexion.

Diagnostic Tests

A. CBC and platelets.
B. Erythrocyte sedimentation rate (ESR).
C. Rheumatoid factor.
D. Antinuclear antibody (ANA).
E. Uric acid level.
F. C-reactive protein (CRP).
G. Synovial fluid (optional).
H. Plain film radiography is used most often to assess and follow the progression.

Differential Diagnoses

A. Rheumatoid arthritis
B. Osteoarthritis
C. Psoriatic arthritis
D. Crystalline arthritis (gout and pseudogout)
E. Polyarthritis
F. Reiter's syndrome
G. Acute viral/infectious process
   1. Lyme disease
   2. Hepatitis B
   3. Hepatitis C
   4. Parvovirus B19
H. Systemic lupus erythematous
I. Sjögren's syndrome: keratoconjunctivitis sicca, splenomegaly, and lymphadenopathy
J. Sarcoidosis
K. Polymyositis
L. Felty's syndrome: rheumatoid arthritis, splenomegaly, and neutropenia

Plan

A. General interventions
   1. Focus on exercise and joint mobility to maintain functional abilities.
   2. Encourage stopping smoking, especially females on glucocorticoids due to the risk of increased bone loss/fracture.
B. Patient teaching
   1. Counsel patients that alcohol should be avoided when using methotrexate due to the risk of hepatotoxicity.
   2. Stress the importance of returning for laboratory follow-up while on DMARDs.
   3. Discuss vaccinations: pneumonia and influenza vaccines.
C. Pharmaceutical therapy
   1. Early disease: anti-inflammatory medications
      a. Daily anti-inflammatory drugs
         i. Ibuprofen 3,200 mg in divided doses
         ii. Naproxen 1,000 mg in divided doses
         iii. Piroxicam (Feldene) 20 mg daily
      b. Comorbid conditions, such as a history of heart failure, renal disease, and ulcers should be considered before starting NSAID therapy.
      c. Be aware of other medications and consider possible drug-to-drug interactions such as NSAIDs with antacids, anticoagulants, oral hypoglycemic agents, antihypertensive/diuretics, lithium, methotrexate, and diphenylhydantoin (Dilantin).
   2. Moderate to severe RA disease:
      a. Oral glucocorticoids, prednisone up to 7.5 mg/day may be added for active joint inflammation. Prednisone may be used up to 6 months and should be tapered over a period of a few months and then completely discontinued if possible.

b. Intra-articular of long-acting glucocorticoid injections are used for the reduction of synovitis in inflamed joints.

c. Gold salt therapy may be implemented by physicians. Patients receiving gold therapy need to be monitored for skin or oral lesions and urinary changes.

d. Disease-modifying antirheumatic drugs (DMARDs) are recommended by the American College of Rheumatology if early RA manifestations have been present for less than 6 months. Adding DMARDs depends on the number of inflamed joints, severity of inflammation, functional impairment, and the number of poor prognostic signs (bony erosions and extra-articular disease).

   i. Methotrexate (MTX) given on a weekly basis starting with 7.5 mg/week and is increased as tolerated to control symptoms. Titration: increase the dose after 4 weeks at a rate of 2.5 mg/week to a maximum of 25 mg/week. MTX should not be given to patients who desire to become or are pregnant or patients with liver disease.

   ii. Sulfasalazine (Azulfidine) 1,000 mg twice a day or three times daily is used more for active synovitis.

   iii. Hydroxychloroquine (Plaquenil) up to 6.5 mg/kg

   iv. Leflunomide (Arava)

   v. If response is not adequate, biologic agents, tumor necrosis factor alpha inhibitors, may be instituted as a single agent or in combination with other DMARDs.

      (a). Infliximab (Remicade)

      (b). Adalimumab (Humira) 0.8 mL (40 mg) every 2 weeks

      (c). Etanercept (Enbrel) 25 mg subcutaneous once or twice weekly

3. Initiate bisphosphonate therapy as indicated. Use a low threshold for starting with postmenopausal women with RA.

Follow-up

A. Follow-up will be guided by medication therapy. Disease activity and response to therapy should be reassessed every 3–5 weeks.

B. Follow laboratory values with certain medications, including methotrexate with liver function testing, albumin, CBC, platelets, and urinalysis monthly.

C. Assume all patients with RA are at risk for osteoporosis. DEXA scan to evaluate bone loss secondary to glucocorticoid-induced osteopenia.

D. Anti-TNF agents are contraindicated in patients with an active infection and who are at high risk for reactivation of tuberculosis. A TB skin test is required before administration. Patients with a positive skin test should be treated with prophylactic antituberculosis therapy 1 month prior to therapy with anti-TNF agents.

Consultation/Referral

A. Refer all patients to a rheumatologist with early inflammatory arthritis if RA is suspected disease.

B. Aspiration of joint fluid may be referred to a physician.

Individual Considerations

A. Pregnancy
   1. RA activity improves substantially in pregnancy.
      a. 70%–80% improved during pregnancy.
      b. RA flares in the postpartum by approximately 90%. Flares usually occur within the first 3 months postpartum.
   2. Leflunomide, etanercept, adalimumab, and infliximab are contraindicated in pregnancy and while breast-feeding.
   3. Therapy during pregnancy should be coordinated with the perinatologist and the rheumatologist.

B. Pediatrics
   1. In children, consider juvenile-onset rheumatoid arthritis.
   2. If suspected, consider referral to a pediatric rheumatologist for evaluation and diagnosis.

C. Geriatrics
   1. Use NSAIDs with caution, age- and weight-appropriate dosing.

THYROTOXICOSIS/THYROID STORM
by Jill C. Cash

Definition

A. Severe thyrotoxicosis of any cause is called thyrotoxic crisis or storm.

Incidence

A. It is rare; the incidence varies, depending on the cause of the thyrotoxicosis.

Pathogenesis

A. Thyrotoxic crisis or storm usually develops in patients either undiagnosed as being hyperthyroid or those who are known to be severely hyperthyroid and are being treated insufficiently, and are subjected to excessive stress from other causes. Oversecretion of T_3 and T_4 is followed by a release of epinephrine. Metabolism is dramatically increased. The adrenal glands produce excessive corticosteroids, which is a response to stress.

Predisposing Factors

A. Severe, uncontrolled hyperthyroidism
B. Noncompliance with antihyperthyroid medication
C. Inadequate preparation for thyroid surgery

Common Complaints

A. Sudden onset of
   1. Hyperthermia
   2. Tachycardia (usually atrial tachydysrhythmias)
   3. High-output cardiac failure
   4. Altered sensorium (usually agitation, restlessness, delirium)
   5. Nausea, vomiting, and diarrhea

Subjective Data

A. Elicit information regarding the onset, duration, and nature of symptoms.
B. Determine the presence of cardiac symptoms.

C. Take a complete drug history, including whether or not patient has been taking antithyroid medication as prescribed.

D. Rule out any excessive acute stressors such as infection, pulmonary or cardiac problems, dialysis, plasmapheresis, and/or emotional stressors.

Physical Examination

A. Check temperature, pulse, respirations, and blood pressure.

B. Inspect
   1. Inspect the skin.

C. Auscultate
   1. Auscultate the heart and lungs.

D. Palpate the neck carefully for thyroid nodules and enlargement.

Diagnostic Tests

A. Serum T_3 and Free T_4

B. TSH

Differential Diagnoses

A. Thyroid storm

B. Thyrotoxic crisis

Plan

A. General interventions
   1. Closely monitor temperature, pulse, respirations, and blood pressure.

B. Patient teaching
   1. See "Patient Teaching" in the "Hyperthyroidism" section.

C. Medical management
   1. Assess the need to hospitalize the patient for supportive therapy: intravenous fluids, medication, antipyretics, and oxygen.

D. Pharmaceutical therapy
   1. See "Pharmaceutical Therapy" in the "Hyperthyroidism" section.

Follow-up

A. Following resolution of the crisis, see the patient in the office every 3–4 weeks for evaluation and monitoring of serum TSH and Free T_4 levels.

B. See "Follow-up" in the "Hyperthyroidism" section.

Consultation/Referral

A. Refer the patient to a physician immediately for possible hospitalization.

Individual Considerations

A. Pregnancy: See "Individual Considerations" in the "Hyperthyroidism" section.

REFERENCES

AACE Thyroid Task Force. (2006). American Association of Clinical Endocrinologist medical guidelines for clinical practice for the evaluation and treatment of hyperthyroidism and hypothyroidism. Amended Version. *Endocrine Practice, 8,* 457–469.

Ahmad, S., Brakke, M., Marks, J., Singer, P., & Cooper, D. (1995, October 4). Treatment guidelines for hyperthyroidism and hypothyroidism. *Journal of the American Medical Association, 274*(13), 1011–1012.

Alberti, K.G.M. M., Eckel, R. H., Grundy, S. M., Zimmet, P. Z., Cleeman, J. L., Donato, K. A., et al. (2009). Harmonizing the metabolic syndrome: A joint interim statement of the International Diabetes Federation Task Force on Epidemiology and Prevention; National Heart, Lung, and Blood Institutes; American Heart Association; World Heart Federation; International Atherosclerosis Society; and International Association for the Study of Obesity. *Circulation, 120,* 1640–1645.

Alley, D. E., & Chang, V. W. (2007). The changing relationship of obesity and disability, 1988–2004. *Journal of the American Medical Association, 298,* 2020–2027.

American Academy of Pediatrics, Committee on Nutrition. Prevention of Pediatric Overweight and Obesity. (2003). *Pediatrics, 112,* 424–430.

American Association of Clinical Endocrinologists. (1995, February 15). American Association of Endocrinologists releases clinical guidelines for thyroid disease. *American Family Physician, 51*(3), 679.

American Association of Clinical Endocrinologists. (2006). *Hyperthyroidism.* Retrieved March 13, 2009, from http://www.endonurses.org/toolbox/pdf/patient_education/AACE%20Hyperthyroidism.pdf

American College of Cardiology, the American Heart Association, and the European Society of Cardiology. (2001). ACC/AHA/ESC guidelines for the management of patients with atrial fibrillation. *Journal of the American College of Cardiology, 38,* 1266ii–1266lxx.

American Diabetes Association. (1998a). Diabetes mellitus and exercise (Position Statement). *Diabetes Care, 21*(Suppl. 1), S40–S44.

American Diabetes Association. (1998b). Gestational diabetes mellitus (Position Statement). *Diabetes Care, 21*(Suppl. 1), S60–S61.

American Diabetes Association. (1998c). Implications of the diabetes control and complications trial (Position Statement). *Diabetes Care, 21*(Suppl. 1), S88–S90.

American Diabetes Association. (1998d). Screening for type 2 diabetes (Position Statement). *Diabetes Care, 21*(Suppl. l), S20–S22.

American Diabetes Association. (1998e). Standards of medical care for patients with diabetes mellitus (Position Statement). *Diabetes Care, 21*(Suppl. 1), S23–S31.

American Diabetes Association. (1998f). Report of the expert committee on the diagnosis and classification of diabetes mellitus (Committee Report). *Diabetes Care, 21*(Suppl.), S5–S19.

Azziz, R., Carmina, E., Dewailly, D., Diamanti-Kandarakis, E., Escobar-Morreale, H. F., Futterweit, W., et al. (2006). Position Statement: Criteria for defining polycystic ovary syndrome as a predominantly hyperandrogenic syndrome: An Androgen Excess Society Guideline. *The Journal of Clinical Endocrinology & Metabolism, 91,* 4237–4245.

Barbieri, R. L., & Ehrmann, D. A. (2008, October 18). Clinical manifestations of polycystic ovary syndrome in adults. *UpToDate.* Retrieved March 8, 2010, from http://www.uptodate.com/online/content/topic.do?topicKey=r_endo_f/24245&view=print

Barbieri, R. L., & Ehrmann, D. A. (2009, January 21). Treatment of polycystic ovary syndrome in adults. *UpToDate.* Retrieved March 8, 2009, from http://www.uptodate.com/online/content/topic.do?topicKey=r_endo_f/24245&view=print

Barlow, S. E., & Dietz, W. H. (1998). Obesity evaluation and treatment: Expert committee recommendations. *Pediatrics, 102,* E29. Retrieved January 25, 2009, from http://www.pediatrics.org/cgi/content/full/102/3/e29

Bermas, B. L. (2007, September 20). Rheumatoid arthritis and pregnancy. *UpToDate.* Retrieved March 13, 2010, from http://www.uptodate.com/online/content/topic.do?topicKey=rheumart/7405&view=print

Bharaktiya, S., Orlander, P. R., Woodhouse, W. R., & Davis, A. B. (2009, July 23). Hypothyroidism. *emedicine.* Retrieved March 10, 2010, from http://emedicine.medscape.com/article/122393-print

BMI Calculator. (n.d.). *BMI calculator.* Retrieved March 16, 2010, from http://www.bmi-calculator.net/

BMI Calculator. (n.d.). *Waist to hip ratio calculator.* Retrieved March 16, 2010, from http://www.bmi-calculator.net/waist-to-hip-ratio-calculator/

Bray, G. A. (2008, October). Patient information: Weight loss treatments. *UpToDate Online 16.3*. Retrieved January 25, 2009, from http://www.uptodate.com

Centers for Disease Control and Prevention. (2009). *Obesity halting the epidemic by making health easier: At a glance 2009*. Retrieved January 23, 2009, from http://www.cdc.gov/NCCDPHP/publications/AAG/obesity.htm

Centers for Disease Control and Prevention. (n.d.). *Adult BMI calculator: English version*. Retrieved March 16, 2010, from http://www.cdc.gov/healthyweight/assessing/bmi/adult_bmi/english_bmi_calculator/bmi_calculator.html

Centers for Disease Control and Prevention. (n.d.). *BMI calculator of child and teen: English version*. Retrieved January 23, 2009, from http://apps.nccd.cdc.gov/dnpabmi/Calculator.aspx

Centers for Disease Control and Prevention. (n.d.). *BMI percentile calculator for child and teen: English version*. Retrieved March 16, 2010, from http://apps.nccd.cdc.gov/dnpabmi/

Centers for Disease Control and Prevention, NCHS National Center for Health Statistics. (n.d.). *Clinical growth charts*. Retrieved January 23, 2009, from http://www.cdc.gov/growthcharts/

Costa, A. (1995, December). Interpreting thyroid tests. *American Family Physician, 52*(8), 2325–2330.

Daniels, G. (1994, September). A delicate balance. *Harvard Health Letter, 19*(11), 3.

Ernst, D., & Lee, A. (Eds.). (2009, Summer). *NPPR: Nurse practitioners' prescribing reference*. New York: A Haymarket Media Publication.

Freeman, S. B. (2002). Polycystic ovary syndrome: Diagnosis and management. *Women's Health Care: A Practical Journal for Nurse Practitioners, 1*, 15–20.

Grubbs, Laurie. (2009). Winning the battle of the bulge: Practical approaches to weight loss. *Advance for Nurse Practitioners, 17*, 33–38.

Grundy, S. M., Cleeman, J. L., Daniels, S. R., Donato, K. A., Eckel, R. H., Franklin, B. A., et al. (2005). Diagnosis and management of the metabolic syndrome: An American Heart Association/National Heart, Lung, and Blood Institute Scientific Statement: Executive summary. *Circulation, 112*, e285–e290.

Hadley, M. E. (1996). *Endocrinology*. Upper Saddle River, NJ: Prentice-Hall.

Harris, E. D., & Schur, P. H. (2009, June 17). Overview of the systemic and nonarticular manifestations of rheumatoid arthritis. *UpToDate*. Retrieved March 13, 2010, from http://www.uptodate.com/online/content/topic.do?topicKey=rheumart/6403&view=print

Harris, E. D., Schur, P. H., & Maini, R. N. (2009, October 8). Treatment of early, moderately active rheumatoid arthritis in adults. *UpToDate*. Retrieved March 13, 2010, from http://www.uptodate.com/online/content/topic.do?topicKey=rheumart/15723&view=print

Hurley, D., & Gharib, H. (1995, April). Detection and treatment of hypothyroidism and Grave's disease. *Geriatrics, 50*, 41–44.

Kelsey, E., Salley, S., Wickham, E. P., Cheang, K. I., Essah, P. A., Karjane, N. W., et. al. (2007). Position Statement: Glucose intolerance in polycystic ovary syndrome: A Position Statement of the Androgen Excess Society. *Journal of Clinical Endocrinology & Metabolism, 92*, 4546–4556.

King, J. (2008). Shouldering the weight of obesity. *The Nurse Practitioner, 33*, 45–51.

Ladenson, P. W., Singer, P. A., Ain, K. B., Bagchi, N., Bigos, T., Levy, E. G., et al. (2000). American Thyroid Association guidelines for detection of thyroid dysfunction. *Archives of Internal Medicine, 160*, 1573–1575.

LaFranchi, S. (2009, July 22). Clinical manifestations and diagnosis of hyperthyroidism in children and adolescents. *UpToDate*. Retrieved March 13, 2010, from http://www.uptodate.com/online/content/topic.do?topicKey=pediendo/5570&view=print

Lee, S. L., & Ananthakrishnan, S. (2009, June 8). Hyperthyroidism. *emedicine*. Retrieved March 10, 2010, from http://emedicine.medscape.com/article/121865-print

Levi, J., Vinter, S., St. Laurent, R., & Segal, L. M. (2008). *F as in Fat: How obesity policies are failing in America*. (Issue Report 5th ed.). Washington, DC: Trust for America's Health.

Lindebaum, C. (2010). Polycystic ovarian syndrome: Where genetics and environment collide. *Advance for Nurse Practitioners, 18*, 20–27.

Lynn, C. H., & Miller, J. L. (2009). Bariatric surgery for obese adolescents: Should surgery be used to treat the childhood obesity epidemic? *Pediatric Health, 3*, 33–40.

Mantzoros, C. (2009, May 28). Insulin resistance: Definition and clinical spectrum. *UpToDate*. Retrieved March 8, 2010, from http://www.uptodate.com/online/content/topic.do?topicKey=diabetes/14407&view=print

Meigs, J. B. (2009, February 11). The metabolic syndrome (insulin resistance syndrome or syndrome X). *UpToDate*. Retrieved March 8, 2010, from http://www.uptodate.com/online/content/topic.do?topicKey=diabetes/21989&view=print

National Heart Lung and Blood Institute. (n.d.). *Obesity education initiative: Calculate your body mass index*. Retrieved March 16, 2010, from http://www.nhlbisupport.com/bmi/

National Institutes of Health. (2002). Third report of the Expert Panel on Detection, Evaluation, and Treatment of High Blood Cholesterol in Adults (ATP III Final Report). Bethesda, MD: National Institutes of Health.

Rosenfield, R. L. (2008, October 3). Treatment of polycystic ovary syndrome in adolescents. *UpToDate*. Retrieved March 8, 2010, from http://www.uptodate.com/online/content/topic.do?topicKey=pediendo/8697&view=print

Rosenfield, R. L. (2009, October 5). Clinical features and diagnosis of polycystic ovary syndrome in adolescents. *UpToDate*. Retrieved March 8, 2010, from http://www.uptodate.com/online/content/topic.do?topicKey=pediendo/8697&view=print

Ross, D. S. (2008, November 26). Diagnosis and screening for hypothyroidism. *UpToDate*. Retrieved March 8, 2010, from http://www.uptodate.com/online/content/topic.do?topicKey=thyroid/9963&view=print

Ross, D. S. (2009a, September 25). Treatment of hypothyroidism. *UpToDate*. Retrieved March 8, 2010, from http://www.uptodate.com/online/content/topic.do?topicKey=thyroid/2117&view=print

Ross, D. S. (2009b, October 7). Diagnosis and treatment of hyperthyroidism during pregnancy. *UpToDate*. Retrieved March 13, 2010, from http://www.uptodate.com/online/content/topic.do?topicKey=thyroid/7568&view=print

Rubin, D. I. (2009, March 18). Neurologic manifestations of hyperthyroidism. *UpToDate*. Retrieved March 8, 2010, from http://www.uptodate.com/online/content/topic.do?topicKey=medneuro/9866&view=print

Schilling, J. (1997, June). Hyperthyroidism: Diagnosis and management of Graves' disease. *Nurse Practitioner, 22*(6), 72–95.

Singhal, V., Schwenk, W. F., & Kumar, S. (2007). Evaluation and management of childhood and adolescent obesity. *Mayo Clinic Proceedings, 82*, 1258–1264.

Snow, V., Barry, P., Fitterman, N., Qaseem, A., & Weiss, K. (2005). Pharmacologic and surgical management of obesity in primary care: A clinical practice guideline from the American College of Physicians. *Annals of Internal Medicine, 142*, 525–532.

Steinberger, J., Daniels, R., Eckel, R. H., Hayman, L., Lustig, R. H., McCrindle, B., et al. (2009). Progress and challenges in metabolic syndrome in children and adolescents: A scientific statement from the American Heart Association Atherosclerosis, Hypertension, and Obesity in the Young Committee of the Council on Cardiovascular Disease in the Young; Council on Cardiovascular Nursing; and Council on Nutrition, Physical Activity, and Metabolism. *Circulation, 119*, 628–647.

Stoffer, S. S. (1993). Addison's disease: How to improve patients' quality of life. *Postgraduate Medicine, 93*(4), 265–276.

The Hormone Foundation. (2010). PCOS overview. Retrieved March 13, 2010, from http://www.hormone.org/polycystic/overview.cfm

Tsigos, C., & Chrousos, G. P. (1996). Differential diagnosis and management of Cushing's syndrome. *Annual Review of Medicine, 47*, 443–461.

U.S. Department of Health and Human Services. (2008). *2008 physical activity guidelines for Americans*. Retrieved February 18, 2009, from http://www.health.gov/paguidelines/pdf/paguide.pdf

Uwaifo, G. I., & Arloglu, E. (2006). Obesity [Electronic version]. *emedicine.medscape.com*. Retrieved January 31, 2009, from http://emedicine.medscape.com/article/123702-overview

Venables, P.J.W., & Maini, R. N. (2009a, June 15). Clinical features of rheumatoid arthritis. *UpToDate*. Retrieved March 13, 2010, from http://www.uptodate.com/online/content/topic.do?topicKey=rheumart/3022&view=print

Venables, P.J.W., & Maini, R. N. (2009b, June 15). Diagnosis and differential diagnosis of rheumatoid arthritis. *UpToDate*. Retrieved March 13, 2010, from http://www.uptodate.com/online/content/topic.do?topicKey=rheumart/4741&view=print

Wang, S. S. (2010, February 22). Metabolic syndrome. *emedicine*. Retrieved March 16, 2010, from http://emedicine.medscape.com/article/165124-print

Wigley, F. M. (2008, April 4). Nonpharmacologic therapy for Raynaud phenomenon. *UpToDate*. Retrieved March 8, 2010, from http://www.uptodate.com/online/content/topic.do?topicKey=sclerode/10816&view=print

Wigley, F. M. (2009, June 8). Clinical manifestations and diagnosis of the Raynaud phenomenon. *UpToDate*. Retrieved March 8, 2010, from http://www.uptodate.com/online/content/topic.do?topicKey=sclerode/2595&view=print

Wigley, F. M. (2009, October 15). Pharmacologic and surgical treatment of the Raynaud phenomenon. *UpToDate*. Retrieved March 8, 2010, from http://www.uptodate.com/online/content/topic.do?topicKey=sclerode/6308&view=print

Youngkin, E., & Davis, M. (1994). *Women's health: A primary care clinical guide*. East Norwalk, CT: Appleton.

Yusuf, S., Hawken, S., Ounpuu, S., Dans, T., Avezum, A., Lanas, F., et al. (2004). INTERHEART Study Investigators. Obesity and the risk of myocardial infarction in 27,000 participants from 52 countries: A case-control study. *Lancet, 366,* 1640–1649.

CHAPTER 20

Psychiatric Guidelines

Moya Cook, Jill C. Cash, and Cheryl A. Glass

ANXIETY *by Moya Cook and Jill C. Cash*

Definition

Anxiety is a normal reaction to acute stress. It is the "fight or flight" response that is part of the survival instinct. It is apprehension, tension, or uneasiness from anticipated danger. Anxiety is distinguished from fear in that fear is a response to consciously recognized external danger. The source of anxiety is largely unknown or unrecognized.

Normal anxiety allows us to get in touch with developmental learning that is part of our human growth. Anxiety in its chronic form is maladaptive and is considered a psychiatric disorder. Many cases of anxiety disorder in late life are chronic, having persisted from younger years. In its pathologic form, it interferes with developmental learning because it infers significant distress.

When a patient presents with anxiety, it is often comorbid with another psychiatric disorder, particularly depression. Anxiety may act as a predispositional factor to early onset depression (before age 26) and to a greater number of depressive episodes. Patients also present clinically with only anxiety, in one of its many forms such as generalized anxiety disorder, posttraumatic stress disorder, obsessive-compulsive disorder, adjustment disorder with anxious mood, acute anxiety or panic disorder, or anxiety as phobic disorders, or agoraphobia.

Incidence

A. Anxiety is present in many medical illnesses and must be distinguished to treat it appropriately. Generalized anxiety disorder and panic disorder are also associated with frequent suicide attempts.

Pathogenesis

Some degree of familial transmission of generalized anxiety disorder, as well as panic disorder, has been noted. Unconscious conflict is thought to be the underlying cause of anxiety, which signals the ego to be careful expressing unacceptable impulses. Behavioral anxiety is considered a conditioned response to a stimulus associated with danger.

Clinically, however, identifying specific anxiogenic stimuli is difficult. The onset of generalized anxiety disorder is also thought to be the cumulative effect of several stressful life events. Many studies have found that phobic/anxiety symptoms predated clinical alcoholism by a number of years. τ-Aminobutyric acid-benzodiazepine receptor complex, the locus coeruleus-norepinephrine system, and serotonin are three neurotransmitter systems implicated in the biologic basis of anxiety. These systems are thought to mediate "normal" anxiety and pathologic anxiety.

Predisposing Factors

A. Young to middle-aged women, onset usually of 20–30 years at age
B. Non-White
C. Single
D. Lower socioeconomic status
E. A childhood overanxious disorder
F. Excessive worrying
G. Unresolved unconscious conflict

Common Complaints

A. Inability to control worrying
B. Motor tension
C. Autonomic hyperactivity vigilance
D. Sleep disturbance

Statements concerning self-medication with alcohol to help with sleep may indicate a coexistent alcohol abuse/dependence diagnosis that must be treated concomitantly.

E. Shortness of breath
F. Increased heart rate and respirations
G. Feelings of apprehension
H. Dizziness
I. Abdominal disturbances/nausea
J. Increased perspiration
K. Trembling

Other Signs and Symptoms

A. Excessive worry out of proportion to the likelihood or impact of the feared events that occurs for a period of 6 months or longer, during which the person has been bothered more days than not by these concerns.
B. *At least three of the following six symptoms.*

1. Muscle tension
2. Restlessness or feeling keyed up or on edge
3. Easy fatigability
4. Difficulty concentrating or "mind going blank" because of anxiety
5. Trouble falling or staying asleep
6. Irritability

C. If another Axis I disorder is present, such as depression, or bipolar affective disorder, the anxiety may be in response to fear of:
   1. Being embarrassed in public in the presence of a social phobia
   2. Being contaminated in the presence of obsessive-compulsive disorder
   3. Gaining weight in the presence of anorexia nervosa
   4. Having an illness (as in hypochondriasis or somatization disorder)
D. The anxiety, worry, or physical symptoms significantly interfere with the person's normal routine or usual activities or cause marked distress.

Subjective Data

A. Review the onset, course, and duration of symptoms. How often does the anxiety occur (i.e., every day, week, month)?
B. Review any history of anxiety and age of onset. If treated, how was the previous anxiety treated and what was the success of the treatment?
C. Determine whether there is a history of suicide attempts. Does the patient have a current plan or vague ideas of suicide? **Ask the patient, "Have you ever thought of hurting yourself or others?" If there is any concern regarding suicide/homicide, immediately refer the patient to a psychiatrist.**
D. Review drug history for prescription, over-the-counter, and recreational/illicit drug use, and the patient's use of caffeine, which precipitates anxiety symptoms.
E. Review the patient's history of alcohol consumption. Mild or moderate alcohol withdrawal presents primarily with anxiety symptoms. In patients who have developed tolerance to the effects of alcohol or benzodiazepines, abrupt cessation of these agents may produce heightened anxiety over baseline, as well as a risk of seizure.
F. Review the patient's history for major stressors. Are these stressors new or chronic? If chronic problems, ask what made the patient come in today?
G. Determine how the patient has been coping with stress up until today (exercise, medication).
H. Review the patient's history of other medical problems.
I. Does anyone else in the family have the same problem? How are they treated?

Physical Examination

A. Check, pulse, respirations, blood pressure, and weight.
B. Inspect
   1. Observe general appearance; note grooming, dress, ability to communicate, body movements, nail biting, playing with hair, and inability to sit still.
C. Administer mental exam of choice.
D. Physical examination as indicated by somatic complaints.

Diagnostic Tests

A. Blood alcohol
B. Thyroid profile
C. Blood glucose
D. Medication level (e.g., theophylline, etc.) if applicable
E. Urine drug screen
F. Additional testing related to suspected physical pathology

Differential Diagnoses

A. Anxiety
B. Psychiatric syndrome
   1. Depressive disorders
   2. Psychotic disorders
   3. Somatoform disorders (characterized by physical complaints lacking known medical basis or demonstrable physical finding in the presence of psychological factors judged to be etiologic or important in the initiation, exacerbation, or maintenance of the disturbance).
   4. Personality disorders
   5. Alcoholism and drug abuse/dependence
C. Medical conditions. Anxiety syndromes mimic many medical illnesses, including intracranial tumors, menstrual irregularities, hypothyroidism, hyperparathyroidism and hypoparathyroidism, postconcussion syndrome, psychomotor epilepsy, and Cushing's disease.
   1. Consider hypoglycemia if anxiety is chronic.
   2. Hypothyroidism.
   3. Hyperthyroidism: Rapid-onset anxiety could be symptom of hyperthyroidism.
   4. Tumor.
   5. Cushing's disease.
   6. Pheochromocytoma (rare).

Plan

A. General interventions
   1. Treat physical/laboratory findings, that is, dietary changes, nutritional supplements.
   2. Adjunctive psychotherapy is strongly encouraged.
B. Patient teaching: See the Section III Patient Teaching Guides as appropriate if having insomnia, "Sleep Disorders/Insomnia," and substance abuse, "Alcohol and Drug Dependence."
C. Pharmaceutical therapy drug of choice:
   1. *Selective Serotonin Reuptake Inhibitors (SSRIs) or Selective Serotonin Norepinephrine Reuptake Inhibitors (SNRIs)*
      a. Fluoxetine (Prozac), 5–10 mg/day initially; usual dose 20–80 mg a day.
      b. Paroxetine (Paxil), 10 mg/day initially; usual dose 25–50 mg a day.
      c. Sertraline (Zoloft), 25–50 mg/day initially; usual dose 50–200 mg a day.
      d. Venlafaxine (Effexor), 37.5 mg/day initially; usual dose 75–300 mg a day.
      e. These medications can take 4–6 weeks to take effect.
      f. Warn patients that they should not stop these medications abruptly, but taper off gradually.
   2. *Nonbenzodiazepine anxiolytic.* Buspirone (Buspar), 7.5 mg twice a day.
      a. May increase by 5 mg/day every 2–3 days.

b. Usual range: 20–30 mg every day, maximum 60 mg every day.

c. Not recommended for children younger than 18 years.

d. Therapeutic effects are delayed from 1–4 weeks.

e. Thus far, the drug appears to lack abuse potential or withdrawal symptoms with abrupt discontinuation.

3. *Short-acting benzodiazepines:* Alprazolam (Xanax), 0.25 mg to 0.5 mg three times daily.

a. Maximum 4 mg daily in divided doses.

b. Lorazepam (Ativan), 0.5 mg to 10 mg every day in divided doses.

i. Use for initial short-term stabilization while simultaneously prescribing buspirone because therapeutic effects of buspirone are delayed from 1–4 weeks.

ii. Limit use to several weeks to a few months to prevent dependence.

4. *Sedating antihistamines* (not to be used for more than 4 months)

a. Hydroxyzine HCl (Atarax) 50–100 mg four times a day

b. Hydroxyzine pamoate (Vistaril) 50–100 mg four times a day

5. α_2-*Agonist*

a. Clonidine (Catapres) 0.1–0.3 mg twice a day.

b. Monitor blood pressure carefully.

Follow-up

A. Follow up in 1 week to assess the patient's status.

B. Follow up every 2 weeks after that to check the patient's progress.

C. Once positive change is seen, the patient can be seen monthly.

D. Assess suicide potential with every office visit.

E. Refer to medical diagnosis for follow-up recommendations.

Consultation/Referral

A. Refer to a psychiatric clinician for complex medication management and psychotherapy after initial assessment.

B. If the patient expresses suicidal thoughts, immediately refer to ER or psychiatric specialist for continuing psychotherapy.

Individual Considerations

A. Pregnancy

1. Caution should be used in prescribing medications for anxiety during pregnancy; the benefits must be weighed against the risks.

2. If the patient becomes pregnant while taking these medications, taper drugs off instead of ceasing abruptly.

B. Pediatrics

1. Children with suspected anxiety disorders should be immediately referred to a pediatric psychiatrist.

C. Geriatrics

1. Anxiety is often unrecognized and inadequately treated in this population because of concomitant medical illness, overlap with cognitive disorders, and comorbid depression, ageism, and cohort effects.

2. Start with the lowest dose of medication and increase slowly.

D. Partners

1. If available in the community, provide resources for partners, such as the National Alliance for the Mentally Ill (listed in most telephone books).

2. Psychotherapy for the patient and partner is often helpful.

ATTENTION DEFICIT HYPERACTIVITY DISORDER *by Moya Cook and Jill C. Cash*

Definition

A. Attention deficit hyperactivity disorder (ADHD) is a syndrome that consists of a cluster of behaviors that emerges early in a child's life and persists over time. Excessively high levels of motor activity, problems with attention span, concentration, and/or impulsivity characterize ADHD. Up to 50% of patients with ADHD also have other psychosocial disorders such as oppositional defiant disorder, depression or bipolar disorder (develops in 25% of children with ADHD), posttraumatic stress disorder, or Tourette's syndrome.

B. The diagnostic criteria for ADHD include symptoms of inattention and symptoms of hyperactivity/impulsivity (see Table 20.1).

Incidence

A. 3%–5% of all school-aged children.

B. Occurs in all races and socioeconomic groups.

C. Boys are three to six times more likely to have symptoms than girls.

D. Not uncommon for this disorder to persist into adulthood.

Pathogenesis

A. Unknown, but several studies suggest a biochemical basis involving deficits in the availability of neurotransmitters to the frontal-orbital circuits of the neurobehavioral regulatory systems of the brain. ADHD may also be inherited.

B. Other commonly suspected causes, with little or no scientific support, include dietary-related conditions, such as high-sugar diets, food additives (including preservatives and colorings), vitamin deficiencies, chemicals, allergies, poor role models, and poor schools.

Predisposing Factors

A. A close relative with a mood disorder, anxiety, or ADHD.

B. Brain trauma.

C. Selective therapeutic regimens, such as intrathecal chemotherapy.

D. Recent studies have suggested a possible link to maternal smoking, alcohol abuse, or other toxins during pregnancy.

E. Some perinatal influences have been theorized to be connected to ADHD, including fetal distress, prolonged labor, prematurity, and perinatal asphyxia.

TABLE 20.1 Diagnostic Criteria for Attention Deficit Hyperactivity Disorder

The presence of six or more symptoms is used for the diagnosis of ADHD.

A. Symptoms of Inattention
1. Fails to give close attention to details; makes careless mistakes
2. Difficulty sustaining attention
3. Does not seem to listen when spoken to
4. Struggles to follow through on instructions
5. Has difficulty organizing tasks
6. Avoids or dislikes tasks that require sustained mental activity
7. Loses things that are essential for tasks
8. Easily distracted
9. Forgetful in daily activities

B. Symptoms of Hyperactivity/Impulsivity
1. Fidgets or squirms
2. Has difficulty remaining seated
3. Runs or climbs excessively or inappropriately
4. Difficulty engaging in quiet leisure activities
5. Acts "on the go" or as if driven by a motor
6. Talks excessively
7. Blurts out answers before questions have been completed
8. Difficulty awaiting his or her turn
9. Interrupts or intrudes on others

Adapted from the *Diagnostic and Statistical Manual of Mental Disorders* (4th ed.), by the American Psychiatric Association, 1994. Washington, DC: Author.

Common Complaints

A. Hyperactivity, impulsivity, and/or inattentiveness
B. Poor school performance
C. Poor peer relationships

Signs and Symptoms

A. Present before 7 years of age.
B. Some impairment in functioning in two or more settings.
C. Symptoms have continued for at least 6 months.

Subjective Data

A. Determine the presenting symptoms and ascertain when symptoms first began.
B. Note duration of symptoms.
1. Have they been present for at least 6 months?
2. Ask regarding specific behaviors as listed in the diagnostic criteria (refer to Table 20.1).
C. Review settings in which symptoms are present (home, school, day care).
D. Discuss the child's past medical history.
E. Discuss the child's developmental history; did he or she meet all of the developmental milestones?
F. Review the child's family, social, and school histories.
G. Review all current medications, including any over-the-counter and herbals. Specifically review medication history for theophylline, prednisone, and albuterol.
H. Review the child's diet and eating habits.
I. Review the child's sleeping habits.
J. Review the child's stimulation from TV, video, and computer habits.

Physical Examination

A. Check temperature, pulse, respirations, blood pressure, weight, and height.
B. Inspect
C. Observe overall appearance.
1. Note behavior and interactions with others.
2. Inspect the skin, eyes, ears, nose, and throat.
D. Auscultate: Auscultate the heart, lungs, and abdomen.
E. Palpate: Palpate the neck, chest, and abdomen.
F. Perform neurologic examination.
1. Perform hearing/vision evaluation. Evaluate constant, involuntary movement of the eyes (nystagmus).
2. Evaluation coordination difficulties/impaired motor skills.
3. Visual-motor control problems (hand-eye coordination).

Diagnostic Tests

A. Complete blood count (CBC) to rule out iron deficiency anemia.
B. Lead level.
C. Thyroid studies to rule out other organic problems.
D. CBC with differential (if indicated).
E. Administer the NICQH Vanderbilt Assessment Scale available on the Internet at http://www.kidzdoc.com/uploads/files/vanderbilt-assessment-parent.pdf.
F. Psychological tests to measure IQ, social/emotional adjustment, and presence of learning disabilities.
G. Electroencephalogram (EEG) may be considered.
H. Magnetic resonance imaging (MRI) may be considered to rule out organic diagnoses.

Differential Diagnoses

A. ADHD
B. Hyperthyroidism/hypothyroidism
C. Lead poisoning
D. Other behavioral/psychological disorders (pervasive developmental delay, mood disorders, anxiety or personality disorder)
E. Learning disorders
F. Seizure disorder, nonconvulsive
G. Impaired hearing related to chronic or recurrent otitis
H. Adverse reactions to medications (theophylline, prednisone, or albuterol)
I. Mental retardation

Plan

A. General interventions
1. Multimodal and multidisciplinary approach is imperative and includes parent training regarding the nature of ADHD, effective behavioral management, appropriate educational placement and support, family or individual therapy, if indicated.
2. It is important to obtain written reports (which consist of a standardized rating, such as the Connors Tool

and/or the Vanderbilt Screening Tool of ADHD) from teachers, parents, and other adults who have regular contact with the child. The Vanderbilt tools are available over the Internet; see the "Resources" section.

3. The primary care provider, school nurse, school psychologist, or parent may function as the case manager to coordinate services.
4. Behavior management is often effective but is insufficient when used alone.
5. Parent and patient support groups can be helpful.

B. Patient teaching
   1. See the Section III Patient Teaching Guides for this chapter, "Tips for Caregivers: Living (Enjoyably) With a Child Who Has ADHD" and "Coping Strategies for Teens and Adults With ADHD," including "Resources for ADD."
   2. Provide ADHD Resources for parents, children, teens, and adults.

C. Pharmaceutical therapy: The most commonly used medications are:
   1. Methylphenidate (Ritalin): first-line therapy: Starting dose: 0.3–0.6 mg/kg/dose; short half-life (3–6 hours), necessitates two to four doses per day. Safe and effective. A long-acting form is available, but may be less effective.
   2. Dextroamphetamine (Dexadrine): Twice as potent, so use half the dose of methylphenidate. Half-life is longer, so give twice per day.
   3. A combination of dextroamphetamine sulfate, dextroamphetamine saccharate, amphetamine sulfate, and amphetamine aspartate (Adderal): Lasts 8–10 hours, once a day dosing.
   4. Lisdexamfetamine dimesylate (Vyvanse) pediatric dose: children 6–12 years old: 30 mg daily in a single dose in the morning. Maximum dose of 70 mg daily in the morning.
   5. Methylphenidate HCl (Concerta) Not recommended for those younger than 6 years. 6–12 years: 18 mg daily. Increase dose in 18-mg increments weekly as needed. Max 54 mg daily for children and max 72 mg daily for adolescents. Contraindicated with severe anxiety.
   6. Atomoxetine (Strattera): Not a controlled substance. Weight less than 70 kg to less than 0.5 mg/kg per day (maximum 1.4 mg/kg/day). Weight greater than 70 kg to 40 mg/day (maximum 100 mg/day). May take a few weeks to see full effect. Should be taken daily at the same time every day to avoid SNRI effects.

FDA approved indication for adults.

   7. Side effects of these medications include anorexia, insomnia, stomach pain, growth suppression, and tics. If weight loss occurs, give medication after meals.
   8. If psychostimulants are not effective, other medications used include antihistamines, clonidine, and antidepressants.

9. Be cautious when prescribing other medications concurrently.

Follow-up

A. At 1 month: inquire about improvements in each area of life and duration of the medication's actions.
B. Medication frequency may need to be altered.
C. Consider adding a third dose if the duration of action is very short and the child needs better afternoon or evening coverage to successfully complete homework or participate in other extracurricular activities.
D. At 3 months: continue to adjust medication as needed. Consider an extended-release preparation if more continued coverage is needed.
E. When medication schedule is stable, subsequent visits can be every 3 months.

Consultation/Referral

A. Consult with the psychiatrist to help coordinate the medications.
B. Consult the school psychologist if indicated for additional data.
C. Refer the patient for family or individual therapy if indicated.

Individual Considerations

A. Pediatrics
   1. The overall goal of ADHD therapy is to build the child's sense of competence and performance.
   2. Not all behavior issues are ADHD. The diagnosis must be carefully and cautiously established according to the diagnostic criteria of the American Psychiatric Association.
   3. Individualize medications, preparations, and timing; 80% of children respond positively to stimulants.
   4. Instituting routine drug holidays should be done with caution. It is important to occasionally stop medication to compare treated and untreated states.
   5. Discuss with the parents and the child the desirability of medication effects during weekend and holidays. This is an individual decision, but bear in mind that children's ability to concentrate and manage behavior may be as critical during off-school hours as well as during school. This may prevent a "yo-yo" behavior experience for the patient.
   6. Specify exact time for taking medications. Avoid prescribing stimulants at "lunch." Lunchtimes in schools vary widely, from 10:30 AM to 1:30 PM. Avoid school hours if possible. Children and adolescents may have concerns about peer attitudes toward taking medications. Also, not all institutions have a school nurse readily available.
   7. Use caution when medicating children with a personal or family history of Tourette's syndrome. Tics may worsen in these children.
   8. When prescribing psychostimulants to children with seizure disorders who are already on anticonvulsants, closely monitor plasma levels of both medications.

9. Treat the child, not the parents, teachers, day care personnel, or coaches.

10. When the child's behavior improves, give the bulk of the credit to the child.

11. Drug levels may increase when taken concurrently.

B. Adults

1. Up to half of the affected children have some symptoms of ADHD that persist into adulthood. Adults tend to outgrow the "hyperactivity" aspect; however, they may still require treatment for the ADD. Teens and adults benefit from specific coping strategies for attention deficit disorder.

Resources

American Academy of Pediatrics Resource Toolkit for Clinicians: http://www.uthsc.edu/pediatrics/general/clinical/behavior/aap_nichq_adhd_toolkit/01ADHDIntroduction.pdf

NICHQ Vanderbilt Assessment Scale—PARENT Informant: http://www.kidzdoc.com/uploads/files/vanderbilt-assessment-parent.pdf

NICHQ Vanderbilt Assessment Scale—TEACHER Informant: http://www.pedialliance.com/forms/ADHD_Teacher_Assessment42.pdf

NICHQ Vanderbilt Assessment Follow-up—TEACHER Informant: http://www.pedialliance.com/forms/ADHD_Teacher_Follow_Up_Form44.pdf

Scoring Instructions for the NICHQ Vanderbilt Assessment Scales: http://www.uthsc.edu/pediatrics/general/clinical/behavior/aap_nichq_adhd_toolkit/07ScoringInstructions.pdf

ADD Warehouse Catalog, 800-ADD-WARE. *Literature for parents, professionals and educators.*

Attention Deficit Information Network, 617-455-9892, www.addinfon network.com

CHADD (Children With ADD) National Headquarters, 499 NW 70th Ave., Plantation, FL 33322, 305-587-3700, Challenge (ADD Newsletter), PO Box 488, West Newbury, MA 01985, 508-462-0495.

National ADD Association, PO Box 972, Mentor, OH 44061, 800-487-2282, www.92starnet.con-sled

The Parent's Guide to Attention Deficit Disorders, Hawthorne Education Services, Columbia, MO 65205, 314-874-1710

DEPRESSION *by Moya Cook and Jill C. Cash*

Definition

A. Depression is an emotion experienced by almost everyone at some time in their lives. There are many forms of depression, and treatment varies depending on the specific diagnosis. Depression is frequently a concomitant diagnosis with other physical or mental disorders.

Incidence

A. One in 10 adults experiences one or more episodes of depression during his or her lifetime. The lifetime risk is estimated to be as high as 30%. Women have a twofold to threefold higher rate of reported depression than men. Estimated rates of major depression in the elderly are 3%–5% for those living in a community dwelling; 15%–30% for those living in an institutional setting; and 13% for those living in nursing homes.

B. Only 10%–25% of people with depressive disorders seek treatment. There is a high mortality from suicide if untreated (see "Suicide" section).

C. No single causal factor has been identified. Depressive syndromes are so varied in course and symptomatology that a single cause is unlikely. Several factors appear to contribute, including genetics, neurochemical abnormalities (reductions in adrenergic or serotonergic neurotransmission), electrolyte disturbances, and neuroendocrine abnormalities such as hypothalamic, pituitary, adrenal cortical, thyroid, and gonadal functions. Personality and psychodynamic factors include low self-esteem, self-criticism, and interpersonal loss. A childhood history of emotional, physical, and/or sexual abuse can also contribute to adult-onset depression.

Predisposing Factors

A. Elderly.

B. Lack of social support/living alone.

C. A history of early parental loss.

D. Female gender

1. Most common in childbearing years from ages 25–45

2. Premenstrual

3. Perimenopausal

4. Postpartum

E. Family history of depression.

F. Frequent exposure to stressful events.

G. Nutritional disorders

1. Vitamin B_{12} deficiency

2. Pellagra

H. Personality characteristics that include absence of hardiness factors in response to stress (lack of resilience, flexibility, and optimism).

I. Anger not dealt with and turned in on the self.

J. Negative interpretation of one's life experiences.

K. Poor physical health.

L. Postsurgical diagnosis of cancer.

M. Chronic pain.

N. Chronic medical problems such as hypothyroidism and hyperthyroidism, Cushing's syndrome, hypercalcemia, hyponatremia, diabetes mellitus, lupus erythematosus, fibromyalgia, rheumatoid disease, and chronic fatigue syndrome.

O. Neurologic disorders such as stroke, subdural hematoma, multiple sclerosis, brain tumor, Parkinson's disease, epilepsy, dementias, and Huntington's disease.

P. Alcoholism/drug abuse or dependence/withdrawal.

Q. Infectious etiology such as mononucleosis and other viral infections, syphilis, human immunodeficiency virus (HIV), and Lyme disease.

R. Side effect of prescription drugs, such as a-methyldopa, antiarrhythmic, benzocli azepines, barbiturates/CNS depressants, $_\beta$-blockers, cholinergic drugs, corticosteroids, digoxin, H_2-blockers, and reserpine.

Common Complaints

A. Lack of interest in pleasurable activities

B. Digestive problems

C. Chronic aches and pains that are not otherwise explained

Other Signs and Symptoms
A. Vegetative
   1. Changes (increased or decreased) in sleep, appetite, and weight
   2. Changes in appearance: poor grooming and hygiene
   3. Poor eye contact, staring downward, flat affect
   4. Loss of energy
   5. Decreased interest in sex
   6. Psychomotor retardation or agitation
B. Cognitive
   1. Sense of guilt, worthlessness, low self-esteem
   2. Problems with attention span, concentration or memory, frustration tolerance, negative distortions, mild paranoia, and psychosis
C. Impulse control
   1. Suicidal or homicidal thoughts or acts. **Any statements made by the patient that "Life isn't worth living, I wish I were dead, I don't deserve to be alive, I can't deal with this" should be taken seriously. Refer the patient for counseling and assessment and treatment.**
D. Behavioral
   1. Depressed mood, anxiety, and irritability
   2. Isolation, decreased motivation, fatigability, and anhedonia (unable to derive gratification from pleasurable activities)
E. Physical symptoms
   1. Digestion problems, nausea, constipation, diarrhea (less common), and *dry* mouth
   2. Fatigue, but difficulty sleeping
   3. Physical pain, chronic aches and pains that cannot be explained
   4. Recurrent headaches, backaches, or stomachaches that have no cause
   5. Migrating pain that disappears when depression lifts
   6. Increased muscle tension

Subjective Data
A. Review the onset, duration, and course of presenting symptoms.
B. Review any previous history of depression (such as postpartum depression).
C. Determine how the previous depression was treated.
D. Evaluate the patient's suicide potential. Ask: "Have you ever thought of hurting yourself or others?" Does the patient have a current suicide plan or vague ideas of suicide? Has the patient had any previous history of suicide attempts? If so, evaluate how life-threatening they were.
E. Review the patient's medical history (see "Predisposing Factors").
F. Review the patient's drug history for prescription, over-the-counter, and recreational/illicit drug use (how much, how long, how often), and review his or her history of alcohol consumption (how much, how long, how often).
G. Review the patient's history for recent major life changes such as pregnancy, death, divorce, or any loss that may be normal throughout the stages of life. The **patient's perception** of the loss is what is important.
H. Review dietary intake since the symptoms have begun.
I. Establish usual weight, review weight gain/loss, and in what time span.
J. Review the patient's activities of daily living. Does the patient get up and dress daily, perform daily hygiene, put on makeup?
K. Review how many hours of sleep and quality of sleep per day.
L. Review the disruption of usual activities: return to work, return to school, exercise.
M. Review the amount of crying per day, for what length of time (days, weeks).
N. Assess whether the depression is cyclic/seasonal (starts in the fall, ends in the spring).
O. Review occupational/home exposure to lead and lead-based products.
P. Review any exposures to infectious diseases, including Lyme disease (refer to Chapter 15, "Infectious Diseases Guidelines" for specific questions). Does anyone else such as family, friends, or coworkers have similar symptoms?
Q. If female, review for symptoms of menopause (sleep disturbances, irregular menses/amenorrhea, hot flashes, vaginal dryness, dyspareunia).

Physical Examination
A. Check temperature, pulse, respirations, blood pressure and weight.
B. Inspect
   1. Observe overall appearance; note grooming, tone of voice, conduct of patient during communication, and breath (smell of alcohol).
   2. Complete neurologic examination with screening tool of choice.
   3. Complete dermal examination for signs of substance use (refer to "Substance Use Disorders" section).
C. Palpate
   1. Palpate the neck and thyroid; note the goiter.
   2. Palpate the axilla and groin for lymphadenopathy (infectious etiology).
   3. Check the joints for swelling and arthritis and range of motion (rule out musculoskeletal cause).
D. Auscultate
   1. Auscultate the heart, lungs, and abdomen (as applies to physical complaints).

Diagnostic Tests
A. CBC with differential
B. Electrolytes, serum calcium, and phosphorus
C. Thyroid profile
D. Liver profile
E. Lead level
F. Follicle-stimulating hormone/luteinizing hormone (FSH/LH)
G. Viral cultures
H. Blood alcohol
I. Urine drug screen
J. Monospot
K. Computed tomography (CT) and MRI scans
L. Dexamethasone suppression test

Differential Diagnoses

A. Depression.

B. Chronic untreated anxiety disorders such as generalized anxiety disorder, posttraumatic stress disorder, or obsessive-compulsive disorder.

C. Personality disorders.

D. Schizoaffective disorder.

E. Seasonal affective disorder.
   1. Seasonal pattern: starts in the fall, linked to lack of light exposure
   2. Women more than men
   3. Age typically in the 20s

F. Alcoholism and drug abuse/dependence.

G. Early dementia.

H. Endocrine etiologies (see "Predisposing Factors").

I. Infectious etiologies (see "Predisposing Factors").

J. Menopause.

K. Side effect of medication (see "Predisposing Factors").

L. Cancer: **50% of patients with tumors, particularly of the brain and lung, and carcinoma of the pancreas develop symptoms of depression before the diagnosis of tumor is made.**

M. Heavy metal poisoning.

N. Nutritional deficit (see "Predisposing Factors").

Plan

A. General interventions
   1. Keep the patient safe from self-harm.
   2. Treat physical/laboratory findings, that is, dietary change, iron supplements, hormone replacement therapy (see related chapters).

B. Patient teaching
   1. Encourage the patient to take medications as prescribed. Educate the patient that some medications may take time to get into the system to work and time should be allowed to see the effects of the medication. Review side effects.
   2. Encourage the patient to express feelings or worsening of symptoms if this occurs prior to next appointment. Have the patient make a client contract with you that he or she will not hurt himself or others and if he or she begins having these thoughts, the patient will contact you or go to the nearest emergency room.
   3. Encourage exercise on a daily basis for 20–30 minutes to increase energy and enhance a feeling of well-being.
   4. Encourage the patient to get at least 7–8 hours of sleep each night. If sleep is a problem, address this issue with the client.
   5. Avoid caffeine at night and/or watching TV late at night.
   6. Encourage the patient to seek counseling with a professional counselor. Offer local resources to the patient.

C. Pharmaceutical therapy: Table 20.2 presents dosage information.
   1. Drugs of choice: *Selective serotonin reuptake inhibitors (SSRI) antidepressants.* Caution should be used when coadministering SSRIs and drugs with a narrow therapeutic window such as carbamazepine (Tegretol), warfarin, tricyclic antidepressants (TCAs), antiarrhythmics, and some antipsychotic medications (risperidone, haloperidol, and phenothiazine), and other drugs including diazepam (Valium) and monoamine oxidase (MAO) inhibitors.
      a. Most antidepressant therapy takes 3–4 weeks for onset of action to elicit visible changes.
      b. Never prescribe more than a week's supply or a total of 2 g of a TCA if there is a risk of suicide.
      c. Medication should not be changed until it has been given a trial of 6–8 weeks to measure progress.
      d. Before concluding that the antidepressant is ineffective, verify that the patient is taking the medication correctly.
      e. First-line therapy in the elderly is SSRIs. The SSRIs have significantly fewer side effects than the traditional TCAs. Paroxetine and sertraline have short half-lives and can be withdrawn quickly.
      f. Antidepressant therapy should be continued for 6 months to 1 year (up to 5 years if necessary) because of the risk of recurrence of depression.
      g. Taper the medication off instead of abruptly withdrawing.
   2. TCAs: Avoid administration after acute myocardial infarction. **Men with prostatic hypertrophy do best with a nonsedating TCA that has a mild anticholinergic activity, such as desipramine (Norpramin) or nortriptyline (Pamelor).**
   3. *Adrenergic modulators:* A weak inhibitor of norepinephrine, dopamine, and seratonin reuptake: Bupropion hydrochloride (Wellbutrin).
      a. For patients over age 18.
      b. No dosage established for the elderly.
      c. Therapeutic onset in 1–3 weeks.
      d. Serum level peak within 2 hours.
      e. Initially 100 mg twice a day for at least 3 days.
      f. If well tolerated, increase to 375 or 400 mg daily.
      g. After 3 days more, 450 mg daily in four divided doses at least 4 hours apart.
      h. Maximum single dosing 150 mg, maximum 450 mg daily.
         i. Avoid bedtime dosing.
         ii. Do not give to patients with predisposition to seizures.
         iii. Requires reduced dose in patients with renal or hepatic impairment.
   4. *Dual reuptake inhibitors:* Blocks the reabsorption of the norepinephrine and serotonin into the neurons in the CNS. When this occurs, higher levels of norepinephrine and serotonin remain and improve the nerve transmission in the brain, which then improves mood.
      a. Venlafaxine hydrochloride (Effexor)
         i. For patients over age 18.
         ii. No dosage established for the elderly.
         iii. Therapeutic onset unknown.
         iv. Serum level peak and duration unknown.
         v. Initially 75 mg every day in two to three divided doses with food.
         vi. May increase at 4-day intervals in 75 mg/day increments to 150 mg every day. Maximum

TABLE 20.2 Dosages for Common Antidepressant Drugs

Drug	Adults Aged 18–60 Years	Elderly > 60 Years or Renal or Hepatic Patients
Fluoxetine hydrochloride (Prozac) Therapeutic onset occurs in 1–4 wk. Serum levels peak in 4.5–8.5 h.	20 mg daily in AM, dosage increased according to patient response. May be given bid—in the morning and at noon. Maximum dosage is 80 mg/d.	10–20 mg daily in AM with clinical response monitored q 1–2 wk. Gradual dose increases q 6 wk until optimal therapeutic response is obtained.
Sertraline hydrochloride (Zoloft) Therapeutic onset occurs in 2–4 wk. Serum levels peak in 4.5–8.5 h.	50 mg daily in AM. May increase to 100 mg. Dosage adjustments should be made at intervals of no less than 1 wk. Maximum dosage is 200 mg/d.	25–50 mg daily in AM with clinical response monitored q 1–2 wk and gradual increase.
Paroxetine hydrochloride (Paxil) Therapeutic onset occurs in 1–4 wk. Serum levels peak in 2–8 h.	10 mg daily in AM, PM, or @ HS. May increase 10 mg/d increments at weekly intervals. Maximum dosage is 50 mg/d.	10–20 mg daily in AM, PM, or @ HS with clinical response monitored q 1–2 wk and gradual increase.
Nortriptyline hydrochloride (Pamelor) Therapeutic onset occurs in 2–4 wk or longer. Serum levels peak in 7–8.5 h.	25 mg tid or qid initially, gradually increase to maximum dose 150 mg qd.	30–50 mg daily tid or qid or in 1 day's dose.
Desipramine hydrochloride (Norapramin) Therapeutic onset occurs in 2–4 wk or longer. Serum levels peak in 4–6 h.	100–200 mg pd in single or divided dose.	25–100 mg daily in divided doses, increase gradually to maximum of 150 mg qd.
Amitriptyline (Elavil) Therapeutic onset unknown— thought to take several wk. Serum levels peak 2–12 h.	75 mg pd in divided doses initially or 50–100 mg @ HS. Dose not to exceed 150 mg/d.	10–20 mg po tid and 20 mg @ HS daily.

Note. A. Paxil works well for patients who have a component of anxiety to their depression. B. **Monitor prothrombin time for patients taking warfarin, sertraline, and paroxetine.**
bid = twice a day; tid = three times daily; qid = four times a day; q = every; qd = every day; pd = per day; po = by mouth; @ HS = at bedtime.

dosage is 375 mg every day in three divided doses.

vii. With hepatic impairment, reduce dose by 50%.

viii. Withdraw gradually over 2 weeks when discontinuing medication.

ix. Interacts with MAO inhibitors. Do not start venlafaxine within 14 days of discontinuing an MAO inhibitor.

b. Duloxetine (Cymbalta) also blocks reuptake of seratonin and norepinepherine.

i. Usual starting dose is 30 mg/day increasing to 60 mg/day. Maximum dose is 120 mg/day.

ii. Patients should be warned about stopping the medication abruptly and have them taper down slowly.

iii. Duloxetine is also helpful in treating the physical pain that accompanies some depression symptoms.

5. **MAO inhibitors should only be prescribed by a psychiatrist.**

Follow-up

A. Follow up in 1 week to assess patient's status, drug effectiveness, and adverse reactions.

B. Patients can become suicidal after the depression is treated and they begin to have more energy to act on the suicidal ideation. **Assess suicidality with every office visit.**

C. Follow up every 2 weeks afterward to check patient's progress.

D. Once positive change is seen, the patient can be seen monthly.

E. Refer to other applicable medical diagnosis for follow-up recommendations.

Consultation/Referral

A. *If* there is any potential for suicidal/homicidal behavior, refer patient immediately to a psychiatrist for possible emergency admission.

B. Consult with the physician, comanage with the physician, or the patient may need immediate referral/consult for continuing psychotherapy.

C. Patients who fail to respond to antidepressants after 1–2 months of appropriate antidepressant therapy should have a psychiatric consultation.

Individual Considerations

A. Pregnancy

1. A woman with a history of depression or previous postpartum depression is at high risk for postpartum depression (recurrent). Caution should be used in prescribing antidepressants during pregnancy. Review the benefits versus risks.

2. Refer to Chapter 12, "Obstetrics Guidelines," for the section, "Postpartum Depression."

B. Pediatrics

1. Children with depression are more difficult to diagnose and do not necessarily meet adult criteria. The clinical picture can be completely different,

that is, acting out behavior. Children suspected to be depressed should be referred to a child psychiatrist.

C. Adolescence
   1. Teens are at risk for suicide after recent losses from death (especially if one of their friends/family commits suicide). Recent loss includes breaking up with boy/girl friend.
   2. If a teen has had a depressive episode, he or she may be at a higher risk for suicide if he or she is suddenly happy and things are "just fine." He or she may have decided on a suicide plan and may be experiencing a sense of relief because plans have been made.

D. Adults
   1. When prescribing, be sure to consider other existing medical illness for these patients and the impact of prescribing antidepressants. Offer unconditional acceptance and good listening skills to benefit these patients.
   2. Depression related to menopause is generally relieved by estrogen replacement therapy.

E. Partners
   1. If available in the community, provide resources for partners, such as the National Alliance for the Mentally Ill (listed in most telephone books).
   2. Frequently partners will take too much responsibility for the depressed patient's state of mind, and over time also become depressed. Relating to other people with depressed partners will assist them in dealing with their significant other's depression.

F. Geriatrics
   1. Dementia masked as "pseudodepression" is common in the elderly. Check for memory impairment and disorientation because delirium can often be mistaken for depression.
   2. Elderly patients who are depressed may experience agitation rather than retardation in psychomotor function.
   3. White men, age 80, have the highest rate of suicide of any age group in the United States.
   4. Look for depression in caretakers of patients with Alzheimer's disease.

Elderly patients who are suicidal may present with atypical symptoms of depression and may not express their distress directly. Three identified behaviors include impaired ability to communicate, intractable tinnitus, and feelings of helplessness.

FAILURE TO THRIVE *by Moya Cook and Jill C. Cash*

Definition
A. Failure to thrive (FTT) is an abnormality in growth in which an individual fails to gain weight or grow, especially seen in infancy and childhood. In a growing child, a child measuring below the third to fifth percentile on the growth curve, or a drop greater than two percentiles on the growth curve in the past several months, is referred to as FTT. FTT is also seen in adults who have a weight less than 80% of the ideal average body weight for the adult.

B. Failure to thrive in the geriatric population is defined as a deterioration in functional status disproportional to their disease burden.

Incidence
A. Depends on population; however, it is estimated FTT is seen in 5%–10% of low birth weight children and children who live in poverty. Inner-city emergency departments estimate that 15%–30% of their pediatric visits have signs of growth failure.

Pathogenesis
A. Organic causes for FIT include:
   1. Gastrointestinal (reflux, celiac disease, Hirschsprung disease, and malabsorption)
   2. Cardiopulmonary (cardiac diseases, congestive heart failure)
   3. Pulmonary (asthma, bronchopulmonary dysplasia, cystic fibrosis)
   4. Renal (diabetes insipidus, renal insufficiency, urinary tract infections)
   5. Endocrine (hypothyroidism, adrenal diseases, parathyroid disorders, thyroid disorders, pituitary disorders)
   6. Neurologic (mental retardation, cerebral hemorrhages)
   7. Metabolic disorders (inborn errors of metabolism)
   8. Congenital (congenital syndromes such as fetal alcohol syndrome, chromosomal abnormalities, perinatal infections)
   9. Infectious (gastrointestinal infections, tuberculosis, HIV)

B. Inorganic (or psychosocial) causes pertain to family dynamics among the parents, siblings, and the patient. It is common to see both organic and inorganic problems as causative factors for FTT.

C. In geriatrics:
   1. Feel fuller with less food; this may be an endorphin response that decreases the adaptive relaxation of the fundus of the stomach
   2. Increase number of cytokines, which contributes to anorexia
   3. Diminished sense of smell or taste
   4. Dysphagia from stroke, tremors, medication, depression, and poverty

Predisposing Factors
A. Low birth weight
B. Prematurity
C. Poverty
D. Organic conditions with the major organs noted above
E. Parents with psychosocial disorders
F. Altered family processes
G. Geriatrics:
   1. Dementia
   2. Cancer
   3. Chronic infections
   4. Endocrine disorders
   5. Malabsorption syndromes
   6. Psychiatric disorders

Common Complaints
A. Failure to grow and gain weight

Patients do not always present for this problem. Many patients are diagnosed at a routine well-child examination in the ambulatory setting.

Other Signs and Symptoms
A. No growth in height
B. Loss of subcutaneous fat tissue
C. Muscle atrophy
D. Alopecia
E. Dermatitis
F. Marasmus
G. Kwashiorkor

Subjective Data
A. Obtain detailed history of the patient's diet. Note the differences between foods offered and foods eaten. If formula is used, note type, frequency, amount taken each feeding, spits, and so forth.
B. Assess quality of nutrients offered to the patient. Consider knowledge deficit of care provider if inadequate. If breast-feeding, note frequency, duration, milk supply, medications, or foods that would alter breast milk.
C. Query regarding financial resources, and if needed, does the family participate in low-income opportunities (WIC, food stamp programs, etc.)?
D. Evaluate whether religious or unusual dietary beliefs/habits contribute to the food preparation, if inadequate.
E. For children, obtain a detailed perinatal history, noting complications with mother or baby. Obtain height, weight, and head circumference. Plot on growth curve.
F. For infants, determine whether the formula is being prepared correctly (powder, concentrate, ready-to-feed).
G. Rule out any difficulty in swallowing or retaining ingested food.
H. Note regular bowel/bladder habits.
I. Note any recent illness, chronic or acute.
J. Query regarding lead exposure.
K. Rule out family history of cystic fibrosis or lactose intolerance.
L. Note whether a short/small stature runs in the family history.
M. Geriatrics: the best tool to evaluate nutritional screening is the Mini Nutritional Assessment. Obtain accurate weights and heights.

Physical Examination
A. Check temperature, pulse, respirations, blood pressure, height, and weight.
   1. Measure head circumference.
B. Inspect
   1. Observe overall appearance.
   2. Observe oral pathology; for geriatrics check for ill-fitting dentures, dental and gum condition.
   3. Note muscle tone, strength, and movement.
   4. Note social interactions among family members.
   5. Note social skills of the patient.
   6. Perform Denver Developmental II on children.

Note any changes in growth curve, especially if crossing over percentiles, and if height and weight are not concordant. If premature, adjust for gestational age as appropriate.

C. Palpate
   1. Palpate organs and extremities for a complete physical examination.
D. Percuss
   1. Percuss the abdomen for a complete physical examination.
E. Auscultate
   1. Auscultate the heart and lungs for a complete physical examination.

Diagnostic Tests
A. CBC, urinalysis, electrolytes
B. Thyroid panel if indicated
C. Lead screen
D. Sweat test if indicated
E. X-rays if appropriate
F. Serum albumin in geriatrics

Differential Diagnoses
A. FTT inorganic versus organic etiology

Plan
A. General interventions
   1. The plan is based on the cause of FTT. Children with organic etiologies need follow-up regarding the specific problem.
   2. Severe malnutrition requires hospitalization.
B. Patient teaching
   1. Reinforce positive eating habits and encourage dietary meal planning.
   2. Offer nutrition counseling with dietician.
C. Dietary management
   1. Meal suggestions: offer adequate time for meals (20–30 min), offer solid food before drinks/juices, and provide a pleasant environment for eating.
   2. Encourage all family members to sit down and eat at least one meal a day together. This time will also enhance family social interactions.
   3. Provide handout for high-calorie foods (peanut butter, cheese, whole milk, etc.).
   4. Consider exercise sessions for geriatrics to stimulate appetite.
   5. Encourage patients to attend centers where meals are served as a group or have meals delivered to them.
   6. For geriatrics suggest snacks between meals and before bedtime.
D. Pharmaceutical therapy
   1. High-calorie supplements are recommended for some patients (Polycose, Carnation Instant Breakfast, Pediasure, Ensure).

Weight gain with high-calorie supplements is commonly seen with patients who have a psychosocial etiology of FTT.

   2. Geriatrics: Short-term aggressive caloric replacement has been shown to be effective in reversing FTT. Severe malnutrition may require hospitalization with

total parental nutrition. SSRIs and other pharmacotherapy may be necessary to help increase the appetite.

   a. Megestrol 400 mg or 800 mg daily with meal.

Follow-up

A. Two-week evaluation for weight/height measurements and to evaluate compliance with regimen at home. Routine visits recommended every 2–4 weeks to monitor progress.

B. Reevaluate patient in 1–2 months. After 2 months if no improvement, or further loss is noted, refer to a specialist.

Consultation/Referral

A. Consult with a physician if height/weight measurements are noted below the third percentile on graphic chart.

B. For the majority of patients, a nutrition consultation is needed to assist the parents or food provider in providing adequate resources/calories for the patient.

C. Consider social service and visiting nurses for outpatient assistance in the home.

D. Early intervention programs should be considered for children.

Individual Considerations

A. Pediatrics

   1. The prognosis for inorganic etiologies of children in the first year of life is ominous due to the poor brain growth. These children will be at high risk for developmental delay, poor cognitive and emotional development, and social/emotional problems.

   2. Approximately 10% of children are normally small children by genetic makeup. These children are not diagnosed with FTT. FTT is most commonly seen in children younger than 3–5 years.

   3. Consider keeping small children on formula past the 12-month age mark if FTT is diagnosed.

GRIEF *by Moya Cook and Jill C. Cash*

Definition

A. Grief is defined as the normal, appropriate emotional response to loss. It is unique to the individual experiencing it, and there is no general timetable for completing it. Most familiar is grief following the death of a loved one, but grief also follows other losses (e.g., loss of independence, loss of affection, or loss of body parts). Mourning is defined as the process by which grief is resolved. Mourning is very individual and helps in reaching acceptance of a loss.

B. The process through which one resolves grief usually follows a typical course that can be viewed in three phases. These phases are intellectual shock, preoccupation with the deceased, and resolution or recovery.

   1. Phase 1: Shock is present with symptoms such as psychological numbness and distancing of emotional feelings.

   2. Phase 2: Pain, tears, anxiousness, anger, and feelings of guilt may be seen.

   3. Phase 3: The griever begins to rebuild life and can think about the past with pleasure. This is the phase of regaining interest in activities and forming new relationships.

C. It is important to distinguish the normal grief reaction from major depression or pathologic grief. Often, depressive symptoms are a pervasive part of the grief response and a clear delineation of grief versus depression is not always possible.

Incidence

A. Grief is a universal emotional response.

Pathogenesis

A. Abnormal, pathologic grief can occur if the mourner is not encouraged to grieve losses. Normal grief resolution usually takes about 2 years.

Predisposing Factors

A. Sudden or terrible deaths

B. Excessive dependency on the deceased and feelings of ambivalence

C. Traumatic losses earlier in life

D. Social isolation

E. Actual or imagined responsibility for "causing" the death

F. Avoidance of grief and denial of loss

G. Survived a traumatic experience that killed the deceased

Common Complaints

A. Angry feelings at God or medical personnel for not doing more, oneself for not seeing the warning signs, the deceased for not taking better care of himself or herself, being left alone, and not making proper financial/legal preparations

B. Sleeping all the time or inability to sleep without medication

C. Change in eating habits with significant weight loss or gain

D. Fatigue, lethargy, or lack of motivation

E. Decreased concentration and memory, forgetfulness

F. Increased irritability

G. Unpredictable bouts of crying

H. Fears

   1. Of being alone or with people

   2. Of leaving the house

   3. Of staying in the house

Other Signs and Symptoms

A. Normal grief, usually 1–2 months in duration

   1. Protest, disbelief, shock, and denial.

   2. Profound sadness and survivor guilt.

   3. Multiple somatic symptoms without actual organic disease.

   4. Sense of unreality and withdrawal from others.

   5. Disruption of normal patterns of conduct, with restlessness and aimlessness.

   6. Preoccupation with memories of the deceased, dreams of the deceased, hallucinations, fear of going crazy, and transient psychotic symptoms.

   7. Response to support and ventilation improves over time.

B. Pathologic grief, over 2 months in duration
1. Persistence of denial with delayed or absent grief.
2. Depression with impaired self-esteem, suicidal thoughts and impulses with self-destructive behavior.
3. Actual organic disease and medical illness.
4. Progressive social isolation.
5. Persistent anger and hostility, leading to paranoid reactions, especially against those involved in medical care of the deceased, or suppression of any expression of anger and hostility.
6. Continued disruption of normal patterns of conduct, often with a persistent hyperactivity unaccompanied by a sense of loss or grieving.
7. Continued preoccupation with memories of the deceased to the point of searching for reunion (sustained depressive delusions).
8. Conversion symptoms similar to the symptoms of the deceased.
9. Self-blame.
10. Response to support and ventilation shows no change or worsens.

Subjective Data

A. Review onset, duration, and course of presenting symptoms. Review the mourner's grief symptoms.
B. Obtain an in-depth personal history of the mourner and his or her relationship to the identified loss or with the deceased.

Understanding the bereaved's history is critical to understanding the individual's loss.

C. Identify anniversary dates pertinent to the mourner's relationship with the deceased/loss.
D. Determine whether the mourner has suicidal ideation (especially with a plan). **Be sure to ask: "Have you ever thought of hurting yourself or others?"**
E. Assess whether the mourner experiences self-blame.
F. Review the mourner's appetite.
G. Establish usual weight, review weight gain/loss, and in what time span.
H. Review the mourner's activities of daily living. Does the mourner get up and dress daily and perform daily hygiene?
I. Review the mourner's sleep quality.
J. Review the mourner's daily routines; return to work, return to school, and exercise.
K. Review the mourner's amount of crying per day, for what length of time (days, weeks).
L. Review the mourner's drug and alcohol consumption since the loss.

Statements suggesting self-medication with alcohol to facilitate sleep could indicate a coexistent alcohol abuse dependence diagnosis.

M. Review the mourner's usual medical problems and how the loss/grief has affected these problems.

Diagnostic Tests

A. As indicated to rule out other pathology
B. Blood glucose
C. Thyroid studies

Differential Diagnoses

A. Grief
B. Depressive disorder
C. Posttraumatic stress disorder
D. Somatoform disorders (characterized by physical complaints lacking known medical basis or demonstrable physical findings in the presence of psychological factors)
E. Alcoholism and drug abuse/dependence

Plan

A. General interventions
1. Evaluate the nature of the grief and any accompanying psychiatric symptoms.
2. Treat physical/laboratory findings, that is, dietary change and nutritional supplements.
B. Patient teaching: See the Section III Patient Teaching Guide for this chapter, "Grief/Bereavement."
C. Pharmaceutical therapy: Antidepressants should not be prescribed for acute grief, but reserved for a possible subsequent major depression. Clinical data suggests that SSRIs may assist the patient with mobilizing the energy necessary to assist him or her through the grieving process.

Resist sedation of individuals suffering from acute grief because this tends to delay and prolong the mourning process. Refer to the "Depression" section for pharmaceutical therapy.

1. Drug of choice: sedative to help sleep.
   a. Sedative anxiolytic hypnotics may be prescribed for **no more than 2 weeks at a time.** Try initially for 1 week to establish a sleep pattern. If insomnia continues, refer the patient.
   b. Temazepam (Restoril) 7.5–30 mg at bedtime *or* Flurazepam (Dalmane) 15–30 mg at bedtime.
   c. Zolpidem (Ambien) 5–10 mg at bedtime (not to be used for more than 1 month).
2. Sedating antihistamines
   a. Hydroxyzine HCI (Atarax) 50–100 mg at bedtime.
   b. Hydroxyzine pamoate (Vistaril) 50–100 mg at bedtime **(not to be used for more than 4 months).**
3. Antidepressant with sedating properties
   a. Trazodone HCI (Desyrel) 50–100 mg at bedtime
   b. Paroxetine (Paxil) 10–20 mg at bedtime
   c. Mirtazapine (Remeron) 15 mg every day at bedtime. Increase at 1–2 weeks: usual range is 15–45 mg every day at bedtime.

Follow-up

A. Follow up in 1 week to assess the patient's status and symptoms.
B. Then follow up every 2 weeks after that to check the patient's progress.
C. Assess suicidality with every office visit.
D. Once positive change is seen, the patient can be seen monthly.
E. Refer to medical diagnosis for follow-up recommendations.

Consultation/Referral

A. Provide immediate referral/consult for continuing psychotherapy for severe depression and/or suicidal threats.

B. Consult with a physician for evaluation of pharmacologic agents versus referral.

Individual Considerations

A. Pregnancy
1. Miscarriage, stillbirth, and neonatal death should be considered a major loss and treated as a grief reaction.
2. Grief is also seen in pregnancy termination. The woman who terminates a pregnancy (regardless of gestational age and reason for termination) may exhibit a major response to this loss.
3. Hospitals often provide photographs, footprints, and identification bracelets and connect families with perinatal grief support groups.
4. Use the baby's name when discussing feelings about the loss of a child.
5. Suggest that friends and family not put away the baby clothes and bedroom furniture. The couple should do this as part of closure.
B. Pediatrics
1. Grief in children may be delayed or difficult to identify.
2. Children who suddenly experience behavioral problems not present before the death of a significant person should be immediately referred to a child psychiatrist.
3. Children should not be told the deceased person is "asleep" or died because they were "sick"; this may connote fears of falling asleep and becoming sick themselves.
4. Use proper terms: heart attack, stroke, "Your baby brother had a congenital heart defect." Use the correct terms and draw pictures to help explain.
5. Young children do not understand death is forever and may continue to ask to see the deceased.
C. Adults: Grief responses vary from among individuals. Look for behaviors outside the norm.
D. Geriatrics: Grief in the elderly should be closely assessed to rule out medical diagnoses.
E. Partners: Involvement in grief/loss psychotherapy groups is extremely helpful.

SLEEP DISORDERS *by Moya Cook and Jill C. Cash*

Definition

A. In normal sleepers, transient insomnia occurs in those who have traveled to another time zone (i.e., "jet lag"), are under situational stress, or are sleeping in unfamiliar surroundings. Treatment is not required in these situations because time takes care of the problem. Most office visits occur when patients complain of insomnia. With short-term insomnia, the normal sleeper experiences difficulty sleeping that does not resolve within a few days. This can be the result of stress, such as financial difficulty, divorce, and so forth. These patients may require short-term symptomatic relief of insomnia.
B. Long-term insomnia is persistent and disabling. Studies suggest that almost all have an associated psychiatric disorder, especially depression, an associated drug use/abuse/withdrawal problem, or an associated medical disorder.

Incidence

A. Difficulties with sleep are among the most common complaints of medical patients and affect a large percentage of the population. From 10%–20% of all adults express sleep-related complaints they consider to be serious. Sleep disorders also can affect proper mental functioning (53% of chronic insomniacs complain of memory difficulties). Sleep disorders are also implicated in decreased work efficiency, impaired industrial productivity, and increased risk of traffic accidents. They also seem to enhance the propensity for cardiovascular disease and increase the risk of death. Insomniacs are also at increased risk for the development of depression and anxiety disorders. Patients with obstructive sleep apnea syndrome have significant performance impairments on complex motor tasks.

The risk of depression increases with time if insomnia is left untreated.

Pathogenesis

A. Other than situational stress, jet lag, and sleeping in unfamiliar surroundings, difficulty with sleep can be related to psychiatric illness or medical problems. It is most frequently due to chronic depression and/or anxiety. Antisocial and obsessive-compulsive features are also common among these patients. Patients may self-medicate, which produces more insomnia.

Predisposing Factors

A. Alcohol use: initially assists with sleep but produces fragmented sleep.
B. Hypnotic medications can produce tolerance, which causes sleep disruption and rebound insomnia with withdrawal from the medication.
C. Medications such as caffeine, nicotine cigarettes, amphetamines, steroids, methylphenidate; hallucinogens, aminophylline, ephedrine, decongestants, bronchodilators, weight loss/diet pills, thyroid preparations, monoamine oxidase inhibitors, and anticancer agents.
D. Women with fibromyalgia syndrome.
E. Women experiencing menopausal symptoms.
F. Upper respiratory symptoms.
G. Obstructive sleep apnea disorders such as nasal obstruction, large uvula, low-lying soft palate, craniofacial abnormalities, excessive pharyngeal tissue, pharyngeal masses (tumors, cysts), macroglossia, tonsilar hypertrophy, and vocal cord paralysis.
H. Obesity.
I. Hypothyroidism.
J. Acromegaly.
K. Chronic pain.
L. Urinary frequency possibly due to prostatism, diabetes, diuretics, and infection.

Common Complaints

A. Statements regarding impaired sleep pattern
1. Inability to fall asleep
2. Restless throughout the night
3. Early morning awakening with inability to fall back to sleep

4. Feels fatigued after 8 hours of sleep
5. Partner complains of the patient's snoring

Other Signs and Symptoms

A. Excessive daytime sleepiness
B. Feels tense, irritable, and agitated
C. Heightened anxiety and aggressiveness (occasionally)
D. Reports of prolonged pauses in respiration during sleep
E. Weight gain
F. Frontal headaches on awakening
G. Difficulty with short-term recall

Subjective Data

A. Review the onset, course, and duration of problems and symptoms.
B. Take a thorough history of the sleep problem, including the 24-hour sleep-wake cycle: sleep-wake habit history, sleep hygiene history, meal and exercise times, ambient noise, and light and temperature.
C. Identify the pattern: trouble falling asleep, trouble staying asleep (frequent awakenings), and early morning awakenings.
D. Inquire about life stresses, drug and alcohol use, and marital and family problems.

Statements suggesting self-medication with alcohol to facilitate sleep could indicate a coexistent alcohol abuse/dependence diagnosis. In patients who have developed tolerance to alcohol or sleep medications, abrupt cessation of these agents may produce increased insomnia and anxiety.

E. Determine whether the insomnia is simply normal sleep. Some "insomniacs" get ample sleep (pseudoinsomnia) and the problems are psychological.
F. Review the patient's smoking and caffeine intake history.
G. Review all medications, including prescribed and over-the-counter medications, recreational drug use, and weight loss medications.
H. Review the patient's medical history: thyroid problems, hypertension, steroid use, diabetes, and cancer.
I. Conduct an interview with the patient's bed partner to provide information about snoring, breathing pauses, and unusual body positions or movements. Is the partner concerned/frightened about the apneic pauses?
J. Review cardiopulmonary dysfunction: orthopnea, paroxysmal nocturnal dyspnea, or nocturnal angina.
K. If female, establish last menses, rule out pregnancy or menopause. Is there regular menses, vaginal dryness, and/or hot flashes?
L. If male, review for signs of prostatism (> age 50, hesitancy, dribbling, nocturia, frequency, incomplete emptying, etc. See Chapter 11, "Benign Prostatic Hypertrophy [BPH]").

Physical Examination

A. Check temperature, pulse, respirations, blood pressure, and weight.
B. Inspect
   1. Observe general overall appearance; note grooming and behaviors during interview.
   2. Evaluate eyes: pupil dilation/constriction (may indicate recent medication/nonprescription drug use).
   3. Inspect nasal mucosa for erythema, edema, discharge, and nasal patency; look for septal deviation and polyps. Transluminate sinus (if indicated).
   4. Inspect the mouth for erythema, the teeth for uneven surfaces (grinding), and the retropharynx for abnormality.
C. Palpate
   1. Conduct a neurologic examination.
   2. Palpate the neck and thyroid; note goiter.
   3. Check the joints for swelling and arthritis, and range of motion (rule out musculoskeletal cause).
D. Rectal examination if indicated for men with prostate symptoms.
E. Auscultate the heart, lungs, and abdomen.
F. Perform speculum/bimanual examination if indicated to evaluate menopausal atrophy and bladder complaints.

Diagnostic Tests

A. CBG with differential.
B. Electrolytes.
C. Thyroid-stimulating hormone or full thyroid profile FSH, LH.
D. Prostate-specific antigen.
E. Serum creatinine and blood urea nitrogen.
F. Urinalysis: check hematuria.
G. Urine culture (if indicated).
H. Glucose tolerance test.
I. Urine drug screen.
J. Sinus X-rays.
K. Urodynamics tests.
L. Postvoid residual (catheterization or ultrasound).
M. Nocturnal polysomnography.
N. Administer psychiatric evaluation if indicated.

Differential Diagnoses

A. Insomnia/sleep disorder
   1. Inadequate sleep hygiene: habitual behaviors that harm sleep, such as delaying morning awakening time or napping
   2. Insufficient sleep syndrome: curtailing time in bed in response to social and occupational demands, over long periods of time
   3. Adjustment sleep disorder: acute emotional stressors (job loss or hospitalization) resulting in difficulty falling asleep because of tension and anxiety
   4. Psychophysiologic insomnia: anticipatory anxiety over the prospect of another night of sleeplessness and the next day of fatigue
   5. Narcolepsy: persistent daytime sleepiness with brief naps accompanied by vivid dreams
      a. Cataplexy or abrupt paralysis or paresis of skeletal muscles following anger, surprise, laughter, or physical exercise
      b. Hypnagogic hallucinations (vivid and often frightening dreams that occur shortly after falling asleep or on awakening)

c. Sleep paralysis, a transient global paralysis of voluntary muscles that occurs shortly after falling asleep and lasts a few seconds or minutes
d. Disturbed and restless sleep

B. Alcoholism and drug abuse/dependence
C. Major depressive disorder
D. Acute psychosis, mania, and hypomania
E. Medical problems such as chronic pain anxiety, depression, hyperthyroidism, epilepsy, general paresis, diabetes, benign prostatic hypertrophy, urinary problems related to age/diuretic use, cardiopulmonary dysfunction, and menopause

Plan

A. General interventions: Treat physical/laboratory findings, that is, hormone replacement therapy, thyroid medications, glucose tolerance test for diabetes, and so forth, as indicated. See related chapters for plans of care.
B. Patient teaching
1. Have the patient record a 2-week log for sleep-wake habits.
2. See the Section III Patient Teaching Guide for this chapter, "Sleep Disorders/Insomnia."
C. Pharmaceutical therapy
1. Eliminate prescription medications (when possible) and over-the-counter products as part of your management plan *before writing another prescription.*
2. Encourage smoking cessation (see Section III Patient Teaching Guide "Nicotine Dependence").
3. Only after making the assumption that the insomnia cannot be adequately treated by addressing the underlying medical problem responsible for causing the insomnia should medications for sleep be prescribed.

Do not prescribe medications for sleep to patients with alcohol/drug or depressive disorders.

4. Use short-term pharmaceutical therapy.
5. Drug of choice: *Sedative anxiolytic hypnotics:* Try initially for 1 week to establish a sleep pattern.

If insomnia continues for more than 1 month, refer the patient.

a. Temazepam (Restoril) 7.5–30 mg at bedtime (1–2 weeks)
b. Flurazepam (Dalmane) 15–30 mg at bedtime (1–2 weeks)
c. Zolpidem (Ambien) 5–10 mg at bedtime (4 weeks maximum)
d. Eszopiclone (Lunesta) 2–3 mg at bedtime. Start with 1 mg in the elderly.
e. Ramelteon (Rozerem) 8 mg by mouth 30 min before bedtime. Do not take with meals.

Anxiolytic agents such as diazepam (Valium) and alprazolam (Xanax) tend to increase the duration and frequency of sleep apneas and are contraindicated for patients with possible/undiagnosed apnea spells.

6. **Sedating antihistamines not over 4 months**
a. Hydroxyzine HCl (Atarax) 50–100 mg at bedtime
b. Hydroxyzine Pamoate (Vistaril) 50–100 mg at bedtime
7. Antidepressant with sedating properties
a. Trazodone HCl (Desyrel) 50–100 mg at bedtime
b. Paroxetine (Paxil) 10–20 mg at bedtime

Follow-up

A. Follow up in 1 week to assess the patient's status.
B. Then, follow up every 2 weeks to check the patient's progress.
C. Once positive change is seen, the patient can be seen monthly as needed.
D. Assess the patient's potential for suicide with every office visit.
E. Refer to medical diagnosis for follow-up recommendations.

Consultation/Referral

A. Refer to a psychiatric clinician for medication management and psychotherapy after initial assessment if psychiatric differential diagnosis is made.
B. Refer for psychological testing.
C. If insomnia continues for more than 1 month, refer especially if the patient requires sedative anxiolytic hypnotic for more than 4 weeks.

Individual Considerations

A. Pregnancy: Sleep difficulties are more prevalent in second and third trimesters of pregnancy because of the growing size of the uterus and difficulty finding comfortable sleeping positions. Treat with comfort measures.
B. Pediatrics
1. Children normally require about 10 hours of sleep.
2. Children under the age of 18 with sleep problems should be referred to a pediatrician or pediatric psychiatrist, depending on clinical findings.
C. Adults
1. The "right" amount of sleep results in optimal daytime alertness and a sense of mental efficiency and well-being.
2. Daytime naps often interfere with the quality of night sleep.
3. Nocturia and disturbed sleep are the symptoms that cause older men to seek medical help with prostatism.
D. Geriatrics
1. With aging, it is normal for sleep time to decrease (< 7 hours) with a tendency toward sleep fragmentation and an increase in the frequency of awakenings and brief arousals. Explain this to older adults to avoid "worry over sleeplessness."
2. Always assess for depression in elderly patients.
3. Start with the lowest dose of pharmaceutical agents.
4. Chronic pain is a leading cause for sleep disruption in elderly persons with degenerative joint pain.
5. Review elderly patients' medications and dosage for insomnia because of known side effects or as a medication toxicity.
6. Gastroesophageal reflux is commonly seen in geriatric patients at nighttime and causes them to wake up at night. Correcting the reflux with sleeping position, avoiding late night meals and spicy food, medications

(PPIs), and possible weight loss interventions could improve sleep disturbance in these patients.

7. Patients with end-stage renal disease may have nocturnal leg movement disorders and anemia due to renal failure. Improving the anemia will improve the insomnia and will decrease the leg movements.

E. Partners: Those who find it necessary to sleep in another room because of their partner's snoring should refer the snorer to the primary care physician/advanced practice nurse to rule out an obstructive sleep apnea syndrome.

SUBSTANCE USE DISORDERS *by Moya Cook*

Definition

The *Diagnostic and Statistical Manual of Mental Disorders* (*DSM–IV*) (American Psychiatric Association, 1994) lists the following criteria that must be fulfilled to meet the diagnosis for each category:

A. Substance abuse: A maladaptive pattern of substance use leading to clinically significant impairment or distress, as manifested by one (or more) of the following, occurring within a 12-month period:

1. Failure to fulfill major role obligations (work, school, or home)
2. Recurrent substance use in situations in which it is physically hazardous (driving or operating a machine)
3. Recurrent substance-related legal problems (arrest)
4. Continued substance use despite recurrent social or interpersonal problems caused or exacerbated by the effects of the substance (arguments, physical fights)

B. Substance intoxication: The development of a reversible substance-specific syndrome due to recent ingestion of (or exposure to) a substance:

1. Clinically significant maladaptive behavioral or psychological changes that are due to the effects of the substance on the CNS (belligerence, mood lability, impaired judgment, impaired social or occupational functioning).
2. The symptoms are not due to a general medical condition and are not better accounted for by another mental disorder.

C. Substance dependence: A maladaptive pattern of substance use, leading to clinically significant impairment or distress, as manifested by three (or more) of the following, occurring at any time in the same 12-month period:

1. Tolerance as shown by a need for markedly increased amounts of the substance to achieve intoxication or desired effect.
2. Markedly diminished effect with continued use of the same amount of the substance.
3. Withdrawal, as manifested by either of the following:
   a. The characteristic withdrawal syndrome for the substance defined for each specific substance in *DSM–IV.*
   b. The same (or a closely related) substance is taken to relieve or avoid withdrawal symptoms.
4. The substance is often taken in larger amounts or over a longer period than was intended.

5. There is a persistent desire or unsuccessful effort to cut down or control substance use.
6. A great deal of time is spent in activities necessary to obtain the substance (visiting multiple doctors, driving long distances), use the substance (e.g., chain smoking), or recover from its effects.
7. Important social, occupational, or recreational activities are given up or reduced because of substance use.
8. The substance use is continued despite knowledge of having a persistent or recurrent physical or psychological problem that is likely to have been caused or exacerbated by the substance (e.g., current cocaine use despite recognition of cocaine-induced depression, or continued drinking despite recognition that an ulcer was made worse by alcohol consumption).

D. Substance withdrawal: The development of a substance-specific syndrome due to the cessation of (or reduction in) substance use that has been heavy and prolonged:

1. The substance-specific syndrome causes clinically significant distress or impairment in social, occupational, or other important areas of functioning.
2. The symptoms are not due to a general medical condition and are not better accounted for by another medical disorder.

Incidence

A. Statistics indicate the most commonly used legal substances are caffeine, alcohol, and nicotine. The most commonly used illicit drugs are marijuana and cocaine.
B. Approximately 90% of the American population consumes some alcohol (at one time or another). Alcohol use is believed to be involved in 20%–50% of all hospital admissions, but alcohol use disorders are formally diagnosed less than 5% of the time. Five to 7% of Americans have alcoholism in a given year and 13% will have it sometime during their life. Prevalence rates of alcoholism are 5%–6% for men and 1%–2% for women. It is highest in men aged 18–64 and women aged 18–24.
C. Eighty percent of Americans use caffeine-containing beverages or medications.
D. Twenty-five percent of Americans use tobacco products. One study states that there is a link between early nicotine use and alcohol abuse and depression. Smoking before the age of 13 significantly increases the risk of drug dependence.
E. It is estimated that 37% of the population aged 12 or older has used an illicit psychoactive drug at least once in their lifetime.

A substance abuse problem is recognized in as few as 1 in 20 substance-abusing patients seeking medical attention.

Pathogenesis

A. No single gene has been identified as the culprit in the predisposition to substance dependence. Certain biologic features seem to be inherited by first-degree relatives (particularly males) of alcoholics, for example, a resistance to intoxication, a subnormal cortisol rise after drinking, and a subnormal epinephrine release following stress.
B. Some theories postulate alterations in metabolism of alcohol and drugs in people who are dependent. Studies

pertaining to alcohol have included research into genetic heritability, flawed metabolism of alcohol by alcoholics, insensitivity to alcohol inherited by alcoholics (thus tending to increase tolerance or ability to know when to stop), and alterations in brain waves in alcoholics.

C. Although much of the research is specific to only one drug, much of what we know about the research can be applied to other drugs. There appears to be a higher rate of substance dependence, not limited to alcohol, in children of alcoholics.

Predisposing Factors

Factors vary among individuals, and no one factor can account entirely for the risk of substance abuse. Studies indicate a high correlation between substance use and the presence of psychiatric disorders, especially anxiety disorders, depression, schizophrenia, and in women, eating disorders.

A. Genetic
B. Familial
C. Environmental
D. Occupational
E. Socioeconomic
F. Cultural
G. Personality
H. Life stress
I. Psychiatric comorbidity
J. Biologic
K. Social learning and behavioral conditioning

Common Complaints

Patients' complaints will be focused on the symptoms of the problem rather than the substance dependence. The problem itself will be avoided through the use of denial, minimization, blaming, and projection (all signs of the disease of substance dependence).

A. Chronic anxiety and tension
B. Insomnia
C. Chronic depression
D. Headaches and/or back pain

Consider patients who present frequently with somatic complaints, such as back pain or headache, as "drug seeking," especially when the patient knows what drugs work best or asks for specific narcotic analgesics.

E. Blackouts
F. Gastrointestinal problems
G. Tachycardia/palpitations
H. Frequent falls or minor injuries

Substance abuse should be suspected in all patients who present with accidents or signs of repeated trauma, especially to the head.

I. Problems with a loved one, problems at work, or with friends

Other Signs and Symptoms

A. Defensiveness about alcohol/drug use or vagueness with answers.
B. History of problems with family life, marital relationships, work, finances, and physical health.

C. Change in spiritual beliefs (stops attending religious services).
D. Unexplained job changes and multiple traffic accidents.
E. History of impulsive behavior, fighting, or unexplained falls.
F. Arrest for public drunkenness, driving under the influence, or illegal activity when alcohol/drugs were involved.
G. Tremors (shakes).
H. Delirium tremors (DTs).
I. Seizures related to drugs.
J. Hallucinations.
K. History of chronic family chaos and instability.
L. Physical indications of chronic alcohol/drug use include spider angiomas, ruddy nose and face, nasal lesions, bruxism, swollen features, bruises, needle marks/tracks, cutaneous abscesses, malnourished, anemia, jaundice, and severe dental problems such as "meth mouth."
M. Active withdrawal symptoms include nausea and vomiting, malaise, weakness, tachycardia, diaphoresis, tremors, lightheadedness or dizziness, insomnia, irritability, confusion, perceptual abnormalities or hallucinations (auditory, visual, or tactile), paresthesia, blurred vision, diarrhea, anorexia, abdominal cramps, severe depression, severe anxiety, piloerection, fasciculation (muscle twitching), rhinorrhea, fever, elevated blood pressure and pulse, tinnitus, nystagmus, delirium, or seizures.
N. Overdose symptoms related to drug(s) include seizures, cardiovascular depression/collapse, and respiratory depression/collapse. Be prepared to provide cardiovascular and respirator support and supportive care until transport.

Subjective Data

A. Review the onset, duration, and course of presenting complaints.
B. Question the patient regarding relatives with a history of alcohol, tobacco, or drug use or problems pertaining to use.
C. When questioning the patient, assume some use, for example, "At what age did you first start drinking?" Start with the least invasive questions first: cigarettes, over-the-counter medications, prescription medications, then alcohol, marijuana, stimulants, opiates, sedatives, hypnotics, benzodiazepines, barbiturates, hallucinogens, inhalants, steroids, and other drugs.
D. Review use of the following drugs concerning quantity and type (if cigarettes, brand smoked; if alcohol, type of alcohol: beer, wine, hard liquor), and age at initiation. Query regarding previous attempts to stop use.
E. Start with the past and proceed to the present with use; include first use of the mood-altering substance, amounts, and the last use of the particular substance and amount.
F. Follow the CAGE test. The **CAGE** (2 out of 4) is highly predictive of addiction:
   1. Have you ever tried to **Cut** down on your alcohol/drug use?
   2. Do you get **Annoyed** if someone mentions your use is a problem?
   3. Do you ever feel **Guilty** about your use?

4. Do you ever have an **"Eye-opener"** first thing in the morning after you've been drinking or using the night before?

G. If patient admits drinking, or drug use, ascertain specific amounts and last use of each substance.

H. Establish usual weight and recent loss and in what length of time.

I. Determine whether patient experiences suicidal ideation and if there is a history of past attempts. (See section on "Suicide.")

Physical Examination

A. Check temperature, pulse, respirations, blood pressure, and weight.

B. Inspect
   1. Observe general appearance, dress, grooming, breath odor, wasted appearance, attitude, sad affect, psychomotor retardation, or tremors.
   2. Conduct a dermal examination for spider angiomas, bruises, track marks, color, pallor, rash, jaundice, petechiae, and gynecomastia in men (hallucinogens).
   3. Examine the eyes for sclera color and features, pupil size, and reactivity.
   4. Inspect the nasal mucosa for erythema, edema, spider telangiectasis, and discharge; look for septal lesions or perforation, deviation, and polyps.
   5. Inspect the mouth/pharynx: oral lesions, poor dental hygiene, erythema, and teeth for uneven surfaces, tooth decay, and gum erosion.

C. Palpate
   1. Palpate the neck and thyroid.
   2. Palpate the axilla and groin for lymphadenopathy.
   3. Palpate the abdomen; note hepatomegaly/tenderness.

D. Percuss
   1. Percuss the chest; note pulmonary consolidation.
   2. Percuss the abdomen for hepatosplenomegaly.

E. Auscultate
   1. Auscultate the heart for murmur, new S4 gallop, single S2, and arrhythmias.
   2. Auscultate the lungs for rales, effusion, and consolidation.

F. Neurologic examination/mental status.

Diagnostic Tests

A. Blood alcohol level.
B. Cotinine level (nicotine) (where available).
C. Urine drug screen.
D. CBC with differential.
E. Platelet count.
F. HIV or hepatitis.

Intravenous drug use contributes strongly to the spread of acquired immunodeficiency syndrome (AIDS), hepatitis B and hepatitis C, and other infectious diseases. Consider evaluation for sexually transmitted infections.

G. Antinuclear antibody, erythrocyte sedimentation rate, and rheumatoid factor.
H. Electrolytes.
I. Liver panel
   1. Elevated liver enzymes can also be attributed to overuse of acetaminophen (Tylenol), found in combination with opiates.

2. Blood cultures (fever).
3. Bone density studies.

J. Patients who have been drinking for years should have bone density studies done because alcohol increases the risk for osteoporosis.

Differential Diagnoses

A. Substance use disorder
B. Chronic pain syndrome

Plan

A. General interventions
   1. See the patient weekly.
   2. Discuss your concerns about the alcohol, nicotine, or drug use and ask the patient to stop use.
   3. At each office visit, provide support to help prevent relapse. If relapse happens, encourage the patient to try again immediately.
   4. Consider signing a contract with the patient to stop smoking, drinking, or using drugs.
   5. Assess potential for suicide with every office visit.
   6. If possible, obtain confirmation of the patient's abstinence from a family member.
   7. Stress the importance of 12-step meetings, such as Alcoholics Anonymous (AA), Cocaine Anonymous (CA), and Narcotics Anonymous (NA).
   8. Have the patient sign a written release of information so you can speak with a rehabilitation counselor. If the patient is willing, refer to an alcohol and drug treatment facility or smoking cessation program, after initial assessment and differential diagnosis is made.
   9. Treat physical/laboratory findings, that is, caffeine intake reduction and dietary issues.

B. Patient teaching
   1. Educate the patient about the impact of alcohol, tobacco, and drugs on physical/emotional health. Provide information for the patient to read at home.
   2. See the Section III Patient Teaching Guide for this chapter, "Alcohol and Drug Dependence."

C. Pharmaceutical therapy
   1. Consider nicotine replacement for those who smoke more than one pack of cigarettes per day or who smoke their first cigarette within 30 min of waking. Stress that there is NO SMOKING while using the nicotine patch. Nicoderm and Habitrol
      a. 21 mg/24 hours for 4 weeks *then*
      b. 14 mg/24 hours for 2 weeks *then*
      c. 7 mg/24 hours for 2 weeks Prostep
      d. 22 mg/24 hours for 4 weeks *then*
      e. 11 mg/24 hours for 4 weeks Nicotrol
      f. 15 mg/16 hours for 4 weeks *then*
      g. 10 mg/16 hours for 2 weeks *then*
      h. 5 mg/16 hours for 2 weeks
   2. Nonnicotine therapy: Adults: Bupropion (Zyban, Wellbutrin) 150 mg daily for 3 days, then increase to 150 mg twice daily. Treat for 7–12 weeks. The patient may continue to smoke during the first 2 weeks of starting medication. This medication should not be given to patients with seizure disorders.
   3. Varenicline (Chantix): start at 0.5 mg/day for the first 3 days, then for the next 4 days, then 0.5 mg twice

daily. After the first 7 days the dose is 1 mg twice daily.

   a. Encourage the patient to choose a stop date for smoking and start the chantix 1–2 weeks prior to this stop date.

   b. Patients should be encouraged to quit even if they have relapses.

   c. Instruct patients that the most common side effects of Chantix are insomnia, vivid or strange dreams, and nausea, and they are usually transient.

   d. Give precautions to the patient regarding potential side effects of mood swings, aggression, homicidal thoughts, psychosis, anxiety, and panic disorder, which may occur on rare occasions.

   e. See package inserts or *Physicians' Desk Reference* for detailed instructions.

4. Detoxification and methadone maintenance: Should be performed by specially licensed and trained professionals.

5. Disulfiram (Antabuse) therapy is not recommended. Patients who consume alcohol after taking Antabuse can become extremely ill.

Follow-up

A. Make a follow-up appointment weekly. Make contact with the referral source (smoking cessation program, alcohol/drug rehabilitation program) before next follow-up visit to check on the patient's progress. At weekly visit, question the patient regarding compliance.

B. Order blood alcohol, urine drug screen, or nicotine level (as appropriate) with every office visit while in outpatient treatment and throughout the year following treatment.

C. Once positive change is seen, the patient can be seen monthly. Discuss changes the patient has made, past relapses, circumstances under which they occurred, and any special concerns.

D. Refer to the medical diagnosis for other applicable follow-up recommendations.

Consultation/Referral

A. Refer patients with drug and/or alcohol dependence to a community mental health center that has an outpatient alcohol/drug rehabilitation program or to a specialist in the community who deals frequently with substance abuse/dependence.

B. Planning a family meeting to confront the patient is best done with the help of an experienced mental health professional.

C. Have referral numbers at close hand, so that the patient's moment of motivation is not lost.

D. Geriatrics

1. In this population, consumption of as little as 1 oz/day can indicate a problem.

2. Pain medications and benzodiazepines, along with multiple medications for health problems, may create a substance abuse problem.

E. Partners/family members

1. For fear of retribution, the family may remain silent about the problem, even if accompanying the patient.

2. Some studies by corporate business show that per capita, business spends more money on the care of family members of substance-dependent patients than on the employee.

3. Refer family members of alcoholics/drug addicts to Al-Anon, Nar-Anon, Co-dependents Anonymous, or Adult Children of Alcoholics (ACOA) meetings.

Individual Considerations

A. Pregnancy

1. Substance-dependent pregnant women frequently avoid early prenatal care for fear of identification and reprisal.

2. Cocaine use is associated with abruptio placenta and preterm labor. Consider drug screen for emergent admissions for patients in preterm labor and abruption.

3. Notify the hospital nursery personnel/neonatologist before delivery to closely monitor the newborn for withdrawal and seizure precautions.

4. Nicotine/smoking use is associated with intrauterine growth restriction, preterm delivery, and bleeding in pregnancy.

5. Nicotine-dependent pregnant women should be encouraged to stop smoking without pharmacologic treatment. The nicotine patch should be used during pregnancy only if the increased likelihood of smoking cessation, with its potential benefits, outweighs the risk of nicotine replacement and potential concomitant smoking. Similar factors should be considered in lactating women.

6. Pregnant women who use alcohol, tobacco, or drugs should always be classified as substance dependent rather than substance abusive.

B. Pediatrics

1. The diagnosis of substance dependence is more difficult to make in children under age 18. If there is any indication of substance dependence, children should be referred to a pediatrician who deals specifically with this problem.

2. Consider drug use when alienation of friends and family, falling grades, and isolation occur.

3. "Huffing" is common with gasoline, glues, aerosol sprays, and spray paints.

4. Infants of smokers have increased risk of sudden death syndrome (SIDS).

C. Adults

1. With women, tolerance can be established by asking the question, "How many drinks does it take to make you high?" More than two drinks indicates some tolerance.

2. In considering a diagnosis of alcohol dependence, consider the following diagnostic findings: hypertension; nonspecific EKG changes; cardiomyopathy; palpitations; increased mean cell volume; decreased red blood cell count; low platelet count; increased alanine aminotransferase, aspartate aminotransferase, lactic dehydrogenase, γ-glutamyltranspeptidase, alkaline phosphatase; type IV hyperlipoproteinemia; gout; and adult-onset diabetes mellitus.

SUICIDE *by Moya Cook and Jill C. Cash*

Definition

A. Suicide is defined as the intentional destruction of one's own life. It is the most critical consequence of mental illness and occurs in all diagnostic psychiatric categories. Therefore, knowing the risk factors for suicide and eliciting key clinical features that differentiate the truly suicidal patient from the attention-seeker are of utmost importance. **Symptoms are often missed because they can be very subtle. Because there are important legal, social, and religious implications to suicide, the general health care practitioner should not attempt to treat these high-risk patients. This section will focus on identifying the suicidal patient for immediate referral to a psychiatrist or psychiatric inpatient facility.**

Incidence

The Rule of Sevens is helpful in assessment of these patients:

1. **One out of seven** with recurrent depressive illness commit suicide.
2. **Seventy percent** of suicides have depressive illness.
3. **Seventy percent** of suicides see their primary care physician within 6 weeks of suicide.
4. Suicide is the **11th leading cause of death** in the United States; for young people between the ages of 15–24 it is the **third** leading cause of death.

The United States averages 10.6 suicides per 100,000 population annually. Every year between 30,000–35,000 people take their own lives, not including those individuals who die as a result of fatal accidents due to impaired concentration and attention, and death due to illnesses that may be sequelae (e.g., alcohol abuse).

According to the World Health Organization by the year 2010 depression will be the Number 1 disability in the world. Estimates associate 16,000 suicides in the United States annually with depressive disorder. Fifteen percent of those hospitalized for major depressive disorder attempt suicide. Fifteen percent of patients with severe primary major depressive disorder of at least 1 month's duration eventually commit suicide.

The rate of suicide in young adults has more than doubled since 1950. Little is known about midlife suicides compared to adolescent and elderly suicides. Midlife suicide rates tend to be highest among White men, although female suicide rates peak in midlife. Males exceed females in suicide completions but not in attempt. Whites are twice as likely as non-Whites to commit suicide, though in the 25- to 34-year age group they are equal. Rates for widowed, divorced, or separated individuals are higher than for those who are married. Rates are highest in Protestants, intermediate in Jews, and lowest in Catholics.

Pathogenesis

A. Recent studies confirm some changes in the noradrenergic system along with reduced serotonin levels are associated with suicide. In recent studies independent of psychiatric diagnoses, one researcher identified a suicidality syndrome consisting of hopelessness, ruminative thinking, social withdrawal, and lack of activity as core symptoms.

B. Familial, genetic, early life loss experiences, and comorbid alcoholism may be causal factors. In adolescence, depression is the largest single risk factor for suicidal behavior, although family relationship difficulties make a significant independent contribution to this. Environmental stressors in the presence of psychiatric disorders may also be responsible for initiating the impulsive behavior leading to suicide. The risk of suicidal behaviors is higher in those with mental disorders than those with mood disorders.

Predisposing Factors

"SAD PERSONAS"

S = sex
A = age
D = depression

P = previous attempts
E = ethanol abuse
R = rational thinking loss
S = social support loss
O = organized plan
N = no spouse
A = Availability of lethal means
S = sickness

Also consider gender, race and ethnicity, medications and other medical conditions.

Common Complaints

A. Overt or indirect suicide talk or threats: "You won't be bothered by me much longer."

Any mention of dying or ending one's life must be taken seriously.

B. Depressed or anxious mood due to depression

Every depressed patient must be assessed for suicide risk.

C. Significant recent loss such as spouse, job, or self-esteem
D. Unexpected change in behavior such as making a will, intense talks with friends, and giving away possessions
E. Unexpected change in attitude such as suddenly cheerful, angry, or withdrawn
F. Atypical symptoms of depression in the elderly such as impaired ability to communicate, intractable tinnitus, and feelings of helplessness

Other Signs and Symptoms

Indications for Hospitalization of Suicidal Patients

A. Psychosis
B. Intoxication with drugs or alcohol that cannot be evaluated and treated over a period of time in the emergency department
C. No change in affect or symptoms despite the intervention of the physician, family, and friends
D. Command hallucinations
E. Lack of access to, or low availability of, outpatient resources

F. Family exhaustion

G. Escalating number of suicide attempts

H. Uncertainty about the risk of suicide

I. Severe psychic anxiety, anxious ruminations, and global insomnia are acute risk factors

Subjective Data

A. Ascertain the patient's intention. Ask why does he or she want to die?

  1. Asking the patient about suicide does not give the patient any ideas about suicide.

B. Determine whether the patient has thought of a suicide plan. The more specific the plan the more likely the act. A well-worked out, realistic, and potentially lethal plan suggests great risk.

C. Rule out the presence of psychiatric or organic factors such as psychotic depression, thought disorder, or sedative self-medication.

D. Determine whether the precipitating crisis is resolving satisfactorily to the patient.

E. Take an "inventory of loss." Determine the losses the patient has incurred in the last several months or years.

F. Review the patient's plans for the future.

G. Determine whether the patient thinks he or she is going to commit suicide.

H. Evaluate whether the patient has a caring family or other support systems.

Plan

A. General interventions

  1. If the patient is suicidal, refer immediately. Make sure there is someone with the patient at all times.

  2. If the patient came alone, call a family member or friend to accompany the patient to the hospital emergency room.

  3. If you are fearful the patient will try to escape or leave unaccompanied, escort the patient to the hospital emergency room where commitment papers for involuntary hospital admission can be completed.

Be sure to advise the hospital staff of your concerns regarding the patient's suicidal status.

B. Patient teaching:

  1. Educate patient and family regarding treatment with medication for depression. Discuss benefits/risks of medication and side effects.

  2. Encourage the patient to enroll in counseling with a psychologist/therapist to discuss current problems/needs.

  3. Determine if social services need to be contacted for patient for support services.

  4. Provide local resources for counseling and social services as appropriate.

  5. If patient is not hospitalized, make sure that family or friends are aware of the patient's status and that he or she has someone to talk to and monitor his or her condition until the next office appointment.

C. Pharmaceutical therapy: Patients with suicide potential should never be given more than 1 g or 1 week's supply of TCAs.

D. Documentation is critical. Make sure all statements are recorded and the decision-making process followed.

Follow-up

A. After emergency admission for suicidal ideation or threats, patients should be closely observed, especially in the first year after the serious suicide attempt.

B. With each visit, question the patient regarding suicidal ideation or a plan (see "Subjective Data" section for important questions to ask).

Consultation/Referral

A. Consult with the patient's psychiatric practitioner. Obtain a release of information from the patient.

B. Be sure the patient continues to follow up with psychiatric counseling and medication management (see "Depression" section).

Individual Considerations

A. Pregnancy: A woman with a history of depression or previous postpartum depression is at high risk for postpartum depression (recurrent). (See "Postpartum Depression" section in Chapter 12, "Obstetrics Guidelines.")

B. Adolescent

  1. Teens are at risk after recent losses from death (especially if one of their friends/family commits suicide). Recent loss includes breaking up with a boyfriend or girlfriend.

  2. If a teen has had a depressive episode he or she may be at a higher risk if he or she suddenly seems happy and things are "just fine." The teen may have decided on a suicide plan and is experiencing a sense of relief because he or she has made plans.

C. Geriatrics

  1. White men, age older than 80, have the highest rate of suicide of any age group in the United States.

  2. Older persons use the usual means for suicide as well as a slower plan including not eating, stopping prescription drugs or overmedicating, increasing alcohol intake, and refusing treatment.

  3. The elderly population is more susceptible to adverse effects of medications.

  4. Antidepressants should be started at the lowest doses and slowly increased for the elderly. The SSRIs are considered the first line of antidepressant therapy in the elderly population. (See "Depression" section.)

VIOLENCE AGAINST CHILDREN
by Cheryl A. Glass

Definition

The responsibility of the definition of sexual abuse, childhood abuse, and the age of children included in statistics changes with each state in the United States. Any family member, friends, and strangers can perpetrate abuse; however, fathers, mother's boyfriends, female babysitters, and mothers are the most common perpetrators of abuse. Nonaccidental injury/abuse may result in serious physical or emotional harm and may result in failure to thrive, developmental progress, or death. There are four major types of abuse noted in the literature:

A. Physical abuse: infliction of pain/harm producing injuries, including skeletal fractures, skin (i.e., burns), and central nervous system injuries (i.e., abusive head trauma [AHT] and shaken baby syndrome [SBS]/shaking-impact syndrome)

B. Sexual abuse: inappropriate exposure; fondling; sexual stimulation; coercion; oral, genital, buttock, breast contact; anal or vaginal penetration; foreign body insertion; and making and use of child pornography

C. Emotional abuse: rejection, lack of affection or stimulation, ignoring, dominating, describing the child negatively, blaming the child, and verbal (belittle, yell, threats of severe punishment), resulting in impaired psychological growth and development

D. Child neglect: isolation; starvation; lack of medical care; inadequate supervision; failure to provide love, affection, and emotional support; and failure to enroll/attend school

Incidence

A. Childhood abuse occurs worldwide; the exact incidence is not known. It occurs across all cultures and racial, socioeconomic, and educational levels. Approximately 1 million cases of child abuse and/or neglect are reported annually by child protective services (CPS). Sexual abuse is underreported, underrecognized, and undertreated. Approximately 1 in 6 boys are sexually abused before the age of 16 years.

Pathogenesis

A. Societal, environmental, and psychosocial factors contribute to abuse.

Predisposing Factor

A. Children victims
   1. Minority children
   2. Disabled or medically fragile children
      a. Congenital anomalies
      b. Mental retardation
      c. Handicapped
      d. Chronic medical illness
      e. Hyperactive
      f. Adopted children/stepchildren
      g. Poor bonding
   3. Age of children (physical abuse)
      a. Younger than 1 year (67%)
      b. Children younger than 3 years (80%)
B. Parental factors
   1. Young or single parents
   2. Distant or absent extended family
   3. Low educational level of parents
   4. Few role boundaries
   5. Acute or chronic instability and stress in the family
      a. Loss of employment
      b. Divorce/death
      c. Drug/alcohol abuse
      d. Parents with a history of abuse/neglect as a child (learned behavior)
      e. Presence of psychiatric illness
      f. Poverty
      g. Criminal history
C. Sexual abuse risk factors

   1. Male
      a. Younger than 13 years
      b. Non-White
      c. Low socioeconomic status
      d. Not living with the biological father
      e. Disabled
   2. Female
      a. Young age between 7–14 years
      b. Absence of a parent
      c. Appearance of isolation, depression, or loneliness

Common Complaints

A. Oral/facial injuries
   1. Oropharyngeal sexually transmitted infections: sexual abuse
   2. Black eyes
   3. Nasal perforation/septal deviation
   4. Skull fracture
   5. Traumatic alopecia
   6. Retinal hemorrhage
   7. Hearing loss/tympanic injury
B. Burns (6%–20% of injuries)
   1. Cigarette burns are pathognomonic for child abuse.
   2. Scalding/immersion.
   3. Caustic exposure.
   4. Branding.
   5. Microwave burns.
   6. Stun gun burns.
C. Fractures (2nd most common injury)
D. Bruises (most common type of injury)
E. Lacerations
F. Bites
G. Force feeding "bottle jamming"/forced ingestion (water, salt, pepper, poisons)
H. Starvation
I. Sexual abuse
   1. Difficulty with bowel movements
   2. Urinary tract infections
   3. Vaginal infections, itching, or discharge
   4. Complaints of stomachaches
   5. Headaches
   6. Vaginal or rectal bleeding
   7. Difficulty walking or sitting
J. Behavioral signs
   1. Loss of appetite/eating disorder
   2. Clinginess, withdrawn, or aggressive
   3. Nightmares, disturbed sleep pattern, and fear of the dark
   4. Regression (i.e., bedwetting, thumb sucking, crying)
   5. Poor grades/school attendance
   6. Express interest or affection inappropriate for the child's age
   7. Intercourse or masturbation or other sexual acting out
   8. Self-injurious behavior (i.e., cutting, biting, pulling out hair)

Other Signs and Symptoms

A. A caregiver's refusal to allow an interview of the child alone in the examination room is considered a "red flag" for abuse.

B. The history is inconsistent, changes with repeated questioning, conflicts with other family members/caregivers that are interviewed, implausible, or there is a total lack of history (i.e., "I don't know how it happened").

C. History is inconsistent with the child's developmental ability/stage.

D. Caregiver behaviors that may indicate abuse include delay in seeking care, argumentative, lack emotional response, inappropriate, or violent.

E. Radiographs should be obtained for a history of "soft" easily broken bones.

F. The child exhibits inappropriate behavior for his or her developmental age.

Subjective Data

A. Use open-ended questions during the history to evaluate how injuries were sustained. As the interview continues ask specific questions related to responses. If the child can talk, direct questions to him or her before the caregiver.

B. If this is the first clinic visit, ask if the child had routine health care including immunizations.

Physical Examination

The physical examination should be performed with the child totally unclothed; however, clothing can be removed as the physical progresses from head to toe (i.e., upper body, torso, lower body, lastly perineum/rectum). Detailed documentation of history is essential.

A. Blood pressure, pulse, and respiration, temperature if indicated.

B. A forensic examination requires thorough documentation of injuries.
   1. Use color photographs before any treatment is started.
   2. Photograph damaged clothing.
   3. Make at least one full body photograph and a facial photograph.
   4. Make close-up photographs of all injuries.
   5. Use a ruler to identify/document the size of injuries.
   6. Documentation on the back of the photographs should include the patient's name, date, photographer's name, as well as any witnesses to the examination. The photographer should also sign each photograph.

C. General observation
   1. Observe the interactions between the caregiver and the child. Is the child fearful, or reluctant to have the examination? Are there signs of discomfort during the examination with movement such as range of motion?
   2. Evaluate the child's overall appearance: is the child clean, clothes appropriate for the season, poor hygiene, body odor, malnourished, dehydrated, depressed, violent, withdrawn, compliant even during a painful examination of the rectum/genitalia, and level of consciousness?
   3. Dermal examination: evaluate from head to toe, including the palms, soles of the feet, and between toes; observe for injuries in different stages of healing and new trauma, including burns, lesions, swelling, bruises, and signs of pinching. Evaluate the corner of the mouth for signs of being gagged. Examine the head for alopecia from hair pulling. Evaluate bruises and burns for the characteristics of shapes (i.e., iron, handprints, long belt marks, loops, bite marks, ligature marks).
   4. Eye examination: observe for retinal hemorrhages, black eyes, periorbital edema, and papilledema (indicates increased intracranial pressure).
   5. Ear examination: evaluate hearing, hemotympanum or possible laceration to the external canal, and foreign objects.
   6. Nasal exam: evaluate the presence of blood, swelling, and foreign objects.
   7. Mouth and throat: evaluate the presence of caustic ingestion, observe for ligature marks, and cry/voice quality.

D. Auscultate
   1. Heart
   2. Lungs
   3. Abdomen in all four quadrants
   4. Auscultate over the globes of the eyes if warranted (bruit may indicate traumatic carotid-cavernous fistula).
   5. Auscultate the carotid arteries bilaterally if warranted (bruit may indicate carotid dissection).

E. Palpate
   1. Examine for facial fractures, palpate for instability of the facial bones, including the zyogmatic arch.
   2. Abdomen in all four quadrants for guarding, tenderness, and masses (hematoma).
   3. Examine for any trauma to the spine.

F. Neurologic examination
   1. Assess mental status and memory: determine whether the patient is awake, alert, cooperative, and oriented (to person, place, time, and situation). Temporary impairment of memory is one of the most common deficits after a head injury.
   2. Assess cranial nerve function
      a. Opthalmoscopic/visual exam (cranial nerve II)
      b. Pupillary response (cranial nerve III)
      c. Extraocular movements (cranial nerves III, IV, VI)
      d. Facial sensation and muscles of mastication (cranial nerve V)
      e. Facial expression and taste (cranial nerve VII)
   3. Perform a motor examination on all four extremities.
   4. Perform a sensory exam on all four extremities.

G. Genital/rectal examination:
   1. Evaluate genitals/anal for redness, swelling, bruising, hematomas, abrasions, or lacerations.
   2. Evaluate for evidence of sperm.
   3. Evaluate for the presence of condyloma.
   4. Evaluate for the presence of foreign bodies.

Diagnostic Tests

Diagnostic tests and X-rays are ordered dependent on the type of presenting complaints and physical examination.

A. CBC with differential and peripheral smear, bleeding evaluation, including PT/PTT, ALT and AST to evaluate

injury to the liver, serum amylase or lipase to rule out pancreatic injury.
B. Urinalysis.
C. Drug screen/toxicology (urine and serum).
D. Obtain forensic DNA samples from the skin, under nails, vagina, rectum, and saliva from bite marks using sterile cotton-tipped applicators that have been moistened with sterile saline. These should be sent to a crime laboratory as soon as possible.
E. Test for sexually transmitted infections/HIV.
F. Pregnancy test (age appropriate).
G. Radiographs: facial injury, anteroposterior (AP) and lateral radiograph for any areas of bone tenderness, swelling, deformity, or limited range of motion.
H. Neuroimaging CT/MRI for any suspected nonaccidental head injury (i.e., head trauma, history of shaking, and scalp hematoma).

Differential Diagnoses
A. Child abuse (physical, sexual, emotional, and/or neglect)
B. Congenital syphilis
C. Rickets
D. Osteogenesis imprefecta (OI)
E. Mongolian spots
F. Impetigo
G. Dermatitis herpetiformis
H. Folk-healing practices
I. Thrombocytopenia purpura (ITP)
J. Malignancy
K. Meningitis: neurologic signs

Plan
A. General interventions
   1. Your state may also have a requirement for parental permission prior to taking any photographs.
B. Contact child protective services (states differ on reporting).
C. Increase public awareness.
D. Failure to report a suspected case of sexual abuse may incur criminal charges.

Patient Teaching
A. Reinforce that abuse/neglect is not the victim's fault.
B. Elderly abuse is very common and they do not deserve to be abused.
C. Help is available.

Pharmaceutical Therapy
A. Antibiotics to treat sexually transmitted infections or wounds.
B. Antidepressant therapy may be appropriate.

Follow-up
A. Each state mandates reporting child abuse. Refer to your state requirements or laws. Child protective services are responsible for investigations. Depending on your locality, police involvement may be mandatory.
B. Hospitalization may be required, depending on physical findings, child safety, and parental observation.
C. Child victims are at high risk for depression, anxiety, eating disorders, discipline problems, drug/alcohol use, runaway, and low self-esteem. Therapy and follow-up varies for each individual child. Family participation in a recommended treatment program is helpful. The goal of treatment is that the child regains his or her prior state of mental and psychological health. Neglect is the major reason that children are removed from a home, especially with parents with drug/alcohol problems.

Consultation/Referral
A. Consult with other health care providers that have greater experience with abuse (i.e., CPS, physician, psychiatrist or psychologist, social worker).
B. Refer for a nurse in-home assessment if available/indicated.
C. Specialty consultations:
   1. Genetic consultation: osteogenesis imperfecta (OI)
   2. Orthopedic consultation
   3. Plastic surgeon
   4. Child psychiatrist
   5. Ophthalmology

VIOLENCE AGAINST OLDER ADULTS
by Cheryl A. Glass

Definition
Abuse in the older individuals, defined as older than age 65, is associated with loss of functionally capacity, depression, cognitive impairment, increased morbidity, and mortality. Perpetrators include partners, family members (of all ages), as well as strangers. There are several types of mistreatment in this population:

A. Physical abuse: willful unnecessary restraint, the infliction of physical pain, or injury.
B. Sexual abuse: nonconsensual sexual contact.
C. Psychological abuse: infliction of emotional harm, verbal abuse.
D. Neglect: failing to provide for needs and protection of a vulnerable adult.
E. Self-neglect: failure to thrive of the elder is also considered a subset of neglect.
F. Abandonment: desertion.
G. Financial exploitation: misappropriation of resources.

Incidence
A. In 2010 the population age 65 and older is estimated to be 40 million, with an estimated increase to 55 million in 2020. In 2010 the population 85 years and older is estimated to be 5.7 million with an estimated increase to 6.6 million in 2020. The exact incidence of elder abuse, neglect, exploitation, and self-neglect is unknown; however, it is believed to be common. The incidence is underreported due to the reluctance to report abuse, fear of implicating family members, and fear of being removed from the home.
B. The highest rate of abuse is among elderly women older than age 80 with the abuser being the spouse or adult child. In the case of cognitive impairment the victim may not remember or recognize abuse.

Pathogenesis
Mistreatment of vulnerable adults occurs by people that have ongoing relationships with the older person when there is an

expectation of responsibility; this includes paid and unpaid caregivers. There have been several identifying psychopathologies in the abuser:

A. Physical frailty and mental impairment of the victim plays an indirect role. The victim may have a decreased ability to defend or escape.

B. Caregiver stressors from caring for the elderly patient, including the patient's physical and verbal demands. Psychosocial factors of the caregiver, mental illness, and alcohol or drug abuse contribute.

C. The child who was once abused may continue the cycle of violence transferred to the parent.

Predisposing Factors

A. Age: 65 years and older (some studies indicate age 60).

B. Institutionalized.

C. Cognitive impairment/diminished capacity.

D. Decreased capacity performing activities of daily living (ADLs).
   1. Feeding themselves
   2. Bathing and dressing themselves
   3. Going to the toilet and performing hygiene themselves

E. Decreased capacity performing instrumental activities of daily living (IADLs).
   1. Ability to prepare meals
   2. Ability to do household chores
   3. Ability to use the telephone
   4. Ability to manage personal finances

F. Females have a higher incidence of physical/sexual abuse.

G. Male gender is associated with self-neglect associated with impaired ADLs and IADLs.

H. Family stressors involving the caretaker.

Common Complaints

A. Depression
B. Falls
C. History of hip fracture
D. Pressure ulcers
E. Bruises, lacerations, and burns

Other Signs and Symptoms

A. Indications of healing spiral fractures on X-ray

B. Poor nutrition: lack of resources/transportation to obtain food; caregiver not providing adequate nutrition/withholding food

C. Multiple hospitalizations

D. Recurrent urinary tract infections

E. Noncompliance: may not be able to pay for medications, medications may be withheld, or even given in excess by the caregiver

F. Complaints of sexual abuse
   1. Pain or soreness in the genital area
   2. Bruises or lacerations on the perineum/rectum
   3. Vaginal or rectal bleeding

Subjective Data

A. The caregiver often refuses to leave the patient alone and may answer questions for the patient.

B. Ask the patient directly about abuse, neglect, or exploitation.
   1. Has anyone at home threatened or ever hurt you?
   2. Are you afraid of anyone at home?
   3. Are you left alone for long periods of time?
   4. Who cooks your meals? How often and what amounts of food do you eat?
   5. Who handles your financial business? Have you signed any documents that you didn't understand?

C. Assess the patient's living arrangements. Has the patient ever told family or friends, called hotlines, or attempted to leave the caregiver?

Physical Examination

A. Assessment
   1. Observation: If abuse is suspected, enforce the need to do the physical examination in private. Do a full body examination.
      a. Forensic exams need thorough documentation of injuries.
         i. Use color photographs before any treatment is started.
         ii. Make at lease one full body photograph and a facial photograph.
         iii. Make close-up photographs of all injuries.
         iv. Use a ruler to identify/document the size of the injuries.
         v. Documentation on the back of the photographs should include the patient's name, date, photographer's name, as well as any witness to the examination. The photographer should also sign each photograph.
         vi. Use direct quotes of the victim's history.
   2. Blood pressure, pulse, and respirations.
   3. General observation: Observe for depression, withdrawn, flat affect, fearfulness, poor eye contact, and inappropriate dress.
   4. Observe for poor hygiene, presence of urine and feces, matted or lice-infected hair, odors, dirty nails and skin, and soiled clothing.
   5. Assess cognitive abilities, depression, and functional ability of ADLs and IADLs.

B. Inspect
   1. Dermal examination for signs of burns, tears, lacerations, impression marks, and bruises in different stages of healing. Frequent areas of the body involved are the neck, arms, and/or legs. Evaluate for the presence of decubitus/pressure ulcers. Signs of dehydration include dry fragile skin, dry sore mouth, and mental confusion.
   2. Oral examination for poor oral hygiene, absence of dentures, and dry mucus membranes.
   3. Evaluate breasts and genitals for lacerations, and hematomas of the vagina or labia.

C. Auscultate
   1. Auscultate all lung fields.
   2. Auscultate bowel sounds in all four quadrants of the abdomen.

D. Palpate: Evaluate for dislocation, fractures, sprains, and contusions to the wrists, forearms, and shoulders.

E. Percuss: Abdomen and chest (if indicated).

F. Genital/rectal examination:
   1. Evaluate genitals/anal for redness, swelling, bruising, hematomas, abrasions, or lacerations.

2. Evaluate for evidence of sperm.
3. Evaluate for the presence of foreign bodies.

Diagnostic Tests

A. Diagnostic tests and X-rays are ordered dependent on the type of presenting complaints.
B. Obtain a CT for evaluation of injuries to the head and assault to the face, neck, or head. A CT or Doppler may be ordered for abdominal injuries.
C. Laboratory testing to evaluate dehydration, malnutrition, electrolyte imbalance, and medication/substance abuse:
   1. CBC
   2. Chemistry-7
   3. Urinalysis
   4. Calcium, magnesium, and phosphorus
   5. Drug/alcohol screen
   6. Serum levels for relevant medications
D. Obtain DNA samples if sexual abuse is present.

Differential Diagnoses

A. Elder abuse
B. Depression
C. Abdominal trauma
D. Sexual assault
E. Gait disturbance/fall
F. Pathologi fracture
G. Epidural/subdural hematoma

Plan

A. Provide a safe environment.
B. Clearly document the history, physical findings, and interventions.
C. Determine the perpetrator(s).
D. Evaluate the need for emergency room/hospital admission.

Patient Teaching

A. Reinforce that abuse/neglect are not the victim's fault. Elderly abuse is very common and they do not deserve to be abused.
B. Help is available.

Pharmaceutical Therapy

A. Prescriptions are related to physical injuries.
B. Treatment for sexually transmitted infections in the oral-anal-genital areas.

Follow-up

A. Develop a follow-up plan. All states have legislation protecting against abuse, neglect, and exploitation of the older population.
B. Know if your state has mandatory requirements to report any suspect of elder mistreatment.
C. Abuse of a disabled person must be reported to the Disabled Person Protection Commission.
D. Know if your state has additional regulations related to self-neglect. Contact adult protective services or law enforcement agencies.
E. At the present time, there is no recommendation for universal screening of all older adult patients except in nursing facilities.

Consultation/Referral

A. Social work consultation to coordinate an in-home geriatric assessment visit.
B. Facilitate referrals to a shelter, counseling, and legal services.
C. Contact a Sexual Assault Nurse Examiner (SANE) qualified health care provider if indicated.
D. Refer to the community Area Agency on Agency for assistance.
E. Refer for a psychiatric consultation if indicated.
F. Refer for a neurologic or neurosurgical consultation for intracranial injuries or focal neurologic findings.
G. Refer for an orthopedic consultation for fractures.

Resources

American Association of Retired Persons (AARP): http://www.aarp.org
Clearinghouse on Abuse and Neglect of the Elderly (CANE): 302-831-3525.
National Adult Protective Services Administrators (NAPSA): 720-565-0906.
National Association of State Units on Aging: NCEA@nasua.org
National Center on Elder Abuse (NCEA): http://www.elderabuse-center.org

INTIMATE PARTNER VIOLENCE (IPV)
by Cheryl A. Glass

Definition

A. Intimate partner violence (IPV) is defined as intentional controlling or the victimization of a person with whom the abuser has or is currently in an intimate, romantic, or spousal relationship. Domestic-IPV violence crosses all cultures and economic boundaries; encompasses violence between both genders, including gay and lesbian relationships. Elderly abuse is also a significant problem. Abusive behaviors can occur in a single event, sporadically, or be continual.
B. Physical abuse, sexual assault, social isolation, emotional abuse, economic control, and deprivation are associated with intimate partner violence. There is no typical abuser, although they tend to be violent in the home setting and their behavior at work is normal.
C. Forms of physical violence include assault with weapons, pushing, shoving, slapping, punching, choking, kicking, holding, and binding. Psychological abuse includes threats of physical harm to the victim or others, humiliations, intimidation, degradation, ridicule, and false accusations. Cyber stalking is psychological abuse via the Internet.
D. Intimate partner stalking occurs during a relationship or after the relationship ends. Sexual abuse is nonconsensual or painful sexual acts.

Incidence

The exact incidence of intimate partner violence is unknown due to the lack of reporting. The most significant reason for missing the diagnosis of intimate partner violence is failure to ask the patient.

A. An estimated 81% of women stalked by an intimate partner also suffer physical assault.
B. An estimated 4%–15% women presenting in emergency rooms have situations related to domestic violence.
C. Women that separate have a risk of violence approximately three times more than divorced women.

D. Up to 75% of domestic assaults occur after separation; women are most likely to be murdered when reporting abuse or attempting to leave an abusive relationship.

E. Stalking by an intimate partner is estimated at 1 million women and 317,000 men per year.

F. Pregnancy has an increased incidence of violence.
1. One in five young women and 35% of women have experienced pregnancy coercion.
2. 53% of young women have experienced birth control sabotage.
3. It is estimated 5%–20% of intimate partner abuse occurs against pregnant women.

G. Sexual violence, rape, physical assault, or stalking by an intimate partner occurs in 11% of lesbians and in 15% of men with male partners.

H. Among college women, 20%–30% report violence during a date.

Pathogenesis

Intrapartner violence is not associated with an underlying medical condition. The cycle of abuse has three phases:

A. Tension building: the victim tries to avoid violence and is described as "walking on eggs," unsure what will trigger an abusive incident.

B. Explosion and acute battering.

C. "Honeymoon phase," noted for the absence of tension and reconciliation.

Predisposing Factors

A. Gender: Females are predominately the victim.

B. Race: African American, American Indians, Hispanic women, and Alaskan Natives.

C. Higher incidence in interracial couples

D. Pregnancy

E. History of violence
1. Family domestic violence
2. Abuse as a child: 50% report abuse as an adult

F. History of drug use

G. Posttraumatic stress disorder

H. Lack of social support systems

I. Impulse control disorders

J. Poor economic status

Common Complaints

A. Vague complaints

B. Sexual problems

C. Depression

D. Chronic pain inconsistent with organic disease

E. Chronic headaches/migraines

F. Stress
1. Anxiety
2. Panic attacks

G. Alcohol or drug abuse (the batterer, victim, or both)

H. Current or past self-mutilation

I. Gynecologic and obstetric complaints
1. Dyspareunia
2. Frequent vaginal or urinary tract infections
3. Pelvic pain/infection
4. Recurrent sexually transmitted infections
5. Unintended pregnancy
6. Late prenatal care
7. Miscarriage
8. Preterm bleeding/delivery

J. Complaints of falls and other recurrent accidents

K. Eating disorders

L. Gastrointestinal or musculoskeletal complaints

Other Signs and Symptoms

A. Multiple prior visits to the emergency room for traumatic and nontraumatic complaints.

B. A delay between injury and office visits (may result from lack of transportation or the inability to leave the house).

C. Noncompliance with the treatment or missed appointments (lack of access to money or telephones).

D. Suicide attempt (25% higher in women with intimate partner violence).

E. The partner accompanies the patient at all visits.

Subjective Data

A. The batterer often refuses to leave the patient alone and may answer questions for the patient. Translators should not be a member of the patient's or suspected abuser's family.

B. Use direct questions: women-validated Partner Violence Screen (PVS)
1. Have you been hit, punched, kicked, or otherwise hurt by someone in the past year? If yes, by whom and were you injured?
2. Do you feel safe in your current relationship?
3. Is a partner from a previous relationship making you feel unsafe now?
4. Are you here today due to injuries from a partner?
5. Are you here today because of illness or stress related to threats, violent behavior, or fears due to a partner?

C. Assess if the patient has ever told family or friends, called hotlines, or attempted to leave the abuser.

D. Has the patient sought help with law enforcement or legal help, that is, filing a criminal complaint or getting an order of protection?

E. Are there any weapons in the home?
1. Has the abuser ever threatened or tried to kill you?
2. Are you thinking of suicide? Have you ever considered or attempted to commit suicide because of problems in your relationship?
3. Have you ever considered or attempted killing your batterer?
4. Do you have a plan?

Physical Examination

A. Enforce the need to interview and do physical examinations in private. Do a full body examination, including the head/scalp.
1. Most injuries are to the central (breast, chest, and abdomen) area, easily concealed by clothing.
2. Other frequent sites of injury include the head, face, throat, and genitals.
3. Explain the physical examination and touch with permission.
4. Forensic exams need thorough documentation of injuries.
   a. Use color photographs before any treatment is started.

    b. Photograph damaged clothing.

    c. Make at least one full body photograph and a facial photograph.

    d. Make close-up photographs of all injuries.

    e. Use a ruler to identify/document the size of injuries.

    f. Documentation on the back of the photographs should include the patient's name, date, photographer's name, as well as any witnesses to the examination. The photographer should also sign each photograph.

    g. Use direct quotes of the patient's history of the violence.

B. Blood pressure, pulse, and respirations.

C. General observation: Observe for depression/withdrawn, flat affect, anxiousness, fearful, evasive, poor eye contact, and wearing heavy makeup or clothing to conceal signs of abuse. Evaluate voice changes: dysphonia and aphonia. Observe for difficulty breathing.

D. Inspect

    1. Dermal exam for the presence of cigarette burns, impression marks, rope burns, welts, abrasions, scratch marks, claw marks, bite marks, ligature marks, petechiae, and contusions at multiple sites (e.g., back, legs, buttocks).

    2. Eye exam

        a. Observe subconjunctival hemorrhages from strangulation/struggle.

        b. Perform a funduscopic examination (if indicated secondary to trauma).

    3. Evaluate the genitals for lacerations and hematomas of the vagina or labia.

E. Auscultate

    1. Auscultate all lung fields.

    2. Auscultate the bowel sounds in all four quadrants of the abdomen.

F. Palpate

    1. Evaluate skull/facial trauma to the maxillofacial area, eye orbits, mandible, and nasal bones. Facial injuries are reported in 94% of victims.

    2. Evaluate for dislocations, fractures, sprains, and contusions to the wrists and forearms, and shoulders.

G. Percuss: Abdomen, chest, and areas of injury (if indicated secondary to trauma).

H. Neurological examination (if indicated secondary to trauma).

I. Genital/rectal examination:

    1. Evaluate genitals/anal for redness, swelling, bruising, hematomas, abrasions, or lacerations.

    2. Bimanual examination (females).

    3. Anoscopy (if indicated).

    4. Evaluate for evidence of sperm (recto/vaginal).

    5. Evaluate for the presence of condyloma (perineum, rectum, vagina).

    6. Evaluate for the presence of foreign bodies (recto/vaginal).

Diagnostic Tests

Diagnostic tests and X-rays are ordered dependent on the type of presenting complaints and physical examination.

A. Administer a domestic violence tool and have the victim mark a body map of injuries.

B. CBC with differential and peripheral smear, bleeding evaluation, including PT/PTT, ALT and AST to evaluate injury to the liver, serum amylase or lipase to rule out pancreatic injury.

C. Urinalysis.

D. Drug/toxicology screen (urine and blood).

E. Obtain forensic DNA samples from the skin, under nails, vagina, rectum, and saliva from bite marks using sterile cotton-tipped applicators that have been moistened with sterile saline. These should be sent to a crime laboratory as soon as possible.

F. Test for sexually transmitted infections/HIV.

G. Pregnancy test (if indicated).

H. Radiographs: facial injury, anteroposterior (AP) and lateral radiograph for any areas of bone tenderness, swelling, deformity, or limited range of motion.

I. Ultrasounds as indicated.

J. Neuroimaging CT/MRI for any suspected nonaccidental head injury (i.e., head trauma, or scalp hematoma.

Differential Diagnoses

A. Domestic violence

    1. Intimate partner abuse

    2. Elder abuse

    3. Child abuse

B. Rape

C. Other: related to presenting symptoms

Plan

A. Provide a safe environment. Assess for immediate danger.

B. Clearly document the history, physical findings, and interventions.

C. Determine the risk to the victim and any children.

D. Evaluate the need for emergency room/hospital admission.

E. Battery is a crime; assess the victim's readiness for police intervention and need for a court order of protection.

F. Help develop a safety plan.

G. Assess readiness to leave: collection of important papers (e.g., birth certificates, custody papers, divorce papers, and legal agreements, address book, copies of restraining orders), access to money/credit cards, and telling family and friends.

H. Provide contact numbers for shelters. Have the patient hide information in her shoes.

I. Counsel that violence may escalate.

Patient Teaching

A. Reinforce that the violence is not the victim's fault. Intimate partner violence is very common and the victims do not deserve to be abused. Discuss the cycle of abuse.

B. Violence increases in frequency and severity.

C. Help is available.

Pharmaceutical Therapy

A. Prescriptions are related to physical injuries.

B. Treatment for sexually transmitted infections in the oral-anal-genital areas.

C. Tranquilizers may impair the victim's ability to flee or defend herself and should not be prescribed.

ABUSE ASSESSMENT SCREEN

1) Have you ever been emotionally or physically abused by your partner or someone important to you?

Yes ☐   No ☐

If yes by whom? _____

Total number of times _____

2) Within the last year, have you been hit, slapped, kicked or otherwise physically hurt by someone?

Yes ☐   No ☐

If yes by whom? _____

Total number of times _____

3) Since you've been pregnant, have you been hit, slapped, kicked or otherwise physically hurt by someone?

Yes ☐   No ☐

If yes by whom? _____

Total number of times _____

4) Within the last year, has anyone forced you to have sexual activities?

Yes ☐   No ☐

If yes by whom? _____

Total number of times _____

5) Are you afraid of your partner or anyone you listed above?

Yes ☐   No ☐

MARK THE AREA OF INJURY ON A BODY MAP AND SCORE EACH INCIDENT ACCORDING TO THE FOLLOWING SCALE

If any of the descriptions for the higher number apply, use the higher number

1 = Threats of abuse including use of a weapon

2 = Slapping, pushing; no injury and/or lasting pain

3 = Punching, kicking, bruises, cuts, and/or continuing pain

4 = Beating up, severe contusions, burns, broken bones

5 = Head injury, internal injury, permanent injury

6 = Use of weapon; wound from weapon

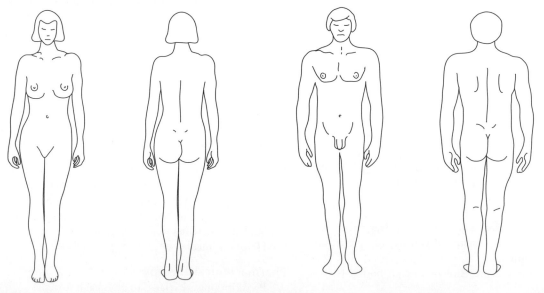

Figure 20.1 Reprinted with permission from The Family Violence Prevention Fund, 383 Rhode Island St., Ste. 304, San Francisco, CA 94103-5133. (415) 252-8900, TTY: (800) 595–4889. HYPERLINK "http://www.endabuse.org" www.endabuse.org.

Follow-up

A. Develop a follow-up plan
  1. What type of help does the patient want?
  2. Does she have a plan for returning; is the batterer home; does she think it is safe?
  3. Does she have a place to stay with family or friends; or does she want to go to a shelter?
  4. Give the telephone numbers for shelters and crises hotlines.
B. Screen the patient for abuse at all subsequent visits.
C. Mandatory reporting
  1. States require reporting when domestic violence involves a child if the child is under the age of 18 and abuse or neglect of the child is suspected.
  2. Abuse of a disabled person must be reported to the Disabled Persons Protection Commission.
  3. Elder abuse reporting may be mandatory in your state.
D. Your state may mandate reporting and intervention with law enforcement. Refer to the Domestic Violence and Sexual Assault Data Resource Center.

Consultation/Referral

A. Facilitate referrals to a shelter, counseling, and legal services.
B. Contact a Sexual Assault Nurse Examiner (SANE) qualified health care provider if indicated.
C. Refer to community or private support groups and agencies.
D. Refer for a consultation with a psychiatrist if the victim is homicidal or suicidal.
E. Refer for a neurological or neurosurgical consultation for intracranial injuries or focal neurological findings.
F. Refer for an orthopedic consultation for fractures.

Individual Considerations

A. Pregnancy is a known period of increased risk of violence.
  1. The genitals, breast, and abdomen are common sites targeted for trauma.
  2. Women may present with a miscarriage or premature labor.
  3. Blunt trauma is a common injury in pregnancy.
  4. Perform universal screening at each trimester since abuse often begins during pregnancy.

Resources

Domestic Violence and Sexual Assault Data Resource Center: http://www.jrsainfo.org/dvsa-drc/state-summaries.shtml
Family Violence Prevention Fund: http://www.endabuse.org/
National Domestic Violence Hotline: 1-800-799-7233

REFERENCES

Administration on Aging (AoA), U.S. Department of Health and Human Services. (2009). *A profile of older Americans: 2009.* Retrieved February 11, 2010, from http://www.aoa.gov/AoARoot/Aging_Statistics/Profile/2009/docs/2009profile_508.pdf

Ahrens, B., & Linden, M. (1996). Is there a suicidality syndrome independent of specific major psychiatric disorder? Results of a split half multiple regression analysis. *Acta Psychiatrica Scandinavia, 94,* 79–86.

American Academy of Bereavement Facilitator Program Syllabus. (1996, April 29–May 3). Tucson, AZ: Carondelet Health Care Corp.

American Academy of Pediatrics Resource Toolkit for Clinicians. Retrieved March 30, 2010, from http://www.uthsc.edu/pediatrics/general/clinical/behavior/aap_nichq_adhd_toolkit/01ADHDIntroduction.pdf

American College of Obstetricians and Gynecologists. (1997, September). Smoking and women's health. *ACOG Educational Bulletin,* Number 240. Washington, DC: Author.

American Psychiatric Association. (1994). *Diagnostic and statistical manual of mental disorders* (4th ed.). Washington, DC: Author.

Ancoli-Israel, S., Benca, R. M., Edinger, J. D., Krystal, A. D., Mendelson, W., Moldofsky, H., et al. (2004). Panel discussion: Changing how we think about insomnia. *Journal of Clinical Psychiatry, 68* (Suppl. 8), 44–46.

Avery, M. E., & First, L. R. (1994). *Pediatric medicine* (2nd ed.). Baltimore: Williams & Wilkins.

Beck, A. T., Guth, D., Steer, R. A., & Ball, R. (1997). Screening for major depression disorders in medical inpatients with the Beck Depression Inventory for Primary Care. *Behavior Research & Therapy, 35,* 785–791.

Bhattacharya, S. K., Satyan, K. S., & Chakrabarti, A. (1997). Anxiogenic action of caffeine: An experimental study in rats. *Journal of Psychopharmacology, 11,* 219–224.

Bonnet, M. H., & Arand, D. L. (1996). The consequences of a week of insomnia. *Sleep, 19,* 453–461.

Brown, G. K., Beck, A. T., Newman, C. F., Beck, J. S., & Tran, G. Q. (1997). A comparison of focused and standard cognitive therapy for panic disorder. *Journal of Anxiety Disorders, 11,* 29–45.

Brown, K., Streubert, G. E., & Burgess, A. W. (2004). Effectively detect and manage elder abuse. *The Nurse Practitioner, 29,* 22–31.

Burnett, L. B., & Adler, J. (2009, August 18). Domestic violence. *emedicine.* Retrieved January 21, 2010, from http://emedicine.medscape.com/article/805546-print

Burns, C., Brady, M., & Starr, N., Blosser, C., Dunn, A. (2004). *Pediatric primary care: A handbook for nurse practitioners* (3rd ed.). St. Louis, MO: Saunders.

Canuso, B. A. (1997). Rethinking behavior disorders: Whose attention has a deficit? *Journal of Psychosocial Nursing, 35,* 24–29.

Castiglia, P. T. (1997). Attention deficit/hyperactivity disorder. *Journal of Pediatric Health Care, 11,* 130–133.

Charlton, R., & Dolman, E. (1995). Bereavement: A protocol for primary care. *British Journal of General Practice, 45,* 427–430.

Crawford, V., Crome, I., & Clancy, C. (2003). Co-existing problems of mental health and substance misuse (dual diagnosis): A literature review. *Drugs, education, prevention and policy, 10,* S1–S74. Retrieved from EBSCOhost Database.

Dadds, M. R., Spence, S. H., Holland, D. E., Barrett, P. M., & Laurens, K. R. (1997). Prevention and early intervention for anxiety disorders: A controlled trial. *Journal of Consulting and Clinical Psychology, 65*(4), 627–635.

Dodge, R., Cline, M. G., & Quart, S. F. (1995). The natural history of insomnia and its relationship to respiratory symptoms. *Archives of Internal Medicine, 55,* 1797–1800.

Dunphy, L., Brown, J., Porter, B., & Thomas, D. (2007). *Primary care: The art and science of advanced practice nursing* (2nd ed.). Philadelphia: F. A. Davis.

Egan, M. P., Rivera, S. G., Robillard, B. R., & Hanson, A. (1997). The "no suicide contract": Helpful or harmful? *Journal of Psychosocial Nursing and Mental Health Services, 35,* 31–33.

Endom, E. E. (2009a, February 10). Physical abuse in children: Epidemiology and clinical manifestations. *UpToDate.* Retrieved February 21, 2010, from http://www.uptodate.com/online/content/topic.do?topicKey=peds_soc/5402&view=print

Endom, E. E. (2009b, October 1). Physical abuse in children: Diagnostic evaluation and management. *UpToDate.* Retrieved February 21, 2010, from http://www.uptodate.com/online/content/topic.do?topicKey=peds_soc/2124&view=print

Flint, A. J., & Rifat, S. L. (1997). Effect of demographic and clinical variables on time to antidepressant response in geriatric depression. *Depression and Anxiety, 5,* 103–107.

Foley, D. J., Monjan, A. A., Brown, S. L., Simonsick, E. M., Wallace, R. B., & Blazer, D. G. (1995). Sleep complaints among elderly persons: An epidemiologic study of three communities. *Sleep, 18,* 425–432.

Giardino, A. P., & Giardino, E. R. (2008, December). Child abuse and neglect, physical abuse. *emedicine*. Retrieved January 21, 2010, from http://emedicine.medscape.com/article/915664-print

Glass, B. C. (1993). The role of the nurse in advanced practice in bereavement care. *Clinical Nurse Specialist, 7,* 62–66.

Gold, M. S. (1993). *Drugs of abuse: A comprehensive series for clinicians.* New York: Plenum Press.

Halphen, J. M., & Dyer, C. B. (2009, August 7). Elder mistreatment: Abuse, neglect, and financial exploitation. *UpToDate*. Retrieved January 21, 2010, from http://www.uptodate.com/online/content/topic.do?topicKey=geri_med/2855&view=print

Hirschfield, R. M., & Russell, J. M. (1997). Assessment and treatment of suicidal patients. *New England Journal of Medicine, 337,* 910–915.

Hughes, D. H. (1995). Can the clinician predict suicide? *Psychiatric Services, 46,* 449–451.

Ilse, S. (1996). *Empty arms: Coping with miscarriage, stillbirth, and infant death.* Maple Plain, MN: Wintergreen Press.

Ilse, S., & Burns, L. H. (1989). *Miscarriage: A shattered dream.* Maple Plain, MN: Wintergreen Press.

Johnston, M., & Walker, M. (1996). Suicide in the elderly: Recognizing the signs. *General Hospital Psychiatry, 18,* 257–260.

Juergens, T. M., & Barczi, S. R. (2007). Sleep. In E. H. Duthie & P. R. Katz (Eds.), *Practice of geriatrics* (3rd ed., Chap. 22, pp. 271–284) Philadelphia, PA: Saunders Elsevier.

Kassel, J. D., & Shiffman, S. (1997). Attentional mediation of cigarette smoking's effect on anxiety. *Health Psychology, 16,* 359–368.

Kirchner, C. G., Davis, S. J., & Jackson, J. A. (Eds.). (1996). *Physician's current procedural terminology: CPT 97.* Chicago: American Medical Association.

La Via, M. F., Munno, L., Lydiard, R. B., et al. (1996). The influence of stress intrusion on immunodepression in generalized anxiety disorder patients and controls. *Psychosomatic Medicine, 58,* 138–142.

Lecrubier, Y., Bourin, M., Moon, C. A., et al. (1997). Efficacy of venlafaxine in depressive illness in general practice. *Acta Psychiatr Scand, 95,* 485–493.

Levenson, J. L. (1994). Psychiatric aspects of medical practice. In A. Stoudemire (Ed.), *Clinical psychiatry for medical students* (pp. 580–600). Philadelphia: Lippincott.

Ludwikowski, K., & DeValk, M. (1998). Attention-deficit hyperactivity disorder: The psychostimulants and beyond. *Advance for Nurse Practitioners, 6,* 55–60.

Lyons-Ruth, K., Easterbrooks, M. A., & Cibelli, C. D. (1997). Infant attachment strategies, infant mental lag, and maternal depressive symptoms: Predictors of internalizing and externalizing problems at age 7. *Developmental Psychology, 33,* 681–692.

MacLeod, A. K., Pakhania, B., Lee, M., & Mitchell, D. (1997). Parasuicide, depression and the anticipation of positive and negative future experiences. *Psychological Medicine, 27,* 973–977.

Mahoney, B., Schwaitzberg, S. D., & Newton, E. R. (2010, January 2). Trauma and pregnancy. *emedicine*. Retrieved January 21, 2010, from http://emedicine.medscape.com/article/435224-print

Manber, R., & Bootzin, R. R. (1997). Sleep and the menstrual cycle. *Health Psychology, 16,* 209–214.

Mathies, R. W. (1997). How to spot depressed patients in your practice. *Postgraduate Medicine, 102,* 219–223.

Merikangas, K. R. (1990). The genetic epidemiology of alcoholism. *Psychological Medicine, 20,* 11–22.

Miller, E., Decker, M. R., McCauley, H. L., Tancredi, D. J., Levenson, R. R., Waldman, J., et al. (2010). Pregnancy coercion, intimate partner violence and unintended pregnancy. *Contraception, 81,* 316–322. Retrieved February 7, 2010, from http://www.sciencedirect.com.proxy.library.vanderbilt.edu/.

National Committee for the Prevention of Elder Abuse (NCPEA). (n.d.). Elder abuse. Retrieved February 12, 2010, from http://www.ncea.aoa.gov/ncearoot/Main_Site/index.aspx

National Institute on Drug Abuse. (2010). *NIDA InfoFacts: Methamphetamine.* National Institute of Health. Retrieved March 19, 2010, from www.drugabuse.gov

Neinstin, L. S. (1996). *Adolescent health care: A practical guide* (3rd ed.). Baltimore: Williams & Wilkins.

NICHQ Vanderbilt Assessment Scale-PARENT Informant. Retrieved March 30, 2010, from http://www.kidzdoc.com/uploads/files/vanderbilt-assessment-parent.pdf

NICHQ Vanderbilt Assessment Scale-TEACHER Informant. Retrieved March 30, 2010, from http://www.pedialliance.com/forms/ADHD_Teacher_Assessment42.pdf

NICHQ Vanderbilt Assessment Follow-up-TEACHER Informant. Retrieved March 30, 2010, from http://www.pedialliance.com/forms/ADHD_Teacher_Follow_Up_Form44.pdf

Persons, R. K., & Nichols, W. (2007). Should we use appetite stimulants for malnourished elderly patients? *Journal of Family Practice, 56,* 761–762.

Prevent Child Abuse America. (n.d.). *Fact sheet: Emotional child abuse.* Retrieved February 25, 2010, from http://member.preventchildabuse.org/site/DocServer/emotional_child_abuse.pdf?docID=122

Prevent Child Abuse America. (n.d.). *Fact sheet: Maltreatment of children with disabilities.* Retrieved February 25, 2010, from http://member.preventchildabuse.org/site/DocServer/maltreatment.pdf?docID=124

Prevent Child Abuse America. (n.d.). *Fact sheet: Sexual abuse of boys.* Retrieved February 25, 2010, from http://member.preventchildabuse.org/site/DocServer/sexual_abuse_of_boys.pdf?docID=127

Prevent Child Abuse America. (n.d.). *Fact sheet: Sexual abuse of children.* Retrieved February 25, 2010, from http://member.preventchildabuse.org/site/DocServer/sexual_abuse.pdf?docID=126

Prevent Child Abuse America. (n.d.). *Fact sheet: The relationship between parental alcohol or other drug problems and child maltreatment.* Retrieved February 25, 2010, from http://member.preventchildabuse.org/site/DocServer/parental_alcohol.pdf?docID=125

Prevent Child Abuse America. (n.d). *Recognizing child abuse: What parents should know.* Retrieved February 25, 2010, from http://www.preventchildabuse.org/publications/All_of_Us/downloads/recognizing_abuse.pdf

Reed, M. D. (1993). Sudden death and bereavement outcomes: The impact of resources on grief symptomatology and detachment. *Suicide and Life-Threatening Behavior, 23,* 204–220.

Reynolds, C. F., III. (1997). Treatment of major depression in later life: A life cycle perspective. *Psychiatric Quarterly, 68,* 221–246.

Robertson, R., & Montagnini, M. (2004). Geriatric failure to thrive. *American Family Physician.* Retrieved March 9, 2010, from www.aafp.org

Romney, D. M., & Bynner, J. M. (1997). A re-examination of the relationship between shyness, attributional style, and depression. *Journal of Genetic Psychology, 158,* 261–270.

Ross, R., Roller, C., & Rusk, T., et al. (2009). The SATELLITE sexual violence assessment and care guide for perinatal patients. *Women's Health Care: A Practical Journal for Nurse Practitioners, 8,* 25–31.

Roy, A. (1994). Recent biologic studies on suicide. *Suicide and Life-Threatening Behavior, 24,* 10–14.

Samuels, S. C. (1997). Midlife crisis: Helping patients cope with stress, anxiety, and depression. *Geriatrics, 52,* 5–63.

Schmidt, B. D. (1992). *Instructions for pediatric patients.* Philadelphia: Saunders.

Scoring Instructions for the NICHQ Vanderbilt Assessment Scales. Retrieved March 30, 2010, from http://www.uthsc.edu/pediatrics/general/clinical/behavior/aap_nichq_adhd_toolkit/07ScoringInstructions.pdf

Sellas, M. I., & Krouse, L. H. (2009, April 20). Elder abuse. *emedicine.* Retrieved January 21, 2010, from http://emedicine.medscape.com/article/805727-print

Shaffer, D., Fisher, P., Hicks, R. H., Parides, M., & Gould, M. (1995). Sexual orientation in adolescents who commit suicide. *Suicide and Life-Threatening Behavior, 25,* S64–S71.

Shneidman, E. S. (1994). Clues to suicide, reconsidered. *Suicide and Life-Threatening Behavior, 24,* 395–397.

Sillman, J. S. (2009, August 25). Diagnosing, screening, and counseling for domestic violence. *UpToDate.* Retrieved January 21, 2010, from http://www.uptodate.com/online/content/topic.do?topicKey=genr_med/9023&view=print

Silverman, M. M., & Marls, R. W. (1995). The prevention of suicidal behaviors: An overview. *Suicide and Life-Threatening Behavior, 25,* 10–21.

Solari-Twadell, P. A., Bunkers, S. S., Wang, C. E., et al. (1995). The pinwheel model of bereavement. *Image, Journal of Nursing Scholarship, 27,* 323–326.

Spangler, D. L., Simons, A. D., Monroe, S. M., et al. (1997). Response to cognitive-behavioral therapy in depression: Effects of pretreatment cognitive dysfunction and life stress. *Journal of Consulting & Clinical Psychology, 65,* 568–575.

Sramek, J. J., Frackiewicz, E. J., & Cutler, N. R. (1997). Efficacy and safety of two dosing regimens of buspirone in the treatment of outpatients with persistent anxiety. *Clinical Therapeutics, 19,* 498–506.

Stahl, S. M. (1996). *Essential psychopharmacology: Neuroscientific basis and practical applications.* New York: Cambridge Press.

Steward, S. H., Taylor, S., & Baker. J. M. (1997). Gender differences in dimensions of anxiety sensitivity. *Journal of Anxiety Disorders, 11,* 179–200.

Stoudemire, A. (1994). *Clinical psychiatry for medical students* (2nd ed.). Philadelphia: Lippincott.

Suicide Awareness Voices of Education (SAVE). (2003). *Suicide facts* Retrieved March 15, 2010, from. www.save.org

Szanto, K., Prigerson, H., Houck, P., Ehrenphreis, L., & Reynolds, C. F. (1997). Suicidal ideation in elderly bereaved: The role of complicated grief. *Suicide and Life-Threatening Behavior, 27,* 194–207.

Taylor, M. A. (1997). Evaluation and management of attention-deficit hyperactivity disorder. *American Family Physician, 55,* 887–894, 897, 901.

Terpstra, T. L., & Terpstra, T. L. (1997). Treating geriatric depression with SSRIs: What primary care practitioners need to know. *The Nurse Practitioner, 22,* 18–123.

Thienhaus, O. J., & Pisecki, M. (1997). Assessment of suicide risk. *Psychiatric Services, 48,* 293–294.

Tomb, D. A. (1998). *Psychiatry for the house officer* (3rd ed.). Baltimore: Williams & Wilkins.

Tower, I. B., Kasl, S. V., & Moritz, D. J. (1997). The influence of spouse cognitive impairment on respondents' depressive symptoms: The moderating role of marital closeness. *Journals of Gerontology, Series B, Psychological Sciences & Social Sciences, 52,* 5270–5278.

Vessey, J. A. (1997). *The child with a learning disorder of ADHD: A manual for school nurses.* Scarborough, ME: National Association of School Nurses, Inc.

Waldinger, R. J. (1989). *Psychiatry Journal for Medical Students.* Washington, DC: American Psychiatric Press.

Walker, K. (1994). Depression. *Professional Nurse, 72,* 872–874.

Weinstein, C. (1994). Cognitive remediation strategies. *Journal of Psychotherapy Practice and Research, 3,* 44–57.

Wetter, D. W., & Young, T. B. (1994). The relation between cigarette smoking and sleep disturbance. *Preventive Medicine, 23,* 328–334.

Williams, G. B., Brackley, M. H., Hibler, T. R., & Prater, S. J. (2008). Screening for intimate partner violence. *Women's Health Care: A Practical Journal for Nurse Practitioners, 7,* 10–26.

Williams, S. A. (1997). Caring in patient-focused care: The relationship of patients' perceptions of holistic nurse caring to their levels of anxiety. *Holistic Nurse Practice, 11,* 61–68.

Woof, W. I., & Carter, Y. H. (1997). The grieving adult and the general practitioner: A literature review in two parts (part D). *British Journal of General Practice, 47,* 443–448.

Zoberi, K., & Pollard, A. (2010). Treating anxiety without SSRIs. *Journal of Family Practice, 59,* 148–154.

Procedures

BEDSIDE CYSTOMETRY *by Cheryl A. Glass*

Description

Bedside cystometry testing is an office procedure to determine bladder capacity, postvoid residual, any fluid leak with stress maneuvers, or inhibited bladder capacity. Urodynamic testing is still considered the gold standard test; however, the cystometry is a good and sensitive screening tool.

Indications

Patients presenting with complaints of urinary incontinence, stress incontinence (leaking), overactive bladder (OAB), and urinary retention (inability to empty bladder) are candidates for cystometry testing.

Precautions

A. A through history should be taken and physical examination.
B. Rule out the presence of a urinary tract infection as a cause of the incontinence prior to cystometry testing.
C. This is a sterile procedure, not to be done when infection or inflammation is present.

Equipment Required

A. Sterile straight catheter (12–14 French catheter)
B. Catheter insertion kit
C. 60 mL sterile syringe
D. 1,000 mL sterile water
E. Sterile measurement container
F. Urine collection device

Procedure

A. Explain the procedure.
B. Obtain consent (if required).
C. Have the patient bear down and/or cough to evaluate urinary incontinence.
D. Have patient void, measure the urine, and collect the specimen for urinalysis.
E. Catheterize using sterile technique.
   1. Measure urine drained from catheter inserted post-voiding; this amount is the "postvoid residual" (PVR).
      a. Normal: less than 100 mL PVR.
      b. Abnormal: more than 100 mL PVR.
      c. Differential diagnostic evaluation: Overflow Incontinence secondary to retention.
F. Attach the 60 cc syringe to the catheter.
   1. Observe if there was any difficulty passing the catheter.
      a. Normal findings: catheter passes with ease.
      b. Abnormal findings: catheter difficult or impossible to pass.
      c. Differential diagnostic evaluation: Overflow Incontinence possibly due to obstruction.

G. Using gravity, fill the bladder slowly through catheter/syringe with sterile water.
   1. Avoid instilling the sterile water too quickly, instill approximately 30 cc amounts at a time.
   2. Measure the amount of water instilled when the patient has the urge to void.
      a. Normal: bladder capacity usually at 300 mL when urge is sensed.
      b. Abnormal: urge at less than 200 mL.
      c. Differential diagnostic evaluation: Urge Incontinence due to small capacity.
   3. Continue to fill, noting if there is any fluctuation of the sterile water in the syringe during filling.
      a. Normal: contractions or fluctuation occurs around 200–250 mL from bladder into syringe (detrusor muscle contraction).
      b. Abnormal: fluid moving into the syringe.
      c. Differential diagnostic evaluation: Urge Incontinence related to bladder spasm.
   4. The instillation of sterile water should be stopped when the patient reports a full bladder.
   5. If the patient has not reported a full bladder prior to the instillation of 600 ccs, the test should be discontinued.
      a. Have patient cough, observe for leaking, clamp catheter.
      b. Normal: normal capacity 400 mL, no leaking with cough.
      c. Abnormal: urge prior to 400 mL, or leaking with pressure.
      d. Differential diagnostic evaluation: Urge Incontinence due to small capacity and/or Stress Incontinence due to leakage with pressure.
   6. Remove catheter after bladder is filled to capacity (strong urge to void); have the patient cough.
      a. Normal: no leakage.
      b. Abnormal: leakage of fluid.
      c. Differential diagnostic evaluation: Stress Incontinence associated with weak pelvic muscles.
   7. Have the patient void; measure output, compare with amount instilled.
      a. Normal: return with a maximum of 100 mL retained (PVR).
      b. Abnormal: greater than 100 mL retained after voiding.
      c. Differential diagnostic evaluation: Overflow Incontinence either from obstruction or an atonic bladder.
H. Discuss treatment options, including pharmaceutical therapy and/or consultation with an urologist.

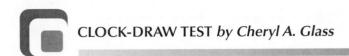

Description

The clock-draw test is a quick screening tool to assess cognitive dysfunction. The tool can be used by itself or as a complement to other screening tests. The clock-draw test is a component of the "7 Minute Neurocognitive Screening Battery." The clock-draw test can be administered repeatedly over time to evaluate deterioration of function.

The test evaluates:

A. Orientation
B. Conceptualization of time
C. Visual spatial organization
D. Visual memory
E. Auditory comprehension
F. Numeric knowledge
G. Concentration
H. Frustration tolerance

Indications

A. Evaluation of dementia
B. Evaluation of delirium
C. Evaluation of neurologic insult
 1. Head trauma
 2. Stroke
 3. Alcohol and drug
D. Evaluation of psychiatric illness
 1. Schizophrenia
 2. Psychotic state

Administering the Clock-Draw Test

There are a number of variations in administering the clock-draw test.

A. Provide the patient with the predrawn circle. See Figure.
B. This is not a timed test. There is no limitation to administration time; however, the test generally takes 1–2 min.
C. Ask the patient to put the numbers in the circle so that it looks like a clock.
D. Ask the patient to add arms to the clock indicating a denoted time such as "ten minutes after eleven."
 1. The time 11:10 has been suggested as useful because of the distraction of "pull" of the numeral 10 on the clock when setting time.
 2. Other variations include 3:00, 8:40, and 2:45.
E. The same time should be used for repeated testing for comparisons.
F. Document the date and time of each test.

Scoring

There are several variations on scoring the clock-draw test. The quickest scoring involves dividing the clock into four quadrants and counting the numbers in the correct quadrant. More complex assessment evaluates up to 20 traits or categorizes errors.

A. A completely normal clock suggests that multiple functions are intact and contributes to the assessment of the patient's ability to continue independently.
B. A grossly abnormal clock is an indicator of potential problems that require immediate attention.
C. The placement of the arms of the clock is the most abstract feature and is useful in evaluating the early dementing process.
D. **Simple scoring involves awarding 1 point for each of the following:**
 1. Approximate drawing of the clock face _____
 2. Presence of numbers in sequence _____
 3. Correct special arrangement of numbers _____
 4. Presence of clock hands _____
 5. Hand showing approximately the correct time _____
 6. Hand depicting the exact time _____
  a. Total Score: _____

Patient's Name: _____   Date: _____

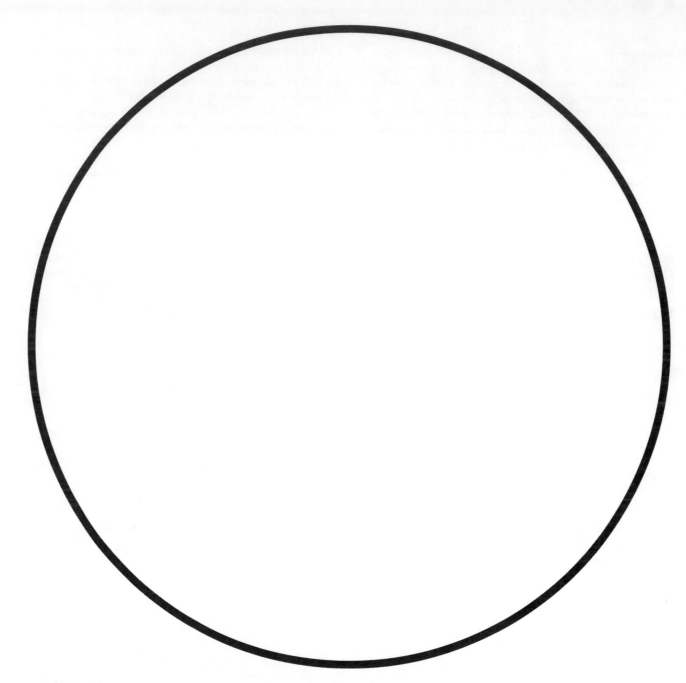

FIGURE Clock-draw test.
Used with permission from Dr. John Wells. http://www.neurosurvival.ca/ClinicalAssistant/scales/ClockDrawingTest.pdf.

Description

Vertigo that occurs with changing position and rapid head movement causes imbalance, disorientation, and nausea. Vertigo is generally benign and positional. Vertigo develops when there is a disturbance of the crystals that are normally evenly distributed in the fluid-filled ear canal and they become clumped together. Often the imbalance can be corrected by the Epley maneuver to redistribute the crystals in the inner ear.

Indications

A. Positional vertigo

Contraindications

A. Testing should never been done in the case of head injury or suspected or confirmed cervical spine injury.

Equipment Required

A. Examination table
B. Stool at the head of the table for the practitioner

Procedure

A. Explain the procedure. See Figure.
B. Have the patient sit on the examination table (Position 1).
   1. Reposition the patient to sitting in the center of the table.
   2. The edge at the head of the table should be at the patient's shoulder height (head will hang off the table).
   3. Your position will be at the head of the examination table, and you use the stool for comfort while holding the patient's head with your hands.
C. Rapidly lay the patient down (Position 2).
   1. The patient's head should be hanging over the table in a slightly downward tilt, supported by both of your hands.
   2. The patient should be instructed to keep his or her eyes open and try to focus on a stationary object on the wall throughout the positions on his or her back and sides.

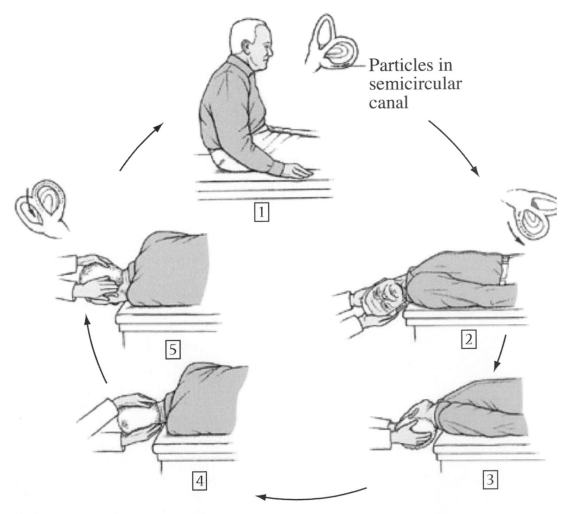

Particles in semicircular canal

FIGURE Epley procedure for vertigo.
Used with permission from *Merck Manual of Health and Aging*.

3. The patient's head is turned to the same side as the affected ear with the provider supporting the head.
   a. If the patient has vertigo affecting both inner ears, turn the patient's head to the dominantly affected side.
   b. As an alternative to just turning the head, the patient may quickly turn and lie down on the affected side while you support the head with both of your hands.
4. After a few minutes the patient will be ready to be repositioned evidenced by his or her lack of nystagmus (rhythmic side-to-side eye movement) and confirmation that the dizziness has stabilized.

D. Turn the patient's head in the opposite direction while you continue to support the head (Position 3). Again the head should be in a slightly downward tilt.
1. If the patient was using the side lying position, have him or her turn to his or her back.
2. Have the patient continue to keep the eyes open and focus on a stationary object on the wall.
3. Again the time lapse to repositioning is evidenced by the lack of nystagmus and subjective confirmation that the dizziness has stabilized/abated.

E. Ask the patient to roll from his or her back to the opposite side (or from the back to the opposition side) (Position 4). The patient's head should be parallel to the floor.
F. With the patient side lying (Position 5), have him or her quickly turn only his or her face to the floor, while you are supporting the head.
G. After the patient verbalized the dizziness has abated from the side lying Position 5
1. The patient is to swing the legs to the edge of the table and quickly sit up.
2. He or she will continue to feel vertigo at this point.
H. Assist the patient off the examination table.
I. The patient should be instructed to be in a sitting position or head no farther back than a 45-degree angle for the next 24 hours.
J. The Epley does not immediately stop the vertigo. The patient may begin to feel better within a few days.
K. If the Epley procedure needs to be repeated, allow 1 week between attempts.

EXPRESSED PROSTATIC SECRETIONS *by Cheryl A. Glass*

Description
A. Obtaining prostatic fluid by prostate massage using the Meares-Stamey 4-Glass urine test.

Indications
A. Expressed prostatic secretion is used to distinguish chronic prostatitis from acute prostatitis or urinary tract infection.

Precautions
A. Do not perform in patients with acute prostatitis (swollen, tender, boggy prostate); may cause septicemia.

Equipment Required
A. Sterile culture specimen cups (4)
B. Labels (4) marked:
    1. Voided bladder 1 (VB$_1$)
    2. VB$_2$
    3. Expressed prostatic secretion (EPS)
    4. VB$_3$
C. Gauze pads or soap sponges (3)

Procedure
A. Patient should retract the foreskin (if applies) and cleanse the glans penis with the 3 soap sponges.
B. Collect first 2 urine specimens without completely emptying the bladder.
    1. VB$_1$ is the first 10 mL of urine.
    2. VB$_2$ is the mainstream urine; again the patient should not empty his bladder. See Table, "Obtaining Prostatic Secretion Specimens."
C. While the patient maintains the foreskin retraction with one hand, prostatic massage is performed with gentle digital pressure moving from the lateral margin of the superior portion of a selected lobe of the prostate toward the apex. Perform the massage for approximately 1 min; longer massage may inhibit the fluid outflow.
D. Several drops of expressed prostatic secretion (EPS) should emerge from the urethra within 2–3 min after the massage is completed.
E. Collect the resulting prostatic fluid and the first 10 mL collected into cup number 3 labeled EPS.

TABLE Obtaining Prostatic Secretion Specimens

Labels for Container	Specimen	Location
VB$_1$	1st 10 mL of urine	Urine from urethra
VB$_2$	Midstream urine: obtain the first 200 mL of urine. *Do not empty bladder.*	Urine from bladder
EPS	Secretions from urethra after massage (may not have any secretions)	Prostatic fluid
VB$_3$	1st 10 mL of urine after massage	Prostate and bladder (100:1 dilution of urine: prostatic fluid)

TABLE Evaluation and Results of Prostatic Secretions

Diagnosis	Microscopic Evaluation	Treatment
Urethritis	WBC, bacteria in VB$_1$; in no other specimens	< 40 years, probably STI RX: Rocephin and doxycycline > 40 years, probably coliform bacteria RX: Bactrim/septra DS po bid × 5–7 days
Cystitis	WBC, RBC, bacteria in VB$_2$	Bactrim DS po bid × 5–7 days
Acute prostatitis	WBC, bacteria in VB$_2$ and/or EPS, VB$_3$	Bactrim DS po bid for 3–4 weeks Alternative: Quinolones: Cipro 500 mg bid for 3–4 weeks May need hospitalization for IV antibiotics
Chronic prostatitis	Bacteria in EPS and/or VB$_3$, but not in VB$_1$ or VB$_2$	Bactrim DS po bid *or* Cipro 500 mg bid for 3–4 months

Note. po = by mouth; bid = twice a day.

1. If no fluid is obtained, the patient is instructed to milk the penis, starting from the base and moving toward the tip of the penis.
2. Finally, if there is no fluid, the patient is told to void another 10 mL into the 3rd sterile container.

F. The last voided specimen is marked VB$_3$.

Treatment
A. See Table, "Evaluation and Results of Prostatic Screening."

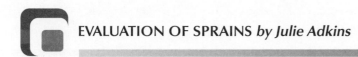

EVALUATION OF SPRAINS *by Julie Adkins*

McMurray Test for Knee Sprains
A. Explain the procedure.
B. Ask the patient to lie down on his or her back (supine).
C. The affected leg, R or L, should have hip flexed 60–70 degrees.
D. The injured knee is flexed 45 degrees.
E. Hold the foot in one hand and place the fingers of the other hand on the joint line.
F. Evaluate the patient's pain level when palpating the joint when the knee is flexed.
G. Apply valgus force by holding the femur steady and slowly move the lower leg laterally while still applying the valgus stress.
H. Then flex the knee to 135 degrees and switch to varus stress.
I. Finally, extend the knee in the varus position.
J. If the test is positive, a meniscus click or pop can be felt, which is characteristic of an anterior cruciate ligament tear or relocation.

Anterior Drawer Test for Evaluation of Lateral Ankle Sprain
A. Explain the procedure.
B. Perform this test on the uninjured ankle first, then repeat on the injured ankle.
C. Ask the patient to position the affected foot in the plantar flexion position (foot slightly at rest).
D. Grasp the lower portion of the uninjured leg for bracing. Use one hand at the shin and attempt to draw the heel anteriorly (forward) with your other hand.
E. Repeat the test on the injured ankle.
F. Anterior drawer test is positive for an ankle sprain if the talus at the injured point slides 4 mm or more than the same bone in the other joint.

Talar Tile Test for Evaluation of Lateral Ankle Sprain
A. Explain the procedure.
B. Perform this test on the uninjured ankle first, then repeat on the injured ankle.
C. To perform the talar test grasp the lower heel with one hand while adducting or inverting the foot with your other hand.
D. The test is positive if the tilt is 5–10 degrees greater around the injured joint.

Description

A. A hernia reduction may be done by a manual technique used for external replacement of the bowel (occasionally omentum) from the hernia back into the abdomen/groin.

Indications

A. Herniation of bowel contents occurs secondary to pregnancy, straining, hard physical labor, or congenital defect.

Precautions

A. **Do not try to reduce a strangulated hernia.** This can cause gangrenous bowel to enter the peritoneal cavity. Strangulation symptoms include tenderness, discoloration, edema, fever, and signs of bowel obstruction.

Equipment Required

A. Gown/drape for the patient
B. Nonsterile gloves

Procedure

A. After doing a complete assessment, explain the reduction procedure to the patient, discussing each step just before performing it.
B. Obtain consent if required by protocol.
C. Ask the patient to void.
D. Apply the gloves.
E. Have the patient lie supine with slight flexion of the hips to relax abdominal muscles.
F. Ask the patient to take deep, slow, relaxing breaths. Hernia reduction should cause minimal discomfort.
   1. *Males:* Gently invaginate the scrotal skin, and replace the herniated contents back through the external/internal inguinal or femoral rings.
   2. *Females:* Gently invaginate the herniated bowel contents back through the external/internal inguinal or femoral rings.
G. Hernias should be easily reducible. Do not force any contents back into the abdominal wall defect.
H. After the reduction, ask the patient to cough and strain to evaluate successful reduction prior to discharge.

Evaluation/Results of Procedure

A. Consult a physician if unable to reduce the hernia. Hernia may be strangulated.
B. Have the patient return in 1 week for reexamination.
C. Tell the patient not to strain with bowel movements, lift heavy objects, or exercise strenuously.
D. Review symptoms of obstruction or strangulation of entrapped bowel: pain, nausea, and vomiting. Warn the patient to seek immediate medical attention for strangulated bowel.
E. Recurrent hernias and congenital defects eventually require surgical repair. Hernias secondary to pregnancy may not require surgery.

INSERTING AN ORAL AIRWAY *by Cheryl A. Glass*

Description

An oropharyngeal airway is a semicircular device used to hold the tongue away from the posterior wall of the pharynx. To insert this device, the mouth and pharynx should first be cleared of secretions, blood, or vomit, using suction tip catheter (if available).

Indications

A. Oral airway insertion can be used to help control the airway, ventilate the patient, and provide oxygenation of the unconscious patient.

Precautions

A. If the patient is conscious, airway insertion may stimulate vomiting and laryngospasm.
B. If the airway is too long, it could press the epiglottis against the entrance of the larynx and produce a complete airway obstruction.
C. If the airway isn't inserted properly, it can push the tongue posteriorly and worsen an upper airway obstruction.
D. If the tongue and/or lips are between the teeth, trauma will result.

Equipment Required

A. An oropharyngeal airway
B. A tongue blade
C. A suction tip and canister (if available)

Procedure

A. Place head/neck in the correct position. See Figure.
B. The best way to insert an oral airway is to turn it backward (upside down) as it enters the mouth.
C. As the airway transverses the oral cavity and approaches the posterior wall of the pharynx, rotate it into proper position.
D. An alternate method is to move the tongue out of the way with a tongue blade before insertion of the airway.

Evaluation/Results of Procedure

A. The airway is in the proper position and of proper size when you hear clear breath sounds on auscultation of the lungs during ventilation.

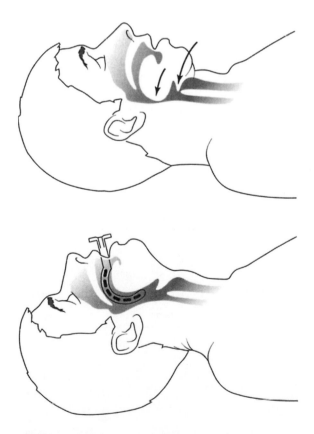

FIGURE Insertion of an oral airway.

Description

A. The bimanual examination is a digital evaluation of the cervix with the index and middle fingers of the examiner's hand.

Indications

To assess cervical dilation, effacement, presentation of the fetus, and position and station of fetal presenting part.

The cervix may be assigned a Bishop score to evaluate cervical change and to determine difficulty/ease with induction of labor. There is an inherent subjective difference between examiners; however, the Bishop score can be used to evaluate preterm labor cervical changes over time. See Table.

Precautions

A. **Bimanual exam should never be performed when there is suspicion of or history of documented placenta previa. Vaginal bleeding in second or third trimester pregnancy should be treated as placenta previa until this is ruled out.**

B. **Suspicion of ruptured membranes with preterm contractions: First perform sterile speculum exam to assess for rupture.** Then, if membranes are intact, proceed with bimanual exam.

C. If membranes are ruptured in the absence of active labor, avoid bimanual examination until frequent, painful uterine contractions are present.

Equipment Required

A. Gloves (nonsterile if membranes are intact; sterile if suspicion of or documented ruptured membranes)

B. Water-soluble lubricant (sterile lubricant required if ruptured membranes)

C. Examination table or bed

Procedure

A. Stand at the foot of the examination table or sit near the foot of the bed and face the patient.

B. Place the patient in lithotomy position, or have the patient draw knees up and allow knees to drop to opposite sides.

C. Suggest relaxation techniques to reduce discomfort. If the patient is in active labor, the cervix will be tender.

D. Place lubricant on the index and middle fingers of examining hand.

E. Inform the patient of each step prior to performance: touch inner thigh first, then touch posterior portion of introitus and introduce gloved fingers into the vagina. Encourage the patient to relax pelvic muscles (a deep breath will often encourage relaxation).

F. Palpate the cervix and lower uterine segment evaluating: (see Figure)
   1. Dilatation.
   2. Effacement.
   3. Station.
   4. Consistency (softness).
   5. Anterior vs. mid-position vs. posterior placement of the cervix.

TABLE **Bishop Scoring**

Score	0	1	2	3
Dilation	0	1–2	3–4	5–6
% Effacement	0%–30%	40%–50%	60%–70%	80% or >
Station	−3	−2	−1 to 0	+1 to +2
Consistency	Firm	Medium	Soft	—
Position	Posterior	Mid	Anterior	—

Total Score: 0–5 Difficult induction; ≥ 6 = Easy induction.

FIGURE Bimanual examination.

6. In cases of preterm uterine contractions, it is helpful to assess the development of the lower uterine segment. A well-developed lower uterine segment (even in the absence of cervical dilation or effacement) is often a sign of preterm labor.

7. Note fetal presentation and station of the presenting part. Use ischial spines as landmarks to determine fetal descent through the pelvis.

8. If the fetus is sufficiently descended into the pelvis, determine the position of the presenting part.

9. If present, note bag of amniotic membranes. A bulging bag, known as a "forebag," may be present, even in the presence of documented ruptured membranes.

G. Following the exam, note if blood or vaginal discharge is on gloves.

Description

A Papanicolaou (Pap) smear is a cytological **screen** that is performed to detect the presence of cancerous and precancerous lesions of the uterine cervix. The procedure involves procuring a sample of both the ectocervix and endocervix. The maturation index (endocrine assessment) is a tool to evaluate atrophic vaginitis/estrogen deficiency.

Indications

According to the American Cancer Society (ACS) and the U.S. Preventative Task Force (USPTS) guidelines, all women should begin cervical cancer screening 3 years after beginning vaginal intercourse and no later than age 21 (whichever comes first).

The ACS recommends that if the conventional Pap test is used, patients should be tested yearly, but if the liquid-based test is used, testing can be done every 2 years. Beginning at age 30, women who have had three normal consecutive Pap tests may decrease Pap test frequency to every 2–3 years. Special conditions that indicate more frequent cervical cytology screening include women with HIV, women who are immunocompromised, women previously exposed to diethylstilbestrol in utero, or women previously treated for CIN2, CIN3, or cancer.

Screening may be discontinued in women ages 65–70 who are at low risk with three consecutive normal screenings. Women in this age group who are at high risk (sexually active with multiple partners or previous abnormal cytology) should continue screening. Screening is not indicated for women who have had a total hysterectomy for benign indications. Screening is indicated for women who have had a hysterectomy with removal of the cervix who have a history of CIN2 or 3 or for whom negative history is not documented.

A Pap smear may be obtained in pregnancy, or at the end of a period in the menses flow if light. If the patient is having a heavy menstrual flow, the procedure should be rescheduled.

A maturation index is obtained to evaluate decreased estrogenization of the vagina. Both liquid-based and conventional methods for collecting cervical cytology are acceptable.

Precautions

A. Ask the woman not to douche, use any antifungal or spermicides, or have intercourse the night prior to the procedure so that there will be nothing to interfere with obtaining a good sample.

B. Practitioners should be aware that some women experience discomfort during the Pap smear procedure and should be sensitive to this possibility.

C. In order to procure an adequate Pap smear, care must be taken to obtain a sample from the entire squamo-columnar junction of the cervical portio. (The squamo-columnar junction is more prominent in teens and women on oral contraceptives.)

D. Blood may obscure an adequate cytology interpretation. It is advisable, therefore, to obtain the endocervical sample following the ectocervical sample. Bleeding from the endocervix is common, particularly if a cytobrush is used. A cytobrush is recommended for sampling the endocervix as more cells are retrieved using this tool as compared to a Q-tip.

Equipment Required

A. Speculum (size appropriate for teen/woman)
B. Warm water for lubrication (excessive K-Y jelly may interfere with the smear and reading)
C. Spatula (wooden or plastic)
D. Q-tip or cytobrush
E. Glass slide (2 if maturation index)
F. Container for slide(s)
G. Cytology fixative

Procedure (Conventional Method)

A. With the patient draped in a lithotomy position, insert the lightly lubricated speculum and visualize the cervix.

B. With the spatula, sample the entire (360-degree sweep) squamo-columnar junction using gentle pressure applied directly to this area (if visualized). The goal of the technique is to scrape exfoliated cells or those cells held loosely on the surface of the cervix. Vigorous scraping that abrades the cervix yields tissue that is virtually uninterpretable in the cytology smear.

C. **Insert the cytobrush or Q-tip until the brush or cotton swab is no longer visible. It is not necessary to insert further to obtain an adequate sample.** A fiber-tipped swab should be introduced in the canal and rotated clockwise several times to obtain cells. A cotton-tipped swab should first be moistened with saline to prevent cells from adhering to the cotton; a synthetic fiber swab is nonabsorbent and can be used without moistening. Pap smears taken with a brush have been found superior in containing endocervical cells.

D. Wipe the sample from the spatula and roll and twist the brush of the cytobrush or the Q-tip on the glass side as quickly as possible. The cytobrush sample can be rolled through the spatula sample. It is not necessary to separate these two areas or obtain two slides.

E. Spray the slide with cytology fixative held at a distance of approximately 12 inches to avoid "blasting" the cells from the slide. If held too far away, inadequate spray reaches the slide and drying distortion could result.

   1. Allow the slide to dry prior to covering in transport container.

   2. To obtain a cytology specimen from the vaginal cuff (posthysterectomy), use a spatula (rounded end) to scrape the upper lateral third of the vaginal wall.

Spread on a slide and fix the slide with cytology fixative.

3. Vaginal pool specimens for a maturation index are often recommended in perimenopausal women; sampling is done by scraping the posterior fornix with the spatula. Spread on a separate slide from the pap smear and fix the slide.

Procedure (Liquid-Based Cytology)

A. With the patient draped in a lithotomy position, insert the lightly lubricated speculum and visualize the cervix.

B. With the spatula, sample the entire (360-degree sweep) squamo-columnar junction using gentle pressure applied directly to this area (if visualized). The goal of the technique is to scrape exfoliated cells or those cells held loosely on the surface of the cervix. Rinse the spatula as quickly as possible in the solution by swirling vigorously 10 times and discard the spatula.

C. Insert the cytobrush until only the bottom-most fibers are visible. Rotate slowly one half-turn in one direction (do not overrotate). Rinse the brush quickly by rotating the brush against the container wall and swirling. Place the cap on the specimen container and label properly. See Figure.

D. Alternatively you may use the broom device instead of the cytobrush. If so, insert the central bristles of the broom device into the endocervical canal (deep enough for the short bristles to contact the ectocervix) and rotate clockwise five times. Rinse the broom by quickly pushing against the bottom of the specimen container and swirling 10 times.

Evaluation/Results of Procedure

A. A Pap smear may be classified as "inadequate" if no endocervical cells are present for interpretation (unless the patient has had a hysterectomy).

B. Pap smear adequacy may be compromised if the slide is allowed to air dry prior to spraying with cytology fixative.

C. A Pap smear reading may be compromised due to the presence of blood, lubricant, or certain vaginal infections creating an increase in vaginal discharge.

D. See Pap Smear Interpretation and American Society for Colposcopy and Cervical Pathology Consensus guidelines on the management of women with abnormal cervical cancer screening tests algorithms on the Internet: http://www.asccp.org/consensus.shtml.

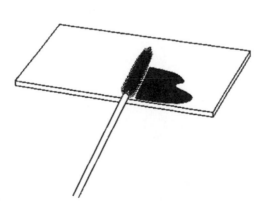

FIGURE Pap smear cytology brush.

TRICHLOROACETIC ACID (TCA)/PODOPHYLLIN THERAPY *by Rhonda Authur*

Description

A. TCA and podophyllin are substances used to eliminate exophytic warts on the external genitalia and perianal area.

Indications

A. External genitalia and perianal warts

Precautions

A. Podophyllin use is contraindicated in pregnancy.

B. Either substance should be applied sparingly to avoid contact with unaffected skin.

Equipment Required

A. Examining table with stirrups for positioning the female client in the lithotomy position.

B. Light source for examining the genitalia and perianal area.

C. Gown/drape for the patient

D. Gloves: Nonsterile glove may be used.

E. Cotton-tipped applicators.

F. Petroleum jelly.

G. Sodium bicarbonate (baking soda) or powder with talc.

H. Plastic medicine cups.

I. Trichloroacetic acid (TCA) 80%–90% *or*

J. Podophyllin 10%–25% in compound tincture of benzoin.

Procedure

A. Assist the female client to the lithotomy position; the male client to a sitting or supine position on the exam table.

B. Inspect the external genitalia and perianal areas for exophytic warts.

C. Pour small amount (0.5–1.0 mL) of solution (TCA or podophyllin) to be used in a plastic medicine cup.

D. Use the cotton-tipped applicator to apply petroleum jelly on unaffected skin surrounding areas identified for therapy.

E. Use the wooden end of the cotton-tipped applicator to apply a small amount of solution (TCA or Podophyllin) to warts.

F. If TCA is used, apply sodium bicarbonate or powder with talc to absorb unreacted acid.

G. If podophyllin is used, instruct the client to thoroughly wash off solution in 1–4 hours.

H. Repeat weekly if necessary. If warts persist after 6 applications, consider other therapeutic methods.

I. Advise the client that mild to moderate pain or local irritation may occur after treatment.

Description

A. The wet mount procedure is a technique used to identify organisms under the microscope for vaginal infections. Any patient complaining of vaginal discharge/irritation should have a wet mount performed to aid in identifying the organism to assist in the diagnosis.

Indications

A. Vaginal discharge
B. Vulvar/vaginal irritation or pain
C. Vaginal discharge with an odor

Precautions

A. Use universal precautions when obtaining specimens.

Equipment Required

A. Examining table with stirrups for positioning the patient in the lithotomy position.
B. Light source for examining the cervix.
C. Gown/drape for the patient.
D. Gloves, 2 pair (nonsterile).
E. Speculum: Always have several different types and sizes of speculums on hand for appropriate sizing, visualization, and comfort.
F. Condoms available if needed.
G. Q-tip/cotton-tipped applicators.
H. Gen-probe, or other collecting tubes for *Neisseria gonorrhoeae* and *Chlamydia* specimens.
I. Small test tube/plastic collection tube.
J. Normal saline and 10% KOH.
K. Glass slides (2): one marked "KOH" and one marked "NS."
L. Cover slips for slides (2).
M. Nitrazine pH test tape.
N. Microscope.

Procedure

A. After the patient has voided and changed into a gown, assist the patient into the lithotomy position.
B. Apply gloves.
C. Prepare the test tube/specimen tube with one millimeter of normal saline. Prepare slides (one marked KOH and one marked NS); apply 1 drop of each solution to a clean slide and set aside.
D. Inspect the perineum for lesions, erythema, condyloma, and lacerations.
E. Gently insert the speculum into the vagina. Do not use lubricant since this may interfere with the quality of the specimen. Use warm water for lubrication.
F. While inserting the speculum, visualize the vaginal vault, walls, and cervix. Note any irregularities such as lesions, masses, and lacerations.
G. If the lateral sidewalls collapse and decrease visualization of the cervix, withdraw the speculum. Apply a condom to the speculum and cut the condom tip. Reinsert the condom-covered speculum to visualize the cervix.
H. Observe for vaginal discharge, noting the amount, color, consistency, and odor.

I. Collect a sample of discharge with the 2 Q-tips.
  1. Place 1 Q-tip into a prefilled test tube/specimen tube and make your slide later *or*
  2. Collect a sample of discharge with the Q-tip and roll the Q-tip into the normal saline–prepared slide cover with a cover slip.
  3. *Then* roll the Q-tip into the KOH-prepared slide.
  4. Note any "musty/fishy" odor prior to placing the cover slip on the slide (Whiff test is positive if amine odor is noted).
J. Using the 2nd Q-tip roll it over a strip of Nitrazine test tape to evaluate pH.
K. Using the Gen-probe, insert the tip onto the cervical os and rotate the tip in the os several times to obtain an adequate specimen (sample for a minimum of about 30 seconds).
L. Withdraw the Gen-probe applicator and place in the appropriate specimen container.
M. Gently remove the speculum and perform a bimanual examination, assessing for cervical motion tenderness and pain.
N. After completing this exam, take the specimens to the lab area for evaluation (while the patient is dressing).
O. Prepare your slides (if you did not follow steps I.1–I.4).
  1. Slide 1: place 1 drop of NS to the slide and roll the Q-tip and apply cover slip.
  2. Slide 2: place 1 drop of KOH to the slide and roll the Q-tip; note any "musty/fishy" odor from the slide prior to placing the cover slide.
P. Observe the NS slide first under the microscope. Start on low power, 10x, and adjust the focus until the specimen is clearly seen under the microscope.
Q. Observe the entire field and note the number of squamous cells.
R. Switch to the high-powered field, 40x, making sure the light source and the visual focus are adequate.
S. Observe the slide for:
  1. Vaginal epithelial cells: appear flat, with clear edges. See Figure.
  2. Clue cells: epithelial cells with irregular borders and a granular appearance; may note the presence of many coccobacilli bacteria. See Figure.
  3. Bacteria.
  4. *Lactobacilli*: appear as large rods. See Figure.
  5. White blood cells (WBCs): a large amount of WBCs is not normal. See Figure.
  6. Trichomonads: appear as ovoid mobile organisms that dart around on the slide. See Figure.
  7. *Candida*: appear as branching pseudohyphae or budding yeast (best seen under the KOH slide). See Figure and Table.

Treatment

A. Refer to specific chapters for treatment recommendations and medication dosages.

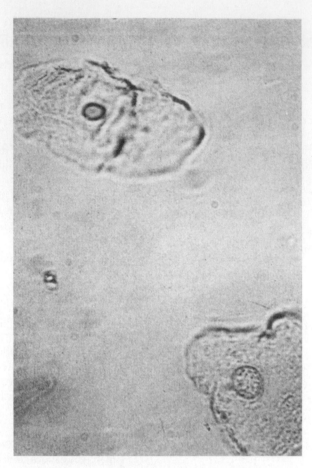

FIGURE Epithelial Cell.
From *Microscopic Procedures for Primary Care Providers,*
by S. Lowe & J. Saxe, 1998. Philadelphia: Lippincott,
Williams & Wilkins.

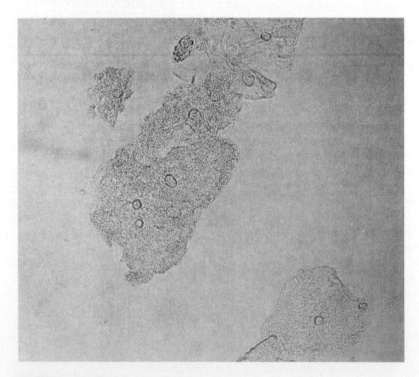

FIGURE Clue cells.
From *Microscopic Procedures for Primary Care Providers,* by S. Lowe & J. Saxe,
1998. Philadelphia: Lippincott, Williams & Wilkins.

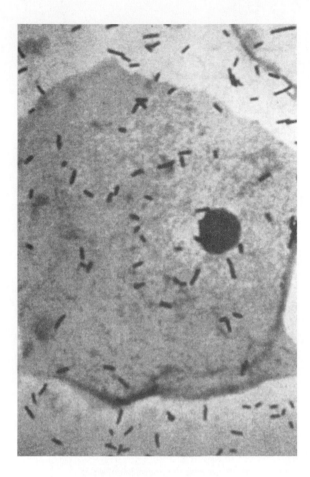

FIGURE *Lactobacilli.*
From *Advanced Assessment of Women,* by H. Carcio, 1998.
Philadelphia: Lippincott, Williams & Wilkins.

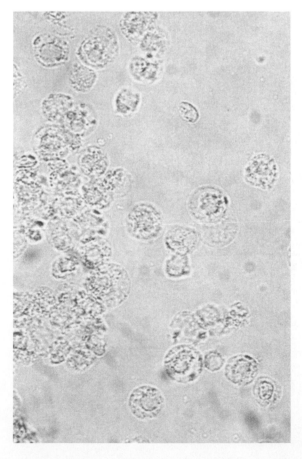

FIGURE White blood cells. These cells have been enlarged to show detail.
From *Microscopic Procedures for Primary Care Providers,* by S. Lowe &
J. Saxe, 1998. Philadelphia: Lippincott, Williams & Wilkins.

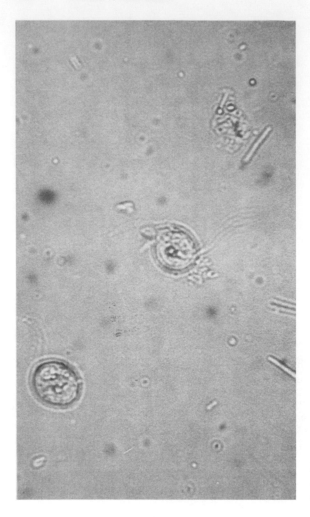

FIGURE *Trichomonas* (1000x). *Note:* Organism is enlarged.
From *Microscopic Procedures for Primary Care Providers,* by S. Lowe &
J. Saxe, 1998. Philadelphia: Lippincott, Williams & Wilkins.

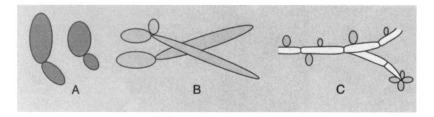

FIGURE (A) Budding yeast cells. (B) Pseudohyphae. (C) Septate hyphae and spores.
From *Microscopic Procedures for Primary Care Providers,* by S. Lowe & J. Saxe,
1998. Philadelphia: Lippincott, Williams & Wilkins.

TABLE **Evaluation and Results of Wet Mount**

Diagnosis	pH	Microscopic Findings
Normal physiologic findings	pH: 3.5–4.0	Rare WBCs, squamous epithelial cells, gram positive rods
Gardnerella (bacterial vaginosis)	pH: 5.0–6.0	Clue cells
Candida	pH: 3.5–4.5	Budding spores, pseudohyphae
Trichomonas	pH: 6.0–7.0	Numerous WBCs, Trichomonads

INTRAUTERINE DEVICE (IUD) INSERTION *by Rhonda Arthur*

Note: **Only trained health care providers who carefully reviewed the selected device's manufacturer's package insert for indications and use as well as specific insertion instructions should place IUDs.**

Description

A. The intrauterine device is a long-acting method of contraception that is inserted into the uterine cavity.
   1. Copper T 380 A (Paragard®)
      a. T-shaped bound in fine copper wire
      b. **Approved for 10 years**
      c. Clear or white knotted double string
   2. Levonorgestrel (Mirena®)
      a. T-shaped polyethylene frame with levonorgestrel reservoir coating
      b. **Approved for 5 years**
      c. Dark monofilament strings
      d. Indications also include use for treatment in women who have heavy menstrual bleeding and choose IUD for contraception

Indications

A. To provide a long-acting method (5–10 years) of contraception.
B. The Mirena® IUD has been therapeutic with severe dysmenorrhea and severe menorrhagia.

Precautions

A. Pregnancy must be ruled out prior to insertion.
B. Risks at the time of insertion include uterine perforation and/or infection and a vagal response.
C. Small amounts of progestins pass into breast milk with Mirena®.
D. To minimize the risk of expulsion, it is advisable to insert an IUD when the woman is *not* on her menstrual cycle.
E. **Removal of an existing IUD should occur *during* the menstrual cycle.**
F. Consent(s) are required by the manufacturer and by individual institutional protocols. The patient should know the type of IUD device and when it should be replaced.

Contraindications

A. Women who have a history of sexually transmitted disease and/or currently have more than one sexual partner may not be good candidates for IUD use.
B. Uterine anomaly.
C. Cervical stenosis (unable to pass an uterine sound).
D. Nulliparous (especially teens) are also not good candidates for the IUD.
E. Active pelvic infection (recent, acute, or subacute).
F. Purulent cervicitis.
G. History of ectopic pregnancy (strong relative risk).

H. Abnormal pap smear/endometrial hyperplasia/cervical inraepithelial neoplasia (CIN)/cancer (review last recent Pap results). Uterine or cervical neoplasm.
I. Concern for future fertility.
J. Allergy to copper (Paragard®) or allergy to component of Mirena® as applies.
K. Valvular heart disease.

Insertion of an IUD may theoretically increase the woman's susceptibility to systemic bacterial endocarditis (SBE). No current evidence supports this. *Optional therapy:* **Some clinicians require antibiotics for valvular coverage. High-risk patients may receive IV ampicillin and gentamicin, and moderate-risk patients may receive oral amoxicillin 2 g before insertion or removal.**

L. Acute liver disease (Mirena®).
M. Known or suspected breast carcinoma (Mirena®).

Equipment Required

A. IUD.
B. Speculum.
C. Iodine solution.
D. Tenaculum.
E. Uterine sound.
F. Scissors.
G. Sterile gloves (2 pair).
H. Urine pregnancy test kit.
I. Atropine 0.5 mg should be available at the time of insertion for severe vasovagal response.

Back-up staff should be available for complications such as vasovagal response and perforation of uterus.

Procedure

A. Perform a urine pregnancy test.
B. Perform a baseline blood pressure and pulse.
C. Obtain the patient's consent after full history, review of last Pap smear, discussion of alternative methods, pros and cons of each method, procedure, side effects, and complications of IUD insertion and device.
D. Perform a bimanual exam to determine uterine position and size.
E. Apply sterile gloves.
F. Cleanse the vagina and cervix with iodine solution.
G. Use the tenaculum to grasp the anterior lip of the cervix approximately 1.5–2.0 cm from the os.
   1. Atropine should be readily available for severe vasovagal response.
   2. Lidocaine (Xylocaine) gel or benzocaine (Hurricane Spray) could be used to decrease discomfort with the application and use of the tenaculum.
H. Insert the uterine sound into the cervix/uterus slowly and gently.
   1. **Moisture mark on the sound will indicate the depth of insertion for the IUD. (Depth less than 6 cm is contraindication.)**

I. Change sterile gloves.

J. Load the IUD as directed by manufacturer.

K. Set indicator for depth of insertion as guided by the uterine sound.

L. While maintaining gentle traction with the tenaculum, insert the IUD gently to the predetermined mark on the guide sheath.
   1. Spasm of the internal cervical os may occur and will resolve by waiting a few minutes.

M. Gently push the IUD through the guide into position. **Excessive pain or bleeding is often a sign of perforation.** *Consult a physician immediately* **(most common perforation sites: fundus, body of uterus, and cervical wall).**

N. Remove the guide sheath.

O. Remove the tenaculum.

P. Cut the IUD strings to approximately 1-inch length past the cervix.

Q. Remove the speculum.

R. Check the patient's blood pressure and pulse to rule out vasovagal potential.

S. Recommend a prostaglandin inhibitor if cramping occurs/persists (Motrin® 400 mg by mouth four times a day).

T. Prophylactic antibiotics may be used for SBE prophylaxis. Amoxicillin is used unless an amoxicillin/penicillin allergy, then erythromycin or clindamycin may be prescribed. Amoxicillin 3.0 g by mouth 1 hour before the procedure, then 1.5 g by mouth 6 hours later.
   1. Erythromycin (EES) 800 mg by mouth 2 hours before the procedure, then 400 mg by mouth 6 hours later.
   2. Clindamycin 300 mg by mouth 1 hour before the procedure, then 150 mg 6 hours later.

U. Instruct the patient regarding string location and periodic checks. The patient should not have vaginal intercourse or use a tampon for 7 days (decreases infection).

Evaluation/Results of Procedure

A. See the patient after first menses to check for expulsion.

B. Two or more missed periods do beta HCG.
   1. Rule out ectopic pregnancy.
   2. Explore the canal for IUD.
   3. Consider ultrasound to rule out pregnancy/expulsion.
   4. Consider flat plate of abdomen.
   5. Consult a physician.

C. Yearly evaluation with Pap smear/annual check-up.

D. Consider hemoglobin for reports of heavy bleeding with Paragard®.
   1. If Hgb is less than 9, remove the IUD, provide an alternative method of contraception, and prescribe iron supplement for 2 months.
   2. Repeat Hgb in 1 month.

IUD Removal Procedure

A. Remove only during menses (cervix is more dilated).

B. Apply gentle, steady traction; remove slowly.

C. **Consider uterine embedding if unable to remove, needs consultation.**

Patient Should Call the Office For

A. A missed period

B. Abdominal pain (severe)

C. Temperature 100.4°F not associated with other problems (sinus infection, UTI)

D. Foul vaginal odor/discharge, especially if bloody or greenish color

E. Heavy bleeding with clots

The first 12 weeks of pregnancy are vital, as the fetal organ systems are developing.

A. Early diagnosis of pregnancy allows counseling about potential risks to the developing fetus.
B. Enables the woman contemplating elective abortion to consider her options.
C. Affords diagnosis/intervention in an ectopic pregnancy.
D. Fosters early entry into prenatal care, which in turn may provide early identification of pregnancy complications.

Obtain Menstrual History

A. Obtain sexual history.
B. Obtain fertility history.
   1. Length of cycles.
   2. Regularity of cycles. Regularity of menstruation is influenced by
      a. Recent previous pregnancy and cycles have not yet reestablished
      b. Breast-feeding
      c. Oral contraceptive pills
      d. Intramuscular contraceptive
      e. Polycystic ovarian syndrome (PCOS)
      f. Comorbid medical conditions
C. Is this a planned pregnancy? If so, how long did it take to conceive?
D. Has the patient been pregnant before? If so, what was the outcome of each pregnancy (miscarriage, stillbirth, live birth), delivery method, and fetal and/or pregnancy complications for each pregnancy?

Initial Assessment/Diagnosis of Pregnancy

A. Is the exact date of the last missed period (LMP) known using the first day of the last period?
B. Was the last missed period (LMP) a normal period? If not, when was most recent normal period?
C. Is there a known isolated sexual incident that could pinpoint a possible conception date?
D. Does the patient know when conception may have occurred?

Pregnancy Testing

Testing includes analysis of maternal blood or urine for the presence of human chorionic gonadotropin (HCG), a hormone produced by the trophoblastic cells of the developing placenta. **Positive testing is not diagnostic of a normal intrauterine pregnancy.**

A. Maternal blood: HCG
   1. Most accurate
   2. Earliest to become positive
   3. Negative test should be repeated in 2 weeks
B. Urine
   1. More commonly used.
   2. Accurate 4–7 days following conception.
   3. Available over-the-counter.
   4. First-voided morning specimen is best (most concentrated).
   5. Negative test should be repeated in 1 week to ensure that the first test was not done too early to detect urine HCG. HCG production decreases after 60–70 days, and thereafter declines below the sensitivity of some tests.

Presumptive Signs of Pregnancy

A. Amenorrhea
B. Has experienced pregnancy before and feels pregnant now
C. Nausea/vomiting: nausea is not limited to "morning sickness"
D. Fatigue
E. Breast tenderness
F. Urinary frequency
G. Enlarging abdomen
H. Unexplained weight gain
I. Constipation

Probable Signs of Pregnancy

A. Positive Chadwick's sign: purplish coloration of vagina and cervix; may be seen on speculum examination
B. Positive Hegar's sign: softening of the lower uterine segment; may be palpated on bimanual examination
C. Uterine enlargement
   1. 8 weeks' gestation = 2 times nonpregnant size
   2. 10 weeks' gestation = 3 times nonpregnant size
   3. 12 weeks' gestation = 4 times nonpregnant size, uterine fundus (size of orange) palpable at symphysis pubis
   4. 16 weeks' gestation = uterine fundus midway between symphysis pubis and umbilicus (size of grapefruit)
   5. 20 weeks' gestation = uterine fundus at umbilicus (size of large honeydew melon)
D. Increased skin pigmentation (face [chloasma], nipples, abdomen [linea nigra])
E. Striae gravidarum: "stretch marks"

Positive Diagnostic Signs

A. Fetal heart tones (FHTs)
   1. 10–12 weeks with ultrasonic Doppler (fetal doptone).
   2. If unable to hear FHTs with doptone at 12 weeks (by size and dates), have the patient return at 14 weeks.
   3. If unable to hear FHTs at 14-week gestation repeat visit, the patient needs ultrasound examination to

confirm fetal viability. Consult with a physician if abnormal ultrasound results.

4. 18–20 weeks with fetoscope (helps verify estimated date of delivery [EDC]).

B. Fetal movements palpated by the mother or health care provider

C. Ultrasound examination
1. Gestational sac visualized by 6 weeks
2. Fetal pole visualized by 8 weeks
3. Fetal cardiac activity visualized by 8 weeks

Estimated Date of Delivery/Estimated Date of Confinement (EDC)

A. 280 days (40 weeks) after last menstrual period (LMP).

B. 266 days (38 weeks) from last ovulation (in a 28-day cycle).

C. **Nagele's Rule** for establishing EDC: First day of the LMP plus 7 days minus 3 months = EDC.

D. Gestational calculator (in the form of a wheel) may be used to determine EDC. **Gestational wheels are based on a 28-day cycle.**

Description

The nonstress test (NST) is a noninvasive test to assess fetal well-being. A fetus with an intact central nervous system with adequate oxygenation will demonstrate transient fetal heart rate accelerations in response to fetal movement. Results of the nonstress test must be evaluated with consideration of gestational age. It is not uncommon for a neurologically intact fetus between the ages of 24–28 weeks' gestation to have a nonreactive nonstress test.

Indications

A. Patients at risk for adverse perinatal outcome.
  1. Maternal indications may include:
     a. Hypertension.
     b. Maternal cardiac disease.
     c. Diabetes (including gestational diabetes).
     d. Renal disease.
     e. Hyperthyroidism.
     f. Collagen vascular disease.
     g. Sickle cell disease.
     h. Previous stillbirth.
  2. Fetal indications may include:
     a. Intrauterine growth restriction (IUGR).
     b. Postdates (> 41 weeks).
     c. Decreased fetal movement.
B. **Frequency of testing:** One must consider prognosis for neonatal survival and severity of maternal disease. In general, most high-risk pregnant women should begin testing by 32–34 weeks' estimated gestational age (EGA). In case of multiple or severe high-risk conditions, testing may begin at 26–28 weeks. Frequency may be weekly or biweekly. If clinical deterioration is noted, reducing the testing interval is prudent.

Precautions

A. **A reactive NST** is reassuring. However, the significance of abnormal results are less clear. Loss of FHR reactivity may be benign, or may be a sign of the metabolic consequences of hypoxemia.

Equipment Required

A. Electronic fetal heart rate monitor (EFM)
B. Reclining chair or bed/stretcher
C. Sphygmomanometer
D. Vibroacoustic stimulator (protocol dependent)

Procedure

A. Place the patient in the semi-Fowler's position in a recliner or on a stretcher. Optimal positioning includes the patient tilted to the left or right side to avoid vena caval compression. The patient is preferably nonfasting and has not recently smoked.
B. Measure the patient's blood pressure.
C. Apply EFM on the maternal abdomen.
D. Record FHR × 20–40 min. Ask the mother to record fetal movements with a marker button, if available. However, all accelerations may be counted as they probably have the same significance whether or not they occur in response to the fetal movement felt by the mother.
E. Interpret FHR tracing as reactive or nonreactive (see below).
F. If the fetus is suspected to be in a sleep state, a vibroacoustic stimulation device may be applied, placed on the maternal abdomen and used for a 3-second stimulation in an attempt to awaken the fetus.

Evaluation/Results of Procedure

A. Reactive NST: Baseline FHR 110–160 bpm with two or more accelerations of greater than or equal to 15 bpm amplitude that last at least 15 seconds or more, within a 10-minute period. (**Note: Before 32 weeks of gestation, accelerations are defined as two accelerations or more greater than 10 bpm amplitude that last at least longer than 10 seconds.**) If these criteria are met prior to 20 min, the test may be declared reactive. The FHR tracing may be continued for at least 40 min to account for the typical fetal sleep-wake cycle.
B. Nonreactive NST: Above criteria are not met.

Treatment

A. If the NST is a reactive, reassuring test, continue obstetrical prenatal care. Further testing is required for maternal and fetal indications as previously noted.

Consultation/Referral

Further evaluation is mandatory for a nonreactive NST. Consult with a physician. Depending on the situation, the patient could be given juice or sent to eat and return later for a repeat NST. She may undergo a modified NST, which includes a single 1–3 second sound (vibroacoustic) stimulation applied to the maternal abdomen plus the assessment of amniotic fluid and/or biophysical profile (BPP). She may also be sent to the hospital for another NST, modified NST, BPP, or a contraction stress test (CST).

The CST should only be preformed in a setting where immediate delivery could occur if indicated for fetal distress.

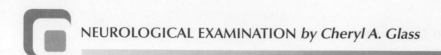
Description

Performance of the neurological examination is a diagnostic component of many physical examinations. Examination of all cranial nerves is not necessary for every patient; it should be performed based on patient-focused presenting complaints. The purpose of this support tool is to review the cranial nerves and review equipment needed for a neurologic examination.

A neurologic examination identifies dysfunction and assists in accurate diagnosis. See Table.

Components of the Neurologic Examination

A. Thorough history
B. Assessment of mental status
C. Assessment of cranial nerve function
D. Assessment of motor function
E. Assessment of sensory function
F. Assessment of gait
G. Assessment of reflexes

Equipment Required

A. Multiple mental examinations are available. The clock-draw test and the Mini Mental examination are two examples.
B. Pen light/ophthalmoscope: light source.
C. Ophthalmoscope.
D. Snellen chart/Rosenbaum pocket card.
E. Items to taste (salt, sugar).
F. Items to smell (vanilla, cinnamon).
G. Tongue depressor.
H. Tuning fork.
I. Ticking watch/clock.
J. Cotton or soft tissue.
K. Pin or other sharp object.
L. Reflex hammer.

TABLE Cranial Nerve Function

Cranial Nerve Number	Cranial Nerve	Functional Test
I	Olfactory	Smell reception and interpretation
II	Optic	Vision: acuity and visual fields
III	Oculomotor	Motor: eye/lid movement, pupil constriction, visual accommodation
IV	Trochlear	Eye movement up/down
V	Trigeminal	Chewing, jaw opening and clenching, facial sensation: corneal, forehead, eyes, nose/mouth mucosa, teeth, tongue, and ears
VI	Abducens	Lateral gaze/eye movement
VII	Facial	Corneal reflex, facial expression, taste to the lateral two-thirds of tongue, and sensation to pharynx, parasympathetic secretion of tears and saliva
VIII	Acoustic	Hearing and equilibrium
IX	Glosso-medulla or Glossopharyngeal	Gag reflex, cough, swallow, taste on posterior third of tongue, and parasympathetic secretion of salivary glands, and carotid reflex
X	Vagus	Laryngeal muscles-muscles of phonation, swallowing, sensation behind ear and part of external canal, parasympathetic secretion of digestive enzymes/peristalsis as well as involuntary action of heart and lungs
XI	Spinal accessory	Head and shoulder movement: shoulder shrug
XII	Hypoglossal	Tongue movement/muscles, swallowing, and sound articulation

Adapted from *Mosby's Guide to Physical Examination* (2nd ed.), by H. M. Seidel, J. W. Ball, J. E. Dains, & G. W. Benedict, 1991. New York: Mosby Year-Book.

RECTAL PROLAPSE REDUCTION *by Cheryl A. Glass*

Description

There are 3 types of rectal prolapse:

A. **Partial.** Anus is inverted; rectal mucosa protrudes 1–3 cm out of rectal sphincter.
B. **Complete.** All layers of rectum have intussuscepted through the anus. (Rare in adults; most often seen in children and the elderly.)
C. **Internal.** Patient complains of a protrusion, but no protrusion is noted on examination.

Indications

Diagnosis of rectal prolapse is made by inspection. Several populations are at risk for rectal prolapse, including infants, women, and the elderly. Other factors associated with rectal prolapse include malnutrition, severe constipation, severe chronic diarrhea, obstetrical injuries, rectal intercourse, and multiple sclerosis as well as other neuromuscular diseases.

Hemorrhoids, mucosal prolapse, polyps, and cancer must be ruled out. Conditions associated with rectal prolapse include cystic fibrosis, ulcerative colitis, intussesception, and Hirschsprung's disease.

Precautions

A. Refer patients with complete prolapse to a physician for evaluation and treatment. After a rectal prolapse reduction by proctoscope, follow-up testing by barium enema or endoscopy is indicated.
B. Surgery may also be indicated, depending on the type of prolapse, recurrence, and risk of strangulation. Children need further assessment for sexual abuse and cystic fibrosis.
C. Patients with a history of surgery for rectal prolapse should be evaluated and assessed for hemorrhage, bowel obstruction, pelvic abscess, fecal impaction, and recurrent prolapse.
D. Instruct the patient on a high-residue diet, and warn him or her to avoid straining to induce a bowel movement.

Equipment Required

A. Sterile gauze
B. Normal saline
C. Anoscope
D. Water-soluble lubricant
E. Gloves
F. Chux pads and tissue
G. Light source
H. Examination table

Procedure

A. Explain the procedure to the patient and discuss all steps just before performing.
B. Obtain the patient's consent.
C. Ask the patient to void. (Urinary stress incontinence is common during the procedure.)
D. Apply gloves.
E. As the procedure is being done, give the patient and/or caregiver instructions on how reduction is done in the event of another prolapse.
   1. Provide the parents with gloves and lubricant for future need.
   2. Prolapses may also reduce spontaneously without any manual reduction.
F. Have the patient lie in left lateral position and give extra tissues for urinary incontinence.
G. Ask the patient to strain (perform Valsalva's maneuver). This allows the health care provider to fully evaluate the prolapse through the anal sphincter. If this does not produce the prolapse, have the patient squat and/or sit on the toilet to strain.
H. With a good light source, do a detailed visual examination to rule out hemorrhoids versus a complete/partial prolapse.
   1. Thrombosed hemorrhoids appear as blue, shiny masses.
   2. A normal hemorrhoid appears as a painless, flaccid skin tag.
   3. Anoscope reveals internal hemorrhoids as bright red to purplish bulges.
   4. Rectal prolapse looks like a pink doughnut or rosette; complete prolapse involving the muscular wall is larger, red, and has circular folds.
I. After visual inspection/evaluation, reposition the patient into a knee-chest position. This allows the bowel to be pulled back into the anus.
J. If after changing positions the prolapse does not reduce with gravity, place a saline-soaked 4 × 4 gauze over the prolapse to prevent drying.
K. Apply gentle pressure with the saline gauze, and replace the rectal prolapse/protrusion back through the anus.
L. Using a lubricated gloved hand, perform a rectal examination to evaluate sphincter tone at rest and with some straining. This rectal exam should be painless. Pain raises suspicion for other pathology, such as incarceration or an unrelated lesion.
M. Apply lubricant to anoscope and slowly insert it anteriorly into the rectum. Remove inner cannula of anoscope, and slowly withdraw it to evaluate and identify any lesions. It is rare to see a polyp or carcinoma. Usually, you will note erythema and edema.

Evaluation/Results of Procedure

A. If reduction of rectal prolapse occurs with minimal discomfort, have the patient return in 1 week to assess sphincter function.
B. If unable to reduce prolapse, send the patient for *immediate* evaluation by a physician. Keep prolapse covered with saline-soaked gauze during transport.
C. If prolapse was partial or complete, refer the patient to a physician after reduction.
D. Further evaluation may include a sigmoidoscope, barium enema, or biopsy.
E. Presence of pain may indicate an incarceration with impending strangulation and requires *immediate* referral.
F. All patients need to follow a high-fiber diet and have instructions on avoiding straining.

Description

A. This is the technique for removing a foreign body that is anterior to the pharynx and can be visualized with a nasal speculum.

Indications

A. Patients with retained nasal foreign bodies often present with unilateral, foul rhinorrhea, nosebleeds, or the request for foreign body removal.

Precautions

A. Try to identify the type of object (e.g., rock, pea, pearl, battery).
B. If you can't identify the object, don't irrigate the nares before removal.
C. Vegetable matter will swell if hydrated, so remove it in a dry environment when possible.
D. When the object is too far into the nasal turbinate/cavity or when in doubt, do not attempt the procedure and refer to an otolaryngologist.
   1. The procedure may need to be done under sedation.
   2. The object may need to be surgically removed.

Equipment

A. Proper lighting (headlight or head mirror).
B. Nasal speculum.
C. Topical anesthetic for use prior to procedure (topical 1% lidocaine with 0.5% phenylephrine).
D. Suction and several suction tips.
E. Other equipment should be available, depending on the type of foreign body: wire loop or curette, alligator or Hartman forceps, bayonet forceps, right-angle hooks and suction.

Procedure

A. Determine the type of object in the nostril during history-taking in order to determine the best approach for removal.
B. Explain the procedure to the patient.
C. Obtain the patient's consent for removal.
D. To best visualize the nasal cavity, have the patient lie down or sit erect with the head slightly tilted.
E. Visualize the nostril with the nasal speculum.
F. If tissue edema is present in the nares, you may use a topical anesthetic with vasoconstrictor to the affected nares to help prevent bleeding.
G. If the patient is willing, have him or her dislodge the foreign body with forceful nose blowing while occluding unaffected nostril and keeping the mouth closed.
H. If forceful blowing is not successful, attempt to remove the foreign object using the most appropriate instrument or technique (wire loop or curette, alligator or Hartman forceps, bayonet forceps, right-angle hooks and suctioning). The choice of instrument for removal is dependent upon the type of object, location, and how well the patient is able to cooperate during the procedure.
I. Simple external pressure should be applied to prevent bleeding.

Evaluation/Results of Procedure

A. Evaluate the other nares and ears if one foreign object is found.
B. Follow-up in 2 days to evaluate the mucosa.
C. Consult a physician if you are unable to dislodge or remove the object.

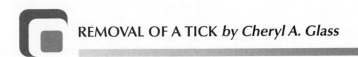

Description

A. Ticks are vectors for Lyme disease, and Rocky Mountain Spotted Fever. Ticks should be removed as soon as possible since they pass bacteria that causes the fevers and rashes.

Indications

A. There are several populations at risk for tick-borne transmission diseases, including hunters, campers, persons in contact with dogs and other animals with ticks, and those in contact with heavy, brushy areas.

Equipment Required

A. Tweezers
B. Antiseptic or rubbing alcohol
C. Gloves, nonsterile may be used
D. Office setting: Scalpel if the tick head remains embedded.

Procedure

A. Use gloves.
B. Remove the tick: refer to the teaching guide.
C. Examine for the entire head and body removal; if the head is embedded, a small incision may be required for the removal.
D. Cleanse the skin with antiseptic or rubbing alcohol.
E. See the Section III Patient Teaching Guide for Chapter 15, "Lyme Disease and Removal of a Tick."

Evaluation/Results of Procedure

A. Examine the rest of the body for other ticks.
B. Try to determine the length of time the tick was on the skin.
C. Assess for symptoms of Lyme disease and Rocky Mountain Spotted Fever.
D. Medications and consultants as applicable.

Blumenfeld, H. (n.d.). Neuroanatomy through clinical cases: Extraocular movements (CN III, IV, VI). Retrieved March 28, 2010, from http://www.neuroexam.com/content.php?p=20

Family Practice Notebook.com. *Orthopedics Book.* (n.d.). Ankle anterior drawer test. Retrieved March 28, 2010, from http://www.fpnotebook.com/Ortho/Exam/AnklAntrDrwrTst.htm

Family Practice Notebook.com. *Orthopedics Book.* (n.d.). McMurray test. Retrieved March 28, 2010, from http://www.fpnotebook.com/Ortho/Exam/McmryTst.htm

Family Practice Notebook.com. *Orthopedics Book.* (n.d.) Talar tilt. Retrieved March 28, 2010, from http://www.fpnotebook.com/Ortho/Exam/TlrTlt.htm

Frank, C., & Brooks, P. (2000). Practice tips: Bedside cystometry, simple diagnostic skill for family physicians. *Canadian Family Physician, 46,* 559–560.

Freidlander, J. A., Mascarenhas, M. R., Garner, L. M., & Cunningham, F. (2008, December 1). Rectal prolapse. *emedicine.* Retrieved March 28, 2010, from http://emedicine.medscape.com/article/931455-print

Merck Sharp & Dohme Corporation. (2009–2010). The Epley maneuver: A possible cure for vertigo? *The Merck manual of health and aging.* Retrieved March 5, 2010, from http://www.merck.com/pubs/mmanual_ha/figures/fg20_1.html

Murray, T. A., Kelly, N. R., & Jenkins, S. (2002). The complete neurological examination: What every nurse should know. *Advance for Nurse Practitioners, 10,* 25–29.

Schraga, E. D. (2009 March 29). Foreign body removal, nose. *emedicine.* Retrieved March 28, 2010, from http://emedicine.medscape.com/article/149299-print

Seidel, H. M., Ball, J. W., Dains, J. E., & Benedict, G. W. (1991). *Mosby's guide to physical examination* (2nd ed.). New York: Mosby Year-Book. Establishing the Estimated Date of Delivery

Patient Teaching Guides

- Health Maintenance
- Pain Management
- Dermatology Conditions
- Eye Disorders
- Ear Disorders
- Nasal Disorders
- Throat and Mouth Disorders
- Respiratory Disorders
- Cardiovascular Disorders
- Gastrointestinal Disorders
- Genitourinary Disorders
- Obstetrics
- Gynecology
- Sexually Transmitted Infections
- Infectious Diseases
- Systemic Disorders
- Musculoskeletal Disorders
- Neurologic Disorders
- Endocrine Disorders
- Psychiatric Disorders

Patient Teaching Guides for Chapter 1: Health Maintenance

- Infant Nutrition
- Childhood Nutrition
- Adolescent Nutrition
- Exercise

INFANT NUTRITION

BREAST-FEEDING

Breast milk is the best choice for feeding infants. Mothers are encouraged to breast-feed for at least 6–12 months. However, if you are unable to breast-feed for this length of time, breast-feeding for the first few weeks is highly beneficial to the newborn. If breast-feeding, you should consult with your practitioner prior to taking any medications.

ADVANTAGES OF BREAST-FEEDING

A. It allows for increased contact with your baby.

B. Breast milk is digested more easily by infants than formula.

C. Breast milk causes fewer spit-ups and stomach problems than formula.

D. There's no preparation, it's ready to feed anytime, it's always the correct temperature.

E. It is inexpensive.

F. Babies who are breast-fed have fewer allergies in childhood.

G. Antibodies in the mother's breast milk protect the newborn against infections.

H. It prevents overfeeding. Breast-fed babies usually feed "on demand."

I. Some women choose to breast-feed and occasionally supplement with formula. This method also works well. For supplementing breast milk, a soy-based formula is usually tolerated by the baby.

J. The diet of a breast-feeding mother requires increased nutrition: 500 kilocalories above normal diet and increased fluids.
   1. Mom's diet should exclude caffeine, chocolate, cabbage, beans, and other gas-forming foods.
   2. Avoid alcohol.
   3. Avoid tobacco.

K. **Fluoride:**
   1. When your child is fed solely breast milk, you should consider adding a vitamin and fluoride supplement.
   2. Fluoride supplementation may also be needed for babies who live in an area where the water is low in fluoride.
   3. Fluoride is important for prevention of dental caries.
   4. Even though your baby does not have any teeth, he or she still needs fluoride for building the developing teeth.
   5. Consult with your practitioner regarding this supplementation.

BOTTLE FEEDING

If breast-feeding is not an option, nutritional formulas are available. Ask your practitioner which is best suited for your baby.

A. It is best to have 6–8 bottles and 6–10 nipples prepared.

B. Formula may be purchased in powder, concentrate, or ready-to-feed forms.

C. Please read the can and be aware of the proper mixing method for each type of formula.

D. When feeding your baby, make sure the nipple is full of milk to avoid getting excess air in the baby's stomach.

E. You should never prop bottles on blankets or other objects when feeding your baby.

ROUTINE SCHEDULE OF FEEDING

A. Newborn:
   1. Give a newborn baby 1–2 ounces of formula every 3–4 hours.
   2. Increase formula by 1 ounce as tolerated by the baby.
   3. Give similar amounts at each feeding. The approximate total amount of formula your baby should take per day is determined by his or her weight (see Table).
   4. If your baby seems dissatisfied with feedings, you may add 1/2 to 1 more ounce of formula. Be careful not to add more than this at a time, because overfeeding may cause the baby to have a "bellyache" or diarrhea.
   5. By 4 months of age, babies usually take 32 ounces of formula per day. At this time, solid foods (e.g., baby cereal) are introduced.

SOLIDS

A. Solid foods are generally introduced to the baby at approximately 4 months.
   1. You may introduce new solid baby food every 3–5 days as tolerated by your baby.
   2. It is necessary to use this 3- to 5-day span between foods in case your baby is allergic or does not tolerate a specific food.
   3. If you have waited after trying a new food, you will be able to determine which food your baby was not able to tolerate.

B. Begin with RICE infant cereal mixed with breast milk or formula.

C. Begin with 1 tablespoon. You may increase the amount to 2–5 tablespoons one to two times a day as tolerated by the baby.

D. Next, introduce fruits followed later by vegetables, increasing the amount as tolerated.

TABLE	Total Formula Needs per Infant Weight
Infant Weight (Pounds)	**Total Infant Formula per Day**
7	19 ounces a day in divided feedings
8	21 ounces a day in divided feedings
9	24 ounces a day in divided feedings
10	27 ounces a day in divided feedings
11	30 ounces a day in divided feedings

1. If your baby does not like one vegetable, wait a few weeks to try to introduce it again.
2. Some babies may be very finicky regarding the texture of solid food. Don't give up! One day the baby may accept the foods he or she used to spit out because of taste or texture.

E. Meats are usually the last food introduced and many babies do not like the texture; however, you should continue to offer them.

F. Juices are usually introduced last at approximately 6 months.

COW'S MILK

A. It is not recommended to feed cow's milk to a baby during the first year of life.

B. Cow's milk may be introduced after your baby turns 1 year old.

HONEY

Honey is not recommended during a baby's first year of life because of the risk of infant botulism.

NUTRITIONAL INFORMATION

Beechnut Nutrition: (800) 523-6633

Carnation's Special Delivery: (800) 782-7766

LaLeche League Helpline: (800) LA-LECHE

CHILDHOOD NUTRITION

TODDLERS

Appetite often decreases during the toddler years. Parents should monitor the child's nutrition by the weekly intake instead of the daily intake. Just like adults, children's appetites change, leaving them hungrier at certain times than others.

Toddlers love to be busy. Therefore, if mealtime tends to be a struggle, after the child tells you he or she is finished with the meal, let the child get up and move around, but continue to offer bites of the meal between the child's activities.

Toddlers also do best with finger foods, which are easy to pick up and eat. Finger food snacks such as crackers, carrots, and celery are great choices. Snacks between meals are important for children. Fresh fruit and vegetables are excellent snacks. Try to limit the amount of sweets and fats the child consumes. Obesity can be a nutritional concern, especially in the early childhood stages. See Table.

FAMILY TEACHING TIPS FOR FEEDING TODDLERS

A. Serve small portions, and provide a second serving when the first has been eaten. Just 1 or 2 tbsp is an adequate serving for the toddler. Too much food on the dish may overwhelm the child.

B. There is no *one* food essential to health. Allow substitution for a disliked food. Food jags in which toddlers prefer one food for days on end are common and not harmful. If the child refuses a particular food, such as milk, use appropriate substitutes such as pudding, cheese, yogurt, and cottage cheese. Avoid a battle of wills at mealtime.

C. Toddlers like simply prepared foods, served warm or cool, *not* hot or cold.

TABLE   Suggested Daily Food Guidelines for Toddlers

Food Items	Daily Amounts[a]	Comments/Rationale
Cooked eggs[b]	3–5 servings a week	Good source of protein; moderate use is recommended because of the high cholesterol content in egg yolks.
Breads, grains, and cereals; whole-grain or enriched	4 or more servings (e.g., ½ slice of bread, ½ cup cereal, 2 crackers, ¼ cup noodles)	Provides thiamine, niacin, and, if enriched, riboflavin and iron. Encourage the child to identify and enjoy a wide variety of foods.
Fruit juices; canned fruit or small pieces of fruit	3 or 4 child-sized servings (e.g., ½ cup juice, ¼–½ cup fruit pieces)	Use those rich in vitamins A and C. Also source of iron and calcium. Self-feeding enhances the child's sense of independence.
Vegetables	1 or 2 child-sized servings (e.g., ¼–½ cup)	Include at least 1 dark-green or yellow vegetable every other day for vitamin A.
Meat, fish, chicken, casseroles, cottage cheese, peanut butter, dried peas, and beans	2 child-sized servings (e.g., 1 oz meat, 1 egg, ½ cup casserole, ¼ cup cottage cheese, 1–2 tbsp peanut butter)	Source of complete protein, iron, thiamine, riboflavin, niacin, and vitamin B_{12}. Nuts and seeds should not be offered until after age 3, when the risk of choking is minimal.
Milk, yogurt, cheese	4–6 child-sized servings (e.g., 4–6 oz milk, ½ cup yogurt, 1 oz cheese)	Cheese, cottage cheese, and yogurt are good calcium and riboflavin sources; also sources of calcium, phosphorus, complete protein, riboflavin, and niacin; also vitamin D if fortified milk is used.
Fats and sweets	In moderation	May interfere with consumption of nutrient-rich foods; chocolate should be delayed until the child is 1 year old.
Salt and other seasonings	In moderation	Children's taste buds are more sensitive than those of adults; salt is a learned taste, and high intakes are related to high blood pressure.

[a] Amounts are daily totals and goals to be achieved gradually.
[b] New food item for the age group.
From "Growth and Development of the Infant: 28 Days to 1 Year. Nutrition," by N. Hatfield, in *Broadribb's Introductory Pediatric Nursing*, 5th ed., pp. 338–341, by M. G. Marks, 2007. Philadelphia: Lippincott-Raven Publishers, p. 249.

D. Provide a social atmosphere at mealtimes; allow the toddler to eat with others in the family. Toddlers learn by imitating the acceptance or rejection of foods by other family members.

E. Toddlers prefer foods they can pick up with their fingers; however, they should be allowed to use a spoon or fork when they want to try.

F. Try to plan regular mealtimes with small nutritious snacks planned between meals. Do not attach too much importance to food by urging the child to choose what to eat.

G. Dawdling at mealtime is common with this age group and can be ignored unless it stretches on to unreasonable lengths or becomes a play for power. Mealtime for the toddler should not exceed 20 minutes. Calmly remove food without comment.

H. Do not make desserts a reward for good eating habits. It gives unfair value to the dessert and makes vegetables or other foods seem less desirable.

I. Offer regularly planned nutritious snacks, such as milk, crackers, and peanut butter, cheese cubes, and pieces of fruit. Plan snacks midway between meals and at bedtime.

J. Remember that the total amount eaten each day is more important than the amount eaten at a specific meal.

Source: "Growth and Development of the Infant: 28 Days to 1 Year. Nutrition," by N. Hatfield, in *Broadribb's Introductory Pediatric Nursing,* 5th ed., pp. 338–341, by M. G. Marks, 2007. *Philadelphia: Lippincott-Raven Publishers, p. 248.*

ADOLESCENT NUTRITION

A. Adolescents need a well-balanced diet. However, requirements vary depending on the build and gender of the adolescent.

B. Adolescents go through a growing spurt and require extra nutrients during this time.
   1. Girls have a growth spurt generally between 10–14 years of age.
   2. Boys have a growth spurt generally between 12–15 years of age.

C. To help prevent obesity, it is important to set a good example.
   1. Limit junk foods.
   2. Limit sugary sodas.
   3. Limit fast food.
   4. Serve regular portions, not "super-sized."
   5. Teens need snacks between meals.
   6. Buy fresh vegetables and fruits for snacking.
   7. Many teens do not get enough vitamins from their regular diet and may need a vitamin supplement. See also Table.

D. Body image is important to teens.

If you are concerned about your child's eating either too much, "binging," or not eating enough to control his or her weight, "anorexia," you need to notify our office.

RESOURCES

United States Department of Agriculture Food Pyramid is located on the Internet at http://www.mypyramid.gov/

TABLE Suggested Number of Servings of Food Groups per Day	
Food Group	**Number of Servings per Day**
Milk/dairy	3 servings
Meat	2–3 servings
Fruits	3–4 servings
Vegetables	4–5 servings
Grains (breads and cereal)	9–11 servings

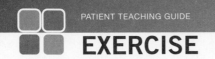

EXERCISE

You have been evaluated and cleared for an exercise program. Your maximum target heart rate during exercise based on your age and physical fitness is _____ beats per minute.

Your goal is to exercise at least three times a week (nonconsecutive days). Your target heart rate should be sustained for 20 to 30 minutes for maximal cardiovascular effect.

A. **Your exercise plan should include four components of activity:**
   1. Warm up
      a. The warm-up phase prepares the body to increase the blood flow to the heart and decreases muscle tension. The **warm-up phase should last 10 to 20 minutes** and may include such exercises as head rotations, arm and shoulder circles, waist circles or bends, and side leg raises.
   2. Stretching
      a. Stretching prepares the major muscles for exercise. Slow stretching and holding repetitions helps to prevent injury. Examples of stretching: sitting hamstring leg stretches and holds, and arm stretches.
   3. Aerobic activity
      a. The aerobic phase of exercise should be continuous. **Your target heart rate should be maintained for 20 to 30 minutes for cardiovascular benefit.** Examples of aerobic activity: brisk walking, running, or swimming.
   4. Cool down phase
      a. **A cool down period for 5 to 10 minutes in length finishes your exercise.** This gradual cool down allows the body temperature to cool and slowly decreases the heart rate, preventing dizziness, fatigue, and nausea. Examples of cool down exercise: walking and cool down stretches.

B. **Exercise should be discontinued if the following symptoms develop:**
   1. Marked increase in shortness of breath (inability to talk while exercising)
   2. Chest pain, including left arm and jaw pain
   3. Irregular heart beat
   4. Nausea or vomiting
   5. Faintness or light-headedness
   6. Injury to muscle or joints (sprains, tears)
   7. Prolonged fatigue
   8. Muscle weakness

Seek immediate medical attention if you experience chest pain. If your shortness of breath or irregular heartbeat does not subside within 1 to 2 minutes of rest, seek help. Return to your health care provider for an evaluation prior to further exercise after you experience any other symptoms.

C. **Other ways exercise can be easily incorporated into daily activities:**
   1. Use the stairs instead of the elevator.
   2. Park away from buildings to add extra walking distance.
   3. Use the walking path and carry golf clubs instead of using golf carts.
   4. Play outdoor games of catch, kick ball, or hopscotch instead of indoor activities.
   5. Push mow your yard instead of riding or hiring others for lawn care.
   6. Take an evening walk in your neighborhood or use the local mall for all-weather exercise.
   7. Shovel snow from the sidewalk instead of using a snow blower.
   8. Sweep the porch patio instead of using a lawn blower.
   9. Rake leaves for composting.
   10. Rent or buy an exercise video on yoga, Tai Chi, or aerobics instead of a movie.
   11. Turn on your radio and dance.
   12. Walk your dog for 20 to 30 minutes at a time.

Patient Teaching Guides for Chapter 2: Pain Management

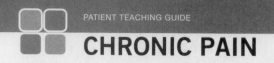

CHRONIC PAIN

RESOURCES

Many patient resources on pain are available at your local library, bookstores, and on the Internet. Look for a local support group in your area to join and learn how other people are coping with your same condition.

An excellent resource book written for patients, families, and physicians is *How to Cope With Chronic Pain,* by Nelson Hendler, MD (Cool Hand Communications, 1993).

There are many pain organizations available to assist patients. Patients may wish to visit these Web sites for further information.

American Academy of Pain Medicine: http://www.painmed.org/

American Chronic Pain Association: http://www.theacpa.org/

American Pain Society: www.ampainsoc.org

Arthritis Foundation: www.arthritis.org

National Fibromyalgia Association: www.fmaware.org

National Chronic Pain Outreach Association: www.chronicpain.org

BACK STRETCHES

You have been approved to do back-stretching exercise to help with your low back pain. Follow the instructions, starting slowly and to build your strength.

EQUIPMENT

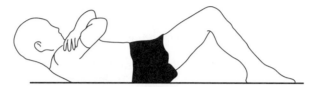

Use a mat or a towel on your floor for extra padding and comfort.

A. In the lying position

1. Lie on your back with knees bent. Cross your arms over your chest.
2. Raise your head and shoulders and curl your trunk upward, no more than 6 inches.
3. Keep the small of your back pressed against the mat.
4. Exhale during the curl up.
5. Hold _____ seconds; do _____ repetitions_____times a day. See Figure A.

Figure A Lie on a mat or towel. Raise head and shoulders as demonstrated.

B. In the standing position

1. Stand with your back against the wall.
2. Place your feet shoulder width apart and 18 inches from the wall.
3. Slowly slide down the wall until you are in the "chair" position.
4. Hold for 10 seconds and relax, then slide back up the wall to a standing position.
5. Do _____ repetitions _____ times a day. See Figure B.

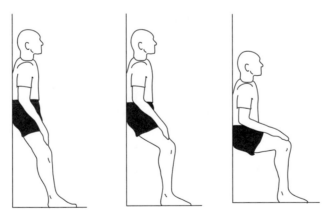

Figure B Place your feet shoulder with apart. Slide down against the wall to the "chair" position.

C. In the lying position

1. Bring your right knee slowly to your chest, holding it in place with your hands on your knee.
2. Relax the buttock and your back muscles.
3. Hold _____ seconds then relax with your right knee down.
4. Repeat with your left knee.
5. Now that you have stretched both legs, pull both of your knees up, holding them in place with your hands on your knees.
6. You will be curled in the fetal position.
7. Hold _____ seconds, then relax with your knees down.
8. Do _____ repetitions, _____ times per day. See Figure C.

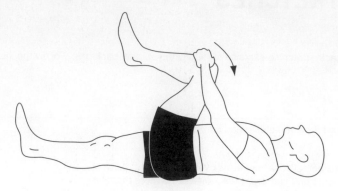

Figure C   Pull your left knee toward you chest to stretch, repeat with your right knee as demonstrated.

D. In the lying position
  1. Lie on you back with your knees bent.
  2. Tighten your abdominal muscles and squeeze. As you squeeze the buttock muscles, flatten your back toward the mat/towel (as shown in Figure D). Relax.
  3. Tighten your buttock muscles and lift your abdomen or "tummy" toward your knees while arching your back. Relax.
  4. Hold _____ seconds; do_____ repetitions _____ times a day. See Figure D.

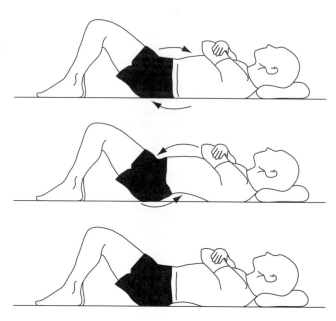

Figure D   Lie with knees bent, flatten your back then lift your tummy toward knees with back arched.

Patient Teaching Guides for Chapter 3: Dermatology Conditions

- Acne Vulgaris

- Dermatitis

- Erythema Multiforme

- Folliculitis

- Eczema

- Herpes Zoster (Shingles)

- Insect Bites and Stings

- Lice (Pediculosis)

- Lichen Planus

- Pityriasis Rosea

- Psoriasis

- Acne Rosacea

- Ringworm (Tinea)

- Scabies

- Seborrheic Dermatitis

- Skin Care Assessment

- Tinea Versicolor

- Warts

- Wounds

- Xerosis (Winter Itch)

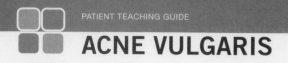

ACNE VULGARIS

PROBLEM

Acne vulgaris is blackheads, whiteheads, or red nodules noted on the face, back, chest, and arms.

CAUSE

Accumulation of cells and bacteria clog the pores and stimulate an inflammatory response, which results in papule or pustule (pimple or blackhead) formation.

PREVENTION/CARE

A. Wash area with mild soap (Purpose or Basis soap) no more than two times per day.

B. Avoid oil-based makeup and creams. Use matte-finished makeup or pore minimizer.

C. Use facial cleansers and moisturizers such as Cetaphil and Moisturel. These prevent the skin from drying out. Benzoyl peroxide 5% lotion or gel may be used at bedtime to help open pores and kill bacteria.

D. To prevent scarring, do not pick lesions.

E. Avoid excessive sun exposure. Use oil-free sunscreen with SPF 15 or greater.

F. Do not get frustrated if lesions return. Do not stop medications without the direction of your provider.

G. Stress can influence outbreaks of lesions. Practice routine exercise programs, stress management tactics, and other measures that decrease stress levels in your daily routine.

Activity: As tolerated: physical activity encouraged.

Diet: Eat a well-balanced diet. Drink 8 to 10 glasses of water a day to help keep your skin well hydrated. Cocoa and chocolate do not have an effect on the development of acne vulgaris.

Medications: Antibiotics may need to be prescribed.

You Have Been Prescribed: _____

You Need to Take: _____

You Need to Notify the Office If:

A. You have a reaction to any of the medications prescribed.

B. You are unable to tolerate the prescribed medications.

Phone: _____

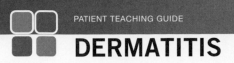

DERMATITIS

PROBLEM

Inflammation of the skin that occurs from contact with an irritant substance (poison ivy, soaps, and so forth).

CAUSE

Skin contact with irritating agent.

PREVENTION/TREATMENT PLAN

A. Avoid aggravating agents.

B. Learn to recognize all plants (poison ivy, poison oak, and so forth).

C. Flare-ups are common.

D. Avoid all known stimuli (poison ivy, soaps, and so forth).

E. Do not wear tight, restrictive clothing.

F. When around irritating substances, wear gloves for protection.

G. For poison ivy

    1. Wash all clothes, shoes, pets, or other substances that may have come in contact with the poison ivy oil.

Activity: As tolerated. Take cool baths as needed for itching. Oatmeal baths (Aveeno Bath) help soothe the itching.

Diet: Regular diet.

Medications: Take Benadryl as needed for itching. Use calamine lotion as needed. Steroid creams may also be prescribed if reaction is severe. Steroid dose packs may be needed if you are not getting better.

You Have Been Prescribed: _____

You Need to Take: _____

You Need to Notify the Office If You Have:

A. Worsening symptoms.

B. Sores on your face, eyes, or ears.

C. More redness, swelling, pain or drainage.

D. Secondary bacterial infection.

E. Fever

F. Other: _____

Phone: _____

ERYTHEMA MULTIFORME

PROBLEM

An acute inflammatory disorder of the skin and mucous membranes, erythema multiforme is usually self-limited and benign.

A severe form is known as Stevens-Johnson syndrome or erythema multiforme majus, and the less severe form is referred to as erythema multiforme minus.

CAUSE

The cause is unknown in 50% of the cases. Erythema multiforme has been associated with viral infections, particularly the herpes simplex virus; bacterial and protozoan infections; an immunologic reaction of the skin; medications (sulfonamides, penicillins, anticonvulsants, salicylates, barbiturates), with reactions occurring up to 7 to 14 days after using the medication; pregnancy; premenstrual hormone changes; malignancy; or radiation therapy. Risk increases with previous history of erythema multiforme.

PREVENTION/CARE

A. Avoid suspected causes.

B. Seek prompt treatment of any illness or infection.

C. Prevent herpes simplex virus outbreaks by avoiding sun exposure and reducing stress.

D. Seek treatment immediately if at any time symptoms seem to be worsening or increasing.

E. Discontinue any implicated medication.

F. Apply wet dressings or soaks, with Burow's solution, or apply lotions to soothe the skin.

G. Bathe in lukewarm to cool water three times a day for 30 minutes.

H. Monitor yourself for any eye involvement and report it to your health care provider immediately.

I. If mouth sores are present, use good oral hygiene (brush two to three times a day using a soft brush) and rinse frequently with cool water.

J. Hospitalization may be required if there is extensive skin involvement.

Activity: As tolerated by the extent of the symptoms. Restrict yourself to bed rest if fever is present.

Diet: Usually no special diet is necessary, although if mouth sores are present, a soft or liquid diet may be better tolerated. Increase fluid intake above the general 8 to 10 glasses per day.

Medications: May be prescribed to control symptoms and pain

You Have Been Prescribed: _____

You Need to Take: _____

You Need to Notify the Office If:

A. You have an adverse reaction to or cannot tolerate any of the prescribed medications.

B. Symptoms worsen during treatment, or the rash does not clear in 3 weeks (usual course: rash evolves over 1 to 2 weeks, usually clears in 2 to 3 weeks, but may take 5 to 6 weeks).

C. New or unexplained symptoms develop.

D. You have any questions or concerns.

Phone: _____

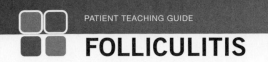

FOLLICULITIS

PROBLEM

A bacterial (or fungal) infection of the hair follicle. Folliculitis is seen when a pustule develops, commonly on the arms, legs, scalp, and face (beard).

CAUSE

A. Bacterial: Infection commonly caused by *Staphylococcus* bacteria.

B. Fungal: May be caused by yeast infection.

PREVENTION/TREATMENT

A. Keep skin clean and dry.

B. Avoid warm, moist conditions.

C. Healing generally occurs in 10 to 14 days after proper treatment with medications.

D. Use good hand washing technique, using antibacterial soaps.

E. Use clean razors daily.

F. Throw old razors away.

G. Do no share razors.

H. Shampoo scalp daily.

I. Folliculitis usually resolves within 4 to 6 weeks after proper treatment.

Activity: As tolerated.

Diet: Regular diet.

Medications: Topical and/or oral antibiotics as prescribed.

You Have Been Prescribed: _____

You Need to Take: _____

You Need to Notify the Office If:

A. You notice lesions worsening or spreading, despite adequate medication treatment.

B. You have a fever higher than 101°F.

C. Your condition is not getting better.

D. You have a reaction to your medication.

Phone: _____

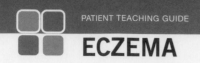

ECZEMA

PROBLEM

Red, itching, scaling, and thickening of skin occurs in patches. You may have papules (bumps) with vesicles (clear fluid) that can be found especially on the hands, scalp, face, back of the neck, or skin creases of elbows and knees.

CAUSE

The cause is unknown. If an allergic reaction, it may be caused by foods such as eggs, wheat, milk, or seafood; wool clothing; skin lotions and ointments; soaps; detergents; cleansers; plants; tanning agents used for shoe leather; dyes; and topical medications. The risk for developing eczema increases with stress, medical history of other allergic conditions, clothing made of synthetic fabric (which traps perspiration), and weather extremes (cold, hot).

PREVENTION/CARE

A. Avoid risk factors.

B. Wear rubber gloves for household cleaning tasks.

C. Wear loose, cotton clothing to help absorb perspiration.

D. Keep fingernails short and wear soft gloves during sleep.

E. Scratching worsens eczema.

F. Bathe less frequently to avoid excessive skin dryness.

G. Use special nonfat soaps (Purpose or Basis soap) and tepid water.

H. Do not use soap on inflamed areas.

I. Lubricate the skin after bathing; avoid lubricants with alcohol in the ingredients.

J. Recommended creams include Eucerin, Keri Lotion, and Lubriderm. Steroid creams may be prescribed.

K. Avoid extreme temperature changes.

L. Avoid anything that has previously worsened the condition.

Activity: No restrictions.

Diet: You may be told to try a special diet. Eliminate any foods known to cause flare-ups.

Medications:

You Have Been Prescribed: _____

You Need to Take: _____

You Need to Notify the Office If:

A. You have a reaction to any of the medications prescribed.

B. You cannot take the medications.

C. New symptoms develop.

Phone: _____

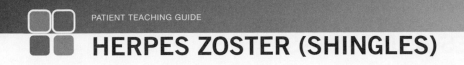

HERPES ZOSTER (SHINGLES)

PROBLEM

Shingles is a reactivation of the viral infection in childhood known as chickenpox. **The virus is contagious for those who have not had the chickenpox.**

CAUSE

Varicella-zoster virus is stimulated and produces a blisterlike rash, commonly seen on the chest and trunk area. The rash is commonly confined to one side of the body.

PREVENTION

Zostavax® is a vaccination for the prevention of shingles. The Centers for Disease Control and Prevention recommends this one-time vaccine for anyone age 60 and older.

TREATMENT

A. Zostavax® cannot be used to treat the shingles breakouts or the painful sensations (postherpetic neuralgia) after you develop shingles.

B. The shingles rash usually lasts 2 to 3 weeks; however, symptoms may persist beyond this period.

C. The goal is to relieve the itching.

D. Apply warm soaks of Burow's solution three times a day to lesions.

E. Notify family and friends of active virus. Advise anyone who has had contact with you that you have shingles, especially pregnant women and those who have never had the chickenpox.

Activity: Avoid touching the shingles. Wash your hands. Your partners should not touch the area especially when blisters are present. Use separate bath towels.

Diet: There is no special diet for shingles.

Medications: Oral and topical medications may be prescribed to soothe the itching. Take acetaminophen (Tylenol) as needed for comfort. Antiviral medications are available to help slow down the virus if started within 48 to 72 hours after the initial outbreak. You may be prescribed medications to help with the painful sensations (neuralgia).

You Have Been Prescribed: _____

You Need to Take: _____

You Need to Notify the Office If You Have:

A. Severe pain at lesion sites.

B. Any new symptoms relating to the shingles, such as excruciating pain, headaches, numbness, tingling sensation, or other symptoms.

C. Any questions regarding the shingles.

Phone: _____

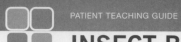

INSECT BITES AND STINGS

PROBLEM

Skin changes and insect bites or stings cause other reactions.

A. **Seek immediate help if you or a family member has any symptoms of allergic reaction or anaphylaxis, either immediately after the bite or in 8 to 12 hours after the bite.**

B. You may need to call 911 or your local emergency response service.

C. If you have had a previous life-threatening allergic reaction, carry an anaphylaxis kit for emergency treatment.
   1. *Local skin reactions* include red bumps in the skin that usually appear within minutes after the bite or sting, but may not appear for 6 to 12 hours. Itching and discomfort may occur at the site.

   2. *Systemic (body) reactions* include nausea or vomiting; headache, fever, dizziness or light-headedness; swelling; or convulsions.

   3. *Allergic reactions* include itchy eyes, facial flushing, dry cough; wheezing; or chest or throat constriction or tightness.

CAUSE

Bites or stings can be caused by mosquitoes, fleas, chiggers, bedbugs, ants, spiders, bees, scorpions, and other insects.

Risk increases with exposure to areas with heavy insect infestation, warm weather in spring and summer, lack of protective measures, use of perfumes or colognes, and previous sensitization.

PREVENTION/CARE

A. **Institute first-aid measures and activate emergency services if severe, life-threatening reactions occur.**

B. Avoid risk factors.

C. Wear protective clothing.

D. Use insect repellents with diethyltoluamide (DEET), avoiding the head, face, eyes, and mouth, especially with children.

E. Products containing DEET are not recommended for children under the age of 2 years.

SPECIFIC INSECT CARE

A. For all stingers: remove stinger.

B. Bee, wasp, yellow jacket, or hornet stings: rub a paste of meat tenderizer and water into the site.

C. Ant bites: rub bite with ammonia, and repeat as often as necessary.

D. Spider and scorpion bites: capture the arachnid if possible and seek medical attention.

E. Mites: apply a petroleum product (Vaseline) until the animal withdraws from the skin.

F. Ticks: remove the tick by following the instructions in the Patient Teaching Guide for Chapter 15, "Lyme Disease and Removal of a Tick."

GENERAL CARE FOR ALL BITES

A. Clean wound with soap and water.

B. Apply ice pack (no ice directly on skin, use towel or cloth to protect skin).

C. Elevate and rest the affected body part.

D. Immerse affected part or apply warm water soaks to site. However, if site itches, cool water feels best.

E. For minor discomfort, you may use nonprescription oral antihistamines (Benadryl) or topical steroid preparations (hydrocortisone cream).

F. Use only low-potency topical steroid products without fluorine on the face and groin area.

G. You may be prescribed more potent, prescription medications.

Activity: No restrictions.

Diet: Eat a regular diet. Maintain adequate hydration with 8 to 10 glasses of water per day.

Medications: You may be prescribed an EPIPEN to use for future major reactions. You need to keep this with you at all times.

You Have Been Prescribed: _____

You Need to Take: _____

You Need to Notify the Office If:

    A. Self-care treatment does not relieve symptoms or if no improvement is noticed after 2 to 3 days.

    B. A bitten area becomes red, swollen, warm, and tender to the touch. These symptoms indicate infection.

    C. You have a temperature higher than or equal to 101°F.

    D. You have a reaction or cannot tolerate any of the prescribed medications.

Phone: _____

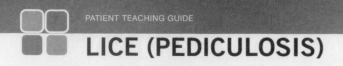

LICE (PEDICULOSIS)

PROBLEM

A parasite called a louse has been found on your body or hair. Lice tend to live on the scalp, eyebrows, or genital area or in warm moist areas of your skin. You may notice you have intense itching, swelling, or reddened areas of the skin and sometimes even enlarged lymph glands.

CAUSE

The lice bite the skin and cause the intense itching. Lice and their eggs (called nits) may be difficult to see on the skin and shafts of hair. Lice look like small, 2- to 3-mm, tan-colored bugs. The eggs are tiny white eggs that stick to the hair shaft.

PREVENTION

You can prevent repeated episodes of lice if you bathe daily; avoid crowded living conditions; change the bed linens frequently; do not share hats, combs, brushes, or other belongings. When your children or other family members have been in contact with others diagnosed with lice, check family members closely for lice and treat as appropriate.

TREATMENT PLAN

A. Use medicated shampoo as directed.

B. Machine wash all linens, stuffed animals, or any other items with which the lice may have come in contact.

C. Wash clothes in hot, soapy water.

D. Dry all linens in a hot dryer for at least 30 minutes.

E. Items that cannot be washed must be taken to the dry cleaner or wrapped and sealed in a plastic bag for 14 days.

F. Boil all hair accessories and clean well.

G. Do not share hats and combs.

H. Spray all furniture with appropriate products that kill all nits and lice.

I. Vacuum.

Activity: There is no activity restriction.

Diet: There is no special diet.

Medications:

You Have Been Prescribed to Use _____ Shampoo.

A. Treat as directed on the bottle.

B. After shampooing as directed, make sure to remove each single nit from each shaft of hair. Any nits left in the hair will hatch and start the cycle over again.

C. Repeat in 24 hours, then again in 1 week.

You Need to Notify the Office If You Have:

A. Any questions regarding the removal of the nits and lice, or if you need any assistance. If other family members need to be evaluated, please let us know. If secondary infection occurs, please call the office.

Phone: _____

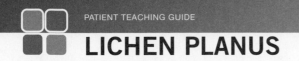

LICHEN PLANUS

PROBLEM

A chronic skin eruption, lichen planus is not cancerous or contagious. It frequently appears as small, slightly raised, itchy, purplish bumps with a whitish surface. Sudden hair loss from the head may occur. Lichen planus may involve the skin of the legs, trunk, arms, wrists, scalp, or penis; the lining of the mouth or vagina; and the nailbeds of the toenails and fingernails.

CAUSE

The cause is unknown, but it may be caused by a virus. In a few cases, this may be an adverse reaction to certain drugs. The risk of developing lichen planus increases with stress, fatigue, or exposure to drugs or chemicals.

PREVENTION/CARE

Currently, there are no known preventive measures.

A. The goal of treatment is to relieve symptoms.

B. Use cool-water soaks to relieve itching.

C. Reduce stress; this may help to prevent recurrences. Learn relaxation techniques or obtain counseling if necessary.

D. Speak with your health care provider if you suspect a drug to be the cause.

Activity: No restrictions.

Diet: Eat a well-balanced diet; drink 8 to 10 glasses of water every day.

Medications:

You Have Been Prescribed: _____

You Need to Take: _____

You Need to Notify the Office If:

A. You have a reaction to any of the prescribed medications.

B. You are unable to tolerate the prescribed medications.

C. Hair loss or nail destruction occur.

D. New lesions appear as old lesions resolve.

E. Other: _____

Phone: _____

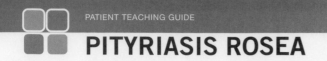

PITYRIASIS ROSEA

PROBLEM

Pityriasis rosea is a very common condition characterized by a rash, which may or may not itch. You may have noticed a large scaly patch prior to breaking out with the more generalized rash. **It is not known to be contagious, and you do not need to isolate yourself.**

CAUSE

The cause of pityriasis rosea is unknown.

PREVENTION

Because the cause of pityriasis rosea is unknown, there are no recommended preventive measures.

TREATMENT PLAN

Good hygiene and avoidance of scratching is recommended to prevent a secondary infection.

Activity: It is not necessary for you to limit your activity.

Diet: No changes are required in your diet.

Medications: You may be prescribed an antihistamine medication to take by mouth and topical steroid creams to apply to the rash itself. If the itching is severe, you may have oral steroids prescribed.

You Have Been Prescribed: _____

You Need to Take: _____

You Need to Notify the Office If You Have:

    A. Any new symptoms.

    B. Any reaction to your medication.

Phone: _____

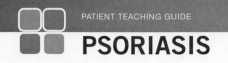

PSORIASIS

PROBLEM

Psoriasis is a chronic, scaly skin disorder with frequent remissions and recurrences. The skin of the scalp, elbows, knees, chest, back, arms, legs, toenails, fingernails, and fold between the buttocks may be involved.

CAUSE

The cause of psoriasis is unknown.

PREVENTION/CARE

A. There is no known prevention, but symptoms can be controlled.

B. Moving to a warmer climate might be beneficial. Severity increases with cold.

C. Maintain good skin hygiene with daily baths or showers.

D. Avoid harsh soaps.

E. Avoid skin injury, including harsh scrubbing, which can trigger new outbreaks.

F. Avoid skin dryness.

G. To reduce scaling, use nonprescription, waterless cleansers and hair preparations containing coal tar (Zetar, T/Gel, Pentrax), emollients (Eucerin Plus lotion or cream, Lubriderm, Moisture Plus, Moisturel), or products containing cortisone (often prescription strength).

H. Expose the skin to moderate amounts of sunlight as often as possible. Avoid long periods in the sun to prevent sunburn.

I. Oatmeal baths may loosen scales. Use 1 cup of oatmeal to a tub of warm water.

J. Stress may increase outbreaks of psoriasis. Consider counseling to assist in lifestyle changes, coping, or any psychological problems caused by psoriasis.

Activity: There are no activity restrictions.

Diet: Eat a well-balanced diet. You may be instructed to try a gluten-free diet. Drink 8 to 10 glasses of water per day.

Medications: You may be prescribed the following types of medications:

A. Ointments containing coal tar. These may stain clothing.

B. Topical cortisone drugs with special dressings.

C. Psoralen plus ultraviolet light (PUVA) (combination of a medication and exposure to ultraviolet A light).

D. Combination of tar baths with ultraviolet B light.

E. Antihistamines to relieve itching.

You Have Been Prescribed: _____

You Need to Take: _____

You Need to Notify the Office If:

A. You have an adverse reaction to or cannot tolerate any of the prescribed medications.

B. Symptoms recur after treatment. Notify your health care provider if during an outbreak, pustules erupt on the skin and/or are accompanied by fever, muscle aches, and fatigue.

C. New, unexplained symptoms develop.

D. Other: _____

Phone: _____

For severe cases, you may be referred to a dermatologist (specialist for skin disorders).

ADDITIONAL RESOURCE

National Psoriasis Foundation
Suite 200
6415 SW Canyon Ct.
Portland, OR 97221
Phone: 800-723-9166
http://www.psoriasis.org/

ACNE ROSACEA

PROBLEM

Acne rosacea appears as red, thickened skin on the nose and cheeks with small blood vessels on the skin surface. You may see flushing associated with facial tenderness.

CAUSE

The cause is unknown. The condition is worsened by stress, warm drinks, hot or spicy foods, and alcohol.

TREATMENT/CARE

A. There are no specific preventive measures.

B. Symptoms can be controlled with treatment.

C. You may have frequent flare-ups.

D. Seek care if you notice evidence of rosacea.

E. Avoid oil-based makeup.

F. Use the thinner water-based makeup preparations.

G. Reduce stress.
1. Seek counseling if symptoms cause distress.
2. Learn and practice relaxation techniques (deep breathing, yoga, listen to music, and visualization).

Activity: No restrictions.

Diet: Eat a well-balanced diet; drink 8 to 10 glasses of water every day.

Medications:

A. Do not use cortisone preparations, including the nonprescription preparations (they may cause the condition to worsen).

B. Antibiotics or topical medications may be prescribed.

C. A special prescription medication may be prescribed. This medication cannot be used if you are pregnant.

You Have Been Prescribed: _____

You Need to Take: _____

You Need to Notify the Office If:

A. You have a reaction to any of the medications prescribed.
B. You are unable to tolerate the prescribed medications.
C. Other: _____

Phone: _____

RESOURCE

National Rosacea Society: http://www.rosacea.org/index.php

RINGWORM (TINEA)

PROBLEM

Ringworm is a fungal infection of the skin, which can be found on any part of the body. A worm does NOT cause ringworm. It gets the name because of the round ring shape that is red on the outside and normal on the inside. It is not uncommon to get more than one time. Other tinea fungal infections are:

A. Tinea pedis (athlete's foot)

B. Tinea cruris (jock itch)

C. Tinea capitis (ringworm on the head)

CAUSE

The fungus is transmitted by direct contact. It can be transmitted from objects, shoes, locker rooms, animals, and people.

PREVENTION/TREATMENT

A. Use good hygiene including not sharing hairbrushes and combs.

B. Keep skin cool and dry.

C. Wear shoes in locker rooms, and pools.

D. Wear loose-fitting clothing.

E. Treat pets' skin problems adequately. Ringworm is often blamed on cats but it can come from almost any animal including horses, rabbits, dogs, and pigs.

F. Infections of fingernails and toenails may require prescription medications.

Activity: As tolerated. Some contact sports may increase getting tinea (football and wrestling).

Diet: There is no special diet.

Medications:

You Have Been Prescribed: _____

You Need to Take: _____   _____

You Need to Notify the Office If:

A. Your symptoms get worse.

B. Other: _____

Phone: _____

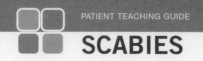

SCABIES

PROBLEM

Scabies is a common condition characterized by severe itching. You may have noticed small burrows between your fingers and in other locations, or you may have some redness and skin irritation that is aggravated by scratching.

CAUSE

Scabies is caused by an infestation of the skin by a mite. You have contracted scabies by coming in close contact with an individual who has the condition.

PREVENTION

You can prevent reinfection of scabies by following these measures:

A. Make sure all close contacts, sexual partners, family, and household contacts are treated.

B. All bedding and clothing that has touched infected skin should be machine washed and machine dried on the highest heat cycle.

C. Any clothing or bedding that cannot be laundered in the above way should be placed in a plastic bag that is securely tied for at least a week. The mites cannot live this long away from human skin.

D. Coats, furniture, rugs, floors, and walls do not require any special cleaning or treatment.

TREATMENT PLAN

A. Most patients with scabies are successfully treated with only one overnight application of a cream known as a scabicide.

B. You should let your practitioner know if you are pregnant or breast-feeding.

C. You may itch for up to a week even with successful treatment.

D. If you still have symptoms after 2 weeks, you should see your practitioner, who will determine if you need a second treatment.

Activity: Affected children in day care or school can return the day after treatment is completed.

Diet: There is no special diet.

Medications: The most common medications used to treat scabies include:

A. Permethrin (Elimite cream), which is applied to all body areas from the neck down and washed off in 8 to 14 hours.

B. Lindane (Kwell cream), which is applied to all skin surfaces from the neck down and washed off in 8 to 12 hours.

C. You may be told to use Benadryl 25 to 50 mg if needed for itching.

D. Do not use it near your eyes.

You Have Been Prescribed: _____

You Need to Apply: _____

You Need to Notify the Office If:

A. You have new symptoms.

B. You have a reaction to the medication.

C. Other: _____

Phone: _____

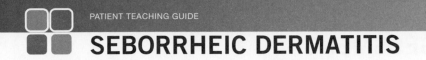

SEBORRHEIC DERMATITIS

PROBLEM

Seborrheic dermatitis is a skin condition characterized by greasy or dry, white, flaking scales over reddish patches on the skin. The scales anchor to the hair shafts and may itch, but they are usually painless unless complicated by infection.

CAUSE

The cause is unknown. The risk of seborrheic dermatitis increases with stress; hot and humid or cold and dry weather; infrequent shampoos; oily skin; other skin disorders such as rosacea, acne, or psoriasis; obesity; Parkinson's disease; use of lotions that contain alcohol; and HIV/AIDS.

PREVENTION/CARE

A. There are no specific preventive measures.

B. The goal of care is to minimize the severity or frequency of symptoms.

1. Shampoo vigorously and as often as once a day. The type of shampoo is not as important as the way you scrub your scalp. To loosen scales, scrub with your fingernails while shampooing, and scrub at least 5 minutes.

2. If you suffer from minor dandruff, you may use nonprescription dandruff shampoos with selenium sulfide (Selsun Blue, Exsel) or zinc pyrithione (Zincon) and lubricating skin lotion.

3. For severe problems, shampoos that contain coal tar or scalp creams that contain cortisone may be prescribed. **Do not use coal tar products on infants or children without specific physician prescription.**

4. To apply medication to the scalp, part the hair a few strands at a time, and rub the ointment or lotion vigorously into the scalp.

5. Topical steroids may be prescribed for other affected parts of the skin.

6. Be sure to dry skin folds thoroughly after bathing.

7. Wear loose, ventilating clothing; avoid constant cap wearing.

Activity: No restrictions. Outdoor activities in the summer may help alleviate symptoms.

Diet: Eat a well-balanced diet. Drink 8 to 10 glasses of water per day. Avoid foods that seem to worsen your condition.

Medications:

You Have Been Prescribed: _____

You Need to Take: _____

You Need to Notify the Office If:

A. You have an adverse reaction to any of the prescribed medications.

B. You are unable to tolerate any of the medications.

C. You have any secondary infection in affected area.

D. Other: _____

Phone: _____

SKIN CARE ASSESSMENT

PROBLEM

Skin cancer is the most common type of cancer. In 2006 the Centers for Disease Control and Prevention notes the rate of skin cancer varies by the state where you live. A state map is located on the Internet at http://www.cdc.gov/cancer/skin/statistics/state.htm.

CAUSE

Skin cancer is frequently caused by damage from the ultraviolet rays of the sun. Some people are at a higher risk for developing skin cancer. These risk factors include:

A. Fair complexion

B. Advanced age with sun-damaged skin

C. A history of a severe sunburn

D. A history of spending long hours outdoors

E. Having a history of X-ray procedures for skin conditions

F. Genetic susceptibility

PREVENTION/CARE

A. Protect yourself and prevent sun exposure to your skin by staying out of the harmful rays as much as possible, especially between the hours of 11:00 AM to 2:30 PM. This time frame accounts for approximately 70% of the harmful ultraviolet radiation.

B. If you are exposed to the sun, wear a sunscreen product with an SPF of 15 or greater at all times.

C. Wear hats that screen your face and neck and your ears.

D. Clothing is available with sun-protective materials. Regular long shirts and long pants also help to protect your skin.

E. Sit in the shade to rest.

F. Do not use a tanning booth.

STEPS TO TAKE TO PREVENT YOURSELF FROM BEING A VICTIM OF SKIN CANCER

A. Examine your skin monthly.

   1. Use a good light source and a mirror to see areas of your skin not clearly visible.

   2. Examine your entire body closely.

   3. Pay particular attention to areas that are frequently exposed to the sun, especially your face, lips, eyes, neck, scalp, and ears.

   4. Monthly screening allows you to familiarize yourself with birthmarks and moles. Note the size, shape, and color of these marks. Note any changes in these marks, using the "ABCDE" method:

      a. *Asymmetry:* The shape of the mark should be noted. Any change in shape or irregularity of the mark needs to be evaluated by your health care provider.

      b. *Border:* Look carefully at the border of the mark. If the border edge is ragged, notched, and not smooth, your health care provider needs to evaluate it.

      c. *Color:* Note the color of moles. If you notice any change in color, or if you notice the mole to have several colors (brown, black, tan, red, and so forth), you need to alert your health care provider.

      d. *Diameter:* Measure the size of the mark and document it. Any change in size, especially if it is greater than 6 mm, should be brought to the attention of your health care provider.

      e. *Elevation:* Note elevation of lesion, change in size, and any evolving changes of the lesion. You need to alert your health care provider if changes occur.

   5. You should also evaluate lesions on your skin for any type of change. If the lesions begin bleeding or hurting or change in texture or in any other way, your health care provider needs to evaluate the change.

   6. Be alerted to any skin ulcers that do not heal within 1 month. Also, any new moles or lesions need to be evaluated by your health care provider for proper diagnosis of the type of lesion.

Activity: As tolerated but protect yourself from sun exposure.

Diet: There is no special diet that will stop skin cancer.

Medications: There are no medications that prevent skin cancer.

You Need to Notify the Office If You Have:

   A. Any of the skin changes mentioned above that need to be evaluated by your health care provider.

Phone: _____

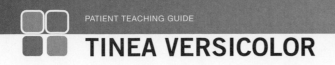

TINEA VERSICOLOR

PROBLEM

A yeast infection of the skin, tinea versicolor may cause color changes of the skin, commonly on the chest, back, shoulders, arms, and trunk. During the summer, these spots usually appear pale and do not tan. During the winter, the spots may appear pinker or darker than the normal skin color.

CAUSE

Tinea versicolor is caused by an increased production of yeast on the skin, which is influenced by warm, moist conditions. It is common to have recurring episodes.

PREVENTION/TREATMENT PLAN

A. Air dry skin as much as possible.

B. Apply medication as directed.

C. Patches on skin (color changes) may take several weeks to be resolved.

D. Monthly treatments may help prevent recurrences.

Activity: There are no activity restrictions with tinea versicolor.

Diet: There is no special diet.

Medications:

A. Apply Selsun Blue shampoo or other medication as directed.

B. Most medications may be washed off of skin 30 minutes after application.

C. Selsun Blue shampoo may be used daily on affected skin for 2 weeks.

D. Keep shampoo out of eyes and genital area.

E. Leave it on skin for about 20 minutes, and then rinse it off.

You Have Been Prescribed: _____

You Need to Take: _____

You Need to Notify the Office If You:

A. Do not see improvement, despite proper treatment.

B. Develop new symptoms.

C. Other: _____

Phone: _____

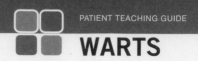

WARTS

PROBLEM

A wart is a raised roughlike growth projecting from the skin, which can be contagious.

CAUSE

Warts are caused by a viral infection that stimulates the cells of the skin to multiply rapidly, which results in an outward growth.

PREVENTION/TREATMENT

A. Wash hands well.

B. Avoid scratching or picking warts. Warts bleed easily.

C. Some warts go away spontaneously without any treatment after time.

D. Medications may be prescribed.

TO ENHANCE DESTRUCTION

A. Soak wart in warm water 10 to 15 minutes a day.

B. After soaking, use an emery board to file wart down.

C. Apply over-the-counter medication as prescribed (Compound W) to site.

D. Duct tape may be applied over wart.

E. Warts may reappear at the same spot or in other areas.

F. Cryotherapy "freezing" is another treatment option. Discuss this with your health care provider.

Activity: There are no activity restrictions for warts.

Diet: There are no special diets for warts.

Medications:

You Have Been Prescribed: _____

You Need to Take: _____

You Need to Notify the Office If:

A. You develop an infection at the site of the wart.

B. Other: _____

Phone: _____

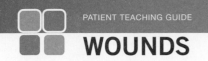

WOUNDS

PROBLEM

A wound is a break in the external surface of the body.

CAUSE

Wounds are often due to an accidental or intentional injury. Wound infection is usually caused by bacterial contamination of the site.

PREVENTION/CARE

A. Prevent accidental or intentional injury.

B. Immediately after injury, cleanse wound well with soap and water.

C. Remove all dirt and foreign material.

D. You may be prescribed antibiotics, if so take all antibiotics until they are completely gone.

E. You may need a tetanus shot.

Activity: No restrictions. If infection is present, you may need to increase rest.

Diet: Eat a well-balanced diet. Drink 8 to 10 glasses of water per day.

Medications:

You Have Been Prescribed: _____

You Need to Take: _____

You Need to Notify the Office If You Have:

A. A reaction or cannot tolerate any of the prescribed medications.

B. A fever and a general ill feeling.

C. A wound/infection that seems to worsen.

D. Any new or unexplained symptoms.

E. Any questions or concerns.

Phone: _____

XEROSIS (WINTER ITCH)

PROBLEM

Xerosis is severely chapped skin that becomes cracked, fissured, and inflamed. It can appear on skin anywhere on the body, but it is seen most commonly on the legs.

CAUSE

Xerosis is caused by insufficient oil on the skin's surface, which allows water to evaporate through the skin. Oil in the skin decreases with aging, excessive bathing, and excessive rubbing of the skin. An environment with low humidity also promotes dryness of the skin.

PREVENTION/CARE

A. Reduce water loss from the skin:

   1. Decrease the frequency and duration of baths or showers; use tepid water.

   2. Use soap sparingly.

   3. Avoid detergent soaps.

   4. Pat skin dry rather than rubbing.

   5. Apply skin lubricants (Lac-Hydrin, Eucerin, and so on) to dry skin before chapped areas become inflamed.

   6. Use ultrasonic, cool-mist humidifiers if the air is very dry.

   7. Clean the humidifier daily.

   8. Oil (such as Nivea) in the bath water may be helpful.

   9. Apply lubricants after bathing when possible to trap additional moisture before evaporation occurs.

B. Apply hand cream 4 to 8 times a day to hands and twice daily on the trunk and extremities.

Activity: No restrictions. Avoid long-term exposure to drying environments.

Diet: Eat a well-balanced diet; drink 8 to 10 glasses of water per day.

Medications:

You Have Been Prescribed: _____

You Need to Take: _____

You Need to Notify the Office If You Have:

   A. Severely chapped skin, and self-care does not relieve the symptoms in 1 week.

   B. Chapped skin that becomes inflamed or if you see any oozing.

   C. Any questions or concerns.

Phone: _____

Patient Teaching Guides for Chapter 4: Eye Disorders

- Conjunctivitis

- How to Administer Eye Medications

CONJUNCTIVITIS

PROBLEM

You have an infection of the eye, or conjunctivitis, that causes redness, itching, drainage from the eye, and crusting on the eyelids.

CAUSE

Bacteria, viruses, or allergies can cause eye infections.

PREVENTION

A. Wash your hands frequently.

B. Avoid persons with conjunctivitis such as pink eye.

C. Avoid known allergens.

TREATMENT PLAN

A. *All types:*

    1. Wash your hands frequently, especially after touching the eyes, to avoid spread.

    2. Use cool compresses on the eyes as needed.

    3. Wash crusting eyelids with baby shampoo daily.

    4. Wipe the eyes from inner to outer corners.

B. *Bacterial:* Bacterial conjunctivitis is contagious until 24 hours after beginning medication.

C. *Viral:* Viral conjunctivitis is contagious for 48 to 72 hours, but it may last up to 2 weeks.

Activity: As tolerated.

Diet: As tolerated.

Medications: No medications are prescribed for viral infections. You will be given instructions on how to use eye drops or eye ointment.

You Have Been Prescribed: _____

You Need to Take: _____

You Need to Notify the Office If You Have:

A. A reaction to your medication.

B. Trouble seeing.

C. New symptoms.

D. Other: _____

Phone: _____

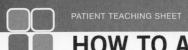

HOW TO ADMINISTER EYE MEDICATIONS

PROBLEM

You have been prescribed a medication for your eye(s). It is very important that you know the correct way to use your eye medication.

CAUSE

You have been diagnosed with _____.

PREVENTION

The health of your eyes is important.

A. Use good hand washing and try not to rub your eyes with your fingers.
B. Clean your contacts regularly with contact cleaning solution. Do not put your contacts in your mouth to moisten.
C. Wear sunglasses in bright sunshine.
D. Use eye goggles when working and playing sports ensures extra protection.
E. Change your eye makeup often. Mascara, eye shadow, and eyeliner grow bacteria. Do not share makeup.

TREATMENT PLAN

A. Correct use of your medication is important.
B. You may or may not require an eye patch or shield.

HOW TO APPLY EYE OINTMENT

A. Always wash your hands before placing medication in your eyes.
B. Gently pull down the lower eyelid.
C. Make a small pocket between the eyeball and the eyelid.
D. If you have someone helping to put your eye ointment in the lower lid pocket, look up and away while he or she puts in the medicine.
E. **Do not let the tube of medicine touch the eye or eyelid.**
F. Squeeze a thin ribbon of the medication into the pocket of the eyelid.
G. Start at the inner fold of the eye **going from the nose to the outer eye.**
H. Let go of the eyelid and blink to spread the medication.

HOW TO INSTILL EYE DROPS

A. Always wash your hands before placing medication in your eyes.
B. Gently pull down the lower eyelid.
C. Make a small pocket between the eyelid and the eyeball.
D. If you have someone helping to put your eye drops in the lower lid pocket, look up and away while he or she puts in the medicine.
E. **Do not let the bottle of medication touch the eye or eyelid.**
F. Squeeze the prescribed number of drops of the medicine into the pocket of the eyelid.
G. Let go of the eyelid and blink (or tell the patient to blink) to spread the medication.

Activity: No restrictions are required unless you require eye surgery; then you will be given specific instructions about the amount of activity allowed.

Diet: No restrictions.

Medications:

You Have Been Prescribed: _____

You Need to Use the Medicine: _____

You Need to Notify the Office If:

A. You are unable to put in the medication yourself or get help from others.

B. You are not better 24 to 48 hours after starting the medication.

C. Your vision is worse after using the medication.

D. You have an allergic reaction to the medicine.

E. Other: _____

Phone: _____

Patient Teaching Guides for Chapter 5: Ear Disorders

- Child With Acute Otitis Media
- Otitis Externa
- Cerumen Impaction (Ear Wax)
- Otitis Media With Effusion

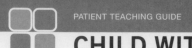

CHILD WITH ACUTE OTITIS MEDIA

PROBLEM

Acute otitis media is infection and swelling of the middle ear with a buildup of fluid.

CAUSE

Bacteria or viruses may cause middle ear infections.

PREVENTION

A. Wash your child's hands often. Always wash their hands before eating and after they play with other children.

B. **Do not smoke.**

C. Children should not be exposed to secondhand smoke.

D. If your child is bottle fed, do not "prop" the bottle. Always hold your baby when bottle feeding.

E. Don't give him or her a bottle in bed.

F. Wean your child from the bottle by his or her first birthday.

TREATMENT PLAN

Follow up with a health care provider as instructed to avoid complications of otitis or permanent hearing loss.

Activity: Your child may not play as much when he or she is sick.

Diet: Your child may not eat well when he or she is sick.

Medications:

A. Children's Tylenol may be used for fever or pain.

B. **Do not use aspirin for children.**

C. Ask for flavored antibiotics.

D. Decongestants may be useful for nasal congestion in older children. Your health care provider will help you decide if your child can take decongestants.

You Child Has Been Prescribed: _____

Your Child Needs to Take: _____

Your child needs to finish all of the antibiotics, even though he or she may start to feel better.

You Need to Notify the Office If You Have:

A. Continued fever or no improvement in symptoms in 48 hours.

B. A child who acts as if he or she has a stiff neck.

C. Continual crying.

D. Rash while taking medicine.

E. Other: _____

Phone: _____

OTITIS EXTERNA

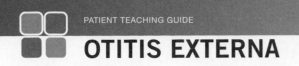

PROBLEM

Your practitioner has diagnosed you with a condition known as otitis externa, sometimes also referred to as "swimmer's ear." This is a common condition characterized by itching in the ear, sometimes followed by ear pain, swelling, and drainage. The eardrum is rarely affected.

CAUSE

The most common causes for otitis externa are frequent swimming and too vigorous cleaning of the wax from your ears. It may involve either a bacterial or a fungal infection.

PREVENTION

You may prevent future problems with otitis externa by following these measures:

A. Clean the outer ear only as needed. Do not use cotton-tipped swabs or any other device to clean down into the ear canal. Usually, wax is just pushed deeper into the canal with this method, and the canal may be traumatized by the instrument used.

B. For swimmers or others susceptible to frequent recurrences of otitis externa, it may be helpful to dry the ear canals with a blow dryer on a low setting after exposure to water. You may also instill a solution of 50% isopropyl alcohol and 50% vinegar in the ear twice daily and after every submersion in water. Over-the-counter eardrops labeled for "swimmer's ear" may also be used as directed.

TREATMENT PLAN

For the most common bacterial infections associated with otitis externa, antibiotic eardrops are usually prescribed. In addition, you should keep water out of your ears for 4 to 6 weeks. (This means no swimming until symptoms are totally resolved and any wick is removed; then swim only with water-resistant earplugs.)

To bathe or shower, first coat cotton balls with petroleum jelly and use them to plug ears.

Activity: The only activity restrictions are those involving submersion in water. Bathing and hair washing are permitted as described above.

Diet: No changes are required in your diet.

Medications:

A. Eardrops are used to treat otitis externa.

B. The drops should be applied down the ear canal's opening, moving the earlobe back and forth to help the eardrops pass downward.

C. In severe cases, antibiotics may be given.

You Have Been Prescribed: _____

You Need to Instill _____ Drops Into the Affected Ear _____ Times per Day.

You Need to Notify the Office If You Have:

   A. Symptoms that have not cleared up in 3 days.

   B. A fever over 100°F.

   C. Severe ear pain.

   D. Other: _____

Phone: _____

CERUMEN IMPACTION (EAR WAX)

PROBLEM

A buildup of earwax causes itching, pain, and temporary hearing loss.

CAUSE

With age, the normal mechanisms of the ear used for removing earwax are decreased. Use of cotton swabs to remove earwax can push wax further into the ear.

PREVENTION

Do not use cotton swabs, paper clips, or other objects to clean your ears. These can damage the ear canal and lead to an external ear infection.

TREATMENT PLAN

A. Clean ears with a wet washcloth.

B. Use Debrox, mineral oil, or olive oil, 2 to 3 drops per day, for 1 week before returning for a follow-up visit.

Activity: As tolerated.

Diet: As tolerated.

Medications:

You Have Been Prescribed: _____

You Need to Take: _____

You Need to Notify the Office If:

A. You are unable to hear.

B. You have colored drainage from your ears.

C. You run a fever.

D. You have dizziness.

E. Other: _____

Phone: _____

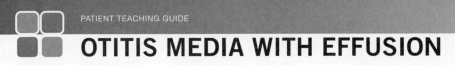

OTITIS MEDIA WITH EFFUSION

PROBLEM

You have inflammation of the middle ear with effusion, which is the presence of fluid in the middle ear without infection.

CAUSE

The middle ear fluid can remain after you have been treated for an ear infection (otitis media).

TREATMENT PLAN

If you or your child has a buildup of fluid in the middle ear for 6 weeks up to 3 months, you should receive a hearing evaluation and possibly medication.

Follow up with a health care provider as instructed to avoid complications and/or permanent hearing loss.

Activity: There is no activity restriction.

Diet: There is no special diet.

Medications: Antibiotics are used to treat this infection.

You Have Been Prescribed: _____

You Need to Take: _____

You need to finish all of your antibiotics.

You Need to Notify the Office If You Have:

    A. Fever.

    B. Decreased appetite.

    C. Decreased activity level.

    D. A rash while on the medication.

    E. No improvement in symptoms in 48 hours.

Phone: _____

Patient Teaching Guides for Chapter 6: Nasal Disorders

- Allergic Rhinitis
- Sinusitis
- Nosebleeds

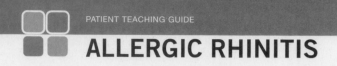

ALLERGIC RHINITIS

PROBLEM

Allergic rhinitis is a chronic or recurrent condition. Common symptoms are nasal congestion, sneezing, and clear nasal discharge. It's not contagious, so you can't catch it from anyone, and you can't spread it to others.

CAUSE

You are having an allergic response after being exposed to an allergen.

PREVENTION

The best prevention is to avoid things you know you're allergic to, for example, smoke (cigarette, cigar, wood smoke); pollens and molds; animal dander; dust mites; and indoor inhalants, such as hair spray and other aerosol spray products.

Target your bedroom as "allergy-free" by removing carpets, damp mopping floors weekly, hanging washable curtains instead of blinds, removing books and stuffed animals, using foam pillows, and encasing the pillows and mattress in plastic.

Do not blow your nose too frequently or too hard. It may cause your eardrum to perforate (tear). Blow through both nostrils at the same time to equalize the pressure.

Use tissues when you blow your nose. Dispose of them and then wash your hands. If no tissue is available do the "elbow sneeze" into the bend of your arm (away from your open hands). Always wash your hands.

TREATMENT PLAN

A. Use the air conditioner in your house and car to decrease exposure to pollens.

B. Use an air filtration system in your house, or buy a small one for your bedroom.

C. Dust your house often, using a cloth and cleaner or polish to keep dust from flying.

D. Allergy testing may need to be done if you've had allergies for a long time. Ask your health care provider about a consultation with an allergist.

Activity: There are no activity restrictions. However, you may want to exercise indoors during the spring, summer, and fall when pollen counts are high.

Diet: Eat well-balanced meals. Drink at least 6 to 8 glasses of liquid a day.

Medications:

You Have Been Prescribed: _____

You Need to Take: _____

You Need to Notify the Office If: _____

A. You experience trouble breathing or catching your breath.

B. If you have asthma call if your symptoms are worse.

C. Your symptoms aren't any better after using the medications for 3 complete days.

D. Your nasal discharge changes to a greenish color.

E. Other: _____

Phone: _____

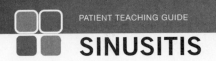

SINUSITIS

PROBLEM

Sinusitis (sinus infection) is classified as acute, subacute, or chronic condition. In acute sinusitis, the infection is resolved after treatment. In subacute sinusitis, there is a persistent, yellow to green nasal discharge despite treatment. In chronic sinusitis, episodes of prolonged inflammation continue longer than 3 months despite treatment.

CAUSE

Sinusitis occurs when the mucus lining in your sinus cavities becomes inflamed and infected with bacteria or allergen. This can occur after a cold or tooth abscess.

PREVENTION

A. If you have a tooth abscess, see your dentist and finish all your antibiotics.

B. Don't blow your nose too frequently or too hard. It may cause your eardrum to perforate (tear). Blow through both nostrils at the same time to equalize pressure.

C. To prevent spreading germs to others, cover your mouth when you cough.

  1. Use tissues when you blow your nose. Dispose of them and then wash your hands.

  2. If no tissue is available do the "elbow sneeze" into the bend of your arm (away from your open hands).

D. Always wash your hands after coughing or using tissues.

TREATMENT PLAN

A. Stop smoking.

B. Use steam inhalation to liquefy secretions.

C. Use a room humidifier. Keep your humidifier clean—it can grow bacteria.

Activity: There are no activity restrictions; however, diving, swimming, and flying may increase the occurrence of symptoms or make them worse.

Diet: Eat a healthy diet. Drink at least 8 to 10 glasses of liquid every day.

Medications: Take all of your prescribed antibiotics, even if you feel better. You may also take the following over-the-counter medications:

A. Ibuprofen (Advil) for facial pain.

B. Ocean saline spray to prevent nasal drying.

C. Nasal decongestants: if you have high blood pressure, ask about the best medication to use.

You Have Been Prescribed: _____

You Need to Take: _____

You Need to Call the Office If:

  A. Your eyelids begin to swell or droop, or you experience decreased vision.

  B. You have stiffness in your neck or increased fever.

  C. You have asthma, and you are getting worse.

  D. You begin vomiting and are unable to keep down your antibiotic.

  E. You are a diabetic and your blood sugars are elevated, or you notice ketones in your urine.

  F. Other: _____

Phone: _____

NOSEBLEEDS

PROBLEM

Most nosebleeds stop within 10 minutes. **If you have trouble breathing with a nosebleed—*call 911.***

CAUSE

Nosebleeds may be caused by several problems:

A. Trauma from nose picking or forcefully blowing the nose

B. Chronic sinus infections

C. Allergies

D. Drugs, including over-the-counter medications such as aspirin and Pepto-Bismol, or street drugs such as snorted cocaine

E. Exposure to irritants

PREVENTION

A. Avoid picking your nose. Keep fingernails trimmed short.

B. Don't blow your nose too frequently or too hard (may also cause eardrum tearing).

C. Blow your nose through both nostrils at the same time to equalize pressure.

D. Use a humidifier in your home, or place a container of water near the radiator.

E. Use a lubricant such as petrolatum, A & D Ointment, or a skin barrier such as zinc oxide to add moisture and promote healing.

TREATMENT PLAN

A. If you experience a nosebleed, take these steps:

   1. Sit up and lean forward.

   2. Apply pressure to the bridge of your nose for 10 to 15 minutes to stop the blood flow.

   3. If the bleeding continues, spray Afrin into your nostril.

   4. If the bleeding still continues, lightly soak a cotton ball with the nasal spray, insert it into your nose, and press.

   5. Apply zinc oxide, petrolatum, or A & D Ointment to prevent further drying and abrasion of the nasal septum (partition between the two nostrils).

B. Gently blowing your nose also decreases or stops a nosebleed.

Activity: Avoid or limit the following activities for 3 to 5 days after a nosebleed:

A. Heavy lifting

B. Straining

C. Bending over from the waist

D. Very hot showers

Diet: Avoid hot, spicy foods for 3 to 5 days after a nosebleed.

Medications: Avoid medications that increase bleeding, such as aspirin and Pepto-Bismol.

You Have Been Prescribed: _____

You Need to Take: _____

You Need to Notify the Office If:

   A. Bleeding doesn't stop with pressure or nasal spray applied to the bleeding site.

   B. You keep having nosebleeds (more than two in a week or four in a month).

   C. Other: _____

Phone: _____

Patient Teaching Guides for Chapter 7: Throat and Mouth Disorders

- Oral Thrush in Children

- Pharyngitis

- Aphthous Stomatitis

ORAL THRUSH IN CHILDREN

PROBLEM

Oral thrush is white patches that coat the inside of the mouth and tongue. It mainly affects bottled-fed infants, although breast-fed infants and debilitated older children may also be affected.

CAUSE

Thrush is caused by a yeast called *Candida* that grows rapidly on the lining of the mouth in areas abraided by prolonged sucking. It may also occur after a course of antibiotic medication.

PREVENTION

A. Don't use large pacifiers and nipples.

B. Boil bottle nipples and pacifiers.

C. Cleanse your nipples well after breast-feeding.

TREATMENT

A. Try to remove any large plaques with a moistened cotton-tipped applicator or gauze pad.

B. Cleanse the infant's mouth before giving medication.

C. Place the medication in the front of the mouth on each side.

D. Rub it directly on the plaques with a cotton swab.

E. Feed the infant temporarily with a cup and spoon.

F. Give a pacifier only at bedtime.

Diet: Decrease sucking time until thrush clears up.

Medications: An antibiotics is used to treat thrush.

You Have Been Prescribed: _____

You Need to Take: _____

You Need to Notify the Office If:

A. The child refuses to eat.

B. Symptoms don't improve or thrush lasts longer than 10 days.

C. Unexplained fever occurs.

D. Secondary infection occurs in the mouth (pain, tenderness, sores).

E. Other: _____

Phone: _____

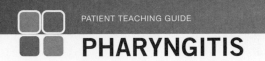

PHARYNGITIS

PROBLEM

Pharyngitis (sore throat) is a condition that occurs when your throat becomes inflamed.

CAUSE

The inflammation can be due to a virus, a bacterial infection, or a fungus. Other noninfectious causes include postnasal drip, allergies, mouth breathing, and trauma.

PREVENTION

A. Avoid sick people and crowds. Stay at home if you are sick.

B. Cover your mouth when coughing.

C. Don't share a drinking glass, kiss, or have close contact with anyone who has an upper respiratory infection.

TREATMENT PLAN

A. Hot tea, soup, and throat lozenges soothe your throat.

B. Use disposable tissues when sneezing. Use tissues when you blow your nose. If no tissue is available do the "elbow sneeze" into the bend of your arm (away from your open hands). Dispose of them and then wash your hands.

Activity: If you have strep throat, don't return to school or work until you have completed a full 24 hours of antibiotic. Rest or nap as often as possible while you're sick.

Diet: Eat a healthy diet. If swallowing is difficult, eat soft foods such as ice cream, Jell-o, pudding, and soup. Increase your fluid intake to 10 to 12 glasses a day.

Medications: You will be prescribed antibiotics if you have a bacterial infection. If your sore throat is due to a virus, antibiotics won't help. Don't share your prescription medications with other family members who are also sick. They need a full prescription, too. Many other medications are available over the counter, such as throat lozenges, cough suppressants, and so forth.

You Have Been Prescribed: _____

You Need to Take: _____

If you are prescribed antibiotics, complete all of the doses.

You Need to Notify the Office If:

A. You have difficulty breathing because of the sore throat or enlarged tonsils.

B. Your symptoms are worse after 24 hours of antibiotics.

C. You are unable to keep down your antibiotic because of vomiting.

D. Your sick child refuses to eat or drink.

E. You develop a rash or itching after starting the antibiotic.

F. You are a diabetic and your blood glucose is high, or you have ketones in your urine.

G. Other:_____

Phone: _____

APHTHOUS STOMATITIS

PROBLEM

Aphthous stomatitis are tender ulcers in the mouth that recur.

CAUSE

The cause is unknown. Possible causes include diet (lack of iron, zinc, or B vitamins), menstrual or hormonal changes, and viruses.

TREATMENT PLAN

A. Use an over-the-counter gel such as Anbesol or Orajel four times daily.

B. You may be prescribed a mouthwash made of diphenhydramine (Benadryl), Maalox, and lidocaine or fluocinonide gel to "swish" in your mouth two to four times daily.

Activity: No restrictions are required.

Diet:

A. Avoiding spicy, salty, or hot foods may help.

B. Using a straw when drinking may decrease pain.

C. Cold foods may be easier to tolerate.

D. Avoid hard or sharp food.

E. Use a soft toothbrush.

Medications:

You Have Been Prescribed: _____

You Need to Take: _____

You Need to Notify the Office If You Have:

A. Worse symptoms than seen at the office visit today.

B. Ulcers that do not heal in approximately 1 to 2 weeks.

C. Other: _____

Phone: _____

Patient Teaching Guides for Chapter 8: Respiratory Disorders

- Acute Bronchitis
- Asthma
- Peak Flow Monitoring and Asthma Action Plan
- How to Use a Metered-Dose Inhaler
- Bacterial Pneumonia: Adult
- Bacterial Pneumonia: Child
- Bronchiolitis: Child
- Chronic Bronchitis
- Common Cold
- COPD
- Cough
- Viral Croup
- Emphysema
- Respiratory Syncytial Virus
- Viral Pneumonia: Adult
- Viral Pneumonia: Child
- Nicotine Dependence

ACUTE BRONCHITIS

PROBLEM

Acute bronchitis is an upper respiratory infection followed by a productive cough.

CAUSE

Respiratory viruses cause acute bronchitis.

PREVENTION

A. Avoid exposure to others with respiratory illnesses.

B. Don't smoke, and avoid secondhand smoke and smoke-filled environments.

C. Avoid other air pollutants, such as wood smoke, solvents, and cleaners.

D. Use good hand washing.

TREATMENT PLAN

A. Humidity and mist may be helpful.

B. Always clean the humidifier daily to prevent bacterial growth.

C. Twenty minutes several times a day in a steamy bathroom may provide relief.

Activity: Rest during early stage of the illness; then increase activity as tolerated when the fever subsides. Children may attend school or day care without restrictions after the fever subsides.

Diet: Eat a nutritious diet. Drink 8 to 10 glasses of water daily.

Medications:

A. Acetaminophen (Tylenol) may be used to relieve discomfort.

B. For a nonproductive cough, take cough suppressants if recommended. You may be prescribed a cough medicine or be told the best kind to buy in the drugstore.

C. Since a virus almost always causes acute bronchitis **antibiotics will rarely be needed to get better.**

You Have Been Prescribed: _____

You Need to Take: _____

You Need to Notify the Office If You Have:

A. No improvement after 48 hours.

B. Worsening symptoms.

C. High fever, chills, chest tightness or pain, shortness of breath.

D. Symptoms that last longer than 3 weeks.

E. Other: _____

Phone: _____

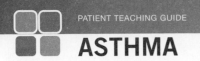

ASTHMA

PROBLEM

Asthma is a chronic condition characterized by wheezing, coughing, breathlessness, and chest tightness.

CAUSE

The most common cause is inflammation that results from exercise or exposure to environmental irritants, allergens, furry animals, cockroaches, dust mites, pollens and molds, cold air, or viral respiratory infections.

PREVENTION

You may be able to prevent frequent recurrences of asthma by following these asthma trigger avoidance strategies:

A. *Dust mite allergens:* Wash bedding weekly in hot water and dry it in a hot dryer. Encase pillows and mattresses in airtight covers. Remove carpets, especially from your bedroom. Avoid use of fabric-covered furniture, especially for sleeping.

B. *Cockroach allergens:* Clean your house thoroughly. Use poison bait or traps. Don't leave food or garbage exposed.

C. *Animal fur allergens:* Avoid keeping house pets, or at least don't allow them in sleeping areas.

D. *Smoke allergens:* Avoid smoking, contact with tobacco smoke, smoke from wood-burning stoves or fireplaces, and unvented stoves or heaters.

E. *Outdoor pollens and molds:* Keep windows closed when pollen or mold counts are high.

F. *Indoor mold:* Reduce dampness in your home by using a dehumidifier. Clean damp areas often. Remove carpets that are laid on concrete.

G. *Other irritants:* Avoid perfumes, cleaning agents, and sprays.

TREATMENT PLAN

See the Patient Teaching Guides, "Peak Flow Monitoring and Asthma Action Plan" and "How to Use a Metered-Dose Inhaler."

Activity:

A. If cold air causes symptoms, wear a scarf over your mouth and nose if you must go outside during the winter.

B. Avoid vigorous exercise if this causes symptoms. Learn to recognize activities that stimulate breathing problems.

C. Make an asthma action plan to follow. Copy the plan and place on the refrigerator, take a copy to school, and give each coach a copy of the action plan.

D. Color code your inhalers with tape or markers, for example, use green tape for quick relief inhalers, and blue tape for long-acting inhalers.

Diet: There are no diet restrictions.

Medications:

You Have Been Prescribed: _____

You Need to Take: _____

You Need to Notify the Office If You Have:

A. A peak flow reading below 60% of your personal best number that doesn't return to the yellow or green zone after taking your medication.

B. Other: _____

Phone: _____

PEAK FLOW MONITORING AND ASTHMA ACTION PLAN

A peak flow meter is a device that measures how well air moves out of your lungs. This measurement is referred to as your "peak expiratory flow," or PER.

HOW TO USE A PEAK FLOW METER

A. Place the indicator at the bottom of the numbered scale.

B. Stand up.

C. Take a deep breath, filling your lungs as deeply as possible.

D. Place the mouthpiece in your mouth and close your lips around it. Don't put your tongue inside the hole.

E. Blow into the mouthpiece as hard and fast as you can. It is important to give this your best effort.

F. Write down the number on the indicator. If you cough or make a mistake, don't record that number—do it over again.

G. Repeat steps A through F two more times.

H. Write down the highest number of the three attempts. This is your PER.

CALCULATING YOUR PERSONAL BEST PEAK FLOW NUMBER

This number is the highest peak flow number you can achieve over a 2- to 3-week period when your asthma is under good control (when you don't have any symptoms). To find this number, take peak flow readings:

A. Twice daily for 2 to 3 weeks.

B. When you wake up and between noon and 2 PM.

C. Before and after taking your quick relief medication.

D. Or as directed by your health care provider.

THE PEAK FLOW ZONE SYSTEM

Once you have determined your personal best peak flow number, your health care provider can give you the numbers that let you know what medications to take based on your PER. The numbers are set up like a traffic light system (red, yellow, and green).

Green Zone (80% to 100% of your personal best number): Signals *good control.* No asthma symptoms are present, and you should take your medication as usual.

Yellow Zone (60% to 80% of your personal best number): Signals *caution.* You may be having an episode of asthma that requires an increase in your medications.

Red Zone (below 60% of your personal best number): Signals a *medical alert.* You must take an inhaled β_2-adrenergic agonist right away and call your health care provider immediately if your peak flow number doesn't return to the yellow or green zone and stay there.

Use the following "Asthma Action Plan," which specifies what medications you should take when you're in each zone and also use the self-assessment diary provided in the Table.

ASTHMA ACTION PLAN

A. My personal best peak expiratory flow (PEF) is _____.

B. When I am in the *green zone,* PEF above _____, I should continue to take my regularly scheduled asthma medications. They are:

    1. _____

    2. _____

    3. _____

C. When I am in the ***yellow zone,*** PEF between _____ and _____ , I should add the following to my regularly scheduled medications:

    1. _____

    2. _____

    3. _____

TABLE	Asthma Diary Self-Assessment

Symptom Codes: Rate your symptoms 1 (mild); 2 (moderate); or 3 (severe)

My Personal Best Peak Expiratory Flow Is _____

DATE	PEAK FLOW ZONES *Green* = Good control *Yellow* = Caution *Red* = Emergency			Symptoms (Use codes) W = Wheeze C = Cough S = Shortness of breath	Quick Relief Medication (include the number of times needed for relief)	Anti-Inflammatory Medication	Additional Medications or Activity
Monday	AM	PM	ZONE				

D. When I am in the ***red zone***, PEF below _____ , I should immediately take the following rescue medication and contact my health care provider:

  1. Rescue Medication: _____

E. Other Directions: _____

_____

_____

HOW TO USE A METERED-DOSE INHALER

USING AN INHALER

To receive the proper dose from your inhaler, you must use good technique. Your health care practitioner may provide you with a drug-free practice inhaler. Practice the following steps until you are comfortable administering your inhalant:

A. Shake the inhaler well immediately before each use.

B. Using a spacer helps to deliver more medication.

C. Remove the cap from the mouthpiece. Hold the inhaler upright. Make sure the medication canister is firmly inserted into the plastic holder (actuator).

D. The first time you use your new inhaler (or if it has been 1 month or longer since the last use), test spray four times into the air.

E. Breathe out through your mouth to the end of a normal breath.

F. Position the mouthpiece about 1 to 2 inches in front of your open mouth. Or you may close your lips in a tight seal around the mouthpiece.

G. Open your mouth widely (unless you are using the second method above), and position your head in a neutral position.

H. While breathing in slowly and deeply, firmly depress the container once.

I. Continue breathing in slowly until your lungs are full.

J. Once you have breathed in fully, hold your breath for 10 seconds or as long as you can.

K. If you need a second puff of the same medication, wait a minimum of 1 minute before repeating steps A through J. If you're using a different inhaler for the second puff, wait at least 5 minutes before using the second inhaler.

OTHER TIPS

A. If you're taking a steroid inhalant, rinse your mouth and throat with water after each dose.

B. When you're short of breath, administer your bronchodilator ("rescue medicine") first; then wait approximately 5 minutes before using your steroid inhaler. The bronchodilator opens your airways so more of the steroid medication reaches your lungs.

C. Keep the inhaler clean. Once a week, remove the medication canister from the actuator and wash the actuator in warm, soapy water. Rinse and allow to air dry. Replace the medication canister in the holder and recap the mouthpiece.

D. Always check the expiration date on your inhaler and make sure to refill your prescription before the medication expires.

E. Color code your inhalers with tape or markers; for example, use green tape for quick relief inhalers, and blue tape for long-acting inhalers.

BACTERIAL PNEUMONIA: ADULT

PROBLEM

Pneumonia is a lung infection that causes fluid to collect in the air sacs. You may have a fever, cough, or trouble breathing.

CAUSE

Respiratory bacteria or viruses cause pneumonia.

PREVENTION

Elderly patients and those with severe lung disease may receive a vaccine to prevent influenza and pneumococcal pneumonia.

TREATMENT PLAN

A. Use a cool mist humidifier. Clean the humidifier daily.

B. Do not smoke, and avoid smoke-filled rooms.

C. Wash your hands frequently.

Activity: Rest during the early phase of the illness.

Diet: Eat a nutritious diet. Drink 8 to 10 glasses of water a day.

Medications: Don't use cough suppressants if your cough produces sputum. Use them only for a dry, nonproductive cough. Acetaminophen (Tylenol) may be used for minor discomfort.

You Have Been Prescribed: _____

You Need to Take: _____

You Need to Notify the Office if You Have:

A. Increased difficulty breathing.

B. Fever after 48 hours on an antibiotic.

C. Blood in your sputum.

D. Worsening discomfort or fatigue.

E. Other: _____

Phone: _____

BACTERIAL PNEUMONIA: CHILD

PROBLEM

Bacterial pneumonia is a lung infection that causes fluid to collect in the air sacs. You may have a fever, cough, or trouble breathing.

CAUSE

Respiratory bacteria cause pneumonia.

PREVENTION

Isolate young infants from people with respiratory illnesses.

TREATMENT PLAN

A. Encourage fluids.

B. Use a vaporizer or humidifier to increase humidity in the child's room. Clean the humidifier or vaporizer daily.

C. Keep the child away from cigarette smoke.

Activity: Have your child rest during the acute phase. Children may return to school after 24 hours of antibiotic therapy and no fever for 24 hours.

Diet: There are no diet restrictions.

Medications:

A. Have child take antibiotics as directed. Finish the antibiotic even though your child may feel well.

B. Acetaminophen (Tylenol) may be given for fever. Children 18 years or younger should not be given aspirin.

C. Don't give your child cough suppressants.

Your Child Has Been Prescribed: _____

Your Child Needs to Take: _____

You Need to Notify the Office Immediately If:

A. The child's breathing becomes more labored or difficult.

B. Retractions (tugging between ribs) become worse.

C. The child's lips become blue.

D. Grunting sounds occur when the child is breathing out.

E. The child starts acting very sick.

F. Other: _____

You Need to Notify the Office Within 24 Hours If:

A. The child is unable to sleep.

B. The child isn't drinking enough.

C. Fever lasts longer than 48 hours on antibiotics.

D. You feel the child is getting worse.

E. Other: _____

Phone: _____

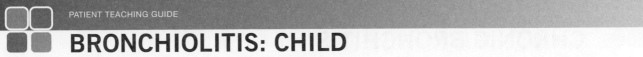

BRONCHIOLITIS: CHILD

PROBLEM

Bronchiolitis is a lung infection that causes respiratory distress, wheezing, coughing, and fever.

CAUSE

Respiratory viruses, usually respiratory syncytial virus (RSV), cause bronchiolitis. The symptoms generally last approximately 7 to 10 days. It usually occurs in fall, winter, and early spring.

PREVENTION

A. Isolate young infants from those with respiratory illnesses.

B. Avoid large crowds.

C. Wash hands frequently if you're a caregiver.

D. Wash toys and surfaces that the child touches.

TREATMENT PLAN

A. Use a cool-mist humidifier in the child's bedroom, and clean the humidifier frequently. If a humidifier is unavailable, promote high humidification in the room. With adult supervision, the child may be placed in a steamy bathroom for 20 minutes 2 to 3 times a day.

B. Use warm water and a bulb syringe to clear an infant's stuffy nose.

C. Children should not be exposed to secondhand smoke.

Activity: Children need rest during early stages of the illness.

Diet: Offer fluids, such as juice and water, frequently. Dilute juice for younger infants. Offer small, frequent feedings.

Medications:

You Have Been Prescribed: _____

You Need to Take: _____

Antibiotics are not prescribed for viral infections.

You Need to Notify the Office Immediately If:

A. The child's temperature is 101°F or greater.

B. Breathing becomes labored or difficult or is faster than 60 breaths/minute.

C. Wheezing becomes severe.

D. Retractions (tugging between ribs) become worse.

E. The child stops breathing or passes out.

F. Lips become bluish.

G. The child starts acting very sick or is difficult to arouse.

H. Other: _____

You Need to Notify the Office Within 24 Hours If:

A. The child is unable to sleep or won't drink enough fluids.

B. The child has a suggestion of an earache or yellow nasal discharge.

C. Fever over 100°F lasts for more than 72 hours.

D. You feel the child is getting worse.

E. Other: _____

Phone: _____

CHRONIC BRONCHITIS

PROBLEM

Chronic bronchitis causes swelling of the bronchial tubes, mucus secretion, and a recurring productive cough.

CAUSE

Chronic bronchitis usually affects patients who smoke cigarettes. Smoke irritates the airways of the lungs, causing mucus formation leading to a cough.

PREVENTION

A. Do not smoke.

B. Avoid smoke-filled environments, environmental pollutants, and crowds.

C. Avoid people with respiratory illnesses.

D. Immunizations against pertussis, diphtheria, and influenza helps to reduce the risk of bronchitis.

TREATMENT PLAN

A. Increase fluid intake.

B. Stop smoking. When you stop smoking, expect an increase in sputum production. If you also have asthma, you may experience wheezing with the return of airway reactivity. Notify the office if you have any questions.

C. Avoid smoke-filled environments.

D. Children may attend school or day care unless they have bronchitis with fevers.

Activity: Rest until your fever subsides; then resume regular activities.

Diet: Eat a nutritious diet. Increase fluids to 8 to 10 glasses of water a day.

Medications: Avoid cough suppressants. Expectorants may be used to loosen secretions, if needed.

You Have Been Prescribed: _____

You Need to Take: _____

You Need to Notify the Office If You Have:

A. No improvement after 3 to 4 days of antibiotics.

B. A fever.

C. Vomiting.

D. A productive cough with blood in sputum.

E. Shortness of breath.

F. Other: _____

Phone: _____

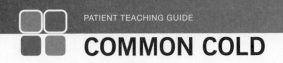

COMMON COLD

PROBLEM

The common cold is an inflammation of the mucous membranes of the respiratory tract. Most people complain of feeling tired, a runny or stopped-up nose, a sore throat, hoarseness, and watery and/or red eyes. You may have a low-grade fever or no fever at all.

CAUSE

A virus usually causes the common cold.

PREVENTION

A. Colds are spread from one person to another through hand-to-hand contact and contact with air droplets from sneezing, coughing, and talking.

B. Use good hand washing with soap and water or hand sanitizers.

C. Do not drink from the same glass after others.

D. Cover your mouth and noise when you sneeze or cough.

E. Use tissues when you blow your nose. Dispose of them and then wash your hands. If no tissue is available do the "elbow sneeze" into the bend of your arm (away from your open hands). Always wash your hands.

TREATMENT PLAN

A. Using a humidifier for your bedroom or inhaling steam helps keep your mucous membranes from drying.

B. As an alternative for nasal decongestants, consider clearing nasal congestion in infants with a rubber suction bulb; secretions can be softened with saline nose drops or a cool-mist humidifier.

C. Follow general cold measures as needed.

D. Secondary infections of the respiratory tract (sinuses, lungs) may occur. If these occur, then antibiotic therapy may be needed.

E. Zinc preparations are not recommended for an acute cough due to the common cold.

Activity: There are no activity restrictions. Frequent rest periods or naps can help with fatigue.

Diet: Eat well-balanced meals and snacks. Drink extra liquids (10 to 12 glasses a day). Warm fluids, such as tea and soups, can increase the rate of mucus flow and provide some symptom relief.

Medications: The American College of Chest Physicians clinical practice guidelines recommend cough suppressants and other over-the-counter cough medications should *not* be given to children younger than 2 years.

A. Antibiotics aren't prescribed for a cold, but they may be prescribed for a secondary infection.

B. All cold medications are available over the counter. Take as directed.

You Have Been Prescribed: _____

You Need to Take: _____

You Need to Notify the Office If:

A. The patient is a child and is listless or hard to wake up, refuses a bottle or won't drink liquids, doesn't want to play, has a fever, or has other symptoms such as shortness of breath.

B. You experience pain that's getting worse in your ears, sinuses, throat, neck, or chest.

C. You have green or yellow nasal drainage.

D. Your temperature is higher than 100.4°F.

E. You are a diabetic and your blood sugars are elevated, or you notice ketones in your urine.

F. Other: _____

Phone: _____

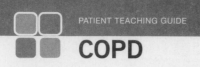

COPD

PROBLEM

COPD is a chronic, progressive, debilitating disease of the lungs that doesn't have a cure. Most people have a combination of emphysema and chronic bronchitis. Persons with COPD usually have some of the following symptoms: cough (usually productive), shortness of breath at rest or with exertion, wheezing, decreased energy level, and weight loss.

CAUSE

COPD is most commonly associated with cigarette smoking and long-term exposure to pulmonary irritants in the environment (e.g., coal dust). Repeated respiratory infections may also contribute to the development of COPD.

PREVENTION

A. Avoid smoking and exposure to secondhand smoke.

B. Avoid exposure to environmental irritants, including pollution, household cleaning products, and smoke from fires.

TREATMENT PLAN

A. Stopping smoking is one of the most important treatments. Talk to your health care provider about support for stopping.

B. Reduce exposure to lung irritants and extremely hot and cold air temperatures.

C. Begin an exercise program with your health care provider's approval. Walking is a good aerobic exercise. Begin with a pace that is tolerable and easy to maintain; then increase the duration and intensity of the exercise as tolerated. Stop if you experience shortness of breath or chest pain. A realistic goal may be 5 to 10 minutes a day, eventually increasing to 30 to 40 minutes a day.

D. Receive the influenza vaccine every fall. The pneumococcal vaccine is recommended every 5 years and may be given at the same time as the influenza vaccine.

E. Use a spacer/holding chamber to help you inhale all of your medicine. Spacers help you place more of your medicine in your lungs instead at the back of your throat and mouth. Keep your spacer clean.

F. Use slow, deep breathing or pursed-lip breathing when you are short of breath. Breathe out like you are blowing out a candle.

G. Ask your health care provider if you are a candidate for low-flow oxygen treatment when shortness of breath occurs at night and causes insomnia and restlessness.

Activity: Group activities together such as planning shopping with going to the post office. Schedule rest periods throughout the day. Exercise programs should help increase activity tolerance.

Diet: Good nutrition is important. Six small, high-calorie meals a day are suggested. Avoid excessive intake of carbohydrates, especially simple carbohydrates like candy, soda, and potato chips. Milk and milk products do not increase the production of mucus. Ask your health care provider to refer you to a dietitian if nutritional problems persist.

Medications:

You Have Been Prescribed: _____

You Need to Take: _____

You Need to Notify the Office If:

A. Your mucus changes color, increases in amount, or if you notice the consistency becoming thicker.

B. After you start your medication, call if your wheezing or shortness of breath is getting worse.

C. You are having trouble walking or talking due to your shortness of breath.

D. Other: _____

Phone: _____

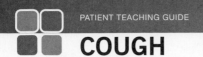

COUGH

PROBLEM

Coughing is an important defense mechanism your body uses to clear your airway of secretions and inhaled particles.

CAUSE

A cough is often associated with other respiratory symptoms and may be a sign of infection. Coughing is often related to environmental or chemical irritants such as smoking.

PREVENTION

A. Coughing can't be prevented, but you do have some voluntary control over it.

B. Occasionally, medications can cause a cough. So review all medications with your health care provider.

TREATMENT PLAN

A. **The American College of Chest Physicians clinical practice guidelines recommend cough suppressants and other over-the-counter cough medications should *not* be given to children younger than 2 years.**

B. Stop smoking, including exposure to secondhand smoke. At the minimum, maintain a smoke-free bedroom.

C. Using a room humidifier may be helpful. Keep your humidifier clean—it can grow bacteria.

D. Change heating and air conditioning filters often to decrease environmental irritants.

E. Coughing for several minutes may tire you, so you may need extra rest.

Activity: No activity restrictions.

Diet: Drink at least 10 to 15 glasses of liquids a day.

Medications:

You Have Been Prescribed: _____

You Need to Take: _____

You Need to Notify the Office If:

A. You have difficulty breathing.

B. Your child makes noises with coughing, such as wheezing, singsong sounds, or crowing sounds.

C. You cough up blood.

D. You develop other symptoms besides coughing, such as green sinus drainage and/or a sore throat.

E. You can't sleep because of coughing.

F. You develop a fever over 101°F.

G. Other: _____

Phone:_____

VIRAL CROUP

PROBLEM

Croup is a childhood illness of the respiratory system involving the voice box, vocal cords, windpipe, and bronchial tubes. The child is hoarse and has a barking cough, which usually gets worse at night. There may be a sore throat, fever, and a harsh sound with each inward breath (stridor). Infants may be irritable, sleepy, and have a poor appetite.

CAUSE

Croup is usually caused by a virus. Occasionally, it's caused by a bacterial infection.

PREVENTION

A. Isolate the child from others who are ill with respiratory symptoms.

B. The virus is most contagious during the first few days of fever.

TREATMENT PLAN

A. Cool mist has not been shown to be effective with croup.

B. Avoid hot steam since it may cause scalding.

C. Cool night air is often helpful, so open the window or take the child outdoors.

D. Croup tents are not generally recommended unless no alternative therapy is available.

E. Do not expose children to tobacco smoke and other irritants.

F. Count the child's respirations, and observe breathing problems, flaring of nostrils, or retractions (pulling in of chest wall while breathing).

Activity: Let your child rest. Handle your child as little as possible. Your child may return to day care or school when his or her temperature is normal and he or she feels better. A lingering cough is no reason to keep the child home.

Diet: The child may have a decreased appetite during the early part of the illness. It's more important to give plenty of fluids, such as juice and water.

Medications:

You Have Been Prescribed: _____

You Need to Take: _____

You Need to Notify the Office Immediately If:

A. The child's breathing becomes difficult or fast, or the lips become blue.

B. The child has difficulty swallowing or begins to drool.

C. Retractions develop.

D. The child can't sleep.

E. Mist from the vaporizer or bathroom doesn't help.

F. You feel the child is getting worse.

G. Other: _____

You Need to Notify the Office Within 24 Hours If:

A. The cough becomes worse.

B. More than three episodes of labored breathing occur.

C. The child isn't drinking enough fluids.

D. Fever is over 104°F.

E. Other: _____

Phone: _____

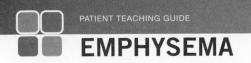

EMPHYSEMA

PROBLEM

Emphysema is a chronic lung disease that is incurable. Emphysema can be managed; the goal of treatment is to improve the activities of daily living and the quality of life by preventing symptoms and by preserving optimal lung function.

CAUSE

Cigarette smoking increases the risk of chronic obstructive pulmonary disease (a blanket term for several lung diseases) by about 30 times. Environmental irritants have also been linked with chronic lung diseases.

PREVENTION

Emphysema can't be prevented once lung changes have taken place.

TREATMENT PLAN

A. **Stop smoking—it causes more lung irritation, sputum production, and coughing. It is never too late to quit smoking.**

B. Eliminate other lung irritants, such as wood smoke; secondhand smoke; hair spray; and paint, bleach, and other chemicals found at home. Avoid sweeping and dusting, and stay indoors when air pollution or pollen counts are high.

C. Pulmonary rehabilitation may be ordered. Exercising is a mandatory component of pulmonary rehabilitation as well as learning breathing techniques.

D. Report respiratory infections to your health care provider as soon as possible.

E. Get a flu shot every year, and get a vaccination for pneumonia.

F. Use postural drainage: lean over the side of the bed, rest your elbows on a pillow placed on the floor, and cough as someone gently pounds on your back.

G. Stay indoors during extremely hot or cold weather. If you must be outside in the cold, cover your nose and face. Use an air conditioner in hot weather.

H. Avoid people who have respiratory illnesses, crowds, and poorly ventilated areas.

I. Oxygen therapy may be ordered if you have trouble breathing.

J. Use community resources such as meals on wheels, handicap tag or parking stickers. Consider a social worker consultation.

Activity:

A. Pace yourself to avoid shortness of breath.

B. Follow a daily exercise plan. Start with three to four sessions a day, each lasting 5 to 15 minutes. Start at half-speed and build up.

C. Sexual dysfunction can occur because of lack of physical energy and trouble breathing. Find other ways to show affection such as kissing, hugging, or massage.

Diet:

A. If you do not have congestive heart failure, drink 3 liters of fluid a day—equal to one and a half large soda bottles.

B. Avoid dairy products; they increase sputum production.

C. Eat five to six small meals a day. Big meals feel like pressure on your stomach and lungs.

D. Avoid foods that cause gas and stomach discomfort.

E. Use oxygen during meals, if necessary; take your time eating, rest between bites, and avoid hard-to-chew foods, because eating may tire you. Rest before and after eating if you have shortness of breath.

F. Eat a high-protein diet with a good balance of vitamins and minerals.

G. Avoid excessively hot or cold foods and drinks that may start an irritating cough.

H. Eat high-potassium foods such as bananas, dried fruit, orange and grape juice, milk, peaches, potatoes, tomatoes, and cantaloupe. Symptoms of low potassium include weakness, leg cramps, and tingling fingers.

Medications:

You Have Been Prescribed: _____

You Need to Take: _____

Use of a spacer/chamber device improves aerosol delivery and reduces side effects.

You Need to Notify the Office If:

    A. You have trouble breathing.

    B. You develop an infection (signs are fever, change in sputum, sinus drainage).

    C. Your inhaler provides no relief.

    D. Your symptoms don't improve within 48 hours of starting medication.

    E. Other: _____

Phone: _____

RESPIRATORY SYNCYTIAL VIRUS

PROBLEM

Respiratory syncytial virus (RSV) causes respiratory distress, wheezing, coughing, and fever.

CAUSE

RSV is a common respiratory virus that affects infants and children in fall, winter, and early spring.

PREVENTION

A. Isolate young infants from people with respiratory illnesses.

B. Wash hands frequently if you're a caregiver.

C. Wash toys and surfaces the child touches.

TREATMENT PLAN

A. Don't smoke around the child.

B. Antibiotics do not help with viral infections.

Activity: The child needs rest during the early stages of the illness.

Diet: Continue to breast-feed. Offer fluids, such as juice and water, frequently. Dilute juice for younger infants. Offer small, frequent feedings.

Medications:

You Have Been Prescribed: _____

You Need to Take: _____

You Need to Call 911 or Call the Office Immediately If:

A. The child's breathing gets labored, difficult, or faster than 60 times a minute.

B. The child's lips become bluish, or he or she stops breathing or passes out.

C. Wheezing becomes severe.

D. Retractions (tugging between ribs) become worse.

E. The child starts acting very sick and lethargic.

F. Other: _____

You Need to Notify the Office Within 24 Hours If:

A. The child is unable to sleep.

B. The child won't drink enough fluids.

C. The child has any suggestion of an earache, a yellow nasal discharge, or a fever over 100°F for more than 72 hours.

D. You feel your child is getting worse.

E. Other: _____

Phone: _____

VIRAL PNEUMONIA: ADULT

PROBLEM

Viral pneumonia is an infection of the lung that causes fluid in the air sacs. You may have fever, cough, or difficulty breathing.

CAUSE

Respiratory viruses cause viral pneumonia.

PREVENTION

A. Avoid contact with people with respiratory illnesses.

B. Get a yearly influenza vaccine.

TREATMENT PLAN

A. Use a cool-mist humidifier, and clean it daily.

B. Take deep breaths and cough frequently to clear secretions from lungs.

C. Avoid smoking and exposure to secondhand smoke.

D. Use good hand washing or the use of hand sanitizers.

Activity: Rest frequently during the early phase of the illness. Fatigue may continue for up to 6 weeks.

Diet: Eat a nutritious diet. Drink 8 to 10 glasses of water a day.

Medications: Take acetaminophen (Tylenol) for fever, discomfort, and headache. Do not take cough suppressants. Antibiotics are not given for a viral infection.

You Have Been Prescribed: _____

You Need to Take: _____

You Need to Notify the Office If You Have:

A. Increased difficulty breathing.

B. Fever over 101°, or fever that persists after 48 hours of antibiotics.

C. Worsening discomfort.

D. Shortness of breath.

E. Blood in sputum.

F. Nausea, vomiting, or diarrhea.

G. Other: _____

Phone: _____

VIRAL PNEUMONIA: CHILD

PROBLEM

Viral pneumonia is an infection of the lung that causes fluid to collect in the air sacs. The child may have fever, cough, or difficulty breathing.

CAUSE

Respiratory viruses cause viral pneumonia.

PREVENTION

A. Isolate young infants from people with respiratory illnesses.

B. Young children should get an influenza vaccine every year.

TREATMENT PLAN

A. Encourage fluids.

B. Use a vaporizer to increase humidity in the child's room.

C. Keep the child away from cigarette smoke.

Activity: Have the child rest during the acute phase. Your child may return to school or day care when he or she is free from fever for 24 hours.

Diet: There is no special diet for viral pneumonia. Follow a regular diet. Increase fluids.

Medications:

A. You may give the child acetaminophen (Tylenol) for fever. Children should never be given aspirin due to the increased risk of Reye's syndrome.

B. Don't give cough suppressants.

C. Only if a bacterial infection is suspected will your child be prescribed antibiotics. Antibiotics are not used for viral infections.

Your Child Has Been Prescribed: _____

Your Child Needs to Take: _____

You Need to Notify the Office Immediately If:

A. The child's breathing becomes more labored or difficult, or his or her lips become blue.

B. Retractions (tugging between ribs) become worse.

C. Grunting sounds occur when the child breathes out.

D. The child starts acting very sick.

E. Other: _____

You Need to Notify the Office Within 24 Hours If:

A. The child is unable to sleep.

B. The child isn't drinking enough.

C. Fever is over 101°F or persists after 48 hours on antibiotics.

D. The child is getting worse.

E. Other: _____

Phone: _____

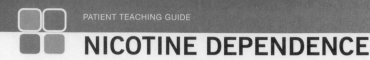

NICOTINE DEPENDENCE

PROBLEM

Cigarette smoking is one of the largest, **preventable causes of death and disability in the United States**. Other forms of nicotine dependence include chewing tobacco and pipe tobacco which can be just as harmful. Risks of lip, tongue oral and throat cancer and problems during pregnancy including bleeding and intrauterine growth restriction. It is well documented that infants and children who are exposed to long term smoke inhalation are at increased risk of **sudden infant death syndrome** and frequent **ear infections and chronic illnesses.**

CAUSE

In adolescence, peer pressure is a big reason why some teenagers begin smoking. By adulthood, the dependence on nicotine has become physical and stopping is difficult. Nicotine also has mood altering effects and can calm the smoker down. The dependence on nicotine becomes emotional as well as physical.

REASONS TO QUIT

Nicotine is a powerful addiction. Quitting will increase your livelihood and increase years to your life. You and your children will have healthier lungs and organs and this will decrease your risk of developing cancer and having a heart attack or stroke. You will also have more energy and feel better physically and mentally. Smoking cessation will also decrease the second hand smoke exposure around your family and friends which will also make them healthier and happier.

TREATMENT PLAN

1. Set a quit date within 2-4 weeks and get information/ treatment from your provider.
2. Throw away all cigarettes, matches, lighters and ashtrays in your home, car and work place.
3. Make smoking very inconvenient.
4. Ask your family/ friends for support and encouragement.
5. Stay in nonsmoking environments and avoid friends/family members that smoke.
6. If you get the urge to smoke, take deep cleansing breaths and try to occupy your time with something else, like chewing gum.
7. Leave the table and change your routine of smoking that you used to have, such as smoking with your coffee after meals, etc.
8. Reward yourself often for staying smoke-free.

Activity:

1. Exercise daily to help alleviate the craving for nicotine.
2. Avoid caffeine if possible.
3. Chew gum or hard candy when you crave a cigarette.
4. Eat celery stick or carrots in place of a cigarette.
5. Drink a lot of water and other fluids to keep hydrated.

Medications:

1. Discuss options available with your health care provider.
2. Oral medications are available and work well for most people. Review side effects and treatment.
3. The nicotine patch, inhaler and gum is available and may be right for you. Discuss these options with your health care provider.

You Have Been Prescribed: _____

You Need To Take: _____

You Need To Notify The Office If You Have:

1. Severe craving and the urge to smoke or chew tobacco
2. Feelings of impulsiveness, like you might do something you will later regret.
3. Begun smoking while using the patch
4. _____

Phone: _____

Patient Teaching Guides for Chapter 9: Cardiovascular Disorders

- Atherosclerosis and Hyperlipidemia
- Peripheral Arterial Disease
- Deep Vein Thrombosis

ATHEROSCLEROSIS AND HYPERLIPIDEMIA

PROBLEM

Hyperlipidemia (excess lipids in the blood) increases your risk of developing atherosclerotic diseases, or "hardening of the arteries." The most common of these diseases are coronary heart disease and heart attack.

CAUSE

Elevated blood cholesterol levels lead to plaque formation in the walls of the major arteries in the body. The higher the level of LDL, or "bad" cholesterol, the greater the chance of getting coronary heart disease. On the other hand, the higher the level of HDL, or "good" cholesterol, the lower the risk of coronary heart disease.

PREVENTION/TREATMENT PLAN

Lowering your risk of atherosclerosis and coronary heart disease involves the following:

A. Diet changes to lower LDL cholesterol and raise HDL cholesterol.

B. Loose weight, if necessary. Start with losing 5 to 10 pounds.

C. Start or increase your physical activity.

D. Modification of other risk factors:

   1. Stop smoking.

   2. Control your blood pressure.

   3. If you are a diabetic it is important to control your blood sugar level.

Activity: Regular exercise, such as walking vigorously for 30 minutes three times a week, increases HDL cholesterol levels, lowers blood sugar, and promotes weight reduction.

Diet: Follow the DASH and Low-Fat/Low-Cholesterol Diet:

A. Decrease total fat calories and cholesterol in diet.

B. Decrease total saturated fats in diet, and replace with monounsaturated fats such as canola oil, olive oil, and margarine.

C. Increase fiber in diet with oatmeal, bran, or fiber supplements.

D. Increase daily intake of fruits and vegetables.

E. Try garlic, soy protein, and vitamin C to help lower LDL cholesterol.

Medications: You may be prescribed a medicine to lower your cholesterol. You will need to come in to have your blood drawn to monitor your liver.

You Have Been Prescribed: _____

You Need to Take: _____

You Need to Notify the Office If You Have:

A. Chest pain.

B. Shortness of breath or trouble breathing while exercising

C. Abdominal pain.

D. Muscle pain or weakness.

E. Other:_____

Phone: _____

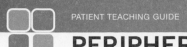

PERIPHERAL ARTERIAL DISEASE

PROBLEM

Peripheral arterial disease makes it difficult for blood to travel to your legs. When a significant amount of fatty deposit collects, symptoms such as pain with exercise begin to appear.

CAUSE

Pain occurs when the oxygen supply doesn't meet the oxygen demand required by the tissue in the legs. This causes less blood to be supplied to the legs, leading to pain in severe cases.

PREVENTION/CARE

A. **Stop smoking.**

1. Talk to your health care provider about using medication or nicotine patches to help you to stop smoking.

B. Keep good care of your feet.

1. Moisturize your feet after bathing.

2. Wear shoes that fit properly.

3. Do not walk barefoot.

4. Keep toenails trimmed and manicured.

5. Avoid injuries to your feet.

6. Inspect your feet for foot ulcers and cracks.

7. Do not try to cut off calluses or corns.

C. It is very important to keep other health problems under control:

1. High blood pressure.

2. Diabetes mellitus: control your blood sugars.

3. High cholesterol.

D. Do not use a heating pad or hot bath water.

Activity:

A. Daily exercise is highly recommended.

B. Walking: warm up 5 to 10 minutes; gradually work up to 30 to 45 minutes of walking daily; cool down for 5 to 10 minutes.

C. This exercise activity must be a part of your daily activity.

Diet: Follow a low-fat, low-salt, high-fiber diet. If you are overweight, consider consulting a dietitian to help you with a weight-loss program.

Medications: You may be prescribed a medicine that helps the blood flow, including a blood thinner and a vasodilator. Make sure to tell your health care provider if you have a history of ulcers if you are placed on one of the medicines that thins your blood.

You Have Been Prescribed: _____

You Need to Take: _____

You Need to Notify the Office If You Have:

A. Severe pain, numbness, or coolness in your legs.

B. Color changes in your legs.

C. Inability to walk.

D. Problems taking your medicine.

E. You develop a foot sore or ulcer.

F. Other:_____

Phone: _____

DEEP VEIN THROMBOSIS

PROBLEM

You have a blood clot in one of the deep veins in your body. Symptoms may include:

A. Pain.

B. Fever.

C. Swelling.

D. Tenderness in the affected leg or arm.

E. The vein in that leg may feel somewhat "hard" to touch.

CAUSE

You developed deep vein thrombosis because your blood-clotting mechanisms were stimulated due to pooling of blood, prolonged bed rest after surgery, a heart attack, a severe illness, a bone fracture, or another cause. The end result is that a clot formed in your vein.

TREATMENT/CARE

A. Most patients require hospitalization and intravenous medications to break up the clots.

B. You will be discharged from the hospital with medications to help break up the clots. Be sure to take them as directed.

C. Don't smoke: this worsens your condition.

D. If you currently take any hormones such as birth control pills, ask your health care provider to tell you about stopping taking them.

Activity:

A. Stay in bed until your health care provider instructs you otherwise.

B. While in bed, continue to perform range-of-motion exercises with your legs.

C. Avoid constrictive clothing such as knee-high hosiery.

D. Wear supportive hosiery as prescribed.

E. Elevate your leg when sitting for long periods, and do not stand for long periods of time when you are off bed rest.

F. Don't sit with your legs crossed.

G. Wear a Medic Alert bracelet during therapy.

H. You will notice that you bruise easier while on your blood thinner.

I. You need to come back to the office to have your labs drawn.

Diet: There is no special diet. Avoid alcohol.

Medications: If you currently take birth control pills, ask your health care provider if you should stop taking them. You may be prescribed a blood thinner by a shot or pills. Take this medicine even if you feel better.

You Have Been Prescribed: _____

You Need to Take: _____

You Need to Notify the Office If You Have:

A. Increased swelling or pain in your affected leg.

B. Fever.

C. Shortness of breath.

D. Chest pain.

E. Difficulty breathing.

F. Bleeding.

    1. Nosebleed that will not stop with pressure

    2. Coughing up blood

    3. Blood in your bowel movements

    4. Heavy periods

G. Any new symptoms not present at your last office visit.

Phone: _____

You can build your own identification bracelets or neck chains from American Medical ID:
http://www.americanmedical-id.com/marketplace/build.php?buildwhat=bracelet.

Patient Teaching Guides for Chapter 10: Gastrointestinal Disorders

- Abdominal Pain: Adults
- Abdominal Pain: Children
- Colic: Ways to Soothe a Fussy Baby
- Crohn's Disease
- Diarrhea: Adults and Children
- Gastroesophageal Reflux Disease (GERD)
- Hemorrhoids
- Irritable Bowel Syndrome
- Jaundice and Hepatitis
- Lactose Intolerance and Malabsorption
- Management of Ulcers
- Roundworms and Pinworms
- Tips to Relieve Constipation

ABDOMINAL PAIN: ADULTS

PROBLEM

Problems relating to abdominal organs may range from simple gas to appendicitis. Suspect a medical emergency if abdominal pain lasts 3 hours or longer, there is fever or vomiting, or the pain is abnormal or unusually sharp or intense. Acute pain is pain that has started recently; recurrent pain is present in three or more separate episodes over at least a 3-month period.

CAUSE

Pain may result from inflammation, ischemia, distension, constipation, or obstruction. Gastroenteritis is the most common cause of acute pain, and chronic stool retention (constipation) is the most common cause of chronic pain. Urinary tract infections can also cause abdominal pain.

A. Males: Torsion of the testicles or a strangulated inguinal hernia may cause abdominal pain.

B. Females: If you have missed a period or suspect you are pregnant, tell your health care provider; ectopic pregnancies are a medical emergency.

PREVENTION

The following suggestions can prevent abdominal pain from constipation:

A. Prompt response to the urge to defecate.

B. Establishing a regular toilet time, such as after breakfast; 15 to 20 minutes after breakfast provides a good opportunity, because spontaneous colonic motility is greatest during that period.

TREATMENT PLAN

Do not take laxatives, use enemas, drugs, food, or liquids (including water) until consulting your health care provider for suspected abdominal pain and the following:

A. Increased or odd-looking vomit or stools

B. Hard, swollen abdomen

C. Lump in scrotum, groin, or lower abdomen

D. Missed period or suspected pregnancy

Activity: Engage in activity as tolerated. Abdominal pain with nausea and vomiting, with fever, or that lasts more than 3 hours and makes you stop doing daily activities should be reported.

Diet: Eat regular foods as tolerated. Do not eat food or drink liquids until you see a health care provider if you have pain with nausea and vomiting, with fever, or that lasts longer than 3 hours.

Medications:

You Have Been Prescribed: _____

You Need to Take: _____

You Need to Notify the Office If You Have:

A. Any change in first symptoms that brought you to the office.

B. Fever higher than _____ degrees.

C. Other: _____

Phone: _____

ABDOMINAL PAIN: CHILDREN

PROBLEM

Problems relating to abdominal organs may range from simple gas to appendicitis. Suspect a medical emergency if abdominal pain lasts 3 hours or longer, there is fever or vomiting, or the pain is abnormal or unusually sharp or intense. Acute pain is pain that has started recently; recurrent pain is present in three or more discrete episodes over at least a 3-month period.

CAUSE

Pain may result from inflammation, ischemia, distension, constipation, or obstruction. Gastroenteritis is the most common cause of acute pain. Chronic pain happens if your child holds in bowel movements and causes constipation. Urinary tract infections can cause abdominal pain, and often the child with a bladder infection does not complain of burning and having to go to the bathroom more often.

PREVENTION

The following can prevent abdominal pain from constipation:

A. Tell your child to go to the bathroom as soon as he or she feels the urge to go.

B. If possible set up a regular toilet time, such as after breakfast; 15 to 20 minutes after breakfast or after school.

TREATMENT PLAN

Do not give laxatives, enemas, drugs, food, or liquids (including water) until consulting your health care provider for suspected abdominal pain and the following:

A. Unusual cry, especially loud crying

B. Increased or odd-looking bowel movements or vomiting

C. Hard, swollen abdomen

D. Lump in scrotum, groin, or lower abdomen

E. If you notice pain symptoms especially when the child bends his or her legs, draws the knees to his or her chest, and/or points to his or her navel.

Activity: Allow activity as tolerated. Children tell you they are in pain with a change in the pitch of crying and making faces (grimacing). For example:

A. Refusing to eat or breast-feed.

B. Drawing their knees to their tummy when you touch their stomach.

Diet: Do not give baby food or liquids until you see a health care provider if you notice a change in the pitch of your baby's crying, facial grimacing, refusal to suck, or your child draws the knees up to his or her stomach especially after you touch him or her.

Medications:

You Have Been Prescribed: _____

You Need to Take: _____

You Need to Notify the Office If You Notice Your Child Has:

A. Any change in first symptoms that brought you to the office.

B. Fever higher than _____ degrees.

C. Other: _____

Phone: _____

COLIC: WAYS TO SOOTHE A FUSSY BABY

PROBLEM

Your baby has been diagnosed with colic: repeated episodes of excessive crying that cannot be explained. Crying may range from fussiness to screaming. Crying follows a pattern:

A. Same time of the day, usually late afternoon or evening.

B. Usually begins at 3 weeks of age and lasts through 3 to 4 months of age.

C. The baby's stomach may rumble, and then the baby may draw up his or her legs as if in pain.

D. No specific disease can be found.

The cause of colic is unknown. Suggested causes are an immature gastrointestinal function, milk allergy, and maternal anxiety.

PREVENTION

There are no specific preventive measures. Remove any causes that can be identified.

TREATMENT PLAN

A. Record time when colic episodes occur. Soothe and comfort the child before the "attack."

B. Don't feed your baby every time he or she cries. Look for a reason, such as a gas bubble, cramped position, too much heat or cold, soiled diaper, open diaper pin, or a desire to be cuddled.

C. Make sure the baby is not overfed or underfed (see "Diet" section below). During an attack of gas, hold the baby securely, and gently massage his or her lower abdomen. Rocking may be soothing.

D. Feed the baby in a vertical position and use frequent burping.

E. Using a collapsible bag/bottle may help to reduce air-swallowing.

F. Do not give your baby any herbal products without a health care provider's approval.

Activity:

A. Overstimulation may cause infant upset. A quiet environment, or being left alone in the crib to work off excess tension may be necessary.

B. Allow the baby to cry if you are certain that everything is all right. Colic is distressing, but not harmful.

C. Take time away from the infant to rest and recoup.

D. Try the following remedies:

1. Rhythmic rocking, use swings.
2. Car rides.
3. Walking the baby in a stroller.
4. Running vacuum or vaporizer for calming noise.
5. Giving the baby a pacifier for sucking.
6. Swaddling and cuddling to soothe the baby.
7. Playing music to quiet the baby.

E. If you are breast-feeding, review all of your medications with your health care provider.

Diet:

A. Your baby should be taking at least _____ ounces of _____ formula at each feeding. Interrupt bottle feedings halfway through the feeding and burp the baby. Burp the baby at the end of the feeding, too.

B. If breast-feeding, do not switch to formula unless you have discussed it with a health care provider. Interrupt breast-feeding every 5 minutes to burp. If breast-feeding, you should avoid eating the following foods: chocolate, cabbage, beans, pizza, or spicy foods.

C. Allow at least 20 minutes to feed the baby. Don't prop the baby for feeding.

D. Do not try a home remedy such as feeding homegrown mint teas to your baby.

You Need to Notify the Office If:

A. The baby has a rectal temperature of 101°F or higher.

B. You fear you are about to loose emotional control.

C. The baby is taking a prescription drug, and new unexplained symptoms develop: the drug may produce side effects.

D. You notice a change in your baby's eating patterns, or he or she has vomiting, diarrhea, or constipation.

E. You notice a change in your baby's pattern of behavior; he or she refuses to suck, his or her crying is high-pitched, he or she draws the legs up when you touch his or her tummy, he or she is limp with no activity.

F. Other: _____

Phone: _____

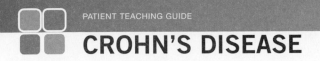

CROHN'S DISEASE

PROBLEM

Crohn's disease (CD) is an inflammatory disorder of the gastrointestinal (GI) tract that produces ulceration, formation of fibrous tissue, and malabsorption. CD is chronic, relapsing, and incurable.

CAUSE

The cause is unknown, but it can be aggravated by bacterial infection or inflammation.

TREATMENT PLAN

A. Adequate nutrition is critical promotion of healing.

B. Vitamin, mineral, and folic acid supplementation is necessary for proper healing and avoidance of secondary complications, such as bone disease and low blood counts.

C. To relieve pain, apply a heating pad or warm compress to your abdomen.

D. Check your bowel movements daily for signs of bleeding. Take any suspicious specimens to the office for evaluation.

E. Surgery may be required to help control symptoms.

Activity: During acute attacks, rest in bed or in a chair. Get up only to go to the bathroom, bathe, or eat. Between attacks, resume normal activities, as tolerated.

Diet:

A. When you have diarrhea, increase the fiber content of your diet.

B. Restricting milk products may stop the diarrhea. Omit milk products for a short time, then try them again in a few weeks.

C. Reducing the amount of fat in your diet may help.

D. Ensure, Sustacal, and Isocal have been found to induce remission and improve symptoms.

E. Severe relapse may require partial bowel rest. Contact the office for instruction.

Medications: You may be prescribed vitamins and minerals, medicine to control pain and relieve diarrhea, and a steroid. Don't stop taking the steroid abruptly. Your health care provider can tell you how to taper the dose over several days.

You Have Been Prescribed the Following Vitamins and Minerals: _____

You Need to Take: _____

You Have Been Prescribed the Following to Relieve Diarrhea: _____

You Need to Take: _____

You Have Been Prescribed the Following Steroid: _____

You Need to Take: _____

Other medications to treat CD include oral medication, intravenous infusions, and injectable medications to control the severity of symptoms. Your health care provider will discuss these with you and the need for close follow-up monitoring.

You Have Been Prescribed: _____

You Need to Take: _____

You Need to Return to the Office for Blood Work: _____

You Need to Notify the Office If You Have:

A. Black, tarry stools or blood in the stool.

B. A swollen abdomen.

C. A temperature of 101.0°F or higher.

D. Other: _____

Phone: _____

RESOURCE

Crohn's and Colitis Foundation of America
800-932-2423
info@ccfa.org

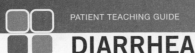

DIARRHEA: ADULTS AND CHILDREN

PROBLEM

Diarrhea is loose, watery stools. Diarrhea is a symptom, not a disease. If you are a diabetic and have more than 1 day of diarrhea, please contact the office.

CAUSE

There are many causes of diarrhea, including viral and bacterial infections and parasites.

PREVENTION

A. Avoid raw seafood and undercooked foods.
B. Store food in the refrigerator within 1 hour of cooking to prevent the growth of bacteria. Especially avoid buffet or picnic foods left out for several hours -and food served by street vendors.
C. Wash your hands well before preparing foods, after going to the bathroom, and after handling diapers.
D. When traveling:
   1. Avoid local water supplies (including ice) when they are in question: drink bottled water instead.
   2. Don't eat fresh vegetables that may have been washed in contaminated water.
E. When hiking or camping, don't drink from streams, springs, or untested wells. Boil all water used for drinking or cooking.
F. Don't allow people with diarrhea to handle food.
G. Don't buy turtles, iguanas, or reptiles for pets: they carry *Salmonella*.
H. Thoroughly cook eggs and other foods of animal origin. Don't eat raw eggs or foods containing raw eggs, such as cookie dough.
I. Keep your child away from child care centers if their diarrhea is too much for a diaper or they are unable to get to the toilet.

TREATMENT PLAN

A. Spontaneous recovery usually occurs in 24 to 48 hours.
B. Keep drinking liquids.
C. If you think a prescription drug is causing diarrhea, consult with the doctor before stopping the medication.
D. Clean toys and hard surfaces with soap and water. Chlorine-based disinfectants inactivate rotavirus and may help prevent disease transmission in child care centers.

Activity: Decrease activities until diarrhea stops.

Diet:

A. If diarrhea is accompanied by nausea, suck ice chips.
B. Drink clear liquids frequently, such as 7-Up, Gatorade, ginger ale, broth, or gelatin, until diarrhea stops.
C. Use popsicles for added liquid.
D. After symptoms disappear, eat soft foods, such as cooked cereal, rice, baked potatoes, and yogurt, for 1 to 2 days.
E. Resume your normal diet in 2 to 3 days after the diarrhea stops.
F. Avoid fruit, alcohol, and highly seasoned foods for several more days.

Medications:

You or Your Child Has Been Prescribed the Following Antidiarrheal Medication: _____

You or Your Child Need to Take: _____

You Need to Notify the Office If:

A. You or your child has diarrhea lasting more than 2 days or chronic diarrhea.
B. You or your child has mucus, blood, or worms in the stool.
C. You have or your child has fever of 101.0°F or higher.
D. You have or your children has severe pain in the stomach or rectum.
E. You have or your child has dehydration symptoms, including dry mouth, wrinkled skin, excessive thirst, little or no urine.
F. Your child:
   1. Becomes listless, refuses to eat, or cries loudly and persistently, even when picked up.
   2. Has abnormal growth and development.

G. Other: _____

Phone: _____

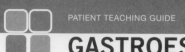

GASTROESOPHAGEAL REFLUX DISEASE (GERD)

PROBLEM

Relaxation of the lower esophageal sphincter causes reflux of gastric acid or a feeling of "heartburn."

CAUSE

Heartburn occurs when reverse peristaltic waves cause regurgitation of acidic stomach contents into the esophagus. Improper diet, pregnancy, and nervous tension are all precipitating factors.

PREVENTION

A. Avoid smoking.

B. Avoid things that increase abdominal pressure:

   1. Wearing tight clothes

   2. Lying down or bending over for 3 hours after eating, which is the time frame of greatest reflux

   3. Coughing

   4. Straining

C. Avoid medications, such as aspirin or ibuprofen, that may irritate your stomach.

TREATMENT

A. Weight loss is advised to relieve symptoms.

B. Stop smoking.

C. You may be instructed to elevate the head of your bed on 6-inch blocks, or sleep on a wedge bolster pillow.

D. Take your medications at the correct times.

Activity: Postpone vigorous exercise until your stomach is likely to be empty, about 2 hours after eating.

Diet:

A. Eat a lower fat, bland diet.

B. Eat four to six small meals a day instead of three larger meals.

C. Don't eat 2 to 3 hours before bedtime.

D. Avoid chocolate, garlic, onions, citrus fruits, coffee (including decaffeinated), alcohol, highly seasoned foods, and carbonated beverages.

E. Eat slowly.

Medications: Sit or stand when taking solid medications (pills or capsules). Follow the drug with at least 1 cup of liquid. When over-the-counter antacids fail to relieve your symptoms, please notify the office for medications that decrease gastric acid secretions. You may require lifelong therapy. Over-the-counter antacids include Mylanta, Rolaids, Turns, Riopan, and Maalox.

You Have Been Prescribed: _____

You Need to Take: _____

You Have Been Prescribed: _____

You Need to Take: _____

You Need to Notify the Office If You Have:

   A. No relief from antacids or second medication, so that we may prescribe the next step of medication therapy.

   B. New symptoms, such as blood in regurgitated stomach contents.

   C. Other: _____

Phone: _____

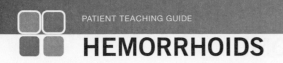

HEMORRHOIDS

PROBLEM

A hemorrhoid is a varicose vein of the rectum. Hemorrhoids may be present for years but go undetected until bleeding occurs. They may cause rectal pain, itching, or a sensation that you have not emptied completely after a bowel movement. Hemorrhoids are often found after painless rectal bleeding with a bowel movement.

CAUSE

Repeated pressure in the anal or rectal veins causes hemorrhoids. They are commonly seen with obesity, pregnancy, constipation, sedentary lifestyle, and liver disease.

PREVENTION

A. Avoid heavy lifting.

B. Try to prevent constipation or straining.

C. Eat a high-fiber diet.

D. Drink 8 to 10 glasses of water a day.

E. Lose weight if you're overweight.

F. Exercise regularly.

TREATMENT PLAN

A. Spend less time sitting on the toilet to reduce pressure in the veins around the anus.

B. Pat with toilet paper instead of rubbing.

C. Take sitz baths or soak in a warm bathtub three or four times a day for comfort.

D. Apply cold packs or witch hazel (Tucks) compresses for symptom relief.

E. Take a stool softener two to three times a day to prevent straining with bowel movements.

F. A hemorrhoid treatment such as ligation, freezing, or surgery may need to be done for severe cases.

Activity: No restrictions are required. Bowel function improves with good physical activity.

Medications:

You Have Been Prescribed the Following Stool Softener: _____

You Need to Take: _____

You Have Been Prescribed the Following Local Cream: _____

You Need to Apply: _____

You Need to Notify the Office If You Have:

A. A hard lump that develops where a hemorrhoid has been.

B. Hemorrhoids that cause severe pain that is not relieved by the above treatment.

C. Excessive rectal bleeding: more than a trace or streak on the toilet paper or bowel movement. **Rectal bleeding may be an early sign of cancer.**

D. Other: _____

Phone: _____

IRRITABLE BOWEL SYNDROME

PROBLEM

Irritable bowel syndrome (IBS) is an irritative and inflammatory disorder of the intestine. You may have diarrhea, you may have constipation, or you may have problems with alternating constipation and diarrhea.

CAUSE

Irritable bowel syndrome is **not contagious,** inherited, or cancerous. It has no known direct cause, but it flares with severe stress and may also be triggered by eating.

PREVENTION

A. Try to reduce stress or modify your response to it. Keep a stress diary to avoid stress triggers.

B. Good food habits also help.

C. No specific food has been identified as responsible for all IBS symptoms. Keep a food diary to identify and avoid your food triggers.

TREATMENT PLAN

A. Quit smoking: nicotine may contribute to the problem.

B. Apply a warm heat compress to your abdomen for comfort.

Activity: Exercise, such as walking 20 minutes a day, improves bowel function and helps reduce stress. Other stress-reduction techniques include self-hypnosis and biofeedback.

Diet:

A. Eat a high-fiber diet. Fiber is good for both diarrhea and constipation.

B. Avoid sorbitol-containing (sugar-free) candies and gum as well as lactose-containing milk products to see if this eases your diarrhea symptoms.

C. Don't eat or drink anything that aggravates your symptoms such as the following:
   1. Coffee may be a major food trigger.
   2. Avoid spicy and gas-producing foods.
   3. Avoid large meals, but eat regularly.
   4. Limit alcohol.

Medications:

You Have Been Prescribed: _____

You Need to Take: _____ _____

You Need to Notify the Office If You Have:

   A. Fever.

   B. Black or tarry-looking bowel movements.

   C. Vomiting.

   D. Unexplained weight loss of 5 pounds or more.

   E. Symptoms that don't improve despite changes in diet, exercise, and medication.

   F. Other: _____

Phone: _____

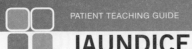
JAUNDICE AND HEPATITIS

PROBLEM

Jaundice is a yellow tinge of the skin or mucous membranes, which are the tissue that lines the mouth and other body cavities. Jaundice is a symptom, not a disease. It occurs when the blood contains too much bilirubin—a yellow pigment found in bile, which is a fluid secreted by the liver.

When the liver is damaged, bilirubin builds up in the body and skin, turning the skin yellow and itchy. Other symptoms that occur with jaundice are dark urine, light-colored bowel movements, fatigue, fever, chills, appetite loss, nausea, and vomiting.

CAUSE

Jaundice usually comes from a liver disorder, such as cirrhosis, hepatitis, or a disease of the gallbladder or pancreas. But it can also be a symptom of other disorders, like anemia or severe heart failure. Sometimes jaundice results from taking a drug that damages the liver.

PREVENTION

Although hepatitis is considered contagious, you don't need to be confined to your home. However, to help prevent the spread of hepatitis:

A. Do not prepare or handle food for others until cleared by your health care provider.
B. Wash your hands well after using the toilet and changing diapers.
C. If you have hepatitis A or B, avoid intimate sexual contact until cleared by your health care provider.
D. If you have hepatitis B or C, don't share razors, toothbrushes, and other personal items.
E. Never donate blood after a hepatitis B or C infection.
F. Your family and sexual partners may need an injection of immune globulin or a vaccination, depending on the type of hepatitis you have.
G. School exposure to hepatitis A does not generally pose a risk to others.
H. Risk of hepatitis B transmission in day care centers appears to be extremely rare.

TREATMENT PLAN

Treatment for jaundice includes the following:

A. Use good hygiene with bathing, using the bathroom, and hand washing.
B. Apply anti-itch lotions, such as calamine.
C. Rest.
D. Alteration of medications if jaundice is from a liver disorder.
E. Surgery may be required to remove the stone or to have a procedure called lithotripsy to crush it, if a stone blocking the bile duct causes jaundice.
F. If you have hepatitis, you may need to be referred to a specialist.
G. The public health department will be notified by your health care provider for acute hepatitis.
H. Your health care provider may discuss the need for a liver biopsy.

Activity: Plan rest periods throughout the day. Avoid strenuous exercise. Gradually resume activities and mild exercise during your convalescent period.

Diet: Eat small, frequent, low-fat, high-calorie meals. You may be instructed to limit protein during acute phases of some types of hepatitis. Sit down to eat to decrease pressure on your liver. Drink 8 to 10 glasses of liquids a day.

Medications:

You Have Been Prescribed: _____

You Need to Take: _____

You Have Been Prescribed: _____

You Need to Take: _____

You Need to Notify the Office If You Have:

A. Mild confusion.
B. Personality changes.
C. Worsening symptoms.
D. Tremors.
E. Other: _____

Phone: _____

RESOURCES

American Liver Foundation: http://www.liverfoundation.org
Hepatitis B Foundation: http://www.hepb.org/

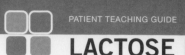
LACTOSE INTOLERANCE AND MALABSORPTION

PROBLEM

You have been diagnosed as having difficulty digesting milk (lactose) products or have problems with malabsorption. Lactose intolerance can cause gas, bloating, abdominal cramps, diarrhea, and nausea or vomiting. You may be able to eat small portions without problems or be unable to tolerate any foods containing lactose.

CAUSE

Lactose is the sugar present in milk. Lactose intolerance is very common; it occurs when the body is not able to appropriately digest this milk sugar content and results in diarrhea.

PREVENTION

Follow a lactose-free or lactose-controlled diet.

Activity: No restrictions are required. Resume normal activities as soon as diarrhea symptoms improve. You may be sent to see a registered dietitian to assist in your dietary plan.

Diet:

A. Limit or omit foods that contain milk, lactose, whey, or casein.

B. Lactose-controlled diets allow up to 1 cup of milk per day for cooking or drinking, if you can tolerate it.

C. If you can't tolerate any lactose, choose lactose-free foods with lactate, lactic acid, lactalbumin, whey protein, sodium caseinate, casein hydrolysates, and calcium compounds. Read labels carefully.

D. You may also choose kosher foods marked "pareve" or "parve," which don't contain lactose. Read labels carefully.

E. A low-fat diet is important if you have fat malabsorption.

F. To help with diarrhea due to malabsorption, avoid more than one serving a day of caffeine-containing drinks.

G. Beverages with high sugar content such as soft drinks and fruit juices may increase diarrhea. Juices and fruits with high amounts of fructose include apples, pears, sweet cherries, prunes, and dates.

H. Sorbitol-containing candies and gums may cause diarrhea.

Medications: You may need the enzyme lactase to help you digest your food. You may need vitamins and minerals if you are having problems with malabsorption/diarrhea.

You Have Been Prescribed: _____

You Need to Take: _____

You Need to Notify the Office If You Have:

A. Severe abdominal pain.

B. Diarrhea causing dehydration.

C. Other: _____

Phone: _____

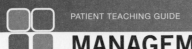

MANAGEMENT OF ULCERS

PROBLEM

An ulcer is a sore in the lining of the stomach or intestine occurring in areas exposed to acid and pepsin. Complications include bleeding ulcer and perforation, and obstruction can be life-threatening.

CAUSE

Although the precise cause of ulcer formation isn't completely understood, the process appears to involve excess acid production, excess pepsin secretion, and mucosal defense mechanisms. *Helicobacter pylori,* an infectious bacterium, and certain anti-inflammatory drugs have also been identified as causes.

PREVENTION

Modify your lifestyle to include health practices that prevent recurrences of ulcer pain and bleeding.

TREATMENT PLAN

A. If aspirin or a nonsteroidal anti-inflammatory drug causes the ulcer, eliminate the drug. If you need the drug for other health problems, discuss other options with your health care provider, such as using the lowest doses and duration.
B. Avoid caffeine, colas, alcohol, and chocolate because they may increase acid production.
C. Stop smoking: it decreases the ulcer's healing rate and increases its recurrence.
D. Be sure to tell health care providers about your history of ulcer and gastrointestinal pain if you need new prescriptions or are sent to the hospital.

Activity: Exercise daily. Plan rest periods, avoid fatigue, and learn to cope with or avoid stressful situations.

Diet:

A. Eat a well-balanced diet with high fiber content.
B. Eat meals at regular intervals. Frequent small feedings are unnecessary. Avoid bedtime snacks.
C. Eliminate foods that cause pain or distress; otherwise, your diet is usually not restricted. Examples of foods that cause worse pain are:
    1. Peppermint
    2. Spicy food
    3. Alcohol
D. Avoid extremely hot or cold food or fluids, chew thoroughly, and eat in a leisurely fashion for better digestion.

Medications:

A. H_2 blockers and proton pump inhibitors (PPIs) reduce stomach acid.
B. Antibiotics fight *H. pylori* infection.
C. Other medications may be prescribed to coat the ulcer area. Antacids can be taken during the ulcer treatment but should not be used 1 hour before or 2 hours after the ulcer treatments because antacids can interfere with absorption.
D. Take the entire prescription: don't stop when you feel better.
E. If you have been prescribed metronidazole (Flagyl) or clarithromycin, you may notice a metallic taste in your mouth.
F. Alcohol (including wine) should be avoided when taking Flagyl. The interaction can cause skin flushing, headache, nausea, and vomiting.
G. If you are prescribed bismuth, you may notice black bowel movements.

You Have Been Prescribed: _____

You Need to Take: _____

You Have Been Prescribed: _____

You Need to Take: _____

You Need to Notify the Office If You Have:

A. Worsening symptoms while taking your medication.
B. Vomiting that is bloody or looks like coffee grounds.
C. Tar-colored or "grape jelly" bowel movements. If this occurs, bring a stool sample to the office.
D. Diarrhea and/or severe pain despite treatment.
E. Unusual weakness or paleness.
F. Other: _____

Phone: _____

ROUNDWORMS AND PINWORMS

PROBLEM

Roundworms and pinworms are intestinal parasites. Roundworms resemble earthworms; pinworms are small, white, and threadlike. Both types of worms thrive in the intestinal tract and are very common in children. They can spread to other family members, so the entire family needs to be treated.

CAUSE

Pinworms live in the human rectum or colon and emerge onto the skin around the anus. Nighttime itching is due to the daily evening migration of the female pinworm downward to deposit eggs on the perianal skin. Pinworms are transmitted from person to person by direct transfer of infective eggs to the mouth, or by indirect transfer through clothing, bedding, food, or other articles contaminated with the eggs.

Roundworm eggs enter the human body by means of contaminated water or food or by transfer from contaminated unwashed hands.

PREVENTION

The following measures help prevent the spread of worms:

A. Remove sources of infection by treating the infected person and family members.

B. Household measures:

1. Wash (132°F) or boil soiled bedsheets, nightclothes, underwear, towels, and washcloths used by infected persons.

2. Soak fabrics that can't be boiled in an ammonia solution: 1 cup of household ammonia to 5 gallons of cold water.

3. After treatment, scrub toilet seats, bathroom floors, and fixtures. Vacuum rugs, and clean table tops, curtains, sofas, and chairs carefully.

C. Practice good personal hygiene. Wash hands before handling foods and eating, and after using the toilet. Wash the anus and genitals with warm water and soap at least twice a day. Rinse well and then wash your hands.

D. Take a morning bath to remove most eggs.

E. Keep fingers away from the mouth. Cut nails and discourage nail biting and scratching the bare anal area.

F. Clean fingernails before meals and after bowel movements.

G. Reduce overcrowding when possible.

H. For roundworms: Have pets treated, and avoid strange animals.

TREATMENT PLAN

Parasitic infection is easily treated with medication. All family members need to be treated.

Activity: Resume normal activities after treatment is complete and symptoms improve.

Diet: No special foods are needed.

Medication:

You Have Been Prescribed: _____

You Need to Take: _____

You Need to Notify the Office If You Have:

A. Reappearance of worms after treatment.

B. New or unexplained symptoms. Drugs used in treatment may produce side effects.

C. Other: _____

Phone: _____

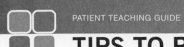

TIPS TO RELIEVE CONSTIPATION

PROBLEM

Constipation is an infrequent and difficult passing of hard stools and sensation of incomplete emptying or straining.

CAUSE

There are many reasons why you have constipation. You may note that you have just one or have a combination of these common causes:

A. Not drinking enough liquids.

B. Eating a low-fiber diet.

C. Sedentary lifestyle, lack of exercise.

D. Ignoring the urge to go to the bathroom.

E. Taking drugs, including blood pressure medications, antidepressants, pain medications and antacids, or overusing laxatives can cause constipation.

F. Depression.

G. Other medical conditions may also cause chronic constipation.

PREVENTION

A. Respond promptly to the urge to. When you feel the urge to go to the bathroom do not wait.

B. Establish a regular toilet time, such as after breakfast; 15 to 20 minutes after breakfast provides a good opportunity because spontaneous colonic motility is greatest during that period.

C. Use a footrest during elimination to provide support and decrease straining.

D. Do not rely on laxatives; use prune juice as a natural substitute.

E. Stimulate the intestine by drinking hot or cold water or prune juice before meals.

F. Decrease the intake of sweets, which increase bacterial growth in the intestine and can lead to gas.

G. Stop taking enemas and nonessential drugs and herbals.

TREATMENT PLAN

A. Follow the suggested prevention tips.

B. Change to a high-fiber diet.

C. Get daily exercise

Activity: Daily exercise such as walking helps to maintain healthy bowel patterns.

Diet:

A. Eat a high-fiber diet.

B. Restrict cheese: it causes constipation.

C. Drink at least 8 glasses of water each day.

D. Avoid refined cereals and breads, pastries, and sugar.

E. Coffee, tea, and alcohol decrease water to the colon. Limit to 2 drinks per day.

Medications: You may be prescribed a stool softener or a laxative for short-term use only. You may be prescribed a bulk-forming agent to take on a regular basis to increase the bulk of your stool.

You Have Been Prescribed: _____

You Need to Take: _____

You Need to Notify the Office If:

A. Constipation persists in spite of the self-care instructions, including diet and exercise.

B. You notice a change in your bowel movements. Changes in bowel patterns may be an early sign of cancer.

C. You develop fever, constipation, or severe abdominal pain.

D. Other: _____

Phone: _____

Patient Teaching Guides for Chapter 11: Genitourinary Disorders

- Benign Prostatic Hypertrophy
- Epididymitis
- Prostatitis
- Testicular Self-Examination
- Urinary Incontinence: Women
- Urinary Tract Infection (Acute Cystitis)

BENIGN PROSTATIC HYPERTROPHY

PROBLEM

Enlargement of the prostate gland causes difficulty urinating; increased urination, especially at night; difficulty starting or stopping; decreased stream; and feeling that your bladder is not empty.

CAUSE

The cause is not known, but it may be due to changes in hormonal levels as you get older.

PREVENTION

None.

TREATMENT PLAN

Treatment depends on how bad the symptoms are. Medications can help, but an operation to fix the obstruction may be needed. Empty your bladder on a schedule every 2 to 3 hours to prevent overfilling of the bladder.

Activity: There are no restrictions. You may need to plan schedules with access to bathrooms in mind.

Diet: Avoid spicy foods that irritate the bladder. Caffeine and alcohol act as diuretics and increase your need to urinate.

Medications:

A. Medications that help relieve the blockage may block hormones or relax the muscles that control urination.

B. Antibiotics are used if there is also an infection in the bladder or prostate.

C. Over-the-counter medications to avoid: cold medications, decongestants, antihistamines (for allergies), and antidiarrheals.

D. Always read labels to check for advice: "Do not take if you have prostate enlargement."

E. Avoid drinking liquids before bedtime or before going out.

F. Double void to empty your bladder more completely.

You Have Been Prescribed: _____

You Need to Take: _____

You Need to Notify the Office If:

A. You cannot urinate.

B. Your symptoms worsen.

C. You have a fever.

D. Other:

Phone: _____

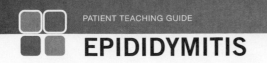

EPIDIDYMITIS

PROBLEM

Epididymitis is infection of the epididymis, the gland that carries sperm.

CAUSE

An infection may be the cause of bacteria from the urethra (urine opening). The infection may be a urinary tract infection or from a sexually transmitted disease, including gonorrhea and chlamydia.

PREVENTION

A. Prevent urinary tract infections with good hygiene:

    1. Clean under foreskin if uncircumcised.

    2. Wash your hands after each time you go to the bathroom (urine and bowel movements).

B. Limit your sexual partners and use a condom to prevent all types of infection.

TREATMENT PLAN

A. Antibiotics to kill bacteria that cause infection.

B. Try one of the following comfort measures:

    1. Intermittent cold compresses for acute swelling and pain relief.

    2. Local heat or sitz bath after the initial discomfort.

C. Athletic supporter or elevation of scrotum on a small rolled washcloth.

Activity: Rest; do not engage in strenuous activity or heavy lifting. Avoid sexual intercourse until you finish the antibiotic and sexual partner(s) have been treated for sexually transmitted disease, too.

Diet: Avoid foods that irritate bladder: caffeine, alcohol, and spicy foods.

Medications:

A. Antibiotics are used to kill bacteria causing infection. Take all of the drugs prescribed; don't stop drugs after symptoms have resolved.

B. Take pain medications or anti-inflammatory drugs such as acetaminophen (Tylenol) or ibuprofen as needed.

You Have Been Prescribed the Following Antibiotic: _____

You Need to Take:_____

Finish all of the antibiotics, even if you feel better.

You Have Been Prescribed the Following for Pain: _____

You Need to Take: _____

You Need to Notify the Office If:

    A. You have a great increase in pain or swelling after going home.

    B. You have worsening symptoms after starting the antibiotics.

    C. You have fever over 101.0°F.

    D. You get very constipated.

    E. Other: _____

Phone: _____

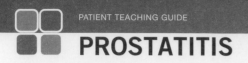

PROSTATITIS

PROBLEMS

Prostatitis is infection and/or inflammation of the prostate. Symptoms can be problems with urinating, increased frequency or painful urination, fever or chills. You may have pain in scrotum and buttocks and blood in the urine or semen. Prostatitis can be treated and does not cause impotence.

CAUSE

An infection may be caused by bacteria from the bladder or reflux of urine, or it may have started from a rectal infection.

PREVENTION

A. Prevent prostate infection with good hygiene:
   1. Clean under foreskin if uncircumcised and wash your hands after each time you go to the bathroom (urine and bowel movements).
   2. Limit your sexual partners and use a condom to prevent all types of infection.
   3. Urinate when you have the urge. Do not hold your urine for long periods of time.
B. Maintaining sexual activity and ejaculation may decrease the incidence.

TREATMENT PLAN

A. Hospitalization may be necessary for severe infections.
B. Try the following comfort measures:
   1. Use a sitz bath or sit in warm bath water or a whirlpool three times a day to provide some relief.
   2. You may find you feel more comfortable when you empty your bladder in a warm water bath when your pelvic muscles relax.
C. Your sexual partner(s) may need to be evaluated and treated, too (ask your health care provider).

Activity: Rest; do not engage in strenuous physical activity or heavy lifting.

Diet: Increase fluid intake. ***Fluid Exception:* Decrease caffeine and alcohol, which can irritate the urethra.**

Medications: Antibiotics cure the infection by killing bacteria. You need to continue taking these drugs until infection is completely cured (usually about 1 month). You need to take all the antibiotics even if your symptoms are gone.

You Have Been Prescribed the Following Antibiotic: _____

You Need to Take: _____

Finish all of the antibiotic even if you feel better.

Pain medications combined with anti-inflammatory drugs to decrease pain are usually taken for 3 to 7 days. Take acetaminophen (Tylenol) to bring down fever.

You Have Been Prescribed the Following for Pain: _____

You Need to Take: _____

You Have Been Prescribed the Following for Fever: _____

You Need to Take: _____

You Need to Notify the Office If You Have:

   A. Symptoms that get worse or do not improve during treatment.
   B. Symptoms that recur after treatment.
   C. Fever over 101.0°F.
   D. Other:_____

Phone:_____

RESOURCES

American Urological Association Foundation: www.UrologyHealth.org
National Kidney and Urologic Disease Information Clearinghouse: www.kidney.niddk.nih.gov
National Urology Health Hotline Toll Free 1-800-828-7866
The Prostatitis Foundation: www.prostatitis.org

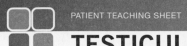
TESTICULAR SELF-EXAMINATION

The testicular self-examination is easy to do and does not take very much time to perform. The monthly examination is an effective way to become familiar with this area of the body and will enable early detection of testicular cancer. Set a date for the same day every month. An easy way to remember your chosen day is to use the first day of the month, last day of the month, or your birth date. The best time to examine your testicles is during or after a hot bath or shower. (Heat makes the testicles relax and descend into the scrotal sac, which is the pouch of skin containing your testicles and parts of the spermatic cords.)

Tumors are palpable and can easily be detected. Ages 15 to 35 are considered the tumor-prone years because they are the most active years for hormonal activity.

PROCEDURE

A. If possible, do the self-examination in front of a mirror.

B. Check for any swelling of the scrotal skin.

C. Support each testicle with one hand and examine it with the other hand (see Figure).

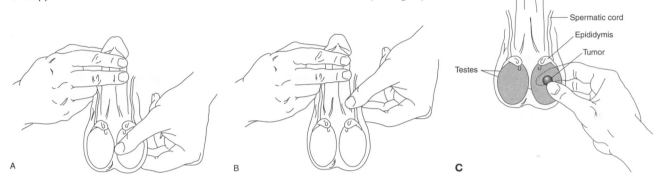

Figure Testicular self-examination. A. Check each spermatic cord. Locate the cordlike structure called the epididymis at the back of your testicle; the spermatic cord extends upward from it. B. Gently squeeze the spermatic cord above your left testicle between your thumb and the first two fingers of your left hand. Check for lumps and masses along the entire cord. C. Palpation for testicular tumor using the thumb, the epididymis, testes, and spermatic cord located bilaterally.

From *The Lippincott Manual of Nursing Practice* (9th ed.), by S. Nettina, 2010. Philadelphia: Wolters Kluwer Health/Lippincott Williams & Wilkins.

D. Use both hands to feel all of the scrotal contents.

   1. With one hand, lift your penis, and check the scrotum with the other hand. Feel any change in shape or size.

   2. Look for reddened or enlarged blood veins.

   3. The left side may hang slightly lower than the right (this is normal).

E. Check each testicle.

   1. Place your left thumb on the front of your left testicle and your index and middle fingers behind it.

   2. Gently but firmly roll the testicle between your thumb and fingers.

   3. Then use your right hand to examine the right testicle the same way.

   4. The testicles should feel smooth, rubbery, oval shaped, and slightly tender. They should move freely.

   5. Locate the epididymis and spermatic cord. The epididymis is the irregular, cordlike structure on the top and the back of the testicle.

      a. Gently squeeze the spermatic cord above your left testicle between you thumb and the first two fingers of your left hand.

      b. Check for lumps and masses along the entire length of the cords.

      c. Repeat on the right side, using your right hand.

F. Consult your health care provider, preferably a urologist, if you notice:

   1. Any lumps, even small pea-sized ones.

   2. Any masses, like a bag of worms.

   3. A dull ache in the lower abdomen or in the groin.

   4. A feeling of heaviness in the scrotum.

   5. A significant loss of size in one of the testicles.

   6. Pain or discomfort in a testicle or in the scrotum.

   7. Any other changes you notice since your last self examination.

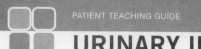

URINARY INCONTINENCE: WOMEN

PROBLEM

Urinary incontinence is the inability to control the release of urine.

CAUSE

Multiple causes have been associated with incontinence, depending on the type of incontinence you have.

PREVENTION

Exercise regularly, and practice pelvic floor exercises, commonly called Kegel exercises. Manage constipation so you do not strain to have a bowel movement. Stop smoking and treat any lung disease especially if you have coughing.

TREATMENT PLAN

Treatment depends on cause and type of incontinence. See Table.

A. Pelvic floor exercises should be done every morning, afternoon, and evening, starting with five repetitions each set, gradually increasing to 10 repetitions each set. To perform these exercises:

   1. Start by doing your pelvic muscles lying down. When your muscles get stronger, do your exercises sitting or standing.

   2. Do not tighten your stomach, leg, or buttock muscles: just squeeze the pelvic muscles you use to stop the flow of urine.

   3. Do not hold your breath or practice while urinating.

   4. Pull in pelvic muscles and hold the contraction for a count of 5.

   5. Repeat five times.

   6. Work up to doing 3 sets of 10 repeats.

   7. Kegel exercises take just a few minutes a day and most women notice an improvement after a few weeks of daily therapy.

B. Empty your bladder frequently.

C. You may be taught relaxation techniques to control the feeling of urgency.

Activity: Try to get daily exercise. Use absorbent undergarments until incontinence is controlled.

Diet: Eat a well-balanced diet. If overweight, consider a weight-loss program. Avoid excessive fluid intake especially caffeinated beverages and alcohol.

Medications: What you take depends on the type of incontinence you have.

You Have Been Prescribed: _____

You Need to Take:_____

You Need to Notify the Office If You Have: _____

Phone: _____

RESOURCES

American Urogynecologic Society www.augs.org
American Urological Association www.UrologyHealth.org
National Association for Continence www.nafc.org
The Simon Foundation for Continence www.simonfoundation.org

TABLE **Bladder Control Diary**

Your Daily Bladder Diary

This diary will help you and your health care team figure out the causes of your bladder control trouble. The "sample" line shows you how to use the diary. Use this sheet as a master for making copies that you can use as a bladder diary for as many days as you need.

Your name: _____

Date: _____

Time	Drinks		Trips to the Bathroom		Accidental Leaks	Did you feel a strong urge to go?	What were you doing at the time?
	What kind?	*How much?*	*How many times?*	*How Much urine? (circle one)*	*How much? (circle one)*	*Circle one*	*Sneezing, exercising, having sex, lifting, etc.*
Sample	Coffee	2 cups	✓✓	sm med lg	sm med lg	Yes No	Running
6–7 a.m.						Yes No	
7–8 a.m.						Yes No	
8–9 a.m.						Yes No	
9–10 a.m.						Yes No	
10–11 a.m.						Yes No	
11–12 noon						Yes No	
12–1 p.m.						Yes No	
1–2 p.m.						Yes No	
2–3 p.m.						Yes No	
3–4 p.m.						Yes No	
4–5 p.m						Yes No	
5–6 p.m.						Yes No	
6–7 p.m.						Yes No	
7–8 p.m.						Yes No	
8–9 p.m.						Yes No	
9–10 p.m.						Yes No	
10–11 p.m.						Yes No	
11–12 midnight						Yes No	
12–1 a.m.						Yes No	
1–2 a.m.						Yes No	
2–3 a.m.						Yes No	
3–4 a.m.						Yes No	
4–5 a.m.						Yes No	
5–6 a.m.						Yes No	

(continued)

(continued)

I used ____ pads today. I used ____ diapers today (write number).

Questions to ask my health care team: _____

_____

_____

_____

_____

Let's Talk About Bladder Control for Women is a public health awareness campaign conducted by the National Kidney and Urologic Diseases Information Clearinghouse (NKUDIC), an information dissemination service of the National Institute of Diabetes and Digestive and Kidney Diseases (NIDDK), National Institutes of Health.

From National Kidney and Urologic Diseases Information Clearinghouse (NKUDIC), National Institutes of Health (NIH). http://kidney.niddk.nih.gov/kudiseases/pubs/bcw_ez/insertB.htm

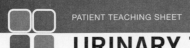

URINARY TRACT INFECTION (ACUTE CYSTITIS)

PROBLEM

You have been diagnosed with a bladder infection. The symptoms include painful, frequent urination and pain over bladder. The symptoms may be mild, moderate, or painful.

CAUSE

Bacteria move up the urethra (tube that connects bladder with the outside of the body), causing infection of the bladder. A bladder infection is more common in women, or in persons who have had a catheter, and men that have prostate problems.

PREVENTION

A. Urinate frequently:
   1. As soon as you feel the urge to go, empty your bladder at that time. Do not hold your urine.
   2. You may need to urinate on a schedule during the day, at least every 2 to 3 hours if you do not urinate this frequently.
B. Wash your hands after going to the bathroom (urine and bowel movements).
C. Good hygiene for females:
   1. Wipe front to back every time you empty your bladder and especially after bowel movements.
   2. Take showers instead of baths; do not take bubble baths.
   3. Empty your bladder before and after sexual intercourse.
   4. Avoid feminine hygiene sprays and douches.
D. Wear cotton underwear. Do not wear tight underwear and clothes. Take off your underwear at night while sleeping.

TREATMENT PLAN

Treatment depends on the severity of the infection. Antibiotics are used to kill bacteria that cause infections. The most important thing is to finish all of your medications even if you feel better.

Activity: Rest; avoid strenuous activity. Avoid sexual activity until you finish the antibiotics.

Diet:

A. Increase fluids; drink at least one large glass of liquid every hour.
B. Avoid foods that irritate the bladder: caffeine, alcohol, and spicy foods.
C. Drink cranberry juice to help fight bladder infections. If you do not like plain cranberry juice, mix it 1:1 with another juice, such as orange juice.

Medications:

A. Antibiotics kill bacteria that cause infection. Make sure you take all of your medications, not just until you feel better.
B. Take acetaminophen (Tylenol) for fever.
C. You may be prescribed a medication to prevent bladder spasms and pain while urinating. This changes the color of your urine to orange.

You Have Been Prescribed the Following Antibiotic: _____

You Need to Take: _____

Take all of your antibiotics, even if you feel better.

You Have Been Prescribed the Following for Discomfort: _____

You Need to Take: _____

You Need to Notify the Office If You Have:

A. Worsening symptoms or symptoms not improving during treatment.
B. Fever higher than 100.4°F.
C. Blood in urine; your urine color will be red-orange with the medication for your bladder discomfort.
D. Recurring symptoms after finishing all of your medications: painful urination, back pain, fever, chills, or nausea.
E. Other:_____

Phone: _____

Patient Teaching Guides for Chapter 12: Obstetrics

- Iron Deficiency Anemia (Pregnancy)

- Preterm Labor

- Gestational Diabetes

- Insulin Therapy During Pregnancy

- Urinary Tract Infection During Pregnancy: Pyelonephritis

- First Trimester Vaginal Bleeding

- Vaginal Bleeding: Second and Third Trimester

- Breast Engorgement and Sore Nipples

- Endometritis

- Mastitis

- Wound Infection: Episiotomy and Cesarean Section

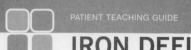

IRON DEFICIENCY ANEMIA (PREGNANCY)

PROBLEM

You have a "low blood count" called iron deficiency anemia. Iron is needed for red blood formation.

CAUSE

This is caused by a deficiency of iron in your diet, and it is very common.

PREVENTION

Anemia may be prevented by increasing iron in your diet and by taking extra iron tablets.

TREATMENT PLAN

A. You need to increase the iron-rich food in your diet.

B. You will be prescribed an iron supplement.

C. Antacids for indigestion and dairy products interfere with iron absorption. Do not take your iron supplements with milk or just before or after an antacid.

D. If you are pregnant, you may be eligible for the WIC program (Women, Infants, and Children), which provides supplemental foods for pregnant women and young children. Ask your health care provider for information about its availability in your community.

Activity: You may feel more tired than usual due to anemia. You may need to rest more than usual; however, try to continue your current exercise routine as tolerated. Alternative exercise includes walking 20 minutes a day or swimming.

Diet: You need to increase the amount of iron in your diet. Generally, the redder the meat and the greener the vegetable, the richer it is as a source of iron. You also need to make sure you have adequate intake of vitamin C (this helps increase the absorption of iron into your body). Vitamin C is found in fresh, dark-green vegetables and citrus fruits. Drink 8 to 10 glasses of liquids every day.

Medications:

You Have Been Prescribed: _____

You Need to Take: _____

Special Instructions About Iron Supplements:

A. Take the iron medication as prescribed; higher doses are not better. You may need to be taking it for a longer time. High doses of iron can be toxic to children and adults.

B. Your body only absorbs a small portion of the iron pills you take.

C. You may notice green or black bowel movements. This is normal.

D. It is best to take the iron pills on an empty stomach.

E. Try taking your iron pill with a glass of orange juice. The vitamin C in the juice helps the iron be absorbed better.

F. You may have nausea or vomiting when you take iron pills, especially during early pregnancy. If this happens, try taking the pill with food. It is better to take your iron with food than to skip your pill altogether.

G. If you are not able to tolerate the iron in the morning, try taking it in the middle of the afternoon or at bedtime.

H. You may become constipated while taking iron pills. Increase your intake of fruits, vegetables, and water to avoid constipation.

You Need to Notify the Office If You Have:

A. Nausea and vomiting while taking the iron supplement even after following the special instructions.

B. Become extremely constipated even after increasing the fiber and liquids in your diet.

C. Other: _____

Phone: _____

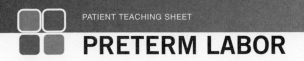

PRETERM LABOR

PROBLEM

Premature contractions and early labor put your baby at risk for premature delivery. Babies born too soon are at risk for breathing problems, bleeding into their brain, infection, and bowel problems, to name a few. Early recognition is the key to stopping premature labor and delivery.

CAUSE

There are several predisposing factors for preterm labor, including previous premature delivery, smoking, incompetent cervix, multiple gestation (twins or triplets), and infection. In most cases, the cause of preterm labor is unknown.

PREVENTION

You can decrease your risk for preterm labor by living a healthy lifestyle with a balanced diet, proper fluid consumption, and no smoking. Please review any previous preterm labor symptoms with your health care provider. Early recognition is a key to success.

TREATMENT PLAN

Treatment depends on the clinical picture. In general, you should remember:

A   Drink at least 8 to 10 glasses of liquid a day; dehydration can increase contractions.

B. Empty your bladder every 2 to 3 hours.

C. Report any bladder infection symptoms, such as burning with urination, to your health care provider.

D. Avoid breast stimulation (including showers where the water stream is on your breasts); this can stimulate contractions.

E. Rest frequently. Rest means lying down on either side, not on your back.

F. Contractions and cramping happen more often in the evening and nighttime after having activity during the day.

G. Do not have intercourse or sexual stimulation without asking your nurse practitioner, certified nurse-midwife, or doctor. If intercourse is okay, use a condom to decrease infection.

H. Try to arrange for help with housework and child care to help you maintain your bed-rest schedule.

I.   Take medications to stop contractions as directed.

Activity: Activity at home is based on how strong your preterm labor has been. You should follow the following activity guidelines:

Level 1: As Tolerated

A. Avoid heavy lifting above 20 pounds.

Level 2: Modified Bed Rest

A. You may be out of bed for breakfast.

B. Rest for 2 hours in the morning with only moderate activity until lunch.

C. Rest for 2 hours with only moderate activity until dinner.

D. Go to bed by 8 PM.

Moderate activity consists of short periods of cooking, light housework (dusting and sweeping).

Level 3: Strict Bed Rest

A. You may be out of the bed only to go to the bathroom or to move to the couch.

B. You may take a shower, use the toilet, brush your teeth, then return immediately to bed.

C. You should not engage in lifting, bending, housework, or lengthy cooking.

D. You should not have sexual intercourse.

E. Perform range-of-motion exercises as directed by your practitioner to avoid muscle weakness and blood clots in your legs. Example: make small circles with your feet, bend and straighten your legs.

Level 4: Hospitalization

Diet: Diet as tolerated, or follow your prescribed diet. Drink 8 to 10 glasses of water each day. Avoid beverages with caffeine. Eat fresh vegetables, fruits, and bran cereal to avoid becoming constipated.

Medications: Continue taking your prenatal vitamin every day.

You Have Been Prescribed the Following to Stop Contractions: _____

You Need to Take: _____

You Need to Notify the Office If You Have:

A. Contractions or cramping more frequent than four in 1 hour.

B. A gush of fluid or blood from your vagina (it is normal to have spotting after vaginal exam or intercourse).

C. Pelvic pressure or low dull backache.

D. Noticed that your baby is not moving as much as usual: less than 10 fetal movements in 1 hour after drinking and resting on your side for 1 hour.

E. Chest pain or difficulty breathing.

F. Other: _____

Phone: _____

GESTATIONAL DIABETES

PROBLEM

Gestational diabetes only develops during pregnancy because of the new hormones being produced. The hormonal influence makes you "insulin resistant," meaning you still produce insulin but the hormones prevent it from working effectively.

Your blood sugar needs to be controlled so that the amount of sugar going to your baby is controlled, too. High blood sugar causes a big baby at delivery, increases your risk of a cesarean birth, causes the baby to have a low blood sugar after delivery, increases jaundice, and causes other problems for the baby such as lung problems.

CAUSE

You are producing new hormones that cause insulin resistance. The likelihood of having gestational diabetes increases with other factors, such as the mother's age, and it is more common in certain groups, such as Latin Americans and American Indians.

PREVENTION

Good control of your diet, exercise, and the possible use of medication and/or possibly insulin will help you to control your blood sugar during your pregnancy.

TREATMENT PLAN

A. You are asked to keep a record of your blood glucose values.

1. You will be shown how to test your blood.

2. You need to test your blood four times a day: first thing in the morning, after lunch, after dinner, and at bedtime.

3. You will be given specific instructions before or after meals.

4. Phone in your blood sugar values every week. Your insulin may be changed weekly.

5. The goal of your fasting blood sugar before breakfast is 60 to 90 mg/dL.

6. Your blood sugar goal before and 2 hours after meals is less than 120 mg/dL.

B. You need to test your urine for ketones every day.

1. You will be shown how to test your urine.

2. You need to test for ketones if you are unable to eat or if you have diarrhea.

3. You need to test for ketones if you feel like you have a urinary tract infection, sinus infection, or any kind of infection.

4. You need to test for ketones if your blood sugar is higher than 150 mg/dL.

5. You must follow the diet given to you by the dietician. If you have questions or do not understand what you should be eating, contact your dietician.

Activity: Exercise lowers blood sugar—gestational diabetes control involves regular exercise. You need to walk at least 20 to 30 minutes a day. Try your local mall for a climate-controlled place to walk. Your heart rate should not get above 140 beats per minute.

Diet: You are placed on a _____ calorie diet. The amount of calories needs to be spread out over three meals and three snacks:

1. Breakfast, mid-morning snack, lunch, mid-afternoon snack, dinner, and a snack at bedtime.

2. The time you eat is as important as what you eat. Try to keep on a regular schedule.

Medications: Depending on your blood sugar, you may require medication to control it. You will be instructed on how to take the medicine. If you are started on insulin you will require extra testing for the rest of your pregnancy.

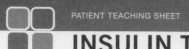

INSULIN THERAPY DURING PREGNANCY

You have been prescribed insulin therapy:

A. Your insulin needs may change weekly because of the change in your hormones (you become more insulin resistant as your pregnancy progresses).

B. Insulin therapy is safe for your baby. Insulin does not cross the placenta like the sugar does.

C. The insulin lowers your blood sugar and therefore controls the amount of sugar that goes to your baby.

D. You have been prescribed Humulin insulin, which works very much like your own body's insulin.

E. Some of the insulin therapies have a mix of short-term regular (clear) insulin with intermediate-acting (cloudy) insulin.

1. You will be instructed how to mix and give yourself your insulin.

2. The first key to insulin therapy is to be able to recognize signs of too much and too little insulin. A chart is included to post on your refrigerator (see Table).

3. The second key is to let people know you are on insulin.

4. You need a Medical Alert bracelet or necklace as well as information to put in your car and billfold.

5. The third key is to have your baby and yourself evaluated more often when on insulin therapy.

   a. You need to be seen twice a week from 32 weeks' gestation to delivery.

   b. You will have extra testing to make sure the baby is doing well, and to make sure you are doing well, too.

F. You need to check your blood sugars 4 times a day. Your blood sugar target is _____

1. Fasting _____.

2. Before lunch _____.

3. Before dinner _____.

4. Before going to bed _____.

G. You will be instructed to check your urine for ketones when you are sick, or if you have high blood sugar.

Activity: It is important to continue to exercise.

Diet: Eat a good healthy diet. You will be instructed on how many calories to eat. Eat 6 smaller meals a day; with insulin it is important to eat snacks.

TABLE   Signs of High and Low Blood Sugar

Blood Sugar	What to Watch For	What to Do	Causes
HYPOGLYCEMIA Low blood sugar	Excessive sweating Feeling faint Feel shaky Headache Impaired vision Hunger Irritable feelings Personality change Trouble awakening	**Call the provider immediately if your blood sugar is below _____** Take glucose tablets or **eat** Do not take your insulin Do not try to force any food or liquids by mouth if patient is not conscious	**Too much insulin** Not eating on time or enough food Unusual amounts of exercise
HYPERGLYCEMIA High blood sugar	Increased thirst Need to urinate more often Large amounts of sugar in your blood or urine Ketones in your urine Weakness and generalized aches Heavy, labored breathing with a fruity breath Nausea and vomiting	Test your blood sugar **Call your provider immediately if your blood sugar is _____** Test your urine for ketones Drink extra water if able to swallow	**Too little insulin** Eating more foods and foods not on your diet Infections and fever Stress

You Need to Notify the Office If:

    A. You have moderate ketones in your urine.

    B. You are unable to eat or you have loose diarrhea stool.

    C. You have insulin reactions (blood sugar is below 50 mg/dL or you feel the symptoms of low blood sugar).

    D. You have blood sugars higher than 175 mg/dL for two readings.

    E. You have any signs of infection.

    F. You have a decrease in fetal movement or do not feel your baby moving.

    G. Other: _____

Phone: _____

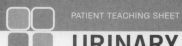

URINARY TRACT INFECTION DURING PREGNANCY: PYELONEPHRITIS

PROBLEM

You have been diagnosed with an infection of the kidney (where urine is made). Bladder infections can spread to the kidney.

CAUSE

Bacteria from the bladder can move up to the kidney and cause a kidney infection. Other causes are blockage in the urine system or having a catheter, or tube, in the bladder.

PREVENTION

A. Urinate frequently. Don't hold urine for long periods of time.

B. Empty your bladder as soon as you feel it is filling.

C. Urinate before and after sexual intercourse.

D. After urinating, always wipe from front to back with toilet tissue.

E. Don't wear tight underwear or pants that can cause increased moistness and warmth in the perineal area.

F. Cotton panties are the best.

G. Wash your hands every time after going to the bathroom.

H. Do not use the same tissue that you blow your nose to wipe after emptying your bladder: this spreads infection.

TREATMENT PLAN

Antibiotics kill the bacteria that cause infection.

Activity: Rest; do not engage in strenuous physical activity.

Diet: Increase fluids; drink at least one large glass of water every hour while you are awake. Drink cranberry juice to help fight and prevent urinary tract infections. If you do not like the taste of cranberry juice, mix cranberry juice with another juice like grape juice.

Medications: You will be prescribed antibiotics to kill the bacteria causing infection. The drugs may be changed if your urine culture results show a different bacteria. You may need mild pain relievers if you have a lot of back pain. Medications such as Tylenol may be used to bring down fever. You may be prescribed a medicine to stop bladder spasm and pain.

You Have Been Prescribed an Antibiotic: _____

You Need to Take: _____

Finish all of your antibiotics even if you feel better.

You Have Been Prescribed the Following for Bladder Spasms: _____

You Need to Take: _____

This medicine will make your urine turn a different color.

You Need to Notify the Office If You Have:

A. Symptoms that worsen or don't get better during treatment.

B. New symptoms that develop during treatment.

C. Symptoms that return after treatment when you finish all of your antibiotics.

D. Difficulty taking your medication (you break out or vomit).

E. Other: _____

Phone: _____

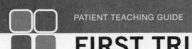

FIRST TRIMESTER VAGINAL BLEEDING

PROBLEM

Vaginal bleeding may occur in the first trimester of pregnancy. The amount of bleeding may range from spotting to a complete miscarriage.

CAUSE

Bleeding may occur for a variety of reasons, including smoking, trauma, abnormal fetus, or fetal chromosomes.

PREVENTION

In most cases, the cause of vaginal bleeding may not be prevented. If bleeding is light, it may lessen or stop. You need to avoid sexual intercourse, tampons, and douches. You may also want to stop smoking.

TREATMENT PLAN

Treatment depends on the cause or suspected cause of your bleeding.

ACTIVITY:

A. Many women experience less bleeding and cramping while on limited activities or bed rest. Unfortunately activity restriction does not prevent miscarriage.

B. Avoid sexual intercourse until at least 2 weeks after the bleeding has stopped, or until your provider tells you.

C. If bed rest is prescribed, perform simple range-of-motion activities as directed by the practitioner. Examples are foot circles and moving legs in bed.

D. Do not use tampons during this period of time. Use pads so that you can evaluate how much you are bleeding.

    1. **Scant amount**: Blood only on tissue when wiped or less than 1-inch stain on peri pad.

    2. **Light amount:** Less than 4-inch stain on peri pad.

    3. **Moderate amount:** Less than 6-inch stain on peri pad.

    4. **Heavy amount:** Saturated peri pad within 1 hour.

Diet: As tolerated. If you are on bed rest, eat fresh vegetables, fruits, and bran cereal to avoid becoming constipated.

Medications: You may not be prescribed any medications.

You Need to Notify the Office If:

A. You develop a fever with your bleeding.

B. You have a gush of blood from your vagina that is more than a period.

C. You pass blood clots or tissue from your vagina.

D. Your vaginal bleeding has a foul odor.

E. You experience abdominal pain or uterine cramping not relieved by taking acetaminophen.

F. Other: _____

Phone: _____

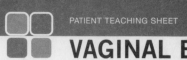

VAGINAL BLEEDING: SECOND AND THIRD TRIMESTER

PROBLEM

Vaginal bleeding may occur during the second and third trimesters of pregnancy (more than 12 weeks). The bleeding may range from spotting of blood on your panties to bleeding like a menstrual period.

CAUSE

A small amount of bloody mucous discharge or spotting may occur for about 1 day following a pelvic examination or sexual intercourse. This is normal if it is not associated with cramping or contractions.

Other causes of vaginal bleeding may be related to the location of the placenta (placenta previa) or premature separation (abruption) of the placenta from your womb. Placental abruptions are associated with cocaine use, cigarette smoking, and trauma (injuries from car wrecks or physical violence).

PREVENTION

There is no known way to prevent most types of vaginal bleeding. If you have been diagnosed with placenta previa, you may be able to prevent bleeding by avoiding sexual intercourse and maintaining bed rest.

There is no known method of preventing placenta previa. Smoking has been associated with placental abruption and placenta previa. You should not smoke or at least try to stop or cut down smoking during pregnancy. Stopping smoking is also good for your baby's health after delivery.

TREATMENT PLAN

A. Treatment depends on the cause of your vaginal bleeding. You may be placed on bed rest.
B. Stop smoking. Ask your provider for a handout on tips to stop smoking.
C. You may need to be on a rest schedule.
D. You may need to stop work.
E. You need to arrange help for child care, grocery shopping, and housework.

Activity: The checked activity restriction(s) are prescribed by the doctor.

_____**Level 1: As tolerated,** avoid heavy lifting above 20 pounds.

_____**Level 2: Modified bed rest.**

You may be out of bed for breakfast; rest (laying down) for 2 hours in the morning with moderate activity until lunch; rest for 2 hours with moderate activity until dinner.

Go to bed by 8 PM.

Moderate activity consists of short periods of cooking and light housework.

_____**Level 3: Strict bed rest.**

You may be out of the bed only to go to the bathroom or to move to the couch.

You may take a shower, use the toilet, and brush your teeth, but then return immediately to bed.

_____No sexual intercourse.

_____Perform range-of-motion exercises as directed by your practitioner.

Diet: Eat fresh vegetables, fruits, and bran cereal to avoid becoming constipated on bed rest. Drinking extra liquids (especially water) also helps to prevent constipation.

Medications: Continue taking your prenatal vitamins every day.

You Need to Notify the Office If You Have:

A. Contractions or cramps, eight in 1 hour or four in 20 minutes.
B. Bloody, mucous discharge not associated with recent sexual intercourse or a pelvic examination.
C. Bright red or dark red vaginal spotting.
D. Bleeding like a period.
E. A gush of fluid or blood from your vagina.
F. Sharp, knifelike pain in your abdomen that does not go away.
G. Pelvic pressure or low backache not relieved with emptying your bladder and resting on one side.
H. Noticed decreased movement of the baby.
I. Other: _____

Phone: _____

BREAST ENGORGEMENT AND SORE NIPPLES

PROBLEM

Engorgement causes swollen, tender breasts, which may have palpable nodular areas.

CAUSE

Engorgement may develop because of inadequate suckling by your baby.

PREVENTION

A. At first, nurse your baby every 2 hours.

B. Make sure your baby latches on to as much as possible of the areola (darkened area around the nipple). The baby suckling on the tip of the nipple does not provide the stimulation necessary to bring down the milk and can make your nipples sore and cracked.

C. If your baby is not well attached to the breast, detach the baby and make sure he or she opens the mouth wide to accommodate most of the areola.

D. Wear a supporting nursing bra (avoid underwire bras as they can exert pressure on certain areas of the breast and cause milk stasis, which is a good medium for bacterial growth and infection); make sure that your bra does not squeeze your breasts too tightly.

E. Making sure that the baby is properly attached to the nipple helps to avoid cracking of nipples that can predispose you to an infection of the breast called mastitis.

F. After the baby feeds, express some milk and apply it to the nipple and areola.

G. Purified lanolin can also be very helpful for sore nipples and can prevent further cracking and infection. Apply routinely after each breast-feeding session for the first several days of nursing and longer if tender or cracked nipples occur. If the lanolin is purified, there is no need to wash it off prior to feedings.

TREATMENT PLAN

A. Engorgement

1. Treatment of engorgement includes the application of heat, breast massage, and expression of milk for comport only.

2. A warm moist washcloth or a warm shower before massaging the breast decreases discomfort.

3. Massage breast by making several gentle but firm stroking movements with the fingertips along the swollen ducts, moving toward the nipple. This should be done around the entire breast.

4. After massaging, milk should be expressed or pumped until the breast softens enough for the baby to latch well. The baby should then be allowed to nurse from both breasts.

5. Best strategy for engorgement is frequent breast-feeding (at least every 1/2 to 2 hours until engorgement resolves).

B. Sore Nipples

1. Sore nipples are usually caused by the improper positioning of the baby on the nipple.

2. Ensure your baby is grasping the areola when sucking and not just the nipple.

3. Continuous suction pressure at the same spot of the nipple can be painful.

4. Change the position of the baby to change the "latching on" position of your baby's mouth.

5. If nipples become sore or cracked, start feeding on the less-affected breast first.

6. Apply purified lanolin to nipples after each feeding.

7. Prevent mastitis with the following personal hygiene measures:

   a. Avoid using soap on nipples.

   b. Avoid decrusting the nipples of dried colostrum or milk.

   c. Change breast pads frequently.

   d. Wash hands before handling your breast and before breast-feeding.

Activity: As tolerated, extra rest is recommended after delivery.

Diet:

A. Breast-feeding mothers need extra liquids for milk production.

B. Drink 10 to 12 glasses of liquid a day.

C. Use caffeine in moderation (eliminate if possible).

D. Continue your regular diet and add about 500 extra calories per day.

E. Avoid gas-producing foods that may upset your baby's stomach.

Medications: Continue your prenatal vitamins while breast-feeding.

You Have Been Prescribed: Acetaminophen 500 mg *or* ibuprofen 600 mg every 3 to 4 hours for discomfort.

You Need to Notify the Office If You Have:

A. Temperature of 100.4°F or higher.

B. Pain that is not controlled with Tylenol or ibuprofen.

C. Flulike symptoms (fever, chills, malaise).

D. Red streaks on breast.

E. Headache with the symptoms above.

F. Other: _____

Phone: _____

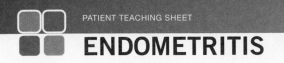

ENDOMETRITIS

PROBLEM

You have an infection of the inside of the uterus.

CAUSE

One or more types of bacteria that invaded damaged tissue following your delivery could cause endometritis. The bacteria may be from the vagina, the bowel, or the environment.

PREVENTION

A. Use careful perineal care:

1. Wipe from front to back after voiding.

2. Remove peri pad from front to back.

3. Change peri pad at least every 4 hours.

4. Use your squeeze bottle filled with warm water to cleanse after each time you urinate or have a bowel movement.

5. Use good hand washing after changing your pads and the baby's diaper.

TREATMENT PLAN

A. You will need to be treated with antibiotic therapy:

B. Take your temperature three times a day for the first 3 days on the antibiotics.

C. Take Tylenol or ibuprofen as needed for fever or discomfort.

Activity: It is very important for you to increase rest with an infection. Try to get a nap when the baby is sleeping. You may continue to breast-feed on some antibiotic therapy. If you don't breast-feed while you are feeling bad, pump your breast milk to keep up your milk supply but dispose of it.

Diet: Eat well-balanced meals. Drink at least 10 to 12 glasses of liquid a day.

Medications: Continue your prenatal vitamins. Take all of your antibiotics even if you start feeling better.

You Have Been Prescribed: _____

You Need to Take: _____

You Need to Notify the Office If You Have:

A. Temperature that rises significantly or reaches 101°F.

B. Foul-smelling vaginal bleeding.

C. Increase in pain or tenderness.

D. Other: _____

Phone: _____

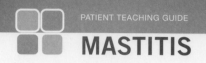

MASTITIS

PROBLEM

You have an infection in your breast tissue, not your breast milk.

CAUSE

The most common organism causing mastitis is *Staphylococcus aureus*. The immediate source of the organism is almost always the nursing infant's nose and mouth. Mastitis often develops in the presence of breast injury, such as cracked nipples.

PREVENTION

A. Prevent injury to the breast:

    1. Avoid overdistension of the breasts; feed infant or use the breast pump frequently (every 2 to 4 hours).

    2. Avoid clogged milk ducts by applying moist heat to the breasts and massage.

    3. Avoid rough manipulation of the breast; pump carefully.

    4. Avoid cracking of nipples by proper positioning of the infant's mouth on the nipple during feeding. The baby's mouth should cover the entire areola (dark brown part of the nipple area).

    5. Read the Patient Teaching Guide, "Breast Engorgement and Sore Nipples."

B. Personal hygiene measures:

    1. Avoid soap on the nipples; cleanse nipples with warm water only.

    2. Avoid decrusting the nipple of dried colostrum or milk.

    3. Use purified lanolin cream after each breast-feeding for sore, cracked nipples. (If lanolin is purified there is no need to remove it prior to the next feeding.)

    4. Use good hand washing before handling the breast and before and after breast-feeding.

TREATMENT PLAN

A. Complete course of antibiotics. Be aware that antibiotics may cause a yeast infection.

B. Continue breast-feeding even on the antibiotics. It is not uncommon for your baby to develop "thrush" (looks like white patches on your baby's mouth and tongue). You may also be prescribed Nystatin cream to apply to your breasts to help prevent thrush.

C. Apply warm soaks to your breast (see the Patient Teaching Guide, "Breast Engorgement and Sore Nipples"). Breast massage may be needed, too.

D. Use Tylenol or ibuprofen for pain (see the Patient Teaching Guide, "Breast Engorgement and Sore Nipples").

Activity: Increased rest is recommended. Try to lie down for a nap when the baby goes to sleep.

Diet: There are no dietary restrictions; continue your regular diet and avoid gas-producing foods that may upset your baby's tummy (cabbage, chocolate, beans, pizza, spicy foods). Increase fluid intake with elevated temperature. Drink at least 10 to 12 glasses of liquid a day. Use caffeine in moderation (eliminate if possible).

Medications: Continue your prenatal vitamins while breast-feeding.

You Have Been Prescribed: _____

You Need to Take: _____

Take all of your antibiotics even if you feel better.

You Have Been Prescribed: Nystatin cream for your breasts and nipples.

You Need to Apply It:

A. After each feeding, apply the Nystatin to each nipple and areola of your breast.

B. Before feeding, wipe off the excess cream with a warm washcloth (do not use soap for your breast because it causes excessive drying and cracking).

You Have Been Prescribed _____ for a yeast infection.

You Need to Use It: _____

You Need to Notify the Office If:

A. You have a temperature that does not decrease within 2 days and resolve within 4 days of taking the antibiotics.

B. You have pain that is not controlled with acetaminophen or ibuprofen.

C. Your baby develops thrush. Notify your baby's health care provider for medication.

D. Other. _____

Phone: _____

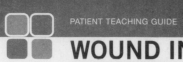
WOUND INFECTION: EPISIOTOMY AND CESAREAN SECTION

PROBLEM

You have an infection of your episiotomy site or cesarean section incision.

CAUSE

The cause is one or more types of bacteria that invaded the tissue following your delivery. The bacteria may be from the vagina, the bowel, or the environment.

TREATMENT

A. Take your temperature if you have fever and chills.

B. Episiotomy:

1. Wash hands before and after changing your sanitary pads and your baby's diaper.

2. Wipe or pat dry from front to back after every urination or bowel movement.

3. Apply and remove perineal pad from front to back.

4. Change perineal pad at least every 4 hours and after each voiding or bowel movement.

5. Use squeeze bottle: position nozzle between legs, empty entire bottle over perineum, blot dry with toilet paper, and avoid contamination from anal area.

6. Use a blow dryer on the lowest setting to "air dry" your stitches.

7. Wash perineum with mild soap and warm water at least once daily.

C. Cesarean section incision:

1. Wash hands before and after dressing change and wound care.

2. Follow all of the above directions (except 6) for your bleeding, too.

3. After showering, gently pat dry your abdomen.

4. If wound is draining, cover it with clean dressing and call the office for instructions. Otherwise, leave it open to air.

5. Cleanse incision with hydrogen peroxide and cotton swab. Do not clean the same area more than once with the same swab.

6. If your incision opens, notify your practitioner for further instructions.

Activity: Increased rest is recommended; try to lie down for a nap when the baby goes to sleep.

Diet: There are no dietary restrictions; eat well-balanced meals. Increase your fluid intake with an infection. Drink at least 10 to 12 glasses of liquid a day.

Medications: Continue your prenatal vitamins. You may take acetaminophen 1 to 2 tablets every 4 to 6 hours for your fever and/or discomfort.

You Have Been Prescribed the Following Antibiotic: _____

You Need to Take: _____

Take all of your antibiotics, even if you feel better, unless you have an adverse reaction to them. Then call our office.

You Need to Notify the Office If You Have:

A. Temperature that rises significantly or reaches 101°F.

B. Foul smelling drainage from the incision or episiotomy site.

C. Increased pain or tenderness.

D. Separation of wound or incision.

E. Other: _____

Phone: _____

Patient Teaching Guides for Chapter 13: Gynecology

- Failure to Have a Menstrual Period (Amenorrhea)
- Atrophic Vaginitis
- Bacterial Vaginosis
- Fibrocystic Breast Changes and Breast Pain
- Cervicitis
- How to Take Birth Control Pills (for 28-Day Cycle)
- Basal Body Temperature (BBT) Measurement
- Emergency Contraception
- Painful Menstrual Cramps or Periods (Dysmenorrhea)
- Pain With Intercourse (Dyspareunia)
- Instructions for Postcoital Testing
- Menopause
- Pelvic Inflammatory Disease (PID)
- Premenstrual Syndrome (PMS)
- Vaginal Yeast Infection

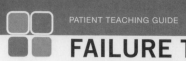

FAILURE TO HAVE A MENSTRUAL PERIOD (AMENORRHEA)

PROBLEM

For some reason that we do not fully understand, you have stopped ovulating, or putting out an egg each month, and you have stopped having menstrual periods. This is a very common problem.

It is not immediately dangerous for you. However, it is not good for you to let this go on for a long period of time because the inside lining of your uterus is still being stimulated by estrogen, and over a long period of time, this could become cancerous.

CAUSE

Although the cause is usually unknown, amenorrhea is often associated with low thyroid activity, excessive exercise such as that of an athlete or dancer, or excessive weight loss.

PREVENTION

There is no specific prevention. However, if you notice a decreased frequency of menstrual periods or absence of menstrual periods when you increase your exercise, you should decrease the intensity of exercise. If you lose too much weight, you could stop having periods. Try to gain some weight.

TREATMENT PLAN

Decrease exercise, increase weight, and replace progesterone.

Activity: Decrease intensity of exercise. Take at least 2 days off each week, and decrease the amount of time during each exercise session.

Sexual Activity: You may have a return of fertility without warning. If pregnancy is undesired, be sure to use an effective birth control prevention method such as condoms and foam to prevent unintended pregnancy.

Diet: Increase calories and try to put on 5 pounds if you have lost a lot of weight.

Medications: Your health care provider will prescribe progesterone to replace what your ovaries are not making at the present time. Progesterone may be prescribed in the form of birth control pills.

You Have Been Prescribed:_____

You Need to Take: _____

You Need to Notify the Office If:

    A. You have any new symptoms.

    B. You have problems taking your medication.

    C. You think you might be pregnant.

    D. Other: _____

Phone: _____

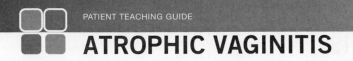

ATROPHIC VAGINITIS

PROBLEM

You have been diagnosed with atrophic vaginitis. This means that the cells lining your vagina are thinner, less pliable, and less lubricated so more prone to tears and abrasion. It does not mean that your sexual organs are "wasting away." This is a natural part of aging, and it is also very common with teens and with breast-feeding.

CAUSE

Atrophic vaginitis is caused by an alteration in estrogen either from premature ovarian failure, delayed puberty, breast-feeding, or from naturally occurring menopause.

PREVENTION

A. This is a physical problem, *not* an emotional problem.
   1. If you are a preadolescent girl, the symptoms will decrease as puberty approaches.
   2. If you are breast-feeding, your symptoms will resolve after weaning the baby.
   3. If you are menopausal or have premature ovarian failure, your symptoms will get better after starting a hormone replacement pill or using a hormonal vaginal cream.
B. You also can help your symptoms by doing the following:
   1. Use good hygiene; wipe yourself from front to back with every urination and bowel movement.
   2. Avoid perfumed hygiene sprays, talcs, and harsh soaps.
   3. Wear cotton underwear.
   4. Sleep without underwear.
   5. Use a water-soluble vaginal lubricant with sexual intercourse, such as K-Y jelly or Astroglide. **Do not use vaseline.** Vaseline can contribute to infections.
   6. Regular sexual activity or masturbation facilitates the natural production of lubricating secretions of your body.
   7. Kegel exercise (using the muscles that start and stop the flow of the urine stream) improves muscle tone and elasticity of the vagina.
   8. The female-superior "on top" or side-lying position for sexual intercourse gives you the ability to control the depth of thrusting with the penis, and this may make sex more comfortable.
   9. Yogurt douches or acidophilus tablets by mouth or inserted into your vagina can help maintain the vaginal pH to prevent vaginitis.

TREATMENT PLAN

A. Vitamin E oil may be used for vaginal dryness.
B. Use K-Y jelly or other water-soluble lubricants for intercourse.
C. You may be prescribed an estrogen cream or hormone replacements for menopause.
D. If you still have your uterus, hormones need to be balanced with estrogen and progesterone to prevent the lining of the uterus from overgrowing. Follow your hormone therapy instructions.
E. You still need regular Pap smears, even if you do not have a period.

Activity: Increase foreplay for increased lubrication. Try the above suggestions on sexual positions for greater comfort and control.

Diet: As tolerated.

Medication:

You Have Been Prescribed: _____

You Need to Take It/Use It: _____

You Need to Notify the Office If You Have:

   A. No relief of symptoms after following the above instructions.
   B. No relief of symptoms after beginning the hormonal replacements.
   C. Vaginal bleeding after intercourse.
   D. A change in your symptoms.
   E. Other: _____

Phone: _____

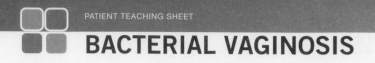

BACTERIAL VAGINOSIS

PROBLEM

You have been diagnosed with a vaginal infection, also known as bacterial vaginosis or BV. This is a very common problem that has a "fishy vaginal discharge." The odor increases after sexual intercourse, but it is not considered a sexually transmitted infection. Recurrence is common, and your partner may also need to be treated.

YOU CAN BE TREATED IN PREGNANCY

BV has been associated with premature rupture of the membranes and preterm labor.

CAUSE

BV is caused by an alteration in the normal flora of the vagina. There are many contributing pathogens and factors, including the routine use of douches, antibiotic use, menses, and pregnancy.

PREVENTION

A. Wear cotton panties or panties with a cotton crotch.
B. Do not wear tight restrictive clothes such as tight jeans.
C. Leave your underwear off during sleep.
D. Limit tub bathing and the use of hot tubs or whirlpools.
E. Avoid the use of bubble bath, feminine deodorant sprays, perfumed sanitary products (sanitary pads, tampons, and toilet paper).
F. Use good hygiene:
   1. Wipe with toilet tissue from front to back after urinating and bowel movements.
   2. Wipe from front to back using clean towels with each bath or shower.
   3. Change your tampons and pads often during your period.
G. Routine douching destroys the normal vaginal flora, causing yeast to overgrow. You may be prescribed a medicated douche to treat yeast infections.

TREATMENT PLAN

A. Try the prevention tips to decrease the recurrence of BV.
B. You may be given a prescription for pills or vaginal creams.
C. Do not use a tampon with vaginal creams because it will absorb the medication.
D. Clindamycin is an oil-based, medicated cream used to treat BV. It can weaken latex condoms for at least 72 hours after stopping the therapy.
E. All treatments (medications and douches) may be used during your period.
F. Metronidazole (Flagyl) oral tablets may be prescribed. The side effects include a sharp, unpleasant metallic taste in the mouth, furry tongue, and some urinary tract symptoms. Please remind your provider if you have a history of seizures or if you are on any blood-thinning drug.

OTHER METHODS OF TREATMENT

A. Vinegar and water douches: 1 tablespoon of white vinegar in 1 pint of water. Douche one to two times a week.
B. *Lactobacillus acidophilus* culture four to six tablets daily.
C. Garlic suppositories: Place 1 peeled clove of garlic wrapped in a cloth dipped in olive oil into your vagina overnight, and change daily. You will not smell like garlic.

Activity: As tolerated.

Diet: When taking the medicine metronidazole (Flagyl), you must **avoid alcohol during the entire week you are taking the medicine and 24 hours after your last dose.** The combination of the medicine and alcohol may cause nausea, vomiting, stomach upset, and a headache.

Medication:

You Have Been Prescribed: _____

You Need to Take It/Use It: _____

You Need to Notify the Office If:

   A. You vomited your medication (Flagyl).
   B. Your vaginal odor and discharge are not relieved after the medications.
   C. You continue to have repeated infections after following the instructions.
   D. Other: _____

Phone: _____

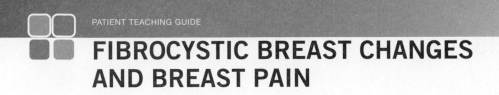

FIBROCYSTIC BREAST CHANGES AND BREAST PAIN

PROBLEM

You are being treated for breast pain or breast lumpiness that is from breast changes that are painful, but not cancerous. You have probably had an extensive examination by your health care provider, perhaps a mammogram, sonogram, and/or a breast biopsy.

CAUSE

The cause is unknown. It is probably related to estrogen changes that occur with menstrual periods.

PREVENTION

None known.

TREATMENT PLAN

Be fitted for a well-fitted bra. This helps to eliminate breast movement as a source of pain. Try ice packs on your breasts for 20 minutes every few hours. Some women find that heat on the breast can also relieve discomfort.

Activity: There are no activity restrictions. When exercising, wear a good, supportive bra.

Diet: Eliminate or decrease salt in your diet to decrease water retention if you have swelling of your breasts near your period.

Medications: There are several medications that have been found to relieve breast pain from fibrocystic breast changes, such as medications that decrease or stabilize estrogen (oral contraceptive pills). Ask your health care provider which is best for you.

Complementary: Recent research has show that flaxseed may reduce cyclic pain. Flaxseed 25 mg a day.

You Have Been Prescribed: _____

You Need to Take It/Use It: _____

Phone: _____

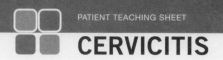

CERVICITIS

PROBLEM

You are being treated for cervicitis. The cervix is the lower section of the uterus that opens into the vagina. Cervicitis is a condition or inflammation of the cervix.

CAUSE

Certain germs such as *C. trachomatis* or *N. gonorrhe a* may cause cervicitis; however, in many cases no specific germ may be identified. In these cases, inflammation may be due to douching, chemical irritants, or altered vaginal flora. In many cases, no cause may be found.

Your health care provider will perform a physical evaluation, including pelvic examination, and obtain certain tests to diagnose the cause of cervicitis. If a sexually transmitted organism is found, you and your partner will need to be treated.

PREVENTION

In cases where cervicitis is caused by sexually transmitted organisms, use of condoms may prevent infection.

Do not douche or use any other chemically irritating products.

TREATMENT PLAN

A. You may be prescribed an antibiotic by your health care provider.

B. **Depending on the cause of cervicitis, your sexual partner(s) may also need medical evaluation and treatment.**

Activity: Avoid sexual activity until treatment is completed.

Medications:

You Have Been Prescribed: _____

You Need to Take It: _____

You need to finish all of your antibiotics even though you may feel good.

You Need to Notify the Office If:

A. You are not able to take your medicine.

B. You have other new symptoms.

C. Other: _____ _____

Phone: _____

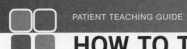

HOW TO TAKE BIRTH CONTROL PILLS (FOR 28-DAY CYCLE)

You have been prescribed an oral contraceptive, also known as a birth control pill. Most birth control pills contain a combination of synthetic estrogen and progestin.

A. Birth control pills suppress ovulation.

B. They make the lining of the uterus unreceptive for an egg to implant and grow. Birth control pills also alter the cervical mucus, making it thicker and harder for sperm to penetrate.

C. **A birth control pill does not prevent any sexually transmitted infection or HIV. A condom must still be used to protect yourself from the HIV virus or other infections.**

D. You will be asked to return to the office in 3 months after starting birth control pills to check your blood pressure and to check for other side effects of the pill, such as your potassium level and nausea.

E. If your blood pressure is normal and you are not having any other problems taking the pills, your prescription for birth control pills may be written for 1 year.

F. At the end of that time, you will need another physical examination and a Pap smear. Then your prescription can be refilled for another year.

You Have Been Prescribed:_____

A. This is a combination pill of estrogen and progestin.

1. Your packet contains 28 pills. Notice that your pills are different colors. **You must take them in the order that they come in the packet.** There are 21 "active" pills, and the last 7 are "inactive or sugar pills" to keep you in the habit of taking a pill every day.

2. You must take a pill **every day** at approximately the same time. Develop the habit of taking the pill with brushing your teeth, for example. You cannot share your birth control pills with anyone else.

3. Start your packet on the Sunday of your period. Take the pill marked "1," "start here," or "Sunday."

4. You take a pill every day for 21 days; when you start the last 7 pills, you will have a period or "withdrawal bleed."

5. Your period may not start for 1 to 2 days into the last week of pills. This is normal. You generally have a shorter, lighter period on birth control pills.

6. When you start your period, it is time to refill your prescription for your next month of pills.

7. If this is your first packet of birth control pills, you are not considered protected and may get pregnant. Use a backup method of birth control for the first packet of pills.

8. **Missed pills instructions:**

   a. If you miss one pill: take it as soon as you remember, then get back on your regular schedule (you take two pills in 1 day).

   b. If you miss two pills: Take two pills as soon as you remember, then get back on schedule (you take three pills in 1 day). You must use a **backup method of birth control** such as a condom until you finish that packet of pills. You may have spotting if you miss two pills. This is normal.

   c. If you miss three pills: you may have a period. Discard that packet of pills and start a new packet on Sunday. You must use a **backup method of birth control** such as a condom for the first 7 days of the new packet.

   d. If one or more birth control pills are missed, no backup method of contraception is used, and you miss your period, you should do a pregnancy test.

9. If you are prescribed antibiotics while taking birth control pills, you must use a **backup method of birth control** such as a condom. You can get pregnant. Antibiotics and other medications such as those used to prevent seizures make birth control pills less effective, making it possible to get pregnant.

You Need to Notify the Office If You:

A. Vomit your birth control pills.

B. Have a severe or migrainelike headache.

C. Are depressed (can't make yourself happy).

D. Have pain in your legs, especially if your calf hurts when walking or flexing your foot.

E. Break your leg and need to have a cast.

F. Think you are pregnant (skipped pills or taking antibiotics).

G. Have blurred vision, loss of vision, or spots before your eyes.

H. Feel chest pain or shortness of breath.

I. Feel severe abdominal pain.

J. Have lots of swelling of the fingers, hands, ankles, or face.

K. Other: _____

Phone: _____

BASAL BODY TEMPERATURE (BBT) MEASUREMENT

DEFINITION

Basal body temperature assessment is done to determine if and when a woman ovulates. It may be used to achieve or prevent pregnancy. During the follicular phase of the normal menstrual cycle (the first 2 weeks), one follicle and the oocyte it contains matures. The normal body temperature during the follicular phase when estrogen dominates ranges from 97.2°F to 97.6°F.

At midcycle, when progesterone dominates, the ovum is extruded from the ovary and may be fertilized any time from 12 to 24 hours later. Ovulation manifests as an increase in BBT from 0.6° to 1°F above your baseline temperature. Some women have a dip in temperature just before the day of ovulation and then their temperature may rise.

Besides taking your temperature to predict ovulation (the best time to try to get pregnant or avoid sexual intercourse), another reason to take it is to check your cervical mucus.

CHECKING YOUR BASAL BODY TEMPERATURE

A. A basal body temperature thermometer must be used. They are easily accessible in the contraceptive section of any pharmacy. If using any other type beside a basal body thermometer, such as a digital thermometer, it must be able to measure to .10 degree due to the slight changes that will be measured.

B. Record your temperature on the temperature chart provided in the thermometer packet or by a health care provider. The chart can be easily copied for as many months as needed.

C. Keeping your BBT calendar

   1. Day ONE (1) of the cycle is the first day of menstruation/bleeding.

   2. Mark the days of bleeding and other discharge, especially mucus, on the calendar.

   3. Mark any days that you are sick, stay up late, or sleep less than 6 hours since this will interfere with your temperature.

   4. Mark the days that you have sexual intercourse.

   5. Mark your medications on your BBT calendar.

D. **Each morning, prior to arising or any activity,** place the thermometer under the tongue, leaving it in for 1 minute. **Take your temperature consistently at the same time every morning.**

E. A temperature elevation of 0.2°F or greater from your last 6 days of temperature (and stays elevated) indicates an ovulatory pattern.

   1. This is the time when you are more likely to get pregnant.

      a. If pregnancy is desired, the standard recommendation is that sexual intercourse should be done 2 days before ovulation is expected and every 2 days thereafter until 2 to 4 days have passed following the rise in body temperature.

      b. If pregnancy is not desired, avoid sexual intercourse.

F. The record should be kept for 2 to 6 months minimum.

CHECKING YOUR CERVICAL MUCUS

Your cervical mucus ranges from thick and tacky feeling to thin and slippery, the consistency of egg whites. The type of mucus you have also signals the time of ovulation.

A. Your mucus can be checked daily by touching yourself on the outside or, to be the most accurate, inserting 1 finger in your vagina to check the cervix.

   1. Wash your hands.

   2. Sit on the toilet and gently insert your finger to feel the cervix.

   3. The cervix feels firm, like the end of your nose.

   4. Check the thickness of the mucus and note it on your BBT temperature chart.

B. After you have your period, the cervical mucus is thick and tacky. It is more difficult to get pregnant when the mucus is thick.

C. As ovulation approaches, you will notice the mucus getting thinner.

D. When the mucus is the consistency feeling of egg whites, that signals ovulation and you are the most fertile.

   1. This is the time to have sexual intercourse/avoid intercourse.

   2. Continue until you see your basal body temperature rise.

   3. You will notice the cervical mucus getting thicker.

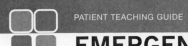

EMERGENCY CONTRACEPTION

You have indicated that you want to use an emergency contraception method. **Plan B®** is an over-the-counter brand of emergency contraceptive that is available without prescription to people who are age 18 and older; however, a prescription is still required for persons under age 18.

TREATMENT PLAN

A. You must start emergency contraception within 72 hours of unprotected sex.

B. It is best if to start within the first 12 to 24 hours.

C. You will be given a prescription or a supply of birth control pills.

D. You take a number of pills two times during 1 day.

E. The number of pills depends on the brand of the pill.

F. Your health care provider will give you clear instructions.

G. The sooner you begin emergency contraception, the more effective it will be.

H. The birth control pills and Plan B® prevent pregnancy because the hormones cause the mucus in the cervix to thicken and the lining of the uterus and tubes to change.

I. You may not ovulate, but if you ovulate, the egg will not be ready to be fertilized by a sperm.

J. Emergency contraception in the form of hormonal pills will *not* interrupt an already established pregnancy.

K. Because you are taking more female hormones than you are used to, you may become sick to your stomach.

L. Your health care provider will tell you what medication to buy or give you a prescription for medicine to keep you from being sick to your stomach.

M. Take this medicine at least 1 hour before you take the hormone pills.

N. You take the birth control pills 12 hours apart.

   1. For example, if you take your first pills at 8:00 AM, then you take the second pills at 8:00 PM.

   2. If you get sick and vomit the pills within 3 hours, take the other dose and call us so that we can get a replacement dose.

O. Other common side effects include breast tenderness, headache, or dizziness. These side effects go away in a day or two.

P. You should have a menstrual period a week or so after you take the pills.

Q. If you have not had a period by 3 weeks, please call our office.

R. It is unlikely that you would get pregnant, but if you do and choose to have a baby, the emergency contraception is *not* associated with any increased chance of birth defects.

Medication:

You Have Been Prescribed the Following Emergency Contraception Medication: _____

You Have Been Prescribed the Following Nausea Medication: _____

You Need to Call Us If You Have and Questions or Problems.

You Need to Notify the Office If You Have:

   A. Serious side effects of medicine.

   B. Severe chest pain.

   C. Severe abdominal pain.

   D. Headache.

   E. Vision changes.

   F. Shortness of breath.

Phone: _____

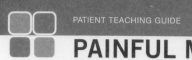

PAINFUL MENSTRUAL CRAMPS OR PERIODS (DYSMENORRHEA)

PROBLEM

Painful menstrual cramps, or dysmenorrhea, can cause occasional diarrhea, nausea or vomiting, and headache with menstrual periods.

CAUSE

A substance called prostaglandin causes most painful menstrual cramps. This substance is made in the uterus and causes the uterus to contract. Most menstrual cramps are normal and are not a sign of anything wrong. However, menstrual cramps may cause you to feel badly enough that you are unable to go to school or work. If that is the case, your health care provider can suggest medication to decrease the painful periods.

TREATMENT/CARE

A. Your health care provider may suggest a medicine such as a prostaglandin inhibitor. This medication helps decrease or eliminate the most likely substance that is causing the cramping of your uterus. The medication most often suggested is ibuprofin (Motrin IB, Advil, Nuprin, or others). Another medication is naproxen (Aleve).

   1. These are available at your local drug store, grocery store, or convenience store.

   2. Take any of these with a snack or meal to protect your stomach lining and prevent nausea.

   3. If you usually have very painful menstrual cramps, begin your medication as soon as your period begins or even the day before your period. This helps stop the production of prostaglandin.

B. If your cramps are not better using over-the-counter medications, your health care provider may write a prescription for a stronger medicine.

C. Many women take oral contraceptive pills to relieve menstrual cramps. A prescription is necessary. **Notify your care provider if you are a cigarette smoker as smoking may increase your chance of side effects with oral contraceptives.**

D. Some women find that exercise such as walking helps ease the cramps.

E. Another idea is a warm bath, shower, or a warm heating pad on your abdomen.

F. General health practices such as regular exercise, yoga, routine sleep habits, and regular sexual activity are beneficial.

Activity: Try to continue your usual activity. Try taking a walk, swimming, or doing yoga. Try a warm bath or shower.

Diet: Eat your normal diet. If you are nauseated, drink a clear carbonated soda (7-Up or Sprite).

Medication:

You Have Been Prescribed: _____

You Need to Take: _____

You Need to Notify the Office If You Have:

   A. Any questions concerning your condition.

   B. Problems taking the medicine.

   C. No relief when taking the medicine, and other measures do not help.

   D. Any signs of infection, such as fever, chills, bad smelling vaginal discharge, or burning sensation when you urinate.

Phone: _____

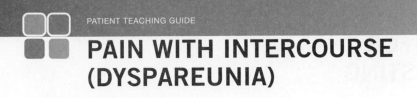

PAIN WITH INTERCOURSE (DYSPAREUNIA)

PROBLEM

As many as 60% of women complain of pain with sexual intercourse, also known as dyspareunia. Pain may occur with insertion of and/or with deep penetration of the penis into the vagina.

CAUSES

There are physical causes, such as episiotomy scars, a short vagina, and infections; musculoskeletal causes such as disk problems; hormonal causes: such as the lack of estrogen in menopause; and poor communication with partners and lack of foreplay.

PREVENTION AND TREATMENT PLANS

A. Inadequate lubrication.

1. More prolonged foreplay increases natural vaginal lubrication.
2. Use a water-soluble lubricant such as K-Y jelly or Astroglide.
3. **Do not use vaseline as a lubricant.**
4. Do not use contraceptive creams for lubrication; they often cause dryness (dehydration) and may worsen soreness.

B. Pain on insertion of penis.

1. Try different positions that give you more control.
2. Guide the penis for insertion.
3. If menopausal, you may be prescribed estrogen cream to use on an intermittent basis.

C. Pain with deep penetration.

1. Use a side-lying position during intercourse; this may be more comfortable so that deep penetration is limited.
2. You may need to be referred to a gynecologist for further treatment and/or surgery if you have any masses or scar tissue noted on a physical examination.

D. If you have or suspect an infection:

1. Inform your provider that you may have an infection.
2. A culture will be done.
3. Antibiotics will be prescribed for you and possibly your partner(s).
4. Refrain from sexual intercourse until all medications are gone (unless otherwise instructed).
5. If you have a Bartholin's duct cyst, it will be drained and you will be treated with antibiotics.

E. If you have a very narrow vaginal opening, you may be referred to a gynecologist for vaginal dilation.

F. Spasm of the muscles upon touching the vaginal area may be treated with medication, relaxation techniques, and Kegel exercises.

G. You and your partner may be referred to a sex counselor.

Medication:

You Have Been Prescribed: _____

You Need to Take/Use It: _____

You Need to Notify the Office If You Have:

A. No relief of your symptoms after your prescribed treatment.

B. Other: _____

Phone: _____

INSTRUCTIONS FOR POSTCOITAL TESTING

PROBLEM

This test is performed during an infertility evaluation to determine the presence of sperm and how they behave in cervical mucus. The postcoital test assists the clinician in determining possible causes for infertility that are often easy to correct. The test is performed about day 14 of the menstrual cycle, or around the time of expected LH surge as determined by the rise of temperature seen on the basal body temperature (BBT) chart.

PROCEDURE

A. You and your partner should abstain from sexual intercourse for 48 hours prior to the test.

    1. Ideally, intercourse should take place the morning of or the night before the office visit.

    2. It is preferable to not use vaginal lubricants. If you must use a vaginal lubricant, use one that is water soluble, such as K-Y jelly or Astroglide.

B. At the office, you will have a speculum inserted into your vagina as if you were getting a Pap test.

C. Your cervix will be evaluated for the presence, amount, and consistency of mucus.

D. Mucus is taken from the cervix with a syringe and placed on a slide.

E. The clinician will evaluate the slide for presence of sperm, number of living sperm, and movement of sperm.

RESULTS

A. A normal test usually reveals the presence of 5 to 10 sperm moving deliberately.

B. A poor test may indicate that intercourse has been mistimed (poor amount of cervical mucus).

C. Sperm should live at least 48 hours in good cervical mucus.

D. If your first test is abnormal, it will be repeated because a common problem is mistimed evaluation.

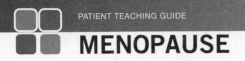

MENOPAUSE

DEFINITION

Menopause is the cessation of menses (stopping of menstrual periods) for 12 consecutive months and is generally experienced in women between 45 and 55 years of age; however, some women may be earlier or later.

A. Menopause before the age of 40 is considered premature.

B. Induced menopause is the abrupt cessation of menses related to chemical or surgical interventions.

Perimenopause is the time proceeding menopause and may last several years. The average age of onset is usually in a woman's 40s but may occur earlier. Symptoms may occur during this time period due to fluctuations in hormone levels. Due to fluctuations in ovarian function, **pregnancy may still occur and unintended pregnancy should be avoided.**

CAUSE

Menopause can be natural or induced. Natural menopause is a normal function of aging. Surgical or chemical intervention can result in induced menopause.

SYMPTOMS

Symptom occurrence and severity vary from very mild to moderate or severe. Symptoms may include:

A. Hot flashes

B. Night sweats

C. Insomnia

D. Vaginal dryness

Treatment

Your care provider will work with you to develop a plan of treatment that is based on your individual symptom pattern. Inform your care provider if you have:

A. Acute liver disease

B. Cerebral vascular or coronary artery disease, MI, or stroke

C. History of or active thrombophlebitis or thromboembolic disorders

D. History of uterine or ovarian cancer

E. Known or suspected cancer of the breast

F. Known or suspected estrogen-dependent neoplasm

G. Pregnancy

F. Undiagnosed, abnormal vaginal bleeding

Activity:

A. Regular physical exercise can be beneficial for weight reduction and symptom control.

B. Dress in layers to accommodate hot flashes and avoid warm areas.

C. Avoid hot showers and baths.

D. Regular sexual intercourse is encouraged and you may find water-soluble vaginal lubricants (K-Y jelly, Astroglide, Replense) helpful for vaginal dryness.

E. Be sure to use a method of **birth control** to prevent undesired pregnancy if you have had a period within one year.

Diet: You need to eat a well-balanced diet (three meals). Supplement your diet to achieve calcium 1,200–1,500 mg/day and vitamin D 400–800 IU/day. Avoid alcohol, caffeine, and spicy food as they may trigger hot flashes.

Medication:

You Have Been Prescribed: _____

You Need to Take/Use It: _____

You Need to Notify the Office If:

A. You experience unexpected vaginal bleeding.

B. Your symptoms worsen.

C. You are on HRT and if you experience calf pain, chest pain, shortness of breath, cough up blood, severe headaches, visual disturbances, breast pain, abdominal pain, or yellowing of the skin.

D. Other: _____

Phone: _____

PELVIC INFLAMMATORY DISEASE (PID)

PROBLEM

You have been diagnosed as having pelvic inflammatory disease, also known as PID. This inflammation can involve the uterus, fallopian tubes, ovaries, broad ligament, and/or the pelvic vascular system or pelvic connective tissue.

CAUSE

Organisms that go up from the vagina and cervix into the uterus cause PID. The two most common organisms cultured from patients with PID are *Chlamydia trachomatis* and *Neisseria gonorrhoeae*. Your period increases the ability of gonococcal invasion into the upper genital tract. Infection and inflammation spread throughout the endometrium to the fallopian tubes. From there, it extends to the ovaries and peritoneal, or abdominal, cavity.

PREVENTION

A. Condoms and a spermicidal foam or cream with nonoxynol 9 is very protective against PID.

B. Condoms must be used with *every* sexual intercourse.

C. Vaginal douching may lead to an increase risk for PID.

    1. Routine douching is *not recommended;* it wipes out the normal vaginal flora.

    2. If you douche, do not douche more than once a month.

D. The more sex partners you have, the greater the chances are of contracting any sexually transmitted infections.

TREATMENT

A. Your partner(s) need to be evaluated and treated with antibiotic therapy, too.

B. Sexual abstinence

    1. **You should not have sexual intercourse until all of your symptoms are gone and your partner(s) have completed antibiotic therapy.**

    2. If you do have sexual intercourse, you should use condoms consistently.

Activity: Limit yourself to bed rest for about 3 to 4 days, then pursue activity as tolerated.

Diet:

A. You need to drink at least 10 to 12 glasses of liquid every day.

B. You need to eat a well-balanced diet (three meals).

C. You need to eat high-protein snacks such as peanut butter sandwiches and milk.

D. If you have been prescribed Flagyl (metronidazole) you must avoid all alcohol ingestion for at least three days after the last dose or you will experience severe nausea and vomiting.

Medications:

A. You will be prescribed *two or more* antibiotics; it is extremely important to **take all of the antibiotics.**

B. You may take acetaminophen (Tylenol) for fever.

C. You may be prescribed some pain medication.

You Have Been Prescribed: _____

You Need to Take: _____

Take all of your antibiotics, even if you feel better.

Your Second Prescribed Antibiotic Is: _____

You Need to Take: _____

You need to take all of both antibiotics, even if you feel better.

You Have Been Prescribed the Following for Your Pain: _____

You Need to Take: _____

You Need to Notify the Office If:

    A. Your fever does not respond to acetaminophen (Tylenol).

    B. Your symptoms worsen, even while taking both antibiotics.

    C. You vomit or cannot tolerate your antibiotics.

    D. You must return to the office 2 or 3 days after the antibiotics have been started for a repeat examination and if you are unable to return for your follow-up office visit.

    E. Other: _____

Phone: _____

Next Appointment: Date _____ **Time** _____

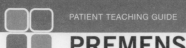

PREMENSTRUAL SYNDROME (PMS)

DEFINITION

Premenstrual syndrome (PMS) is a common problem experienced by women in their reproductive years. You may have some or all of the following symptoms:

A. Cravings for food, particularly chocolate and salty foods
B. Irritability
C. Feelings of depression; crying spells
D. Bloated stomach
E. Weight gain and water retention
F. Difficulty concentrating
G. Tiredness
H. Feelings of faintness
I. Sometimes clumsiness
J. Sore breasts

CAUSE

Although the cause is really not known, PMS is a response of your body to the changes in female hormones during the last half of your menstrual cycle.

PREVENTION

All of your symptoms probably cannot be prevented, but some of them may be made less severe.

TREATMENT PLAN

A. Keep track of your symptoms for at least 3 months so that your health care provider can determine if the symptoms always happen in the last half of your cycle.
B. Eat six small meals each day. Eat breakfast, have a morning snack like fruit or a glass of milk, eat lunch, have an afternoon snack, eat supper, and then have another evening snack. This helps keep your blood sugar even, to avoid low blood sugar.
C. Avoid candy, desserts, and other sugars. They may be associated with episodes of low blood sugar. Complex carbohydrates such as pasta, potatoes, fresh fruit, rice, and bread break down more slowly than sweets and keep your blood sugar more steady.
D. Stay away from salty foods such as chips, fast food, and pickles.
E. Avoid caffeine in soda, coffee, and chocolate. Caffeine makes you irritable and nervous.
F. Exercise daily. It is a good idea to do aerobic exercises or even walking. Exercise increases chemicals in your brain that help with your mood.
G. Join a PMS group so that you can get support from other women who have similar symptoms. You may get ideas of how other women handle PMS, and you can share your ideas, too.
H. If you smoke, try to cut down or quit.
I. Get a good night's rest and take naps during the day if possible.
J. Try stress reduction classes or yoga. Local community organizations usually have classes available.

Medications: There are a number of medications available that your health care provider may suggest for you.

You Have Been Prescribed: _____

You Need to Take: _____

You Have Also Been Prescribed: _____

You Need to Take: _____

You Need to Call to the Office If:

A. You have questions or concerns.

B. You feel that things are not improving.

C. Other: _____

Phone: _____

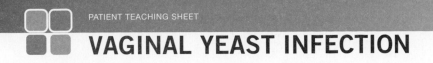

VAGINAL YEAST INFECTION

PROBLEM

You have been diagnosed with a vaginal yeast infection. This is an infection or inflammation of the vagina that is caused by a fungus known as yeast (*Monilia* or *Candida albicans*).

CAUSE

Yeast cells (*Monila*) are normally present on the skin in healthy people. These cells may be found in the vagina or rectal area. However, due to a disturbance in the body's hormones and pH, an overproduction of these cells has occurred and has caused an infection. Several factors can cause this disturbance, which include menstrual periods, pregnancy, diabetes, antibiotics or other medications, increased dietary intake of sugars and alcohol, and an increase in moisture and warmth in the vaginal or rectal area by wearing tight restrictive clothing.

PREVENTION

A. Keep the vaginal and rectal areas clean and dry.

B. Shower daily and avoid tub baths.

C. Avoid tight, restrictive clothing such as tight jeans and underwear.

D. Wear cotton panties that allow air to circulate. At bedtime, do not wear underwear with your pajamas.

E. Obesity can contribute to this problem too. If you have gained an excessive amount of weight, try to lose these extra pounds.

F. Avoid douching because this changes the normal flora and pH of the vagina, which can contribute to causing yeast infections.

TREATMENT PLAN

A pelvic exam may have been necessary to identify the source of your infection. Practice preventive tips to speed your recovery.

Activity: Avoid excessive exercise and activities that produce excessive sweating, also avoid sexual intercourse until your infection is gone. Your partner may also need to be treated for this same infection.

Diet: Drink plenty of water and other liquids. Avoid alcohol and excessive sugars. Increase the intake of yogurt and buttermilk in your diet.

Medications: Antifungal medications may be prescribed for you.

1. Over-the-counter medications may include Monistat vaginal suppositories and cream. This is also known as miconazole nitrate, which you may find in the drug store at a much lower price and which can be just at effective.

2. You must use the full days of the over-the-counter medication. If you stop too early the yeast can regrow.

If you have also been diagnosed with a bacterial infection of the vagina, other medications may also be prescribed. If your provider has prescribed Flagyl (metronidazole), **please do not drink any alcohol while taking this medication and for the next 3 days following this medication. The combination of this medication and alcohol can make you very sick.**

You Have Been Prescribed: _____

You Need to Take: _____

You Need to Notify the Office If You:

A. Over-the-counter medications do not help your symptoms.

B. You develop other symptoms.

C. Other: _____

Phone: _____

Patient Teaching Guides for Chapter 14: Sexually Transmitted Infections

- Chlamydia
- Gonorrhea
- Herpes Simplex Virus
- Human Papillomavirus (HPV)
- Syphilis
- Trichomoniasis

CHLAMYDIA

PROBLEM

Chlamydia is a sexually transmitted infection. Often, no problems are present, but you may notice a yellowish discharge from the penis or vagina, burning during urination, frequent and urgent urination, or pelvic pain.

Untreated chlamydia in females may lead to a condition called pelvic inflammatory disease (PID). PID is a leading cause of infertility, increased ectopic pregnancies, and chronic pelvic pain in women.

CAUSE

Chlamydia is caused by a bacterium called *Chlamydia trachomatis*. This bacterium is spread through sexual contact and may infect the eyes, throat, vagina, penis, or rectum.

PREVENTION

A. Limit sexual partners.

B. Have routine screening tests for chlamydia prior to beginning a new sexual relationship.

C. Use condoms with sexual activity.

TREATMENT PLAN

Abstain from sexual activity until you and your partner(s) have completed your prescribed medication. Your health care provider is required to report this disease to the public health department. They may contact you.

Diet: As desired.

Medications: Chlamydia can be cured by the prescribed antibiotics.

You Have Been Prescribed: _____

You Need to Take: _____

You need to take all of your antibiotics.

You Need to Notify the Office If:

    A. You are unable to take your antibiotics because of nausea, vomiting, or a reaction.

    B. Other: _____

Phone: _____

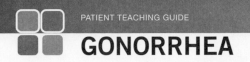

GONORRHEA

PROBLEM

Gonorrhea is a sexually transmitted infection. You may have the following symptoms: burning during urination, yellowish discharge from the penis or vagina, heavier menstrual periods, or pelvic pain.

Untreated gonorrhea in females can lead to a condition called pelvic inflammatory disease (PID). PID is a leading cause of infertility, increased ectopic pregnancies, and chronic pelvic pain in women.

CAUSE

Gonorrhea is caused by an organism called *Neisseria gonorrhoeae*. This organism is spread through sexual contact and may infect the eyes, throat, vagina, penis, or rectum.

PREVENTION

A. Limit sexual partners.

B. Have routine screening tests for gonorrhea prior to beginning a new sexual relationship.

C. Use condoms when having intercourse.

TREATMENT PLAN

Your health care provider is required to report this disease to the public health department. They may contact you. **Abstain from sexual activity until you and your partner(s) have completed your prescribed medications.**

Diet: There is no special diet that needs to be followed.

Medications: Gonorrhea can be cured by the prescribed antibiotics.

You Have Been Prescribed: _____

You Need to Take: _____

All of the antibiotics need to be taken.

You Need to Notify the Office If:

A. You have any new symptoms.

B. You are unable to take all of the antibiotics due to nausea or vomiting or a reaction.

C. Other: _____

Phone: _____

HERPES SIMPLEX VIRUS

PROBLEM

You may experience oral or genital bumps or lesions (often painful), burning, itching, sensation of pressure, painful urination, painful lymph nodes (bumps along underwear line), flulike symptoms (fever, headache, muscle aches, tired feeling).

CAUSE

A. The herpes simplex virus (HSV) is spread by direct contact with the secretions of someone who has the virus.

B. Viruses cannot be cured, but the problems or symptoms caused by them can often be managed with medication.

C. It is possible for someone to have HSV and have no symptoms. The first outbreak after contact with an infected individual usually occurs within 2 to 10 days, but it may take up to 3 weeks.

D. More severe symptoms are experienced with the first outbreak of HSV. The symptoms usually peak 4 to 5 days after the onset of infection and resolve after 2 to 3 weeks without medication.

E. Medication may decrease the severity and duration of the symptoms. Recurrent outbreaks usually last 5 to 7 days.

F. The virus may be spread even when symptoms are not present. This is known as viral shedding. Medication may also decrease the time of viral shedding.

G. Often, individuals with HSV experience itching, burning, or a feeling of pressure at the site 24 to 48 hours prior to an outbreak. This is known as prodrome.

H. Sexual activity should be avoided during this time because the viral shedding is occurring, which means the infection may be spread.

TREATMENT PLAN

A. Avoid sexual activity when lesions are present or when you feel the prodrome.

B. Use condoms with sexual activity.

C. Limit sexual partners.

D. Do not use any creams, lotions, or powders on lesions unless instructed to do so by your health care provider.

E. If urination is painful, pour water over genital area while urinating.

F. Dry affected area thoroughly.

Activity: Stress is a trigger for an outbreak. Exercise may help with keeping your stress level down.

Diet: There is no special diet.

Medications: Antiviral medications are used to suppress the virus. They do not cure it but decrease the viral outbreaks.

You Have Been Prescribed: _____

You Need to Take It: _____

You Need to Call the Office If:

A. You are unable to empty your bladder when you have an outbreak.

B. Other: _____

Phone: _____

HUMAN PAPILLOMAVIRUS (HPV)

PROBLEM

Human Papillomavirus (HPV), also known as condyloma, or genital or venereal warts, is a sexually transmitted infection.

A. You may experience "bumps" or lesions on genitals or perianal area. They may be raised and rough appearing or flat and smooth. They are often wartlike in appearance.

B. Lesions may appear singly or in clusters and may be small or large. They are usually soft, painless, and pale pink to grayish in color, and they may itch.

C. **It is very important to get regular Pap smears.**

D. There are several treatment options that your health care provider will discuss.

CAUSE

HPV is acquired by having genital contact or intercourse with someone who has the infection.

PREVENTION/TREATMENT PLAN

There is no cure for HPV, but the following may decrease the spread of HPV:

A. Do not have genital contact or intercourse without a condom when the lesions are present. Some people who have the infection never have symptoms (bumps or warts). It is possible to spread the infection even when no symptoms are present.

B. Limit sexual partners and openly discuss the need to use a condom.

C. Examine new partners for bumps or warts.

D. Obtain Garadasil vaccine now available for adolescent females and males for preventing four strains of HPV.

Medications:

You Have Been Prescribed: _____

You Need to Take: _____

You Need to Notify the Office If:

A. You have any new symptoms.

B. It is time for your Pap smear.

C. Other: _____

Phone: _____

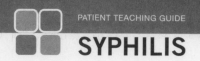

SYPHILIS

PROBLEM

You may have round or oval painless lesions, most commonly in the genital region, but they may occur anywhere on the body where transmission occurred.

A. You may experience a rash covering your body, including palms and soles.

B. **Flulike symptoms** include fever; headache; sore throat; swollen, tender lymph nodes; decreased appetite.

CAUSE

Syphilis is contracted by genital or oral contact with someone who has the infection. The infection Is spread when lesions are present.

PREVENTION

A. Use condoms.

B. Limit sexual partners.

C. Screen new sexual partners by asking about any known infections.

TREATMENT PLAN

Do not engage in sexual activity while lesions are present. Notify all partners of the need for treatment. Keep follow-up appointments to determine if treatment has been effective.

Diet: There is no special diet.

Medications: Penicillin is the drug of choice for treating syphilis. Other antibiotics can be used if you are allergic to penicillin. Within 24 hours of treatment of antibiotic treatment, you may experience a fever or headache. Aspirin, acetaminophen (Tylenol), or ibuprofen may be taken if these symptoms occur.

You Have Been Prescribed: _____

You Need to Take: _____

You need to finish all of your antibiotics. [emphasis added]

You Need to Notify the Office If You Have:

A. Any new symptoms.

B. Any reaction to your antibiotics.

C. Any other concerns about syphilis.

Phone: _____

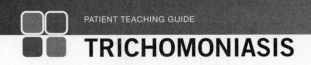

TRICHOMONIASIS

PROBLEM

You may experience increased vaginal discharge, yellow-green or watery gray in color. It may have a foul odor. You may also have vaginal itching or irritation, burning during urination, discomfort during sexual intercourse, spotting or bleeding during or after sexual intercourse, or abdominal discomfort.

CAUSE

Trichomonas vaginalis is acquired by having sex with someone who has the infection.

PREVENTION

A. Condom use with each act of intercourse.

B. Limiting the number of sexual partners.

C. Screening new sexual partners.

TREATMENT PLAN

Do not have sexual activity until you and your partner have both completed medications. There are no limitations in other physical activity.

Diet: Do not drink alcohol during the use of medication and for 3 days after taking the last dose of your medicine. Alcohol use while taking this medication may result in nausea, vomiting, and severe upset stomach. You may have a metallic taste from the medicine that may slightly alter the taste of food. No other limitations in diet are required.

Medications: Metronidazole (Flagyl) is used to treat the infection.

You Have Been Prescribed: _____

You Need to Take: _____

Finish all of the medication.

You Need to Notify the Office If:

A. You are unable to tolerate the medicine.

B. Any new symptoms develop.

C. Other: _____

Phone: _____

Patient Teaching Guides for Chapter 15: Infectious Diseases

- Influenza (Flu)
- Lyme Disease and Removal of a Tick
- Mononucleosis
- Rocky Mountain Spotted Fever and Removal of a Tick
- Prevention of Toxoplasmosis
- Chickenpox (Varicella)

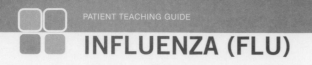

INFLUENZA (FLU)

PROBLEM

Influenza (flu) is an acute, self-limiting, febrile illness of the respiratory tract. Respiratory droplets and direct contact spread it. You are contagious for 24 to 48 hours before feeling symptoms and you are contagious up to 7 days after symptoms begin.

CAUSE

There are many flu viruses and they can mutate easily. Stress, excessive fatigue, poor nutrition, recent illness, crowded places, and immunosuppression from drugs or illness lower your resistance to these viruses.

PREVENTION

A. Influenza vaccine should be taken yearly (in the fall) if you are at high risk:

   1. Health care worker

   2. Immunocompromised (transplant patients, HIV-positive patients, etc.)

   3. Pregnant (after the first trimester)

   4. Elderly (>65 years of age)

   5. Children with severe asthma

B. Avoid unnecessary contact with sick persons, including in crowded areas.

C. Use droplet and secretion precautions.

   1. Cover your mouth when coughing or sneezing.

   2. Use tissues when you blow your nose. Dispose of them and then wash your hands. If no tissue is available do the "elbow sneeze" into the bend of your arm (away from your open hands). Always wash your hands.

   3. Do not share drinking glasses.

   4. Wash your hands with soap and water or use hand sanitizer.

TREATMENT PLAN

A. Rest.

B. Force fluids.

C. Run cool-mist vaporizer.

D. Take tepid sponge baths in warm water to prevent chilling and shivers.

E. Gargle with warm salt water for a sore throat.

F. Use warm compresses or heating pad on low for aching muscles.

Activity: Maintain bed rest for a minimum of 24 hours after fever subsides.

Diet: Eat regular diet; you may not be hungry. Drink plenty of liquids (at least 10 glasses a day).

Medications: Antibiotics *do not* help the flu. Do not use aspirin for a child due to the risk of Reye's syndrome.

You Have Been Prescribed for Your Fever: _____

You Need to Take: _____

For Your Respiratory Symptoms, You Have Been Prescribed: _____

You Need to Take: _____

For Your Respiratory (Cough Suppressant) Symptoms, You Have Been Prescribed: _____

You Need to Take: _____

You Need to Notify the Office If You Have:

A. Thick, purulent (green) nasal drainage.

B. Ear pain.

C. Increase in fever or cough.

D. Shortness of breath or chest pain.

E. Blood in your sputum.

F. Neck pain or stiffness.

G. New or unexplained symptoms. (Drugs in treatment may produce side effects.)

H. Other: _____

Phone: _____

LYME DISEASE AND REMOVAL OF A TICK

PROBLEM

Ticks are vectors for Lyme disease and Rocky Mountain spotted fever. You have been diagnosed with Lyme disease.

CAUSE

Lyme disease is caused by a spirochete, *Borrelia burgdorferi.*

PREVENTION

A. Avoid areas with large deer populations.

B. Wear light-colored clothes to make ticks easier to spot. Wear long sleeves, and tuck pants into the socks to form a barrier.

C. Stick to hiking trails. Avoid contact with overgrown foliage. Ticks prefer dense woods with thick growth of shrubs and small trees as well as along the edge of the woods.

D. Check for ticks after each outdoor activity, especially hairy regions of the body and beltline where ticks often attach. Check for ticks prior to bathing, especially at the back of the neck, knees, and ears.

E. Remove ticks promptly. See Precautions below for instructions to remove a tick.

F. Inspect pets daily and remove ticks when present.

G. Some manufacturers currently offer permetrin-treated clothing that is effective for up to 20 washings. There is no safety data on clothing treated with permetrin. This clothing is not recommended for children.

H. Use tick repellant with DEET (except for small children younger than 2 years). As an alternative, picaridin and oil of eucalyptus preparations have been approved for use as repellents by the U.S. Environmental Protection Agency (EPA).

PRECAUTIONS

A. Do not hold a lighted match or cigarette to the tick. Do not apply gasoline, kerosene, or oil to the tick's body.

B. Care should be taken to avoid squeezing the body of the tick.

C. It should be grasped with a fine-tip tweezer close to the skin. Remove by gently pulling the tick upward straight out without using any twisting motions. See Figures.

D. In the home, if fingers are used to remove ticks, they should be protected with facial tissue or gloves and washed after removal of the tick.

E. Do not crush the tick during removal.

F. **Save the tick for identification in case you become ill. Write the date of the tick bite on paper and place the paper and the tick in a resealable baggie and place it in the freezer.**

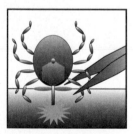

Grasp the tick's body as close to the skin using a
fine-tip tweezer. Avoid squeezing the body.

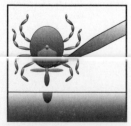

Remove by pulling the tick straight
upward without using twisting motions.

TREATMENT PLAN

A. Antibiotics are effective against *B. burgdorferi* and Lyme disease.

B. If you are prescribed doxycycline, avoid exposure to the sun, because a rash may develop.

Activity: As tolerated.

Diet: Eat regular diet.

Medications: Acetaminophen may be taken for body aches. You may be given an antibiotic for infection.

You Have Been Prescribed: _____

You Need to Take: _____

Take all of your antibiotics even if you feel better.

You Need to Notify the Office If You Have:

1. No signs of improvement with antibiotic therapy.

2. Other: _____

Phone: _____

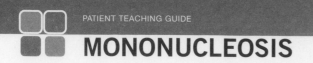

MONONUCLEOSIS

PROBLEM

Mononucleosis is an acute, infectious, viral disease with three classic symptoms: fever, sore throat, and swollen lymph glands.

CAUSE

Epstein-Barr virus, the causative agent, is spread to other persons by kissing, sharing food, and coughing without covering your mouth.

PREVENTION

Avoid contact with persons diagnosed with mononucleosis. Cover your mouth and nose when you cough or sneeze to prevent the spread of infection.

TREATMENT PLAN

There is no specific cure. Gargle with warm salt water for a sore throat.

Activity: Bed rest with gradual return to activity. Children may require home schooling for long convalescences. You should have no social contact until the acute phase is over. You should not do any physical activity, especially contact sports (football, soccer, basketball, and so on), if an enlarged spleen is present.

Diet: Eat a high-caloric diet. Drink plenty of liquids (at least 8 glasses a day).

Medications: Acetaminophen may be taken for body aches. You may be given an antibiotic for infection if indicated.

You Have Been Prescribed: _____

You Need to Take: _____

Take all of your antibiotics even if you feel better.

You Need to Notify the Office If You Have:

- A. Fever over 102°F.
- B. Severe pain in the upper left abdomen (rupture of the spleen is a medical emergency).
- C. Swallowing or breathing difficulty from a severe throat inflammation.
- D. Rash: a rash may follow the use of antibiotics.
- E. Other _____

Phone: _____

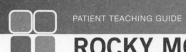

ROCKY MOUNTAIN SPOTTED FEVER AND REMOVAL OF A TICK

PROBLEM

Ticks are vectors for Lyme disease and Rocky Mountain spotted fever. You have been diagnosed with Rocky Mountain spotted fever.

CAUSE

Rocky Mountain spotted fever is caused by a bacterium, *Rickettsia rickettsii.* The tick passes the bacterium that causes a fever and a rash.

PREVENTION

A. Avoid areas with large deer populations.

B. Wear light-colored clothes to make ticks easier to spot. Wear long sleeves, and tuck pants into the socks to form a barrier.

C. Stick to hiking trails. Avoid contact with overgrown foliage. Ticks prefer dense woods with thick growth of shrubs and small trees as well as along the edge of the woods.

D. Check for ticks after each outdoor activity, especially hairy regions of the body and beltline where ticks often attach. Check for ticks prior to bathing, especially at the back of the neck, knees, and ears.

E. Remove ticks promptly. See Precautions below for instructions to remove a tick.

F. Inspect pets daily and remove ticks when present.

G. Some manufacturers currently offer permetrin-treated clothing that is effective for up to 20 washings. There is no safety data on clothing treated with permetrin. This clothing is not recommended for children.

H. Prophylactic antibiotic therapy for Rocky Mountain spotted fever is not recommended for tick exposure. Instead, inform your health care provider if any symptom, especially fever and headache, occurs in the following 14 days.

I. Use tick repellant with DEET (except for small children younger than 2 years). As an alternative, picaridin and oil of eucalyptus preparations have been approved for use as repellents by the U.S. Environmental Protection Agency (EPA).

PRECAUTIONS

A. Do not hold a lighted match or cigarette to the tick. Do not apply gasoline, kerosene, or oil to the tick's body.

B. Care should be taken to avoid squeezing the body of the tick.

C. It should be grasped with a fine-tip tweezer close to the skin. Remove by gently pulling the tick upward straight out without using any twisting motions. See Figures.

D. In the home, if fingers are used to remove ticks, they should be protected with facial tissue or gloves and washed after removal of the tick.

E. Do not crush the tick during removal.

F. **Save the tick for identification in case you become ill. Write the date of the tick bite on paper and place the paper and the tick in a resealable baggie and place it in the freezer.**

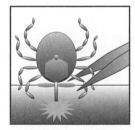

Grasp the tick's body as close to the skin using a fine-tip tweezer. Avoid squeezing the body.

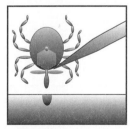

Remove by pulling the tick straignt upward without using twisting motions.

TREATMENT PLAN

Activity: As tolerated, regular activity. Tepid sponge baths may also reduce fever.

Diet: Eat regular diet. Drink 8 to 10 glasses of water daily.

Medications: Acetaminophen (Tylenol) may be taken for body aches. You may be given an antibiotic for secondary infection if needed.

You Have Been Prescribed: _____

You Need to Take: _____

Take all of your antibiotic even if you feel better.

You Need to Notify the Office If You Have:

A. No improvement while on antibiotic therapy.

B. Decreased urinary output, or dryness in your skin or mouth.

C. Other: _____

Phone: _____

PREVENTION OF TOXOPLASMOSIS

PROBLEM

Toxoplasmosis is an infection acquired through contact with infected cat feces, by eating raw or undercooked meat, or by transfusions or organ transplant. Toxoplasmosis is dangerous for AIDS patients and during pregnancy.

CAUSE

Toxoplasma gondii is an intracellular protozoan parasite that is the causative agent. Cats are the primary host, and humans are the intermediate host. **You do not need to destroy your cat.**

PREVENTION

A. Avoid uncooked eggs and unpasteurized milk.

B. Wash hands after handling raw meat.

C. Meat should be thoroughly cooked at 152°F or higher, or frozen for 24 hours in a household freezer before eating (smoked meats and meats cured in brine are considered safe). Avoid tasting meat while cooking.

D. Wash fruits and vegetables before consumption.

E. Wash all kitchen surfaces that come into contact with uncooked meats.

F. Avoid drinking unfiltered water in any setting.

G. Use care in gardening where cats have access.

H. Wear gloves for gardening and landscaping.

I. Wear gloves for handling kitty litter, and wash hands after contact with cats. **Change kitty litter daily:** oocysts are not infective during the first 1 to 2 days after being passed by cats.

J. Keep outdoor sandboxes covered.

K. Domestic cats can be protected from infection by feeding them commercially prepared cat food and preventing them from eating undercooked kitchen scraps and hunting wild rodents.

L. Nonpregnant infected women should delay pregnancy for at least 6 months.

TREATMENT PLAN

A. If you are pregnant, you may be referred to a specialist.

B. Because the most serious fetal effects occur if the disease is contracted during the first 20 weeks of pregnancy, abortion may be presented as an option for you to consider.

C. If you have AIDS, you will be referred to a specialist.

Activity: No activity restriction.

Diet: Avoid uncooked eggs and unpasteurized milk. Meat should be thoroughly cooked.

Medications: Depending on your risk status, you may be prescribed one or two medications. You may be required to take the medication for several weeks for lifelong prophylaxis to prevent recurrence.

You Have Been Prescribed: _____

You Need to Take: _____

You Need to Notify the Office If You Have:

A. Headache, dull and constant, with no relief from acetaminophen.

B. Abnormal speech.

C. Seizures.

D. Loss of visual acuity.

E. Poor concentration, forgetfulness.

F. Personality changes.

G. Other: _____

Phone: _____

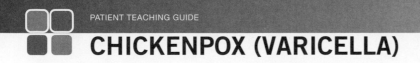

CHICKENPOX (VARICELLA)

PROBLEM

Chickenpox is a viral disease with a vesicular rash that occurs in crops. The varicella virus that is responsible can be reactivated and is known as "shingles." The virus can affect all ages, but usually affects children and older adults.

CAUSE

Varicella-zoster virus is a herpes virus that is highly contagious. It is spread by direct person-to-person contact and occasionally by airborne means from respiratory secretions.

PREVENTION

A. Avoid contact with anyone with chickenpox.

B. If infected, remain in strict isolation until lesions are all crusted over.

C. Sores "lesions" should be covered by clothing or a dressing until they have crusted. **Covering sores prevents invasion of bacteria causing secondary infection and helps to prevent scarring.**

D. Thorough hand washing is warranted whenever there is contact with fluid from the sores.

TREATMENT PLAN

A. Remain in strict isolation.

B. Children may return to daycare or school after all lesions have dried and crusted.

C. Care for skin with daily cool-water bathing or soaks.

D. Keep fingernails short and clean; try to prevent scratching.

E. Alleviate itching with cornstarch bath, baking soda, or oatmeal (Aveeno) or topical lotions such as calamine (follow package instructions).

F. Change bed linens and clothes often.

G. **Aspirin should never be used for a fever; it may contribute to the development of Reye's syndrome (a form of encephalitis) when given to children during a viral illness.**

Activity: Bed rest is not necessary. Quiet play activity in a cool room or outside in the shade during nice weather is permitted. Keep all ill children away from others and away from school and day care, until all blisters have crusted and there are no new ones.

Diet: No special foods are needed.

Medications: Acetaminophen may be administered for fever. Your child may have a medication prescribed for itching.

You Have Been Prescribed: _____

You Need to Take: _____

You Need to Notify the Office If You Have or Your Child Has:

A. Symptoms of chickenpox.

B. Lethargy, headache, sensitive to bright light.

C. Fever over 101°F.

D. Chickenpox sores that contain pus or otherwise appear infected.

E. A cough that occurs during a chickenpox infection.

F. Other: _____

Phone: _____

Patient Teaching Guides for Chapter 16: Systemic Disorders

- Lupus

- Pernicious Anemia

- Reference Resources for Patients With HIV/AIDS

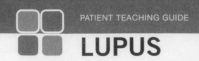

LUPUS

PROBLEM

You have been diagnosed with a condition called lupus. Lupus is a chronic, inflammatory, autoimmune disorder. There is currently no cure for lupus; however, it can be managed and can go into remission, or a dormant state. Rashes, hair loss, arthritislike joint pain, and fatigue are very common problems with lupus.

CAUSE

Lupus causes your body to attack its own cells. The exact cause is unknown. Lupus tends to run in families, but it is not contagious.

PREVENTION

There is no known prevention, only long-term management.

TREATMENT PLAN

A. Avoid sun exposure:
   1. Many lupus patients' eyes are sensitive to light; wear sunglasses and avoid direct exposure.
   2. Light exposure can make your rash worse.
   3. Apply a protective lotion or sunscreen to your skin while outside.
   4. Wear long sleeves and use hats.
B. You may be given steroids for your skin rashes or lesions.
C. Avoid exposure to drugs and chemicals:
D. Please review all of your medications and over-the-counter drugs with your health care provider.
E. Avoid hair sprays and hair coloring agents.
F. Mouth ulcers may occur with lupus:
   1. Avoid hot or spicy foods that might cause irritation to ulcers.
   2. Use good oral hygiene:
      a. Get regular dental exams.
      b. Floss your teeth daily.
      c. Brush your teeth at least twice a day.
G. Rest and drugs called nonsteroidal anti-inflammatory drugs (NSAIDs) are used for minor joint pain.
H. It is very important for you to have your eyes examined **twice** a year to monitor eye changes.
I. Talk to your health care provider if you are planning a pregnancy.

Activity: You may get tired more easily; plan rest periods. However, you should still get some exercise as tolerated. Many people gain some weight from steroids.

Diet: Eat a regular diet as tolerated; you do not need any special foods.

Medications:

You Have Been Prescribed the Following Steroid: _____

You Need to Take: _____
   A. Do not stop taking your steroid abruptly.
   B. **Steroid medication should be tapered off (decreased until you are off of it).**

You Need to Notify the Office If:
   A. You are unable to tolerate your medication.
   B. You have any sign of infections, sinusitis, bronchitis, flu, urinary tract infections, and so forth.
   C. You are getting worse or do not feel better.
   D. You are planning a pregnancy or think you are pregnant.
   E. Other: _____

Phone: _____

RESOURCES

Lupus Foundation of America, 800-558-0121 or www.lupus.org/, Livestrong.com/American Lupus Society, http://www.live strong.com/american-lupus-society/, Terri Gotthelf Lupus Research Institute, 800-825-8787, 9 AM to 7:30 PM eastern time, Monday through Friday

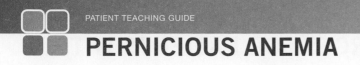

PERNICIOUS ANEMIA

PROBLEM

You have been diagnosed with a condition called pernicious anemia. It is a condition in which vitamin B_{12} is not well absorbed. Vitamin B_{12} is necessary for red blood cell function.

CAUSE

Pernicious anemia is a common problem in pregnancy, with vegetarian diets, with previous stomach problems, and as you get older. Your condition may be due to the lack of a special factor in your stomach juices whereby your body cannot absorb the vitamin, or it may be from an autoimmune reaction.

PREVENTION

Pernicious anemia cannot always be prevented. But pernicious anemia is treatable once the cause is identified.

TREATMENT PLAN

A. You will need vitamin B_{12} injections for the rest of your life. This cannot be given in pill form.

   1. After you have been on the shots for a while, the nurses can teach you or a family member to give the shot. Please ask your health care provider about this.
   2. Common side effects of vitamin B_{12} shots include:
      a. Pain and burning at the place the shot is given. This does not last very long.
      b. Some people experience diarrhea after taking the shot.

B. You may need to take iron tablets too.

C. You may be sent to see a nutritionist to help you review your diet and how you prepare foods.

Activity: Pernicious anemia may cause the loss of some senses and give you numbness and tingling, memory loss, loss of coordination, and some depression or irritability.

A. It is important to avoid extremely hot foods and drinks.

B. It is important to use caution in your home such as:

   1. Do not use loose "scatter" rugs to prevent slips.
   2. Install shower or tub rails to help get in and out and toilet rails to get up and down easier.
   3. Use hand rails going up and down stairs.
   4. Do not use extremely hot water for bathing, showers, and doing dishes.
   5. Use nonslip surfaces in the tub and shower.

   6. **Do not to use a heating pad if you do not have all your sensations in order to avoid burns.**

A home safety evaluation should be done to reduce the risk of falls. A checklist can be obtained from:

National Safety Council: 1250 Eye Street, NW Suite 1000, Washington, DC 20005; http://www.homesafetycouncil.org/

Diet: A balanced, healthy diet is important. Increase your liquids to 8 to 10 glasses a day; iron supplements tend to cause constipation. Increase the fiber in your diet.

Medication:

You Have Been Prescribed the Following Iron Supplement: _____

You Need to Take It: _____

Your next vitamin B_{12} shot is due: _____

You Need to Notify the Office If: _____

   A. You feel worse the first week after the shot or have symptoms such as chest pain and shortness of breath.

   B. You have worsening symptoms such as problems with balance and walking.

   C. You have leg pain, especially when you put your weight on it.

   D. You would like to make arrangements for home injections.

   E. Other:_____

Phone: _____

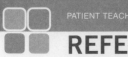

REFERENCE RESOURCES FOR PATIENTS WITH HIV/AIDS

AIDS HEALTHCARE Foundation
http://www.aidshealth.org/

A Positive Life
Features real people telling their stories.
http://www.apositivelife.com/

Centers for Disease Control and Prevention (CDC)
Provides general information on HIV.
http://www.cdc.gov/hiv/default.htm

HIVandHepatitis.com
Provides the latest information about coinfection with hepatitis B and hepatitis C.
http://www.hivandhepatitis.com/

National Association of People with AIDS
POZ AIDS Services Directory is a comprehensive guide to HIV care and services.
http://directory.poz.com/napwa/

Project Inform (includes Spanish resources)
Provides multiple topics including the latest treatment options.
http://www.projectinform.org/info/

The AIDS InfoNet
http://www.aidsinfonet.org/

The Body
The most-visited Internet site about HIV.
http://www.thebody.com/

The Well Project
Designed for HIV-positive women.
http://www.thewellproject.org/en_US/

Treat HIV
Provides information about your treatment options.
http://www.treathiv.com/

Patient Teaching Guides for Chapter 17: Musculoskeletal Disorders

- Fibromyalgia

- Gout

- RICE Therapy and Exercise Therapy

- Osteoarthritis

- Osteoporosis

- Ankle Exercises

- Knee Exercises

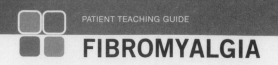

FIBROMYALGIA

PROBLEM

You have inflammation or pain in the muscles and connective tissues, usually noted in the low back, shoulders, neck, chest, arms, hips, and thighs.

CAUSE

The cause is unknown.

TREATMENT/CARE

A. Get regular exercise.

B. Get adequate amounts of sleep.

C. For symptoms of discomfort, you may try applying heat to the areas of pain, such as hot showers, heating pad, and whirlpools.

D. Gentle massages by a massage therapist may help with comfort.

E. Try to eliminate the daily stress in your life.

F. Consider alternatives to relieving stress, such as biofeedback, relaxation techniques, and yoga.

Activity: Regular exercise is recommended. Exercise at least 30 minutes for 3 to 5 times a week if possible. Even 5 minutes is better than no exercise. Establish a regular sleep time. Adequate and sound sleeping may decrease symptoms. You may require naps during the day.

Diet: Eat a nutritious regular diet. Avoid foods, caffeine, and alcohol that interfere with your normal sleep.

Medications: There are medications to help with your fibromyalgia. They may cause swelling of your legs.

You Have Been Prescribed: _____

You Need to Take: _____

You Need to Notify the Office If You Have:

A. New or unexplained symptoms that have developed,

B. Fever higher than 100.0°F.

C. Other: _____

Phone: _____

RESOURCE

The National Fibromyalgia Association: http://www.fmaware.org/

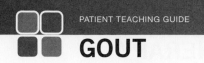

GOUT

PROBLEM

Gout is caused from high uric acid deposits in the joints, which cause pain and swelling at the joint. Gout commonly occurs in the big toe; however, other joints may be affected too. Other signs/symptoms include red, hot, and swollen joints, which may be tender to touch.

PREVENTION/CARE

A. The goal is to prevent recurrences of the attacks.

B. Acute attacks: You may use warm or cool compresses to affected areas for comfort.

C. Avoid weight-bearing objects on the affected joint.

D. Take your medication as prescribed.

Activity: When you have an attack, resting the joint is the best treatment. Drinking large amounts of water will keep your urine diluted to help prevent kidney stones.

Diet:

A. Drink 10 to 12 glasses of water a day.

B. Refrain from alcohol (beer, wine, liquor). These will worsen your symptoms or trigger a new attack.

C. If overweight, you need to begin a weight loss program appropriate for you.

D. Avoid crash diets. These will also precipitate an acute attack.

E. Foods to avoid: sardines, kidneys, anchovies, liver, and sweet bread.

Medications: Medications to avoid: Salicylates (aspirin).

You Have Been Prescribed: _____

You Need to Take: _____

You Need to Notify the Office If You Have:

A. Acute attacks.

B. Fever higher than 101°F.

C. Rash.

D. Swelling of extremities.

E. Vomiting/diarrhea.

F. Signs/symptoms not improving within 3 to 4 days after starting therapy.

G. Any adverse effects occur from your medication.

Phone: _____

RICE THERAPY AND EXERCISE THERAPY

RICE therapies are used for muscle injuries. RICE stands for rest, ice, compression, and elevation.

REST

A. Take it easy, eliminate abuse; reduce regular exercise or activities of daily living as needed, but do not eliminate them.

B. Change activity or components of activity, for example, change running to walking.

C. Stop sports; restrict squatting, kneeling, and repetitious bending.

D. Limit weight bearing; immobilize with crutches for partial weight bearing.

ICE

A. Use cold in the acute phase of the injury (first 72 hours) to reduce pain and swelling.

B. Use cold in the form of ice in a plastic bag, or even use frozen peas in a bag.

C. Apply cold four to eight times a day for 20 minutes at a time, with 45 to 60 minutes between applications.

COMPRESSION

A. Use elastic bandages, dry or wet, or open basket weave tape.

B. Avoid trying to provide support with elastic bandages; use a brace, overlap taping, or a cast may be needed.

ELEVATION

A. Elevate the joint above the level of the heart to reduce swelling.

B. Apply cold compresses while the joint is elevated.

EXERCISE THERAPY

A. Begin exercise therapy after initial 48-hour period if pain and swelling begin to resolve.

B. Do gentle range-of-motion exercises several times a day within limits of pain for 7 to 10 days after knee ligament strain.

C. Exercise after 6 minutes of icing to take advantage of the cold's numbing effect.

D. Start with nonresistive, non-weight-bearing exercises.

E. Use exercises that improve range of motion and strength.

F. Maintain fitness of the extremity.

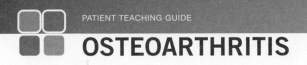

OSTEOARTHRITIS

PROBLEM

Osteoarthritis is a very common disorder that affects the weight-bearing and movable joints. Osteoarthritis (OA) damages the cartilage tissue in the joint. The joints most commonly involved are the finger and toe joints, knees, hips, and spine.

CAUSES

There are many different causes of osteoarthritis. A previous injury to the joint, repeated stress to the joint (like a bricklayer's hands), genetics, obesity that may cause additional injury to the knee, and other diseases (such as diabetes or infections) may cause OA.

TREATMENT

A. The goal of treatment of osteoarthritis is to prevent further joint damage.

B. Learn as much as you can about this disorder and ask your health care provider lots of questions.

C. Heat and massage may increase joint movement and decrease pain.

D. Physical or occupational therapy may be needed.

E. Heat or ice packs may be used for localized relief.

Activity: Exercise:

1. Range-of-motion exercises increase the movement of the joint.

2. Careful exercise may also strengthen the muscles around the joint.

3. Ask your provider what's the best type of exercise for you.

Joint protection:

1. Don't overuse a joint.

2. If you work with your hands and have OA of the fingers, take frequent rest periods. This applies to all the other joints as well.

Diet: Low-fat, low-cholesterol diet may be suggested. Losing weight may help if you have OA of the knees, hips, or spine.

Medications: Your health care provider may recommend that you take acetaminophen or an anti-inflammatory drug. This should help relieve the pain and stiffness. Special creams also sometimes help joint pain. In cases of severe OA, your health care provider may recommend an injection to the joint or surgery. *Remember* to take only the medicines prescribed for you.

You Have Been Prescribed:_____

You Need to Take: _____

You Need to Notify the Office If You Have:

A. Increased pain despite medication.

B. Fever higher than 100.4°F

C. Abdominal pain or discomfort after taking medicine.

Phone: _____

RESOURCE

Arthritis Foundation
800-283-7800
www.arthritis.org/

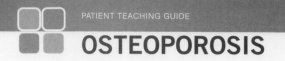

OSTEOPOROSIS

PROBLEM

Osteoporosis is a condition in which the bone loses its normal density, mass, and strength, which makes it weak and more vulnerable to fracture (break).

CAUSES

The weakening of the bone can be caused by several factors. Some of these include:

A. Inadequate amounts of calcium, protein, and vitamin D in the diet
B. Decreased exercise
C. Thyroid disease
D. Cancer
E. Smoking
F. Low estrogen levels (menopause)

PREVENTION

A. Be sure to get adequate calcium intake daily (1,500 mg/day).
B. Food sources are best absorbed.
C. Calcium supplements may also be needed to meet the daily recommendation.
D. Get daily exercise, such as walking, jogging, or running.

TREATMENT PLAN

A. If osteopororsis is suspected, your provider may order a bone density study of your bones. Goals are to prevent the disease from occurring.
B. If you have been diagnosed with osteoporosis, you need to prevent the disease from progressing and take measures to prevent all bone fractures.
C. Use caution when walking on wet, slippery surfaces.
D. Heat or ice may ease pain.

Activity:

A. Physical activity is vital to maintain and prevent further bone loss.
B. Weight-bearing activity is the best activity, such as walking or running.
C. Avoid high-impact sports and activity such as jumping and high-impact aerobics to prevent fracturing the bones.
D. Avoid any risk of falls.
E. Do not use throw rugs.
F. Bathtubs should have nonskid protection.

Diet:

A. Eat a regular well-balanced diet. Increase food sources rich in calcium, protein, and vitamin D.
B. Sources of vitamin D include milk, some fish (salmon), drinks, and cereals with added vitamin D and minerals.
C. You can also get vitamin D from spending 20 to 30 minutes in the summer sunlight, exposing your skin to the sun without wearing sunscreen for this length of time.
D. Sources of calcium include dairy products, green leafy vegetables (broccoli), almonds, tofu, and drinks fortified with calcium such as orange juice and soy milk.
E. If you are overweight, a low-fat, low-cholesterol diet is suggested to lose weight.

Medications:

A. You may be prescribed nonprescription medications like acetaminophen (Tylenol) as needed for pain.
B. Supplements: calcium, vitamin D, and hormone replacement for women who are menopausal.
C. If prescribed bisphosphonate, take medication with a full glass of water.
D. Wait approximately 30 to 60 minutes before reclining or consuming other medications, beverages, or food to lower the risk of regurgitation or a burning sensation.

You Have Been Prescribed: _____

You Need to Take It: _____

You Need to Notify the Office If You Have:

A. Been experiencing any pain; you need to have your provider assess this pain.

B. Other: _____

Phone: _____

RESOURCES

National Osteoporosis Foundation: http://www.nof.org/
The National Women's Health information Center: www.4women.gov/FAQ/osteoporosis.cfm

ANKLE EXERCISES

A. Education

1. Exercise in your bare feet or in stocking feet.

2. Count slowly (1001, 1002, and so on) when you must hold a position and count.

3. Do each exercise 10 times the first day, and increase the repetitions by 5 each following day until you reach a maximum of 30, unless otherwise instructed.

4. Repeat prescribed exercises three times a day.

5. Exercise slowly and get the greatest stretch possible.

6. Stop any exercise that causes new, unusual, or intense pain.

7. You need to perform daily stretching exercises and toning to speed your recovery.

8. It takes months to adequately heal these types of injuries. Therefore, do not be discouraged that it takes time for your ankle to heal.

9. Sports to avoid: stop and go activity, basketball, running, and impact aerobics.

10. You may need to wear a velcro ankle brace or high-top tennis shoes for support.

B. Toe and Foot Bend (Floor)

1. Sit on the floor or bed with legs out straight.

2. Bend the injured foot back toward the head and curl toes.

3. Then point injured foot away and bend toes back.

C. Toe Rise and Foot Slide (Chair)

1. Sit in a chair with knees bent at a right angle and feet flat on the floor.

2. Raise all toes on the injured foot and slide the foot back 3 to 4 inches.

3. Relax.

4. Continue the sliding and toe raising until heel can no longer be kept on the floor.

D. Toe and Foot Bends (Chair)

1. Sit in a chair with knees bent at a right angle and feet flat on floor.

2. Slide the foot on the injured side forward as far as possible while keeping the toes and heel in contact with the floor.

3. From the straight-leg position, bend the foot toward the head as far as possible.

4. Lower your foot back onto the floor.

5. Bend the foot back and forth from the straight-leg position.

E. Heel-Cord Stretch

1. Stand straight and face a wall with feet together, arms straight out, and palms flat against the wall.

2. Lean toward the wall, bending the elbows, to stretch the cords above the heels.

3. Continue leaning to a count of five, and then straighten up again.

F. Inner-Tube Stretch (1)

1. Sit with feet dangling side by side at a right angle to your legs.

2. Tie stretch bands around your feet until they are snug.

3. Keeping ankles together, move toes as far apart as possible.

4. Hold the stretch for a count of five.

G. Inner-Tube Stretch (2)

1. Sit with feet dangling.

2. Cross your feet at the ankles.

3. Tie bands snugly around feet.

4. Move toes as far apart as possible.

5. Hold the stretch for a count of five.

KNEE EXERCISES

CARE FOR YOUR KNEE

Please follow the type of exercises recommended for your knee. You may begin straight leg raises after the pain resolves. Continue to wear your brace with activities as directed. It may take months for your knee to completely heal. You may gradually resume normal activity as directed by your provider. If you are not sure what activities you may perform, ask your provider before performing the activity.

A. Quad Sets

   1. Exercise may be done while standing, sitting, or lying down.

   2. Straighten knee with intensity.

   3. Hold for 10 counts then relax.

   4. Repeat the exercise three to four times per day.

   5. If a cast or splint is in place, straighten the knee until the front of the thigh and the cast pinch together.

   6. If the knee is bent, keep the foot planted and use the floor to push against.

B. Co-Contractions

   1. Similar to quads, but the difference is to tighten the entire thigh while straightening the knee.

   2. Hold for 10 counts then relax.

   3. Repeat the exercise approximately three to four times a day.

C. Hamstring Sets

   1. Pull the leg back against other foot, floor, or cast.

   2. Hold approximately 10 counts then relax.

   3. Perform these three to four times a day.

D. Heel Lifts

   1. Lie on back with support under the knee.

   2. Lift the heel while resting the knee on support.

   3. Make the knee as straight as possible.

   4. Hold for 10 counts then relax.

   5. Do not use weights.

   6. Perform these three to four times a day.

E. Straight Leg Raises

   1. Straighten the knee.

   2. Lift and pause for 5 to 10 counts then relax.

   3. Lower leg and relax then repeat.

   4. Do three to five sets, three to four times a day. Rest between each set.

   5. Start with _____ pounds of ankle weight and work up to _____ pounds.

   6. Gradually increase weight used.

F. Hip Flexors

   1. While sitting, lift the knee toward the chest.

   2. Hold for 10 counts then relax.

   3. Lower the leg and relax. Repeat.

   4. Do 10 times, three to four times a day.

   5. Start with _____ pounds of weight and work up gradually to _____ pounds.

   6. The weights should be on the knee or ankle.

G. Hamstring Stretches

   1. While seated on a sturdy table with the foot of your injured leg resting on the floor, lean forward with chin directed toward toes.

   2. Hold for at least 10 counts then relax.

   3. The knee should be straight from your hips.

   4. **Do not do this exercise with bouncing or violent movements.**

   5. Do _____ minutes, _____ times a day.

Patient Teaching Guides for Chapter 18: Neurologic Disorders

- Bell's Palsy
- Dementia
- Febrile Seizures (Child)
- Managing Your Parkinson's Disease
- Mild Head Injury
- Myasthenia Gravis
- Transient Ischemic Attack (TIA)

BELL'S PALSY

PROBLEM

Bell's palsy is a disorder that can occur at any age, but most frequently occurs between the ages of 20 and 60. The disorder affects the muscles associated with expression on one side of the face, including the muscles that allow smiles, the eyes to close, and the eyebrows to raise.

The exact cause of Bell's palsy remains unknown. Possible causes may include viral infections or a type of inflammatory process. Another explanation is that other diseases may play a role, such as autoimmune diseases.

PREVENTION/CARE

A. Bell's palsy is usually treated with a steroid, such as prednisone.

B. Pain is usually managed with acetaminophen (Tylenol) or another over-the-counter pain medication.

C. Sometimes it is helpful to use gentle massage, moist heat, or electrical stimulation of the nerve to help with the pain.

D. Protection of the eye is very important if there is loss of lid function. Eye drops and lubricating ointment may be recommended along with taping of the eyes while sleeping.

E. Physical therapy may also be helpful.

F. Symptoms usually resolve within 3 or 4 weeks to a few months. Occasionally, patients have symptoms lasting longer than this. The degree of paralysis varies in each person.

Activity: Engage in activities as tolerated. Use caution when performing activities requiring visual demands such as depth perception (driving, walking, and so on).

Diet: Eat regular diet as tolerated.

Medications:

You Have Been Prescribed: Prednisone _____

You Need to Take: _____

You Have Been Prescribed: _____

You Need to Take: _____

You Need to Notify the Office If You Have:

A. No relief in symptoms in 4 weeks.

B. New symptoms such as headaches, visual changes, or other problems such as trouble walking.

C. Other: _____

Phone: _____

RESOURCE

The Bell's Palsy Network: http://www.bellspalsy.net/

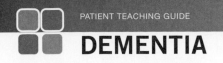

DEMENTIA

PROBLEM

Dementia is mental impairment due to a variety of disorders.

CAUSES

Dementia is caused by degeneration and loss of the gray matter from the brain; common causes are Alzheimer's disease, inadequate blood supply to the brain, alcoholism, chronic infections, inherited conditions, brain injury, or brain tumors.

PREVENTION

Early medical treatment is required for reversible causes of dementia. Prevention includes protection from head injury, eating a balanced diet, preventing alcoholism, avoiding drug abuse, and preventing atherosclerosis.

TREATMENT PLAN

A. Minimize changes in daily routines.

B. Provide simple memory reminders such as notes, calendars, and clocks.

C. Encourage social contacts.

D. Treat with respect.

E. Provide a safe environment.

    1. Remove scatter rugs.

    2. Install handrails and stairs.

    3. Discourage driving.

    4. Install stove cut-off switch.

    5. Lock closets.

    6. Lock up matches and firearms.

F. Encourage "thinking" games such as puzzles, word games, and reading.

G. Provide frequent gentle reorientation to surroundings.

Activity: Patient may engage in as much activity as possible with *supervision and direction.*

Diet: Eat a well-balanced diet low in saturated fat.

Medications: A variety of medications are available to treat symptoms.

You Have Been Prescribed: _____

You Need to Take: _____

You Need to Notify the Office If:

    A. The symptoms/behaviors are getting worse.

    B. You are unable to tolerate the medications due to side effects.

    C. You need help with social services.

    D. Other: _____

Phone: _____

RESOURCE

Alzheimers's Association: http://www.alz.org/contact_us.asp; 24/7 Helpline 1-800-272-3900

FEBRILE SEIZURES (CHILD)

PROBLEM

Convulsions or seizures may occur with an illness with a fever.

CAUSE

The cause of seizures with a febrile illness is not certain. Some families have seizures with fever that runs in the family.

CARE

A. Contact the office when your child gets sick with a fever.

1. Aspirin is not given to a child because of the risk of Reye's syndrome.

2. You may be instructed to give Tylenol or Motrin by your health care provider to help comfort your child. These medications do not prevent febrile seizures.

3. Be sure that your child gets plenty of fluids and rest.

4. You do not need to take your child's temperature on a strict schedule if he or she is not getting/feeling worse. For children ages 0 to 5 years, the rectal and oral (mouth) is *not routinely* used to measure fever.

5. Do not use the old thermometers with mercury in the glass. Use electronic/digital, infrared/tympanic, or chemical dot thermometers. The mouth, rectum, forehead (chemical dots), ears, or in the armpit are common areas for taking temperatures in children, depending on the age of your child. Always hold the thermometer while taking your child's temperature.

B. Care during a seizure:

1. Make sure that your child is breathing without difficulty.

2. Lie the child down on a safe surface and position the head to the side so that he or she does not spit up and get vomit into his or her lungs.

3. Try not to restrain your child, but protect him or her from hurting himself or herself.

4. Do not try to open his or her mouth or put your fingers in the mouth.

5. Seizures from fever generally last less than 5 minutes.

6. If the seizure lasts longer than 5 to 7 minutes, or if your child is not breathing or looks blue, call 911 for an ambulance.

7. After the seizure, your child may be sleepy. This is normal, and it's OK to let him or her rest.

Activity: When your child is not sick, there should be no restrictions on normal activity. When your child has a fever, try to keep him or her quiet and avoid strenuous play activity. Follow your child's day care/school policy about when to return after having a fever/illness.

Diet: There is no special diet for a child with a fever; a regular diet is fine. While your child has a fever, offer fluids to make sure he or she gets plenty of fluids, including formula and breast milk. I appropriate use juices or water, and if directed use Pedilyte. If your child is old enough, try Popsicles for extra fluids.

Medications: You may be directed to use Tylenol or Motrin for your child's fever. These medications do no *prevent* febrile seizures.

Your Child Has Been Prescribed: _____

Take the Medications on This Schedule: _____

You Need to Notify the Office If:

A. Your child develops seizures lasting longer than 10 minutes.

B. Your child continues to have a high fever.

C. Your child is unable to keep fluids down due to nausea, vomiting, or diarrhea.

D. Other: _____

Phone: _____

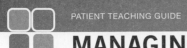

MANAGING YOUR PARKINSON'S DISEASE

PROBLEM

Parkinson's disease (PD) is a problem with the central nervous system that causes progressive muscle rigidity and tremors.

CAUSE

The brain is not able to produce or use the correct amount of dopamine required by the body, and therefore the nervous system reacts by producing the muscle rigidity and tremors.

TREATMENT/CARE

A. People with PD can be very sensitive to heat. During hot weather stay outside for very short periods of time, stay inside during the hottest part of the day, and increase your fluid intake.

B. Balance problems are common with PD and increase the risk of falls. Some ways to avoid injury are no loose rugs or other floor coverings; grab bars around the tub and toilet; a sturdy rail on stairs; adequate lighting so you can see where you are going; and straight-backed, firm chairs with arms.

C. Tremor increases the risk of accidents. Use sturdy plastic cups instead of glasses, use an electric razor to shave, and be cautious with sharp objects and power tools.

D. For clothes, Velcro fasteners, zippers, and snaps are easier to fasten than buttons. Loose clothing is also easier to put on and take off.

E. To avoid sleep problems, stay busy during the day and avoid naps. Discuss any problems you have with your neurologist; sometimes changes in your medication schedule can help.

F. If you have speech problems, work on ways to make your needs known. Practice speech exercises or consider speech therapy with a speech therapist.

G. Stay active in your daily work, hobbies, and other daily activities you enjoy.

Activity: Regular exercise helps maintain muscle flexibility and may reduce medication needs. Exercises to improve face, jaw, and tongue movement are encouraged.

Diet: Your diet should include plenty of fluids and adequate fiber to prevent or manage constipation. Have bran cereal in the morning and eat five or more servings of fruits and vegetables throughout the day. Bananas are low in fiber and should be avoided.

Plan medication schedules so you are functioning well at meal times. Be sure you allow plenty of time to finish your meal.

If you need help planning your meals, your health care provider can suggest a dietitian with whom you can talk about food choices.

Alcoholic beverages are discouraged as alcohol can interfere with the effectiveness of your medications.

If you are having difficulty with swallowing, let your provider know. Take your time with eating meals. Sit upright. Thick liquids are easier to swallow than thin liquids.

Medications:

A. The medicines you are taking can improve your ability to carry out everyday activities, but they cannot totally eliminate your symptoms. It is important that you know why you are taking each medication as well as possible side effects from each.

B. Check with your neurologist before starting any new medicine to be sure it does not interact with your PD medicines. Even vitamins can be a problem, so take only those recommended by your neurologist.

C. In case of emergency, keep with you a list of your medicines, including the amounts you take and your schedule for taking them.

You Have Been Prescribed: _____

You Need to Take: _____

You Need to Notify the Office If:

A. You have a reaction to your medication.

B. You are unable to tolerate your medication due to side effects.

C. Your symptoms become worse.

D. Other: _____

Phone: _____

RESOURCES

Parkinson's Disease Foundation: http://www.pdf.org/
National Parkinson Foundation: http://www.parkinson.org/
The Michael J. Fox Foundation for Parkinson's Research: http://www.michaeljfox.org/index.cfm

MILD HEAD INJURY

PROBLEM

Mild head injury is trauma to the head that results in no loss of consciousness or a brief loss of consciousness.

GUIDELINES FOR CARE AT HOME

Activity:

A. Remain in the company of a person to observe you for the next 24 hours.

B. Limit your physical activities, especially sports or heavy lifting.

C. Slowly increase your activities.

D. Do not drive or operate heavy machinery during the next 24 hours.

E. You may be instructed to stay off work or out of school.

F. Coaches should be aware of any head injury.

Diet: Do not eat or drink if you feel nauseated. Once the nausea resolves, you can eat or drink anything with the exception of alcohol until the observation period is over and you have returned to your normal state of health.

Medications: You should not take any medications, including those regularly taken, unless approved by your primary care provider.

INSTRUCTIONS FOR OBSERVATION AFTER HEAD INJURY

Check the patient every 2 hours for the first 24 hours after discharge. If he or she is asleep, awaken him or her for testing.

HOW TO TEST THE PATIENT

A. Test orientation: Ask the patient to tell you his or her name, where he or she is, the year, and who you are.

B. Test the patient's strength: Ask the patient to squeeze one or two of your fingers as hard as he or she can, checking both hands at the same time and compare them. Also, have the patient lift one leg at a time off the bed and hold it up for a few seconds.

C. Have the patient open both eyes at the same time and check his or her pupils to make sure they are the same size. (The pupil is the black circular part in the center of your eye.)

D. If there are any questions about the results of these tests, repeat them every 5 minutes until you are sure of the results.

WARNING SIGNS

You need to notify the office or go to the emergency room if:

A. The patient cannot be easily awakened or sleeps constantly in between tests for no apparent reason.

B. The patient cannot answer orientation questions correctly or appears to be confused.

C. The patient has weakness of arms or legs.

D. The patient becomes very restless, agitated, or has other behavior changes.

E. One pupil is larger than the other.

F. You cannot understand what the patient is saying, or the patient is having difficulty understanding what you have said.

G. The patient complains of a severe or worsening headache.

H. The patient has continued episodes of nausea or repeated vomiting.

I. The patient develops a fever over 101.4°F.

J. The patient has a convulsion or seizure, or passes out.

K. The patient has drainage of fluid from nose or ear.

If any of the above signs are present or you have any questions regarding any of the tests, please notify your primary care provider or return the patient to the emergency room or clinic as soon as possible.

Phone: _____

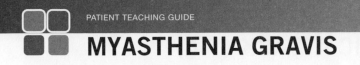

MYASTHENIA GRAVIS

PROBLEM

Myasthenia gravis, or MG, is a chronic disorder in which the body's immune system mistakenly attacks and destroys proteins that help muscles respond to nerve impulses. This causes people to have muscle weakness that is worse with use and better with rest.

Eye muscles and muscles that help with chewing, swallowing, and talking tend to be affected the most. MG can be treated but not cured.

People with myasthenia generally have to take medicine for the rest of their lives to control the disorder. Surgery to remove their thymus gland may be necessary.

TREATMENT/CARE

A. Wear a Medic Alert tag and keep a list of medicines and the dosing schedule, along with the name and telephone number of your neurologist in case of emergency.

B. Dentists and any other health care providers should know that you have MG because many medicines can make your MG worse. Some examples of medicines that can be problems for people with MG are birth control pills, some antibiotics, and some local anesthetics. There are many medicines that can be problematic, so you should *never* start a new medicine without talking to your neurologist first, even if you took it in the past without having problems.

C. Any time you feel worse, particularly if you are having trouble with chewing and swallowing, you should contact your neurologist and plan to go to the hospital, because MG could possibly affect your breathing. You should have a plan for emergencies that includes how you will get to a hospital, childcare arrangements, and how to contact your neurologist.

D. An annual flu shot is recommended because infections can make MG worse.

E. Emotional upset and stress are other things that can make MG worse. Your health care provider can supply you with information on handling stress effectively or assist in referring you to a counselor.

F. Surgery can make MG worse so it should, when possible, be planned with your neurologist. Some changes in your medication schedules in the weeks before the surgery can make problems less likely.

Activity: It is best to plan your activities to take advantage of the peak effects of your medicine and to avoid getting overtired.

Diet: A diet high in potassium-rich foods has been found by some to be helpful because low body potassium is associated with muscle weakness.

Medications:

You Have Been Prescribed: _____

You Need to Take: _____

You Need to Notify the Office If:

A. You have worsening or new symptoms.

B. You are unable to tolerate your medicines due to side effects.

C. Other: _____

Phone: _____

RESOURCES

Myasthenia Gravis Foundation of America, Inc.: http://www.myasthenia.org

You can build your own identification bracelets or neck chains from American Medical ID:
http://www.americanmedical-id.com/marketplace/build.php?buildwhat=bracelet

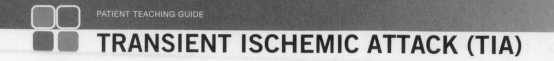

TRANSIENT ISCHEMIC ATTACK (TIA)

PROBLEM/CAUSE

A transient ischemic attack is a temporary loss of brain function due to a decrease of blood flow to the brain. It is considered a mini stroke.

RISK FACTORS FOR TIAS

A. High blood pressure

B. Irregular heart beat (atrial fibrillation)

C. Smoking

D. High cholesterol

E. Being overweight

WARNING SIGNS OF A TIA

A. Weakness or numbness of face, arm, or leg on one side of the body

B. Trouble talking or understanding others when they talk

C. Changes in eyesight such as dimness, double vision, or loss of vision

D. Dizziness, unsteadiness, or sudden falls

E. Sudden severe headaches

If you experience any of the above signs, seek medical attention (call 911) immediately.

PREVENTION/CARE

A. A full workup is necessary to decide why you are having TIAs.

B. You may be referred to a neurologist, a doctor who specializes in medical problems involving the brain.

C. Special tests may be done to evaluate your heart and blood vessels.

D. Treatment starts with modifying your own individual risk factors. Other treatment depends upon your test results.

E. Do not smoke or use any tobacco products.

F. You may be prescribed a blood thinner. Some require regular laboratory testing.

G. If you are taking a blood thinner get a Medic Alert bracelet/necklace, or carry a card in your wallet and car in case you are in an accident.

Activity: You need to exercise at least 30 minutes daily three to four times a week.

Diet: Eat a low-fat, low-cholesterol, and low-sodium diet.

Medications:

You Have Been Prescribed: _____

You Need to Take: _____

Phone: _____

Patient Teaching Guides for Chapter 19: Endocrine Disorders

- Addison's Disease
- Cushing's Syndrome
- Diabetes

ADDISON'S DISEASE

PROBLEM

Addison's disease has many symptoms, including weakness and fatigue, fainting or dizziness, poor appetite, weight loss, nausea, vomiting, diarrhea, abdominal discomfort, skin discoloration and low blood pressure, as well as cravings for salty foods.

CAUSE

Addison's is most commonly caused by your body's unusual ability to attack its own tissues, called autoimmunity. This results in inadequate amounts of cortisol and/or aldosterone produced by the adrenal glands.

TREATMENT/CARE

A. Wear your identification band stating that you have Addison's disease and that list treatment, and your health care provider's name and phone number.

B. Increased medication dosage will be required during any significant illness, especially with vomiting and/or diarrhea, before dental extractions, and before major surgical procedures. **These issues need to be discussed with your health care provider so you will know the correct dosage of medication to take.**

C. Have injectable cortisol available for emergencies when you are unconscious or otherwise unable to take pills.

Activity: As tolerated, avoid overexertion.

Diet: High-sodium, low-potassium, high-protein diet.

Medications:

You Have Been Prescribed: _____

You Need To Take: _____

You Need to Notify the Office If:

A. You have a reaction to your medications.

B. You cannot tolerate the prescribed medications.

C. You are having dental procedures or surgery to discuss adjusting your medicines.

D. You are sick with nausea and vomiting to discuss adjusting your medicines or coming into the office.

E. Other: _____

Phone:_____

RESOURCES

National Adrenal Diseases Foundation (NADF): http://www.nadf.us/

You can build your own identification bracelets or neck chains from American Medical ID:
http://www.americanmedical-id.com/marketplace/build.php?buildwhat=bracelet

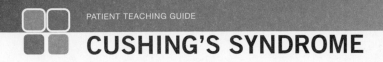

CUSHING'S SYNDROME

PROBLEM

Cushing's syndrome has many symptoms, including weight gain, obesity, moon-shaped face, excessive hair growth, easy bruising, thin skin, muscle weakness, decreased or no menstrual periods, increased blood pressure, osteoporosis, and impaired wound healing.

CAUSE

Cushing's syndrome is caused by excessive cortisol production.

TREATMENT/CARE

A. Take medications precisely as directed.

B. Avoid excessive alcohol.

C. You may be instructed to purchase a Medic Alert bracelet or necklace for any emergencies. This can be used to list your treatment and health care provider's name and phone number.

Activity: Exercise is encouraged.

Diet: Low-sodium, high-potassium, high-calcium diet.

Medications:

You Have Been Prescribed: _____

You Need to Take: _____

You Need to Notify the Office If You Have:

A. A reaction to the medications.

B. If you cannot tolerate the prescribed medicines.

C. Other _____

Phone: _____

RESOURCES

National Adrenal Diseases Foundation (NADF): http://www.nadf.us/

You can build your own identification bracelets or neck chains from American Medical ID:
http://www.americanmedical-id.com/marketplace/build.php?buildwhat=bracelet.

DIABETES

PROBLEM

You have been diagnosed as having diabetes. Diabetes does not go away, you have to manage it every day. It is a condition in which your body cannot use the glucose from food properly. Some signs that your blood sugar is too high and too low are listed here.

A. *Hyperglycemia* (high blood sugar) signs/symptoms: fruity breath odor, abnormal breathing pattern, rapid, weak pulse, confusion or stupor.

B. *Hypoglycemia* (low blood sugar) signs/symptoms: hunger, weakness, sweating, headache, shaking, rapid heartbeat, paleness, fainting, seizures or coma.

CAUSE

Your body has an organ close to the stomach called a pancreas. Your pancreas is not making enough insulin or your body is not using the insulin it is making properly.

TREATMENT/CARE

A. Lifestyle changes—exercise, stop smoking, follow your diet, and lose some weight—are necessary to control your diabetes.

1. Stop smoking. Smoking doubles your risk of developing heart or blood vessel disease.

2. Weight loss of even 5 to 10 pounds helps to control your diabetes.

3. You need to wear an identification tag that tells others you have diabetes in case of an emergency.

B. Foot care is very important.

1. Check feet every day.

2. Wash with mild soap and lukewarm water.

3. Apply lotion.

4. File or clip nails after washing and drying.

5. Do not tear skin around calluses.

6. Wear clean socks daily.

7. Wear well-fitted shoes at all times: no bare feet. You may not be able to feel or detect damage.

8. Avoid crossing your legs.

9. Take shoes off at every office visit.

C. Blood glucose monitoring: You will be instructed on how to check your blood sugar at home.

Goals of Glycemia Control

1. Fasting blood sugar: 80–120 mg/dL

2. 2-h postprandial glucose: <180 mg/dL

3. Bedtime glucose: 100–140 mg/dL

4. Hemoglobin A1c: <7%

D. For low blood sugar you need to follow the 15:15 rule:

1. After having low blood sugar you need to check your blood every 4 hours for next 24 hours.

2. 15:15 rule: choose one to follow:

   a. Take 3 glucose tabs

   b. Drink 1/2 cup orange juice

   c. Drink 1/2 cup apple juice

   d. Drink 1/3 cup grape juice

   e. Drink 6 oz of regular coke

3. If your blood sugar drops less than 59, then you need to follow the 15:15 rule, drinking juice or taking glucose tablets and then follow with 1/2 cup of milk and a starch and 1 ounce of protein.

4. **If you have severe low blood sugar you could pass out and go into a coma. You need to have Glucagon for emergencies.**

   a. Glucagon is not glucose, but helps the liver raise your blood glucose.

   b. Glucagon is prescription and is given by injection; it usually works within 15 minutes.

   c. If you do not respond with the first shot of glucagon, your family needs to call 911.

    d. A second dose of glucagon should be given by your family if you do not awaken in 15 minutes.

    e. After receiving glucagon and you respond, you need to eat a snack.

REGULAR CARE

A. You will need to come to the office at regular time to have your diabetes checked and make sure you do not have any complications. Your provider will follow national standards of care, including:

    1. Order a dilated eye examination every year.

    2. Check your blood pressure and keep it less than 130/80.

    3. Check your cholesterol at least once a year.

    4. Do a special foot examination at least once a year.

    5. Check your A1c every 3 months to see if your blood sugar is under control.

    6. Check your urine for protein/kidney problems.

    7. Give you a flu vaccine every year.

    8. If you are older, give you need a pneumonia vaccine, too.

SICK DAY RULES

You will also need a special plan in the event you are sick or have a special occasion.

A. Test blood sugar more often up to every 2 to 4 hours.

B. Increase your fluids, even if you don't feel like eating.

C. Follow a meal plan if you can.

D. Call your health care provider if your blood sugar is less than 70 or greater than 240 for two readings in a row that can't be explained; if you are unable to retain food/fluids, and spilling ketones.

E. Check your ketones if your blood sugar is greater than 240. If your ketones are negative, keep testing if your blood sugar stays up.

F. Continue to take your usual insulin dose.

G. **Do not take glucophage if you are dehydrated.**

Activity: Exercise is very important in controlling your diabetes. It not only improves blood sugar by helping your insulin to work, it reduces your risk of heart attack and stroke and helps with losing weight.

Talk with your health care provider before starting an exercise plan. If you are currently doing some form of exercise, please continue; however, avoid any strenuous exercise.

Moderate exercise (walking, cycling, and swimming) is the best exercise. Your goal will be to develop a consistent exercise activity three to four times a week for 20 to 45 minutes. Drink plenty of fluids before and after you exercise to prevent dehydration.

Exercise causes a decrease in your blood sugar for up to 24 hours. Do not exercise if your fasting blood sugar is greater than 250 or your sugar at any time is over 300. Exercise is not recommended if you have ketones (burning fat instead of sugar).

Diet:

A. You will be seeing a dietitian to develop a nutritional plan that is suited for you.

B. Consistency with meal times and amounts and food from all the six major food groups is important.

C. Even though we stress carbohydrate counting, diabetes has abnormalities in carbohydrate, fat, and protein metabolism that cause hyperglycemia.

D. Dietary control includes control of fats such as cholesterol and saturated fat to help control blood lipid levels and prevent cardiovascular disease.

E. Eat a balanced diet, eat at regular times, and try not to skip meals; eat about the same amount of food at meal/snack times.

F. Use portion control, decrease the fats that you eat, and decrease fast simple sugars.

G. Decrease your alcohol consumption.

Medications:

A. You may need a combination of medications or insulin to help control your blood sugar to prevent complications.

B. If you use insulin injections or the insulin pump, the best place to give it is your stomach.

C. The American Diabetes Association recommends that you take an ACE inhibitor (blood pressure medicine) to help protect your kidneys.

D. You may be told to take an aspirin every day (if you are not allergic).

You Have Been Prescribed: _____

You Need to Take: _____

You Have Been Prescribed: _____

You Need to Take: _____

You Have Been Prescribed: _____

You Need to Take: _____

You Need to Notify the Office If:

    A. You are sick and unable to keep foods/fluids down (vomiting) or have severe diarrhea.

    B. You intend to take over-the-counter medications, because they could react with your diabetes medication.

    C. You are using Metformin (glucophage) and are going to have X-rays using any dyes. You must stop your medicine.

Phone: _____

Remember to carry ID and carbohydrate source. Glucagon should be available for severe low blood glucose due to risk of aspiration and/or inability to swallow.

RESOURCES

American Diabetes Association (ADA): http://www.diabetes.org/

You can build your own identification bracelets or neck chains from American Medical ID: http://www.americanmedical-id.com/marketplace/build.php?buildwhat=bracelet.

Patient Teaching Guides for Chapter 20: Psychiatric Disorders

- Alcohol and Drug Dependence

- Coping Strategies for Teens and Adults With ADHD

- Tips for Caregivers: Living (Enjoyably) With a Child Who Has ADHD

- Grief/Bereavement

- Sleep Disorders/Insomnia

ALCOHOL AND DRUG DEPENDENCE

PROBLEM

Dependence on alcohol or drugs is a disease with signs and symptoms and a progressive course that requires treatment, just like diabetes or cancer.

CAUSES

Factors that contribute to dependence on alcohol and drugs may include inherited traits, the environment, occupation, socioeconomic status, family and upbringing, personality, life stress, and emotional stress. These factors vary among individuals, but no one factor can account entirely for the risk.

PREVENTION

The only way to prevent alcohol and/or drug abuse and dependence is not to start. Warning signs for needing help are not always dramatic. The following questions can help identify dependence.

A. **Are you or someone you know experiencing any of the following:**

1. Steadily drinking or using more at a time or more often?
2. Setting limits on how much, how often, when, or where you will drink or use other drugs and repeatedly violating your limits?
3. Keeping a large supply on hand or becoming concerned when you run low?
4. Drinking or using other drugs before going to activities where they won't be available (e.g., class or work)?
5. Drinking or using other drugs alone? Drinking or using other drugs every day?
6. Spending more money than you can afford on alcohol or other drugs?
7. Doing or saying things when you're under the influence that you regret later, or don't remember?
8. Lying to friends and family about your drinking or other drug use?
9. Becoming accident prone when you're under the influence (spilling, dropping, or breaking things)?
10. Regularly hung over the morning after drinking?
11. Worrying about your drinking or other drug use?
12. Having work or school problems, such as tardiness or absenteeism?
13. Reducing contact with friends, or experiencing increasing problems with important relationships?

B. **If you answered, "yes" to any of these questions, it suggests your drinking or drug use may be a problem.**

TREATMENT PLAN

A. There are no "quick cures" for alcohol and drug dependence, but early intervention is of utmost importance because it helps avoid the harmful affects of long-term alcohol or other drug use.

B. Your health care provider will be suggesting a plan of action for you to consider. You are strongly encouraged to follow the recommendations.

C. Don't hang around your drinking/drug-using friends. Instead, go to new areas, play new sports, and develop new hobbies.

D. Talk to your provider about seeking professional rehab treatment.

E. Ask about a support group in your area.

Activity: Daily exercise is helpful in alleviating the craving for alcohol and drugs. Walking daily and increasing your tolerance for distance is recommended.

Diet:

A. Avoid caffeine and nicotine, if possible.

B. Try to eat three meals a day and three snacks.

C. You may be given vitamin supplements to help restore the vitamins and minerals that have been depleted as a result of your alcohol or drug dependence.

Medications: Usually, medications are not prescribed because they may make the problem worse. If you are prescribed any medications, take them exactly as directed by your health care provider.

You Have Been Prescribed the Following: _____

Vitamins/Minerals: _____

You Need to Take Them: _____

You Need to Notify the Office If You Have:

    A. Severe craving and the urge to use alcohol or drugs.

    B. Any thoughts of hurting yourself or others.

    C. Impulsive feelings, like you might do something you will later regret.

Phone: _____

RESOURCES

Al-Anon Family: 888-4AL-ANON and http://www.al-anon.alateen.org/

American Council for Drug Education: 800-488-3784

Alcohol Help Line 24 hours a day, 7 days a week: 800-345-3552 and www.adcare.com

Cocaine Anonymous: 800-347-8998 and www.cawso.org

Cocaine Hotline 24 hours a day, 7 days a week 800-262-2463 and www.acde.org

Families Anonymous: 800-736-9805 and familiesanonymous.org

New Life (Women for Sobriety): 800-333-1606

Mothers Against Drunk Driving (MADD) 24 hours a day, 7 days a week 800-438-6233

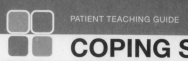

COPING STRATEGIES FOR TEENS AND ADULTS WITH ADHD

A. Clarify all assignments and tasks.

B. Keep simple lists of your chores for the day.

C. Attach reminder notes to logical items, for example, put a self-adhesive note on your bathroom mirror to remind yourself to do something.

D. Organize your things in a logical way. For example, put your medication bottle with your toothbrush so you will be sure to take it in the morning.

E. Establish a daily routine and stick to it.

F. Keep your environment as quiet and peaceful as possible. Seek out work and study sites that are quiet and peaceful.

G. Be good to yourself: eat well, get enough rest, and exercise.

RESOURCES FOR ADD

Children and Adults with Attention Deficit Hyperactivity Disorder (CHADD): www.chadd.org

The National Attention Deficit Disorder Association: www.add.org

National Resource Center for ADHD: www.help4adhd.org

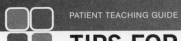

TIPS FOR CAREGIVERS: LIVING (ENJOYABLY) WITH A CHILD WHO HAS ADHD

A. A child with ADHD may not respond to your direction and discipline as easily as other children. Here are a few ways you can organize your home and your child to try to help him or her.

1. Accept your child's limitations. Understand that his or her activity and inattention are intrinsic. Be as tolerant, low-key, and patient as you can possibly be.

2. Provide an outlet for the release of excess energy, such as active games, especially outdoors or in open spaces.

3. Keep your home well organized. Have routines for the usual activities for the day. This will help your child to anticipate activities. Eliminate extraneous noise and clutter, such as having the TV on or piling your kitchen table high with newspapers.

4. Be sure your child gets plenty of rest and good nutrition.

5. Avoid formal gatherings or other places where you and your child will have added stress to behave well.

6. Establish discipline that is firm, reliable, and nonphysical.

7. Stretch your child's attention span by quietly and regularly reading to or playing with him or her. Praise whenever possible.

8. Medications may be very helpful. *Often* they will allow your child to attend to his or her schoolwork, and school performance and experience may be much improved.

9. Be active with your child's school. *You* are his or her most interested advocate.

10. Make sure that his or her school placement and program are appropriate. Enlist the support of the school nurse, school psychologist, or principal if needed.

11. Most important, enjoy your child as much as possible. Try to take breaks whenever possible.

GRIEF/BEREAVEMENT

PROBLEM

Normal grief resolution may take as long as 2 years.

CAUSES

Grief can follow the death of a loved one, but grief also follows other losses such as a loss of independence, loss of affection, or loss of body parts after an accident.

TREATMENT PLAN

It is important that you talk about your loss, and how it affects you. The more you are able to talk about your feelings related to the loss you are experiencing, the more you will be able to work through your feelings.

You may be encouraged to seek supportive therapy in the form of divorce groups, loss groups, or groups dealing specifically with death and dying.

Activity: Moderate exercise such as daily walking is encouraged. Vigorous, prolonged exercise, however, may precipitate anxiety attacks.

Diet: Avoid caffeinated beverages, including coffee, tea, and carbonated colas that do not specify "decaffeinated." Try to eat healthy food and avoid overeating or skipping meals.

Medications: Medications for loss and grief are usually avoided at first because the use of drugs can prolong the time it takes to work through your grief. However, your health care provider will discuss medications in more depth.

You Have Been Prescribed: _____

You Need to Take It: _____

Do not stop antidepressants quickly. Talk to your health care provider if you want to discontinue them.

You Need to Notify the Office If:

   A. You feel like you can't stop crying.

   B. You are not eating and are losing weight.

   C. You feel like you have no one to turn to and talk about your feelings.

   D. You have difficulty sleeping after several weeks.

   E. You have thoughts of hurting yourself or others.

   F. You don't think you are getting better on the prescribed medication.

Phone: _____

Local Support Group: _____

SUGGESTED BOOKS

Empty Arms: Coping With Miscarriage, Stillbirth, and Infant Death by Sherokee Ilse (Wintergreen Press, Inc. 2008).
A Child Dies: A Portrait of Family Grief, 2nd ed., by Joan Hagan, Arnold and Penelope B. Gemma (Charles Press, 1994).
The Anguish of Loss by Julie Fritsch and Sherokee Ilse (Wintergreen Press, 1992).
Empty Chair: Handling Grief on Holidays and Special Occasions by Susan Zonnebelt-Smeenge and Robert C. De Vries (Baker Books, 2001).
A Decembered Grief: Living with Loss while Others are Celebrating by Harold Ivan Smith (Beacon Hill Press of Kansas City, 1999).

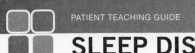
SLEEP DISORDERS/INSOMNIA

PROBLEM

Continued loss of sleep over a long period of time (several days to weeks) can produce a decrease in daytime awareness and functioning, as well as work impairment.

CAUSE

Most sleep difficulties are related to situational problems and are best treated without medications. **Medical illness may also predispose you to a sleeping disorder.**

PREVENTION

A. Practice good "sleep hygiene." Here are a few tips:

   1. Try to get to bed at the same time every night (even on weekends).
   2. Plan for 8 hours of sleep.
   3. Maintain the same waking time every morning (even on weekends).
   4. Reserve the bedroom for sleeping. Do not do your work/homework in the bed. Do not watch TV in the bedroom, unless you sit in a chair. Do not read in bed.
   5. Put your children in their own bed/bedroom.
   6. Try a small bedtime snack.
   7. Do not drink any liquids for at least 1 hour before going to bed. This helps prevent getting up to go to the bathroom during the night.
   8. Review all of your prescription medications and over-the-counter drugs with your health care provider to evaluate if the drugs are making you stay awake.
   9. Avoid alcohol and tobacco.

TREATMENT PLAN

A. Develop a "sleeping ritual": wear you favorite pajamas and use your favorite pillows.
B. Keep the room dark and quiet. Try not to use a nightlight.
C. Run a small fan for background noise.
D. Arise promptly in the morning.
E. Avoid sleeping medication if possible.
F. Try some relaxation exercises, like yoga, self-hypnosis, or meditation. There are many books on these subjects that will assist you in developing good sleep hygiene. (Try your local library or bookstore.)

Activity: Regular exercise during the day helps. (Do not exercise vigorously 1 hour before your bedtime—this could keep you awake.)

Relaxation techniques such as progressive relaxation, biofeedback, self-hypnosis, and meditation are helpful when done before bedtime. Avoid vigorous mental activities late in the evening.

Diet:

A. Avoid caffeinated drinks including coffee, tea, and soda.
B. Avoid large meals in the evening.
C. Eat a nutritious balanced diet.
D. Limit your liquids to early evening. Do not drink water after 8 PM.

Medications: Discuss the need for medications to help your sleep.

You Have Been Prescribed: _____

You Need to Take It: _____

You Need to Notify the Office If You Have:

   A. No relief in your symptoms, and you are following the above recommendations.
   B. No relief in your symptoms, and you are taking your medications as directed.
   C. Feelings of depression or thoughts of hurting yourself or others.
   D. Noticeable physical symptoms that were not mentioned in your office visit, or any new symptoms that you are concerned about.

Phone: _____

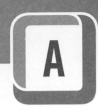

Normal Laboratory Values

Normal laboratory values are presented here. However, laboratory values reference ranges differ from laboratory to laboratory. Values differ because of age and gender. Different values presented; all normal values are listed under the Females column. Male and children values are the same unless otherwise noted. Legend: 10^6 = 1,000,000, 10^3 = 1,000.

Normal Laboratory Values

	FEMALES	MALES	CHILDREN
Complete Blood Count			
Red Blood Cells (RBC)	3.5–5.0 10^6/µL	4.3–5.9 10^6/µL	3.5–5.0 10^6/µL
Hemoglobin (Hgb) ↑ Polycythemia, dehydration, ↓ blood loss, severe anemia, low production or death of blood cell	12–16 g/dL	13.6–18 g/dL	10–14 g/dL Newborn 15–25 g/dL
Hematocrit (Hct) ↓ anemia, massive blood loss ↑ dehydration or hemoconcentration with shock	37%–47%	40%–54%	30%–42%
Mean Corpuscular Volume (MCV) RBC size: normocytic, microcytic, macrocytic	76–100 fL		
Mean Corpuscular Hemoglobin (MCH) RBC color: normochromic, hypochromic	27–33 pg		
Mean Corpuscular Hemoglobin Concentration (MCHC)	33–37 g/dL or %		
Reticulocyte Count Measures the number of new RBCs produced by the bone marrow	33–137 x 10/uL		
White Blood Cells (WBC) ↑ bacterial infections, infectious diseases (mononucleosis), ↓ stress, tissue death, leukemia, cancer, hemorrhage	4.0–11.0 million/mm	3.8–11.0 10^3/mm³	5.0–10.0 10^3/mm³
Differential: Segmented Neutrophils ↑ stress, trauma, inflammatory disorders, ↓ viral infections, severe bacterial infections, aplastic anemia	54%–62%		
Band Neutrophils	3%–5%		
Lymphocytes ↑ chronic bacterial infection, viral infections, ↓ leukemia, AIDS, Lupus erythematosus	20%–40%		
Monocytes ↑ chronic inflammatory disorders, viral infections, chronic conditions, ↓ steroid therapy	0%–7%		
Eosinophils ↑ allergies, parasite infections, leukemia	1%–3%		

Normal Laboratory Values (*continued*)

	FEMALES	MALES	CHILDREN
Basophils ↑ leukemia ↓ allergic reactions, stress, hyperthyroidism	0%–0.75%		

Platelets
↓ thrombocytopenia, acute leukemia/aplastic anemia
   during chemotherapy, interferon, infections and
   drug reactions
↑ myeloproliferatve disease, cancer, and RA
	150,000–400,000/
	mm		

Serum Iron concentration of iron bound to transferrin	60–160 µg/dL	80–180 µg/dL	
Total Iron Binding Capacity (TIBC) Amount of iron transferrin can bind	250–460 µg/dL		
Erythrocyte Sedimentation Rate (ESR) ↑ pregnancy, inflammatory conditions, ↓ sickle cell anemia	Women < 50 < 20 mm/h Women > 50 < 30 mm/h	Males < 50 < 15 mm/h Males > 50 < 20 mm/h	

BUN/Creatinine-Renal function tests

	FEMALES	MALES
Blood Urea Nitrogen (BUN)	8–22 mg/dL	
Creatinine: (Cr)	0.6–1.5 mg/dL	
Creatine	0.6–1.0 mg/dL	0.2–0.6 mg/dL
Uric Acid	2.5–6.6 mg/dL	3.5–7.7 mg/dL

Thyroid Studies

	FEMALES
Thyroid Stimulating Hormone (TSH) ↑ hypothyroidism, ↓ hyperthyroidism	2.0–10.5 µ/mL
T3 ↑ pregnancy & oral contraceptive use	0.8–1.1 µ/dL
Thyroxine (T4) ↑ hyperthyroidism, ↓ hypothyroidism	4.5–12.5 µ/dL

Aminotransferases

	FEMALES	MALES
↑ liver damage & medications	4–35 U/L	7–46 U/L
ALT	8–20 U/L	10–20 U/L
AST		

Bilirubin (measures bile salt conjugation and excretion) 0.1–1.0 mg/dL
3.0 mg/dL indicates
hepatic disease,
jaundice is visible

Glucose
Fasting 65–110 mg/dL
2 hour postprandial 65–140 mg/dL

Serum Albumin (measures protein synthesis)
4.0–6.0 g/dL
↑ Dehydration, inflammatory illness, liver insufficiency, malnutrition, and cancer

Lipid Profile
Fasting Cholesterol: < 200 mg/dL:
   200 – 239 mg/dL: borderline CHD
   > 240 mg/dL: high risk for CHD
Triglycerides: 30–175 mg/dL
HDL: > 45 mg/dL, desirable levels higher than 50 mg/dL
LDL: < 130 mg/dL
   130–159 mg/dL: borderline CHD
   > 160 mg/dL: high risk for CHD

Sickle Cell Disease
HgbS: normal, none present
Homozygous HgbS: sickle cell disease
Heterozygous HgbS: sickle cell trait
Hemoglobin electrophoresis: determines hemoglobin types and percentages

Hepatitis B
Hepatitis B Surface Antigen: negative
Positive: acute or chronic infection, further liver function tests needed
Hepatitis B Surface Antibody: Positive indicates immunity to infection (previous infection or HBV vaccine)

PSA (males)
0–4.0 mg/mL normal

Serum Alkaline Phosphatase (ALP) (marks liver disease)
30–120 IU/L
Pregnancy value 30–200 IU/L
↑ bile stones, biliary and pancreatic CA, viral hepatitis, cirrhosis, Paget's disease, osteomalacia, bone metastasis

Urinalysis
Color: pale yellow/straw to amber
Clarity: Clear
Specific gravity: 1.001–1.035
pH: normal 4.6–8.0 (acidic)
Glucose: absent
Ketones: absent
Protein: negative

Urine Dipstick U/A
Nitrites: negative (positive = bacteria, infection)
Leukocytes Oxidase: negative (positive = WBCs)

HIV
ELISA: negative
ELISA: positive: repeat, if second ELISA postive perform Western blot
Western blot negative: no evidence of HIV
Western blot positive: evidence of HIV

Rubella
Titer: > 1:10 Immune
Titer: < 1:8 Nonimmune administer Rubella vaccine

Female Hormone Levels

	FSH	*LH*	*Progesterone*	*Prolactin*
Follicular phase:	2–25 mIU/mL	5–30 mIU/mL	0.2–6.0 mIU/mL	< 23 ng/mL
Midcycle phase:	10–90 mIU/mL	75–150 mIU/mL	6–30 mIU/mL	< 28 ng/mL
Luteal phase:	2–25 mIU/mL	3–40 mIU/mL	5.7–28.1 mIU/mL	5–40 ng/mL
Postmenopausal:	40–350 mIU/mL	30–200 mIU/mL	0–0.2 mIU/mL	< 12 ng/mL

Diet Recommendations

Cheryl A. Glass

You have been prescribed a bland diet. This diet provides adequate nutrition along with the treatment of gastrointestinal problems, such as ulcerative conditions or inflammatory problems of the stomach and intestines. It is intended to decrease irritation in the lining of the stomach and intestines.

Food Tips

Foods to Avoid

Garlic, onions, alcohol, fatty foods, fried foods, chocolate, cocoa, coffee (even decaffeinated), dried fruits, citrus fruit and juices (orange, pineapple, and grapefruit), tomato products, peppermint, whole grain breads and cereals, pre-spiced foods such as processed lunch meats and ham, pepper, and chili powder. Avoid pepper, chili powder, and cocoa spices.

General Instructions

A. Eat at least 3 small meals a day.
B. Avoid alcohol and beer.
C. Avoid caffeinated drinks/colas.
D. Avoid fried, greasy foods; bake or broil your foods.
E. Trim the fat from meats before cooking.
F. Bake, broil, mash, or cream potatoes.
G. Avoid raw fruits and vegetables such as corn on the cob and other gas-forming vegetables such as cabbage, dried beans, and peas.
H. Avoid rich desserts.
I. Avoid bedtime snacks—they may increase acid production and cause discomfort at night.
J. Ask your health care provider if nutritional supplements are necessary.

Approved Foods by Food Group

A. Dairy Products
  1. Whole milk
  2. Low fat or 2% milk
  3. Skim milk
  4. Evaporated milk
  5. Buttermilk
  6. Cottage cheese
  7. Yogurt
  8. Cheese

B. Meat
  1. Beef
  2. Veal
  3. Fresh pork
  4. Turkey
  5. Chicken
  6. Fish (canned or fresh)
  7. Liver
  8. Egg (as a meat substitute)

C. Breads/Grains
  1. Enriched breads (plain toast)
  2. Oats
  3. Cereal
  4. Tortillas
  5. English muffins
  6. Saltine crackers
  7. Pasta (all types)

D. Fruits/Vegetables
  1. All vegetables
  2. All fruits and juices (except citrus)

E. Desserts
  1. Custard
  2. Pudding
  3. Sherbet
  4. Ice cream (except peppermint and chocolate)
  5. Gelatin
  6. Angel food cake
  7. Pound cake
  8. Sugar cookies
  9. Jams and jellies
  10. Honey

F. Drinks
  1. Decaffeinated tea
  2. Juices (except citrus)
  3. Caffeine-free sodas

G. Spices
  1. Salt
  2. Thyme
  3. Sage
  4. Cinnamon
  5. Paprika
  6. Apple cider vinegar
  7. Prepared mustard
  8. Lemon and lime juices

DASH DIET: DIETARY APPROACHES TO STOP HYPERTENSION

The Dietary Approaches to Stop Hypertension (DASH) diet is based on a combination of different types of foods and is recommended to help control high blood pressure. It is a food plan that is based foods that are low in cholesterol and high in dietary fiber, potassium, calcium, and magnesium; it is moderately high in protein. DASH eating has a reduction in lean red meats, added sugar, and sugar-containing sodas. The DASH diet's dairy food portions make the diet high in calcium and vitamin D. Overall, Americans, especially African Americans, are deficient in vitamin D.

The DASH diet along with weight loss and exercise are used control other health problems such as, type 2 diabetes and heart disease. If your ethnic background is Hawaiian, American Indian, Eskimo, Hispanic, or African American, you are at higher risk for high blood pressure. Following a DASH eating plan also will help in lowering the bad cholesterol, or LDL, which can reduce heart disease.

A major way the DASH diet helps lower blood pressure is to limit the amount of salt (sodium). The recommendations are limiting sodium to 1,100 to 3,000 mg a day or less. If you have high blood pressure you may be limited to 1,500 mg or less a day. **One teaspoon of salt contains 2,000 mg of sodium.**

Foods high in sodium make you retain extra fluid. If you notice that your hands are swelling (rings are tight) or your feet and legs swell (sock rings or shoes feel tight) you are getting too much salt. Fluid retention is bad if you have heart failure. This diet is rich in potassium, which can help you get rid of the extra sodium and decrease the fluid retention.

Sea salt, even though it may contain less sodium, is not low enough in sodium to use as a substitute for regular salt. Salt substitutes contain potassium chloride; this can cause more fluid retention. Potassium chloride salt substitutes may also interfere with your blood pressure medications, so check with your health care provider before using them.

Tips for Reducing Sodium

A. Slowly cut back on your salty foods and begin to use healthier products. Take the salt shaker off the table.
B. Eat fresh foods.
  1. Avoid prepackaged foods.
  2. Eat fresh vegetables instead of canned vegetables. If you use canned vegetables choose the low sodium option and/or rinse the vegetables.
C. Read food labels.
  1. Sodium is in almost all processed foods, including milk.
  2. **Focus on the amount of sodium *per food serving.***
  3. Don't forget to read labels on soda and sports drink bottles.
  4. Choose your favorite food brand with low salt or low-sodium labels on the package instead of the same product with more salt.

D. Avoid salty snacks and foods, including:
  1. Crackers, chips, and pretzels
  2. Cheeses
  3. Olives, pickles, pickled okra, and other foods
  4. Processed foods, including jerky, hot dogs, bacon, deli meats, canned fish, and canned meats, which contain a large amount of sodium.
E. Limit using soy sauce, seasoned salts, and meat tenderizers.
F. Many seasonings, including ketchup and sauces, contain a lot of sodium. Substitute with other flavors such as fresh herbs (e.g., rosemary, thyme, oregano, cilantro, and basil). Use garlic powder, lemon and lime juice, crushed red peppers, as well as ginger.
G. Try making your own salt-free herb blend to use on your foods. Ingredients that can add flavor without adding salt include:
  1. Peppers such as cayenne, black pepper, and lemon pepper
  2. Dried herbs such as thyme
  3. Garlic powder
  4. Paprika
  5. Celery seed
H. Helpful websites for salt-free herb blend, products, and recipes are:
  1. Salt-Free season recipes:
    a. http://busycooks.about.com/od/homemade mixes/r/nosaltmix.htm
    b. http://www.tasteofhome.com/Recipes/Salt-Free-Seasoning-Mix
  2. Web sites with low-salt recipes:
    a. http://homecooking.about.com/library/archive/blhelp13.htm
    b. McCormick: http://www.mccormick.com/
    c. Mrs. Dash: http://www.mrsdash.com/

Tips on Eating the DASH Way

A. Start small. Make gradual changes in your eating habits, such as eating smaller portions.
B. Center your meal around carbohydrates, such as pasta, rice, beans, or vegetables.
C. Treat meat as only part of a whole meal instead of the main focus of the meal.
D. Use fruits or low-fat, low-calorie foods such as sugar-free gelatin for desserts and snacks.
E. Choose "whole" grains in breads and cereals.
F. Choose to eat vegetables without butter or sauce.
G. Choose lean cuts of meat. Use fresh poultry, for example, skinless turkey and chicken.
H. Choose ready-to-eat breakfast cereals that are lower in sodium.
I. Eat fruits for dessert. Use fruits that are canned in their own juice.

J. Add fruit to plain yogurt.
K. To increase vegetables have stir-fry with 2 ounces of chicken and use 1½ cups of raw vegetables.
L. Snack on vegetables, bread sticks, graham crackers, or unbuttered/unsalted popcorn.
M. Drink water or club soda.

RESOURCES

DASH for Health http://www.dashforhealth.com/index.php

DASH diet recipes http://www.mayoclinic.com/health/dash-diet-recipes/RE00089

The DASH Diet Eating Plan http://dashdiet.org/dash_diet_recipes.asp

TABLE B.1 Serving Portion Sizes

Food	Portion Size	Food	Portion Size
1 baked potato 1 cup of flaked cereal	Fist	½ cup of fresh fruit (½ of baseball) ½ cup of pasta, rice or potato (½ of baseball) ½ cup of ice cream	Baseball
1½ ounces cheese (4 dice) 1 tsp of margarine (1 dice)	Dice		
¼ cup of raisins	Egg	3 ounces of meat, includes fish, meat and chicken	Deck of cards
¼ cup almonds	Golf ball	1 pancake	Compact disc (CD)
2 tbsp peanut butter	Ping Pong ball	1 piece of cornbread	Bar of soap
1 cup of salad 1 cup of popcorn (unbuttered)	Baseball	3 ounces of grilled or backed fish	Checkbook

Adapted from the 2010 NHLBI Portion Distortion.

TABLE B.2 DASH Diet Daily Servings

Food Group	Daily Servings	Serving Sizes	Examples and Notes	Significance of Each Food Group to the DASH Diet Pattern
Grains and grain product	6–8	1 slice bread ½ C dry cereal ½ C cooked rice, pasta, or cereal	Whole wheat bread, English muffin, pita bread, bagel, cereals, grits, oatmeal, couscous	Major sources of energy and fiber
Vegetables	4–5	1 C raw leafy vegetables ½ C cooked vegetables 6 oz vegetable juice	Tomatoes, potatoes, carrots, peas, squash, broccoli, turnip greens, collards, kale, spinach, artichokes, beans, sweet potatoes	Rich sources of potassium, magnesium, and fiber
Fruits	4–5	6 oz fruit juice 1 medium fruit ¼ C dried fruit ¼ C fresh, frozen, or canned fruit	Apricots, bananas, dates, grapes, oranges, orange juice, grapefruit, grapefruit juice, mangoes, melons, peaches, pineapples, prunes, raisins, strawberries, tangerines	Important sources of potassium, magnesium, and fiber
Low-fat or fat-free milk and dairy foods	2–3	1 C milk 1 C yogurt 1.5 oz cheese	Skim or 1% milk, skim or low-fat buttermilk, non-fat or low-fat yogurt, part-skim mozzarella cheese, non-fat cheese	Major sources of calcium and protein
Lean meats, poultry and fish	6 or less	1oz cooked meats, poultry, or fish 1 egg	Select only lean; trim away visible fat; broil, roast or boil instead of frying. Remove skin from poultry	Rich sources of protein and magnesium
Nuts, seeds, and legumes	4–5 per week	⅓ C or 1⅓ oz of nuts ½ oz or 2 Tbsp seeds 2 Tbsp of peanut butter ½ C cooked legumes	Almonds, filberts, mixed nuts, peanuts, walnuts, sunflower seeds, kidney beans, lentils	Rich sources of energy, magnesium, potassium, protein, and fiber
Sweets and added sugars	5 or less per week	1 Tbsp sugar 1 Tbsp jelly or jam ½ C sorbet or gelatin 1 C lemonade	Fruit-flavored gelatin, fruit punch, hard candy, jelly, maple syrup, sugar	Sweets should be low in fat

Adapted from the NHLBI DASH Diet Eating Plan.

TABLE B.3 Total Number of Servings in 2000 Calories/Day

Food Group	Servings
Grains	7–8
Vegetables	5
Fruits	5
Fat-free or low-fat milk and dairy foods	3
Lean meats, poultry, and fish	2
Nuts, seeds, and legumes	1
Fats and oils	2.5
Sweets and added sugars	1

TABLE B.4 DASH Example Menu (2000 calorie)

Food	Amount	Servings Provided
Breakfast		
Orange juice	6 oz	1 fruit
1% low-fat milk	8 oz (1 C)	1 dairy
Corn flakes (with 1 tsp sugar)	1 C	2 grains
Banana	1 medium	1 fruit
Whole wheat bread (with 1 Tbsp jelly)	1 slice	1 grain
Soft margarine	1 tsp	1 fat
Lunch		
Chicken salad	¾ C	1 poultry
Pita bread	½ large	1 grain
Raw vegetable medley:		
Carrot and celery sticks	3–4 sticks each	
Radishes	2	1 vegetable
Loose-leaf lettuce	2 leaves	
Part-skim mozzarella cheese	1.5 slice (1.5 oz)	1 dairy
1% low-fat milk	8 oz (1 C)	1 dairy
Fruit cocktail in light syrup	½ C	1 fruit
Dinner		
Herbed baked cod	3 oz	1 fish
Scallion rice	1 C	2 grains
Steamed broccoli	½ C	1 vegetable
Stewed tomatoes	½ C	1 vegetable
Spinach salad:		
Raw spinach	½ C	
Cherry tomatoes	2	1 vegetable
Cucumber	2 slices	
Light Italian salad dressing	1 Tbsp	½ fat
Whole wheat dinner roll	1 small	1 grain
Soft margarine	1 tsp	1 fat
Melon balls	½ C	1 fruit
Snacks		
Dried apricots	1 oz (¼ C)	1 fruit
Mini-pretzels	1 oz (¾ C)	1 grain
Mixed nuts	1.5 oz (½ C)	1 nuts
Diet ginger ale	12 oz	0

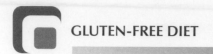

Gluten-Free Diet Tips

The symptoms from celiac disease are triggered from glutens in your diet. Three cereals that contain gluten are: wheat, rye, and barley. Glutens are also in other products, such as food additives, so it is **very important to read all the ingredients on food labels** (see Table).

Dietary Recommendation for Celiac Disease

A. You may also be told to follow a lactose-free diet for a short time to help your symptoms.
B. Most bread sold in the grocery aisle is not allowed on a gluten-free eating plan.
C. All vegetables and fruits are gluten-free. However, frozen and canned fruits and vegetables may contain an additive with gluten.
D. Although you should not enjoy beer, wine is still on the menu when you go to dinner.
E. Specialty bakeries are able to make gluten-free cakes for special occasions. Plain hard candy, marshmallows, and other candies are usually gluten-free.
F. Caution should be taken when ordering any breaded foods such as chicken nuggets or breaded fish.
G. Deli meats may also contain gluten.

RESOURCES

Celiac Disease Foundation: www.celiac.org
www.celiac.com
www.chex.com/glutenfree
www.BettyCrocker.com/glutenfree
http://www.celiacdisease.net/gluten-free-diet
Gluten-Free Recipes: http://allrecipes.com/Recipes/Healthy-Cooking/Gluten-Free/Main.aspx

---

TABLE B.5 Examples of Foods That Are Avoided on a Gluten-Free Diet

Allowed	Avoid
Fresh fruits and vegetables without any processing or additives	Wheat, wheat berry, wheat bran, wheat germ, wheat grass, whole wheat berries
Meat	Flours, bread flour
Soy, soybean, tofu	Bulgur (bulgur wheat, bulgur nuts)
Brown rice	Rye
Enriched rice/instant rice/wild rice	Barley
Buckwheat	Barley malt/barley extract
Millet	Oats, oat bran, oat fiber
Sorghum	Cereals
Alfalfa	Matzo
Almond	Beer, ale, porter, stout
Canola	Farina
Chickpea	Croutons
Corn, corn flour, cornmeal	Bran
Brown rice flour	Tabbouleh
Tapioca	Soy Sauce

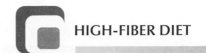

Fiber is a plant cell-wall component that is not broken down by the digestive system. An old term for fibers is *roughage* because it absorbs fluid and moves waste faster through the intestines in a bulky mass. The Food and Drug Administration defines as high-fiber those products that contain 20% of the daily fiber value. High-fiber diets are used to help prevent constipation as well as diarrhea. Fiber has been used to help several medical conditions such as diabetes, diverticulosis, irritable bowel syndrome (IBS), high cholesterol, as well as weight loss. If you have a chronic health condition, check with your health care provider about starting any new dietary change.

Fiber provides a full feeling that can help with spacing meals further apart (3–4 hours). Fiber recommendations change with your age (see Table B.6).

Tips for Increasing Fiber in Your Diet

A. Read the Nutrition Facts food labels for fiber content per food serving.
   1. Cereals that provide 5 grams of fiber per serving give you 20% of your daily fiber.
   2. Look for "whole grain" on the label. Just because bread is brown does not mean it is whole grain.
B. Increase fiber in your diet gradually to prevent gas. Adding too much fiber too quickly may give you abdominal pain, bloating, and constipation. Increase you fiber over several weeks so that it gives time for you to adjust.
C. As you increase fiber, it is also important to increase the amount of fluids your drink up to 6–8 glasses a day, including tea, milk, fruit juices, coffee, and even soft drinks. The extra fluids that you drink along with the extra fiber makes you feel more full, which can help control snacking.
D. Keep a food diary and review it periodically to decide of other diet adjustments need to be made.
E. Several fiber supplements are available over the counter to help you get your daily recommendation of fiber.

Good Food Sources of Fiber

A. Bran: Add 1 teaspoon of whole-grain bran to food 3 times a day, or take an over-the-counter fiber supplement such as psyllium (Metamucil), as directed.
B. Whole-grain cereals and breads: Eat oat, bran, multigrain, light, wheat, or rye breads rather than pure white bread or breads that list eggs as a major ingredient. Grains are not only a good source of fiber but also contain vitamins and minerals. Folic acid has been added to breads and cereals to help reduce neural tube defects.
C. Fresh or frozen fruits and vegetables: Citrus fruits are especially good sources of fiber. Eat raw or minimally cooked vegetables, especially squash, cabbage, lettuce other greens, and beans. Leave the skins on fruits and vegetables; eating the whole fruit is better than drinking the juice. Whole tomatoes offer more fiber than peeling the skin off. The more colorful the fruit and vegetable (dark green, reds, blue, yellow) the better; they provide a good source of antioxidants that are good for the heart and the prevention of some cancers. Apples are a good source of both fiber and water.
D. Legumes (pods): Peas and beans are a good source of fiber. Add chickpeas and kidney beans to salads for extra fiber and flavor. Add baked beans as a delicious side item to your meal.
E. Coffee is another source of fiber.
F. Nuts are an excellent source of fiber. They are considered nutrient-dense and are a good source of vitamins and folic acid. Sprinkle sunflower seeds on a salad to add flavor and fiber. The amount of nuts eaten should be to be limited to 1 to 2 ounces because they are also high in calories.
G. If you have diverticulosis: Avoid foods with seeds or indigestible material that may block the neck of a diverticulum, such as nuts, corn, popcorn, cucumbers, tomatoes, figs, strawberries, and caraway seeds.

TABLE B.6	Fiber Recommendations by Age	
Group/Gender	**Age**	**Fiber Recommendations**
Children	1 to 3 years	19 grams of fiber each day
Children	4 to 8 years	25 grams of fiber each day
Boys	9 to 13 years	31 grams of fiber each day
Girls	9 to 13 years	26 grams of fiber each day
Men	Under age 50 years	38 grams of fiber each day
Women	Under age 50 years	25 grams of fiber each day
Men	Over age 50 years	30 grams of fiber each day
Women	Over age 50 years	21 grams of fiber each day

Adapted from the 2008 ADA Position Paper on Nutrition for Health Children.

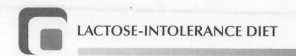

Lactose is the sugar present in milk. Lactose intolerance is very common; it occurs when the body is not able to appropriately digest this milk sugar content and results in diarrhea. You have been diagnosed as having difficulty digesting milk (lactose) products or have problems with malabsorption. Lactose intolerance can cause gas, bloating, abdominal cramps, diarrhea, and nausea or vomiting. You may be able to eat small portions without problems or you may be unable to tolerate any foods containing lactose (see Table B.7).

Tips for Following a Lactose-Intolerance Diet

A. Limit or omit foods that contain milk, lactose, whey, or casein.

B. Lactose-controlled diets allow up to 1 cup of milk per day for cooking or drinking, if you can tolerate it.

C. If you can't tolerate any lactose, choose lactose-free foods with lactate, lactic acid, lactalbumin, whey protein, sodium caseinate, casein hydrolysates, and calcium compounds. Read labels carefully.

D. You may also choose kosher foods marked "pareve" or "parve," which do not contain lactose. Read labels carefully.

E. A low-fat diet is important if you have fat malabsorption.

F. To help with diarrhea due to malabsorption, avoid more than one service a day of caffeine-containing drinks.

G. Beverages with high sugar content, such as soft drinks and fruit juices, may increase diarrhea. Juices and fruits with high amounts of fructose include apples, pears, sweet cherries, prunes, and dates.

H. Sorbitol-containing candies and gums may cause diarrhea.

TABLE B.7 Recommended Foods for Lactose Intolerance

Foods	Recommended	Not Recommended
Milk	Soybean milk, milk treated with lactase, nondairy creamers, whipped topping. Up to 1 cup/day of buttermilk, yogurt, sweet acidophilus milk, whole, low-fat, or skim milk	Milk products in excess of 1 cup/day, malted milk, milk shakes, hot chocolate, cocoa
Meat and protein foods	All meats, fish, poultry, eggs, peanut butter, tofu, hard, aged, and processed cheese, if tolerated	Sandwich meat, hot dogs that contain lactose, cottage cheese, any meat prepared with milk products
Vegetables	All fresh, frozen, canned, buttered and/or breaded vegetables	Any vegetable prepared with milk or milk products in excess of allowance (1 cup)
Fruits	All fresh, frozen, or canned fruits	Any fruits processed with lactose
Breads, cereal, and starchy food	White, wheat, rye, or other yeast breads, crackers, macaroni, spaghetti, popcorn, dry or cooked cereals	Commercial bread products (French toast, bread mixes, pancakes, biscuits), cakes/cookies containing milk or milk products
Fats and oils	Butter/margarine, salad dressing, mayonnaise, all oils, nondairy creamers, bacon	Sour cream, salad dressings with milk products in excess of 1 cup allowance
Soups	Vegetable and meat soups, broth, and bullion	Dried soups, creamed soups made with milk
Desserts	Plain and fruit flavored gelatins, sherbet, fruit pies, cakes, pudding, pastries, angle food cake, sponge cake	Ice cream, ice milk, cream pie, puddings, custards, cakes, and pastries with milk (unless count as day's allowance)
Beverages	Coffee, tea, soft drinks, fruit juices, carbonated and mineral waters	Beverages with milk over the 1 cup allowance
Miscellaneous condiments	Catsup, mustard, soy sauce, vinegar, steak sauce, Worcestershire sauce, chili sauce	None
Seasonings	Salt, pepper, spices, herbs, and seasonings	None
Sweets	Sugar, jelly, honey, molasses, preserves, marmalade, syrups, hard candy, baker's cocoa, carob powder, artificial sweeteners	Cream or chocolate candies containing milk or milk products (unless count as day's allowance), caramels, toffee, and butterscotch

The connection between fat in the diet and heart attack is cholesterol. Cholesterol is a fatlike substance produced by your liver and also found in many foods. Too much cholesterol causes heart attacks by clogging the arteries that deliver blood to your heart.

Exercising and following a low-fat/low-cholesterol diet can help control your blood cholesterol and reduce your risk of heart attack.

Tips

A. Read food labels. Use the ingredient list on labels to identify products containing saturated fat. High-fat ingredients may have many names. Remember: Foods can say "no cholesterol" and still be high in saturated vegetable fat and calories.
B. Train yourself to think "low fat" in your food and cooking methods.
   1. Bake
   2. Broil
   3. Grill
   4. Stir-fry
C. Eat less fried food, fast food, and baked products.
D. Eat more fruits and vegetables.
E. Organize your shopping around low-fat foods.
F. Add flavor to foods by using herbs and spices instead of butter and sauces.
G. Choose cole slaw, sliced tomatoes, or a dill pickle instead of fries and chips.

Foods to Avoid or Limit

A. Proteins/Meats
   1. Shrimp
   2. Fried meats, fish, or poultry
   3. Fatty ground meat
   4. Prime or heavily marbled meats
   5. Bacon, sausage, high-fat deli meats, and cheeses
   6. Liver and organ meats
B. Breads/Cereals
   1. High-fat baked foods, such as Danish, croissants, and doughnuts
   2. Fried rice, crispy chow mein noodles
   3. Granola bars with coconut or coconut oil
   4. Chips, cheese, or butter crackers
   5. High-fat cookies and cakes
C. Fruits and Vegetables
   1. Coconut
   2. Fried vegetables such as onion rings and breaded fried pickles, mushrooms, and okra
   3. Cream, cheese, or butter sauces on vegetables
D. Milk/Dairy Products
   1. Whole or 2% milk

   2. Cream, half-and-half, nondairy creamers
   3. Ice cream, whipped cream, nondairy whipped toppings
   4. Whole-milk yogurt, sour cream
   5. Cheeses: cheddar, American, Swiss, cream cheese, Brie, Muenster
E. Very High-Fat Foods
   1. Butter or margarine made with partially hydrogenated oils
   2. Lard, meat fat, and coconut or palm oils
   3. Salad dressings made with sour cream or cheese
   4. Chocolate
   5. Beef tallow
   6. Hydrogenated or partially hydrogenated vegetable shortening
   7. Cream
   8. Cocoa butter

Foods That Are Allowed

A. Proteins/Meats
   1. Fish and shellfish
   2. Chicken and turkey cooked without the skin
   3. Ground turkey
   4. Eggs: Limit to 2 yolks per week
   5. Dried beans, lentils, tofu
   6. Small amounts of meat and seafood
B. Breads/Cereals
   1. Plain bread and English muffins and bagels
   2. Plain pasta, rice
   3. Cereals, oatmeal
   4. Pretzels, air-popped popcorn, rice cakes, Melba toast
   5. Low-fat baked goods: angel food cake, graham crackers, fruit cookies, and gingersnaps
C. Fruits and Vegetables
   1. Eat several servings per day of high-nutrition, low-fat fruits and vegetables.
   2. Prepare vegetables by steaming, broiling, baking or stir-fry.
D. Milk/Dairy Products
   1. Skim or 1% milk
   2. Low-fat milk, evaporated milk, nonfat dry milk powder
   3. Frozen yogurt, ice milk, sherbet, sorbet
   4. Low-fat yogurt
   5. Low-fat cheeses: 1% cottage cheese, skim-milk ricotta, mozzarella, and American cheeses
E. Allowed High-Fat Foods
   1. Margarine made with liquid safflower, corn, or sunflower oils
   2. Olive, canola, or peanut oils
   3. Nut snacks in moderation (high fat and calories)
   4. Salad dressings made with saturated oils

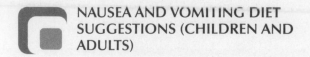

For simple nausea and vomiting accompanied by an upset stomach, follow these steps.

Step 1: Replace Lost Fluids
A. Rest your stomach for 1–2 hours.
B. Infants and small children: Pedialyte or Ricelyte are recommended because children become dehydrated quickly.
C. Infants: Resume breast- or bottle-feeding as soon as possible.
D. Young children: Give very small sips every 10–20 minutes until they keep the fluid down.
E. Older children: Give Gatorade or Pedialyte.
F. Older child and adults
   1. After vomiting stops, take sips of clear liquids at room temperature, such as flat ginger ale, flat cola, or gelatin.
   2. Suck on lollipops or Popsicles.
   3. Gradually increase amount of liquids. If 4 hours pass without vomiting, progress to Step 2.

Step 2: Dry Diet
The foods in this diet don't meet all daily food requirements and should be used only for a short period before adding foods or advancing to Step 3, More Advanced Carbohydrates.

A. Cheerios
B. Crackers
C. Cornflakes
D. Graham crackers
E. Rice Krispies
F. Vanilla wafers
G. Toast
H. Dinner rolls

Step 3: More Advanced Carbohydrates
A. Oatmeal
B. Grits, unseasoned
C. Rice, unseasoned
D. Mashed potatoes
E. Baked potato
F. Noodles
G. Peanut butter
H. Pudding

Step 4: Bland Foods With Limited Odors
After tolerating dry and more complex carbohydrates, a trial of bland foods may be attempted. Foods with little or no odors are more easily tolerated after experiencing nausea and vomiting (see Table B.8).

BRAT Diet
You may be told to use a BRAT Diet. This is a combination of foods that make up a bland diet and help with nausea and vomiting: **B**ananas, **R**ice, **A**pplesauce, and **T**oast as tolerated.

TABLE B.8 Bland Foods With Limited Odors

Baked chicken	Chicken noodle soup	Canned peaches
Baked turkey	Apple sauce	Canned pears
½ turkey sandwich	Fresh banana	Ice cream
Cottage cheese	Fresh apple	Sherbet
Apple juice	Iced tea	Low-fat milk

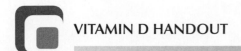

VITAMIN D HANDOUT

Vitamin D Enriched Foods

Food Source	Serving Size	Food International Units (IU)
Fish liver oils, cod liver oil	15 mL	1,360
Mushrooms	3 oz	2,700
Fortified milk	8 oz	100
Herring	3 oz	1,383
Catfish	3 oz	425
Mackerel (cooked)	3.5 oz	345
Salmon (cooked)	3.5 oz	360
Sardines (canned in oil, drained)	1.75 oz	250
Fortified orange juice	8 oz	100
Fortified cereal	1 serving	100
Fortified cheese	3 oz	100

Sunlight exposure to the skin is also recommended for approximately 20–30 minutes without sunscreen. Sun exposure provides an adequate source of vitamin D. Care should be taken not to burn skin.

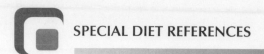
American Dietetic Association. (2010, January 5). *Tip of the day: Cereal + fiber = A good breakfast.* Retrieved March 7, 2010, from http://www.eatright.org/Public/content.aspx?id=3188&terms=high+fiber

American Dietetic Association. (2010, February 10). *Tip of the day: Food and the prevention of colon cancer.* Retrieved March 7, 2010, from http://www.eatright.org/Public/content.aspx?id=6442451024&terms=high+fiber

American Dietetic Association. (2009, February 11). *Tip of the day: Start your day with fiber.* Retrieved March 7, 2010, from http://www.eatright.org/Public/content.aspx?id = 3629&terms=high+fiber

American Dietetic Association Reports. (2008). Position of the American Dietetic Association: Nutrition guidance for healthy children ages 2 to 11 years. *Journal of the American Dietetic Association, 108,* 1038–1047.

Banks, D. (n.d.). Salt: Too much of a good thing. *University of Illinois Extension: Thrifty Living.* Retrieved March 6, 2010, from http://urbanext.illinois.edu/thriftyliving/tl-salt.html

The DASH diet and African American heart health. (n.d.). Retrieved March 6, 2010, from http://dashdiet.org/dash_diet_and_african_american.asp

The DASH diet eating plan. (n.d.). Retrieved March 6, 2010, from http://dashdiet.org/default.asp

DASH diet FAQ. (n.d.). Retrieved March 6, 2010, from http://dashdiet.org/dash_diet_faq.asp

Dietary Fiber Guide Web Site: http://dietaryfiberguide.com/

Low salt and the DASH diet. (n.d.). Retrieved March 6, 2010, from http://dashdiet.org/low_salt_diet.asp

National Heart Lung and Blood Institute. (2010). *Keep an eye on portion size: What is the difference between portions and servings?* Retrieved March 27, 2010, from http://hp2010.nhlbihin.net/portion/servingcard7.pdf

NHLBI. (n.d). *Tips for reducing sodium in your diet.* Retrieved March 6, 2010, from http://www.nhlbi.nih.gov/hbp/prevent/sodium/tips.htm

NHLBI. (n.d.). *Tips on how to make healthier meals.* Retrieved March 6, 2010, from http://www.nhlbi.nih.gov/hbp/prevent/h_eating/tips.htm

The University of Chicago Celiac Disease Center. (n.d.). *Gluten free diet.* Retrieved October 3, 2009, from http://www.celiacdisease.net/gluten-free-diet

U.S. Department of Health and Human Services, National Institutes of Health, National Digestive Diseases Information Clearinghouse. (2009, June). *Lactose intolerance* (NIH Publication No. 09–2751). Retrieved March 6, 2010, from http://digestive.niddk.nih.gov/ddiseases/pubs/lactoseintolerance/Lactose_Intolerance.pdf

U.S. Department of Health and Human Services, National Institutes of Health, National Heart, Lung, and Blood Institute. (2003, May). *Facts about the DASH eating plan* (NIH Publication No. 03–4082). Retrieved March 6, 2010, from http://www.hhs.state.ne.us/hew/hpe/cvh/docs/new_dash.pdf

U.S. Department of Health and Human Services, National Institutes of Health, National Heart, Lung, and Blood Institute. (2006, April). *Your guide to lowering your blood pressure with DASH, DASH eating plan, Lower your blood pressure* (NIH Publication No. 06–4082). Retrieved March 6, 2010, from http://www.nhlbi.nih.gov/health/public/heart/hbp/dash/new_dash.pdf

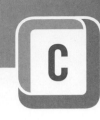

Tanner's Sexual Maturity Stages

SEXUAL MATURITY STAGES IN FEMALES

Stage	Breasts
1	Preadolescent—Only papilla is elevated above level of chest wall
2	Breast budding—Breast and papilla elevated as small mound, increased diameter of areola
3	Continued breast and areola enlargement, no contour separation
4	Areola and papilla form secondary mound
5	Mature—Nipple projects, areola is part of general breast contour

Stage	Pubic Hair
1	Preadolescent—None or vellous hair in pubis area
2	Sparse, straight, lightly pigmented along medial border of labia
3	Darker, coarser, curlier, and in increased amount
4	Abundant but has not spread to medial surface of thighs
5	Adult feminine, inverse triangle, spread to medial surface of thighs

SEXUAL MATURITY STAGES IN MALES

Stage	Penis, Testes, and Scrotum
1	Preadolescent—All are size and proportion seen in early childhood (testes 1 cm)
2	Slight enlargement, with alteration in color (more reddened) and texture of scrotum (testes 2.0–3.2 cm)
3	Further growth and enlargement (testes 3.3–4.0 cm)
4	Penis significantly enlarged in length and circumference; further development of glans; enlargement of testes and scrotum with darkening of scrotal skin (testes 4.1–4.9 cm)
5	Genitalia of adult size (testes 5.0 cm)

Stage	Pubic Hair
1	Preadolescent—None or vellous hair in pubis area
2	Sparse, straight, lightly pigmented at base of penis
3	Darker, coarser, curlier and in increased amount
4	Abundant but less quantity than adult type
5	Adult distribution, spread to medial surface of thighs

Used with permission from the Child Growth Foundation
www.childgrowthfoundation.org

Teeth

DECIDUOUS (BABY)

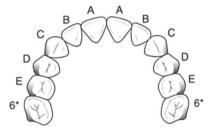

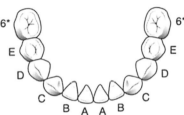

A,B Incisors
     6–9 months

C   Cuspid (eyetooth)
     16 months

D   1st Molar
     14 months

E   2nd Molar
     26 months

When They Are Lost

A   6–8 years
B   7–9 years
C   9–13 years
D   8–12 years
E   8–12 years

Expected number of teeth up to 24
months = age of child in months – 4
(e.g., 18-month-old should have 14 teeth)

PERMANENT

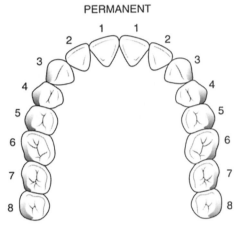

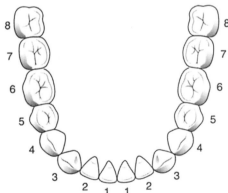

1, 2 Incisors
      7–9 years

3   Cuspid (eyetooth)
      11–13 years

4   1st Bicuspid
      9–11 years

5   2nd Bicuspid
      10–12 years

6   6th Year Molar*
      1st permanent tooth

7   2nd Molar
      12–14 years

8   3rd Molar (wisdom)
      16–20 years

787

Index